2nd Edition

HARRISON'S™
M A N U A L   O F
O N C O L O G Y

W0082174

NOTICE

Medicine is an ever-changing science. As new research and clinical experience broaden our knowledge, changes in treatment and drug therapy are required. The authors and the publisher of this work have checked with sources believed to be reliable in their efforts to provide information that is complete and generally in accord with the standards accepted at the time of publication. However, in view of the possibility of human error or changes in medical sciences, neither the authors nor the publisher nor any other party who has been involved in the preparation or publication of this work warrants that the information contained herein is in every respect accurate or complete, and they disclaim all responsibility for any errors or omissions or for the results obtained from use of the information contained in this work. Readers are encouraged to confirm the information contained herein with other sources. For example and in particular, readers are advised to check the product information sheet included in the package of each drug they plan to administer to be certain that the information contained in this work is accurate and that changes have not been made in the recommended dose or in the contraindications for administration. This recommendation is of particular importance in connection with new or infrequently used drugs.

2nd Edition

HARRISON'S™
MANUAL OF
ONCOLOGY

Bruce A. Chabner, MD

Professor of Medicine
Harvard Medical School
Director of Clinical Research
Massachusetts General Hospital Cancer Center
Boston, Massachusetts

Dan L. Longo, MD

Professor of Medicine
Harvard Medical School
Senior Physician
Brigham and Women's Hospital
Deputy Editor
New England Journal of Medicine
Boston, Massachusetts

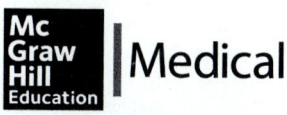

Mc
Graw
Hill
Education | Medical

New York   Chicago   San Francisco   Athens   London   Madrid
Mexico City   Milan   New Delhi   Singapore   Sydney   Toronto

Harrison's Manual of Oncology, Second Edition

Copyright © 2014 by McGraw-Hill Education. All rights reserved. Printed in the United States. Except as permitted under the United States Copyright Act of 1976, no part of this publication may be reproduced or distributed in any form or by any means, or stored in a data base or retrieval system, without prior written permission of the publisher.

1 2 3 4 5 6 7 8 9 0   DOC/DOC   18 17 16 15 14 13

ISBN 978-0-07-179325-4
MHID 0-07-179325-9

This book was set in Minion Pro by Cenveo® Publisher Services.
The editors were James F. Shanahan and Kim J. Davis.
The production supervisor was Catherine H. Saggese.
Project management was provided by Vastavikta Sharma of Cenveo Publisher Services.
RR Donnelley was the printer and binder.

Library of Congress Cataloging-in-Publication Data

Harrison's manual of oncology / [edited by] Bruce A. Chabner, Dan L. Longo. — Second edition.
    p. ; cm.
    Manual of oncology
    Complemented by: Harrison's principles of internal medicine / editors, Dan L. Longo ... [et al.]. 18th ed. 2012.
    Includes bibliographical references and index.
    ISBN 978-0-07-179325-4 (pbk. : alk. paper) — ISBN 0-07-179325-9 (pbk. : alk. paper)
    I. Chabner, Bruce, editor of compilation.   II. Longo, Dan L. (Dan Louis), 1949- editor of compilation.   III. Harrison's principles of internal medicine. Complemented by (work):   IV. Title: Manual of oncology.
    [DNLM: 1. Neoplasms—drug therapy. 2. Antineoplastic Agents—therapeutic use. QZ 267]
    RC271.C5
    616.99'4061—dc23
                                                                    2013022638

International Edition ISBN 978-1-25-925561-8; MHID 1-25-925561-1. Copyright © 2014. Exclusive rights by McGraw-Hill Education, for manufacture and export. This book cannot be re-exported from the country to which it is consigned by McGraw-Hill Education. The International Edition is not available in North America.

McGraw-Hill Education books are available at special quantity discounts to use as premiums and sales promotions, or for use in corporate training programs. To contact a representative, please visit the Contact Us pages at www.mhprofessional.com.

CONTENTS

INTRODUCTION Considerations for Cancer Pharmacotherapy

SECTION 1 Classes of Drugs

SECTION 2 Hormonal Agents

CONTRIBUTORS

JEREMY S. ABRAMSON, MD, MMSc
Assistant Professor of Medicine, Harvard Medical School
Director, Center for Lymphoma, Massachusetts General Hospital Cancer Center
Boston, Massachusetts

PHILIP C. AMREIN, MD
Assistant Professor of Medicine, Harvard Medical School
Physician, Massachusetts General Hospital
Boston, Massachusetts

EYAL C. ATTAR, MD
Assistant Professor of Medicine, Harvard Medical School
Attending Physician, Massachusetts General Hospital Cancer Center
Boston, Massachusetts

KAREN BALLEN, MD
Director, Leukemia Program, Massachusetts General Hospital Cancer Center
Boston, Massachusetts

ADITYA BARDIA, MD, MPH
Instructor in Medicine, Harvard Medical School
Attending Physician, Massachusetts General Hospital Cancer Center
Boston, Massachusetts

JEFFREY A. BARNES, MD, PhD
Instructor, Harvard Medical School
Attending Physician, Center for Lymphoma
Massachusetts General Hospital Cancer Center
Boston, Massachusetts

LAWRENCE S. BLASZKOWSKY, MD
Instructor in Medicine, Harvard Medical School
Assistant Physician, Massachusetts General Hospital Cancer Center
Boston, Massachusetts

JAMES BRADNER, MD
Assistant Professor of Medicine
Dana-Farber Cancer Institute
Harvard Medical School
Associate Member, Chemical Biology Program, Broad Institute
Boston, Massachusetts

PAUL M. BUSSE, MD, PhD
Associate Professor of Radiation Oncology, Harvard Medical School
Clinical Director, Department of Radiation Oncology
Massachusetts General Hospital
Boston, Massachusetts

STEPHEN M. CARPENTER, MD
Clinical and Research Fellow, Division of Infectious Disease
Massachusetts General Hospital and Brigham and Women's Hospital
Harvard Medical School
Boston, Massachusetts

BRUCE A. CHABNER, MD
Professor of Medicine, Harvard Medical School
Director of Clinical Research, Massachusetts General Hospital Cancer Center
Boston, Massachusetts

YI-BIN CHEN, MD
Assistant Professor of Medicine, Harvard Medical School
Director of Clinical Research, Bone Marrow Transplant Unit
Massachusetts General Hospital Cancer Center
Boston, Massachusetts

ANDREW S. CHI, MD, PhD
Assistant Professor of Neurology, Harvard Medical School
Attending Physician, Stephen E. and Catherine Pappas Center for Neuro-Oncology
Massachusetts General Hospital Cancer Center
Boston, Massachusetts

EDWIN CHOY, MD PhD
Assistant Professor of Medicine, Harvard Medical School
Attending Physician, Division of Hematology/Oncology
Massachusetts General Hospital Cancer Center
Boston, Massachusetts

TESSA CIGLER, MD, MPH
Assistant Professor of Medicine, Weill Cornell Medical College
Attending Physician, New York Presbyterian Hospital
New York, New York

JEFFREY W. CLARK, MD
Associate Professor, Harvard Medical School
Massachusetts General Hospital Cancer Center
Boston, Massachusetts

AMY COMANDER, MD, MA
Instructor in Medicine, Harvard Medical School
Massachusetts General Hospital Cancer Center
Boston, Massachusetts

TANJA BADOVINAC CRNJEVIC, MD, PhD
Avon International Breast Cancer Research Program
Massachusetts General Hospital
Boston, Massachusetts

DOUGLAS M. DAHL, MD, FACS
Associate Professor of Surgery, Harvard Medical School
Attending Urologist, Massachusetts General Hospital
Boston, Massachusetts

MARCELA G. DEL CARMEN, MD, MPH
Associate Professor, Harvard Medical School
Division of Gynecologic Oncology
Massachusetts General Hospital
Boston, Massachusetts

THOMAS F. DELANEY, MD
Professor of Radiation Oncology, Harvard Medical School
Radiation Oncologist, Department of Radiation Oncology
Medical Director, Francis H. Burr Proton Therapy Center
Co-Director, Center for Sarcoma and Connective Tissue Oncology
Massachusetts General Hospital Cancer Center
Boston, Massachusetts

DANIEL G. DESCHLER, MD, FACS
Professor, Department of Otology and Laryngology
Harvard Medical School
Director, Division of Head and Neck Surgery
Director, Norman Knight Hyperbaric Medicine Center
Massachusetts Eye and Ear Infirmary
Director, Head and Neck Surgical Oncology
Massachusetts General Hospital
Boston, Massachusetts

JORG DIETRICH, MD, PhD
Assistant Professor of Neurology, Harvard Medical School
Attending Physician, Massachusetts General Hospital
Boston, Massachusetts

DON S. DIZON, MD, FACP
Medical Gynecologic Oncology
Gillette Center for Women's Cancers
Director, Oncology Sexual Health Clinic
Massachusetts General Hospital Cancer Center
Boston, Massachusetts

JASON A. EFSTATHIOU, MD, DPhil
Assistant Professor of Radiation Oncology, Harvard Medical School
Attending Radiation Oncologist, Massachusetts General Hospital
Boston, Massachusetts

APRIL F. EICHLER, MD, MPH
Assistant Professor of Neurology, Harvard Medical School
Assistant Neurologist, Massachusetts General Hospital
Boston, Massachusetts

JEFFREY ENGELMAN, MD, PhD
Associate Professor of Medicine, Harvard Medical School
Director of Thoracic Oncology, Massachusetts General Hospital Cancer Center
Boston, Massachusetts

ANNA F. FARAGO, MD, PhD
Clinical Fellow in Medicine, Harvard Medical School
Fellow in Hematology/Oncology
Dana-Farber/Partners CancerCare
Boston, Massachusetts

AMIR T. FATHI, MD
Instructor, Harvard Medical School
Massachusetts General Hospital Cancer Center
Boston, Massachusetts

CARLOS G. FERNANDEZ-ROBLES, MD
Instructor, Harvard Medical School
Attending Psychiatrist, Massachusetts General Hospital
Boston, Massachusetts

PANOS FIDIAS, MD
Associate Professor of Medicine, Harvard Medical School
Attending Physician, Thoracic Oncology Clinic
Massachusetts General Hospital
Boston, Massachusetts

TITO FOJO, MD, PhD
Senior Investigator, Center for Cancer Research
National Cancer Institute, National Institutes of Health
Bethesda, Maryland

OLIVIA FOLEY, BA
Williams College
Williamstown, Massachusetts

JAMES W. FRASER, BSc
Clinical Research Manager, Division of Leukemia and Bone Marrow
Transplantation
Research Technician/Tumor Bank Manager, MGH Center for Regenerative
Medicine
Massachusetts General Hospital
Boston, Massachusetts

JUSTIN GAINOR, MD
Instructor, Harvard Medical School
Attending Physician, Massachusetts General Hospital Cancer Center
Boston, Massachusetts

JENNIFER GAO, MD
Internal Medicine Resident
Massachusetts General Hospital
Boston, Massachusetts

TIMOTHY GILLIGAN, MD
Hematology/Oncology Fellowship Program Director
Cleveland Clinic Taussig Cancer Institute
Cleveland, Ohio

PAUL E. GOSS, MD, PhD, FRCPC, FRCP (UK)
Professor of Medicine, Harvard Medical School
Director of Breast Cancer Research
Co-Director Breast Cancer Disease Program, DF/HCC
Director, Avon Breast Cancer Center of Excellence
Massachusetts General Hospital Cancer Center
Boston, Massachusetts

PHILLIP J. GRAY, MD
Resident in Radiation Oncology, Harvard Radiation Oncology Program
Boston, Massachusetts

REBECCA SUK HEIST, MD, MPH
Assistant Professor of Medicine, Harvard Medical School
Attending Physician, Massachusetts General Hospital Cancer Center
Boston, Massachusetts

EPHRAIM PAUL HOCHBERG, MD
Assistant Professor of Medicine, Harvard Medical School
Clinical Director, Inpatient Medical Oncology
Attending Physician, Center for Lymphoma
Massachusetts General Hospital Cancer Center
Boston, Massachusetts

THEODORE S. HONG, MD
Assistant Professor of Radiation Oncology, Harvard Medical School
Director, Gastrointestinal Radiation Oncology
Massachusetts General Hospital
Boston, Massachusetts

FRANCIS J. HORNICEK, MD, PhD
Associate Professor Orthopaedic Surgery, Harvard Medical School
Chief, MGH Orthopaedic Oncology Service
Director, MGH Sarcoma and Connective Tissue Oncology Group
Director, MGH Stephan L. Harris Chordoma Center
Co-Leader, Dana Farber/Harvard Cancer Center Sarcoma Program
Boston, Massachusetts

STEVEN J. ISAKOFF, MD, PhD
Instructor in Medicine, Harvard Medical School
Division of Hematology and Oncology
Massachusetts General Hospital Cancer Center
Boston, Massachusetts

BENJAMIN IZAR, MD, PhD
Resident, Department of Medicine
Massachusetts General Hospital
Boston, Massachusetts

VICKI JACKSON, MD, MPH
Assistant Professor of Medicine, Harvard Medical School
Chief, Palliative Medicine Division, Massachusetts General Hospital
Boston, Massachusetts

JULIET JACOBSEN, MD, DPH
Assistant Professor of Medicine, Harvard Medical School
Harvard Palliative Medicine Fellowship Program Director
Massachusetts General Hospital
Boston, Massachusetts

PASI A. JÄNNE, MD
Associate Professor of Medicine
Harvard Medical School
Lowe Center for Thoracic Oncology
Belfer Institute for Applied Cancer Science
Dana-Farber Cancer Institute
Boston, Massachusetts

LEE M. KRUG, MD
Associate Professor of Medicine, Weill Cornell Medical College
Associate Attending Physician, Memorial Sloan-Kettering Cancer Center
New York, New York

ANN S. LACASCE, MD
Assistant Professor of Medicine, Harvard Medical School
Attending Physician, Dana-Farber Cancer Institute
Boston, Massachusetts

DONALD P. LAWRENCE, MD
Instructor in Medicine, Harvard Medical School
Assistant Physician, Massachusetts General Hospital Cancer Center
Boston, Massachusetts

RICHARD J. LEE, MD, PhD
Assistant Professor of Medicine, Harvard Medical School
Attending Physician, Massachusetts General Hospital Cancer Center
Boston, Massachusetts

DAN L. LONGO, MD
Professor of Medicine, Harvard Medical School
Senior Physician, Brigham and Women's Hospital
Deputy Editor, New England Journal of Medicine
Boston, Massachusetts

ANUJ MAHINDRA, MD
Assistant Clinical Professor, Division of Hematology/Oncology
University of California, San Francisco
San Francisco, California

M. DROR MICHAELSON, MD, PhD
Associate Professor of Medicine, Harvard Medical School
Massachusetts General Hospital Cancer Center
Boston, Massachusetts

BEVERLY MOY, MD, MPH
Assistant Professor of Medicine, Harvard Medical School
Attending Physician, Massachusetts General Hospital Cancer Center
Boston, Massachusetts

HAMZA MUJAGIC, MD, MrSc, DrSc
Former Visiting Scholar and Ribakoff Fellow
Massachusetts General Hospital Cancer Center
Boston, Massachusetts

JANET E. MURPHY, MD, MPH
Instructor in Medicine, Harvard Medical School
Assistant Physician, Massachusetts General Hospital Cancer Center
Boston, Massachusetts

SARAH NIKIFOROW, MD, PhD
Clinical Instructor, Dana-Farber Cancer Institute, Harvard Medical School
Boston, Massachusetts

RICHARD T. PENSON, MD, MRCP
Associate Professor of Medicine, Harvard Medical School
Physician, Massachusetts General Hospital
Boston, Massachusetts

WILLIAM F. PIRL, MD, MPH
Associate Professor of Psychiatry, Harvard Medical School
Attending Psychiatrist, Massachusetts General Hospital
Boston, Massachusetts

MARK C. POZNANSKY, MD, PhD
Associate Professor of Medicine, Harvard Medical School
Director, Vaccine and Immunotherapy Center
Massachusetts General Hospital
Boston, Massachusetts

NOOPUR RAJE, MD
Associate Professor of Medicine, Harvard Medical School
Director, Center for Multiple Myeloma
Rita Kelley Chair in Oncology, Massachusetts General Hospital Cancer Center
Massachusetts General Hospital
Boston, Massachusetts

RACHEL P.G. ROSOVSKY, MD, MPH
Assistant in Medicine, Massachusetts General Hospital
Instructor in Medicine, Harvard Medical School
Department of Hematology/Oncology
Boston, Massachusetts

KRISTA M. RUBIN, MS, FNP-BC
Nurse Practitioner, Center for Melanoma
Massachusetts General Hospital Cancer Center
Boston, Massachusetts

DAVID P. RYAN, MD
Associate Professor of Medicine, Harvard Medical School
Chief, Division of Hematology/Oncology
Clinical Director, Massachusetts General Hospital Cancer Center
Boston, Massachusetts

PAULA D. RYAN, MD, PhD
Associate Professor, Medical Oncology
Fox Chase Cancer Center
Philadelphia, Pennsylvania

JENNIFER SHIN, MD
Instructor in Medicine, Harvard Medical School
Assistant Physician, Massachusetts General Hospital
Boston, Massachusetts

AMY SIEVERS, MD, MPH
Instructor in Medicine, Harvard Medical School
Associate Physician, Dana-Farber Cancer Institute
Boston, Massachusetts
Staff Physician, Portsmouth Regional Hospital
Portsmouth, New Hampshire

MATTHEW R. SMITH, MD, PhD
Professor of Medicine, Harvard Medical School
Director, Genitourinary Malignancies Program
Massachusetts General Hospital Cancer Center
Boston, Massachusetts

THOMAS R. SPITZER, MD
Professor of Medicine, Harvard Medical School
Director, Bone Marrow Transplant Program
Massachusetts General Hospital Cancer Center
Boston, Massachusetts

JERRY L. SPIVAK, MD
Professor of Medicine and Oncology
Director, The Johns Hopkins Center for the Chronic Myeloproliferative Disorders
Johns Hopkins University School of Medicine
Baltimore, Maryland

RYAN J. SULLIVAN, MD
Instructor of Medicine, Harvard Medical School
Assistant Physician, Massachusetts General Hospital Cancer Center
Boston, Massachusetts

JENNIFER TEMEL, MD
Associate Professor of Medicine, Harvard Medical School
Associate Physician of Medicine, Massachusetts General Hospital Cancer Center
Boston, Massachusetts

ZUZANA TOTHOVA, MD, PhD
Fellow in Hematology and Oncology, Dana-Farber Cancer Institute
Boston, Massachusetts

FABRIZIO VIANELLO, MD
Assistant Professor in Medicine, Department of Medicine
Padova University School of Medicine
Padova, Italy

SRINIVAS R. VISWANATHAN, MD, PhD
Resident in Internal Medicine, Massachusetts General Hospital
Boston, Massachusetts

LORI J. WIRTH, MD
Assistant Professor of Medicine, Harvard Medical School
Attending Physician, Massachusetts General Hospital
Boston, Massachusetts

JENNIFER WO, MD
Assistant Professor of Radiation Oncology, Harvard Medical School
Attending Physician, Massachusetts General Hospital
Boston, Massachusetts

SAM S. YOON, MD
Associate Attending Surgeon, Gastric and Mixed Tumor Service
Memorial Sloan-Kettering Cancer Center
New York, New York

ANDREW X. ZHU, MD, PhD, FACP
Associate Professor of Medicine, Harvard Medical School
Director, Liver Cancer Research
Massachusetts General Hospital Cancer Center
Boston, Massachusetts

PREFACE

We produced the first edition of this handbook in 2008 and were gratified by its reception. Accordingly, we have undertaken a thorough revision and updating for 2013 and are happy that such extensive revision was necessary given the remarkable progress in cancer treatment over the last 5 years. We have again enlisted help from our colleagues at Massachusetts General Hospital and Dana-Farber Cancer Center and from other outstanding physicians around the country. Our goal was to provide in a hand-held source (either book or electronic) a source of information useful in the management of patients. The front sections deal with classes of agents used to treat cancer and review their pharmacology and mechanisms of action. A section is dedicated to symptom management including pain, nausea and vomiting, anemia, febrile neutropenia, metabolic emergencies, venous thrombosis, psychological issues in cancer patients, and end-of-life care. The remaining sections are dedicated to particular tumor types. Each chapter provides what is known about pathogenesis, incidence, prognostic factors, staging, and management.

The pace of discovery outstrips the pace of writing and producing a textbook; therefore, you will find that some of the information in this book will have been superseded by very recent research results. Thus, we encourage readers to supplement what they learn here with information from peer-reviewed publications in the medical literature.

As a companion to *Harrison's Principles of Internal Medicine*, we expect this volume to provide more detailed and expanded coverage suitable for use in managing patients with cancer. It is envisioned as a tool for physicians in practice and in various levels of training both within the subspecialty of medical oncology and for internal medicine in general.

We are grateful to the many contributors whose undercompensated but greatly appreciated labor produced this text. Laura Collins helped us keep track of the process of inviting authors, maintaining deadlines, tracking and editing manuscripts, and boosting us through to the finish. Kim Davis and James Shanahan at McGraw-Hill provided essential help getting the book edited and published. Our families were generous in letting us spend too much of our "free" time on this labor of love. Finally, we are grateful for the lessons in medicine and life that our mentors, patients, and students have taught us and for the privilege of working together to pass some of those lessons onto others.

Bruce A. Chabner, MD
Dan L. Longo, MD

Introduction

Considerations for Cancer Pharmacotherapy

Aditya Bardia, Bruce Chabner

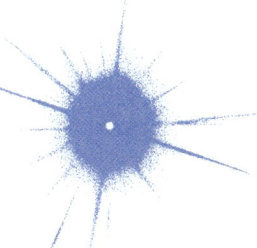

INTRODUCTION

Since the first use of intravenous nitrogen mustard as a chemotherapeutic agent to treat cancer in the 1940s, a number of chemotherapy agents have been successfully developed over the past half century with improved efficacy and toxicity profile. The advent of targeted therapies has further increased the arsenal of available cancer therapies.

Surgery and radiation play a primary role in control of localized tumors, and as adjuncts to chemotherapy in relieving symptoms in metastatic disease, and need to be considered in developing the overall treatment plan.

With the multitude of cancer therapies and treatment modalities, the decision to choose the best therapeutic regimen for an individual can be complex. Conceptually, both host and tumor-related factors need to be carefully considered in the decision-making process and personalizing therapy (1). The general principles involved in deciding the optimal cancer pharmacotherapy for an individual are reviewed in this introductory chapter.

■ HOST FACTORS

1. Goal of therapy

In general, the goal of treatment of localized disease is different from metastatic disease. Therapy in metastatic disease is directed toward improvement in quality of life and prolongation of survival, while in localized disease the overarching goal is cure. For localized disease one is willing to take "higher toxicity" for the price of potential cure. However, for metastatic disease quality of life is an important consideration. Multiple studies in various solid tumors have shown that, with certain exceptions (lymphomas, testicular cancer, choriocarcinoma, and others), combination chemotherapy can improve response rates but with only modest or incremental improvement in survival and at the cost of significantly increase in toxicity (2, 3). Therefore, while combination chemotherapy is the norm for localized tumor, sequential therapy with single agent chemotherapy may be preferred for metastatic disease (4, 5).

Besides stage, the location of tumor can also influence the decision for chemotherapy. For example, while endocrine therapy (such as tamoxifen or an aromatase inhibitor) is the mainstay for management of metastatic hormone receptor (HR) positive breast cancer, chemotherapy is preferred among patients who have a widespread visceral disease where rapid control of disease burden is needed.

The location of tumor can influence the decision for adjunctive therapy. Patients with bone metastasis routinely get bone strengthening

1

such as bisphosphonates, in additional to chemotherapy. These agents have been shown to improve bone pain and reduce risk of pathological fractures among patients with bone metastasis (6).

Other factors such as social support systems, economic considerations, and cultural attitudes may also influence the choice of therapy for an individual, and need to be carefully weighed.

2. Organ dysfunction

While patients receiving any medication require careful assessment of organ function, particularly hepatic and renal function, the assessment is particularly important for those receiving chemotherapy due to the narrow therapeutic window and potential for significant toxicity. For example, administering a regular dose of a chemotherapeutic agent predominantly metabolized by the liver, without appropriate dose reduction in the presence of hepatic dysfunction, could result in higher levels of the drug and life-threatening toxicity (7). Indeed, the degree of liver or renal function can affect the dose, schedule, and choice of chemotherapy (8–10). Table 1 lists the dose-modification(s) required for common

TABLE 1 IMPACT OF HEPATIC AND RENAL DYSFUNCTION ON DOSE-MODIFICATION FOR COMMON CHEMOTHERAPY AGENTS

Chemotherapy (Alphabetical Order)	Dose Reduction Required in Hepatic Dysfunction	Dose Reduction Required in Renal Dysfunction
5-FU	No	No
Capecitabine	No	Yes
Carboplatin	No	Yes
Cisplatin	No	Yes
Cyclophosphamide	Yes	Consider at high doses
Doxorubicin	Yes	No
Docetaxel	Yes	No
Epirubicin	Yes	Yes
Eribulin	Yes	Yes
Etoposide	Yes	Yes
Gemcitabine	Yes	No
Irinotecan	Yes	No
Ixabepilone	Yes	No
Methotrexate	Consider	Yes
Oxaliplatin	No	Yes
Paclitaxel	Yes	No
Pemetrexed	Yes	Yes
Vincristine	Yes	No
Vinorelbine	Yes	No

chemotherapeutic agents in the setting of hepatic and renal dysfunction. The dose modification(s) required for common targeted therapies is covered in Chapter 10.

3. **Host genotype**

The inherent genetic variations among individuals (genotype) can alter the expression and functional activity of the encoded protein and lead to a different functional outcome (phenotype). These genetic variations, including single nucleotide polymorphisms (SNPs), can alter the metabolism, and thus efficacy and toxicity, of a drug for a particular individual. For example, tamoxifen, a selective estrogen receptor modulator, is a prodrug that gets metabolized to its active metabolite, endoxifen, predominantly by hepatic enzyme CYP2D6 (11). The enzymatic activity of CYP2D6 is variable among individuals due to genetic polymorphisms in the CYP2D6 genes, which can influence the concentration of endoxifen. Specific genetic polymorphisms can reduce metabolic inactivation and increase the toxicity of certain chemotherapeutic agents such as 5-FU and 6-MP. DNA repair mechanisms are also subject to polymorphic variability. The expression of variants of ERCC1, a component of nucleotide excision repair, influences the effectiveness and toxicity of platinum drugs in treating lung cancer, although reliable tests for enzyme expression are not generally available (12). The only variant in routine clinical use is thiopurine methyltransferase, which is tested in children receiving 6-MP.

4. **Drug interactions**

Concomitant drugs that affect the enzymatic activity of the hepatic enzymes can influence the concentrations of drugs metabolized by the liver. In this regard, the CYP (P450) microsomal system of hepatic enzymes is extremely important as they metabolize up to 90% of all clinically prescribed drugs, including most targeted small molecules. Thus, drugs that increase (phenantoin, barbiturates) or decrease (antifungal imidazoles, proton pump inhibitors, macrolide antibiotics) their activity can alter the metabolic processing of several chemotherapeutic agents and produce lack of therapeutic effect or toxicity. For example, antidepressants are often used to mitigate hot flashes associated with tamoxifen or to treat depression, and may affect the metabolism of tamoxifen by inhibiting CYP2D6. Among the various antidepressants, paroxetine and fluoxetine are strong inhibitors of CYP2D6, whereas sertaline and venlafaxine are weak inhibitors (13). A detailed list of drugs affecting P450 is available at http://medicine.iupui.edu/clinpharm/DDIs/table.aspx.

Besides concomitant medications, interactions of chemotherapy with other therapies such as radiation must be considered in developing the treatment plan. For example, while platinum drugs and 5-FU integrate well with irradiation and enhance response, gemcitabine and anthracyclines significantly enhance local toxicity when used with irradiation.

5. **Age, concomitant illnesses, and performance status**

Age and concomitant comorbidities can have a profound effect on drug metabolism, response, and toxicity (14, 15). In aging, activity of hepatic microsomes decreases, serum protein binding decreases, and renal blood flow decreases, all leading to higher drug concentrations. It is recommended that for an elderly cancer patient, management decisions should consider the physiological age, life expectancy, potential risks versus absolute benefits, treatment tolerance, patient preference, and potential barriers to treatment (16). For example, the majority of elderly patients diagnosed with prostate cancer are more likely to die *with* prostate cancer, than *due to* prostate cancer. Several prognostic algorithms can help with the decision-making process and should be considered as appropriate.

Performance status (PS), a measure of the general state of activity, can be helpful in determining the prognosis as well as tolerability of chemotherapy for an individual. In general, intensive chemotherapy should be used with extreme caution, if at all, in an individual with ECOG PS > 2, unless the tumor is known to be highly responsive or curable. There are several methods to calculate the PS. The two most prominent scoring systems, namely the Karnofsky score and the ECOG/WHO score, are listed in Table 2.

TABLE 2 SCORING SYSTEMS TO ASSESS PERFORMANCE STATUS

Karnofsky Scale	ECOG Performance Status
• 100—Normal no complaints; no evidence of disease	• 0—Fully active, able to carry on all pre-disease performance without restriction
• 90—Able to carry on normal activity; minor signs or symptoms of disease	• 1—Restricted in physically strenuous activity but ambulatory and able to carry out work of a light or sedentary nature, e.g., light house work, office work
• 80—Normal activity with effort; some signs or symptoms of disease	
• 70—Cares for self; unable to carry on normal activity or to do active work	
• 60—Requires occasional assistance, but is able to care for most of his personal needs	• 2—Ambulatory and capable of all self-care but unable to carry out any work activities. Up and about more than 50% of waking hours
• 50—Requires considerable assistance and frequent medical care	
• 40—Disabled; requires special care and assistance	• 3—Capable of only limited self-care, confined to bed or chair more than 50% of waking hours
• 30—Severely disabled; hospital admission is indicated, although death not imminent	
• 20—Very sick; hospital admission necessary; active supportive treatment necessary	• 4—Completely disabled. Cannot carry on any self-care. Totally confined to bed or chair
• 10—Moribund; fatal processes progressing rapidly	• 5—Dead
• 0—Dead	

■ TUMOR FACTORS

1. **Pathological characteristics**

   The pathological characteristics of the tumor, including size, grade, proliferation index, and histology, are the crucial determinants for choice of therapy, and for localized tumors, the decision to give adjuvant therapy. In general, tumors with higher proliferation index (Ki-67 score) are more aggressive and have a greater chance of recurrence after local therapy, but also respond better to chemotherapy. Small cell lung cancers, testicular cancer, and diffuse large B-cell lymphomas, which are characterized as having a high rate of proliferation, show excellent response to chemotherapy agents. Pathological grade is an important surrogate marker for tumor proliferation and prognosis, which can be helpful in therapeutic decision making (17). For example, one would recommend adjuvant chemotherapy for high grade, hormone receptor (HR) positive breast cancer, but would be hesitant to recommend chemotherapy for a grade 1 HR+ tumor. Adjuvant hormonal therapy alone would be more appropriate for the latter.

   Tumor histology can also influence the chemotherapy decision. For example, non-small cell lung cancers with squamous histology are poorly responsive to pemetrexed, but tumors with non-squamous histology respond well (18). Similarly, breast cancers with lobular features have a lower response to chemotherapy than ductal breast cancers.

2. **Molecular characteristics**

   Large-scale genome-wide tumor analysis efforts, such as the Cancer Genome Atlas Network, have provided key insights into molecular heterogeneity of cancers, and have opened doors to new therapeutic opportunities (19–21). Indeed, molecular profiling of the tumor can help identify specific actionable mutations and amplified receptors that could be inhibited by targeted therapies, and should be routinely incorporated in clinical practice, particularly for breast, melanoma, colon, and lung cancer treatment (22, 23). For example, in breast cancer, it is a standard practice to assess for presence of the HR and human epidermal growth factor receptor 2 (HER2) overexpression, as the presence of these factors will determine the choice of treatment of both localized and metastatic disease. Treatment with the BRAF inhibitor, vemurafenib, is the most effective choice for metastatic melanoma harboring a BRAF mutation (24). Targeted therapies, alone or in combination with chemotherapy, have better response rates and lesser toxicity than chemotherapy regimens alone for cancers with actionable mutations (23, 25, 26). Table 3 lists the common FDA-approved targeted therapies based on mutation profile of the tumor. Targeted therapies are discussed in detail in Chapters 10 and 15.

3. **Risk stratification algorithms**

   Gene signatures and risk stratification algorithms that predict risk of recurrence and/or sensitivity to chemotherapy can be valuable tools in decision making. For example, the decision to use (or not to) use adjuvant chemotherapy for localized stage I-II, HR+, grade 2, breast cancer can be difficult one. The risk of recurrence is low and benefit of chemotherapy marginal for the majority of patients, but not for all.

TABLE 3 FDA APPROVED TARGETED THERAPIES BASED ON MUTATION PROFILE OF TUMOR

Targeted Therapy	Mutation Profile	FDA Approval
Trastuzumab	HER2 amplification	Breast cancer
Pertuzumab	HER2 amplification	Breast cancer
Erlotinib	EGFR	Non-small cell lung cancer
Geftinib	EGFR	Non-small cell lung cancer
Crizotinib	ALK rearrangement	Non-small cell lung cancer
Vemurafenib	BRAF	Melanoma
Cetuximab	Wild type KRAS	Colorectal cancer
Panitumumab	Wild type KRAS	Colorectal cancer
All-trans retinoic acid (ATRA)	t(15;17) translocation	Acute promyelocytic leukemia
Imatinib	bcr-abl translocation, c-kit	Chronic myeloid leukemia, Philadelphia positive acute lymphoblastic leukemia
		Gastrointestinal stromal tumor

Predictive biomarkers, such as the 21-gene expression assay (Oncotype Dx®), 70-gene assay (Mammaprint), and the breast cancer index (BCI), provide an estimate of risk of recurrence and relative benefit of chemotherapy, and can be helpful in the therapeutic decision making (27–29). Similar predictive algorithms have been developed for other cancers, such as colon cancer, although less validated (30, 31). The detection and molecular characterization of circulating tumor cells after definitive surgery is a promising research strategy to predict prognosis, guide type of adjuvant therapy, and provide molecular information about mechanisms of drug resistance (32–36), but is not ready for routine clinical use.

SUMMARY

The decision to choose a particular chemotherapeutic regimen is complex and should be personalized for an individual considering the various host and tumor factors. A multidisciplinary team approach is critical to integrate drug treatment with the total treatment plan. It is important to communicate the choices available clearly and involve the patient in the therapeutic decision making. One suggested strategy, practiced at our institution, is the utilization of a treatment plan and chemotherapy consent sheet that outlines the goals of treatment, the regimen, the schedule, and the expected side effects. The consent is signed both by the patient and the treating physician. The treatment plan and consent are included in the patient's medical record, and a copy provided to the patient. Such a strategy could enhance communication, reinforce key therapeutic elements, and improve patient satisfaction.

REFERENCES

1. Bardia A, Stearns V. Personalized tamoxifen: a step closer but miles to go. *Clin Cancer Res.* 2010; 16: 4308–4310.

2. Joensuu H, Holli K, Heikkinen M, et al. Combination chemotherapy versus single-agent therapy as first- and second-line treatment in metastatic breast cancer: a prospective randomized trial. *J Clin Oncol.* 1998; 16: 3720.

3. Wilcken N, Dear R. Chemotherapy in metastatic breast cancer: a summary of all randomised trials reported 2000-2007. *Eur J Cancer.* 2008. 44: 2218.

4. Heidemann E, Stoeger H, Souchon R, et al. Is first-line single-agent mitoxantrone in the treatment of high-risk metastatic breast cancer patients as effective as combination chemotherapy? No difference in survival but higher quality of life were found in a multicenter randomized trial. *Ann Oncol.* 2002; 13: 1717–1729.

5. Huober J, Thürlimann B. The role of combination chemotherapy in the treatment of patients with metastatic breast cancer. *Breast Care (Basel).* 2009; 4: 367–372.

6. Wong MH, Stockler MR, Pavlakis N. Bisphosphonates and other bone agents for breast cancer. *Cochrane Database Syst Rev.* 2012; 2: CD003474.

7. Koren G, Beatty K, Seto A, et al. The effects of impaired liver function on the elimination of antineoplastic agents. *Ann Pharmacother.* 1992; 26: 363.

8. Floyd J, Mirza I, Sachs B, Perry MC. Hepatotoxicity of chemotherapy. *Semin Oncol.* 2006; 33: 50.

9. Janus N, Thariat J, Boulanger H, et al. Proposal for dosage adjustment and timing of chemotherapy in hemodialyzed patients. *Ann Oncol.* 2010; 21: 1395.

10. Launay-Vacher V, Oudard S, Janus N, et al. Prevalence of renal insufficiency in cancer patients and implications for anticancer drug management: the renal insufficiency and anticancer medications (IRMA) study. *Cancer.* 2007; 110: 1376.

11. Stearns V, Johnson MD, Rae JM, et al. Active tamoxifen metabolite plasma concentrations after coadministration of tamoxifen and the selective serotonin reuptake inhibitor paroxetine. *J Natl Cancer Inst.* 2003; 95: 1758–1764.

12. Friboulet L, Olaussen KA, Pignon JP, et al. ERCC1 isoform expression and DNA repair in non-small-cell lung cancer. *N Engl J Med.* 2013; 368: 1101–1110.

13. Sideras K, Ingle JN, Ames MM, et al. Coprescription of tamoxifen and medications that inhibit CYP2D6. *J Clin Oncol.* 2010; 28: 2768–2776. Review.

14. Lichtman SM, Wildiers H, Launay-Vacher V, et al. International Society of Geriatric Oncology (SIOG) recommendations for the adjustment of dosing in elderly cancer patients with renal insufficiency. *Eur J Cancer.* 2007; 43: 14.

15. Chen RC, Royce TJ, Extermann M, Reeve BB. Impact of age and comorbidity on treatment and outcomes in elderly cancer patients. *Semin Radiat Oncol.* 2012; 22: 265–271.

16. Biganzoli L, Wildiers H, Oakman C, et al. Management of elderly patients with breast cancer: updated recommendations of the International Society of Geriatric Oncology (SIOG) and European Society of Breast Cancer Specialists (EUSOMA). *Lancet Oncol.* 2012; 13: e148–e160.

17. Cuzick J, Dowsett M, Pineda S, et al. Prognostic value of a combined estrogen receptor, progesterone receptor, Ki-67, and human epidermal growth factor receptor 2 immunohistochemical score and comparison with the genomic health recurrence score in early breast cancer. *J Clin Oncol.* 2011; 29: 4273–4278.

18. Syrigos KN, Vansteenkiste J, Parikh P, et al. Prognostic and predictive factors in a randomized phase III trial comparing cisplatin-pemetrexed versus cisplatin-gemcitabine in advanced non-small-cell lung cancer. *Ann Oncol.* 2010; 21: 556.

19. Banerji S, Cibulskis K, Rangel-Escareno C, et al. Sequence analysis of mutations and translocations across breast cancer subtypes. *Nature.* 2012; 486: 405–409.

20. Cancer Genome Atlas Network. Comprehensive molecular portraits of human breast tumours. *Nature.* 2012; 490: 61–70.

21. Cancer Genome Atlas Research Network. Integrated genomic analyses of ovarian carcinoma. *Nature.* 2011; 474: 609–615.

22. Sequist LV, Heist RS, Shaw AT, et al. Implementing multiplexed genotyping of non-small-cell lung cancers into routine clinical practice. *Ann Oncol.* 2011; 22: 2616–2624.

23. Von Hoff DD, Stephenson JJ Jr, Rosen P, et al. Pilot study using molecular profiling of patients' tumors to find potential targets and select treatments for their refractory cancers. *J Clin Oncol.* 2010; 28: 4877–4883.

24. Chapman PB, Hauschild A, Robert C, et al. BRIM-3 Study Group. Improved survival with vemurafenib in melanoma with BRAF V600E mutation. *N Engl J Med.* 2011; 364: 2507–2516.

25. Kwak EL, Bang YJ, Camidge DR, et al. Anaplastic lymphoma kinase inhibition in non-small-cell lung cancer. *N Engl J Med.* 2010; 363: 1693–1703.

26. Flaherty KT, Infante JR, Daud A, et al. Combined BRAF and MEK inhibition in melanoma with BRAF V600 mutations. *N Engl J Med.* 2012; 367: 1694–1703.

27. Paik S, Shak S, Tang G, et al. A multigene assay to predict recurrence of tamoxifen-treated, node-negative breast cancer. *N Engl J Med.* 2004; 351: 2817.

28. Marchionni L, Wilson RF, Wolff AC, et al. Systematic review: gene expression profiling assays in early-stage breast cancer. *Ann Intern Med.* 2008; 148: 358–369. Review.

29. Nagaraj G, Ma CX. Adjuvant chemotherapy decisions in clinical practice for early-stage node-negative, estrogen receptor-positive, HER2-negative breast cancer: challenges and considerations. *J Natl Compr Canc Netw.* 2013; 11: 246–251.

30. O'Connell MJ, Lavery I, Yothers G, et al. Relationship between tumor gene expression and recurrence in four independent studies of patients with stage II/III colon cancer treated with surgery alone or surgery plus adjuvant fluorouracil plus leucovorin. *J Clin Oncol.* 2010; 28: 3937.

31. Salazar R, Roepman P, Capella G, et al. Gene expression signature to improve prognosis prediction of stage II and III colorectal cancer. *J Clin Oncol.* 2011; 29: 17.

32. Criscitiello C, Sotiriou C, Ignatiadis M. Circulating tumor cells and emerging blood biomarkers in breast cancer. *Curr Opin Oncol.* 2010; 22: 552–558. Review.

33. Iinuma H, Watanabe T, Mimori K, et al. Clinical significance of circulating tumor cells, including cancer stem-like cells, in peripheral blood for recurrence and prognosis in patients with Dukes' stage B and C colorectal cancer. *J Clin Oncol.* 2011; 29: 1547.

34. Markopoulos C. Overview of the use of OncotypeDX® as an additional treatment decision tool in early breast cancer. *Expert Rev Anticancer Ther.* 2013; 13: 179–194.

35. Miyamoto DT, Lee RJ, Stott SL, et al. Androgen receptor signaling in circulating tumor cells as a marker of hormonally responsive prostate cancer. *Cancer Discov.* 2012; 2: 995–1003.

36. Yu M, Bardia A, Wittner BS, et al. Circulating breast tumor cells exhibit dynamic changes in epithelial and mesenchymal composition. *Science.* 2013; 339: 580–584.

CHAPTER **1**

Antimetabolites: Nucleoside and Base Analogs

Bruce A. Chabner

ANALOGS OF DNA PRECURSORS; GENERAL CONSIDERATIONS

The synthesis of new DNA is an essential step in the replication of normal and malignant cells. Accordingly, the four bases that comprise DNA (the pyrimidines: cytosine, thymine; and the purines: adenine, and guanine) have provided a rational target for synthesis of analogues that inhibit the function of DNA, including its replication. These bases become active substrates for DNA synthesis through the attachment of deoxyribose sugars to form a *deoxynucleoside*. Three phosphate molecules must then be attached to the 5′-OH position of the nucleoside's sugar, forming a metabolically active *deoxynucleotide*. These synthetic reactions, which lead to formation of the *triphosphates* required for making DNA, occur within the cancer cell, as well as within normal proliferating tissues, such as bone marrow and epithelium.

Normal as well as tumor cells do not have to synthesize bases for DNA. They can take up certain bases (guanine and uracil) as well as nucleosides (deoxycytidine, thymidine, adenosine, guanosine) from the circulation. Alternatively, these bases or their nucleosides can be synthesized by tumor cells de novo, in a complex, multistep system of reactions. Many of the earliest effective anticancer agents were designed as analogs of these bases or nucleosides. These analogs are transported into cells and converted to active triphosphates by the same transporters and enzymes that activate physiologic bases and deoxynucleosides.

FLUOROPYRIMIDINES

5-Fluoro-uracil (5-FU) and its prodrug, capecitabine (4-pentoxycarbonyl-5′-deoxy-5′-fluorocytidine), are central agents in the treatment of epithelial cancers. They have synergistic interaction with other cytotoxic agents, such as cisplatin or oxaliplatin, and with radiation therapy. As a component of adjuvant and anti-metastatic therapy, fluoropyrimidines have improved survival in patients with colorectal cancer (1).

■ MECHANISM OF ACTION AND RESISTANCE

The first agent of this class, 5-FU (Figure 1-1), was synthesized in 1956 by Heidelberger, based on experiments that demonstrated the ability of tumor cells to salvage uracil for DNA synthesis. Later work showed that 5-FU is converted by multiple different routes to an active deoxynucleotide, FdUMP, a potent inhibitor of thymidylate synthase (TS), and thereby, DNA synthesis (Figure 1-1).

11

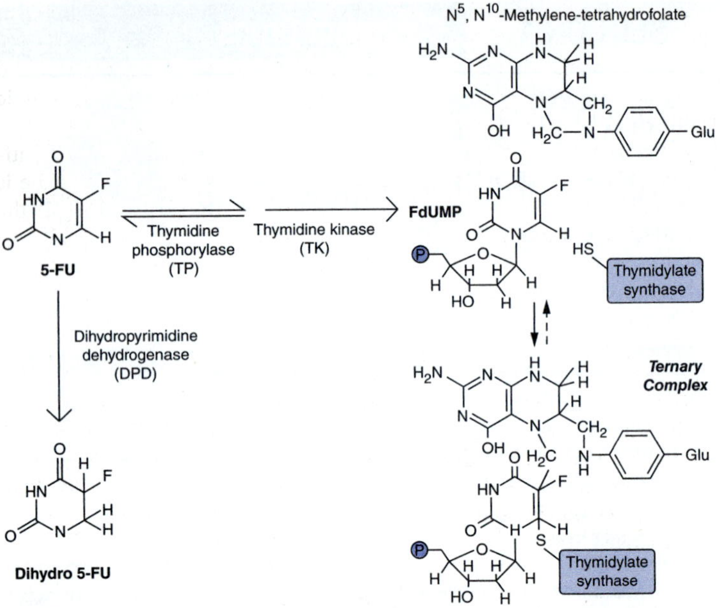

FIGURE 1-1 Routes of activation (via TP and TK) and inactivation (via DPD) of 5-fluorouracil (5-FU). Note that TP is a reversible reaction.

The active product, FdUMP, forms a tight tripartite complex with TS in the presence of the enzyme's cofactor, 5-10-methylene tetrahydrofolic acid. It thereby blocks the conversion of dUMP to dTMP, a necessary precursor of dTTP (2). dTTP is one of four deoxynucleotide substrates required for synthesis of DNA. An exogenous folic acid source such as leucovorin (5-formyl-tetrahydrofolate) enhances formation of the TS-F-dUMP-folate complex and increases the response rate in patients with colon cancer (3).

5-FU also forms 5-FUTP, and becomes incorporated into RNA, where it blocks RNA processing and function. Inhibition of TS predominates as the mechanism of antitumor action.

Resistance to fluoropyrimidines arises through several mechanisms (4). Increased expression of TS, or amplification of the TS gene, occurs both experimentally and in a patient's tumors after exposure to FU, and probably represents the primary mechanism. Some resistant tumors fail to convert 5-FU to its active nucleotide form through decreased expression of activating enzyme(s). Increased expression of degradative enzymes (thymidine phosphorylase [TP] and dihydropyrimidine dehydrogenase [DPD]; Figure 1-1 has been found in resistant cells. Increased expression of TP reduces the cellular pool of fluorodeoxyuridine, an intermediate in the activation pathway, and increases resistance. Upregulation of the AKT, RAS, and HER2 pathways may also contribute to resistance. Finally, anti-apoptotic changes, such as increased expression of bcl-2 or mutation of the cell cycle checkpoint, p53, are associated with resistance in experimental systems. A signature for resistance in patients treated with cisplatin and 5-FU for gastric cancer demonstrates increased expression of embryonic stem cell and PI-3-kinase pathway genes (5).

Capecitabine, an orally active prodrug of 5-FU, has demonstrated anti-tumor efficacy equal to 5-FU in breast and colon cancer. Capecitabine is activated by three sequential metabolic steps: (1) esterase cleavage of the aminoester at carbon 4 to yield fluoro-5′-deoxycytidine (F-5′-dC); (2) deamination of F-5′-dC, yielding fluoro-5′-deoxyuridine (ftorafur); and (3) cleavage of the inactive 5′-deoxy sugar of ftorafur by TP, releasing 5-FU (Figure 1-2). Steps 1 and 2 are believed to occur in the liver and plasma, while step 3, release of active 5-FU, takes place in tumor cells. Tumor cells with high TP are sensitive to capecitabine but resistant to 5-FU.

Two other preparations of fluoropyrimidines, UFT and S-1, not available in the United States, incorporate ftorafur with inhibitors of DPD, yielding an orally active product that produces a long 5-fluorouracil half-life (2 h for S-1) in plasma, and somewhat increased epithelial toxicity (6). Both products are widely used (with leucovorin) in Japan but are not approved in the United States.

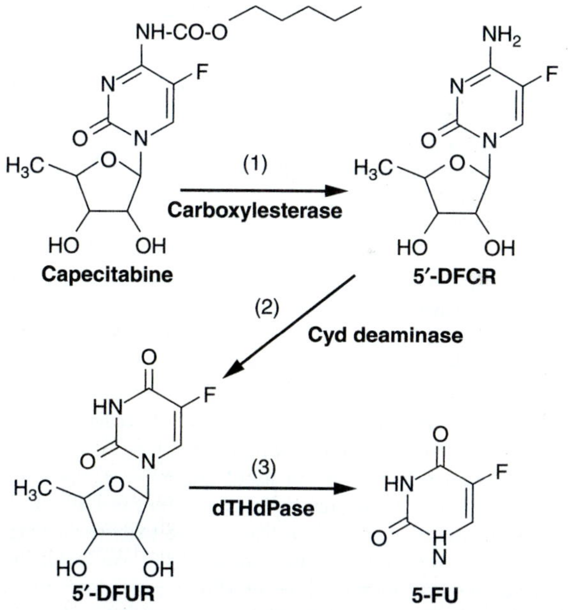

FIGURE 1-2 Metabolic activation of capecitabine by 1, carboxylesterase; 2, cytidine deaminase; 3, thymidine phosphorylase. 5-FU: 5-fluorouracil; 5′-DFCR: 5′-deoxy-5-fluoro-cytosine riboside; 5′-DFUR, 5′-deoxy-5-fluorouracil riboside.

■ **CLINICAL PHARMACOLOGY**

5-FU is administered intravenously in several different regimens. It was originally given in doses up to 450 mg/m^2/day × 5 days, and leucovorin, 25–500 mg/day orally, was later added to enhance efficacy. 5-FU given once weekly causes less neutropenia and diarrhea, and is probably equally effective. More recent and more effective regimens employ a bolus of FU on day 1, followed by 48-h infusion of up to 1000 mg/m^2/day for 2 days. Bolus and infusion doses vary according to other drugs in the combination regimen and the use of radiation therapy concomitantly.

The parent drug is not readily bioavailable by the oral route due to rapid first-pass metabolism in the liver. Following intravenous administration, plasma concentrations of 5-FU decline rapidly, with a $t_{1/2}$ of 10 min, due to the conversion of 5-FU to dihydro-5-FU by DPD. Intracellular concentrations of 5-FdUMP and other nucleotides build rapidly, and decay with a half-life of approximately 4 h. Little intact 5-FU appears in the urine. Drug doses do not have to be altered for abnormal hepatic or renal function.

Capecitabine, given in total doses of 2500 mg/m^2/day for 14 days, is readily absorbed, converted to 5-fluoro-5'-deoxyuridine (5-F-5'-dU) by the liver, and peak levels of metabolites appear in plasma about 2 h after a dose. Food taken with capecitabine protects the drug from degradation and leads to higher active metabolite concentrations in plasma. 5-F-5'-dU, the primary active precursor of 5-FU, exits plasma with a $t_{1/2}$ of 1 h. There is no evidence that leucovorin enhances the activity of capecitabine. Because the clearance of 5-F-5'-dU is delayed in patients with renal dysfunction, capecitabine should not be used in patients with severe renal failure (7). Patients with moderately impaired renal function (CCr of 30–50 ml/min) should receive 75% of a full dose.

In fluoropyrimidine therapy, doses should be adjusted according to white blood cell count, gastrointestinal symptoms, and cutaneous (palmar plantar dysesthesia) toxicity.

■ **TOXICITY**

Fluoropyrimidines cause significant acute toxicity to the gastrointestinal tract and bone marrow. Of primary concern are mucositis and diarrhea, which may lead to dehydration, sepsis, and death. The risk is greatest in the presence of myelosuppression. Persistent watery diarrhea should alert the patient to receive immediate medical attention. Women are more often affected than men, and elderly patients (above 70 years) are particularly vulnerable to 5-FU toxicity. Myelosuppression follows a typical pattern of an acute fall in white cell and platelet count over a 5–7 day period, followed by recovery by day 14. Occasional patients deficient in DPD due to inherited polymorphisms may display overwhelming toxicity to first doses of the drug (8). A test for DPD in white blood cells is now available, and can confirm this deficiency, which, if present, should preclude further attempts to use fluoropyrimidines. Other toxicities encountered with 5-FU include cardiac vasospasm with angina and rarely myocardial infarction and cerebellar dysfunction, the latter predominantly after high-dose intravenous or intracarotid infusion.

Capecitabine has the additional significant toxicity of palmar-plantar dysesthesias, with redness, extreme tenderness, and defoliation over the palms and plantar surfaces.

A third fluoropyrimidine, 5-F-deoxyuridine (5-F-dU), is used almost exclusively in regimens of hepatic artery infusion (0.3 mg/kg/day for 14 days) for metastases from colon cancer, in which setting it has a greater than 50% response rate (9). Given in this manner it has the advantage of achieving higher intratumoral concentrations. It is cleared by hepatic parenchyma and, by this route, produces modest systemic toxicity. Intrahepatic arterial infusion may lead to serious hepatobiliary toxicity, including cholestasis, hepatic enzyme elevations, and ultimately biliary sclerosis. Glucocorticoids given with 5-F-dU decrease the incidence of biliary toxicity. Thrombosis, hemorrhage or infection at the catheter site, and ulceration of the stomach or duodenum may further complicate this treatment approach.

CYTOSINE ARABINOSIDE

The first of these analogs, cytosine arabinoside (ara-C) (Figure 1-3), was isolated from a fungal broth and proved to be the single most effective drug for inducing remission in acute myelogenous leukemia (AML).

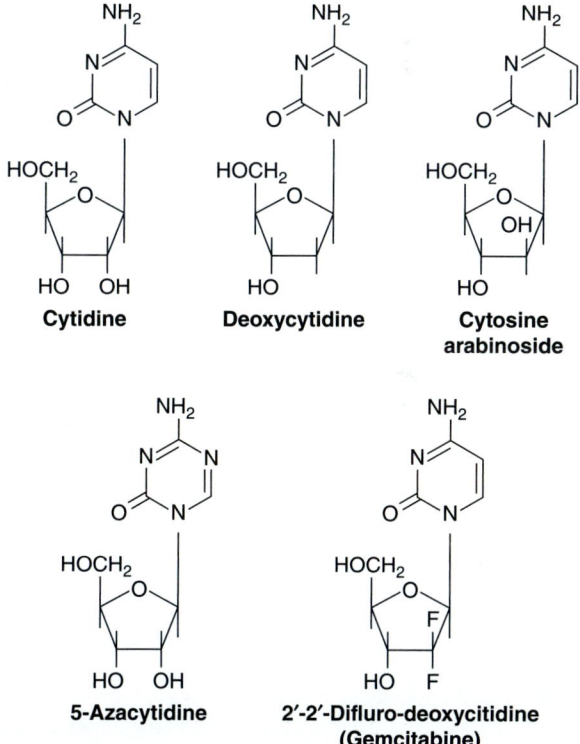

FIGURE 1-3 Structure of cytidine analogs.

It differs from the physiological substrate deoxycytidine in having an arabinose sugar rather than a deoxyribose, with a 2′-OH group in the abnormal beta configuration, rather than the 2′-H found on deoxyribose. The presence of the beta-2′-OH does not inhibit entry into cells or its further metabolism to an active triphosphate, or even its subsequent incorporation into the growing DNA strand. However, incorporation of a very few molecules of ara-C blocks further elongation of the DNA strand by DNA polymerase, and initiates apoptosis (programmed cell death) (10).

The steps leading from polymerase inhibition to cell death are not clearly understood. Exposure of cells to ara-C induces a complex set of reactive signals, including induction of the transcription factor AP-1, and the damage response factor, NF-κB. At low concentrations of ara-C, some leukemic cell lines in culture may differentiate, while others activate the apoptosis pathways. Exposure to ara-C leads to stalling of the replication fork for cells undergoing DNA synthesis, and this event activates checkpoint kinases, ATR and Chk 1, which block further cell cycle progression, activate DNA repair, and stabilize the replication fork. Loss of ATR or Chk 1 function sensitizes cells to ara-C. Levels of pro-apoptotic and anti-apoptotic factors within the leukemic cells also influence survival (11).

The specific steps in ara-C uptake and activation to a triphosphate within the cancer cell are important (Figure 1-4). It is taken into cells by an equilibrative cell membrane transporter, hENT1, which also transports physiologic nucleosides (12). Ara-C is then converted to its monophosphate by

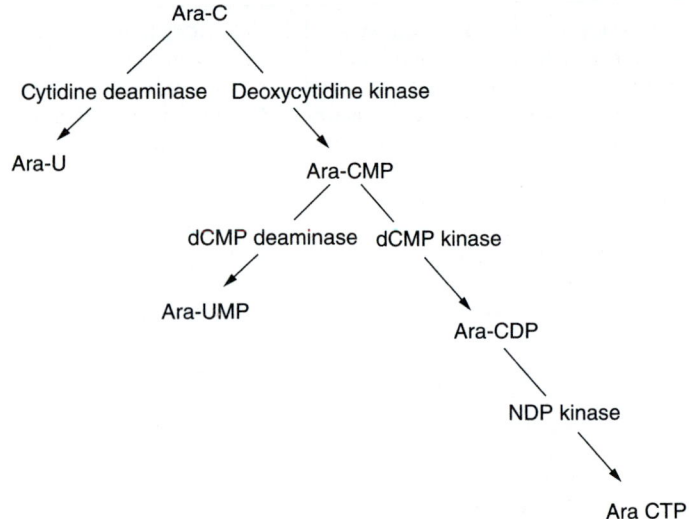

FIGURE 1-4 Metabolic pathway for conversion of deoxycytidine and its anticancer analog, cytosine arabinoside, to a triphosphate. Ara-CMP: ara-C monophosphate; ara-CDP: ara-C diphosphonate; ara-CTP: Ara-C triphosphate; ara-U: ara-uracil; dCMP: deoxycytidine monophosphate; NDP: nucleoside diphosphate.

deoxycytidine kinase, a key rate-limiting step in its activation and antitumor action. Ara-CMP requires further conversion to its triphosphate, but the enzymes involved are found in abundance and do not limit its activity.

The drug and its monophosphate, ara-CMP, are both subject to degradation by deamination. The resultant products, ara-U and ara-UMP, are inactive as a substrate for either RNA or DNA synthesis. Cytidine deaminase (CDA) is found in most human tissues, including epithelial cells of the intestine, the liver, and even in plasma. Elevated concentrations of CDA have been implicated as the cause of ara-C resistance in AML, but the evidence is as yet not convincing. Polymorphic variants of CDA (C-451T) decrease enzyme levels and are associated with greater toxicity and poorer survival (13). The most important cause of resistance appears to be a deletion of deoxycytidine kinase activity. Other evidence suggests that the pharmacokinetics (degree of formation and the duration of persistence) of ara-CTP in leukemic cells determine the therapeutic outcome. The intracellular half-life of ara-CTP is about 4 h. Exporters, particularly MRP 8, may reduce the intracellular drug levels and promote resistance (14).

High-dose ara-C has become the standard for consolidation of remission in AML, following remission induction. Cure rates for patients under 60 years of age now approach 30%–40%, but vary with patient age and with cytogenetics, the poorest results coming in older patients who have leukemia with complex karyotypes, leukemia secondary to cytotoxic therapy, or leukemia following a period of myelodysplasia.

■ CLINICAL PHARMACOLOGY

Ara-C, in doses of 100–200 mg/m²/day × 7 days, by continuous infusion, is commonly used with a topoisomerase 2 inhibitor (daunomycin or idarubicin) for remission induction in AML. Once remission has been induced, high-dose ara-C is given in doses of 1–3 g/m² for consolidation therapy (15). Doses are repeated every 12 h twice daily on days 1, 3, and 5 in a commonly used schedule. Continuous infusion regimens are designed to maintain cytotoxic levels (above 0.1 μM) of drug throughout a several-day period, in order to expose dividing cells during the DNA synthetic phase of the cell cycle.

Ara-C disappears rapidly from plasma, with a half-life of 10 min, due primarily to its rapid deamination by CDA (see above). High-dose ara-C follows similar kinetics in plasma, although a slow terminal phase of disappearance becomes apparent, and may contribute to toxicity. The primary metabolite, ara-U, has no known toxicity, but, in patients with renal dysfunction, through feedback inhibition of deamination ara-U, may contribute to the slower elimination of high-dose ara-C from plasma, resulting in greater risk of toxicity. High-dose regimens provide cytotoxic drug concentrations in the cerebrospinal fluid, but direct intrathecal injection of 50 mg, either as a standard formulation of drug or in a depot form of ara-C immersed in a gel suspension for slow release (DepoCyt), is the preferred treatment for lymphomatous or carcinomatous meningeal disease. Ara-C has comparable intrathecal activity to methotrexate in these settings. DepoCyt produces sustained CSF concentrations of ara-C above 0.4 μM for 12–14 days, thus avoiding the need for more frequent lumbar punctures (16).

TOXICITY

Ara-C primarily affects dividing tissues such as the intestinal epithelium and bone marrow progenitors, leading to stomatitis, diarrhea, and myelosuppression, all of which peak at 7–14 days after treatment. In addition, ara-C may cause pulmonary vascular/epithelial injury, leading to a syndrome of non-cardiogenic pulmonary edema. Liver function abnormalities and rarely jaundice may occur as well, and are reversible with discontinuation of therapy.

High-dose ara-C may cause cerebellar dysfunction, seizures, dementia, and coma; this neurotoxicity is most common in patients with renal dysfunction and those over 60 years, thus leading to recommendations that highest dose consolidation (3 g/m^2) not be used in such patients. The same neurotoxicities, as well as arachnoiditis, may follow intrathecal drug injection.

GEMCITABINE

A second deoxycytidine analog, gemcitabine (2′-2′-difluoro-deoxycytidine, dFdC, GEM), has become an important component of treatment regimens for pancreatic cancer, non-small cell lung cancer, and other solid tumors. Its metabolic pathways are similar to those of ara-C (Figure 1-4), although its triphosphate has a much longer intracellular half-life, perhaps accounting for its solid tumor activity. In vitro, sensitive tumor cells are killed by exposure to GEM concentration of 0.01 μM for 1 h or longer, levels achieved by usual intravenous doses.

Gemcitabine uptake and activation in tumor cells mimic that of ara-C, requiring the hENT1 transporter, initial phosphorylation to dFdCMP by deoxycytidine kinase (dCK), conversion to the triphosphate, and incorporation into DNA. It has additional sites of action. Its diphosphate forms an inhibitory complex with ribonucleotide reductase (RNR) (17), and thereby it lowers intracellular levels of its physiologic competitor, dCTP, allowing greater incorporation of dFdC into DNA. Experimental findings suggest that RNR inhibition is an important contributor to the toxicity of GEM. Incorporation into DNA leads to chain termination and apoptosis. Exposure of cells to GEM activates the same ATR/Chk 1 kinases that block further cell cycle progression after ara-C treatment, but, in addition, it activates ATM, a checkpoint pathway that responds to double-strand breaks, and thus its action may differ from the single break pathway activation by ara-C.

Resistance in experimental tumors arises by several mechanisms, including deletion of the hENT1 transporter, deletion of dCK, increased phosphatase activity, or increased expression or amplification of either the large, catalytic subunit of RNR or its smaller tyrosyl-containing subunit. In clinical studies, higher dCK activity may predict improved survival in pancreatic cancer patients treated with GEM (18).

CLINICAL PHARMACOLOGY

The standard regimen of administration is 1000 mg/m^2 given as a 30-min infusion on days 1, 8, and 15 of a 28-day cycle. More prolonged periods of infusion, up to 150 min, may produce higher intracellular levels of dFdCTP, but also greater toxicity, and perhaps greater antitumor effects. Comparative trials of short- and long-infusion strategies are ongoing.

Doses may be modified for myelosuppression. GEM markedly sensitizes both normal and tumor tissues to concurrent radiation therapy, thus requiring drug dose reductions of 70%–80%. The mechanism of radiosensitization appears to be related to inhibition of repair of double-strand breaks and to inhibition of cell cycle progression. The drug is cleared rapidly from plasma by the ubiquitous cytoplasmic enzyme, CDA, and has a half-life of 15–20 min. Patients with the CDA variant, 27A>C, have delayed drug clearance and improved survival (19). Women and elderly patients may clear the drug more slowly, and all patients should be watched carefully for extreme myelosuppression.

■ TOXICITY

The primary toxicity of GEM is myelosuppression, which peaks in the third week of a 4-week schedule, blood counts usually recovering rapidly thereafter. Mild liver enzyme abnormalities may appear with longer term use. Pulmonary toxicity, with dyspnea and interstitial infiltrates, may occur in up to a quarter of patients treated with multiple cycles of the drug. In addition, patients on repeated cycles of GEM experience progressive anemia, which appears to have several components, including the direct effects of drug on red cell production, and the induction of hemolysis. After multiple cycles of treatment, a small but significant fraction of patients will experience a hemolytic-uremic syndrome (HUS), including anemia, edema and effusions, and a rising BUN (20). The HUS reverses with drug discontinuation, but in patients with pancreatic cancer, there may be no alternative effective therapy, and careful reinstitution of GEM at lower doses may be tried.

Severe toxicity has been reported in Japanese patients with an inactivating polymorphism of the CDA gene at position 208 was found (21), a variant associated with a fivefold slower clearance of the parent drug, as compared to nontoxic controls.

5-AZACYTIDINE (5AZAC)

5-Azacytidine (5azaC) (Figure 1-3) is both a cytotoxic and a differentiating agent, and has become a standard drug for treatment of myelodysplasia (22). Decitabine (DazaC), the closely related deoxy analog of 5azaC, is also approved for treatment of MDS and has the same mechanism of action. In MDS, which is characterized by refractory cytopenias and diverse chromosomal abnormalities, 5azaC reduces blood transfusion requirements and improves the platelet and mature granulocyte count in one-quarter to one-third of patients. While both analogs inhibit DNA synthesis and cause myelosuppression, their favorable effects on MDS are believed to be due to inhibition of DNA methyltransferase (DMT) and thereby activation of genes that induce maturation of hematopoietic cells.

5azaC and DazaC are transported into cells by nucleoside transporters, and are then converted to a nucleoside monophosphate by cytidine or deoxycytidine kinase, respectively. After further conversion to a triphosphate, they become incorporated into DNA, and act as a suicide inhibitor of the

DMT, inducing expression of silenced genes (23). Thus, in non-cytotoxic concentrations in tissue culture, both analogs promote differentiation of both normal and malignant cells. In patients with sickle-cell anemia, 5azaC induces synthesis of hemoglobin F and thereby reduces the frequency of sickle-cell crisis and acute chest syndrome. However, DNA synthesis inhibitors, such as hydroxyurea (HU), have a similar effect on patients with sickle-cell anemia; thus it is unclear whether 5azaC's beneficial effects are mediated by DNA demethylation or by inhibition of DNA synthesis (24).

The mechanism of 5azaC action in MDS likely relates to gene demethylation and induction of differentiation. Both global DNA demethylation and induction of specific genes follow azaC and DazaC treatment. An unfavorable response to DazaC correlates with an unfavourable (high) ratio of CDA to dCK activity, and to a lack of demethylation of selected genes (25). The pretreatment level of global methylation does not predict response.

■ CLINICAL PHARMACOLOGY

The elimination of both aza analogs occurs through their rapid deamination in plasma, liver, and other tissues by CDA. The plasma half-life of parent drugs is brief, 20–25 min. The primary metabolites, 5-azauridine and 5-deaza-deoxyuridine, undergo spontaneous hydrolysis and are inactive.

Toxicity of both aza analogs is primarily myelosuppression, with recovery 10–14 days after treatment. 5azaC causes significant nausea and vomiting when administered in high doses as antileukemic therapy. In occasional patients, hepatic dysfunction, rash, fever, or myalgias may be reported. In the usual regimen for myelodysplasia, 5azaC doses of 75 mg/m^2/day × 7 days are repeated every 4 weeks. The drug has minimal side effects aside from leukopenia.

DazaC has more potent cytotoxic and differentiating properties, and causes leukopenia and thrombocytopenia as its major toxicities. Doses of 10 mg/m^2/day × 5 days, in some regimens repeated on days 8–12, as tolerated, are given every 4 weeks in MDS treatment, but may induce prolonged neutropenia in patients with low WBC counts (25).

HYDROXYUREA

Hydroxyurea (HU), an inhibitor of RNR (26), is a useful agent for acutely lowering the white blood cell count in patients with myeloproliferative disease, especially acute or chronic myelogenous leukemia (CML). It also effectively lowers the platelet count in essential thrombocythemia. It has little value as a remission-inducing agent. Prior to imatinib, HU was a component of the maintenance regimen for CML but is now rarely employed for that purpose. Its effects on myelopoiesis are seen within 24 h, and reverse rapidly thereafter. Because of its minimal side effects and predictable and reversible action, it is commonly used to lower high white blood cell counts at the time of initial presentation of leukemia. It is also a potent radiosensitizer, and has been used with radiation therapy in experimental protocols for treatment of cervical cancer and head and neck cancer. It strongly induces fetal hemoglobin expression, and has become the standard agent for prevention of sickle-cell crisis (27). It has multiple effects on sickling, including an induction of fetal Hb, a reduction of adhesion of red cells to vascular endothelium, and a lowering of the white cell count, all of which may contribute to its beneficial action.

$$H_2N - \overset{\overset{\displaystyle O}{\|}}{C} - \overset{\overset{\displaystyle H}{|}}{N} - OH$$

Hydroxyurea

HU inhibits RNR by binding to the iron required for catalytic reduction of nucleoside diphosphates. Through deoxynucleotide depletion, it blocks progression of cells through the DNA synthetic phase of the cell cycle. Through its effects on deoxynucleotide pools, it enhances incorporation of other antimetabolites into DNA, and inhibits repair of alkylation. Resistance arises through outgrowth of cells that amplify or overexpress the catalytic subunit of RNR.

In addition to its effects on DNA synthesis, HU stimulates production of nitric oxide by neutrophils; NO in turn may function as an inducer of differentiation and a vasodilator, effects that may contribute to its control of sickle-cell crisis.

■ CLINICAL PHARMACOLOGY

HU is well absorbed after oral administration, but is available for intravenous infusion as well for emergent situations. Usual daily oral doses are 15–30 mg/kg, although higher doses are used for acute lowering of the white cell count. It is cleared by renal excretion, and its plasma half-life is approximately 4 h in patients with normal renal function. Doses should be adjusted according to creatinine clearance in patients with abnormal renal function.

Its toxicity is manifest primarily as acute myelosuppression, affecting all three lineages of blood cells. It may also cause a mild chronic gastritis, an interstitial pneumonitis, skin hyperpigmentation, ulcerations on the lower extremities, and neurologic dysfunction. It is a potent teratogen and should not be used without contraception in women of childbearing age. It has uncertain potential as a carcinogen, a concern in patients with nonmalignant disease and in chronic myeloproliferative syndromes such as polycythemia vera.

PURINE ANTAGONISTS

At least three general classes of purine antagonists have proven useful for treatment of cancer. The first were the thiopurines, 6-mercaptopurine (6-MP), and 6-thioguanine (6-TG), which were introduced as antileukemic drugs in the early 1950s (**Figure 1-5**). 6-MP remains a standard drug for maintenance of remission in childhood acute lymphocytic leukemia, in combination with methotrexate. 6-MP, the active metabolite of Imuran, is a potent immunosuppressive agent and is commonly used for Crohn's disease. The second group (**Figure 1-6**) of purine analogs consists of halogenated adenosine derivatives, fludarabine, clofarabine, and cladribine. Unlike adenosine, these drugs are resistant to deamination, and are toxic to both normal and malignant lymphoid cells. Cladribine is highly effective,

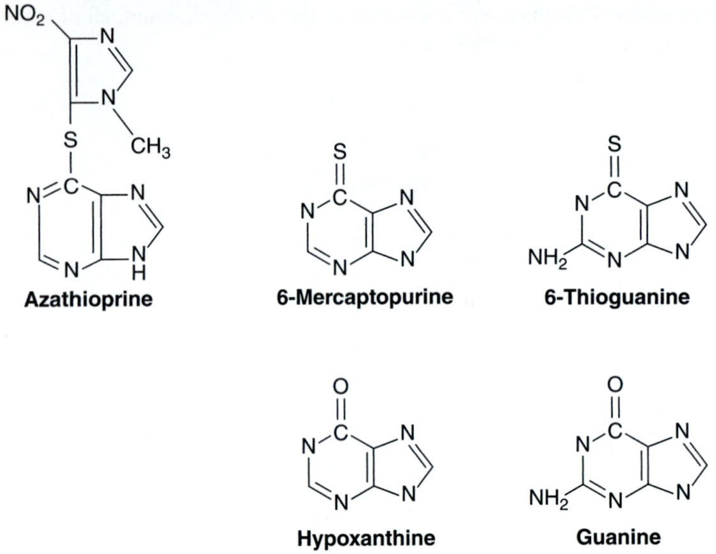

FIGURE 1-5 Structure of the naturally occurring purines, hypoxanthine and guanine, and related antineoplastic agents 6-mercaptopurine and 6-thioguanine, and the immunosupressive agent azathioprine.

and possibly curative for hairy cell leukemia, while fludarabine has become a first-line agent for chronic lymphocytic leukemia and for follicular lymphomas (28). Fludarabine suppresses T-cell function and is effective against graft versus host disease when used with low dose irradiation in allogeneic bone marrow transplantation. Finally, nelarabine, an arabinosyl guanine (ara-G), is specifically effective against T-cell lymphoid tumors (29).

The purine analogs are readily activated to nucleotides (mono-, di-, and triphosphates) in lymphoid tumors, and the active purine nucleotides are long lived ($t_{1/2}$ up to 16 h) and only slowly degraded intracellularly. T-cell-related immunosuppression is a common feature of the purine analogs.

■ CLINICAL PHARMACOLOGY OF 6-MP

6-MP is converted to 6-thioinosine monophosphate (6-IMP) by hypoxanthine-guanine phosphoribosyl transferase (HGPRT'ase). 6-IMP has multiple actions. It inhibits the first step in de novo purine synthesis. It is also converted to a triphosphate, which is incorporated into RNA and DNA, inhibiting RNA and DNA synthesis. Resistance to 6-MP arises through loss of HGPRT'ase, or by increased degradation of the active nucleotides.

6-MP is administered in doses of 50–100 mg/m²/day, and is titrated according to the degree of leukopenia. Oral absorption is erratic, and may contribute to therapeutic failure, further strengthening the need for titration of dose to leukopenia (30).

6-MP is cleared by two pathways, leading to a half-life in plasma of 90 min. The first step is its oxidation by xanthine oxidase (XO), a ubiquitous

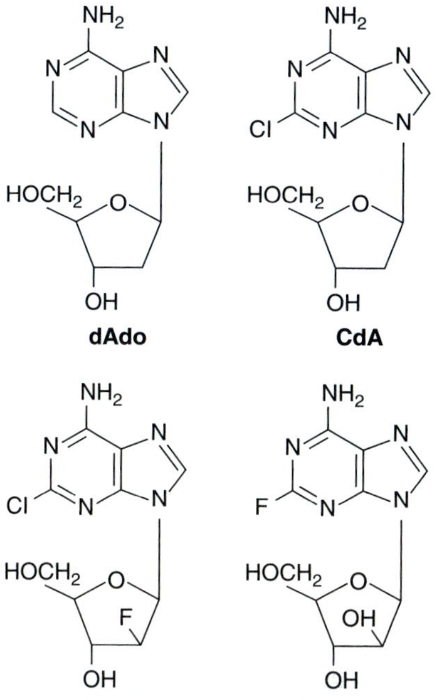

FIGURE 1-6 Structures of deoxyadenosine, cladribine (CdA), clofarabine (ClFdA), and fludarabine (Fara-A). Substitution with a chloro or fluoro atom at the 2-position of the adenine ring makes the compounds resistant to deamination by adenosine deaminase. At the 2′-arabino position, ClFdA has a fluoro atom and Fara-A has a hydroxy group.

enzyme. In the presence of allopurinol, a potent XO inhibitor used for treating gout, breakdown of orally administered 6-MP is inhibited by 75%, and thus the dose of 6-MP must be reduced by 75% in that circumstance. In the second degradative pathway, the sulfhydryl (SH) group undergoes methylation by thiopurine methyltransferase (TPMT) to the less potent 6-methyl MP. Polymorphisms of the TPMT gene are found with reasonable frequency (31). Fewer than 1% of the Caucasian population is homozygous for inactive forms of the enzyme, but these affected individuals become severely toxic with standard doses of 6-MP. About 10%–15% of Americans are heterozygotes for one allele of a relatively less active form of TPMT and often require reduction of 6-MP dose during maintenance therapy. Heterozygotes may have a lower relapse rate than patients with wild-type TPMT. A hyperactive polymorphism of methyltransferase has been identified in rare individuals of African descent; these patients may require increased doses of 6-MP, again titrated to produce modest leukopenia. While direct genetic testing of patients is not routinely available, many larger pediatric cancer centers test for TPMT variants or measure the erythrocyte enzyme or 6-thioguanine nucleotide content after 6-MP in order to detect patients at risk of over- or under-treatment.

The principal toxicities of 6-MP, as mentioned above, are myelosuppression and immunosuppression. 6-MP predisposes patients to opportunistic infection and causes biliary stasis and serum hepatocellular enzyme elevations in up to one-third of patients on treatment, although these effects rarely lead to permanent discontinuation of treatment. The drug is teratogenic, and is associated with an increased incidence of squamous cell carcinomas of the skin.

■ CLINICAL PHARMACOLOGY OF FLUDARABINE AND CLADRIBINE

Fludarabine is administered as a water-soluble monophosphate that is rapidly hydrolyzed to a nucleoside in plasma, while cladribine, clofarabine, and nelarabine are administered as the parent nucleoside in solution. The cellular uptake of the fludarabine nucleoside, cladribine, clofarabine, and nelarabine proceeds via nucleoside transporters. Inside the cell, fludarabine, clofarabine, and cladribine are activated to the monophosphate by deoxycytidine kinase, while nelarabine is activated by guanosine kinase. All four are then converted to their active triphosphate, and inhibit DNA synthesis. In addition, fludarabine diphosphate inhibits RNR, thereby depleting the physiologic deoxyadenosine triphosphates and enhancing the analog's incorporation into DNA. The triphosphates have long intracellular half-lives of 12–16 h. All four analogs lead to apoptosis, an effect that, in the case of fludarabine, depends on activation of cytochrome c released by the intrinsic apoptosis pathway. Loss of deoxycytidine kinase leads to resistance to fludarabine, clofarabine, and cladribine.

Fludarabine and cladribine share many common pharmacological features. Both are cleared by renal excretion of the parent drug, leading to plasma half-lives of 7 h for cladribine and 10 h for fludarabine. Both cause prolonged immunosuppression (low CD4 counts) and moderate and reversible myelosuppression at therapeutic doses. Opportunistic infection is common, particularly in CLL patients who are hypogammaglobulinemic prior to treatment. Fludarabine also causes a host of autoimmune phenomena, including hemolytic anemia, pure red cell aplasia, idiopathic thrombocytopenic purpura, arthritis, and antithyroid antibodies (32). It may also cause peripheral neuropathy, renal dysfunction, and altered mental status. Rare cases of AML, with deletion of the long arm of chromosome 7, in fludarabine-treated patients have been reported.

Doses of both fludarabine and cladribine should be reduced in proportion to the reduction in creatinine clearance in patients with abnormal renal function. The usual dose and schedule of fludarabine is 25 mg/m²/day intravenously for 5 days, repeated every 4 weeks for 6 cycles of treatment. Lower doses may be given in combination with cyclophosphamide and with rituximab in treating CLL. Fludarabine is well absorbed (60% bioavailability) and probably equally active when given orally in doses of 40 mg/m²/day, and preliminary results indicate equal activity by this route (33). Cladribine is administered in a single course of 0.09 mg/kg/day for 7 days to patients with hairy cell leukemia.

Resistance to fludarabine in CLL patients is associated with 17p13 chromosomal deletion, but it is uncertain whether loss of p53 function (located on this chromosome) is responsible (34).

NELARABINE

Nelarabine, a 6-methoxy prodrug of ara-G (Figure 1-7), has received approval for treatment of relapsed T-cell acute leukemia and for lympho-blastic lymphoma, for which it gives a complete response rate of approximately 20%, but with a few long-term remissions (35).

The mechanism of action of nelarabine proceeds through its activation by adenosine deaminase, which rapidly removes the 6-methoxy group in blood and tissues, generating the active ara-G. Ara-G is resistant to purine nucleoside phosphorylase, an enzyme essential for regulation of T-cell function, and the primary mechanism of protecting T-cells against buildup of toxic purine nucleotides. Intracellular ara-G is converted to its monophosphate by either deoxycytidine kinase or deoxyguanosine kinase, and then further to its triphosphate. Incorporation of ara-GTP into DNA terminates DNA synthesis and induces apoptosis in a manner similar to the effects of other ara nucleotides (36). T-lymphocytes, either normal or malignant, accumulate greater concentrations of ara-GTP, and retain the triphosphate for longer periods, than do B-cells, perhaps explaining its preferential effects on T-cell malignancy. Maximal cellular concentrations of ara-GTP are reached within 4 h of the end of infusion, declining thereafter with a $t_{1/2}$ of up to 24 h, and $t_{1/2}$ in individual patients closely correlates with complete response.

The conversion of nelarabine to ara-G occurs rapidly, in plasma, with a $t_{1/2}$ of 15 min. Ninety-four percent of the parent drug is converted to ara-G in 1 h. The active metabolite, ara-G, is then cleared from plasma, predominantly by hydrolysis to guanine, with a $t_{1/2}$ of 2–3 h (36). No modification of dose is required in patients with renal dysfunction.

Adults receive 1500 mg/m^2/day infused over 2 h on days 1, 3, and 5, while pediatric patients are given 650 mg/m^2/day for 5 days. Courses are repeated every 21 days until remission. Almost half of adult patients experience serious neurologic side effects, including somnolence, confusion, lethargy, or peripheral neuropathy. Other significant side effects include neutropenia and transaminase elevations. However, neurologic side effects are in general dose-limiting, may progress to an ascending neuropathy resembling the Guillain-Barré syndrome and may be irreversible.

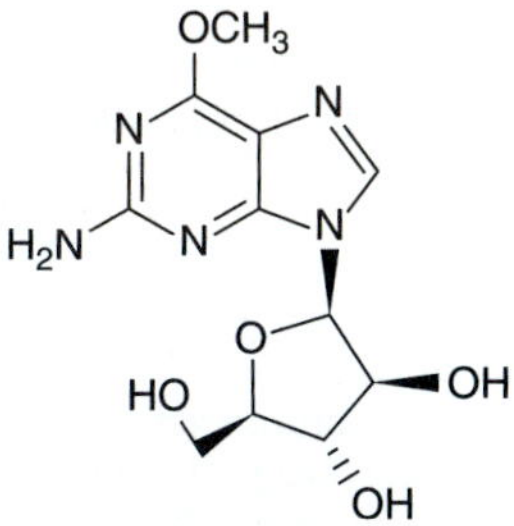

Nelarabine

FIGURE 1-7 Molecular structure of nelarabine.

CLOFARABINE

The newest antipurine is clofarabine. It contains a chlorine substitution at position 2 of the adenosine ring, as found in cladribine, and a fluorine in the beta-2′ position of the arabinose sugar (37), as in fludarabine (Figure 1-6). It thus has the general properties of both. It becomes incorporated into DNA, thereby inhibiting DNA synthesis; it also inhibits RNR and is resistant to adenosine deaminase. The 2′-fluorine confers resistance to purine nucleoside phosphorylase, and probably increases the stability of the intracellular nucleotide pool. It has the additional feature of promoting apoptosis through mitochondrial toxicity. Clofarabine is approved for treatment of relapsed or refractory pediatric ALL, but other indications including combination therapies in adult AML and myelodysplasia are being explored. Oral administration is associated with an acceptable bioavailability of 50%, and is under evaluation for lymphomas, but is not approved by the FDA.

Clofarabine is administered as a 1-h infusion of 30–40 mg/m^2 daily for 5 consecutive days in the treatment of AML and ALL. The drug is eliminated primarily by renal excretion. Its half-life in plasma varies from 4 to 10 h, having the shortest half-life in children, and slower clearance in adolescents and adults (38). Intracellular clofarabine triphosphate levels reach a maximum at doses of 40 mg/m^2/day, and at steady state, plasma clofarabine concentrations peak at 2–3 μM. The intracellular triphosphate persists at near peak levels (10 μM or higher) for longer than 24 h and accumulates with each dose. The mechanism of resistance of clofarabine has not been defined, but may result from decreased expression of deoxycytidine kinase, its initial activating enzyme (39).

The primary toxicity encountered at low doses (2–5 mg/m^2/day for 5 days) in nonleukemic patients is prolonged (30- to 40-day) myelosuppression. However, in patients with leukemia, treated with much higher doses, hepatic dysfunction (enzyme elevations and increased bilirubin) develops in 50%–75%. Hepatic function tests normalize within 14 days after drug discontinuation.

A skin rash is noted in 50% of leukemia patients receiving clofarabine, and palmo-plantar dysesthesia may also develop.

It is not known whether clofarabine treatment is associated with long-term immunosuppression, as occurs after fludarabine and cladribine.

REFERENCES

1. Meyerhardt JA, Mayer RJ. Systematic therapy for colorectal cancer. *N Engl J Med.* 2006; 352: 476–487.

2. Santi DV, McHenry CS, Sommer H. Mechanism of interaction of thymidylate synthetase with 5-fluorodeoxyuridylate. *Biochemistry.* 1974; 13: 471–481.

3. Grogan L, Sotos GA, Allegra CJ. Leucovorin modulation of fluorouracil. *Oncology.* 1993; 7: 63–72.

4. Washtein WL. Thymidylate synthetase levels as a factor in 5-fluorodeoxyuridine and methotrexate cytotoxicity in gastrointestinal tumor cells. *Mol Pharmacol.* 1982; 21: 723–728.

5. Kim HK, Choi IJ, Kim CG, et al. A gene expression signature of acquired chemoresistance to cisplatin and fluorouracil combination chemotherapy in gastric cancer patients. *PLoS One.* 2011; 6: e16694, 1–11.

6. Koizumi W, Boku N, Yamaguchi K, et al. Phase II study of S-1 plus leucovorin in patients with metastatic colorectal cancer. *Ann Oncol.* 2010; 21: 766–771.

7. Milano G, Ferrero JM, Francois E. Comparative pharmacology of oral fluoropyrimidines: a focus on pharmacokinetics, pharmacodynamics and pharmacomodulation. *Br J Cancer.* 2004; 91: 613–617.

8. Milano G, Etienne MC, Pierrefite V, et al. Dihydropyrimidine dehydrogenase deficiency and fluorouracil-related toxicity. *Br J Cancer.* 1999; 79: 627–630.

9. Kemeny N, Huang Y, Cohen AM, et al. Hepatic arterial infusion of chemotherapy after resection of hepatic metastases from colorectal cancer. *N Engl J Med.* 1999; 341: 2039–2048.

10. Kufe DW, Munroe D, Herrick D, et al. Effects of 1-beta-D-arabinofuranosylcytosine incorporation on eukaryotic DNA template function. *Mol Pharmacol.* 1984; 26: 128–134.

11. Campos L, Rouault J, Sabido O, et al. High expression of bcl-2 protein in acute myeloid leukemia cells in association with poor response to chemotherapy. *Blood.* 1993; 81: 3091–3096.

12. Wiley JS, Taupin J, Jamieson GP, et al. Cytosine arabinoside transport and metabolism in acute leukemias and T cell lymphoblastic lymphoma. *J Clin Invest.* 1985; 75: 632–642.

13. Mahlknecht U, Dransfeld CL, Bulut N, et al. SNP analysis in cytarabine metabolizing enzymes in AML patients and their impact on treatment response and patient survival: identification of CDA SNP C-451T as an independent prognostic parameter for survival. *Leukemia.* 2009; 23: 1929–1932.

14. Guo Y, Kock K, Ritter CA, et al. Expression of ABC-type nucleotide exporters in blasts of adult acute myeoloid leukemia: relation to long-term survival. *Clin Cancer Res.* 2009; 15: 1762–1769.

15. Bishop JF, Matthews JP, Young GA, et al. A randomized study of high-dose cytarabine in induction in acute myeloid leukemia. *Blood.* 1996; 87: 1710–1717.

16. Cole BF, Glantz MJ, Jaeckle KA, et al. Quality-of-life-adjusted survival comparison of sustained-release cytosine arabinoside versus intrathecal methotrexate for treatment of solid tumor neoplastic meningitis. *Cancer.* 2003; 97: 3053–3060.

17. Wang J, Lohman GJS, Stubbe J. Enhanced subunit interactions with gemcitabine-5'-diphosphate inhibit ribonucleotide reductases. *Proc Nat Acad Sci USA.* 2007; 104: 14324–14329.

18. Marachal R, Mackey JK, Lai R, et al. Deoxycytidine kinase is associated with prolonged survival after adjuvant gemcitabine for resected pancreatic adenocarcinoma. *Cancer.* 2010; 116: 5200–5206.

19. Tibaldi C, Giovannetti E, Vasile E, et al. Correlation of CDA, ERCC1, and XPD polymorphisms with response and survival in gemcitabine/cisplatin-treated advanced non-small cell lung cancer patients. *Clin Cancer Res.* 2008; 15: 1797–1803.

20. Humphreys BD, Sharman JP, Henderson JM, et al. Gemcitabine-associated thrombocytic microangiopathy. *Cancer.* 2004; 100: 2664–2670.

21. Sugiyama E, Kaniwa N, Kim SR, et al. Population pharmacokinetics of gemcitabine and its metabolite in Japanese cancer patients: impact of genetic polymorphisms. *Clin Pharmacokinet.* 2010; 49: 549–558.

22. Kaminskas E, Farrell AT, Wang YC, Sridhara R, Pazdur R. FDA drug approval summary: azacitidine (5-azacytidine, VidazaTM) for injectable suspension. *The Oncologist.* 2005; 10: 176–182.

23. Issa J-P, Kantarjian HM. Targeting DNA methylation. *Clin Cancer Res.* 2009; 15: 3938–3946.

24. Galanello R, Stamatoyannopoulos G, Papayannopoulous T. Mechanism of Hb F stimulation by s-phase compounds: in vitro studies with bone marrow cells exposed to 5-azacytidine, Ara-C or hydroxyurea. *J Clin Invest.* 1988; 81: 1209–1216.

25. Qin T, Castoro R, Ahdab SE, et al. Mechanisms of resistance to decitabine in the myelodysplastic syndrome. *PLoS One.* 2011; 6: e23372.

26. Elford HL. Effect of hydroxyurea on ribonucleotides reductase. *Biochem Biophys Res Commun.* 1968; 33: 129–135.

27. Cokic VP, Smith RD, Belesin-Cokic BB, et al. Hydroxyurea induces fetal hemoglobin by the nitric oxide-dependent activation of soluble guanylyl cyclase. *J Clin Invest.* 2003; 111: 231–239.

28. Keating MJ, O'Brien S, Albitar M, et al. Early results of a chemoimmunotherapy regimen of fludarabine, cyclophosphamide, and rituximab as initial therapy for chronic lymphocytic leukemia. *J Clin Oncol.* 2005; 23: 4079–4088.

29. Kisor DF. Nelarabine: a nucleoside analog with efficacy in T-cell and other leukemias. *Ann Pharmacother.* 2005; 39: 1056–1063.

30. Balis FM, Holcenberg JS, Zimm S, et al. The effect of methotrexate on the bioavailability of oral 6-mercaptopurine. *Clin Pharmacol Ther.* 1987; 41: 384–387.

31. Schmiegelow K, Foresterier F, Kristinsson J, et al. Thiopurine methyltransferase activity is related to the risk of relapse of childhood acute lymphoblastic leukemia: results from the NOPHO ALL-92 study. *Leukemia.* 2009; 23: 557–564.

32. Fujimaki K, Takasaki H, Koharazawa H, et al. Idiopathic thrombocytopenic purpura and myasthenia gravis after fludarabine treatment for chronic lymphocytic leukemia. *Leuk Lymphoma.* 2005; 46: 1101–1102.

33. Rossi JF, Van Hoof A, De Boeck K, et al. Efficacy and safety of oral fludarabine phosphate in previously untreated patients with chronic lymphocytic leukemia. *J Clin Oncol.* 2004; 22: 1260–1267.

34. Zenz T, Habe S, Denzel T, et al. Detailed analysis of p53 pathway defects in fludarabine-refractory chronic lymphocytic leukemia (CLL): dissecting the contribution of 17p deletion, TP53 mutation, p53-p21 dysfunction, and miR34a in a prospective clinical trial. *Blood.* 2009; 114: 2589–2597.

35. Kurtzberg J, Ernst TJ, Keating MJ, et al. Phase I study of 506U78 administered on a consecutive five day schedule in children and adults with refractory hematologic malignancies. *J Clin Oncol.* 2005; 23: 3396–3403.

36. Kisor D, Plunkett W, Kurtzberg J, et al. Pharmacokinetics of nelarabine and 9-beta-D-arabinofuranosyl guanine in pediatric and adult patients during a phase I study of nelarabine for the treatment of refractory hematologic malignancies. *J Clin Oncol.* 2000; 18: 995–1003.

37. Faderl S, Gandhi V, Keating MJ, Jeha S, Plunkett W, Kantarjian HM. The role of clofarabine in hematologic and solid malignancies— development of a next-generation nucleoside analog. *Cancer.* 2005; 103: 1985–1995.

38. Bonate PL, Cunningham CC, Gaynon P, et al. Population pharmacokinetics of clofarabine and its metabolite 6-ketoclofarabine in adult and pediatric patients with cancer. *Cancer Chemother Pharmacol.* 2001; 87: 875–890.

39. Mansson E, Flordal E, Liliemark J, et al. Down-regulation of deoxycytidine kinase in human leukemic cell lines resistant to cladribine and clofarabine and increased ribonucleotide reductase activity contributes to fludarabine resistance. *Biochem Pharmacol.* 2003; 65: 237–247.

CHAPTER **2**
Antifolates

Bruce A. Chabner

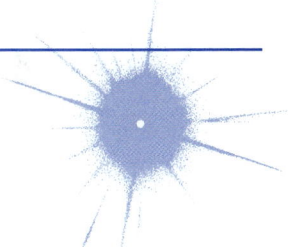

The antifolates were introduced as antileukemic drugs in 1948; in landmark experiments treating children with acute lymphocytic leukemia (ALL), Sidney Farber produced the first evidence that chemotherapy with a folate analogue, aminopterin, could lead to complete remissions (1). Methotrexate subsequently became the standard antifolate in treatment of ALL. It has since gained an important role in regimens for lymphomas, and choriocarcinoma, and as an immunosuppressive following allogeneic bone marrow transplantation. It is also a standard agent for treating rheumatoid arthritis, Wegener's granulomatosis, and other inflammatory/autoimmune diseases. Pemetrexed (Alimta), a closely related structure but with a different site of action, is widely used for non-small cell lung cancer, mesothelioma, and ovarian cancer. Pralatrexate, the newest antifolate similar in action to methotrexate, is highly active against peripheral T-cell lymphoma and cutaneous T-cell lymphoma.

The structures of antifolates are shown in Figure 2-1. The analogues closely resemble naturally occurring folates, but contain substitutions in the basic pteridine ring system, as in pralatrexate and pemetrexed, which enhance binding and transport. The key addition of the amino group on the C-4 position of the pteridine ring, as found in methotrexate, enhances inhibition of dihydrofolate reductase. Changes in the bridge system connecting

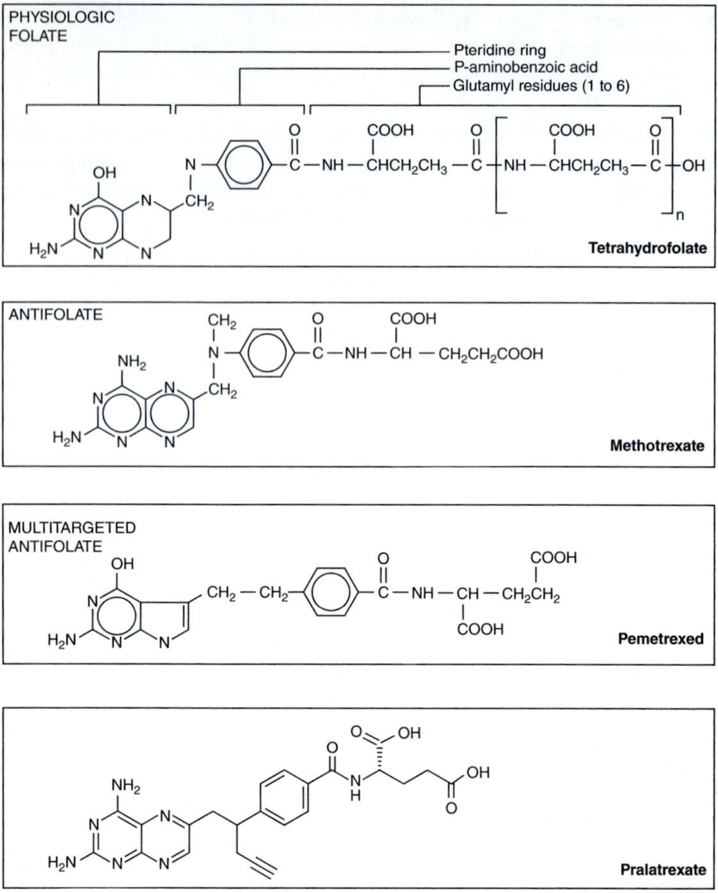

FIGURE 2-1 Molecular structure of folic acid, methotrexate, pemetrexed, and pralatrexate.

the unsaturated rings to para-aminobenzoyl glutamate (PABG) enhance the active uptake and polyglutamation of pemetrexed and pralatrexate. Because of their strong electronegative charge at physiologic pH, the parent antifolates, like physiologic folates, require active transport into cells via the reduced folate carrier (2). In selected cells, such as choriocarcinomas, a second carrier, the folate binding protein, mediates folate and methotrexate transport, and becomes the preferred transporter. Pemetrexed is also transported by a third carrier, the proton-coupled folate carrier, which may be responsible for its unique activity against epithelial cancer and mesothelioma (3). Inside the cell, the analogues, like the physiologic folates, are converted at their PABG terminus to highly charged, long-chain polyglutamates. These polyglutamate metabolites are retained preferentially within cells and inhibit, with increased affinity, a number of folate-dependent enzymes

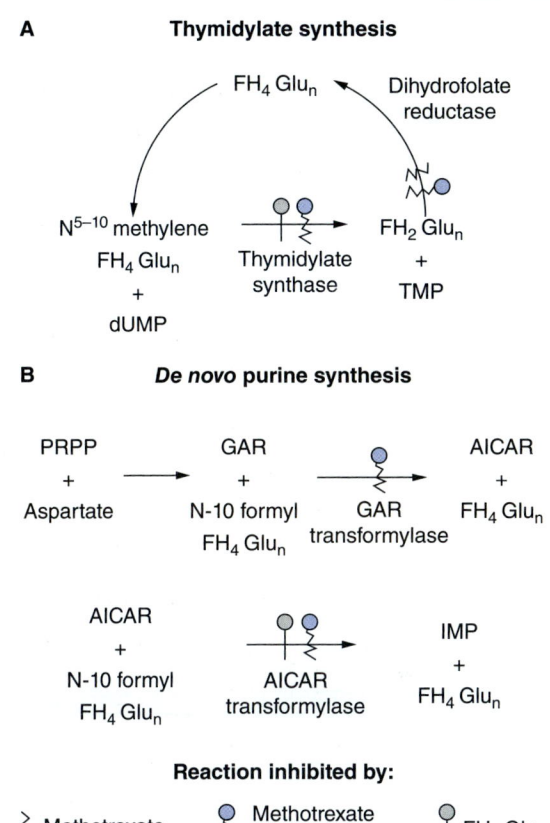

A **Thymidylate synthesis**

B *De novo* **purine synthesis**

Reaction inhibited by:

FIGURE 2-2 Multiple sites of inhibitory action of methotrexate, its polyglutamate metabolites, and dihydrofolate polyglutamates, the substrate that accumulates when dihydrofolate reductase is inhibited. AICAR: aminoimidazole carboxamide; TMP: thymidine monophosphate; dUMP: deoxyuridine monophosphate; FH_2Glu_n: dihydrofolate polyglutamate; FH_4Glu_n: tetrahydrofolate polyglutamate; GAR: glycinamide ribonucleotide; IMP: inosine monophosphate; PRPP: 5-phosphoribosyl-1-pyrophosphate. Pralatrexate acts in a very similar fashion, while the polyglutamates of pemetrexed primarily act as direct inhibitors of TS.

critical for both thymidine and purine biosynthesis (Figure 2-2). Through their inhibition of dihydrofolate reductase, methotrexate and pralatrexate deplete intracellular folates, leading to a block in both purine and pyrimidine biosynthesis. The primary action of pemetrexed is its inhibition of another folate-dependent enzyme, thymidylate synthase.

PHARMACOLOGIC CONSIDERATIONS

Methotrexate and Pralatrexate antifolates kill cells through depletion of thymidylate and purine precursors of DNA, and are thus most effective against rapidly growing tumors, such as leukemias and lymphomas. Cell kill by methotrexate depends on both drug concentration and duration of exposure. Its threshold concentration for drug toxicity for normal cells lies in the range of 10 nM. Methotrexate-resistant cells arise through loss of the reduced folate transporter, loss of the ability to polyglutamate antifolates, or amplification of the gene coding for dihydrofolate reductase, all of which have been demonstrated in ALL cells in association with relapse (4, 5). High levels of TS expression are associated with poor response to pemetrexed (4), while resistance to pralatrexate likely parallels that of methotrexate but is incompletely understood.

Inherited genetic variants modify folate metabolism (6, 7). The methylene tetrahydrofolate reductase variant C677T increases the intracellular level of 5–10 methylene tetrahydrofolic acid, the substrate for TS, and is associated with an increased rate of relapse in childhood ALL (7). Attempts to relate response and toxicity to variations in transporter and polyglutamate synthase genes have been inconclusive.

Pemetrexed and pralatrexate are more avidly transported and converted to a polyglutamate than is methotrexate (8). Because of its mild and predictable toxicities, pemetrexed has become a preferred agent for first- or second-line treatment of adenocarcinoma of the lung. Unlike methotrexate, pemetrexed and pralatrexate are given with folic acid (0.4–1.0 mg/day, beginning 1 week prior to treatment, and continuing throughout therapy) and with vitamin B_{12} (1 µg on day 1 i.m. and thereafter with each cycle of therapy), as these vitamins ameliorate toxicity to bone marrow (9).

CLINICAL PHARMACOLOGY

Methotrexate is well absorbed orally in doses of 25 mg/m^2 or less, and is used by that route in maintenance therapy of ALL. In higher doses (50–500 mg/m^2) it is given primarily by the intravenous route, or in higher dose regimens (1–20 g/m^2) with leucovorin (5-formyl-tetrahydrofolic acid) rescue. Individual drug regimens vary considerably, and are tailored to specific indications. Careful adherence to proven regimens is critical, with particular attention to the status of the patient's pretreatment renal function, which may drastically alter clearance of the drug and its toxicity.

Methotrexate is cleared primarily by renal excretion. Small amounts are metabolized to a nontoxic 7-OH derivative. In patients with normal renal function, it has a primary elimination half-life from plasma of 2–4 h, followed by a secondary elimination phase of 8–10 h (10). The terminal phase of disappearance determines the duration of exposure to cytotoxic concentrations of drug, and becomes much longer in patients with compromised renal function. Doses should be modified in proportion to the reduction in renal function for patients with a creatinine clearance of less than 60 ml/min. Nonsteroidal anti-inflammatory drugs reduce renal blood flow and displace methotrexate from plasma protein binding, thereby slowing clearance and increasing unbound drug concentrations in plasma, and should not be used in conjunction with methotrexate. Proton pump inhibitors may displace the drug from albumin binding and increase its toxicity. Penicillins reduce methotrexate secretion by renal tubules and may also increase the risk of toxicity.

■ HIGH-DOSE METHOTREXATE

High doses of methotrexate are administered to patients with ALL, osteosarcoma, and central nervous system lymphoma, and high-grade non-Hodgkin lymphoma in order to increase intracellular drug concentration, polyglutamate formation, and penetration into the central nervous system. These potentially lethal doses ($1-20$ g/m^2) are infused over $6-24$ h, and are followed by intravenous or oral leucovorin (5-formyl-tetrahydrofolate), $15-100$ mg/m^2, which restores the intracellular pool of tetrahydrofolates and rescues normal tissue from drug toxicity. Various regimens have proven safe and effective, and should be followed strictly to assure avoidance of toxicity. Methotrexate is relatively insoluble at acid pH, a property that may cause its precipitation in renal tubules in acidic urine, leading to acute renal dysfunction, a failure to excrete drug at normal rates, and overwhelming bone marrow and epithelial toxicity. Thus, patients require alkalinization of the urine prior to drug administration, and aggressive hydration and diuresis during methotrexate infusion (10). Drug levels in plasma and renal function should be monitored in the $24-48$ h post-infusion to assure normal rates of clearance. Concentrations of methotrexate above 1 μM at 24 h after the completion of infusion, particularly in conjunction with a rise in serum creatinine levels, should alert clinicians to impending serious toxicity. In such patients, the first step should be to increase and extend leucovorin administration (up to 500 mg every 6 h for 48 h IV), along with continued hydration. In extreme cases, when drug levels remain above 10 μM after 48 h, and show a very slow decline, leucovorin may be ineffective. In this setting, continuous flow hemodialysis is able to reduce drug levels at a clearance rate of 50 ml/min, and may avoid prolonged myelosuppression and mucositis.

Very rapid clearance of methotrexate and effective rescue from toxicity can be achieved for patients with delayed drug clearance through the intravenous administration of a recombinant bacterial folate-cleaving enzyme, carboxypeptidase G-2 (glucarpidase), which is now available for general clinical use (11). Greater than 95% clearance of drug from plasma is achieved within 15 min of administration of 50 units/kg given as a 5-min intravenous infusion, and life-threatening toxicity will be avoided in patients with plasma methotrexate levels in the range of $1-50$ μM. For patients with levels above 50 μM, reductions in plasma methotrexate, although substantial, do not reach the critical rescue level of 1 μM, probably due to reentry of drug from tissue compartments. Drug levels should be monitored after glucarpidase administration to determine the necessity of further measures, such as leucovorin or dialysis. Leucovorin is also cleaved by glucarpidase and is ineffective if used concurrently with the enzyme.

■ INTRATHECAL METHOTREXATE

Methotrexate is routinely administered intrathecally in doses of 12 mg for prevention or treatment of meningeal lymphoma, leukemia, or meningeal carcinomatosis. In patients with no evidence of meningeal tumor, the drug clears with a half-life of 2 h from the cerebral spinal fluid. In patients with active meningeal tumor, after lumbar intrathecal administration, its clearance may be slow and it may penetrate poorly into the ventricular space, requiring the placement of a reservoir for direct intraventricular therapy. Intrathecal methotrexate, particularly in patients with active meningeal disease, in whom drug clearance is slow, may lead to arachnoiditis, seizures, coma, and death. High-dose methotrexate regimens do produce cytotoxic drug concentrations in the spinal fluid, and appear to be sufficient for prophylaxis of CNS leukemia in average-risk ALL patients (12). High-dose systemic methotrexate rarely causes CNS toxicity. Oral or intravenous leucovorin is not an effective antidote to CNS toxicity.

■ PEMETREXED AND PRALATREXATE PHARMACOKINETICS

Pemetrexed pharmacokinetics closely follow those of methotrexate, with a 3-h terminal half-life in plasma, clearance by renal excretion, and dose adjustment for renal dysfunction. The usual dose of pemetrexed administration is 500 mg/m^2 every 3 weeks, with vitamin B$_{12}$ and folate supplementation. Higher doses, up to 900 mg/m^2 may be tolerated well by individual patients, but the therapeutic benefit of dose escalation is not established. Pralatrexate, given in doses of 30 mg/m^2/week with folate and vitamin B$_{12}$ supplementation, undergoes renal elimination, with a half-time in plasma of 4–8 h.

■ TOXICITY

Virtually every organ system may be affected by antifolate toxicity. Acutely, bone marrow suppression, mucositis, and gastrointestinal symptoms are the primary side effects of all 3 antifolates, and usually resolve within 10–14 days of completion of therapy. In most patients, high-dose methotrexate may be accompanied by very minimal evidence of toxicity, aside from acute reversible elevations in hepatic enzymes in serum. In toxic patients who develop renal failure, myelosuppression, severe mucositis, and desquamation may supervene. Cirrhosis is occasionally reported in psoriasis or rheumatoid arthritis patients on long-term oral methotrexate, and is heralded by elevations in plasma type III procollagen aminopeptide (PIIIAP). Patients with elevated PIIIAP levels in plasma are at 20% risk of drug-related cirrhosis and should undergo a liver biopsy (13). An interstitial pneumonitis, likely related to hypersensitivity to the drug, with eosinophilic infiltrates, is occasionally seen with methotrexate.

Pemetrexed is toxic to bone marrow and gastrointestinal and oral mucosa. Toxicity tends to be predictably mild in patients receiving concurrent folic acid and vitamin B$_{12}$. Early trials without vitamin protection witnessed a significant (15%–20%) incidence of severe toxicity, primarily in patients with high levels of homocysteine in plasma, an indicator of folate deficiency, prior to treatment. Pulmonary toxicity, manifested as an interstitial pneumonitis, may complicate therapy in 3%–5% of patients (14). Another important but uncommon side effect is peripheral edema, and in rare cases, pleural effusions (15). Up to 40% of patients may experience a bothersome erythematous rash, which can be largely prevented by oral dexamethasone, 4 mg twice daily on days –1, 0, and +1.

Pralatrexate is given in doses of 30 mg/m^2/week for 6 of 7 weeks. Myelosuppression and mucositis may lead to delays in treatment or dose adjustment.

REFERENCES

1. Farber S, Diamond LK, Mercer RD, et al. Temporary remission in acute leukemia in children produced by folic acid antagonist 4-amethopteroylglutamic acid (aminopterin). *N Engl J Med.* 1948; 238: 787–793.

2. Moscow JA, Gong M, He R, et al. Isolation of a gene encoding a human reduced folate carrier (RFC1) and analysis of its expression in transport deficient, methotrexate-resistant human breast cancer cells. *Cancer Res.* 1995; 55: 3790–3794.

3. Zhao R, Qui A, Jansen M. The proton-coupled folate transporter: impact on pemetrexed transport and on antifolate activities compared with the reduced folate carrier. 2008; 74: 854–862.

4. Takezawa I, Ikamoto I, Okamoto W, et al. Thymidylate synthase as a determinant of pemetrexed sensitivity in non-small cell lung cancer. *Brit J Cancer.* 2011; 104: 1594–1601.

5. Whitehead VM, Shuster JJ, Vuchich MJ, et al. Accumulation of methotrexate and methotrexate polyglutamates in lymphoblasts and treatment outcome in children with B-progenitor-cell acute lymphoblastic leukemia: a Pediatric Oncology Group study. *Leukemia.* 2005; 19: 533–536.

6. Buikhuisen WA, Burgers JA, Vincent AD et al. Pemetrexed pathway-associated germline polymorphisms: a useful tool for treatment individualization? *J Clin Oncol.* 2010; 28: e482–e483.

7. Aplenc R, Thompson J, Han P, et al. Methylenetetrahydrofolate reductase polymorphisms and therapy response in pediatric acute lymphoblastic leukemia. *Cancer Res.* 2005; 65: 2482–2487.

8. Izbicka E, Diaz A, Streeper R, et al. Distinct mechanistic activity profile of pralatrexate in comparison to other antifolates in in vitro and in vivo models of human cancers. *Cancer Chemother Pharmacol.* 2009; 64: 993–999.

9. Scagliotti GV, Shin DM, Kindler HL, et al. Phase II study of pemetrexed with and without folic acid and vitamin B12 as front-line therapy in malignant pleural mesothelioma. *J Clin Oncol.* 2003; 21: 1556–1561.

10. Stoller RG, Hande KR, Jacobs SA, et al. Use of plasma pharmacokinetics to predict and prevent methotrexate toxicity. *N Engl J Med.* 1977; 297: 630–634.

11. Buchen S, Ngampolo D, Melton RG, et al. Carboxypeptidase G2 rescue in patients with methotrexate intoxication and renal failure. *Br J Cancer.* 2005; 92: 480–487.

12. Glantz MJ, Cole BF, Recht L, et al. High-dose intravenous methotrexate for patients with nonleukemic leptomeningeal cancer: is intrathecal chemotherapy necessary? *J Clin Oncol.* 1998; 16: 1561–1567.

13. Chalmers RJ, Kirby B, Smith A, et al. Replacement of routine liver biopsy by procollagen III aminopeptide for monitoring patients with psoriasis receiving long-term methotrexate: a multicentre audit and health economic analysis. *Br J Dermatol.* 2005; 152: 444–450.

14. Cohen MH, Johnson JR, Wang YC, et al. FDA drug approval summary: pemetrexed for injection (Alimta) for the treatment of non-small cell lung cancer. *The Oncologist.* 2005; 10: 363–368.

15. D'Angelo SP, Kris MG, Paetanza, MC, et al. A case series of dose-limiting peripheral edema observed in patients treated with pemetrexed. *J Thoracic Oncol.* 2011; 6: 624–626.

CHAPTER **3**

The Taxanes, Vinca Alkaloids, and Their Derivatives

Bruce A. Chabner

INTRODUCTION

In the past decade, the taxanes have emerged as one of the most powerful classes of anticancer drugs (1). Two unmodified taxanes, paclitaxel and docetaxel, are approved for clinical use in multiple tumors. An albumin-stabilized paclitaxel (abraxane) is also available for treatment of breast cancer (2), and a new analogue, cabazitaxel, is approved for hormone refractory prostate cancer. Despite their similar structures and a common mechanism of action (disruption of microtubule function), the taxanes differ in their pharmacological profiles, toxicity, and their patterns of clinical activity. Taxanes are predominantly employed in solid tumor chemotherapy in combination with platinum derivatives, with other cytotoxics, or with monoclonal antibodies such as Herceptin (trastuzumab). Both unmodified taxanes act synergistically with trastuzumab against HER2/neu overexpressed breast cancer cells in vitro and in vivo, and the combination of taxane and trastuzumab improves survival against HER2/neu amplified breast cancer in the adjuvant setting. The two original taxanes differ in their interaction with doxorubicin, paclitaxel potentiating the anthracycline's cardiac toxicity, while docetaxel and doxorubicin are well tolerated and highly active in combination (3). The taxanes are also primary agents for treating other malignancies, including ovarian, lung, and bladder cancer.

A closely related antimitotic agent, ixabepilone, is approved for second-line breast cancer treatment after taxanes, and differs from taxanes in its greater neurotoxicity and its lack of cross-resistance in MDR-positive tumors.

STRUCTURE

Paclitaxel was first isolated from the bark of the Pacific yew, *Taxus brevifolia*. Paclitaxel and its analogue, docetaxel, are now synthesized from 10-deacetylbaccatin III, a precursor found in the leaves of the European yew, *Taxus baccata* (4). Both molecules are composed of a 15-member taxane ring system linked to a 4-member oxetan ring at the C-4 and C-5 positions of the molecule. The structures of paclitaxel and docetaxel differ in substitutions at the C-10 ring position and in the configuration of an ester side chain attached at C-13. Docetaxel is slightly more water soluble than paclitaxel and a more potent inhibitor of tubulin in cell-free systems. The side chain substitutions at C-13 position are essential for antimicrotubule activity. The chemical structures of paclitaxel and docetaxel are shown in Figure 3-1. Abraxane is identical to paclitaxel, but is formulated within a microalbumin particle that eliminates the hypersensitivity caused for the lipid excipient used to deliver paclitaxel. Cabazitaxel retains the taxane nuclear ring system but has multiple side chain modifications to increase its solubility and decrease susceptibility to multidrug resistance.

MECHANISM OF ACTION

The taxanes stabilize microtubules. They bind to the interior surface of the β-microtubule chain and enhance microtubule assembly by promoting the nucleation and elongation phases of tubulin polymerization. In solution they reduce the critical tubulin subunit concentration required for microtubule assembly. Unlike the vinca alkaloids, which *prevent* microtubule assembly, the taxanes decrease the lag time to assembly and dramatically shift the dynamic equilibrium from tubulin dimers to microtubule polymers (5).

The taxane binding site on β-tubulin is distinct from those of vinca alkaloids, podophyllotoxin, colchicines, maytansine, and the maytansine-like antimitotic attached to anti CD30 antibody (brevituximab vendotin). Paclitaxel and docetaxel bind reversibly to both the N-terminal residues and the internal amino acid residues at 217–233 positions. This binding increases the rate of tubulin polymerization, disrupts the orderly formation of mitotic spindles and segregation of chromosomes, halts progression through mitosis, and promotes apoptosis. Taxanes block the anti-apoptotic effects of the BCL-2 gene family, and induce p53 gene activation with consequent mitotic arrest, formation of multinucleated cells, and cell death.

In addition to their direct cytotoxic effects, taxanes potently inhibit vascular endothelial cell proliferation, and enhance the cytotoxic effects of radiation at clinically achievable concentrations.

DRUG RESISTANCE

Two major mechanisms of taxane resistance have been characterized in cells selected in vitro (6). Taxanes are one of many natural product drugs affected by multidrug resistance (MDR) as mediated through increased expression of the 170-kD p-glycoprotein, an efflux pump encoded by the MDR-1 gene. The p-glycoprotein promotes rapid efflux of taxanes, anthracyclines, and vinca alkaloids, as well as other natural products. MDR resistance can be reversed in vitro and in animal test systems by calcium channel blockers, tamoxifen, hormones, cyclosporine A, and even cremaphor, the principal lipid used to formulate paclitaxel. The precise role of MDR-1 in conferring resistance to the taxanes in the clinical setting is not firmly established. For example, clinical observations to date suggest that in breast cancer, there is

(a) Paclitaxel

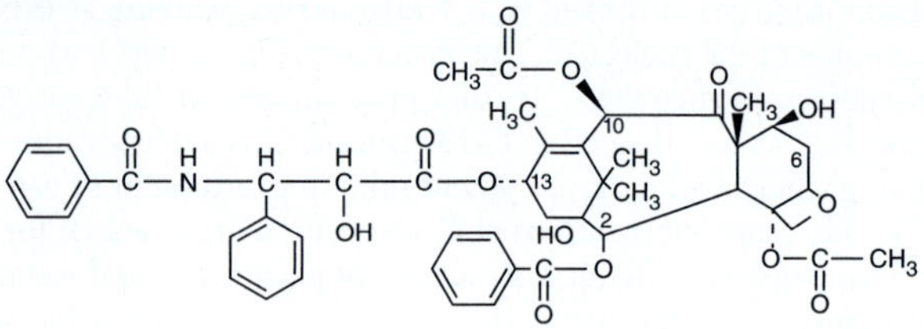

(b) Docetaxel

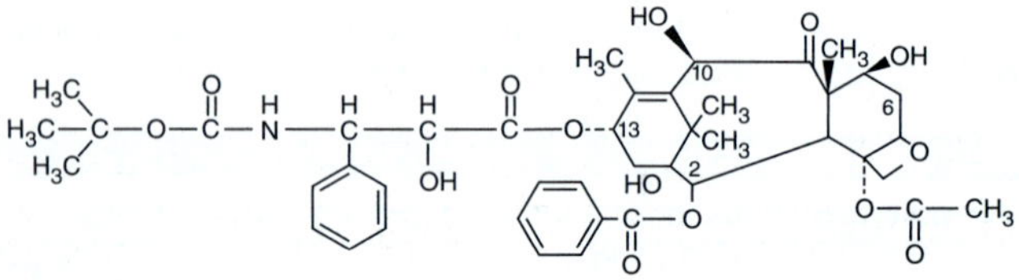

(c) Cabazitaxel

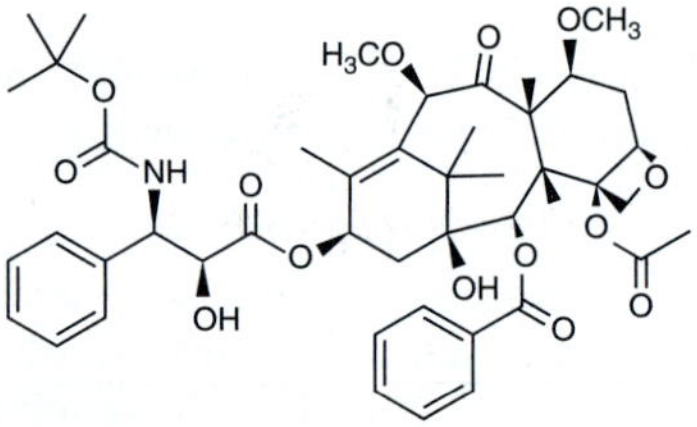

(d) Ixabepilone

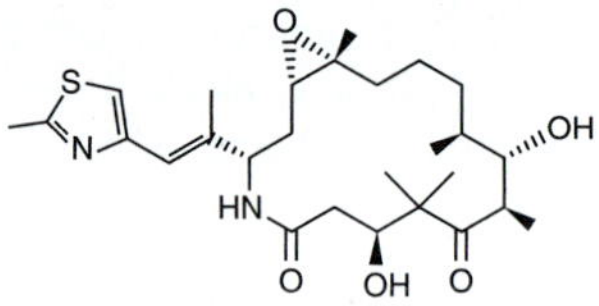

(e) Eribulin

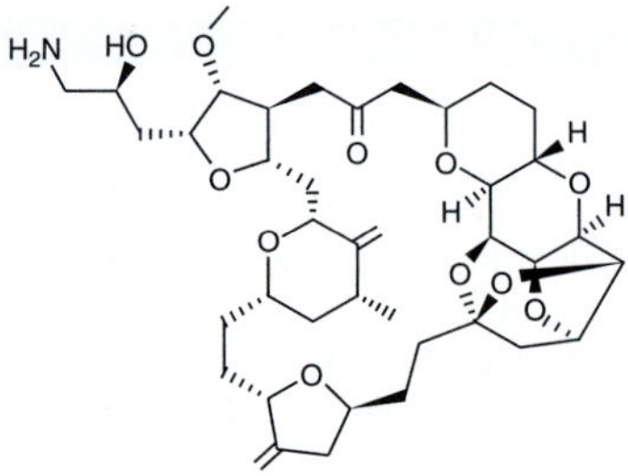

FIGURE 3-1 The chemical structure of antimitotics: (A–C) taxanes, (D) ixabepilone, and (E) eribulin.

incomplete cross-resistance between taxanes and anthracyclines, implying that MDR-1 expression is not responsible for drug resistance in all cases. A second form of resistance to taxanes is seen in cells that express an altered β-tubulin phenotype, either through mutations or due to minor polymorphisms that modify taxane binding. Paclitaxel-resistant, β-tubulin mutant cells have an impaired ability to polymerize tubulin dimers into microtubules. Amplification of β-tubulin encoding genes, mutation of the β-tubulin binding sites, and isotype switching of β-tubulin all have been reported in taxane-resistant cell lines.

An additional mechanism responsible for taxane resistance has been attributed to increased expression of MCL-1 and BCL-2, both of which inhibit apoptosis. Ixabepilone and cabazitaxel are less susceptible to MDR-mediated resistance, as compared to the original taxanes. β-Tubulin mutations have been linked to ixabepilone resistance in preclinical experiments.

CLINICAL PHARMACOLOGY AND METABOLISM

The taxanes are active only in their parent form, and all are administered intravenously. Oral bioavailability of either paclitaxel or docetaxel is poor due to high-level expression of p-glycoprotein and other ATP-binding cassette (ABC) transporters in intestinal epithelium, and first-pass drug metabolism in the liver.

The metabolism of all clinically approved taxanes is mediated through hepatic cytochrome p450 mixed-function oxidases. Paclitaxel is inactivated to hydroxylated metabolites through stepwise catalysis by cytochrome 2C8, producing 6α-OH, and CYP3A4, producing 6α-OH-3′OH, and finally to the dihydroxyl product (7). Docetaxel is oxidized at C13 by CYP3A4. The involvement of cytochrome enzymes in taxane biotransformation has two important implications: first, co-medications capable of inducing or inhibiting cytochromes influence the rate of inactivation and the metabolic fate of taxanes (8). Second, polymorphisms affecting enzymatic function have been described for both CYP2C8 and CYP3A4, thereby leading to interpatient variability of pharmacokinetics. Pharmacokinetic data for paclitaxel and docetaxel are shown in Table 3-1.

■ PACLITAXEL

Pharmacokinetic studies have disclosed substantial interpatient variability and nonlinearity of the relationship between paclitaxel dose and drug concentration in plasma (Table 3-2). Nonlinearity is particularly prominent with shorter (1- to 3-h) drug infusion schedules, and may indicate variability of tissue binding and clearance mechanisms.

The pharmacokinetics of this drug have been evaluated in doses ranging from 100 to 300 mg/m² infused in time periods of 1, 3, and 24 h. Following intravenous administration, the drug exhibits a biphasic decline in plasma concentration, reaching peak concentrations between 5 and 10 μM for 1-3 h infusions, and remaining in the inhibitory range for myelopoiesis (above 50 nM) for 12–24 h. Both the terminal half-life of 10-24 h and the mean clearance of paclitaxel appear to either remain unchanged or slightly increase as the infusion time is increased. Approximately 80% of paclitaxel is excreted in feces in the form of CYP2B8

TABLE 3-1 COMPARATIVE PHARMACOKINETIC CHARACTERISTICS OF TAXANES

Characteristic	Paclitaxel	Docetaxel
Dose and schedule	135–175 mg/m^2, 3-h infusion every 3 weeks	75–100 mg/m^2, 1-h infusion every 3 weeks
Pharmacokinetic behavior	Nonlinear	Linear
Volume of distribution	182 l/m^2	74 l/m^2
Plasma protein binding	>95%	>90%
Peak plasma concentration	5–10 μM (175 mg/m^2/3 h)	2–5 μM (100 mg/m^2/1 h)
Average terminal plasma half-life/h	11.5	12
Tissue distribution	Extensive except CNS and testes	Extensive except CNS
Clearance	~350 ml/min/m^2	300 ml/min/m^2
Primary route of clearance	Hepatic metabolism and biliary elimination	Hepatic metabolism and biliary elimination
Renal clearance	<10%	<10%

and 3A4 metabolites, the 6α-hydroxy-paclitaxel, the C3′-hydroxy paclitaxel, and the dihydroxy products accounting for the bulk of the dose. Renal clearance of paclitaxel and its metabolites is minor, accounting for about 15% of administered dose and only 5% is excreted unchanged. The dose should be reduced by 50% in patients with a bilirubin greater than 1.5 mg/dl, and the drug should be withheld in patients with severe hepatic dysfunction.

■ DOCETAXEL

The pharmacokinetic behavior of docetaxel on a 1-h schedule at doses of 75–115 mg/m^2 or less displays a linear relationship between dose and drug concentrations in plasma. The terminal half-life is about 17 h. As with paclitaxel, docetaxel is cleared by CYP-mediated metabolism and is widely distributed among tissues except for central nervous system.

TABLE 3-2 PHARMACOKINETIC PARAMETERS FOR PACLITAXEL

Dose Range (mg/m^2)	Infusion Duration (h)	Peak Plasma Concentration (μM)	AUC (ng/ml/h)	Terminal Half-Life (h)	Clearance (l/h/m^2)
100–135	1	6.0–19.3	9,918–35,018	10.6–15.8	8.05–11.64
135–175	3	1.3–4.3	6,568–15,007	6.3–20.2	12.2–17.2
135–175	24	0.2–0.4	6,300–7,993	15.7–24.6	21.7–23.8

DRUG INTERACTIONS

Because of its reliance for clearance upon the cytochrome system, taxanes have pharmacokinetic interactions with other cancer drugs (Table 3-3).

Paclitaxel preceding doxorubicin increases the frequency of mucositis, cardiotoxicity, and neutropenia than would be anticipated from additive effects of the two drugs. Pharmacokinetic studies indicate that paclitaxel decreases doxorubicin clearance. Administration of these drugs 24 h apart may ameliorate this effect.

Alternating sequences of paclitaxel and cyclophosphamide revealed that cytopenias were profound when paclitaxel was infused prior to, but not after, cyclophosphamide. Docetaxel given before ifosfamide increases the clearance of the alkylator, and dose-limiting toxicity occurred at lower doses of docetaxel when ifosfamide preceded the taxane (9).

Enzyme-inducing anticonvulsants increase CYP3A4 activity, accelerate taxane clearance, and markedly increase the dose of paclitaxel required to reach a maximum tolerated dose. CYP3A inhibitors, such as ketoconazole, profoundly slow taxane clearance.

TOXICITY

Neutropenia is the principal and dose-limiting toxicity of both taxanes, docetaxel being the most myelosuppressive. The severity and frequency of paclitaxel-induced neutropenia increases when infusion is prolonged from

TABLE 3-3 CLINICALLY SIGNIFICANT TAXANE-DRUG INTERACTION

Paclitaxel and Doceel	Interacting	Mechanism	Comment
	Doxorubicin	Increased C_{max} and decreased clearance of doxorubicin	Administer doxorubicin before paclitaxel
	Cisplatin	Decreased taxane clearance	Administer taxane 24 h before cisplatinum
	Carboplatin	Increased carboplatin clearance, decrease in thrombocytopenia	
	Anticonvulsants	CYP induction decreases plasma concentration and increases clearance of paclitaxel	Increase dose of taxane
	Warfarin	Taxane displaces coumadin from protein-binding sites	Decrease dose of coumadin
	Gemcitabine	Increased level of gemcitabine triphosphate by unknown mechanism	Decrease dose of gemcitabine

3 to 24 h and at doses above 175 mg/m^2. However, neutropenia is non-cumulative, and its duration even in heavily pretreated patients is usually brief. Weekly treatments with lower doses of 80–100 mg/m^2 of paclitaxel yield antitumor activity at least equivalent to higher doses given every 3 weeks in breast cancer, with less acute toxicity. Severe thrombocytopenia and anemia are uncommon except in heavily pretreated patients.

In the absence of antihistamines and glucocorticoids, paclitaxel administration causes a high incidence of acute hypersensitivity reactions, primarily related to the cremaphor solvent. The incidence and the intensity of hypersensitivity to paclitaxel formulations are significantly diminished by pretreatment with dexamethasone, diphenhydramine, and ranitidine.

Cardiac arrhythmias, especially asymptomatic bradycardias, are seen after paclitaxel. Paclitaxel should be used with EKG monitoring in patients with a history of cardiac conduction disturbances. As discussed previously, paclitaxel increases the incidence of anthracycline-induced congestive heart failure (CHF), when the two drugs are used together. There is no conclusive evidence for an increased rate of CHF in patients receiving docetaxel/anthracycline combinations. Neither taxane increases the cardiac toxicity of trastuzumab. Dose-related myalgia and neuropathy, especially an increase in neurosensory symptoms (numbness in a symmetrical glove and stocking distribution), may become significant complaints with paclitaxel, particularly with higher doses, after multiple cycles, and in combination with cisplatin.

Neurotoxicity is more frequently associated with shorter (1–3 h) infusion schedules and with weekly, "dose-dense" schedules commonly used in ovarian and breast cancer, indicating that peak plasma concentrations and dose density are principal determinants. Mild to moderate peripheral neurotoxicity occurs in approximately 40% of patients receiving every 3 week paclitaxel, especially with those who have previously received cisplatin, but neurotoxicity, asthenia, and muscular weakness become prominent complaints from patients who have received large cumulative doses and those treated on a long-term weekly schedule (10).

The toxicity of docetaxel closely mimics that of paclitaxel with several important exceptions. Docetaxel is more myelosuppressive and stomatitis is more frequent. Nausea, vomiting, and diarrhea have been observed with both taxanes, but severe gastrointestinal toxicity is uncommon.

During its early phases of development, docetaxel treatment led to a cumulative fluid retention syndrome in approximately 50% of patients after three to five cycles of therapy. Ankle edema, pleural effusions, and even ascites may become dose limiting. Premedication with dexamethasone, 8 mg twice daily for 3–5 days, beginning 1 day before drug administration, significantly decreases the incidence and severity of the fluid retention syndrome.

FORMULATION AND ADMINISTRATION

■ PACLITAXEL

Taxanes are insoluble in water. Paclitaxel is formulated in 50% alcohol and 50% polyoxyethylated castor oil derivative (cremaphor). An initial dose of 135 mg/m^2 of paclitaxel on a 24-h schedule was approved for patients with refractory or recurrent ovarian cancer, but later regulatory approval was obtained for a dose of 175 mg/m2 infused over 3 h every 3 weeks in ovarian cancer as well as for other indications. In ovarian and breast cancer patients treated on different schedules of 3-, 24-, and 96-h infusion every 3 weeks, the various schedules may be equally effective (11), although the 96-h infusion produces less myelosuppression and systemic complaints. In children, higher doses may be well tolerated.

In ovarian cancer treatment, a "dose-dense" weekly schedule of 70–90 mg/m^2 with carboplatin, AUC 3, was more effective than every 3-week infusions of paclitaxel with carboplatin, AUC 5 (12). Paclitaxel, even in low doses of 20 mg/m^2 weekly, reduces the thrombocytopenic effect of carboplatin. An alternative regimen in ovarian cancer employs a combination of intravenous, day 1, and intraperitoneal, day 8, paclitaxel with intraperitoneal cisplatin (see Ovarian Cancer, Chapter 54), but is associated with catheter-related toxicity and significant systemic toxicity.

◼ DOCETAXEL

Docetaxel is formulated in polysorbate 80, and it can be administered after dilution in 0.9% saline, or 5% dextrose solution to a concentration of between 0.3 and 0.9 mg/ml. It is administered in doses of 60–100 mg/m^2 over 1 h every 3 weeks. Weekly schedules of 30–40 mg/m^2 cause a higher incidence of cumulative muscular weakness and neurotoxicity. This toxicity was especially noticeable with docetaxel doses exceeding 36 mg/m^2 weekly.

◼ ABRAXANE

The newest approved taxane is abraxane, a formulation of paclitaxel in 3%–4% human albumin. This formulation of paclitaxel causes markedly less hypersensitivity than either paclitaxel or docetaxel, and is administered without premedication. The presence of the albumin particle surrounding the taxane enhances uptake in tumor cells that have an albumin receptor complex (SPARC) (13), which is found on many breast cancers and some normal tissues. The abraxane formulation leads to greater tissue penetration of paclitaxel (a much larger volume of distribution), a longer plasma half-life (27 h), and a greater free drug concentration in plasma. In clinical trials, the drug has at least equivalent activity to paclitaxel as second-line therapy in metastatic breast cancer, but produces greater myelosuppression, sensory neuropathy, and asthenia. The recommended dose and schedule are 260 mg/m^2 infused over 30 min every 3 weeks.

◼ CABAZITAXEL

Cabazitaxel (a dimethyloxy derivative of docetaxel, see Figure 3-1) was selected for clinical development because of its lack of substrate affinity for the p-glycoprotein export pump. It is approved for treatment of prostate cancer refractory to docetaxel and hormonal inhibitors, based on an improvement of 2.1 months in overall survival, compared to survival in patients receiving mitoxantrone (14). The drug is administered in doses of 25 mg/m^2 as a 60-min infusion every 3 weeks, in combination with prednisone 10 mg daily throughout treatment. It has a prolonged terminal half-life of 92 h and is primarily cleared by hepatic CYP3A4 metabolism.

At this dose, its primary toxicities are grade 3 or greater neutropenia in 20% of patients. G-CSF use in prostate patients is recommended in high-risk patients (age greater than 65 years, comorbidities), and after the first cycle of therapy if patients develop severe neutropenia. It also causes a mild neuropathy in 10% of patients. Ongoing studies are evaluating a lower and potentially less toxic dose (20 mg/m^2), and are comparing cabazitaxel to docetaxel as initial therapy for castration-resistant prostate cancer (13).

■ CLINICAL PHARMACOLOGY OF OTHER ANTIMITOTICS

Ixabepilone

The epothilones, an entirely new class of antimitotics with action similar to the taxanes (stabilization of tubulin polymers, mitotic arrest), were isolated from a fungal fermentation broth. Ixabepilone (a derivative of epothilone B, see Figure 3-1), in combination with capecitabine, is approved for treating breast cancer patients whose tumor is resistant to taxanes or anthracyclines. The drug has a large volume of distribution, limited protein binding, a long terminal half-life in plasma of 52 h, and is cleared predominantly by CYP3A4 metabolism, a pathway inhibited by imidazole antifungals. The recommended dose is 40 mg/m^2 in a 3-h infusion every 3 weeks.

Ixabepilone, like other epothilones, produces a potent but usually reversible sensory neurotoxicity (burning, hypesthesias, neuropathic pain), which becomes increasingly prominent with successive cycles of therapy and may lead to drug delay or discontinuation. Patients with hepatic dysfunction or preexisting neuropathy should be treated with extreme caution. Dose reduction is recommended for patients with hepatic enzyme or bilirubin elevation. It also causes myelosuppression, and with its castor oil formulation, hypersensitivity reactions. Histamine antagonists (benadryl, 50 mg, and ranitidine, 150–300 mg) are recommended for premedication, and for patients experiencing hypersensitivity symptom, glucocorticoids should be given with succeeding doses (15).

Eribulin

The newest antimitotic to receive FDA approval is eribulin (Figure 3-1), a macrocyclic ketone derivative of halichondrin B, a natural product of a marine sponge. The halichondrins are extremely potent mitotic inhibitors in a manner distinct from the taxanes, but competitive with vinca alkaloids. They bind to the plus end position of β-tubulin and prevent microtubule extension, with no effect on shortening at the minus end of the polymer. The result is an aggregation of tubulin dimers, and arrest in G$_2$-M. Eribulin is a weak substrate for the p-glycoprotein transporter. It was approved for taxane and anthracycline-resistant metastatic breast cancer, based on a positive phase III study showing an overall survival advantage of 2.5 months in comparison to physician's choice of standard treatment. The primary toxicities were grade 3/4 neutropenia in 52% and peripheral neuropathy in fewer than 10%. In this heavily pretreated population, pharmacokinetic analysis revealed a long terminal half-life of 36–48 h, and slow clearance by hepatic metabolism, with dose adjustment of 50% indicated in patients with hepatic dysfunction (16).

VINCA ALKALOIDS

The vinca alkaloids, derived from the vinca rosea plant, have been a mainstay of the treatment of hematologic malignancies for almost 50 years. They were first discovered in an in vitro antileukemic screen at Eli Lilly and Co. in the early 1950s, and reached prominence in the combination therapy of childhood acute lymphocytic leukemia and Hodgkin disease a decade later. They continue as part of curative regimens for the lymphomas and testicular cancer, and a third derivative, vinorelbine, has proven active in breast and lung cancers. The vinca alkaloids share a common structure and have similar pharmacologic properties, but differ in their profiles of toxicity and specific disease indications (**Figure 3-2**).

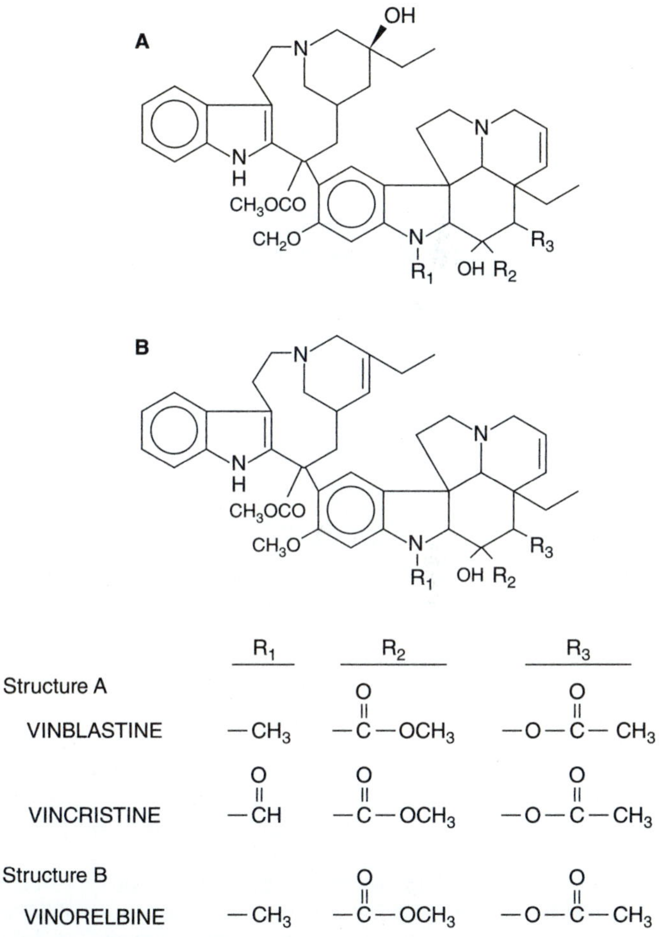

	R_1	R_2	R_3
Structure A			
VINBLASTINE	$-CH_3$	$-\overset{O}{\overset{\|}{C}}-OCH_3$	$-O-\overset{O}{\overset{\|}{C}}-CH_3$
VINCRISTINE	$-\overset{O}{\overset{\|}{C}}H$	$-\overset{O}{\overset{\|}{C}}-OCH_3$	$-O-\overset{O}{\overset{\|}{C}}-CH_3$
Structure B			
VINORELBINE	$-CH_3$	$-\overset{O}{\overset{\|}{C}}-OCH_3$	$-O-\overset{O}{\overset{\|}{C}}-CH_3$

FIGURE 3-2 Metabolic structures of vinca alkaloids.

■ MECHANISM OF ACTION

The vincas bind to a common site on β-tubulin and prevent dimerization of tubulin alpha and beta subunits to form microtubules (17). They block cells in mitosis due to the absence of a microtubular apparatus required for chromosomal segregation. Apoptosis follows. An acute cell death dependent on jun kinase activation and potentiated by downregulation of the anti-apoptotic protein, Mcl-1, has also been demonstrated experimentally (18).

Resistance to vincas arises through upregulation or amplification of one of several drug exporters, including the MDR gene product (p-glycoprotein) and the breast cancer resistance protein. Resistant cells may manifest a mutation in the vinca binding site on β-tubulin, a mutation that stabilizes microtubules and slows their rate of disassembly. In contrast mutations that destabilize microtubules confer sensitivity to taxanes and resistance to taxanes (19).

■ CLINICAL PHARMACOLOGY

The vincas share a common pharmacokinetic pattern of rapid clearance from plasma, extensive distribution into tissues, slow inactivation through hepatic metabolism by P-450 isoenzymes (primarily CYP3A4) and long half-lives in plasma of up to several days. Vincristine has the longest terminal plasma $t_{1/2}$ (up to 85 h), while vinorelbine is intermediate (46 h) and vinblastine is the most rapidly cleared ($t_{1/2}$ of 24 h). Vinblastine induces CYP3A4 activity. While there is no clear relationship of vinca clearance to any single liver function test, patients with abnormal hepatic function (bilirubin >1.5 mg/dl or >2-fold AST or ALT levels in serum) should receive no more than 50% of a full dose for their initial infusion, as prolonged ileus, myelosuppression, and neurotoxicity may result (20). No adjustment for renal dysfunction is required. The drugs are given intravenously as bolus infusions every 1–3 weeks, depending on the regimen employed. Usual single doses of the vinca alkaloids are vincristine, 1–2 mg/m²; vinorelbine, 20–30 mg/m²; and vinblastine, 6–8 mg/m².

■ TOXICITY

All vinca alkaloids cause neurotoxicity, primarily a peripheral sensory neuropathy. Vincristine, the most highly neurotoxic, may cause significant motor weakness of the hands and feet in severely toxic patients, and should not be given to patients with significant neurologic dysfunction due to other drugs, diabetes, stroke, or inherited neurologic disease. Neurotoxicity due to vinorelbine occurs with repeated cycles of therapy, but is usually mild and reversible. Vinblastine causes minimal neurotoxicity, but like vinorelbine, is a potent myelosuppressant, with rapid recovery of blood counts in 10–14 days. At usual doses, vincristine has little effect on the bone marrow. In high doses (not used in common practice) vincristine causes abdominal distention and ileus.

Because the vinca alkaloids depend for their clearance on CYP3A4, drug interactions are likely if the vincas are given with inducers or inhibitors of this isoenzyme (21). Thus phenytoin induces vinca clearance, and vincas may accelerate phenantoin metabolism and lead to seizures in patients receiving both drugs. Imidazole antifungal drugs, such as ketoconazole or itraconazole, inhibit CYP3A4 and slow vinca clearance, leading to severe toxicity if the dose of vinca alkaloid is not reduced.

REFERENCES

1. Eisenhauer EA, Vermorken JB. The taxoids: comparative clinical pharmacology and therapeutic potential. *Drugs.* 1998; 55: 5–30.

2. Gradishar WJ, Tjulandin S, Davidson N, et al. Phase III trial of nanoparticle albumin-bound paclitaxel compared with polyethylated castor oil-based paclitaxel in women with breast cancer. *J Clin Oncol.* 2005; 23: 7794–7803.

3. Crown J, O'Leary M, Wei-Seong O. Docetaxel and paclitaxel in the treatment of breast cancer: a review of clinical experience. *The Oncologist.* 2004; 9 (Suppl 2): 24–32.

4. Wani MC, Taylor HL, Wall ME, et al. Plant antitumor agents. VI. The isolation and structure of taxol, a novel antileukemic and antitumor agent from Taxus brevifolia. *J Am Chem Soc.* 1971; 93: 2325–2327.

5. Dumontet C, Sikic BI. Mechanism of action of and resistance to antitubulin agents; microtubule dynamics, drug transport and cell death. *J Clin Oncol.* 1999; 17: 1061–1070.

6. Wertz IE, Kusam S, Lam C, et al. Sensitivity to antitubulin chemotherapeutics is regulated by MCL1 and FBW7. *Nature.* 2011; 471: 122.

7. Gianni L, Kearns CM, Gianni A, et al. Nonlinear pharmacokinetics and metabolism of paclitaxel and it pharmacokinetic/pharmacodynamic relationship in humans. *J Clin Oncol.* 1995; 13: 2127–2135.

8. Baker AF, Dorr RT. Drug interactions with the taxanes: clinical implications. *Cancer Treat Rev.* 2001; 27: 221–233.

9. Viganol L, Locatelli A, Granelli G, Gianni L. Drug interactions of paclitaxel and docetaxel and their relevance for the design of combination chemotherapy. *Invest New Drugs.* 2001; 19: 179–196.

10. Rowinsky EC. Taxanes: paclitaxel (taxol) and docetaxel (taxotere). In *Cancer Medicine,* 6th edition, BC Decker, Hamilton, Canada, 2003.

11. Ghersi D, Wilcken N, Simers RJ. A systematic review of taxanecontaining regimens for metastatic breast cancer. *Br J Cancer.* 2002; 93: 293–301.

12. Katsumata N, Yasuda M, Takahashi F, et al. Dose dense paclitaxel once a week in combination with carboplatin every 3 weeks for advanced ovarian cancer: a phase 3, open-label, randomized controlled trial. *Lancet.* 2009; 374: 1331–1338.

13. Gradishar WJ, Tjulandin S, Davidson N, et al. Phase III study of nanoparticle albumin-bound paclitaxel compared with polyehtylated castor oil–based paclitaxel in women with breast cancer. *J Clin Oncol.* 2005; 23: 7784–7803.

14. Pean E, Demolis P, Moreau A, et al. The European Medicines Agency review of cabazitaxel (Jevtana) for the treatment of hormone refractory metastatic prostate cancer: summary of the scientific assessment of the Committee for Medicinal Products for Human Use (CHMP). *The Oncologist.* 2012; 17(4): 543–549.

15. Rivera E, Gomez H. Chemotherapy resistance in metastatic breast cancer: the evolving role of ixabepilone. *Breast Canc Res.* 2010; 12 (Suppl 2): 52–64.

16. Jain S, Cigler T. Eribulin mesylate in the treatment of metastatic breast cancer. *Biologics.* 2012; 6: 21–29.

17. Jordan MA, Wilson L. Microtubules as a target for anticancer drugs. *Nat Rev Cancer.* 2004; 4: 253–265.

18. Salemi BL, Bates DJ, Albershardt TC, et al. Vinblastine induces acute, cell phase-independent apoptosis in some leukemias and lymphomas and can induce acute apoptosis in others when Mcl-1 is suppressed. *Mol Cancer Therap.* 2011; 9: 791–802.

19. Cheung CHA, Wu S, Lee T, et al. Cancer cells acquire mitotic drug resistance properties through beta 1-tubulin mutations and alterations in expression of beta-tubulin isotypes. *PLoS One.* 2010; 5: 1–11.4.

20. Robieux I, Sorio R, Borsatti E, et al. Pharmacokinetics of vinorelbine in patients with liver metastases. *Clin Pharmacol Ther.* 1996; 59: 32–40.

21. Villikka K, Kivisto KT, Maenpaa H, et al. Cytochrome p450-inducing antiepileptics increase the clearance of vincristine in patients with brain tumors. *Clin Pharmacol Ther.* 1999; 66: 589–593.

CHAPTER 4

Topoisomerase Inhibitors: Camptothecins, Anthracyclines, and Etoposide

Bruce A. Chabner

Topoisomerases carry out the important function of unwinding DNA by creating temporary breaks in DNA, promoting passage of single strands of DNA through breaks, and then resealing the breaks. This function is critical in allowing access of repair and replication complexes to linear strands of DNA. Similar enzymes are found throughout the eukaryotic and prokaryotic world, a testament to their essential function. Likewise, they are one of the most common targets of naturally occurring poisons. Two classes of topoisomerases (topos) are found in human cells: topo I does not require ATP for strand breakage and resealing, and creates single strand breaks, while the several isoforms of topo II require ATP and create double strand breaks.

TOPOISOMERASE I INHIBITORS: CAMPTOTHECINS

The camptothecins are inhibitors of topo 1 with broad activity against epithelial cancers. Camptothecin was isolated from the Chinese tree *Camptotheca acuminata* in 1966 and had potent antitumor effects in

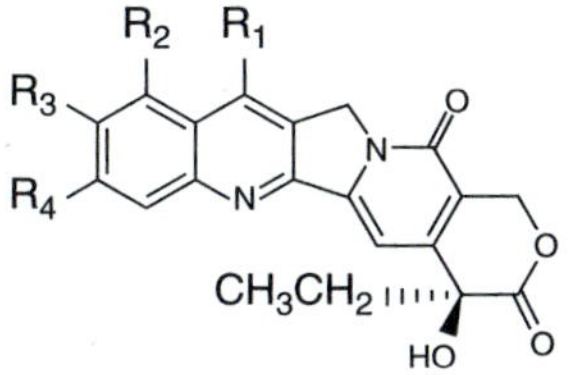

Compound	Molecular weight	R_1	R_2	R_3	R_4
Camptothecin	348.36	–H	–H	–H	–H
Topotecan	421.46	–H	–CH$_2$N(CH$_3$)$_2$	–H	–H
Irinotecan	586.69	–CH$_2$CH$_3$	–H	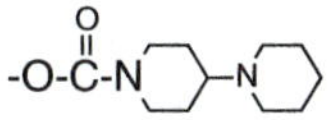 -O-C-N⬡-N⬡	–H
SN-38	392.42	–CH$_2$CH$_3$	–H	–OH	–H

FIGURE 4-1 Structure of the camptothecins.

animal systems. Topotecan (Hycamptin) and irinotecan (Camptosar), two synthetic agents in this class, have been subsequently approved for clinical use in the United States. Topotecan is currently used as second-line chemotherapy for ovarian cancer and small cell lung cancer (SCLC). Irinotecan is indicated for the treatment of metastatic colon cancer, both in first-line and salvage combination therapy, and has been incorporated into regimens to treat small cell lung cancer, gynecologic, and upper gastrointestinal malignancies.

■ STRUCTURE

The camptothecins consist of a five-ring structure in which a quinolone moiety is joined to a terminal α-hydroxy-δ-lactone ring (Figure 4-1). The electrophilic center of the lactone subunit is responsible for the camptothecins' biological activity. At the same time, the lactone is also vulnerable to reversible hydrolysis to a less active carboxylate species at neutral and alkaline pH. Substitutions on the C-9 and C-10 positions on the quinolone ring stabilize the lactone and enhance antitumor activity by preventing its conversion to the inactive carboxylate form in human blood and tissues (1).

■ MECHANISM OF ACTION

Camptothecin and its analogs exert their antitumor activity by inhibiting the enzyme DNA topo I, a nuclear enzyme that relieves torsional strain in supercoiled DNA during replication, repair, and transcription (Figure 4-2). The enzyme forms a transient, intermediate complex with single-stranded DNA that opens the DNA strand and allows passage of an intact single strand through the nick. The strand break also allows for rotation about the intact strand. Camptothecins bind to and stabilize the otherwise transient

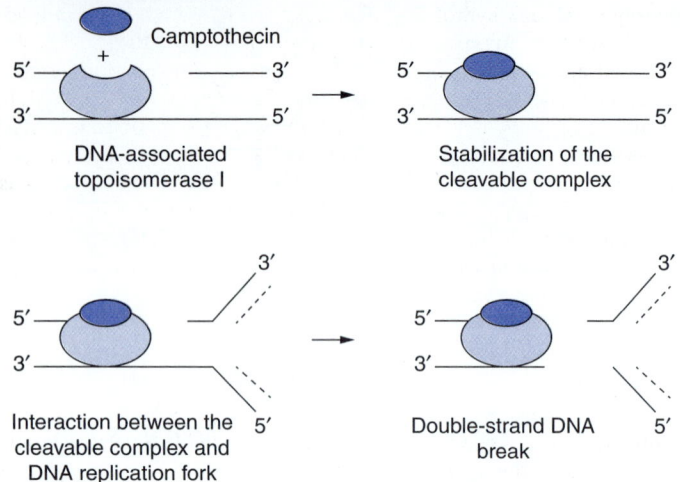

FIGURE 4-2 Mechanism of the camptothecins. (Used with permission from www. scielo.br.)

DNA-enzyme complex and prevent resealing of the broken strand. The single strand break, when it encounters a replication complex, leads to a double-stranded break, and an accumulation of double strand breaks leads to apoptosis. Active synthesis of DNA is a prerequisite for this interaction (1). In addition to strand breakage, irinotecan causes a downregulation of HIF1-alpha, a transcription factor critical to cell survival in the presence of hypoxia; angiogenesis is inhibited as a result (2). The mechanism of drug effects on HIF1-alpha is not known.

■ MECHANISMS OF RESISTANCE

In preclinical studies, resistance to the camptothecins may result from multiple mechanisms: increased expression of the multidrug resistance (MDR) efflux pump, p-glycoprotein, and a related transporter, ABCG2, the breast cancer resistance transporter; downregulation of topo I expression; mutations in the catalytic or DNA binding sites of topoisomerase I; upregulation of topoisomerase II; upregulation of NFκB; and inhibition of apoptosis. The clinical significance of these mechanisms of resistance is unproven.

CAMPTOTHECINS: CLINICAL PHARMACOLOGY

■ TOPOTECAN

Pharmacokinetics

Topotecan is usually given as a 30-min intravenous infusion. Plasma concentrations of the inactive carboxylate species begin to predominate over the active lactone form within 5–10 min after the end of infusion. The plasma half-life of topotecan is 2.4–4.3 h. Topotecan is eliminated primarily by plasma hydrolysis to the inactive carboxylate form, followed by renal excretion. Approximately one-third to one-half of a dose of drug is excreted unchanged in the urine. The clearance of topotecan and the carboxylate metabolite is reduced by 33% in patients with renal dysfunction and a creatinine clearance between 40 and 59 ml/min, and by 75% in patients with a creatinine clearance between 20 and 39 m/min. There is no significant change in elimination or toxicity in patients with liver disease, even in patients with total bilirubin levels up to 10 mg/dl. Administration of cisplatin decreases topotecan clearance, presumably through renal tubular damage. Topotecan pharmacokinetics are not altered when it is combined with anthracyclines, cyclophosphamide, or cytarabine (1).

Dosing and Schedule

The standard dosing schedule for topotecan is 1.5 mg/m^2 given as a 30-min intravenous infusion on 5 consecutive days, repeated every 21 days. Continuous infusion regimens up to 21 days in duration have attempted to take advantage of the in vitro observation that prolonged exposures of low concentrations are more efficacious than intermittent exposures to high concentrations. Results have been equivocal.

Toxicity

Neutropenia is the most significant dose-limiting toxicity for all schedules of topotecan administration, with grade 4 neutropenia in up to 81% of patients and febrile neutropenia in 26%. Renal dysfunction requires a dose reduction as indicated above. There is no dose modification required for patients with hepatic dysfunction. Non-hematologic toxicities of topotecan include nausea, vomiting, mucositis, elevated transaminases, fatigue, and rash. These side effects are generally minimal and easily managed (1).

■ IRINOTECAN

Pharmacokinetics

Irinotecan (Camptosar) is a congener of camptothecin specifically designed to facilitate generation of its lactone-stabilized metabolite, the 7-ethyl-10-hydroxy analog, SN-38, which is a 1000-fold more potent inhibitor of topo I than the parent drug. Irinotecan is primarily eliminated through the liver via two clinically relevant mechanisms (**Figure 4-3**). First, irinotecan is a substrate of the cytochrome p450 system and is metabolized to inactive derivatives by CYP2B6 and CYP3A4. These inactivation pathways are inducible by phenobarbital or phenytoin (1). Second, irinotecan is converted to SN-38 by ubiquitous esterases, and SN-38 is then cleared by glucuronidation and excreted in the biliary system. The half-life of the active lactone form of SN-38 is 11.5 h (1).

SN-38 undergoes glucuronidation by the polymorphic enzyme uridine diphosphoglucuronosyl-transferase (UGT1A1), which is also responsible for bilirubin glucuronidation. The activity of this enzyme is significantly reduced in patients homozygous for the allele UGT1A1*28, the same defect seen in subjects with Gilbert's syndrome. This homozygous deficiency is found in approximately 10% of patients. When treated with standard doses

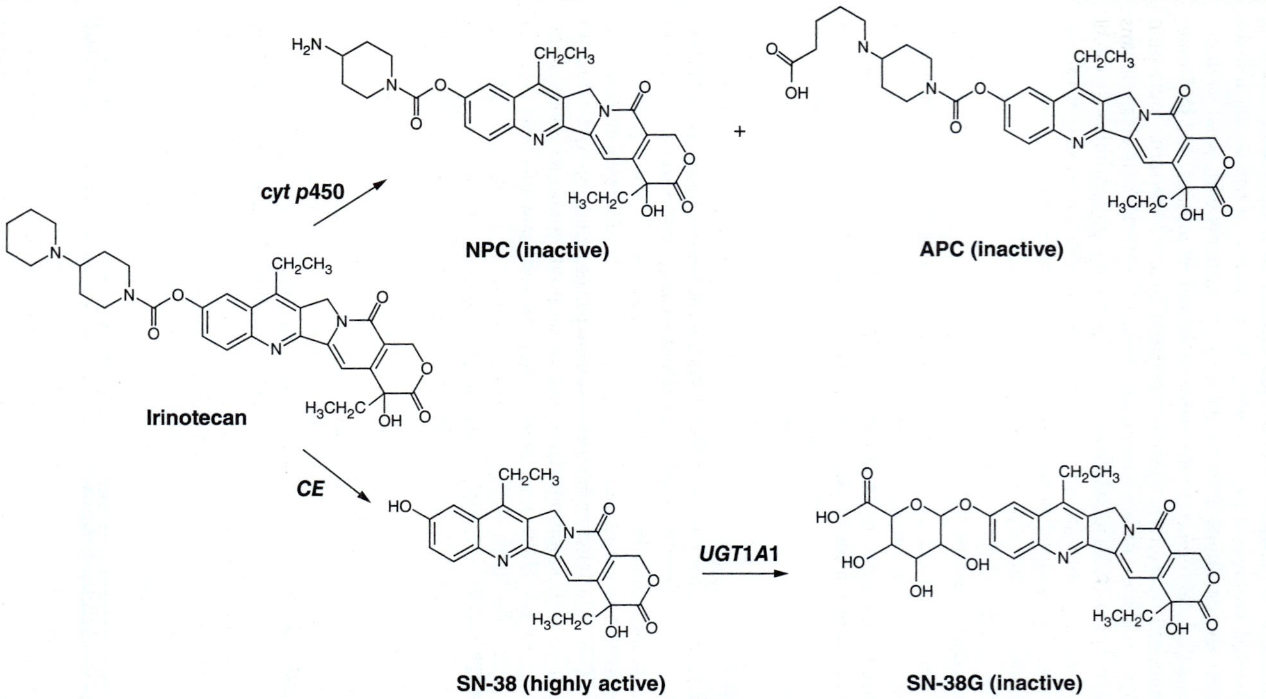

FIGURE 4-3 Metabolic pathway for irinotecan showing the conversion to inactive metabolites NPC and APC via cytochrome p450 enzymes and the conversion by liver carboxyxylesterase (CE) to the active form, SN-38, and its subsequent inactivation to SN-38G by the enzyme UGT1A1.

of irinotecan, such patients have slower clearance of the parent drug and higher levels of plasma SN-38 and encounter higher rates of toxicity, particularly neutropenia (3, 4). In patients with Gilbert's syndrome, or with an unexplained elevated indirect bilirubin level, lower starting doses of irinotecan should be used. A commercially available test for the UGT1A1*28 polymorphism (Invader UGT1A1*28 Molecular Assay) can be used, although it has not been widely accepted in clinical practice. Common polymorphisms in ABC cassette drug transporters, which export the parent drug and SN-38 from intestinal epithelium, may account for the severe gastrointestinal toxicity that affects 20%–30% of patients (5).

Dosing and Schedule

Irinotecan, as a single agent, can be given at a dose of 125 mg/m^2 over a 90-min intravenous infusion every week for 4 of 6 weeks or at a dose 350 mg/m^2 over a 90-min intravenous infusion every 3 weeks. The weekly schedule appears to be equally effective, although there are lower rates of diarrhea with the every 3-week regimen (6).

Toxicity

The most common adverse effects of irinotecan are diarrhea, which can be life-threatening in some instances, myelosuppression, and an acute cholinergic syndrome of nausea, vomiting, mucositis, diarrhea, and flushing. The latter responds to atropine. Interstitial pneumonitis has been reported in Japanese patients receiving irinotecan. Grade 3–4 diarrhea was observed in up to 35% of patients in early clinical studies. Irinotecan, when given at 125 mg/m^2 on a weekly basis for 4 of 6 weeks in combination with 5-FU and leucovorin (7), led to toxic deaths due to severe diarrhea and neutropenia. An alternative and better tolerated schedule of biweekly irinotecan at 180 mg/m^2, whether as single agent or combined with 5-FU and leucovorin (FOLFIRI), has been widely adopted. Loperamide starting at 4 mg should be given at the first sign of diarrhea, and repeat doses of 2 mg every 2 h may be given until resolution of the diarrhea.

Myelosuppression is common with irinotecan; grade 3–4 neutropenia occurs in 14%–47% of patients.

Clinical Indications

Irinotecan is most commonly used in advanced colorectal cancer. As first-line therapy in metastatic disease, it is combined with 5-FU and leucovorin, with or without bevacizumab. It can also be given in the second-line therapy as a single agent, or in patients with k-ras wild-type tumors, it may be combined with cetuximab (8).

TOPOISOMERASE II INHIBITORS: ANTHRACYCLINES

Drugs of this class, derived from the fungal culture broths of *Streptomyces peucetius*, have become critical components of treatment for acute leukemias, lymphomas, breast cancer, and sarcomas. The two original members of this family, daunorubicin (DN) and doxorubicin (DX), remain in active clinical practice: DN for acute myelogenous leukemia (AML), and DX for lymphomas and solid tumor chemotherapy. Two semisynthetic derivatives, idarubicin (IDA) and epirubicin (EPI), have made inroads as valuable agents for leukemia and breast cancer, respectively. Doxil, a liposomal formulation of DX has found limited use, primarily for ovarian cancer, and a similar liposomal DN preparation is indicated for Kaposi's sarcoma.

■ MECHANISM OF ACTION

The anthracyclines share a rigid planar four-ring structure complemented by a glycosidic substitution on the D ring and variable side groups on the A and D rings (**Figure 4-4**). The planar configuration allows anthracyclines to intercalate between strands of DNA, and this action was originally thought to be responsible for its inhibition of DNA synthesis. However, the anthracyclines possess other important features. The quinone on ring C readily undergoes oxidation/reduction cycling in the presence of Fe^{++}, producing free radicals from oxygen and/or lipids (9). These free radicals are responsible for the cardiac toxicity inherent in this class of agents. The anthracyclines bind to and inhibit topo II, an enzyme that promotes DNA strand unwinding essential for DNA synthesis and repair. In its normal function, topo II binds to DNA and creates a double strand break that allows strand passage. The enzyme then reseals the break. Anthracyclines bind to and stabilize the DNA-topo II complex, preventing the resealing of the strand break. An accumulation of strand breaks signals the p53 system to halt cell cycle progression, and to initiate DNA repair. If the breaks are sufficiently numerous, the cell undergoes apoptosis. High levels of topo II expression correlate positively with response to DX in patients with breast cancer (10, 11). Cells become resistant to anthracyclines through diminished expression of topo II activity or through topo II

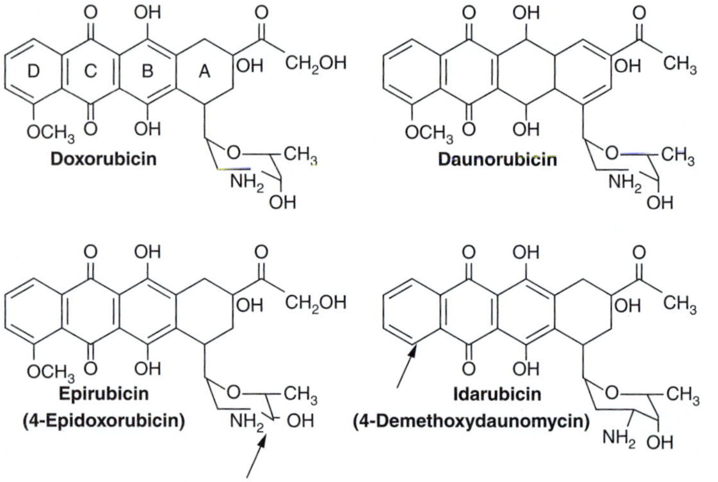

FIGURE 4-4 Anthracyclines in current clinical use. For epirubicin and idarubicin, arrows point to the sites where these new drugs differ from doxorubicin and daunomycin, respectively.

mutations that decrease binding affinity of the enzyme for the drugs of this class. An interesting correlation has been observed between amplification of the isoenzyme topo IIa and the HER2/neu receptor. The topo IIa gene is located on chromosome 17 adjacent to the gene coding for the HER2/neu. HER2/neu amplification is found in one quarter of breast cancers. In one-third of patients with amplified HER2, topo IIa is co-amplified, and this subset of breast cancer patients has a higher response rate to DX.

■ DRUG RESISTANCE

Transporters that export anthracyclines and other natural products influence response to this class of agents. Expression of the MDR gene, which codes for the membrane transporter p-glycoprotein, increases resistance to anthracyclines, and confers drug resistance in patients with AML, multiple myeloma, and lymphomas. Other membrane exporters, including the MRP family, and the breast cancer resistance transporter (ABCG2) cause resistance in cell lines, but their clinical role is uncertain. IDA is less affected by the presence of MDR than is DX (12).

Other intracellular processes that recognize DNA strand breaks and initiate apoptosis may influence sensitivity to anthracyclines. High levels of BCL-2 expression, an anti-apoptotic factor, render cells insensitive to anthracyclines, as does a loss of function of the mismatch repair complex that recognizes defective strand pairing. Mutations in p53, mutations in ATM (a sensor of strand breaks), and high levels of MDM2 (an antagonist of p53) also confer resistance to DX (13).

■ CLINICAL PHARMACOLOGY

To a variable extent, anthracyclines are converted to an active alcohol (-ol) intermediate by the ubiquitous enzyme, aldoketoreductase, but for DX and EPI, the parent compounds are believed to be more potent and are responsible for their clinical efficacy. IDA is rapidly converted to its alcohol metabolite, and the alcohol becomes the predominant species in plasma 1–4 h after drug administration. The metabolite is slightly less potent than the parent drug and likely contributes to the drug's antitumor activity in vivo.

The important pharmacokinetic features of the various anthracyclines are shown in Table 4-1. The parent compounds (DX, DN, and EPI), or in the case of idarubicin, the active alcohol metabolite, have a prolonged terminal half-life in plasma of 1 day or longer, thus allowing intermittent dosing once every week to once every 3 weeks. Clearance occurs primarily through hepatic non-microsomal conversion to sulfates, aglycones, and other inactive metabolites. Anthracycline semiquinone radicals may also be inactivated by enzymatic or chemically mediated conjugation with sulfhydryls such as glutathione. Because of the importance of hepatic enzymatic clearance of parent compounds and alcohol metabolites, hepatic dysfunction, with bilirubin greater than 1.5 mg/dl, is associated with delayed drug clearance and a probable increased risk of toxicity (9). In this case, most regimens call for a 50% dose reduction, with subsequent escalation if the dose is well tolerated. Renal dysfunction (creatinine clearance less than 60 ml/min) also slows DX and IDA clearance, probably through changes in hepatic blood flow or diminished hepatic clearance of parent drug.

TABLE 4-1 ANTHRACYCLINE PHARMACOKINETICS

Drug	Route of Elimination	Plasma $t_{1/2}$ (h)	Primary Metabolites	Typical Dose and Schedule
Doxorubicin	Hepatic metabolism, biliary excretion of metabolites	30	13-Alcohol (minor), aglycone, conjugates	45–60 mg/m² q3w
Daunorubicin	"	20–50	13-Alcohol (predominant), conjugates	30–45 mg/m² qd × 3 90 mg/m² qd × 3 may improve response rate and survival in AML (27)
Epirubicin	"	18	13-Alcohol, glucuronide of parent and alcohol	90–110 mg/m² q3w
Idarubicin	Hepatic conversion to 13-alcohol, urinary excretion of alcohol	13–18 (parent) 40–60 (alcohol)	13-Alcohol predominates	10–15 mg/m² q3w

High doses of DN (90 mg/m² vs. 45 mg/m², both qd × 3) have improved complete response rates and survival in patients with AML, without an increase in life-threatening toxicity (15).

■ TOXICITY

All anthracyclines cause myelosuppression, mucositis, and alopecia. Recovery of peripheral blood counts occurs within 10–14 days. Their most significant late toxicity is cardiac injury. Initial clinical experience with DX, as documented by sequential endomyocardial biopsy, disclosed myocardial necrosis, both in animals and in patients receiving multiple doses of drug. Subsequent studies in children have revealed elevations of troponin T in the days following drug administration and an elevated risk of late cardiac events in patients demonstrating such elevations. Cardiac function is ordinarily monitored through tests of left ventricular ejection fraction (scans or echocardiography). Decreases of greater than 10% from baseline values, or a fall below 40%, signal a high risk of later congestive failure. These changes should prompt discontinuation of anthracycline treatment. Symptomatic cardiac disease, manifested primarily as congestive heart failure, usually does not occur until total doses of DX exceed 450 mg/m², with a marked increase in risk above 550 mg/m². However, in DX-treated children receiving a total dose of 300 mg/m² or less, a significantly elevated risk of cardiac disease (arrhythmias, sudden death, myocardial infarcts, or congestive failure) emerges later in adult life (16).

EPI appears to be less cardiotoxic than DX in studies of breast cancer patients receiving adjuvant chemotherapy (17). The incidence of congestive failure following adjuvant therapy reaches 1%–1.5% of patients treated with EPI and is slightly higher (approximately 2%) for DX-containing regimens. It appears that cardiac toxicity may be less in patients receiving DX by continuous infusion over 4 days, or in small weekly doses, but the convenience of single bolus doses every 2–3 weeks has led to the use of this schedule in standard adjuvant therapy.

In both children and adults, oncologists usually limit total doses of DX to 300 mg/m². In children, dexrozoxane, an iron chelating drug, clearly decreases the frequency of acute troponin T elevations and lessens the risk of late cardiac toxicity, and is routinely administered with DX to children.

Radiation therapy to the chest delivered with chemotherapy increases the risk of cardiotoxicity. Other chemotherapy drugs potentiate anthracycline cardiotoxicity. Paclitaxel, administered with DX, decreases the rate of DX clearance and significantly enhances the rate of DX cardiotoxicity, an effect attributed to inhibition of DX metabolism and/or biliary excretion (18). Trastuzumab, the anti-HER2/neu antibody, increases the risk of DX cardiotoxicity. Sequential administration of DX and cyclophosphamide (19), followed by trastuzumab, is associated with a more than twofold increase in heart failure, as compared to the heart failure risk of either drug alone. EPI given with trastuzumab or DX with docetaxel leads to no obvious increase in cardiotoxicity, although less data are available for these regimens (20).

In addition to cardiac toxicity, the anthracyclines as a class increase the risk of AML, and less commonly, acute promyelocytic leukemia (PML) (21). The onset of myelodysplasia (MDS) occurs within 1–3 years of treatment in patients receiving cyclophosphamide/EPI as adjuvant therapy, and the risk increases markedly in patients receiving greater than 720 mg/m² EPI or 6300 mg/m² cyclophosphamide. With alkylating agents and EPI, leukemias displayed either chromosome 5 or 7 deletions, or more commonly balanced translocations involved 11q23, a finding characteristic of leukemia secondary to topo II inhibitors. EPI also leads to (15:17) acute promyelocytic leukemia, perhaps due to a specific "hot spot" sensitive to topo II in exon 6 of the PML gene (22).

■ OTHER ANTHRACYCLINES AND ANTHRACENEDIONES

Mitoxantrone is a planar multi-ring quinine similar to anthracyclines but lacks the sugar linkage. It is less cardiotoxic, and is a less potent antileukemic agent than DN, but shares pharmacological properties with the anthracyclines: hepatic metabolism, long terminal half-life in plasma, myelosuppression as its major toxicity, susceptibility to MDR and other ABC cassette transporters, and a risk of causing acute AML and PML as a late toxicity (14, 22). It is rarely used in clinical oncology practice. The recommended doses are 12 mg/m²/day for 3 days for acute leukemia and 14–16 mg/m² every 3 weeks for solid tumor therapy.

LIPOSOME ENCAPSULATED ATHRACYCLINES

In an effort to increase drug uptake selectively in tumor cells and to decrease cardiac toxicity, both DX and DN have been reformulated in lipid spheres (liposomes). In this form, the drug has a half-life in plasma of greater than 50 h. Liposomal DX (Doxil) has proven useful in platinum-refractory ovarian cancer, while liposomal DN is approved for treatment of Kaposi's sarcoma. These preparations have less cardiotoxicity than the parent drugs. Late side effects of Doxil have included renal failure and oral-pharyngeal carcinomas (23).

ETOPOSIDE

Topo II inhibitors are found in nature as potent cellular poisons. Etoposide, etoposide phosphate (rarely used), and teniposide (**Figure** 4-5) are semi-synthetic derivatives of podophyllotoxin, a plant product, which itself is

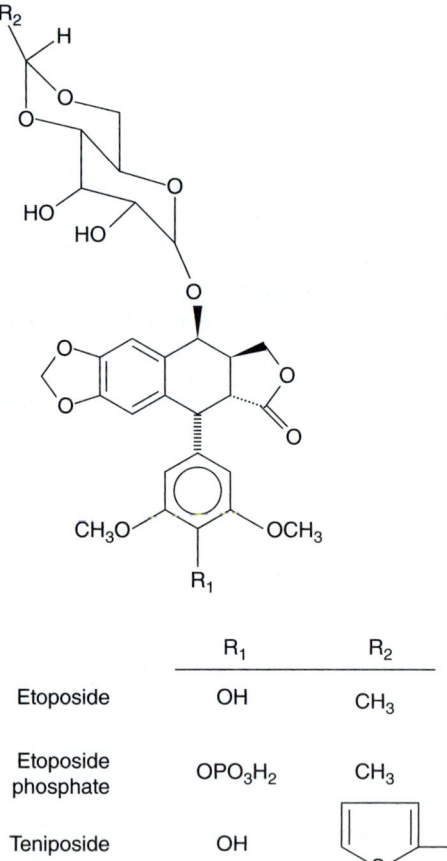

	R_1	R_2
Etoposide	OH	CH_3
Etoposide phosphate	OPO_3H_2	CH_3
Teniposide	OH	(thiophene)

FIGURE 4-5 Molecular structure of etoposide, etoposide phosphate, and teniposide.

an antimitotic without topo II inhibitory activity. Etoposide has been a valuable agent for the treatment of leukemias, lymphomas, and germ cell tumors in both conventional and high-dose regimens, while teniposide is used primarily for the treatment of AML in children.

■ MECHANISM OF ACTION AND RESISTANCE

As described above, topo II cleaves a DNA strand in a reaction mediated by ATP hydrolysis. Etoposide and teniposide bind to the complex of DNA and enzyme, inhibiting the resealing activity of the enzyme and perpetuating strand breaks (**Figure 4-6**) (24). Through p53, these strand breaks signal a halt to cell cycle progression and, if breaks are sufficiently numerous, prompt apoptosis.

As natural products, the epipodophyllotoxin derivatives are subject to transport from tumor cells by the p-glycoprotein, a product of the MDR gene. Resistance may also arise through deletion of topo II (via methylation of the gene or loss of promoter activity) or through mutation of its binding site for these drugs. Finally, disruptions of apoptotic pathways, and the capacity to repair double strand breaks, may also determine the outcome of therapy.

■ CLINICAL PHARMACOLOGY

Etoposide is eliminated by both renal excretion and hepatic metabolism, and doses should be adjusted for dysfunction of either organ (25). Approximately 40% of a dose of etoposide is excreted unchanged in the urine, and dose should be reduced in proportion to changes in creatinine clearance. The remainder is eliminated by glucuronidation. A smaller fraction of drug undergoes CYP3A4 metabolism through demethylation, producing a cytotoxic catechol metabolite and other quinine derivatives of

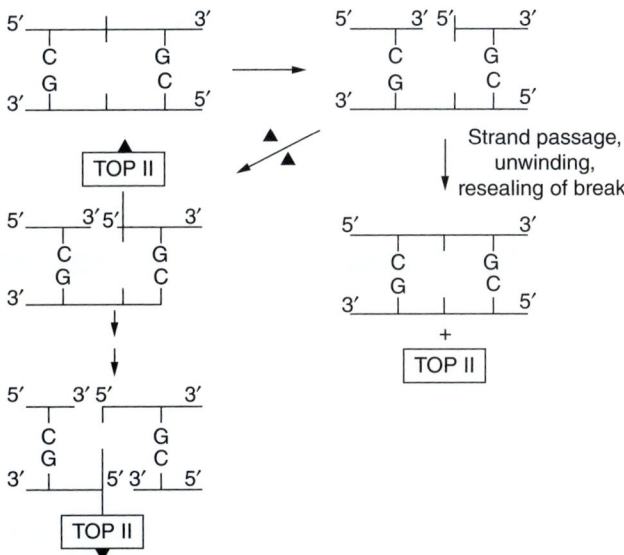

FIGURE 4-6 Formation of single and double strand breaks by topoisomerase II (TOP II), and prevention of break resealing in the presence of etoposide (▲).

uncertain significance. The drug has a terminal half-life of 8 h in plasma in patients with normal renal and hepatic function. In patients with elevated serum bilirubin of 1.5–3.0 mg/dl, the dose should be reduced by 50%, while in those with higher bilirubin, the drug should be used with extreme caution and in lesser doses, and alternative therapies should be considered.

High-dose etoposide (1.5 g/m^2 or above) is used alone, or in combination with cyclophosphamide, ifosfamide, or carboplatin (26). It is the only topo II agent that can be significantly escalated in dose without encountering irreversible nonmyeloid toxicity. At these high doses, mucositis and hepatic enzyme elevations become dose limiting. Its pharmacokinetics remain linear at these high doses.

Teniposide is eliminated primarily by the liver, with a variety of microsomal and other metabolites appearing in bile. Its half-life in plasma is 10–21 h. Very little drug is excreted unchanged in the urine, and no dose adjustment for renal dysfunction is needed.

■ TOXICITY

At usual doses of 100 mg/m^2 per day for 3 days every 3 weeks, bone marrow suppression is the primary toxicity of etoposide, with recovery 10–14 days after treatment. Hypotension, fever, and asthmatic episodes may follow drug infusion, probably a response to the cremophor diluent in which the drug is administered. Liver function abnormalities and mucositis supervene at higher doses.

Etoposide causes acute myelogenous leukemia as a later toxic event, usually 2–3 years after treatment. The leukemia often involves a translocation (at 11q 23) in the MLL gene on the long arm of chromosome 11 at AT-rich sites favored for topo II cleavage. The leukemia may be preceded by a period of myelodysplasia. Less commonly, acute promyelocytic leukemia has also been reported following etoposide. The risk of AML increases with cumulative doses >6 g/m^2 and with schedules of weekly or biweekly administration (27).

Tenoposide side effects follow the same pattern as these of etoposide; myelosuppression and mucositis are common toxicities. The incidence of acute hypersensitivity reactions is higher for teniposide, probably related to the greater concentration of lipid diluent used in its formulation. Like etoposide, it causes secondary AML.

REFERENCES

1. Garcia-Carbonero R, Supko JG. Current perspectives on the clinical experience, pharmacology, and continued development of the camptothecins. *Clin Cancer Res.* 2002; 8: 641–661.

3. Massacesi C, Terrazzino S, Marcucci F, et al. Uridine diphosphate glucuronsyl transferase 1A1 promoter polymorphism predicts the risk of gastrointestinal toxicity and fatigue induced by irinotecan-based chemotherapy. *Cancer.* 2006; 106: 1007–1016.

4. Zhou Q, Sparreboom A, Tan E-H, et al. Pharmacogenetic profiling across the irinotecan pathway in Asian patients with cancer. *Br J Clin Pharmacol.* 2005; 59: 415–424.

5. Di Martino MT, Arbitrio M, Leone E, et al. Single nucleotide polymorphisms of ABCC5 and ABCG1 transporter genes correlate to

irinotecan-associated gastrointestinal toxicity in colorectal cancer patients. A DMET microarray profiling study. *Cancer Biol Ther.* 2011; 12: 780–787.

6. Fuchs CS, Moore MR, Harker G, et al. Phase III comparison of two irinotecan dosing regimens in second-line therapy of metastatic colorectal cancer. *J Clin Oncol.* 2003; 21: 807–814.

7. Saltz LB, Cox JV, Blanke C, et al. Irinotecan plus fluorouracil and leucovorin for metastatic colorectal cancer. *N Engl J Med.* 2000; 343: 905–914.

8. Cunningham D, Humblet Y, Siena S, et al. Cetuximab monotherapy and cetuximab plus irinotecan in irinotecan-refractory metastatic colorectal cancer. *N Engl J Med.* 2004; 351: 337–345.

9. Doroshow JH. Anthracyclines and anthracenediones. In BA Chabner, DL Longo (eds.), *Cancer Chemotherapy and Biotherapy: Principles and Practice.* Lippincott, Williams and Wilkins, Philadelphia, PA, 2011; 356–391.

10. Durbecq V, Paesmans M, Cardoso F, et al. Topoisomerase-II expression as a predictive marker in a population of advanced breast cancer patients randomly treated either with single-agent doxorubicin or single-agent docetaxel. *Mol Cancer Ther.* 2004; 3: 1207.

11. Brase E, Schmidt M, Fischbach T, et al. ERBB2 and TOP2A in breast cancer: a comprehensive analysis of gene amplification, RNA levels, and protein expression and their influence on prognosis and prediction. *Clin Cancer Res.* 2010; 16: 2391–2401.

12. Kroschinsky R, Schleyer E, Renner U, et al. Increased myelotoxicity of idarubicin: is there a pharmacological basis? *Cancer Chemother Pharmacol.* 2004; 53: 61.

13. Chrisanthar R, Knappskog S, Lokkevik E, et al. Predictive and prognostic impact of TP53 mutations and MDM2 promoter genotype in primary breast cancer patients treated with epirubicin or paclitaxel. *PLoS One.* 2011; 1–10.

14. Camaggi CM, Strocchi E, Carisi P, et al. Idarubicin metabolism and pharmacokinetics after intravenous and oral administration in cancer patients: a crossover study. *Cancer Chemother Pharmacol.* 1992; 30: 307.

15. Lowenburg B, Ossenkoppele GJ, van Putten W, et al. High dose-daunorubicin in older patients with acute myeloid leukemia. *New Engl J Med.* 2009; 361: 1235–1248.

16. Nysorn K, Holm K, Lipsitz SR, et al. Relationship between cumulative anthracycline dose and late cardiotoxicity in childhood acute lymphoblastic leukemia. *J Clin Oncol.* 1998; 16: 545.

17. Smith LA, Cornelius VR, Plummer CJ, et al. Cardiotoxicity of anthracycline agents for the treatment of cancer: systematic review and meta-analysis of randomised controlled trials. *MBMC Cancer.* 2010; 10: 337–351.

18. Partridge AH, Burstein HJ, Winer EP. Side effects of chemotherapy and combined chemohormonal therapy in women with early-stage breast cancer. *J Natl Cancer Inst Monogr.* 2001; 30: 135.

19. Bowles EJA, Wellman R, Feigelson HS, et al. Risk of heart failure in breast cancer patients after anthracycline and trastuzumab treatment: a retrospective cohort study. *J Natl Cancer Inst.* 2012; 104: 1293–1306.

20. Buzdar AU, Ibrahim NK, Francis D, et al. Significantly higher patho-logic complete remission rate after neoadjuvant therapy with trastuzu-mab, paclitaxel, and epirubicin chemotherapy: results of a randomized trial in human epidermal growth factor receptor 2-positive operable breast cancer. *J Clin Oncol.* 2005; 23: 3676.

21. Praga C, Bergh J, Bliss J, et al. Risk of acute myeloid leukemia and mye-lodysplastic syndrome in trials of adjuvant epirubicin for early breast cancer: correlation with doses of epirubicin and cyclophosphamide. *J Clin Oncol.* 2005; 23: 4179.

22. Mays AN, Osheroff N, Xiao Y, et al. Evidence for direct involvement of epirubicin in the formation of chromosomal translocations in t(15;17) therapy-related acute promyelocytic leukemia. *Blood.* 2010; 14: 326–330.

23. Muggia F, Cannon T, Safra T, Curtin J. Delayed neoplastic and renal complications in women receiving long-term chemotherapy for recur-rent ovarian cancer. *J Natl Cancer Inst.* 2011; 103: 160–161.

24. Minford J, Pommier Y, Filipski J, et al. Isolation of intercalator-dependent protein-linked DNA strand cleavage activity from cell nuclei and identification as topoisomerase II. *Biochemistry.* 1986; 25: 9–16.

25. D'Incalci M, Rossi C, Zucchetti M, et al. Pharmacokinetics of etoposide in patients with abnormal renal and hepatic function. *Cancer Res.* 1986; 46: 2566–2571.

26. Beyer J, Kramar A, Mandanas R, et al. High-dose chemotherapy as salvage treatment in germ cell tumors: a multivariate analysis of prog-nostic variables. *J Clin Oncol.* 1996; 14: 2638–2645.

27. Le Deley MC, Leblanc T, Shamsaldin A, et al. Societe Francaise d'Oncologie Pediatrique. Risk of secondary leukemia after a solid tumor in childhood according to the dose of epipodophyllotoxins and anthracyclines: a case-control study by the Societe Francaise d'Oncologie Pediatrique. *J Clin Oncol.* 2003; 21: 1074–1081.

CHAPTER **5**

Adduct-Forming Agents: Alkylating Agents and Platinum Analogs

Bruce A. Chabner

Since the first clinical experiments with nitrogen mustard at Yale in the early 1940s, alkylating agents have played a primary role in cancer treatment (1). The early mustards have gradually been replaced by platinum-based compounds in most regimens for treating epithelial cancers, but remain pri-mary components in the treatment of childhood solid tumors, lymphomas, and adult sarcomas, and in high-dose chemotherapy. As a class, they have the features of the prototypical cytotoxic drugs, with broad antitumor activity, but they adversely affect many normal tissues as well. They share common characteristics of a significant increase in response as doses are escalated: acute toxic effects on bone marrow, epithelium of the gastrointestinal tract, and hair follicles; significant toxicity to lung, heart, and central nervous systems at bone marrow ablative doses; and late induction of myelodysplasia and acute leukemia.

MECHANISM OF ACTION

Three general classes of DNA adduct-forming agents have found clinical application. The first are the chloroethyl nitrogen mustards, exemplified by cyclophosphamide, ifosfamide, melphalan, and chlorambucil (**Figure 5-1**). These drugs become active through formation of a highly reactive imonium intermediate, which transfers its ethyl group to nucleophilic (electronegative) sites on DNA (amino, hydroxyl, or phosphate sites) and to sulfhydrils on amino acids and glutathione (**Figure 5-2**). These drugs contain two chloroethyl groups and can cross-link DNA, creating a lesion that is difficult to repair. The classical nitrogen mustard was a highly unstable molecule, while the current agents of this type, such as cyclophosphamide and melphalan, have been modified by conjugation with electronegative groups that reduce their reactivity. The single strand adducts are repaired by nucleotide excision repair, while double strand breaks require the complex homologous recombination system. The newest agent of this class, bendamustine (Figure 5-1), consists of a purine-like ring, to which is attached a classical bifunctional nitrogen mustard. This bulky molecule forms adducts that are more slowly repaired. The drug is incompletely cross-resistant with traditional alkylators and is highly effective for chronic lymphocytic leukemia and follicular lymphomas (2).

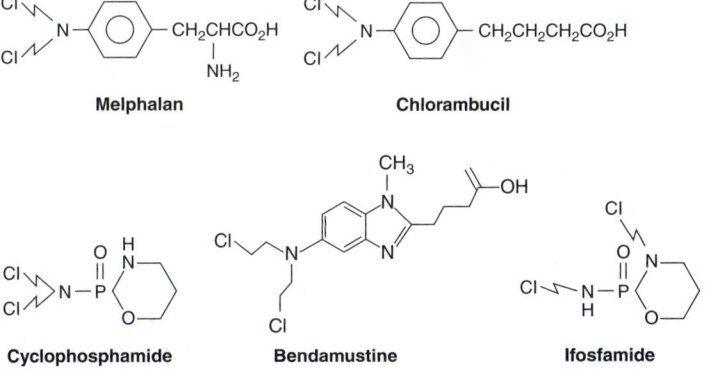

FIGURE 5-1 Molecular structures of melphalan, chlorambucil, cyclophosphamide, ifosfamide, and bendamustine.

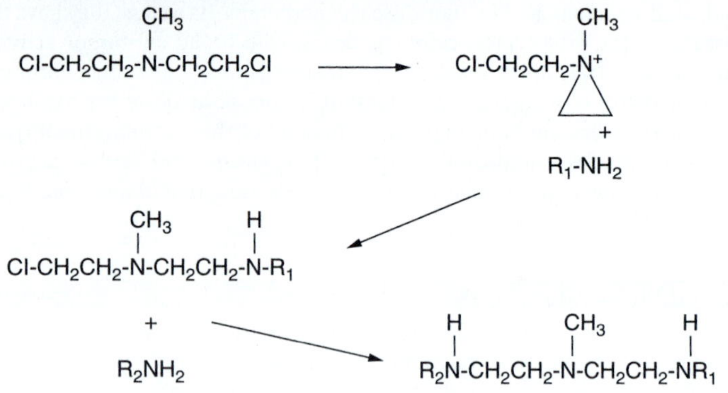

FIGURE 5-2 Nitrogen mustard undergoes spontaneous chemical rearrangement in aqueous solution to form a highly reactive, positively charged, three-member aziridinium ring, which reacts with nucleophilic sites on DNA such as amines and hydroxyl groups. (R_1NH_2 and R_2NH_2 represent reactive sites on DNA bases.)

The second group consists of drugs that transfer single methyl radicals to DNA. This second class—which includes procarbazine, dimethyl triazinoimidazolecarboxamide (DTIC); its close congener, temozolomide; and busulfan—requires more complex activation, either enzymatic or chemical. The methylating drugs preferentially attack the O-6 position of guanine, as well as other reactive sites on purines and pyrimidines. The methylation of O-6 guanine is repaired by methyl guanine-O-6 methyltransferase, (MGMT). The activity of MGMT in cancer cells determines the response of primary brain tumors to this group of drugs.

The third group of drugs, platinum complexes, closely mimic alkylators, as they form reactive intermediates that attack the same nucleophilic sites on DNA. The activation of these analogs begins with the displacement of chloride or other leaving groups by water, with the formation of a reactive hydroxyl intermediates (**Figure 5-3**). The platinum analogs have two leaving groups, either chlorides or an oxalate group, and thus are capable of cross linking DNA. Their adducts are repaired in a manner similar to the chloroethyl alkylators.

■ CELLULAR PHARMACOLOGY OF ALKYLATING AGENTS

As a class, most alkylating agents are lipid soluble and easily cross cell membranes. Two members of the class, nitrogen mustard and melphalan are actively transported into cells, the former by the choline transporter and the latter by amino acid transporters. Resistance may arise experimentally by deletion of these transporters.

Following uptake, most alkylating agents, and in particular the chloroethyl mustards, spontaneously undergo activation to an unstable, electrophilic intermediate. Some agents, such as DTIC, require metabolic activation, but

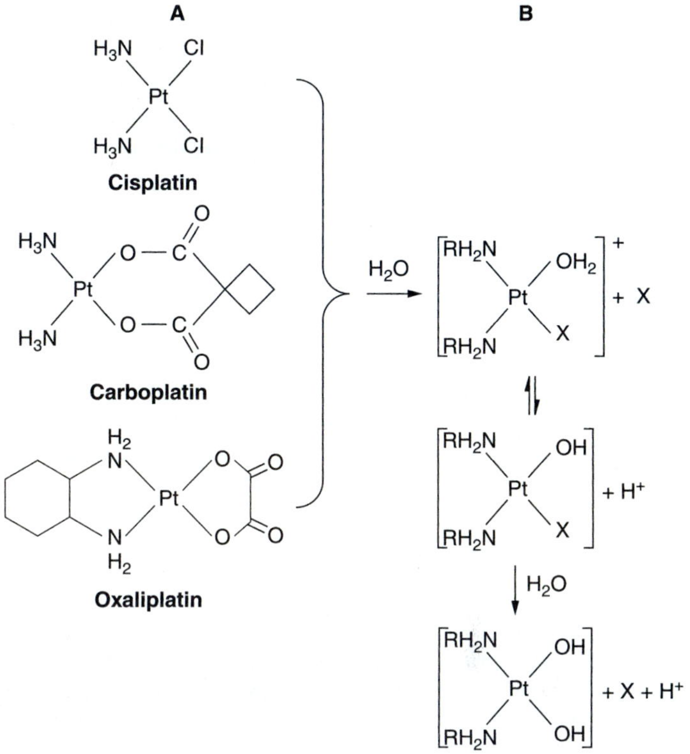

FIGURE 5-3 Activation of platinum analogs.

the closely related temozolomide generates the same unstable methyltriazino derivative spontaneously, and has become the standard agent for treating gliomas. Cyclophosphamide and ifosfamide require prior p450 oxidative activation in the liver in order to generate their chemically reactive end products, which are phosphoramide mustards (**Figure 5-4**).

Once inside cells, chloroethyl alkylating agents form reactive imonium ions (Figure 5-2), which attack sites such as sulfhydryl groups on proteins and glutathione (the sulfhydryl found in highest concentration within cells). They also react with electron-rich sites on nucleic acids, including the N-2 and N-7 groups on guanine, the O-6 on guanine, and the N-3 on adenine. Single-base alkylations are recognized by the DNA nucleotide excision repair (NER) complex, while cross-links must be repaired by a more complex process of excision of the alkylated bases and adjoining segments, and accurate repair of the resulting double stand break through homologous recombination. An accumulation of cross-links and strand breaks, particularly interstrand breaks, signals p53 to initiate apoptosis (3).

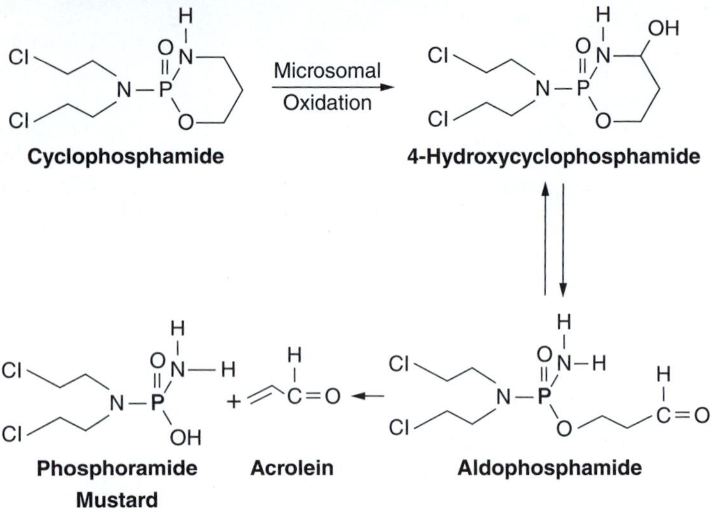

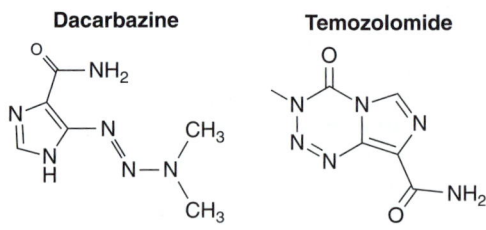

Cyclophosphamide → Microsomal Oxidation → **4-Hydroxycyclophosphamide**

Phosphoramide Mustard + **Acrolein** ← **Aldophosphamide**

FIGURE 5-4 Microsomal activation of cyclophosphamide.

Specific enzymes may be critical to the process of DNA repair and survival. Methylating agents and the nitrosoureas have a particular propensity for alkylation of the O-6 position of guanine, and this alkylation is removed by MGMT. The MGMT gene is methylated and silenced in 20% of primary brain tumors, and these tumors have greater sensitivity and a better prognosis when treated with procarbazine, temozolomide, or the nitrosoureas.

The ability to repair alkylating damage is likely an important determinant of antitumor response. Repair capacity varies among tumors. This variation may result from inherited polymorphisms in NER components, notably ERCC1. Low levels of expression of ERCC1 have correlated with greater response in lung, ovarian, and head and neck cancers (4), but results are inconsistent in other studies. Polymorphisms of enzymes in the NER pathway have also been correlated with greater host toxicity in lung cancer patients (5). Inherited or somatic changes in the double strand break repair

Dacarbazine

Temozolomide

FIGURE 5-5 Dacarbazine, Temozolomide

pathway may also influence response. BRCA1- or BRCA2-deficient cells have impaired double strand break repair and exhibit heightened sensitivity to platinum analogs (6), a finding confirmed in some breast cancer trials with triple negative tumors (7).

Mismatch DNA repair (MMR), which is initiated by a multi-protein system that recognizes distortions created by mismatched bases in double stranded DNA, is required for recognition of alkylated DNA bases due to methylating agents (temozolomide, procarbazine), the platinum analogs, and nitrosoureas. Deletion of MSH6, a component of MMR, leads to resistance to temozolomide after treatment of gliomas (8).

■ RESISTANCE

Any one of the several critical steps in the action of alkylating agents may present an opportunity for development of resistance. In experimental systems, tumor cell resistance can arise through increased levels of sulhydrils, increased activity of glutathione transferases, and increased expression of MGMT or NER enzymes. Competence of the double strand break repair sequence, which includes BRCA1, Rad-51, and other proteins, is required for effective elimination of potentially lethal cross-links. Finally, changes that interfere with apoptosis, including mutation of p53 or increased expression of BCL-2, may alter the threshold for cell death. On the clinical level, the understanding of alkylating resistance is incomplete. Bendamustine is incompletely cross-resistant with other alkylators, perhaps because its adducts are less efficiently repaired by NER.

■ CLINICAL PHARMACOLOGY

In general, because of their reactivity in aqueous solution, the parent alkylators and particularly their reactive metabolites have a brief residence time in plasma. Because their decomposition is primarily through chemical reactivity, doses of most alkylating agents (cyclophosphamide, bendamustine, temozolomide, busulfan) are not modified for renal or hepatic dysfunction. Bendamustine has a short (40-min) plasma half-life, undergoes spontaneous hydrolysis, and is well tolerated by patients with mild to moderate hepatic or renal impairment. Melphalan is partially cleared by renal excretion and requires dose modification in patients with renal dysfunction. Busulfan is eliminated by hepatic CYP3A4 and glutathione S-transferase in sequential steps and is affected by drugs that induce or inhibit CYP3A4.

The pharmacokinetics of busulfan, a drug used frequently in high doses with bone marrow stem cell rescue, are highly variable, being influenced by patient age and weight. In adults, its half-life averages about 2.5 h in plasma, while in children it is cleared more rapidly (half-life of 2 h). Underdosing may lead to poor allogeneic bone marrow engraftment, while overdosing increases risk of veno-occlusive disease of the liver. Typical pediatric transplant doses are in the range of 0.8 mg/kg given intravenously over 2 h every 6 h for 4 days. Dose adjustment of busulfan is based on pharmacokinetic (PK) monitoring in the pediatric transplantation setting (9). Typically, the area under the PK curve (AUC) is calculated after the first dose, and proportional adjustment of dose is made to achieve an AUC between 900 and 1350 μM·min. A common dose for adult patients is 0.8 mg/kg intravenously for the first infusion, with dose adjustment based on PK monitoring.

The intravenous formulation of busulfan yields more predicatable PK than oral busulfan, which is given in 25% higher doses. Busulfan, the nitrosoureas, temozolomide, thiotepa, and the active metabolite of procarbazine penetrate into the central nervous system well. Busulfan causes seizures in high-dose regimens, and because it accelerates the metabolism of phenytoin, the latter must be used in higher-than-average doses to prevent breakthrough seizures.

▪ TOXICITY

The alkylating agents as a class inhibit hematopoiesis. They suppress the immune system and injure intestinal epithelium and gonadal tissue. Multiple cycles of treatment may lead to epithelial pulmonary injury, pneumonitis, and pulmonary fibrosis (especially after treatment with busulfan and the nitrosoureas, and other agents in high doses), as well as renal tubular injury (nitrosoureas) and bladder toxicity (cyclophosphamide and ifosfamide). In high-dose regimens, busulfan, carboplatin, cyclophosphamide, and melphalan all cause veno-occlusive disease of the liver, due to endothelial damage, while high doses of cyclophosphamide may produce hemorrhagic myocarditis and heart failure.

Bone marrow recovers 10–14 days after conventional doses, except in the case of nitrosourea treatment, which produces a nadir in neutrophil and platelet count 5–6 weeks after administration. Busulfan typically causes a prolonged suppression of the white blood count, probably due to its toxicity to marrow stem cells, and is used in high doses to produce host marrow ablation. Cyclophosphamide tends to have modest effects on platelet production in conventional doses.

Male spermatogenesis is typically lost after a complete course of chemotherapy for lymphomas in adults, and sperm banking prior to treatment may be indicated. Younger women (15–35 years) often remain fertile after alkylating agent treatment but may experience an early menopause.

Acrolein, an alkylating metabolite of both cyclophosphamide and ifosfamide, causes injury to the bladder mucosa and renal tubules, necessitating the use of a sulfhydryl, MESNA (2-mercaptoethanesulonate), in patients receiving high doses of these drugs. MESNA is an inactive disulfide at neutral pH in plasma or tissues but becomes a reactive sulfhydryl in acid urine. Hemorrhagic cystitis may become life threatening in patients receiving continuous low-dose or single high-dose cyclophosphamide without MESNA, and may require cystectomy to control bleeding. The nitrosoureas cause interstitial renal fibrosis and renal failure when used in higher doses and for multiple cycles of treatment.

All alkylating agents cause leukemia, often preceded by a myelodysplastic phase. Cytogenetic studies of bone marrow cells reveal a deletion of portions of chromosome 5 or 7. Full-blown leukemia appears on average 3–5 years after chemotherapy administration and responds poorly to anti-leukemic treatment (10). There is also an increased risk of solid tumors after alkylating agent chemotherapy, most obvious in the second decade after treatment. Concomitant radiation therapy increases the risk of leukemia and of solid tumors.

PLATINUM ANALOGS: MECHANISM OF ACTION

The cytotoxic effects of the platinum analogs result from the formation of adducts with purine bases in DNA. A reactive platinum intermediate is formed by the replacement of the dichloride arms of the platinum complex with two –OH groups (Figure 5-4), and subsequently, the –OH groups are displaced by formation of adducts at sites such as the N-7 position of guanine or adenine. A variety of single DNA adducts, as well as intrastrand and interstrand cross-links, results from reaction of the platinum analogs with DNA. The intrastrand adducts formed between adjacent bases in d(GpG) or d(ApG) sequences appear to be important in blocking DNA and RNA polymerase activity and promoting apoptosis. Adducts cause a bending of the DNA strand, a distortion recognized by DNA repair complexes. Mismatch repair and HMG proteins recognize the adducts and are required for full expression of the cytotoxicity of cisplatin and carboplatin; these proteins trigger attempts to excise the adduct-bearing sequence, creating DNA strand breaks and apoptosis. p53 initiates the process of apoptosis.

■ RESISTANCE

Resistance to platinum analogs has been studied experimentally, and has been ascribed to: (1) failure of DNA damage recognition due to defective mismatch repair, (2) increased detoxification of reactive platinum species by glutathione, (3) increased efflux of platinum complexes by active transport, (4) increased NER capacity, (5) loss of p53, and (6) overexpression of anti-apoptotic genes such as BCL-2. It is unclear which of these responses leads to clinical resistance, although tumors that recur after extensive platinum-based chemotherapy often show cross-resistance to alkylating agents, irradiation, and loss of p53 function. In colorectal cancer treatment, oxaliplatin has greater antitumor activity than the other platinum analogs, perhaps due to the unique properties of the adduct formed by its bulky diaminocyclohexyl group. Additionally, oxaliplatin cytotoxicity does not depend on recognition of adducts by mismatch repair and by HMG proteins (11).

■ CLINICAL PHARMACOLOGY

The three clinically useful analogs differ in their reactivity, pharmacokinetics, and toxicity profiles. Cisplatin is highly reactive at neutral pH and in aqueous solution. It rapidly disappears from plasma, as it forms adducts with protein sulfhydryls in the extracellular space, and reacts with nucleic acids and glutathione intracellularly. Little of the parent compound is found in plasma within a few hours after its administration. Carboplatin, by virtue of its more stable dicarboxylate leaving group, persists in plasma as unchanged drug with a $t_{1/2}$ of 2 h and is eliminated by renal excretion. Carboplatin doses should be adjusted according to creatinine clearance, as calculated by the Calvert formula:

$$\text{Dose (mg)} = \text{target AUC (5–6 mg/ml} \times \text{min)} \times \text{(glomerular filtration rate (ml/min)} + 25)$$

Oxaliplatin is rapidly eliminated through its reaction with nucleophilic targets. No dose adjustment is required for patients with a creatinine clearance of greater than 20 ml/min.

■ TOXICITY

The toxicity profiles of the three analogs differ significantly. Cisplatin causes severe acute nausea and vomiting, which is modified by pretreatment with antiemetics and glucocorticoids. Parent drug excreted in the glomerular filtrate causes renal tubular damage that can be averted by a chloride diuresis. A high chloride concentration in urine converts the drug to its unreactive dichloride form. Cisplatin also causes a progressive high-tone hearing loss. It is only mildly myelosuppressive, but with repeated doses, patients develop a progressive anemia that responds to erythropoietin. Renal tubular toxicity of cisplatin may lead to calcium and magnesium wasting and tetany, but hydration during drug administration and electrolyte replacement mitigate this problem. Intraperioneal therapy with 75–100 mg/m² cisplatin produces intraperitoneal drug levels that are 10- to 20-fold higher than in plasma and improves outcomes of combination therapy of ovarian cancer. However, intraperitoneal therapy is associated with abdominal pain and catheter complications, and many patients are unable to complete the protocol (12).

Carboplatin is less nephrotoxic and otototoxic than cisplatin but causes greater myelosuppression, particularly thrombocytopenia. Oxaliplatin is minimally nephrotoxic but causes moderate leukopenia and thrombocytopenia. Its most bothersome toxicities are an acute neuropathic throat pain, and a progressive peripheral sensory neuropathy in 20% of patients on prolonged treatment. Carboplatin and cisplatin may also cause a disabling peripheral motor and sensory neuropathy after multiple cycles of therapy, especially in combination with taxanes. In high-dose regimens, carboplatin may be associated with interstitial pneumonitis, hepatic veno-occlusive disease, and pulmonary fibrosis.

All three platinum derivatives may cause allergic reactions, including rash, wheezing, and diarrhea, in up to 10% of patients, but usually only after multiple cycles of treatment. Pretreatment with glucocorticoids and antihistamines may allow continued treatment in patients displaying mild allergy. Desensitization is successful in a majority of patients with moderate or severe allergic symptoms (13).

The platinum analogs have been associated with myelodysplasia and acute myelogenous leukemia as a late complication of therapy.

REFERENCES

1. Chabner BA, Roberts TG Jr. Timeline: chemotherapy and the war on cancer. *Nat Rev Cancer.* 2005; 5: 65–72.

2. Chesin BD, Rummel MJ. Bendamustine: rebirth of an old drug. *J Clin Oncol.* 2009; 27: 1–9.

3. Leong CO, Vidnovic N, DeYoung MP, et al. The p63/p73 network mediates chemosensitivity to cisplatin in a biologically defined subset of primary breast cancers. *J Clin Invest.* 2007; 117: 1370–1380.

4. Chiu T-J, Chen C-H, Li S-H, et al. High ERCC1 expression predicts cisplatin-based chemotherapy resistance and poor outcome in unresectable squamous cell carcinoma of head and neck in a betel-chewing area. *J Transl Med.* 2011; 9: 31–39.

5. Suk R, Gurubhagavatula S, Park S, et al. Polymorphisms in ERCC1 and grade 3 or 4 toxicity in non-small cell lung cancer patients. *Clin Cancer Res.* 2005; 15: 1534–1538.

6. Rottenberg S, Nygren AO, Pajic M, et al. Selective induction of chemotherapy resistance of mammary tumors in a conditional mouse model for hereditary breast cancer. *Proc Natl Acad Sci USA.* 2007: 104: 12117–12122.

7. Silver DP, Richardson AL, Eklund AC, et al. Efficacy of neoadjuvant cisplatin in triple-negative breast cancer. *J Clin Oncol.* 2010; 28: 1145–1153.

8. Cahill DP, Codd PJ, Batchelor TT, et al. MSH6 inactivation and emergent temozolomide resistance in human glioblastomas. *Clin Neurosurg.* 2008; 55: 165–171.

9. Gaziev J, Nguyen L, Puozzo C, et al. Novel pharmacokinetic behaviour of intravenous busulfan in children with thalassemia undergoing hematopoietic stem cell transplantation: a prospective evaluation of pharmacokinetic and pharmacodynamic profile with therapeutic drug monitoring. *Blood.* 2010; 115: 4597–4604.

10. Tucker MA, Coleman, CN, Cox RS, et al. Risk of second cancers after treatment for Hodgkin's disease. *N Engl J Med.* 1988; 318: 76–81.

11. Bhattacharyya D, Ramachandran S, Sharma S, et al. Flanking bases influence the nature of DNA distortion by platinum 1,2-intrastrand (GG) cross-links. *PLoS One.* 2011; 6: 1–13.

12. Mackay HJ, Prvencheur D, Heywood M, et al. Phase II/III study of intraperitoneal chemotherapy after neoadjuvant chemotherapy for ovarian cancer. *Current Oncol.* 2011; 18: 84–90.

13. Lenz HJ. Management and preparedness for infusion and hypersensitivity reactions. *The Oncologist.* 2007; 12: 601–609.

CHAPTER **6**

Immunomodulatory Drugs and Proteasome Inhibitors

Anuj Mahindra, Hamza Mujagic, Bruce A. Chabner

The therapeutic options for the treatment of multiple myeloma (MM) have expanded over the past decade with the introduction of novel biologically targeted agents, which in turn have resulted in significantly improved outcomes (1). The use of the immunomodulatory drug thalidomide in the 1990s and subsequently its analogue lenalidomide and more recently pomalidomide has been a major advance in the field. The proteasome inhibitor, bortezomib, was FDA approved in 2003, and the next-generation proteasome inhibitors are now undergoing evaluation in clinical trials. Antibodies targeting membrane-bound receptors are another promising class of agents.

IMMUNOMODULATORY DRUGS (IMiDs)

Thalidomide was originally developed as an antihistamine, but produced significant sedation and was marketed as a hypnotic. It alleviated symptoms of morning sickness due to pregnancy. However, in 1963 it was withdrawn when its use was associated with stunted limb growth (dysmelia) in children born of women exposed to the drug during pregnancy. Three decades later it was found to improve signs and symptoms of erythema nodosum leprosum. This approval reawakened interest in its antiangiogenic and immunomodulatory effects and led to its successful trial for the treatment of patients with refractory MM (2).

Lenalidomide was developed as a thalidomide analogue that more effectively inhibited TNF-α. Pomalidomide is the newest IMiD.

■ STRUCTURE

Thalidomide is piperidinyl isoindole ([±]-α-[*N*-phthalimido]) glutarimide. It is a neutral racemic compound derived from glutamic acid, and is structurally related to the analeptic drug bemegride (α-ethyl-α-methyl-glutarimide, $C_{18}H_{13}NO_2$), and to a sedative and antiepileptic drug, glutethimide (β-ethyl-β-phenyl-glutarimide, $C_{15}H_{23}NO_4$). It has two ring systems: a left-sided phthalimide, and a right-sided glutarimide with an asymmetric carbon atom at position 3′ of the glutarimide ring. The drug consists of equimolar amounts of (+)-R- and (–)-(S)-enantiomers. Thalidomide is sparingly soluble in water (<0.1 g/l) and spontaneously hydrolyses in solution at pH 6.0 or higher to produce at least 12 different products. The structure of thalidomide was modified through the addition of an amino group at the 4 position of the phthaloyl ring, to generate pomalidomide and with the further removal of a carbonyl on the ring to form lenalidomide (**Figure 6-1**).

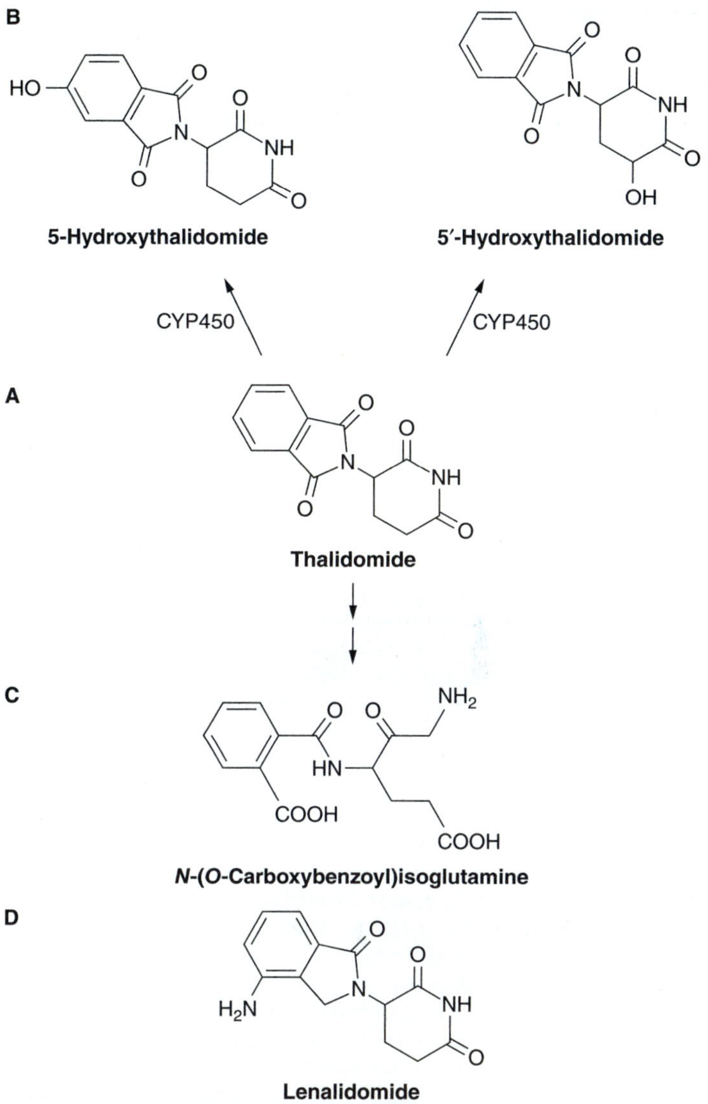

FIGURE 6-1 The structure of thalidomide, hydroxylated metabolites with their hydrolytic products and analogs lenalidomide and pomalidomide. (A) Thalidomide, (B) its p450 hydroxylation product, (C) a spontaneous hydrolytic breakdown product, and (D) its analog, lenalidomide.

■ MECHANISM OF ACTION

IMiDs are hypothesized to act through multiple mechanisms including:

1. A direct antiproliferative/proapoptotic effect probably mediated by downregulation of TNFα, a tumor stimulating and immunomodulatory cytokine, and a suppressive effect on nuclear factor kappa B (NF-κB), a transcription factor that promotes a protective response to cell injury.
2. An indirect antitumor effect mediated by downregulation of tumor cell adhesion molecules (I-CAM 1) and stimulatory cytokines such as IL-6.
3. Inhibition of secretion of angiogenic cytokines such as basic FGF and VEGF.

Its teratogenic activity is attributed to its binding to and inactivating a ubiquitin ligase, cereblon, the suppression of which aborts limb development in zebrafish (3). The presence of cereblon is required for the antimyeloma activity of the IMiDs (4).

■ METABOLISM AND CLINICAL PHARMACOLOGY

Thalidomide is slowly absorbed from the gastrointestinal tract of human subjects due to its poor aqueous solubility, with peak levels in plasma at 3–6 h after ingestion. Absorption at doses at or below 200 mg is variable but becomes linear as doses increase to 800–1200 mg. Thalidomide is loosely bound to serum albumin and to $α_1$-acidic glycoprotein and is widely distributed throughout the body. It is mainly broken down through nonenzymatic hydrolytic cleavage, but about 20% of the drug is also metabolized by hepatic CYP2C19 to form hydroxylated metabolites (Figure 6-1).

The extent of hydrolysis has been estimated to be 80% by 24 h. Hydrolysis cleaves the two-imide bonds of both enantiomers, opening the glutarimide and phthalimide rings, and yielding a series of 12 products, 11 of which are chiral (5). These products are further broken down to yield numerous optically active compounds.

Thalidomide disappears from plasma with an apparent half-life of 4.7 h for both the (S)- and (R)-enantiomers, which are rapidly interconvertible in vivo. Thalidomide and its metabolites are excreted in the urine, while the nonabsorbed portion of the drug is excreted unchanged in feces. Clearance of the parent compound is primarily metabolic and non-renal. Studies of multiple oral doses in healthy subjects showed that thalidomide capsules 200 mg/day over 18–21 days did not produce accumulation and the AUCs on days 1 and 21 were equivalent. It is not known if accumulation occurs with higher daily dosages, although pharmacokinetic simulations of 400 and 800 mg once daily suggest that this would not occur (6).

Lenalidomide is absorbed rapidly after oral intake, reaches maximum plasma concentration after 1–1.5 h, and disappears from plasma with a half-life of 3.1–4.2 h. Approximately two-thirds of the drug are excreted intact in the urine; its renal clearance exceeds glomerular filtration. The remainder of the drug is excreted unchanged in feces, with little evidence for metabolism. Dose adjustments are required in the presence of renal insufficiency (Table 6-1) (7).

■ TOXICITY

Sedation and constipation are the most important side effects of thalidomide and become dose limiting at daily doses of 400 mg or greater.

TABLE 6-1 RECOMMENDED DOSE ADJUSTMENTS OF LENALIDOMIDE FOR PATIENTS WITH MM WITH IMPAIRED RENAL FUNCTION

Renal Impairment	Dose
Moderate (30 ≤ CLcr < 60 ml/min)	10 mg every 24 h
Severe (CLcr < 30 ml/min, not requiring dialysis)	15 mg, every 48 h
End-stage renal disease (CLcr <30 ml/min, requiring dialysis)	5 mg once daily. On dialysis days, administer the dose following dialysis

Other side effects include dizziness, mood changes, headaches, skin rash, and, rarely, neutropenia. Peripheral neurotoxicity, primarily peripheral sensory changes, is reported in up to one-third of patients, usually at doses of 400 mg or greater. Hematologic toxicity, primarily a decrease in the neutrophil and platelet counts, is modest and seen only at doses of 400 mg or greater. As a single agent, thalidomide causes a 5% incidence of deep vein thromboses, but both lenalidomide and thalidomide in combination with dexamethasone cause major thrombotic events in up to 15% of patients, especially in these receiving 400 mg doses of thalidomide or greater (8).

Lenalidomide does not cause significant sleepiness, or constipation, and neuropathy is infrequent. However, it causes neutropenia and thrombocytopenia in approximately 20% of patients. It enhances myelosuppression caused by concomitant chemotherapy, and predisposes to venous thrombosis and embolism when used with dexamethasone.

Prophylactic anticoagulation should be considered in all patients receiving an IMiD particularly in combination with glucocorticoids. The International Myeloma Working Group panel recommends the use of aspirin in patients with one risk factor for VTE. Low-molecular-weight heparin (equivalent to enoxaparin 40 mg/day) is recommended for patients with two or more risk factors for VTE (8).

In clinical trials, second malignancies are more common in patients receiving lenalidomide maintenance compared to patients receiving placebo. McCarthy et al. reported 8 new hematologic cancers and 10 solid-tumor cancers (excluding nonmelanoma skin cancers) among the 231 patients in the lenalidomide group (3.5% and 4.3%, respectively) compared to 1 new hematologic and 5 solid-tumor cancers among the 229 patients in the placebo group (0.4% and 2.2%, respectively) (9). Factors predisposing to second malignancies are being evaluated (10).

The major toxicity of pomalidomide is neutropenia. Grade 3 or greater neutropenia has been seen in 26%–66% of patients, depending on the dose and intensity of prior treatment (11–13). Thromboembolic complications occur with a frequency similar to lenalidomide. Neuropathy is infrequent, with some worsening reported in heavily pretreated patients, most of whom had neuropathy at baseline. Noninfectious acute lung injury is a rare but serious complication that responds well to glucocorticoids (14).

CLINICAL EFFECTIVENESS

Thalidomide is approved for the treatment of newly diagnosed MM patients. Because of thalidomide's known teratogenicity, the FDA restricts marketing of thalidomide in the United States via the System for Thalidomide Education and Prescribing Safety (S.T.E.P.S.®) program.

Lenalidomide is approved by the U.S. Food and Drug Administration for use in combination with dexamethasone in patients with MM who have received one prior therapy. It is also approved for patients with 5q-myelodysplastic syndrome. Lenalidomide is available under a special restricted distribution program, called RevAssist[SM].

Pomalidomide is approved for treatment of relapsed or refractory myeloma.

There is emerging data supporting the use of lenalidomide as maintenance treatment after autologous stem cell transplantation (9, 15, 16).

Selected clinical trials with the above drugs are summarized in **Table 6-2**.

PROTEASOME INHIBITORS

■ MECHANISM OF ACTION

Bortezomib, the first in class boronate peptide proteasome inhibitor, reversibly inhibits chymotrypsin-like activity of the 20S core of the 26S proteasome, which degrades ubiquitinated proteins and thus maintains cellular homeostasis (17). More potent inhibitors of chymotryptic activity, including carfilzomib an irreversible proteasome inhibitor in the epoxyketone category, are being evaluated in clinical trials (Table 6-2).

NF-κB, a key transcription regulator, is found mainly in the cytosol bound to IkB; in this form, NF-κB is restricted to the cytosol and cannot enter to the nucleus to regulate transcription. Bortezomib (**Figure 6-2**) blocks proteasomal degradation of IκB, thereby preventing the transcriptional activity of NF-κB and downregulating survival responses. Bortezomib also disrupts the ubiquitin-proteasomal degradation of p21, p27, p53, and other key regulators of the cell cycle and initiators of apoptosis (17).

■ METABOLISM AND CLINICAL PHARMACOLOGY

The recommended starting dose of bortezomib is 1.3 mg/m^2 given as an intravenous bolus on days 1, 4, 8, and 11 of every 21-day cycle (with a 10-day rest period per cycle) or days 1, 8, 15, and 22 of every 35-day cycle. At least 72 h should elapse between doses.

After intravenous administration of 1–1.3 mg/m^2 of bortezomib, the drug exhibits a terminal $t_{1/2}$ in plasma of 5.5 h (18). Peak proteasome inhibition reaches 60% within 1 h and declines thereafter, with a $t_{1/2}$ of ~24 h.

Bortezomib is cleared by deboronation of 90% of the parent compound, followed by hydroxylation of the boron-free product by CYP3A4 and CYP2D6; administration of this drug with potent inducers or inhibitors/substrates of CYP3A4 requires caution. No dose adjustment is required for patients with renal dysfunction. Patients with moderate (bilirubin more than $1.5 \times - 3 \times$ ULN) or severe (more than $3 \times$ ULN) hepatic dysfunction should start treatment at a reduced dose of 0.7 mg/m^2 per injection during the first cycle. A subsequent dose escalation to 1.0 mg/m^2 or further dose reduction to 0.5 mg/m^2 may be considered based on patient tolerance.

TABLE 6-2 SUMMARY OF SELECTED CLINICAL TRIALS EVALUATING IMiDs AND PROTEASOME INHIBITORS

Reference	Dosing Schedule	Disease Status/ Phase	N (enrolled/ evaluable)	Response rates, %	Median Time-to-Event
Rajkumar et al. (23)	Thal 200 mg on days 1–28 Dex 40 mg oral on days 1, 8, 15, 22 28-Day cycles	ND Ph III ThalDex vs. Dex	TD 235 D 235	ORR 63% vs. 46%	TTP 22.6 vs. 6.5 mo
Facon et al. (24)	Mel 0.25 mg/kg oral on days 1–4 (0.2 mg/kg/day days 1–4 in patients >75 y) Pred 2 mg/kg oral on days 1–4 Thal 100–200 mg on days 1–28 Repeated every 6 wk	ND (age 65–75 y) Ph III MP vs. Mel100 vs. MPT	MP196 Mel100 126 MPT 125	ORR MP 35% Mel100 65% MPT: 76%	OS MP: 33.2 mos Mel100: 38.3 mos MPT: 51.6 mos
Cavo et al. (25)	Bort 1.3 mg/m² on days 1, 8, 15, 22 Thal 100–200 mg on days 1–21 Dex 20 mg oral on day of and day after bortezomib 28-Day cycles	ND Ph III Thal/Dex vs. Bort/ Thal/Dex	TD 238 Bort TD 236	ORR 79% vs. 93%	PFS 40 mo vs. not reached
Weber et al. (26)	Len 25 mg on days 1–21 Dex 40 mg on days 1–4, 9–12, 17–20 Days 1–4 only from cycle 5	RR Ph II	170	ORR 61% CR/nCR: 13%	TTP: 11.1 mo OS: 29.6 mo

(continued)

TABLE 6-2 SUMMARY OF SELECTED CLINICAL TRIALS EVALUATING IMiDs AND PROTEASOME INHIBITORS (CONTINUED)

Reference	Dosing Schedule	Disease Status/ Phase	N (enrolled/ evaluable)	Response rates, %	Median Time-to-Event
Dimopoulos et al. (27)	Len 25 mg on days 1–21 Dex 40 mg on days 1–4, 9–12, 17–20 Days 1–4 only from cycle 5	RR Ph II	176	ORR 60.2% CR/nCR 15%	TTP: 11.3 mo OS: NR
Morgan et al. (28)	Len 25 mg on days 1–21 Cy 500 mg on days 1, 8, 15, 21 Dex 40 mg on days 1–4 and 12–15 4-week cycles for 9 cycles	RR Ph II	21/20	ORR: 65 CR: 5 VGPR: 15	NR
Richardson et al. (29)	Bort 1.3 mg/m² on days 1, 4, 8, 11 Len 25 mg on days 1–14 Dex 20 mg oral on day of and day after bortezomib 3-week cycles	ND Ph II	66	ORR 100% ≥ VGPR 74%	Estimated 18 mo PFS 75% OS 97%
Vij et al. (30)	Carfilzomib i.v. on days 1, 2, 8, 9, 15, 16 of 28-d cycle Cohort 1: 20 mg/m² for all treatment cycles Cohort 2: 20 mg/m² for cycle 1 and then 27 mg/m² for all subsequent cycles	RR Ph II	Cohort 1: 59 Cohort 2: 70	ORR Cohort 1: 42.4% Cohort 2: 52.2%	TTP Cohort 1: 8.3 mos Cohort 2: Not reached

				ORR	OS at 6 mo
Lacy et al. (31)	Pomalidomide Cohort 1: Pom 2 mg daily; Dex 40 mg weekly Cohort 2: Pom 4 mg daily; Dex 40 mg weekly	RR Ph II	35 each cohort	Cohort 1: 49% Cohort 2: 43%	Cohort 1: 78% Cohort 2: 67%

Drugs: Bort, bortezomib; Cy, cyclophosphamide; Dex, dexamethasone; Len, lenalidamide; Mel or M, melphalan; Pom, pmalidomide; Thal, thalidomide

Response: CR, complete response; nCR, near complete response; NR, not reported; ORR, overall response rate; OS, overall survival; PFS, progression free survival; PR, partial response; TTP, time to progression; VGPR, very good partial response

Patient category: ND, newly diagnosed; RR, relapsed or refractory

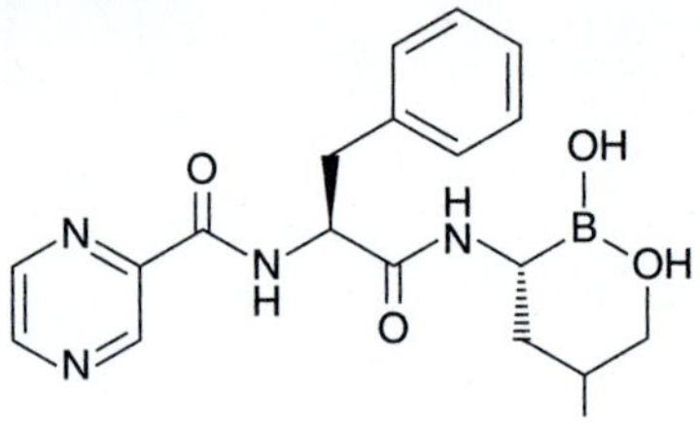

Bortezomib

FIGURE 6-2 Structure of bortezomib.

■ TOXICITY

Peripheral neuropathy, thrombocytopenia, and gastrointestinal symptoms, although manageable, are important side effects (19, 20). Peripheral neuropathy is less frequent with once weekly as opposed to twice weekly bortezomib and the subcutaneous rather than the intravenous route (21, 22). Dose reductions or discontinuation of bortezomib ameliorates the neuropathic symptoms. Reactivation of herpes zoster has been observed, and routine prophylaxis with acyclovir is recommended.

■ CLINICAL EFFECTIVENESS

Bortezomib is approved for treatment of patients with MM both as initial therapy and at relapse. Bortezomib is generally used in combination with other active agents in MM including dexamethasone, lenalidomide, and melphalan. Selected clinical trials are summarized in Table 6-2.

Carfilzomib is not yet approved by the U.S. Food and Drug Administration.

In addition, other promising agents include monoclonal antibodies targeting CS-1—a cell surface glycoprotein, CD 138, CD 38, HDAC-6 inhibitors, and HSP-90 inhibitors.

REFERENCES

1. Kumar SK, Rajkumar SV, Dispenzieri A, et al. Improved survival in multiple myeloma and the impact of novel therapies. *Blood*. 2008; 111: 2516–2520.

2. Singhal S, Mehta J, Desikan R, et al. Antitumor activity of thalidomide in refractory multiple myeloma. *N Engl J Med*. 1999; 341: 1565–1571.

3. Ito T, Ando H, Suzuki T, et al. Identification of a primary target of thalidomide teratogenicity. *Science*. 2010; 327: 1345–1350.

4. Zhu YX, Braggio E, Shi CX, et al. Cereblon expression is required for the antimyeloma activity of lenalidomide and pomalidomide. *Blood*. 2011; 118: 4771–4779.

5. Eriksson T, Bjorkman S, Roth B, et al. Hydroxylated metabolites of thalidomide: formation in-vitro and in-vivo in man. *J Pharm Pharmacol*. 1998; 50: 1409–1416.

6. Teo SK, Colburn WA, Tracewell WG, et al. Clinical pharmacokinetics of thalidomide. *Clin Pharmacokinet*. 2004; 43: 311–327.

7. Dimopoulos MA, Terpos E, Chanan-Khan A, et al. Renal impairment in patients with multiple myeloma: a consensus statement on behalf of the international myeloma working group. *J Clin Oncol.* 2010; 28: 4976–4984.

8. Palumbo A, Rajkumar SV, Dimopoulos MA, et al. Prevention of thalidomide- and lenalidomide-associated thrombosis in myeloma. *Leukemia.* 2008; 22: 414–423.

9. McCarthy PL, Owzar K, Hofmeister CC, et al. Lenalidomide after stem-cell transplantation for multiple myeloma. *N Engl J Med.* 2012; 366: 1770–1781.

10. Thomas A, Mailankody S, Korde N, et al. Second malignancies after multiple myeloma: from 1960s to 2010s. *Blood.* 2012; 119: 2731–2737.

11. Lacy MQ, Hayman SR, Gertz MA, et al. Pomalidomide (CC4047) plus low-dose dexamethasone as therapy for relapsed multiple myeloma. *J Clin Oncol.* 2009; 27: 5008–5014.

12. Lacy MQ, Hayman SR, Gertz MA, et al. Pomalidomide (CC4047) plus low dose dexamethasone (Pom/dex) is active and well tolerated in lenalido-mide refractory multiple myeloma (MM). *Leukemia.* 2010; 24: 1934–1939.

13. Leleu X, Attal M, Moreau P, et al. Phase 2 study of 2 modalities of pomalidomide (CC4047) plus low-dose dexamethasone as therapy for relapsed multiple myeloma. IFM 2009-02. *ASH Annual Meeting Abstracts.* 2010; 116: 859.

14. Geyer HL, Viggiano RW, Lacy MQ, et al. Acute lung toxicity related to pomalidomide. *Chest.* 2011; 140: 529–533.

15. Ludwig H, Durie BG, McCarthy P, et al. IMWG consensus on mainte-nance therapy in multiple myeloma. *Blood.* 2012; 119: 3003–3015.

16. Attal M, Lauwers-Cances V, Marit G, et al. Lenalidomide maintenance after stem-cell transplantation for multiple myeloma. *N Engl J Med.* 2012; 366: 1782–1791.

17. Hideshima T, Mitsiades C, Akiyama M, et al. Molecular mechanisms mediating antimyeloma activity of proteasome inhibitor PS-341. *Blood.* 2003; 101: 1530–1534.

18. Papandreou CN, Daliani DD, Nix D, et al. Phase I trial of the protea-some inhibitor bortezomib in patients with advanced solid tumors with observations in androgen-independent prostate cancer. *J Clin Oncol.* 2004; 22: 2108–2121.

19. Richardson PG, Sonneveld P, Schuster MW, et al. Bortezomib or high-dose dexamethasone for relapsed multiple myeloma. *N Engl J Med.* 2005; 352: 2487–2498.

20. San Miguel JF, Schlag R, Khuageva NK, et al. Bortezomib plus melpha-lan and prednisone for initial treatment of multiple myeloma. *N Engl J Med.* 2008; 359: 906–917.

21. Bringhen S, Larocca A, Rossi D, et al. Efficacy and safety of once-weekly bortezomib in multiple myeloma patients. *Blood.* 2010; 116: 4745–4753.

22. Moreau P, Pylypenko H, Grosicki S, et al. Subcutaneous versus intrave-nous administration of bortezomib in patients with relapsed multiple

myeloma: a randomised, phase 3, non-inferiority study. *Lancet Oncol.* 2011; 12: 431–440.

23. Rajkumar SV, Blood E, Vesole D, et al. Phase III clinical trial of thalidomide plus dexamethasone compared with dexamethasone alone in newly diagnosed multiple myeloma: a clinical trial coordinated by the eastern cooperative oncology group. *J Clin Oncol.* 2006; 24: 431–436.

24. Facon T, Mary JY, Hulin C, et al. Melphalan and prednisone plus thalidomide versus melphalan and prednisone alone or reduced-intensity autologous stem cell transplantation in elderly patients with multiple myeloma (IFM 99-06): a randomised trial. *Lancet.* 2007; 370: 1209–1218.

25. Cavo M, Tacchetti P, Patriarca F, et al. Bortezomib with thalidomide plus dexamethasone compared with thalidomide plus dexamethasone as induction therapy before, and consolidation therapy after, double autologous stem-cell transplantation in newly diagnosed multiple myeloma: a randomised phase 3 study. *Lancet.* 2010; 376: 2075–2085.

26. Weber DM, Chen C, Niesvizky R, et al. Lenalidomide plus dexamethasone for relapsed multiple myeloma in North America. *N Engl J Med.* 2007; 357: 2133–2142.

27. Dimopoulos M, Spencer A, Attal M, et al. Lenalidomide plus dexamethasone for relapsed or refractory multiple myeloma. *N Engl J Med.* 2007; 357: 2123–2132.

28. Morgan GJ, Schey SA, Wu P, et al. Lenalidomide (revlimid), in combination with cyclophosphamide and dexamethasone (RCD), is an effective and tolerated regimen for myeloma patients. *Br J Haematol.* 2007; 137: 268–269.

29. Richardson PG, Weller E, Lonial S, et al. Lenalidomide, bortezomib, and dexamethasone combination therapy in patients with newly diagnosed multiple myeloma. *Blood.* 2010; 116: 679–686.

30. Vij R, Wang M, Kaufman JL, et al. An open-label, single-arm, phase 2 (PX-171-004) study of single-agent carfilzomib in bortezomib-naive patients with relapsed and/or refractory multiple myeloma. *Blood.* 2012; 119: 5661–5670.

31. Lacy MQ, Allred JB, Gertz MA, et al. Pomalidomide plus low-dose dexamethasone in myeloma refractory to both bortezomib and lenalidomide: comparison of 2 dosing strategies in dual-refractory disease. *Blood.* 2011; 118: 2970–2975.

CHAPTER 7
Natural Products: Bleomycin and Trabectedin

Bruce A. Chabner

Natural product research has yielded many active anticancer compounds acting as inhibitors of topoisomerases (Chapter 4) and as antimitotics (Chapter 4). Others, such as bleomycin and trabectedin, interact directly with DNA and exhibit unusual mechanisms of action.

BLEOMYCIN

Traditional fermentation research has been the backbone of efforts to discover anti-infective and antitumor agents. From this research has come bleomycin, a drug important in the curative combination therapy of Hodgkin disease and testicular germ cell tumors. Among the exquisite cytotoxics designed by nature, the most unique is bleomycin, which was isolated from the broth of the fungus, *Streptomyces verticillus*. The clinical bleomycin preparation consists of a family of peptides that share a common C-terminal metal binding core, attached to a variable DNA binding portion with different substitutions on the amino-terminal end of the molecule (**Figure 7-1**). The various bleomycin peptides have a molecular weight of about 1500, and differ in their potency for DNA cleavage, but share a common chemistry. The predominant peptide, bleomycin A2, comprises 70% of the clinical preparation.

■ MECHANISM OF ACTION

The bleomycin peptides function as carriers for a catalytic metal that undergoes rapid cycles of oxidation/reduction (1). The metal may be copper, iron, cobalt, zinc, or others. The metal ligand is bound in a coordination complex of amine groups contributed by the unusual amino acids of the peptide. All metals but the cobalt species are readily exchangeable; thus 57-Co (II) bleomycin is sufficiently stable to be used as a tumor-imaging agent. The clinical preparation of bleomycin is metal free, but upon administration rapidly acquires Cu (II) or Fe (II), the latter probably representing the active form of the drug. Bleomycin binds to DNA by intercalation of its C-terminal bithiazole groups between guanine bases in adjacent DNA strands. Intercalation brings the bleomycin metal group into proximity with the deoxyribose backbone of DNA. The radicals released by cycles of oxidation/reduction of the metal core oxidize adjacent deoxyribose groups at the 3′-4′ bond, releasing propenal or propenal-thymine as its most frequent products (**Figure 7-2**). DNA single and double strand breaks (in the ratio of 10:1) result and must be repaired if the cell is to survive. If double strand breaks are sufficient in number, the cell undergoes apoptosis.

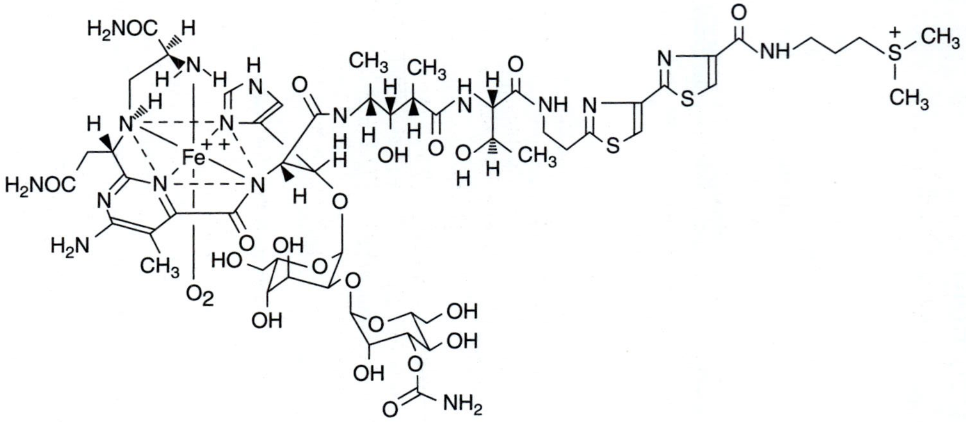

FIGURE 7-1 Bleomycin A$_2$.

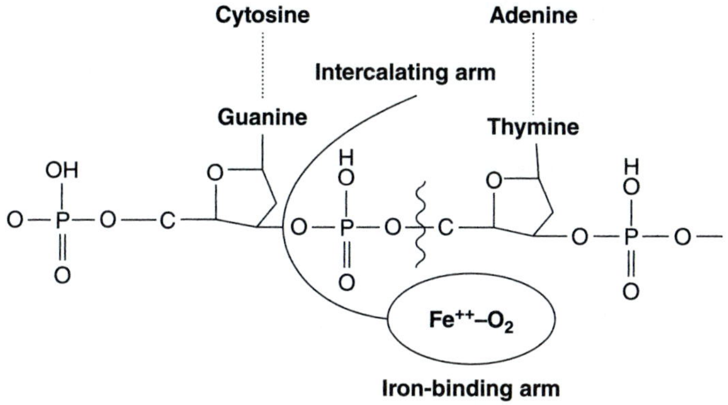

FIGURE 7-2 Intercalation of bithiazole groups between DNA strands in which one strand has the preferred sequence of GpT or GpC. The $Fe^{++}-O_2$ complex bound to bleomycin comes in opposition to the deoxyribose of DNA, abstracting a proton and cleaving the deoxyribose phosphate bond.

Cells deficient in double strand break repair, such as those from tumors with BRCA1 mutation, are highly sensitive to bleomycin (2).

Bleomycin, a large, positively charged molecule, crosses the cell membrane slowly, possibly entering through vesicles. In the cytoplasm it is subject to cleavage by a specific aminohydrolase (AH), found in both malignant and normal tissues. AH may play a role in determining both response and toxicity (3). AH is found in low concentrations in lung tissue and skin, both of which are highly susceptible to bleomycin toxicity. Mice deficient in AH are extremely susceptible to the drug's toxicity, while tumor cells with high levels of AH are resistant to the drug.

Other factors contribute to bleomycin sensitivity in experimental studies. Defective double strand break repair leads to hypersensitivity to the drug (3). Resistant cell may have increased capacity for detoxification of free radicals (4).

■ CLINICAL PHARMACOLOGY

Bleomycin is administered i.v. or i.m. in doses of 10–20 units/m^2 every 2 weeks. Higher doses are associated with an increased risk of pulmonary toxicity. The disposition of bleomycin is characterized by its slow uptake in tissues and selective hydrolysis in certain tissues, including liver and kidney. Most of an administered dose is excreted in the urine as an intact molecule. After intramuscular or intravenous administration, it disappears from plasma with a half-life of 2–3 h. Patients with renal dysfunction exhibit much delayed clearance and may develop overwhelming systemic toxicity (see below). Doses should be reduced at least 50% in patients with moderately reduced renal function (creatinine clearance 30–80 ml/min), and bleomycin should not be given to patients in severe renal failure (creatinine clearance below 30 ml/min) (5).

Bleomycin is also instilled intrapleurally (60 mg or greater, dissolved in 50–100 ml of saline) to ablate the pleural space. Given in this way it has a 75% success rate for ablation of effusions and has little systemic toxicity (6).

■ TOXICITY

The primary *acute* toxicity of bleomycin is cutaneous erythema, tenderness, and ulceration over the joints or the distal extremities. It may cause frank Raynaud's phenomenon in occasional patients. Hyperpigmentation, nail changes, and alopecia may occur after prolonged use.

The most serious *long-term* toxic effects damage the lung. Pulmonary toxicity is dose related and most frequent (10% or greater) in patients receiving total doses of 450 mg or more, but may appear at lower total doses in selected patients, especially in those over 70 years of age, in those treated with single doses above 20 mg/m^2, in those who are receiving chest irradiation or other pulmonary toxins such as gemcitabine (7) or the armed monoclonal antibody, SGN-35 (breituximab). Pulmonary function may deteriorate acutely in patients exposed to high concentrations of inspired O_2, as during surgery, subsequent to bleomycin treatment. In patients undergoing surgical resection of residual tumor after chemotherapy for germ cell tumors of the testis, oxygen must be used sparingly. In patients receiving a full course of therapy for Hodgkin disease, 20% have a greater than 20% decrease in diffuse capacity but most remain asymptomatic (8).

The pathophysiology of bleomycin pulmonary toxicity is not well understood. Experimental intertracheal injection of small doses of bleomycin or its terminal amine fragment evokes an acute inflammatory response and subsequent pulmonary fibrosis in mice and hamsters. Bleomycin induces macrophage and endothelial secretion of pro-inflammatory cytokines such as interleukins 1 and 6, TNF-alpha, and TGF-beta, and toxic lipid products such as phosphatidic acid. Mice deficient in metalloproteinases or plasminogen activators are resistant to bleomycin pulmonary fibrosis, suggesting that inhibitors of these enzymes might be useful in preventing fibrosis. A number of other experimental treatments block or ameliorate pulmonary toxicity of bleomycin, but as yet there are no clinical antidotes (9).

Bleomycin pulmonary toxicity initially manifests as a dry cough and shortness of breath, with or without fever. Alveolar infiltrates are seen on chest x-ray. Computerized tomography may reveal extensive infiltrates, even in patients with minimal evidence on routine chest x-rays, as well as pleural thickening and even cavitation. In later stages, there is evidence of extensive pulmonary parenchymal fibrosis. The acute syndrome must be distinguished from opportunistic infection or other causes of pulmonary infiltrates in cancer patients. In such patients, biopsy discloses inflammatory alveolar infiltrates, hyaline membrane formation, and fibrosis. Patients on bleomycin experience a steady decrease in pulmonary diffusion capacity with increasing total dose of drug, and, in later stages, develop evidence of restrictive disease and desaturation. There is no proven therapy for bleomycin pulmonary toxicity other than discontinuation of the drug. Glucocorticoids may produce temporary improvement of symptoms, but there is no evidence that glucocorticoids prevent or reverse pulmonary fibrosis. With discontinuation of the drug, the inflammatory component may resolve and pulmonary function may improve. Approximately a quarter of patients who develop extensive bleomycin toxicity, with symptoms, hypoxia, and bilateral infiltrates, will have a fatal outcome.

Limitation of total doses to less than 250 units, selection of patients without risk factors (see above), and careful clinical monitoring for evidence of toxicity have reduced the incidence of serious pulmonary injury to less than 5% in patients treated for Hodgkin disease or testicular cancer. The drug remains a unique and important component of their treatment.

TRABECTEDIN

Trabectedin belongs to a class of highly toxic natural products that bind to the minor groove of DNA and alkylate guanine at the N-2 position (Figure 7-3). Its DNA binding stabilizes double-stranded DNA, and stalls replication and transcription. It was isolated from the marine tunicate *Ecteinacscidia turbinate* and has a multi-ring structure with an isoquinoline group that interacts with transcription factors (TFs) and with the XPG component of nucleotide excision repair (NER). This interaction may contribute to its activity against NER proficient cells (10). In Europe, it is approved for second-line treatment of soft tissue sarcomas and, with Doxil, for treatment of ovarian cancer, and is available for compassionate use in the United States. A more potent and potentially less toxic analogue, xalypsis, which lacks the side chain and does not interact with NER (11), is in clinical development and appears to have lesser hepatic toxicity in early trials.

Trabectedin is believed to function as a DNA intercalator and alkylator, and inhibits transcription factors; however, it has other actions that may contribute to its antitumor activity: Downregulation of the MDR protein and HSP70 and inhibition of sarcoma-related transcription factors, such as the FUS-CHOP fusion protein found in myxoid liposarcomas (10), may explain its utility in sarcomas.

Resistance is poorly understood but, in experimental cell lines, has been related to loss of NER proficiency. Cells deficient in double strand break repair are hypersensitive.

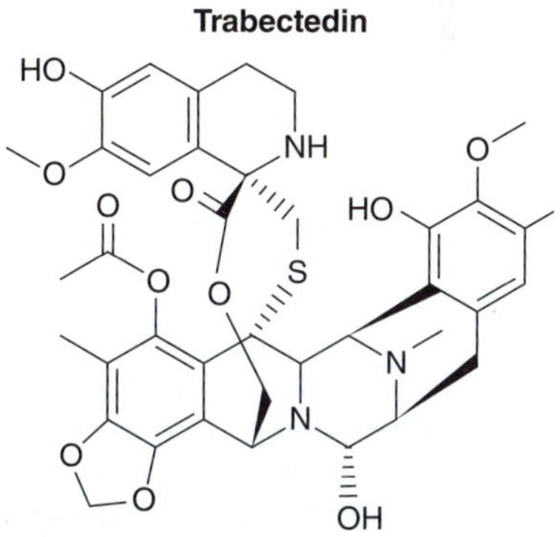

Trabectedin

FIGURE 7-3 Trabectedin.

◼ CLINICAL PHARMACOLOGY

Infusions of 1, 3, and 24 h have been tested in trials. The 24-h infusion of 1.5 mg/m² appears the most active and is well tolerated over multiple cycles of treatment for soft tissue sarcomas. A 3-h infusion of 1.1 mg/m² with Doxil, 30 mg/m², has been approved in Europe for second-line ovarian cancer (12). The drug has a large volume of distribution and a long terminal half-life in plasma of 40–50 h (13). It is slowly metabolized by CYP3A4, with minimal urinary excretion of parent drug. Metabolites are inactive. It is administered after premedication with a 20-mg infusion of dexamethasone to lessen hepatic enzyme elevations.

◼ TOXICITY

The primary toxicities of trabectedin are neutropenia, occurring 5–12 days after drug administration, hepatic enzyme elevations, hand-foot syndrome, and mucositis. If hepatic enzyme elevations exceed grade 2 but recover by the start date of the next cycle of treatment, doses are reduced to 0.9 mg/m². If recovery from grade 2 or greater hepatic toxicity is incomplete, treatment with trabectedin should be terminated. Approximately 10% of patients will require termination of treatment.

REFERENCES

1. Lazo JS, Chabner BA. Bleomycin. In BA Chabner, DL Longo (eds.), *Cancer Chemotherapy & Biotherapy Principles and Practice*, 4th edition. Lippincott Williams & Wilkins, Philadelphia, 2011, 323–341.

2. Quinn JE, Kennedy RD, Mullan PB, et al. BRCA1 functions as a differential modulator of chemotherapy-induced apoptosis. *Cancer Res.* 2003; 63: 6221–6228.

3. Li HR, Shagisultanova EI, Yamashita K, et al. Hypersensitivity of tumor cell lines with microsatellite instability to DNA double strand break producing chemotherapeutic agent bleomycin. *Cancer Res.* 2004; 64: 4760–4767.

4. Atienza JM, Roth RB, Rosette C, et al. Suppression of RAD21 gene expression decreases cell growth and enhances cytotoxicity of etoposide and bleomycin in human breast cancer cells. *Mol Cancer Ther.* 2005; 4: 361–368.

5. O'Sullivan JM, Huddart RA, Norman AR, et al. Predicting the risk of bleomycin lung toxicity in patients with germ-cell tumors. *Ann Oncol.* 2003; 14: 91–96.

6. Sartori S, Tassinari D, Ceccotti P, et al. Prospective randomized trial of intrapleural bleomycin versus interferon alfa-2b via ultrasound-guided small-bore chest tube in the palliative treatment of malignant pleural effusions. *J Clin Oncol.* 2004; 22: 1228–1233.

7. Bredenfeld H, Franklin J, Nogova L, et al. Severe pulmonary toxicity in patients with advanced-stage Hodgkin's disease treated with a modified bleomycin, doxorubicin, cyclophosphamide, vincristine, procarbazine and gemcitabine (BEACOPP) regimen is probably related to the combination of gemcitabine and bleomycin: a report of the German Hodgkin's Lymphoma Study Group. *J Clin Oncol.* 2004; 22: 2424–2429.

8. Martin WG, Ristow KM, Habermann TM, et al. Bleomycin pulmonary toxicity has a negative impact on the outcome of patients with Hodgkin's lymphoma. *J Clin Oncol.* 2005; 23: 7614–7620.

9. Scotton CJ, Chambers RC. Bleomycin revisited: towards a more representative model of IPF? *Am J Physiol Lung Cell Mol Physiol.* 2010; 299: 439–441.

10. D'Incalci M, Galmarini CM. A review of trabectedin (ET-743): a unique mechanism of action. *Mol Cancer Therap.* 2010; 9: 2157–2163.

11. Guirouilh-Barbat J, Antony S, Pommier Y. Zalypsis (PM00104) is a potent inducer of gamma-H2AX foci and reveals the importance of the C ring of trabectedin for transcription-coupled repair inhibition. *Mol Cancer Ther.* 2009; 8: 2007–2014.

12. Monk BJ, Herzog, TJ, Kaye SB, et al. Trabectedin plus pegylated liposomal doxorubicin in recurrent ovarian cancer. *J Clin Oncol.* 2010; 28: 3107–3114.

13. Forouzesh B, Hidalgo M, Chu Q, et al. Phase I and pharmacokinetic study of trabectedin as a 1- or 3-hour infusion weekly in patients with advanced solid malignancies. *Clin Cancer Res.* 2009; 15: 3591–3599.

CHAPTER **8**

L-Asparaginase

Bruce A. Chabner

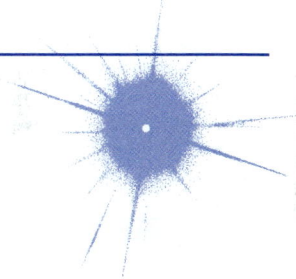

Most anticancer drugs are small synthetic molecules designed to inhibit enzymes or to interact with DNA. Newer drugs may also be proteins, such as monoclonal antibodies or cytokines (interferon, IL-2) that interact with cell surface receptors. L-asparaginase (L-ASP) is unique as a bacterial enzyme that hydrolyzes an essential amino acid, L-asparagine, and through that action, kills tumor cells. Its efficacy is based on the observation that some lymphoid malignancies are unable to synthesize asparagine and must derive it from the blood stream. Enzyme purified from *Escherichia coli* (1) is now an essential component of the regimen for remission induction and consolidation for childhood acute lymphocytic leukemia (ALL). While enzymatic activity is highly specific for asparagine hydrolysis, asparagine depletion not only kills tumor cells but also leads to a broad range of toxicities resulting from inhibition of the synthesis of clotting factors, insulin, and other essential proteins.

L-ASP is a 144,000 tetrameric protein that catalyzes the deamination of the circulating blood pool of L-asparagine. Enzyme from *E. coli* and an alternative protein from *Erwinia chrysanthemi* are highly specific for L-asparagine but retain minor cleaving activity against glutamine. The two enzymes lack immunologic cross-reactivity; therefore, the *Erwinia* enzyme may be used with relative safety in patients hypersensitive to *E. coli* enzyme, but because of its short plasma half-life of 16 h, must be administered in higher doses to produce prolonged asparagine depletion. A third form of L-ASP, the *E. coli* enzyme conjugated to polyethylene glycol (pegaspargase— PEG L-ASP), has a much long plasma $t_{1/2}$ of 6 days, is less immunogenic than native L-ASP, and is particularly useful in patients hypersensitive to the unconjugated enzymes, 70% of whom will not react to the pegylated enzyme (2). PEG L-ASP is as effective as native *E. coli* enzyme in first-line use. A recombinant *E. coli* L-ASP, which is free of the immunogenic oligomers of the native bacterial enzyme preparation, is undergoing clinical evaluation and may prove to be a superior product (2).

CLINICAL PHARMACOLOGY

A comparison of the primary features of the three drugs is shown in Table 8-1. No single dosing schedule of the various L-ASP preparations has been established. The native L-ASP drug is primarily administered by intramuscular injection, a route associated with a lesser risk of anaphylaxis, although PEG L-ASP appears safe by the intravenous route (3). Higher doses are associated with more complete and prolonged asparagine depletion, but cause a higher incidence of side effects, particularly thrombotic events, and more frequent hypersensitivity responses. In general, most regimens strive to maintain a trough level of enzyme activity in plasma of 0.1 units/ml for the duration of therapy (for 7–21 days). This level is associated with total asparagine depletion in plasma but not in the cerebrospinal fluid.

Clinical effectiveness of L-ASP requires the continuous depletion of asparagine during a cycle of treatment, but its activity is compromised by the development of neutralizing antibodies and side effects. Cellular resistance to L-ASP arises by induction of asparagine synthetase in tumor cells.

TOXICITY

Anaphylaxis occurs in less than 5% of patients. In ALL patients, antibodies are detected in up to 50% of patients receiving single agent L-ASP, but in only 20% of patients receiving L-ASP with immunosuppressive drugs, such as methotrexate, 6-mercaptopurine, or glucocorticoids. About half of patients with neutralizing antibodies will have clinical evidence of hypersensitivity,

TABLE 8-1 COMPARISON OF THE PRIMARY FEATURES OF THREE DRUGS

Preparation	Typical Dose/Schedule IU/m²/Dose	Elimination from Plasma (Half-Life)	Antibody Positive Patients (%)*
E. coli	10,000 IU/m² 3 d/wk × 2–4 wk 25,000 IU/m² qwk × 3	30 h	45–75
Erwina	10,000 IU/m² qd × 7	16 h	30–50
Pegaspargase	2,500 IU/m² q2wk	6 d	5–18

*Following completion of a course of therapy, with no prior asparaginase exposure, and with no concurrent glucocorticoids.

but some asymptomatic patients will have "silent inactivation," more rapid clearance of L-ASP, and incomplete depletion of asparagine in plasma, and will be at increased risk of leukemic relapse (4). Monitoring of L-ASP levels during therapy is recommended to assure achievement of trough levels. In relapsed patients, PEG L-ASP may be less effective than native enzyme in depleting asparagine, a finding that prompts the use of higher and more frequent doses (3500 IU/m^2 weekly) of PEG L-ASP in these patients (5). Other toxicities of L-ASP include its effects on coagulation and protein synthesis. It depletes both antithrombotic (protein C and protein S, antithrombin III) and procoagulant (prothrombin) factors, and is associated with a significant risk of stroke related to cortical sinus thrombosis. The risk of thrombosis seems highest in adolescent and adult patients, in patients receiving concomitant glucocorticoids, and in those with underlying inherited defects in anticoagulant factors, such as homocystinemia, factor V Leiden deficiency, or prothrombin mutations (6). Low-molecular-weight heparin reduces the incidence of venous thrombosis in high-risk individuals. Protein synthesis inhibition may cause extreme hypertriglyceridemia (levels of 5000 mg/dl or greater) and pancreatitis due to lipoprotein lipase deficiency, as well as hypoalbuminemia, hyperglycemia (insulin deficiency), and, infrequently, hemorrhage (prothrombin, factor IX, and factor X deficiency). The same spectrum of side effects occurs in patients receiving PEG L-ASP, although the frequency of hypersensitivity reactions is significantly reduced.

Considerable uncertainty remains regarding the best regimen, including dose and schedule (Table 8-1), for treating ALL, and the best use of the various L-ASP preparations. Alternative regimens employing higher doses, more extended periods of treatments, and new drug combinations are undergoing clinical evaluation for childhood ALL.

REFERENCES

1. Cooney DA, Handschumacher RE. L-asparaginase and L-asparaginase metabolism. *Annu Rev Pharmacol.* 1970; 10: 421–440.

2. Peters R, Appel I, Kuehnel H-J, et al. Pharmacokinetics, pharmacodynamics, efficacy and safety of a new recombinant asparaginase preparation in children with previously untreated acute lymphoblastic leukemia: a randomized phase 2 clinical trial. *Blood.* 2008; 112: 4832–4838.

3. Silverman LB, Supko JG, Stevenson KE, et al. Intravenous PEG-asparaginase during remission induction in children and adolescents with newly diagnosed acute lymphoblastic leukemia. *Blood.* 2010; 115: 1351–1353.

4. Panetta JC, Gajjar A, Hak LJ, et al. Comparison of Native *E. coli* and PEG asparaginase pharmacokinetics in pediatric acute lymphoblastic leukemia. *Clin Pharmacol Therap.* 2009; 86: 651–658.

5. Rytting M. Peg-asparaginase for acute lymphoblastic leukemia. *Expert Opin Biol Ther.* 2010; 10: 833–839.

6. Nowak-Gottl U, Wermes C, Junker R, et al. Prospective evaluation of the thrombotic risk in children with acute lymphoblastic leukemia carrying the MTHFR TT 677 genotype, the prothrombocin G20210A variant, and further prothrombotic risk factors. *Blood.* 1999; 93: 1595–1599.

CHAPTER 9
Differentiating Agents

Bruce A. Chabner

An obvious feature of malignant cells is their failure to differentiate, and to acquire the histologic, biochemical, and functional features of the mature cells of the tissue from which they arise. Thus, leukemia cells resemble in appearance, surface markers, and molecular profile the more primitive normal progenitors of the myeloid or lymphoid series. Indeed it has been possible to isolate a small fraction of continuously self-renewing cells (called tumor stem cells) from frankly malignant tissues. These tumor cells are able to reproduce multiple differentiated cell lineages when appropriately stimulated by "differentiating" agents such as 5-azacytidine (see Chapter 1) or retinoids. The progression from mature cell phenotype to an undifferentiated malignancy is recapitulated in serial observations of chronic myelogenous leukemia and in experimental models of malignant transformation.

Research efforts have defined pathways responsible for a block in differentiation in malignant cells and have suggested strategies for pharmacologic intervention. Vitamin A and related retinoids were the first compounds to show differentiating effects in cell culture, and all-trans retinoic acid (ATRA) (Figure 9-1) was subsequently found to be highly effective in inducing remission in promyelocytic leukemia, a disease characterized by a translocation involving the retinoic acid receptor, RAR-alpha (1). Subsequently, other pathways have been exploited as targets for development of differentiating agents, including histone deacetylase (HDAC), DNA cytosine methyltransferase (CMT), and vitamin D signaling pathways. CMT is targeted by both 5-azacytidine and decitabine, as discussed in the section on antimetabolites, while HDAC inhibitors and vitamin A analogs are useful agents in peripheral T-cell lymphoma and acute promyelocytic

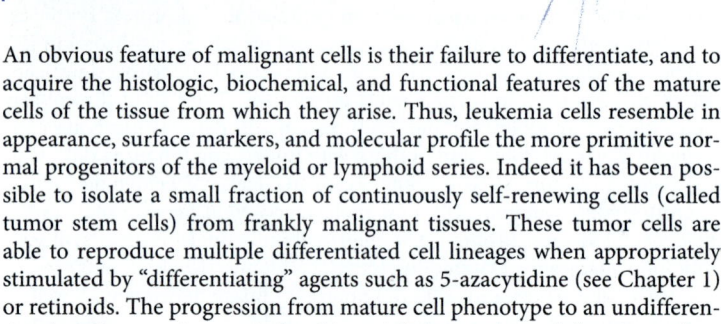

FIGURE 9-1 Differentiating agents useful in APL therapy. (A) All-trans retinoic acid (ATRA) and (B) arsenic trioxide.

leukemia (APL), respectively. Here we will consider four clinically useful agents that promote differentiation: ATRA and arsenic trioxide (ATO), both of which are effective in APL, and vorinostat and rhombedepsin, which are approved for treatment of cutaneous T-cell lymphoma (CTCL).

ATRA

Retinoids (vitamin A and its derivatives) induce differentiation of malignant cells in cell culture systems. Early work showed that retinoids caused promyelocytic leukemia (APL) (HL-60) cells to undergo maturation into granulocytes at drug concentrations easily achievable in humans. In normal cells, RAR-alpha forms homodimers as well as heterodimers with retinoid X receptor, and the dimer in turn complexes with the PML transcription factor. The RAR-alpha homodimer in complex with PML in turn binds ATRA, leading to chromatin modification and transcription of genes that induce differentiation (2). In APL cells, the normal pathway for vitamin A action is disrupted by a translocation fusing portions of the RAR-alpha gene on chromosome 15 and the PML gene on chromosome 17. The fusion protein acts as a repressor of differentiation and, through the FOS gene, promotes proliferation. The RAR-alpha/PML fusion protein has low affinity for ATRA and requires pharmacologic concentrations of retinoid to activate differentiation in APL cells. High concentrations of ATRA lead to multiple effects on leukemic cell differentiation: degradation of the fusion protein, chromatin modification, and upregulation of transcription factors (CEBP beta, OCT-1, and most importantly, PU1) required for myeloid differentiation (2). Resistance to ATRA arises through mutation of the fusion protein to decrease its binding affinity, and possibly by induction of the ATRA metabolizing p450 isoenzyme (CYP26A1) in the liver or in APL cells after prolonged exposure to the drug (3).

■ CLINICAL PHARMACOLOGY

ATRA induces complete remission in more than 90% of patients with APL, alone or in combination with an anthracycline (1). The initial clinical experience with ATRA revealed clear evidence of leukemic cell maturation in bone marrow and peripheral blood. Remission duration for single agent ATRA tends to be brief, and the recurrent tumor is usually refractory to a second cycle of treatment due to further mutation in the RAR-alpha gene. However, when ATRA is used in combination with anthracyclines as primary therapy, the regimen is curative for 70% or more of patients with this disease. It is effective in all patients with the PML/RAR-alpha translocation, including those with a masked translocation, only detectable by PCR. The "long" form of the translocation is more sensitive to APL and has a greater disease-free survival after remission than does the "short" form (4).

ATRA is given in daily intravenous doses of 45 mg/m^2/day until remission is achieved. It is now used as the initial therapy in APL in combination with an anthracycline. ATRA has the additional advantage of quickly aborting the life-threatening coagulopathy associated with this disease. In patients with significant comorbidities or in elderly patients, it efficiently induces remission when used with arsenic trioxide, without a cytotoxic agent. It may also be effective in maintenance therapy, but its continuous use leads to cutaneous toxicity and elevated plasma triglycerides. Therefore, intermittent schedules of maintenance ATRA, given with methotrexate and 6-mercaptopurine, may be better tolerated and equally efficacious. ATRA concentrations in plasma reach 400 ng/ml, and ATRA is rapidly eliminated by p450-mediated metabolism. The half-life in plasma is less than 1 h, and the rate of clearance increases markedly with repeated doses.

■ TOXICITY

ATRA's primary side effects are cutaneous and pulmonary. Retinoids cause a redness, dryness, and sensitivity of the skin and cracking of the lips (cheilosis). A more important, and at times lethal, toxicity is its tendency to cause pulmonary dysfunction. Through its differentiating effects on APL cells, it causes an accumulation of leukemic myeloid precursors in pulmonary vessels, leading to hypoxia, pleural and pericardial effusions, peripheral edema, fever, and, in extreme cases, respiratory failure and death. Concurrent glucocorticoids and cytotoxic chemotherapy (anthracyclines), given with ATRA, control the increase in leukemic granulocytes in the peripheral blood, decrease their adhesion to endothelium, and greatly lessen the risk of the "retinoic acid syndrome." Prophylactic dexamethasone should be given to patients with a presenting white blood cell count of 5×10^9/l or higher (5).

Other ATRA toxicities include pseudotumor cerebri, with headaches, changes in mental status, and papilledema; liver function test abnormalities; bone tenderness; hypercalcemia and renal failure; myocarditis; and elevated plasma triglycerides, all of which reverse with cessation of therapy.

■ ARSENIC TRIOXIDE (ATO)

A second unique therapy, ATO (Figure 9-1) effectively treats APL, with differentiating action that mimics ATRA. ATO induces a high rate of complete response in patients refractory to ATRA and chemotherapy, and is effective as a component of consolidation therapy (6) and in elderly patients during remission induction (7). It promotes differentiation and apoptosis of cultured APL cells. It causes the degradation of RAR-alpha/PML through production of reactive oxygen species, which induce intramolecular disulfide linkages in the PML portion of the fusion protein. ATO binds directly to the disulfide-linked PML, and the complex transfers to the nuclear matrix, where it undergoes sumoylation, ubiquitination, and degradation (8). ATO also promotes degradation of NF-κB, an antiapoptotic transcription factor, and suppresses key transcription factors in the hedgehog signaling pathway (9). The contribution of each of these properties to the antileukemic action of APL is not clear.

■ CLINICAL PHARMACOLOGY

The standard regimen for ATO administration as a single agent is a 1- to 2-h infusion of 0.15 mg/kg/day for up to 60 days or until achievement of a complete response. Further treatment is given after a 3-week break. Alternative schedules of a 5-day loading dose, followed by twice weekly drug infusions until remission, are being explored. Its use in combination with ATRA and cytotoxic chemotherapy for primary therapy of APL is evolving. Early trials indicate that it is highly effective in inducing remission when used with

ATRA, both in low-risk and high-risk patients (WBC count > 5 × 10⁹/l), with minimal toxicity (7).

Peak concentrations of total arsenic achieved during the 2-h infusion reach 5 μM. The parent compound is eliminated through interaction with sulfhydrils and through enzymatic methylation. The concentration of parent drug in plasma, the active principle, is probably lower than 1 μM (10).

■ TOXICITY

ATO causes a long list of side effects, the most important of which is a leukemic cell maturation syndrome similar to that caused by ATRA, with pulmonary distress, pleural and pericardial effusions, and alteration in mental status. This syndrome is effectively prevented and treated with dexamethasone, 10 mg, which should be administered concurrently with ATO in patients with white blood cell counts greater than 5 × 10⁶/ml at presentation. ATO may cause hyperglycemia, hepatic enzyme abnormalities, and rarely acute hepatic failure. Myositis manifested as muscle tenderness and muscle swelling, accompanied at times by fever, has also been reported. ATO inhibits ion channels in the cardiac conduction system, causing a prolongation of the QT interval and predisposing to atrial and ventricular arrhythmias (torsade de pointes). During ATO therapy, a weekly EKG should be monitored for signs of QT prolongation greater than 500 ms and for arrhythmias. Serum K^+ and Mg^{2+} should be monitored weekly and replenished as necessary to maintain concentrations above 4 meq/l (K^+) and 2 meq/l (Mg^+), respectively. An absolute QT interval of > 500 ms should lead to drug discontinuation and immediate repletion of electrolytes.[*]

HISTONE DEACETYLASE (HDAC) INHIBITORS

■ VORINOSTAT

The most recent additions to the list of differentiating agents approved for clinical use are two HDAC inhibitors, vorinostat (12) and romidepsin (13). HDACs are a large family of enzymes that remove acetyl groups from amino groups of the lysines found in chromatin and thereby produce compaction of chromatin, blocking gene transcription and differentiation. Inhibitors of HDACs reverse this process, promoting the transcription of DNA, blocking cell cycle progression, and leading to terminal differentiation and apoptosis. These inhibitors also alter the stability of a broad class of cell cycle checkpoint proteins and DNA repair proteins by blocking their deacetylation. HDAC inhibitors are indicated for treatment of cutaneous and peripheral T-cell lymphomas.

Vorinostat was approved based on its ability to cause partial or complete responses in 30% of patients with CTCL after failure of at least two prior regimens (11). Responses were achieved after a median of 55 days of treatment on a schedule of 400 mg per day, and lasted a median of

---

[*]On a historical note, Napoleon appears to have been the victim of arsenic cardiac toxicity. An analysis of Napoleon's hair has demonstrated high levels of arsenic, indicating chronic arsenic poisoning; it is believed his acute fatal episode was a ventricular arrhythmia (torsades de pointes) induced by hypokalemia that resulted from treatment with emetics and cathartics (11) given for his chronic gastrointestinal symptoms. At autopsy he was discovered to have a gastric carcinoma.

5.5 months. Vorinostat has a plasma half-life of 1.5–2 h. It is eliminated by glucuronidation and by hydrolysis and beta-oxidation. Asian patients with the UDP-glucuronyltransferase 2B17 genotype have delayed drug clearance and a higher rate of toxicity (14). Its primary toxicities are mild to moderate fatigue, anorexia, nausea, diarrhea, thrombocytopenia, and anemia. Serious or dose delaying side effects are uncommon, the most notable being thrombocytopenia in 6%. While the HDAC inhibitors as a class cause lengthening of the QT interval, there is no consistent evidence for cardiotoxicity or arrhythmias related to vorinostat.

■ ROMIDEPSIN

Romidepsin (depsipeptide), a complex natural product composed of unusual amino acids in a cyclic peptide linkage, also inhibits HDACs and is approved for treatment of CTCLs. It is similar to if not more potent and more clinically active than vorinostat, but it has consistent effects on the electrocardiogram (flattening of T-waves, modest prolongation of the QT interval). While in early trials two patients died, possibly due to drug-induced arrhythmias, further trials found that the drug is safe in routine clinical use at a dose of 400 mg per day. Monitoring of serum K^+ and Mg^+, repletion of electrolytes, and monitoring of the QT interval prior to drug administration are advised. Mild myelosuppression may also occur during prolonged use. Other toxicities are nausea, anorexia, and diarrhea. The drug has a plasma half-life of 3 h and is eliminated by CYP3A4 metabolism.

   Both vorinostat and romidepsin may inhibit warfarin clearance and prolong the prothrombin time.

REFERENCES

1. Sanz MA, Tallman MS, Lo-Coco F. Practice points, consensus, and controversial issues in the management of patients with newly diagnosed acute promyelocytic leukemia. *The Oncologist*. 2005; 10: 806–814.

2. Mueller B, Pabst T, Fos J, et al. ATRA resolves the differentiation block in t(15; 17) acute myeloid leukemia by restoring PU l expression. *Blood*. 2006; 107: 3330–3338.

3. Idres N, Marill J, Chabot G. Regulation of CYP26A1 expression by selective RAR and RXR agonists in human NB4 promyelocytic leukemia cells. *Biochem Pharmacol*. 2005; 10: 1595–1601.

4. Tussie-Luna MI, Rozo L, Roy AL. Pro-proliferative function of the long isoform of PML-RARα involved in acute promyelocytic leukemia. *Oncogene*. 2006; 25: 3375–3386.

5. Wiley JS, Firkin FC. Reduction of pulmonary toxicity by prednisolone prophylaxis during all-trans-retinoic acid treatment of acute promyelocytic leukemia. Australian Leukaemia Study Group. *Leukemia*. 1995; 9: 774–778.

6. Powell BL, Moser B, Stock W, et al. Arsenic trioxide improves event-free and overall survival for adults with acute promyelocytic leukemia: North American Leukemia Intergroup Study C9710. *Blood*. 2010; 116: 3751–3757.

7. Hu J, Lio Y-F, Wu C-F, et al. Long-term efficacy and safety of all-trans retinoic acid/arsenic trioxide-based therapy in newly diagnosed acute promyelocytic leukemia. *Proc Nat Acad Sci USA*. 2009; 196: 3342–3347.

8. Jeanne M, Lallemand-Breitenback V, Ferhi O, et al. PML/RARA oxidation and arsenic binding initiate the antileukemia response of As_2O_3. *Cancer Cell*. 2010; 18: 88–98.

9. Platanias LC. Biological responses to arsenic compounds. *J Biol Chem*. 2009; 284: 18583–18587.

10. Fukai Y, Hirata M, Ueno M. Clinical pharmacokinetic study of arsenic trioxide in an acute promyelocytic leukemia patient: speciation of arsenic metabolites in serum and urine. *Bio Farm Bull*. 2006; 29: 1022–1027.

11. Mari F, Bertol E, Fineschi V, Karch S. Channelling the emperor: what really killed Napoleon? *J R Soc Med*. 2004; 97: 397–399.

12. Lane AA, Chabner BA. Histone deacetylase inhibitors in cancer therapy. *J Clin Oncol*. 2009; 27: 5459–5468.

13. Bertino EM, Otterson GA. Romidepsin: a novel histone deacetylase inhibitor for cancer. *Expert Opin Investig Drugs*. 2011; 20: 1151–1158.

14. Wong NS, Seah EZ, Wang ILZ, et al. Impact of UDP-glucuronyltrasferase B17 genotype on vorinostate metabolism and clinical outcomes in Asian women with breast cancer. *Pharmacogenet Genomics*. 2011; 11: 760–768.

CHAPTER **10**
Molecular Targeted Drugs

Benjamin Izar, Jeffrey W. Clark, Bruce A. Chabner

INTRODUCTION

Important discoveries have revealed the molecular basis for the transformation, proliferation, and survival of cancer cells. These advances have revealed new targets for cancer drug design, and have produced agents that inhibit the signaling molecules and pathways responsible for cancer (**Figure 10-1**) (1). These inhibitors of cancer-associated targets include monoclonal antibodies (mAbs) either alone or coupled with cytotoxic agents or radioisotopes; modified proteins and peptidomimetic molecules; and small-molecular-weight drugs. Still in the development stage are small interfering RNAs (siRNA), antisense oligonucleotides, gene therapy approaches, and ribozymes or DNAzymes. In this chapter we will consider the small molecules that have been approved for clinical use. Monoclonal antibodies and their conjugates will be considered elsewhere (Chapter 15) (see **Table 10-1**) (2-9).

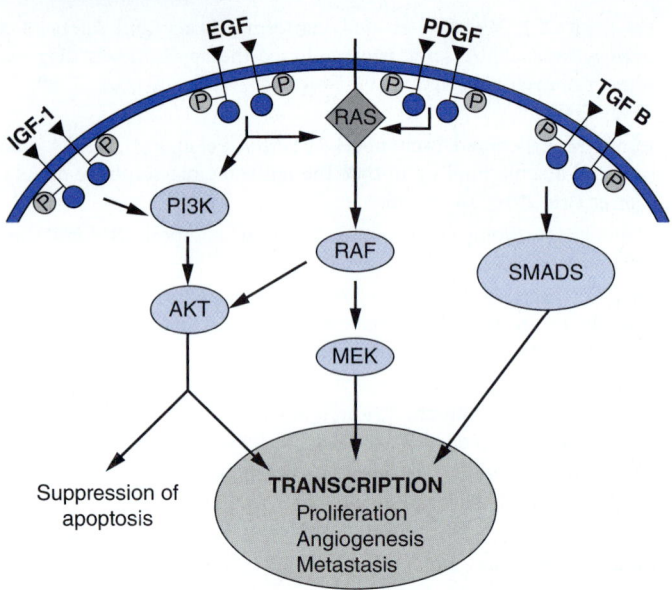

FIGURE 10-1 Schematic of growth factor receptor signaling in tumor cells.

MOLECULAR TARGETS IN CANCER

A rational approach to therapeutic discovery is based on our rapidly growing knowledge of pathways and proteins essential for cancer cell survival, growth, and metastasis. These pathways may be qualitatively unique to cancer (Figure 10-1), or may be simply overexpressed or amplified wild-type proteins. Mutant genes, unique to cancer cells, are particularly attractive in that they alter critical cellular functions and lead to uncontrolled growth, inhibition of apoptosis, escape from growth suppression, invasion of surrounding normal tissues, modifications of the tumor microenvironment including angiogenesis, and metastasis. Inhibition of these mutant functions leads to cancer cell death.

Alterations in a number of fundamental cellular processes may lead to malignant transformation and uncontrolled growth. Malignancy may result from overexpression or amplification of growth factors or their receptors, such as activating mutations or amplifications of the epidermal growth factor receptor (EGFR) family; activation of critical intracellular phosphorylating enzymes such as B-RAF (e.g., by mutation); modulation of the tumor microenvironment such as by activation of angiogenic pathways (e.g., vascular endothelial growth factors [VEGFs] and their receptors); changes in metabolism such as occur with mutations in glucose utilization (such as mutations in the IDH1 or IDH2 genes); epigenetic changes; or activation of anti-apoptotic pathways such as overexpression of Bcl-2 or decreased BAX expression.

TABLE 10-1

| | | | Dose Adjustment (% Reduction of Recommended Dose if Available) | | | Drug Interactions | | |
Agent	Target of Inhibition	Plasma T 1/2	Pharmacokinetics	Liver Dysfunction[2]	Renal Dysfunction (CrCl in mL/min)	Severe Toxicities (BBW in Bold)	CYP Inh.*	CYP Ind.#	Inh. CYP**	Others
Monoclonal antibodies										
Trastuzumab	HER2	5.8 d	Likely eliminated via RES	None	None	**Cardiotoxicity, reduced LVEF, serious infusion reactions, pulmonary toxicities, nephrotic syndrome (rare)**	No	No	No	Anthracyclines, paclitaxel and cyclophosphamide—increased cardiotoxicity. Paclitaxel—increased levels
Pertuzumab	HER2	18 d		None (not studied)	CrCl > 30: none CrCl < 30: none (not studied)	**Cardiotoxicity, reduced LVEF, serious infusion reactions, embryo-fetal toxicity**	No	No	No	None reported

(continued)

99

TABLE 10-1 (CONTINUED)

Agent	Target of Inhibition	Plasma T 1/2	Pharmacokinetics	Dose Adjustment (% Reduction of Recommended Dose if Available)		Severe Toxicities (BBW in Bold)	Drug Interactions			
				Liver Dysfunction	Renal Dysfunction[2] (CrCl in mL/min)		CYP Inh.*	CYP Ind.#	Inh. CYP**	Others
Ibritumomab Tiuxetan Y-90	CD20. Tiuxetan links the antibody and Y-90, a high-energy beta emission	27–30 h	6–11% renal excretion, 7.2% parent compound	None	None	**Serious infusion reactions, severe cytopenias, cut. and mucocut. reactions,** radiation injury	No	No	No	Several medications (including, but not limited to, aspirin, clopidogrel, warfarin, heparin, enoxaparin, dalteparin, fondaparinux)—bleeding
Tositumomab I131	CD20. Binding of the I131 loaded antibody and beta emission	8 d		None	None	**Infusion-related reactions, prolonged and severe cytopenias,** anaphylactic reactions	No	No	No	None reported

Rituximab	CD20	5–78 d		None	None	Serious infusion reactions, TLS, severe mucocut. Reactions, PML	No	No	No	Cisplatin—renal failure. Infection by live vaccines. Inadequate immunologic response to influenza and pneumococcal vaccine
Alemtuzumab	CD52 on several immune cells	12 d		None	None	Cardiotoxicity, serious infusion reactions, infections, cytopenias	No	No	No	Increased risk of infection by live vaccines
Ofatumumab	CD20	12–14 d		None	None	Infusion-related reactions	No	No	No	None reported
Brentuximab Vedotin	CD30. Internalization and disruption of microtubules by MMAE inhibiting cancer cell growth	4–6 d	Metabolizaed by CYP3A4/5. 24% renal excretion	None (not determined for MMAE)	None (not determined for MMAE)	Neutropenia, PNP, PML	Yes	No	No	Bleomycin—increased lung toxicity

(continued)

TABLE 10-1 (CONTINUED)

Agent	Target of Inhibition	Plasma T 1/2	Pharmacokinetics	Dose Adjustment (% Reduction of Recommended Dose if Available)		Severe Toxicities (BBW in Bold)	Drug Interactions			
				Liver Dysfunction²	Renal Dysfunction (CrCl in mL/min)		CYP Inh.*	CYP Ind.#	Inh. CYP**	Others
Ipilimumab	CTLA4	14.7 d		None	None	Rare (enterocolitis, hepatitis, dermatitis, TEN, PNP and endocrinopathy)	No	No	No	None reported
Bevacizumab	VEGF	20 d		None	None	Clotting (arterial and venous), bleeding, proteinuria, surgery and wound healing complications, GI perforation, PRES	No	No	No	None reported
Cetuximab	EGFR	3–7 d	Internalization in liver and skin	None	None	Serious infusion reactions, ILD, acneform rash, cardiopulmonary arrest and/or sudden death	No	No	No	None reported
Panitumumab	EGFR	7.5 d		None	None	Infusion related reactions, dermatologic toxicities	No	No	No	None reported

	Target	Half-life	Metabolism	Hepatic	Renal	Toxicity / Precautions				
Vegfr-1 and 2 Fusion										
Ziv-aflibercept	Binds VEGFR-1 and 2 ligands	6 d		Mild-mod: none, severe (not studied)	None	Clotting (arterial), bleeding, compromised wound healing, GI perforation, PRES, neutropenia, HTN	No	No	No	None reported
Peptide Immunotoxins										
Denileukin diftitox	Cells that express high affinity form IL-2 receptor (CD25, CD122, CD152)	70–80 min		None	None	Severe infusion reactions, capillary leak syndrome, loss of visual acuity, avoid in hypoalbuminemia <3 g/dL	No	No	No	None reported
Proteasome Inhibitors										
Bortezomib	26S proteasome	9–15 h	Metabolized by CYP3A4, 2D6, 2C19, 2C9, 1A2. Extent of renal excretion unclear	Mild: none Mod-sev: ~45%	None Dialysis: administer postdialysis	Thrombocytopenia, PNP	Yes	Yes	No	None reported

(continued)

TABLE 10-1 (CONTINUED)

Agent	Target of Inhibition	Plasma T 1/2	Pharmacokinetics	Liver Dysfunction[2]	Renal Dysfunction (CrCl in mL/min)	Severe Toxicities (BBW in Bold)	CYP Inh.[*]	CYP Ind.[#]	Inh. CYP[**]	Others
Carfilzomib	Similar to Bortezomib	< 1 h	Possibly metabolized by CYP3A4/5. Metabolized by P-glycoprotein. Extent of renal excretion unclear	Not studied	None	PAH, hepatotoxicity, cardiotoxicity, thrombocytopenia	N/A	N/A	N/A	None reported
Histone deacetylase inhibitors										
Vorinostat	Histone deacetylases that are overexpressed in some cancer cells	2 h	Metabolism through glucuronidation, hydrolysis and beta-oxidation. 52% renal excretion, less than 1% parent compound	Mild-mod: not sufficiently studied, caution. Sev: contraindicated	Not sufficiently studied, caution	Severe thrombocytopenia and leukopenia	No	No	No	Warfarin and valproic acid—bleeding
Romidepsin	Same as Vorinostat	3 h	Metabolizaed by CYP3A4	Mild: none. Mod-sev: not studied, caution	None. ESRD: not studied, caution	Neutropenia, thrombocytopenia	Yes	Yes	No	None reported

TABLE 10-1

Agent	Target of Inhibition	Plasma T 1/2	Primary Metabolism CYP	Primary Metabolism Other	Renal Excretion % total[1]	Par. Comp.	Liver Dysfunction[2]	Renal Dysfunction (CrCl in mL/min)	Severe Toxicities, (BBW in Bold)	Drug Interactions CYP Inh.*	Drug Interactions CYP Ind.#	Drug Interactions Inh. CYP**	Others
Kinase inhibitors													
Imatinib	BCR-ABL, KIT, pdgfr	18 h (aM=40 h)	CYP3A4, 1A2, 2D6, 2C9 and 2C19. aM=N-demethylated piperazine		13	5	Sev: 25%	CrCl 40–59: limit to 600 mg/d CrCl 20–39 mL/min: 50% CrCl<20: caution	Neutropenia, thrombocytopenia	Yes	Yes	Yes	Acetaminophen: increased hepatotoxicity. Hypothyroidism: increase Levothyroxine dose
Dasatinib	BCR-ABL, KIT, pdgfr	3–5 h	CYP3A4		4		None	None	Neutropenia, thrombocytopenia	Yes	Yes	No	QT prolonging agents. PPIs/antacids—decr. absorbtion

(continued)

105

TABLE 10-1 (CONTINUED)

Agent	Target of Inhibition	Plasma T 1/2	Primary Metabolism		Renal Excretion		Dose Adjustment (% Reduction of Recommended Dose if Available)		Severe Toxicities (BBW in Bold)	Drug Interactions			
			CYP	Other	% total¹	Par. Comp.	Liver Dysfunction²	Renal Dysfunction (CrCl in mL/min)		CYP Inh.*	CYP Ind.#	Inh. CYP**	Others
Nilotinib	BCR-ABL, KIT, pdgfr	17 h	CYP3A4				Mild, mod or sev.: 25%–33%	None	Neutropenia, thrombocytopenia, QT prolongation, lipase/amylase elev	Yes	Yes	No	QT prolonging agents. PPIs/antacids—decr. absorbtion
Ponatinib	BCR-ABL (including T315I), vegfr, pdgfr, fgfr, src, KIT, ret, tie-2, flt-3	24 h	CYP3A4 and 2C8, 2D6, and 3A5	Esterases and/or amidases	5		Not studied	Not studied	Arterial thrombosis, hepatotoxicity, GI perforation, wound healing complications, hemorrhage, cytopenias, cardiac arrhythmias, pancreatitis	Yes	Yes	No	Ponatinib inhibits ABCG2 and P-gp
Bosutinib	BCR-ABL, src, lyn, hck	22.5 h	CYP3A4		3		Mild, mod or sev: 60%	None	Neutropenia, thrombocytopenia, QT prolongation, hepatotoxicity	Yes	Yes	No	PPIs/antiacids—decr. absorption

Axitinib	Vegfr1-3	2.5–6.1 h	CYP3A4, 2C19 and A2	23	Mod: 50%. Sev: not studied	None	HTN, HTN-associated seizures, proteinuria, bleeding, surgery	Yes	Yes	No	None reported
Pazopanib	Vegfr1-3, pdgfr, fgfr1 and 3, C-KIT, ltk, lck, c-fms	31 h	CYP3A4, 1A2 and 2C8	<4	Mod: 75% Sev: do not use	None	**Hepatotoxicity**, HTN, proteinuria, surgery	Yes	Yes	Yes (weak)	QT prolonging agents
Sorafenib	Vegfr2, vegfr3, pdgfr-a, flt3, C-KIT, p38-alpha, B-raf	1–2 d	CYP3A4 aM=pyridine n-oxide UGT1A9	19	None Sev: not studied	None Dialysis: not studied	Recurrent/persistent skin toxicity, high grade HTN, dyspnea and rash, desquamation	Yes	Yes	No	QT prolonging agents
Sunitinib	Pdgfr-a, pdgfr-b,vegfr 1-3, C-KIT	40–60 h (aM= 80–110 h)	CYP3A4	16	None Sev: not studied	None Dialysis: higher dose (up to 200%)	**Hepatotoxicity**, surgery, reduced LVEF	Yes	Yes	No	QT prolonging agents
Everolimus	Complex formation with fkbp-12 that inhibits mTOR signaling, torc-1 complex	30 h	CYP3A	5	Mod: 50% Sev: not studied	None	Pneumonitis, serious infections, development of lymphoma	Yes	Yes	No	None reported

(continued)

TABLE 10-1 (CONTINUED)

| Agent | Target of Inhibition | Primary Metabolism | | Renal Excretion | | Dose Adjustment (% Reduction of Recommended Dose if Available) | | | Drug Interactions | | | |
		CYP	Other	% total[1]	Par. Comp.	Liver Dysfunction[2]	Renal Dysfunction (CrCl in mL/min)	Severe Toxicities, (BBW in Bold)	CYP Inh.	CYP Ind.*	Inh.# CYP**	Others
Temsirolimus	Same as everolimus	CYP3A4. aM= sirolimus		4.6		Mild: 40%. Mod/sev: do not use	None	Neutropenia, thrombocytopenia, thrombosis, ILD, bowel perforation, seizures, psychosis	Yes	Yes	No	Increased risk of infection by live vaccines
Crizotinib	Alk, ros-1, met	CYP3A4/5		22	2.3	Not studied, caution	CrCl > 30: none. Not studied in CrCl < 30, caution	Transaminits/bilirubinemia, QT prolongation	Yes	Yes	Yes (weak)	QT prolonging agents
Erlotinib	HER1/egfr	CYP3A4, 1A2 and 1A1		8	<1	None	None (not studied)	Skin reactions, severe diarrhea, rash, transaminitis/bilirubinemia	Yes	Yes	Yes	Warfarin and NSAIDs— bleeding. PPIs/antacids—decr. absorbtion. Statins— rhabdomyolysis

Plasma T 1/2:
- Temsirolimus: 17.3 h (aM= 54 h)
- Crizotinib: 42 h
- Erlotinib: 36.2 h

Gefitinib	HER1/egfr	6–49 h	CYP3A4	4	<1	None	Hepatotoxicity, ILD	Yes	Yes	No	Gefitinib is a CYP inducer. Warfarin—bleeding
Lapatinib	HER1 and HER2	14.2–24 h	CYP3A4/5	<2	Sev: 33% Sev, met. breast cancer: 40%	None (not studied)	Hepatotoxicity, ILD/pneumonitis, reduced LVEF, QT prolongation	Yes	Yes	No	QT prolonging agents
Regorafenib	Ret, vegfr1-3, KIT pdgfra, pdgfrb, fgfr1-2, tie2, ddr2, Trk2A, Eph2A, Raf-1, BRAF, BRAFV600E, sapk2, ptk5 and abl	25–51 h	CYP3A4	UGT1A1 17	Mild-mod: None Sev: not studied	Mild: none Mod-sev: not studied	Hepatotoxicity, bleeding, cardio-toxicity, PRES, GI perforation, fistula, wound healing complications, dermatolicgal toxicities	Yes	Yes	No	Inhibits UGT1A9, UGT1A1
Cabozantinib	Ret, met, vegfr-3, KIT, trkb, flt-3, axl, and tie-2	55 h	CYP3A4 and 2C9 aM=XL184 N-oxide	27	Not studied	CrCl > 30: none CrCl < 30: not studied	GI perforation and fistulas, hemorrhage, wound healing compli-cations, PRES, thrombembolism, PPES	Yes	Yes	Yes	Cabozantinib is a CYP inducer

(continued)

109

TABLE 10-1 (CONTINUED)

Agent	Target of Inhibition	Plasma T 1/2	Primary Metabolism CYP	Primary Metabolism Other	Renal Excretion % total[1]	Renal Excretion Par. Comp.	Dose Adjustment (% Reduction of Recommended Dose if Available) Liver Dysfunction[2]	Dose Adjustment (% Reduction of Recommended Dose if Available) Renal Dysfunction (CrCl in mL/min)	Severe Toxicities, (BBW in Bold)	Drug Interactions CYP Inh.*	Drug Interactions CYP Ind.#	Drug Interactions Inh. CYP**	Drug Interactions Others
Ruxolitinib	Dysregulated jak-1 and jak-2	2.8–5.8 h	CYP3A4		74		Mild, mod, sev + platelets 100–150: 33%–50%. Mild, mod, sev + platelets <100: do not use	CrCl 15–59 + platelets 100–150: 30%–50% CrCl 15–59 + platelets <100: do not use CrCl <15: do not use. Dialysis + platelets 100–200: 50%–62.5%. Dilaysis + platelets >200: 33%–50%	Thrombocytopenia, anemia	Yes	Yes	No	

Drug	Target	$t_{1/2}$[1]	Metabolism	FMO		Hepatic adjustment[2]	Renal adjustment	Toxicity				Drug interactions
Vandetanib	egfr and vegf	19 d	CYP3A4. aM=N-desmethyl-vandetanib and vandetanib-N-oxide	FMO	25	None Mod-sev: do not use	CrCl <50: 33%	QT prolongation, torsades de points, sudden death	Yes	Yes	No	QT prolonging agents
Vemurafenib	B-raf	57 h	Unknown		1	None Sev: not sufficiently studied	None CrCl <30: not sufficiently studied	QT prolongation	Yes	Yes	Yes	Vemurafenib is a CYP inducer. Warfarin—bleeding. QT prolonging agents
Pathway inhibitors that are not kinase inhibitors												
Vismodegib	Hedgehog pathway via inhibition of Smoothened	4–12 d	(Likely) CYP2C9 and 3A4/5		4.4	Not sufficiently studied	Not sufficiently studied	Embryo-fetal death/severe birth defects	No	No	No	PPIs/antiacids—decr. absorbtion

[1]Including parent compound and active metabolites.
[2]Most studies use the child pugh classification.
*Cyp inhibitors resulting in increased concentrations of drug.
#Cyp inducers resulting in decreased drug concentration.
**Drug inhibits cyp, leading to increased concentration of drugs metabolized by cyp.

ESRD, end stage renal disease; HTN, hypertension; ILD, interstitial lung disease; PNP, peripheral neuropathy; PRES, posterior reversible encephalopathy syndrome; LVEF, left ventricular ejection fraction; TLS, tumor lysis syndrome; TEN, toxic epidermal necrolysis; MMAE, monomethyl auristatin E; PML, progressive multifocal leukencephalopathy; GI, gastrointestinal; Sz, seizure; PAH, pulmonary artery hypertension; PPES, palmar-plantar erythrodysesthesia syndrome; PPI(s), proton pump inhibitor(s); NSAIDs, non-steroidal anti-inflammatory drugs.

(continued)

acc.	accelerated
ADCC	antibody dependent cytotoxicity
adv.	advanced
ALK	anaplastic lymphoma kinase
ALL	acute lymphocytic leukemia
aM	active metabolite(s)
ASCT	autologous stem cell transplant
BCC	basal cell carcinoma
B-raf	v-raf murine sarcoma viral oncogene homolog B1
BRAF V600+	positive for V600 mutation of BRAF
cCML	chronic phase CML
CDCC	complement dependent cytotoxicity
c-Fms = CSF-1R	colony stimulating factor 1 receptor
CLL	chronic lymphocytic lymphoma
CML	chronic myeloid leukemia
CRC	colorectal cancer
CSF-1R	colony stimulating factor 1 receptor
CTLA4	cytotoxic T-lymphocyte-associated antigen 4
cut.	cutaneous
CVP	cyclophosphamide, vincristine, and prednisone
CYP	p450 cytochrome enzymes
d	day(s)
d/c	discontinue
DLCBL	diffuse large-B-cell lymphoma
DP	dermatofibrosarcoma protuberans
EGFR	epidermal growth factor receptor
Fe	fecal
FGFR	fibroblast growth factor receptor
FKBP-12	FK506 binding protein 12
FLT3	fms-related TK 3
FMO	flavinmonooxidases
GBM	glioblastoma multiforme
GI	gastrointestinal
GIST	gastrointestinal stromal tumor
h	hour(s)
H	hepatic
HI	hepatic impairment
HTN	hypertension
IL-2	Interleukin 2
ILD	interstitial lung disease/pneumonitis
ind.	induce(r)
inh.	inhibit(or)
int.	interrupt
intol.	intolerant or intolerance
Itk	IL-2-inducible T-cell kinase
JAK	Janus kinase
KIT = C-KIT	v-kit Hardy-Zuckerman 4 feline sarcoma viral oncogene homolog
Lck	lymphocyte-specific protein TK
LVEF	left ventricular ejection fraction
MDD	myelodysplastic disorder
met.	metastatic
min	minute(s)
MMAE	monomethyl auristatin E
mod.	moderate
mTOR	mechanistic target of rapamycin (serine/threonine kinase)
NHL	non-Hodgkin lymphoma
NSAIDs	non-steroidal anti-inflammatory drugs
NSCLC	non-small cell lung cancer
NSNSCLC	non-squamous non-small cell lung cancer
PDGFR	platelet-derived growth factor receptor
pers.	persistent
Ph+	Philadelphia chromosome-positive
PML	progressive multifocal leukoencephalopathy
PNP	polyneuropathy
PPIs	proton pump inhibitors
progr.	progressive
Raf-1	v-raf-leukemia viral oncogene 1
RCC	renal cell carcinoma

Re	renal		Th	therapy, therapies
recurrent	rec.		TK	tyrosine kinase
red.	reduce		TLS	tumor lysis syndrome
ref.	refractory		TSS	tuberous sclerosis syndrome
rel.	relapsed		uc	unchanged
RES	reticuloendothelial system		ULN	upper limit of normal
RET	ret proto-oncogene		unresec.	unresectable
RI	renal impairment		VEGF	vascular endothelial growth factor
sev.	severe		VEGFR	vascular endothelial growth factor receptor
Sz	seizures			

[a]Generally consider treatment interruption/dose reduction/discontinuation of treatment if high grade adverse effects and toxicities occur.

*Medications that are metabolized by CYP enzymes may require dose adjustment based on the interaction with other medications that lead to inhibition or induction of CYP enzymes.

#severe toxicity: consider high variability in toxicity may be related to extent to which it was investigated for each drug. Listed are severe toxicities, BBW and adverse effects that were observed at high and supratherapeutic doses.

CYP inhibitors include erythromycin, clarithromycin, itraconazole, ketoconazole, voriconazole, nefazodone, nelfinavir, ritonavir, grapefruit juice, mifepristone.

CYP inducers include rifampin, St. John's wort, phenytoin, phenobarbital, dexamethasone, carbamazepine, rifabutin, rifapentine.

Medications that are metabolized by CYP include warfarin, domperidone, pimozide, fentanzyl, clozapine, ergotamine, dihydroergotamine, simvastatin, alfentanol, tacrolimus, cyclosporine, sirolimus, nimodipine, quinidine, alfuzosin, ivacaftor.

[1]Limited to hematologic/oncologic indications.

Bibliography

Apperley JF, Cortes JE, Kim DW, et al. Dasatinib in the treatment of chronic myeloid leukemia in accelerated phase after imatinib failure: the START a trial. *J Clin Oncol.* 2009; 27(21):3472–3479.

Azzoli CG, Temin S, Aliff T, et al. 2011 Focused Update of 2009 American Society of Clinical Oncology Clinical Practice Guideline Update on Chemotherapy for Stage IV Non–Small-Cell Lung Cancer. *J Clin Oncol.* 2011.

Bang YJ, Van Cutsem E, Feyereislova A, et al. Trastuzumab in combination with chemotherapy versus chemotherapy alone for treatment of HER2-positive advanced gastric or gastro-oesophageal junction cancer (ToGA): a phase 3, open-label, randomised controlled trial. *Lancet.* 2010; 376(9742):687–697.

Baselga J, Cortes J, Kim SB, et al. Pertuzumab plus trastuzumab plus docetaxel for metastatic breast cancer. *N Engl J Med.* 2012; 366(2):109–119.

Baselga J, Tripathy D, Mendelsohn J, et al. Phase II study of weekly intravenous recombinant humanized anti-p185(HER2) monoclonal antibody in patients with HER/neu-overexpressing metastatic breast cancer. *J Clin Oncol.* 1996; 14:737–744.

(continued)

Blanke CD, Rankin C, Demetri GD, et al. Phase III randomized, intergroup trial assessing imatinib mesylate at two dose levels in patients with unresectable or metastatic gastrointestinal stromal tumors expressing the KIT receptor TK: S0033. *J Clin Oncol.* 2008; 26(4):626–632.

Bonner JA, Harari PM, Giralt J, et al. Radiotherapy plus cetuximab for squamous-cell carcinoma of the head and neck. *N Engl J Med.* 2006; 354(6):567–578.

Burtness B, Goldwasser MA, Flood W, et al. Phase III randomized trial of cisplatin plus placebo compared with cisplatin plus cetuximab in metastatic/recurrent head and neck cancer: an Eastern Cooperative Oncology Group study. *J Clin Oncol.* 2005; 23(34):8646–8654.

Cameron D, Casey M, Oliva C, et al. Lapatinib plus capecitabine in women with HER2-positive advanced breast cancer: final survival analysis of a phase III randomized trial. *The Oncologist.* 2010; 15(9): 924–934.

Chapman PB, Hauschild A, Robert C, et al. Improved survival with vemurafenib in melanoma with BRAF V600E mutation. *N Engl J Med.* 2011; 364(26):2507–2516.

Coiffier B, Pro B, Prince HM, et al. Results from a pivotal, open-label, phase II study of romidepsin in relapsed or refractory peripheral T-cell lymphoma after prior systemic therapy. *J Clin Oncol.* 2012; 30(6):631–636.

Cortes J, Rousselot P, Kim DW, et al. Dasatinib induces complete hematologic and cytogenetic responses in patients with imatinib-resistant or -intolerant chronic myeloid leukemia in blast crisis. *Blood.* 2007; 109(8):3207–3213.

Crino L, Dansin E, Garrido P, et al. Safety and efficacy of first-line bevacizumab-based therapy in advanced non-squamous non-small-cell lung cancer (SAiL, MO19390): a phase 4 study. *Lancet Oncol.* 2010; 11(8):733–740.

DeMatteo RP, Ballman KV, Antonescu CR, et al. Adjuvant imatinib mesylate after resection of localised, primary gastrointestinal stromal tumour: a randomised, double-blind, placebo-controlled trial. *Lancet.* 2009; 373(9669):1097–1104.

Demetri GD, VanOosterom AT, Garrett CR, et al. Efficacy and safety of sunitinib in patients with advanced gastrointestinal stromal tumour after failure of imatinib: a randomised controlled trial. *Lancet.* 2006; 368:1329–1338.

Druker BJ, Guilhot F, O'Brien SG, et al. Five-year follow-up of patients receiving imatinib for chronic myeloid leukemia. *N Engl J Med.* 2006; 355(23):2408–2417.

Druker BJ, Sawyers CL, Kantarian H, et al. Activity of a specific inhibitor of the BCR-ABL TK in the blast crisis of chroni myeloid leukemia and acute lymphoblastic leukemia with the Philadelphia chromosome. *N Engl J Med.* 344(14):1038–1042.

Druker BJ, Talpaz M, Resta DJ, et al. Efficacy and safety of a specific inhibitor of the BCR-ABL TK in chronic myeloid leukemia. *N Engl J Med.* 344(14):1031–1037.

Duvic M, Talpur R, Ni X, et al. Phase II Trial of Oral Vorinostat (Suberoylanilide Hydroxamic Acid, SAHA) for Refractory Cutaneous T-cell Lymphoma (CTCL). *Blood.* 2006.

Escudier B, Bellmunt J, Negrier S, et al. Phase III trial of bevacizumab plus interferon alfa-2a in patients with metastatic renal cell carcinoma (AVOREN): final analysis of overall survival. *J Clin Oncol.* 2010; 28(13):2144–2150.

Foon KA, Boyiadzis M, Land SR, et al. Chemoimmunotherapy with low-dose fludarabine and cyclophosphamide and high dose rituximab in previously untreated patients with chronic lymphocytic leukemia. *J Clin Oncol.* 2009; 27(4):498–503.

Friedman HS, Prados MD, Wen PY, et al. Bevacizumab alone and in combination with irinotecan in recurrent glioblastoma. *J Clin Oncol.* 2009; 27(28):4733–4740.

Habermann TM, Weller EA, Morrison VA, et al. Rituximab-CHOP versus CHOP alone or with maintenance rituximab in older patients with diffuse large B-cell lymphoma. *J Clin Oncol.* 2006; 24(19): 3121–3127.

Hallek M, Fischer K, Fingerle-Rowson G, et al. Addition of rituximab to fludarabine and cyclophosphamide in patients with chronic lymphocytic leukemia: a randomised, open-label, phase 3 trial. *Lancet.* 2010; 376(9747):1164–1174.

Hillmen P, Skotnicki AB, Robak T, et al. Alemtuzumab compared with chlorambucil as first-line therapy for chronic lymphocytic leukemia. *J Clin Oncol.* 2007; Epub.

Hochster H, Weller E, Gascoyne RD, et al. Maintenance rituximab after cyclophosphamide, vincristine, and prednisone prolongs progression-free survival in advanced indolent lymphoma: results of the randomized phase III ECOG1496 Study. *J Clin Oncol.* 2009; 27(10):1607–1614.

Hodi FS, O'Day SJ, McDermott DF, et al. Improved survival with ipilimumab in patients with metastatic melanoma. *N Engl J Med.* 2010; 363(8):711–723.

Hudes G, Carducci M, Tomczak P, et al. Temsirolimus, interferon alfa, or both for advanced renal-cell carcinoma. *N Engl J Med.* 2007; 356(22):2271–2281.

Hurwitz H, Fehrenbacher L, Novotny W, et al. Bevacizumab plus irinotecan, fluorouracil, and leucovorin for metastatic colorectal cancer. *N Engl J Med.* 2004; 350(23):2335–2342.

Johnston S, Pippen J, Pivot X, et al. Lapatinib combined with letrozole versus letrozole and placebo as first-line therapy for postmenopausal hormone receptor-positive metastatic breast cancer. *J Clin Oncol.* 2009; 27(33):5538–5546.

Jonasch E, Corn P, Pagliaro LC, et al. Upfront, randomized, phase 2 trial of sorafenib versus sorafenib and low-dose interferon alfa in patients with advanced renal cell carcinoma: clinical and biomarker analysis. *Cancer.* 2010; 116(1):57–65.

Jonker DJ: Randomized phase III trial of cetuximab monotherapy plus best supportive care (BSC) versus BSC alone in patients with pretreated metastatic epidermal growth factor receptor (EGFR)-positive colorectal carcinoma: a trial of the National Cancer Institute of Canada Clinical Trials Group (NCIC CTG) and the Australasian Gastro-Intestinal Trials Group (AGITG). *Cancer Res.* 2007.

Kaminski MS, Zelenetz AD, Press OW, et al. Pivotal study of iodine I-131 tositumomab for chemotherapy-refractory low-grade or transformed low-grade B-cell non-Hodgkin's lymphomas. *J Clin Oncol.* 2001; 19(19):3918–3928.

Kantarjian H, Sawyers C, Hochhaus A, et al. Hematologic and cytogenetic responses to imatinib mesylate in chronic myelogenous leukemia. *N Engl J Med.* 2002; 346:645–652.

Kantarjian H, Shah NP, Hochhaus A, et al. Dasatinib versus imatinib in newly diagnosed chronic-phase chronic myeloid leukemia. *N Engl J Med.* 2010; 362(24):2260–2270.

Kantarjian HM, Giles F, Gattermann N, et al. Nilotinib (formerly AMN107), a highly selective BCR-ABL TK inhibitor, is effective in patients with Philadelphia chromosome-positive chronic myelogenous leukemia in chronic phase following imatinib resistance and intolerance. *Blood.* 2007; 110(10):3540–3546.

Keating MJ, O'Brien S, Albitar M, et al. Early results of a chemoimmunotherapy regimen of fludarabine, cyclophosphamide, and rituximab as initial therapy for chronic lymphocytic leukemia. *J Clin Oncol.* 2005; 23(18):4079–4088.

Kreis TN, Kim L, Moore K, et al. Phase II trial of single-agent bevacizumab followed by bevacizumab plus irinotecan at tumor progression in recurrent glioblastoma. *J Clin Oncol.* 2009; 27(5):740–745.

Krueger DA, Care MM, Holland K, et al. Everolimus for subependymal giant-cell astrocytomas in tuberous sclerosis. *N Engl J Med.* 2010; 363(19):1801–1811.

le Coutre PD, Giles FJ, Hochhaus A, et al. Nilotinib in patients with Ph+ chronic myeloid leukemia in accelerated phase following imatinib resistance or intolerance: 24-month follow-up results. *Leukemia.* 2011.

Lenz HJ, VanCutsem E, Khambata-Ford S, et al. Multicenter phase II and translational study of cetuximab in metastatic colorectal carcinoma refractory to irinotecan, oxaliplatin, and fluoropyrimidines. *J Clin Oncol.* 2006; 24(30):4914–4921.

Llovet JM, Ricci S, Mazzaferro V, et al. Sorafenib in advanced hepatocellular carcinoma. *N Engl J Med.* 2008; 359(4):378–390.

Marcus R, Imrie K, Solal-Celigny P, et al. Phase III study of R-CVP compared with cyclophosphamide, vincristine, and prednisone alone in patients with previously untreated advanced follicular lymphoma. *J Clin Oncol.* 2008; 26(28):4579–4586.

Margolin K, Ernstoff MS, Hamid O, et al. Ipilimumab in patients with melanoma and brain metastases: an open-label, phase 2 trial. *Lancet Oncol.* 2012; Epub.

(continued)

115

Moore MJ, Goldstein D, Hamm J, et al. Erlotinib plus gemcitabine compared with gemcitabine alone in patients with advanced pancreatic cancer: a phase III trial of the National Cancer Institute of Canada Clinical Trials Group. *J Clin Oncol.* 2007; 25(15):1960–1966.

Morschhauser F, Radford J, Van Hoof A, et al. Phase III trial of consolidation therapy with yttrium-90-ibritumomab tiuxetan compared with no additional therapy after first remission in advanced follicular lymphoma. *J Clin Oncol.* 2008; 26(32):5156–5164.

Motzer RJ, Escudier B, Oudard S, et al. Efficacy of everolimus in advanced renal cell carcinoma: a double-blind, randomised, placebo-controlled phase III trial. *Lancet.* 2008; 372(9637):449–456.

Motzer RJ, Hutson TE, Tomczak P, et al. Sunitinib versus interferon alfa in metastatic renal-cell carcinoma. *N Engl J Med.* 2007; 356(2):115–124.

O'Brien SG, Guilhot F, Larson RA, et al. Imatinib compared with interferon and low-dose cytarabine for newly diagnosed chronic-phase myeloid leukemia. *N Engl J Med.* 2003; 348(11):994–1004.

Olsen E, Duvic M, Frankel A, et al. Pivotal phase III trial of two dose levels of denileukin diftitox for the treatment of cutaneous T-cell lymphoma. *J Clin Oncol.* 2001; 19(2):376–388.

Osterborg A, Dyer MJS, Bunjes D, et al. Phase II multicenter study of human CD52 antibody in previously treated chronic lymphocytic leukemia. *J Clin Oncol.* 1997a; 15(4):1567–1574.

Ottmann O, Dombret H, Martinelli G, et al. Dasatinib induces rapid hematologic and cytogenetic responses in adult patients with Philadelphia chromosome positive acute lymphoblastic leukemia with resistance or intolerance to imatinib: interim results of a phase 2 study. *Blood.* 2007; 110(7):2309–2315.

Pegram MD, Lipton A, Hayes DF, et al. Phase II study of receptor-enhanced chemosensitivity using recombinant humanized anti-p185(HER2/neu) monoclonal antibody plus cisplatin in patients with HER2/neu-overexpressing metastatic breast cancer refractory to chemotherapy treatment. *J Clin Oncol.* 1998; 16:2659–2671.

Pfreundschuh M, Trumper L, Osterborg A, et al. CHOP-like chemotherapy plus rituximab versus CHOP-like chemotherapy alone in young patients with good-prognosis diffuse large-B-cell lymphoma: a randomised controlled trial by the MabThera International Trial (MInT) Group. *Lancet Oncol.* 2006; 7(5):379–391.

Piccart-Gebhart MJ, Procter M, Leyland-Jones B, et al. Trastuzumab after adjuvant chemotherapy in HER2-positive breast cancer. *N Engl J Med.* 2005; 353(16):1659–1672.

Piekarz RL, Frye R, Turner M, et al. Phase II multi-institutional trial of the histone deacetylase inhibitor romidepsin as monotherapy for patients with cutaneous T-cell lymphoma. *J Clin Oncol.* 2009.

Press OW, Eary JF, Appelbaum FR, et al. Phase II trial of 131I-B1 (anti-CD20) antibody therapy with autologous stem cell transplantation for relapsed B cell lymphomas. *Lancet.* 1995; 346:336–340.

Product Information: ADCETRIS(TM) IV injection, brentuximab vedotin IV injection. Seattle Genetics, Inc. (per FDA), Bothell, WA, 2011.

Product Information: GLEEVEC(R) oral tablets, imatinib mesylate oral tablets. Novartis Pharmaceuticals Corporation, East Hanover, NJ, 2011.

Product Information: Herceptin(R), trastuzumab. Genentech, Inc., South San Francisco, CA, 2003.

Raymond E, Dahan L, Raoul JL, et al. Sunitinib malate for the treatment of pancreatic neuroendocrine tumors. *N Engl J Med.* 2011; 364(6):501–513.

Rini BI, Escudier B, Tomczak P, et al. Comparative effectiveness of axitinib versus sorafenib in advanced renal cell carcinoma (AXIS): a randomised phase 3 trial. *Lancet.* 2011; 378(9807):1931–1939.

Rini BI, Halabi S, Rosenberg JE, et al. Phase III trial of bevacizumab plus interferon alfa versus interferon alfa monotherapy in patients with metastatic renal cell carcinoma: final results of CALGB 90206. *J Clin Oncol.* 2010; 28(13):2137–2143.

Robak T, Dmoszynska A, Solal-Celigny P, et al. Rituximab plus fludarabine and cyclophosphamide prolongs progression-free survival compared with fludarabine and cyclophosphamide alone in previously treated chronic lymphocytic leukemia. *J Clin Oncol.* 2010; 28(10):1756–1765.

Robert C, Thomas L, Bondarenko I, et al. Ipilimumab plus dacarbazine for previously untreated metastatic melanoma. *N Engl J Med.* 2011; 364(26):2517–2526.

Rutkowski P, Van Glabbeke M, Rankin CJ, et al. Imatinib mesylate in advanced dermatofibrosarcoma protuberans: pooled analysis of two phase II clinical trials. *J Clin Oncol.* 2010; 28(10):1772–1779.

Saglio G, Kim DW, Issaragrisil S, et al. Nilotinib versus imatinib for newly diagnosed chronic myeloid leukemia. *N Engl J Med.* 2010; 362(24):2251–2259.

Salles G, Seymour JF, Offner F, et al. Rituximab maintenance for 2 years in patients with high tumour burden follicular lymphoma responding to rituximab plus chemotherapy (PRIMA): a phase 3, randomised controlled trial. *Lancet.* 2011; 377(9759):42–51.

Saltz LB, Clarke S, az-Rubio E, et al. Bevacizumab in combination with oxaliplatin-based chemotherapy as first-line therapy in metastatic colorectal cancer: a randomized phase III study. *J Clin Oncol.* 2008; 26(12):2013–2019.

Sandler A, Gray R, Perry MC, et al. Paclitaxel-carboplatin alone or with bevacizumab for non-small-cell lung cancer. *N Engl J Med.* 2006; 355(24):2542–2550.

SanMiguel JF, Schlag R, Khuageva NK, et al. Bortezomib plus melphalan and prednisone for initial treatment of multiple myeloma. *N Engl J Med.* 2008; 359(9):906–917.

Shah NP, Kantarjian HM, Kim DW, et al. Intermittent target inhibition with dasatinib 100 mg once daily preserves efficacy and improves tolerability in imatinib-resistant and -intolerant chronic-phase chronic myeloid leukemia. *J Clin Oncol.* 2008; 26(19):3204–3212.

Shaw AT, Yeap BY, Solomon BJ, et al. Effect of crizotinib on overall survival in patients with advanced non-small-cell lung cancer harbouring ALK gene rearrangement: a retrospective analysis. *Lancet Oncol.* 2011; 12(11):1004–1012.

Slamon D, Eiermann W, Robert N, et al. Adjuvant trastuzumab in HER2-positive breast cancer. *N Engl J Med.* 2011; 365(14):1273–1283.

Sosman JA, Kim KB, Schuchter L, et al. Survival in BRAF V600-mutant advanced melanoma treated with vemurafenib. *N Engl J Med.* 2012; 366(8):707–714.

Sternberg CN, Davis ID, Mardiak J, et al. Pazopanib in locally advanced or metastatic renal cell carcinoma: results of a randomized phase III trial. *J Clin Oncol.* 2010; 28(6):1061–1068.

van Oers MH, Klasa R, Marcus RE, et al. Rituximab maintenance improves clinical outcome of relapsed/resistant follicular non-Hodgkin lymphoma in patients both with and without rituximab during induction: results of a prospective randomized phase 3 intergroup trial. *Blood.* 2006; 108(10):3295–3301.

van Oers MH, Van Glabbeke M, Giurgea L, et al. Rituximab maintenance treatment of relapsed/resistant follicular non-Hodgkin's lymphoma: long-term outcome of the EORTC 20981 phase III randomized intergroup study. *J Clin Oncol.* 2010; 28(17):2853–2858.

VanCutsem E, Peeters M, Siena S, et al. Open-label phase III trial of panitumumab plus best supportive care compared with best supportive care alone in patients with chemotherapy-refractory metastatic colorectal cancer. *J Clin Oncol.* 2007; 25(13):1658–1664.

Vermorken JB, Mesia R, Rivera F, et al. Platinum-based chemotherapy plus cetuximab in head and neck cancer. *N Engl J Med.* 2008; 359(11):1116–1127.

Verstovsek S, Mesa RA, Gotlib J, et al. A double-blind, placebo-controlled trial of ruxolitinib for myelofibrosis. *N Engl J Med.* 2012; 366(9):799–807.

Verweij J, Casali PG, Zalcberg J, et al. Progression-free survival in gastrointestinal stromal tumours with high-dose imatinib: randomised trial. *Lancet.* 2004; 364:1127–1134.

Vredenburgh JJ, Desjardins A, Herndon JE, et al. Bevacizumab plus irinotecan in recurrent glioblastoma multiforme. *J Clin Oncol.* 2007; 25(30):4722–4729.

Wierda WG, Kipps TJ, Mayer J, et al. Ofatumumab as single-agent CD20 immunotherapy in fludarabine-refractory chronic lymphocytic leukemia. *J Clin Oncol.* 2010; 28(10):1749–1755.

Wilke H, Glynne-Jones R, Thaler J, et al. Cetuximab plus irinotecan in heavily pretreated metastatic colorectal cancer progressing on irinotecan: MABEL Study. *J Clin Oncol.* 2008; 26(33):5335–5343.

Wiseman GA, Gordon LI, Multani PS et al. Ibritumomab tiuxetan radioimmunotherapy for patients with relapsed or refractory non-Hodgkin lymphoma and mild thrombocytopenia: a phase II multicenter trial. *Blood.* 2002; 99(12):4336–4342.

Wolchok JD, Neyns B, Linette G, et al. Ipilimumab monotherapy in patients with pretreated advanced melanoma: a randomised, double-blind, multicentre, phase 2, dose-ranging study. *Lancet Oncol.* 2010; 11(2):155–164.

Yao JC, Shah MH, Ito T, et al. Everolimus for advanced pancreatic neuroendocrine tumors. *N Engl J Med.* 2011; 364(6):514–523.

■ MUTATIONS AND IMPLICATIONS OF "DRIVER GENES" IN CANCER CELLS

Certain mutations in cancer cells, particularly those that activate cell receptor tyrosine kinases or downstream proteins involved in signaling within cells, can provide the primary stimulus for cell proliferation and survival. Examples of mutations or translocations in receptors leading to uncontrolled cancer cell proliferation include *C-KIT* mutations in gastrointestinal stromal tumors (GIST), and EGFR mutations or *EML-4/ALK* translocations in subsets of non-small cell lung cancer (NSCLC), primarily with adenocarcinoma histology. Mutations of genes in intracellular signal transduction pathways can also become drivers for malignant cell growth or survival. The prototypic example of this is the *BCR-ABL* translocation in chronic myelogenous leukemia (CML). Another cogent example is the constitutive activation of B-RAF, a protein in the RAS-RAF-MEK pathway, by mutation in melanoma (3, 4). These mutations create "addiction" to the continuous signaling, so that when signaling is blocked, the cancer cells die. In experimental settings, siRNAs directed against these mutant genes turn off the survival signals and lead to cell death, while small molecular inhibitors of the offending kinase cause tumor cell death (3, 4, 8, 9) in human subjects. The first agent to target the RAS-RAF-MEK pathway in human cancer is vemurafenib, which inhibits the V600E mutant form of the B-RAF kinase in melanoma (3, 8, 9). Interestingly, activating mutations of *B-RAF* are also found in colon, lung, and a number of other cancers, although these mutations have not been as responsive to vemurafenib as melanomas, indicating that the cellular context matters. Inhibitors of PI-3 kinase and its downstream signaling partner mTOR have led to beneficial treatment of renal cancers and neuroendocrine tumors (4). Multiple agents specific for isoenzymes of PI-3 kinase itself are undergoing evaluation in breast cancer, lymphoma, and endometrial cancer.

Mutations in tumor suppressor genes such as p53, retinoblastoma (RB), or the phosphate and tensin homolog (PTEN) that regulates the PI-3 kinase pathway can produce loss of important brakes on proliferation and enhance cell survival, leading to transformation of normal cells as well as contributing to the prolonged survival of cancer cells. These changes have proved harder to target because it is more difficult to return normal function to a protein than to inhibit aberrant function. However, new approaches are being explored aimed at indirectly reversing adverse effects of suppressor gene mutations such as by modulating downstream effectors of the mutant proteins or by targeting epigenetic factors or miRNAs important in control of functions of the tumor suppressor gene (10).

In the following, we discuss several specific examples of clinically effective targeted therapies.

1. *Inhibitors of growth factor receptors or their ligands.* Growth factor receptors and their ligands are overexpressed or amplified in many epithelial malignancies and are mutated in others (2, 3, 6-8). They are essential for promoting proliferation, survival, and metastasis of various kinds of cancer. The expression of mutated receptors on the cell surface and the presence of their ligands in the circulation make these altered pathways

accessible to monoclonal antibodies. Examples of growth factors and receptors currently being effectively targeted include the following:

- *EGFR family, including HER1 (EGFR), HER2, and HER3.* EGFRs are present on normal epithelium and overexpressed in many cancers and mutated in a subset of NSCLC. The majority of NSCLC with mutated *EGFR* respond to anti-EGFR therapy, either drugs or antibodies. Anti-EGFR therapy with antibodies has also proved useful in colorectal and head and neck cancers in which the *EGFR* is not mutated. Amplified and overexpressed *HER2* is a major target for a subset of breast and gastric cancers.

- *ALK:* Activating translocations were originally identified in anaplastic large cell lymphoma. Subsequently the mutated and translocated receptor was shown to respond to crizotinib in a subset of NSCLC adenocarcinomas as well as in patients with inflammatory myofibroblastic sarcoma. Activating mutations of *ALK* are also present in a subset of patients with neuroblastoma. A closely related receptor, ROS1 kinase, is translocated in a small subset of NSCLC and is susceptible to inhibition by crizotinib.

    C-KIT mutations are frequently found in GIST tumors and uncommonly in several other neoplasms, including mucosal melanomas and mast cell disease.

- *VEGF/VEGFR:* These play an important role in tumor-associated angiogenesis for many epithelial and mesenchymal tumors, and for primary brain tumors.

    Various strategies have been employed to inhibit function of these receptor pathways. Responses are well documented in patients treated with mAbs to HER2 (e.g., trastuzumab) or EGFR (e.g., cetuximab), and small-molecular-weight inhibitors (e.g., erlotinib for EGFR mutated NSCLC) (2, 3, 6). Bevacizimab, a monoclonal antibody directed against VEGF, is effective either alone for the treatment of renal cell cancer (RCC) or glioblastomas or combined with chemotherapy for colorectal or lung cancer (7). Small molecular inhibitors (such as axitinib or pazopanib) of VEGFRs have also proved effective in RCC (7) and in treating soft tissue sarcomas, while numerous small-molecular-weight drugs effectively block receptor tyrosine kinases.

2. *Inhibitors of signal transduction.* A number of signaling pathways downstream of growth factor receptors transmit aberrant growth signals and play essential roles in malignancies. These include the RAS-RAF-MEK pathway, the PI-3 kinase pathway, and the NF-κB pathway. Targeting of mTOR (in the PI-3 kinase pathway) is useful in treating renal cancer, breast cancer, and neuroendocrine tumors of gastrointestinal origin. PI-3 kinase inhibitors, some with broad activity against multiple PI3K isoenzymes while others that are specific for specific isoenzyme, are in active clinical development. Inhibitors of the mutated JAK2 oncoprotein, an important signal mediator in myeloid malignancies, are effective in myeloid metaplasia and other myeloproliferative diseases.

3. *Inhibitors of cell cycle control.* Many of the currently available cytotoxic agents inhibit DNA synthesis, and cell division, but display limited

specificity for cancer. Approaches targeting specific overexpressed or otherwise aberrant cyclin-dependent kinases and other cell cycle regulatory proteins are currently being evaluated based on better understanding of the roles that these play in specific malignant cells.

4. *Promoters of apoptosis.* Apoptosis, or cell death, is dependent on the balance of activity of pro- and anti-apoptotic proteins. This balance is shifted in favor of anti-apoptotic proteins in many neoplastic cells, as for example the BCL-2 protein activated in follicular lymphoma. Inhibitors of the BH3 family of anti-apoptotic proteins have demonstrated activity against chronic lymphocytic leukemia, and continue in clinical evaluation, alone, combined with other targeted agents, and in combinations with chemotherapy.

5. *Restoration of the function of tumor suppressor proteins.* Research continues on approaches aimed at restoring normal functions of these critical proteins (p53, p21) to cancer cells (5, 11). Since restoration of the function of the proteins themselves has so far proved intractable, most of the current emphasis is aimed at indirectly modulating this function (see above for further discussion).

7. *Inhibition of telomerase.* Although much has been learned about the role of telomerase in maintaining telomeres in neoplastic cells and thus allowing continued survival and proliferation, significant preclinical work is needed to translate this into a useful anticancer approach. The furthest along of the approaches directed at telomerase is a vaccine targeting a portion of the telomerase protein. This vaccine is currently being evaluated in a phase III trial in combination with chemotherapy for metastatic pancreatic cancer (12).

8. *Inhibitors of chromatin modifiers and epigenetic factors.* Methylation of DNA or histones, acetylation of histones, and production of micro-RNAs, and long noncoding RNAs all modify gene expression and differentiation in normal and malignant cells (5, 11). Examples of approved agents targeting epigenetic factors include the histone deacetylase inhibitors (vorinostat, romidepsin), which have activity against cutaneous T-cell lymphoma (CTCL), and inhibitors of DNA methylation (azacytidine) in myelodysplasia.

9. *Inhibitors of metabolism.* Abnormal dependence on glycolysis has long been known to be an important aspect of malignant cells. The past decade has revealed other dramatic metabolic differences in tumors, including enhanced utilization of glycine or glutamine and activation of a number of enzymes (e.g., IDH-1 and 2, DNA methyltransferase, altered pyruvate kinase). These and other metabolic processes have become targets for drug development (13).

While single specific targets may initiate malignant transformation, whole genome sequencing of tumors has revealed that most cancers contain multiple mutations. In most cases, the role of these additional mutations in drug resistance and survival is unknown. In addition there are important influences on tumor biology coming from the tumor microenvironment. Thus, targeting multiple genes and their protein products may be necessary in order to kill the heterogeneous clones of cells within any given cancer. Recent studies have confirmed the marked heterogeneity of mutations and other changes in different cells within the same malignancy (14). Thus, targeting multiple proteins or pathways, either through multitargeted single inhibitors, such as sunitinib, sorafenib, or regorafenib, or through combination strategies (the combination of B-RAF and MEK inhibitors in melanoma) (15), will likely be required to maximize antitumor efficacy. In addition, targeting the environment is also important, as demonstrated by activity of antiangiogenic agents (5, 7).

CURRENTLY APPROVED TARGETED AGENTS IN CANCER THERAPY (USA)
■ SMALL MOLECULES

Because they can easily be subjected to high throughput screening and readily modified to incorporate favorable pharmacologic properties, small molecules remain the most attractive and straightforward class of agents for targeted therapy (3, 4, 6-9). High-throughput screening against recombinant proteins allows identification of lead compounds with affinity for the specific target of interest. Subsequent preclinical evaluation, using crystallography and in vitro testing, and analogue chemistry, yields compounds of high target affinity and specificity, with favorable drug properties (e.g., oral bioavailability, extended plasma half-life, decreased toxicity). The major pharmacological properties of representative approved targeted small molecules (grouped by target) are discussed below and are summarized in Table 10-1, which provides information of targets, pharmacokinetics, toxicity, and drug interactions.

TARGET: BCR-ABL

Mechanism of action: The 9:22 translocation in CML places the ABL tyrosine kinase gene on chromosome 9 in juxtaposition to the breakpoint cluster region (BCR) of chromosome 22 with a resultant protein that has constitutive phosphorylating activity, activating multiple downstream signaling pathways and leading to enhanced cell proliferation and survival. Like most other kinase inhibitors, imatinib competes for the ATP binding site of its target protein leading to potent inhibition of the tyrosine kinase activity (8). It binds to the enzyme in the protein's inactive conformation and prevents its catalytic activity. Imatinib also potently inhibits C-KIT kinase, which is frequently mutated in GIST, and PDGFR-alpha, which is mutated in a smaller percentage of GIST tumors, but is also overexpressed in eosinophilic leukemia and hypereosinophilia (8). Resistance arises most commonly through one of several different mutations in the BCR-ABL protein (especially mutations that affect access to the ATP catalytic binding domain [e.g. T315I mutations, or so-called gatekeeper mutations] and those that hold the enzyme in an active configuration), leading to decreased drug binding.

Toxicity: Usually well tolerated. Potential toxicities include neutropenia, thrombocytopenia, anemia; hepatotoxicity (usually manifested by elevated liver enzymes but rarely severe); fluid retention/edema; musculoskeletal pains/cramps; rash; diarrhea; GI irritation; bleeding (GI tract or intratumoral); hypophosphatemia; and, rarely, congestive heart failure.

Pharmacokinetics: As is true for most tyrosine kinase inhibitors, imatinib is metabolized by hepatic CYP3A4. It is therefore important to monitor the dose when given with CYP3A4 inhibitors (e.g., itraconazole, erythromycin) or inducers (phenytoin, barbiturates) and alter dose as necessary. Its plasma $t_{1/2}$ is approximately 18 h. Doses should be reduced in patients with hepatic and renal dysfunction (see package insert).

Clinical indications:

1. Newly diagnosed PH+ chronic phase CML (cCML)
2. Myelodysplastic/myeloproliferative diseases (MDS/MPD) with *PDGFR* gene re-arrangements
3. Aggressive systemic mastocytosis (ASM) without the *D816V C-KIT* mutation or with unknown C-KIT mutational status
4. Hypereosinophilic syndrome (HES) and/or chronic eosinophilic leukemia (CEL)
5. Unresectable, recurrent and/or metastatic dermatofibrosarcoma protuberans (DFSP)
6. C-KIT+ unresectable and/or metastatic GIST

■ DASATINIB

Mechanism of action: In comparison to imatinib, dasatinib is a more potent inhibitor of the tyrosine kinase activity of BCR-ABL (8). It inhibits the active, or open, conformation of the enzyme. It also inhibits a number of other kinases, including *src* family members, C-KIT, EPHA 2, and PDGFR. In CML, resistance arises through the selection of cells with resistance point mutations in the BCR-ABL protein catalytic site (e.g., the T315I mutation), but is unaffected by the numerous possible mutations that hold the enzyme in an active configuration.

Toxicity: Similar to imatinib, including neutropenia, thrombocytopenia, anemia; hepatotoxicity (usually manifested by elevated liver enzymes); fluid retention/edema; musculoskeletal pains/cramps; headaches; fatigue; rash; diarrhea; GI bleeding; hypophosphatemia; and, rarely, congestive heart failure. It also can cause prolongation of the QT interval and should thus not be used in patients with hypokalemia, hypomagnesemia, or prolonged QTc syndrome.

Pharmacokinetics: Similar to imatinib, it is metabolized by CYP3A4. It is therefore important to monitor the dose when given with CYP3A4 inhibitors or inducers. Doses should be reduced in the presence of hepatic dysfunction.

Clinical effectiveness (CML): Dasatinib has activity against untreated CML but also produces clinical hematologic responses in many of the CML or PH+ ALL patients who have become resistant to imatinib therapy through mutation of binding to the ATP-catalytic site on the enzyme (8). The *BCR-ABL* kinase gene containing T315I mutations is resistant. FDA-approved indications are:

1. Newly diagnosed PH+ chronic phase, accelerated phase, or blastic crisis phase CML
2. PH+ ALL

■ NILOTINIB

Mechanism of action: Similar to dasatinib, nilotinib is a potent inhibitor of the active conformation of the tyrosine kinase activity of BCR-ABL (8). It is approximately 30 times more potent than imatinib in vitro and retains activity against most mutations except T315I.

Toxicity: Similar to imatinib and dasatinib, including neutropenia, thrombocytopenia, anemia; hepatotoxicity (elevated liver enzymes); fluid retention/edema; musculoskeletal pains/cramps; headaches; fatigue; rash; diarrhea; GI irritation; bleeding; hypophosphatemia; and, rarely, congestive heart failure. It also can cause prolongation of the QT interval, predisposing to ventricular arrhythmias, and should not be used in patients with hypokalemia, hypomagnesemia, or prolonged QTc syndrome.

Pharmacokinetics: It is metabolized by CYP3A4, with a plasma half-life of 17 h. It is therefore important to monitor the dose when given with CYP3A4 inhibitors and inducers. Dose modifications are recommended in patients with liver dysfunction.

Clinical effectiveness (CML): Nilotinib produces clinical hematologic responses in both untreated CML or PH+ ALL patients as well as many of those who have become resistant to imatinib therapy through mutations that affect imatinib binding to the ATP-catalytic site on the enzyme (8). Nilotinib is FDA approved for following indications:

1. PH+ cCML, AP-CML, BC-CML

■ BOSUTINIB

Mechanism of action: Similar to imatinib, dasatinib, and nilotinib, it is an effective inhibitor of BCR-ALB kinase. Bosutinib also exhibits strong activity against kinases of the SRC family, including SRC, Lyn, and HCK.

Pharmacokinetics: It is metabolized by CYP3A4. Use with CYP inducers or inhibitors should be avoided if possible and may require dose modification when their use is necessary. Its plasma $t_{1/2}$ is approximately 22.5 h.

Toxicity: Bosutinib can cause thrombocytopenia, anemia, neutropenia; hepatotoxicity; fluid retention and edema; gastrointestinal toxicities, including diarrhea, abdominal pain, nausea, vomiting; rash; and QT prolongation.

Clinical effectiveness: Bosutinib is indicated for the treatment of chronic, accelerated, or blast phase PH+ CML with resistance or intolerance to one or more TKIs, including imatinib, dasatinib, or nilotinib. It lacks activity against the T315I and V299L mutations in *BCR-ABL* that are among the mutations that confer resistance to imatinib.

■ PONATINIB

Mechanism of action: Similar to imatinib, dasatinib, nilotinib, and bosutinib, it is an effective inhibitor of the tyrosine kinase activity of BCR-ABL. In contrast, it contains a linker that allows it to retain activity against the T315I mutation, and against other mutations. Ponatinib also inhibits a number of other tyrosine kinases including fibroblast growth factor receptors 1-4, FLT-3, PDGFRA, and C-KIT.

Pharmacokinetics: Its plasma $t_{1/2}$ is approximately 24 h. It interacts with CYP3A4 and the dose needs to be modified when used with strong CYP3A4 inhibitors. It is also an inhibitor of the multidrug resistance transporter.

Toxicity: Ponatinib can cause thrombocytopenia, anemia, neutropenia; gastrointestinal toxicities, including pancreatitis, constipation, abdominal pain, nausea; rash, dry skin; fever; arthralgia; hypertension; fluid retention;

and headache. The most common potentially serious toxicities include hepatotoxicity and arterial thrombosis. Less common potentially serious toxicities include congestive heart failure, cardiac arrhythmias, venous thrombosis, and hemorrhage.

Clinical effectiveness: Ponatinib is indicated for the treatment of chronic, accelerated, or blast phase PH+ CML with resistance or intolerance to one or more TKIs, including imatinib, dasatinib, or nilotinib.

TARGET: EGFR FAMILY

■ ERLOTINIB

Mechanism of action: Erlotinib (Tarceva) is a potent specific inhibitor of the ATP-binding pocket of the EGFR (HER1) tyrosine kinase (6, 8). It targets the ATP binding site of the protein. Resistance arises by a number of mechanisms, including through selection of resistance mutations of the target protein (e.g., T790M, a gatekeeper mutation), by activation of alternate growth factor signaling pathways, especially the C-MET pathway, or by tumor conversion to a small cell cancer histology.

Pharmacokinetics: It has a plasma $t_{1/2}$ of approximately 17 h, is metabolized by CYP3A4 and other CYP enzymes, and requires dose modification when used with CYP inducers or inhibitors.

Toxicity: Rash, dermatitis, and pruritus in the majority of patients, diarrhea (although uncommonly severe), nausea, fatigue, uncommon bleeding or clotting, and, uncommonly, interstitial pneumonitis.

Clinical effectiveness: Erlotinib has its most potent single agent activity against NSCLC with activating mutations in the EGFR kinase domain. Specifically, erlotinib is indicated for:

1. EGFR mutant NSCLC
2. Maintenance treatment in locally advanced or metastatic NSCLC without progression after 4 cycles of platinum-based first-line chemotherapy
3. Locally advanced or metastatic NSCLC after failure of at least one prior chemotherapy regimen
4. In combination with gemcitabine in locally advanced, unresectable or metastatic pancreatic cancer

■ LAPATINIB

Mechanism of action: Lapatinib is a potent specific inhibitor of both the EGFR (ErbB1) and the HER2 (ErbB2) tyrosine kinases (6, 8). It targets the ATP binding sites of the proteins. Resistance arises by a number of mechanisms, including (but not limited to) selection of resistance mutations of the target protein or by activation of alternate signalling pathways (the PI-3 kinase pathway).

Pharmacokinetics: It has a plasma $t_{1/2}$ of approximately 24 h, is metabolized by CYP3A4 and other CYP enzymes, and requires dose modification when used with CYP inducers or inhibitors.

Toxicity: Common toxicities include rash, nausea/vomiting, diarrhea, fatigue, mucosal irritation, palmar-plantar erythrodysesthesia, and elevated liver function tests. Serious but uncommon toxicities include decreased left ventricular ejection fraction, hepatic toxicity, interstitial pneumonitis, severe diarrhea, and QTc prolongation.

Clinical effectiveness: Lapatinib is approved in combination with capecitabine for patients with HER2-amplified metastatic breast cancers that have progressed on prior therapies, or in combination with letrozole for postmenopausal women with hormone receptor positive breast cancers.

TARGET: ALK

■ CRIZOTINIB

Mechanism of action: Crizotinib (Xalkori) is a specific inhibitor of the ALK tyrosine kinase by targeting the ATP binding site (8). It also has significant activity against ROS1 and MET kinases. Similar to erlotinib (see above), resistance arises through a number of mechanisms including target gene amplification, induction of other growth factor receptor pathways, or selection of cells with resistance mutations in the gatekeeper mutations in the ATP-binding domain of the enzyme.

Pharmacokinetics: It is slowly metabolized by CYP3A4, and has a $t_{1/2}$ of approximately 50 h in plasma.

Toxicity: Nausea, vomiting, diarrhea, and visual changes (temporary changes in visual acuity: trailing lights seen in transitions between light and dark) are the most common and usually manageable side effects. Fatigue, edema, elevated liver function tests, neuropathy, dysgeusia, rash, development of renal cysts, and asthenia can be seen. Uncommon but potentially serious toxicities include liver function test elevations with hyperbilirubinemia, and rarely liver failure, and interstitial pneumonitis that can be life-threatening or fatal.

Clinical effectiveness: It has activity against approximately 3%-5% of NSCLC that have translocations of the *ALK* gene, most commonly with *EML4* as a partner (8, 9, 16). It also has potent clinical activity against NSCLC with *ROS1* translocations.

TARGET: JAK 2 KINASE

■ RUXOLITINIB

Mechanism of action: Ruxolitinib is a specific inhibitor of the JAK 1 and 2 tyrosine kinases by targeting the ATP binding site.

Pharmacokinetics: It has a short $t_{1/2}$ of approximately 2-3 h.

Toxicity: Bruising, dizziness, headache, elevated LFTs, anemia, thrombocytopenia, and leukopenia. All of these toxicities tended to be mild and controllable.

Clinical effectiveness: It is approved for the treatment of myelofibrosis, in which it decreases spleen size and relieves symptoms, and is under investigation for other myeloproliferative syndromes.

TARGET: HEDGEHOG PATHWAY

■ VISMODEGIB

Mechanism of action: Vismodegib is an inhibitor of smoothened, a transmembrane protein in the sonic hedgehog (SHH) pathway. Basal cell carcinoma is associated with activation of the SHH pathway through smoothed activation.

Pharmacokinetics: It has a plasma $t_{1/2}$ of approximately 4 days. Although it interacts with CYP enzymes, it doses do not need to be altered in presence of CYP3A4 inhibitors. It is an inhibitor of the multidrug resistance exporter.

Toxicity: Common toxicities include diarrhea, constipation, nausea/vomiting, mucosal irritation, altered taste, decreased appetite, weight loss, fatigue, muscle spasms, arthralgias, alopecia, amenorrhea, lower levels of potassium/sodium, and elevated creatinine.

Clinical effectiveness: It is approved for metastatic or surgically unresectable basal cell carcinomas that are not candidates for radiation therapy.

TARGET: VEGFR AND OTHER KINASES

■ SORAFENIB

Mechanism of action: Sorafenib is an orally available multitargeted kinase inhibitor, with activity against RAF (C-RAF and B-RAF) kinases, VEGFR-2, VEGFR-3, PDGFR-beta, FLT3, and C-KIT (8). Its activity against the VEGF receptors is believed to be primarily responsible for its clinical activity against renal and hepatic cancers. Determinants of resistance are not known.

Pharmacokinetics: It is metabolized by CYP3A4 and by UGT 1A9 and has a plasma $t_{1/2}$ of approximately 24-48 h. Doses should be modified in the presence of inducers or inhibitors of CYP enzymes.

Toxicity: Rash, hand-foot syndrome, hypertension, diarrhea, elevated amylase/lipase (usually without clinical pancreatitis), alopecia, myalgias, arthralgias, mild bone marrow suppression, and uncommonly bleeding or clotting.

Clinical effectiveness: Sorafenib is indicated for patients with unresectable hepatocellular carcinoma and advanced renal cell cancers.

■ REGORAFENIB

Mechanism of action: Regorafinib is an inhibitor of multiple kinases (similar to sorafenib to which it is closely related structurally), including VEGFR-1-3, KIT, PDGFR-alpha and beta (B-RAF and C-RAF), FGFR1/2, and others. As is the case for sorafenib, its most relevant antitumor activity is believed to be related to its antiangiogenic effects.

Pharmacokinetics: It is metabolized by CYP3A4 and has a $t_{1/2}$ of approximately 28 h. It is subject to drug interactions with inducers/inhibitors of the CYP system and requires dose modification in their presence.

Toxicity: Hepatotoxicity (rarely fatal, LFTs should be monitored frequently), hemorrhage, gastrointestinal perforation, asthenia, fatigue, pain, fever, anorexia, rash, diarrhea, mucositis, dysphonia, headache, infection, weight loss, hypertension.

Clinical effectiveness: Regorafenib is indicated for the treatment of metastatic colorectal cancer in patient who failed all other standard treatment with fluoropyrimidine-, oxaliplatin-, and irinotecan-based chemotherapy, and targeted therapy, including an anti-VEGF/VEGFR therapy and, in KRAS wild-type disease, after failure of anti-EGFR therapy (8).

■ SUNITINIB

Mechanism of action: Sunitinib is an orally available small-molecular-weight inhibitor of multiple kinases including the tyrosine kinase activity of the VEGFR-2, PDGFR, and C-KIT receptors (8). In the treatment of GIST, resistance is related to emergence of mutations in the *C-KIT* gene.

Pharmacokinetics: It is metabolized by CYP3A4, with a plasma $t_{1/2}$ of approximately 40-60 h, and doses must be modified in the presence of inducers or inhibitors of CYP3A4.

Toxicity: Cytopenias, bleeding, skin discoloration, diarrhea, mucocutaneous inflammation, altered taste, asthenia, left ventricular dysfunction (uncommon), GI perforation (rare), and pancreatitis (rare).

Clinical effectiveness: It has shown sufficient activity to be approved for treatment of GIST (either intolerant of or after progression on imatinib), advanced RCC, and unresectable or metastatic peripheral neuroendocrine tumors (PNET).

■ CABOZANTINIB

Mechanism of action: Cabozantinib is an inhibitor of multiple kinases including the tyrosine kinase activity of the VEGFR-2, MET, and RET receptors. These receptors are involved in a number of cellular processes critical for tumor growth or maintenance, including tumor cell proliferation, invasion, angiogenesis, and maintenance of the tumor microenvironment.

Pharmacokinetics: It is metabolized by CYP3A4, with a plasma $t_{1/2}$ of approximately 91 h, and doses must be modified in the presence of inducers or inhibitors of CYP3A4.

Toxicity: Common toxicities include diarrhea, constipation, mucocutaneous inflammation, nausea/vomiting, altered taste, decreased appetite, abdominal pain, fatigue, asthenia, hypertension, elevated transaminases and bilirubin, lower levels of calcium/phosphorous/magnesium/potassium/sodium, palmar-plantar erythrodysesthesia syndrome, changes in hair color or skin pigmentation, and rash. Rare but potentially serious toxicities include visceral perforation or fistula formation, altered wound healing, hemorrhage, arterial thrombosis, nephritic syndrome, osteonecrosis of the jaw, and reversible posterior leukoencephalopathy syndrome.

Clinical effectiveness: It is approved for treatment of medullary thyroid cancer (MCT). It is actively being evaluated for efficacy against a number of other malignancies including metastatic prostate cancer.

■ PAZOPANIB

Mechanism of action: Pazobanib is an inhibitor of multiple kinases including the tyrosine kinase activity of the VEGFR-1-3, PDGFRs, C-KIT, and cFMS receptors as well as downstream signaling molecules LCK and ITK kinases. Its antitumor activity is likely related to its antiangiogenic effect.

Pharmacokinetics: It is metabolized by CYP3A4, with a plasma $t_{1/2}$ of approximately 31 h, and doses must be modified in the presence of inducers or inhibitors of CYP3A4.

Toxicity: Common toxicities include diarrhea, nausea/vomiting, altered taste, decreased appetite, abdominal pain, fatigue, asthenia, hypertension, elevated transaminases and bilirubin, lower levels of phosphorous/

magnesium/potassium/sodium/glucose, palmar-plantar erythrodysesthesia syndrome, hypothyroidism, and changes in hair color. Less common but potentially serious toxicities include hemorrhage, arterial thrombosis, hepatotoxicity, and prolonged QTc.

Clinical effectiveness: It has shown sufficient activity to be approved for treatment of metastatic renal cancer. It is actively being evaluated against a number of other malignancies, including neuroendocrine cancers.

■ AXITINIB

Mechanism of action: Axitinib is an inhibitor of multiple kinases including VEGFR-1-3, PDGFRs, and C-KIT. Its major antitumor activity is believed to be mediated by inhibition of VEGF receptors.

Pharmacokinetics: It is metabolized by CYP3A4, with a plasma $t_{1/2}$ of approximately 2.5-6.1 h, and doses must be modified in the presence of inducers or inhibitors of CYP3A4.

Toxicity: Common toxicities include diarrhea, nausea/vomiting, mucosal irritation, rash, altered taste, decreased appetite, abdominal pain, fatigue, asthenia, hypertension, elevated transaminases, elevated amylase/lipase, lower levels of calcium/phosphorous/potassium/sodium, elevated or decreased glucose levels, palmar-plantar erythrodysesthesia syndrome, hypothyroidism, and changes in hair color. Less common but potentially serious toxicities include hemorrhage, arterial/venous thrombosis, hepatotoxicity, hypertensive crisis, prolonged QTc, gastrointestinal perforation or fistula formation, decreased wound healing, and reversible posterior leukoencephalopathy syndrome.

Clinical effectiveness: It is approved for treatment of metastatic renal cancer after failure of one systemic therapy.

TARGET: mTOR

■ TEMSIROLIMUS

Mechanism of action: An intravenous inhibitor of the mTORC1 complex, a critical enzyme in the PI-3 kinase-AKT pathway, important in modifying tumor metabolism, inducing glycolysis, and promoting cell survival and proliferation (4, 8).

Pharmacokinetics. The drug has a plasma $t_{1/2}$ of approximately 17.3 h. Its active metabolite has a $t_{1/2}$ of 54 h. It is eliminated by CYP3A4, and is subject to drug interactions with inducers or inhibitors of the CYP system.

Toxicity: Rash, edema, anorexia, nausea, asthenia, fatigue, mucositis, cough, pneumonitis, diarrhea, hyperglycemia, hyperlipidemia, elevated liver function tests, bone marrow suppression, increased risk of infections, and renal dysfunction.

Clinical effectiveness: It is approved for the treatment of advanced renal cell carcinoma.

■ EVEROLIMUS

Mechanism of action: An oral inhibitor of mTOR, a critical enzyme in the PI-3 kinase-AKT pathway (see temsirolimus, above).

Pharmacokinetics: It is metabolized by CYP3A4 and is subject to drug interaction with inhibitors or inducers of this enzyme. It has a plasma $t_{1/2}$ of approximately 30 h.

Toxicity: Rash, edema, anorexia, nausea, asthenia, fatigue, mucositis, cough, pneumonitis, diarrhea, hyperglycemia, hyperlipidemia, elevated liver function tests, bone marrow suppression, increased risk of infections, and increased serum creatinine.

Clinical effectiveness: It has activity against advanced RCC and is approved for use after progression on either sunitinib or sorafenib. It is also approved for the treatment of peripheral neuroectodermal tumors, hormone positive breast cancer (combined with exemestane), and subependymal giant cell astrocytoma.

TARGET: B-RAF

■ VEMURAFENIB

Mechanism of action: An oral inhibitor of activated B-RAF kinase carrying a V600E mutation. B-RAF is a serine/threonine kinase in the RAS-RAF-MEK signaling pathway. Mutations in this pathway are frequently found in melanoma, colon cancer, lung cancer, and thyroid cancer.

Pharmacokinetics: Vemurafenib is metabolized by CYP3A4 and is subject to drug interaction with inhibitors or inducers of this enzyme as well as several CYP2 substrates such as warfarin. It has a plasma $t_{1/2}$ of approximately 57 h.

Toxicity: Rash, photosensitivity, pruritis, dry skin, hyperkeratosis, alopecia, joint pain, nausea, diarrhea, fatigue, elevated liver function tests, prolonged QTc interval, skin papillomas, and cutaneous squamous cell carcinomas.

Clinical effectiveness: It is approved for treatment of melanomas carrying a *B-RAF* V600E mutation.

FUTURE OF TARGETED THERAPY FOR TREATING CANCER

Many additional agents targeting proteins (primarily kinases) of interest as drivers of malignancy are currently undergoing clinical investigation. In addition to development of agents targeted against cell surface receptors, much current interest involves inhibitors of steps in signal transduction pathways from cell surface to nucleus, including steps in the PI3K-mTOR and RAS-RAF-MEK pathways (2-4, 6-9). Recent studies have shown significant activity of MEK inhibitors, either alone or in combination with B-RAF inhibitors, against melanoma (11, 15). Clearly, there are many other potential targets within cells, including proteins involved in other signaling pathways, proteins involved in survival, regulatory proteins such as transcription factors, enzymes involved in intermediary metabolic processes, epigenetic modifiers, and proteins that enhance antitumor immune function by blocking inhibitory proteins (e.g., anti-PD1, anti-PDL1, anti-CTLA4) (5, 10, 12, 13). Certain agents under development have greater specificity for one protein or gene, whereas others have activity against a number of proteins. It is not known whether having agents with highly specific activity (and potentially combining different agents each with specific activity) or having broader activity within one agent will be more clinically effective against any specific cancer. This will likely vary depending on disease indications, targets, and agents.

Given the complexity of genetic, epigenetic, and tumor microenvironment changes in most cancers, it is unlikely that modulation of single targets will have long-term antitumor efficacy against most cancers. Thus, combinations of target approaches are being explored. Strategies to inhibit multiple sequential steps in a given pathway (such as a signal transduction pathway) or multiple receptors or pathways in parallel are being evaluated. Strategies for combining different classes of targeted agents (e.g., mAbs and small molecules, which tend to have fewer overlapping toxicities than two agents of the same class) are also being pursued. In some instances, a combination of monoclonal antibodies targeting different sites on the same molecule may be more effective than single agents. Other approaches, such as specifically delivering cytotoxic compounds to malignant cells by coupling them to mAbs (e.g., TDM1, which contains the mAB trastuzumab coupled with the antimitotic agent emtansine, targeted against HER2) are attracting increasing attention because of the success of the antibody-drug conjugate brentuximab vedotin against Hodgkin disease and anaplastic large cell lymphoma.

To date, clinically useful targeted compounds have come from one of three classes of agents (mABs, small molecules, or modified proteins or peptides). However, other classes of compounds are likely to have utility as anticancer agents, such as RNA interference with small inhibitory RNA (siRNA) (5, 10). siRNAs bind to complementary RNA molecules leading to their cleavage and produce post-transcriptional gene silencing (PTGS), a powerful tool for studying the effects of silencing specific genes, and in fact represents a potential therapy modality if barriers in the delivery of the molecule can be solved.

Biomarkers are essential to define the population of patients who represent appropriate candidates for specific targeted therapy. Biomarkers are also needed for monitoring the effectiveness of that therapy. Therefore, a significant effort is being devoted to identifying the most useful biomarkers for different agents and malignancies. Given the critical need to have a uniform, standard, and widely available test to select patients that will benefit from the agent, the FDA is now mandating that, when it is feasible, the appropriate diagnostic test must be developed at the same time that the drug is being evaluated and the test must be validated at the time of approval. Both vemurafenib (with a companion pcr test for the V600E *B-RAF* mutation) for melanoma and crizotinib (with a companion FISH analysis for presence of *EML4-ALK* translocation for NSCLC) were codeveloped with biomarker tests that were available at the time of approval (3, 9). There remain certain targeted agents (e.g., angiogenesis inhibitors including VEGF and VEGFR inhibitors, histone deacetylase inhibitors, proteosome inhibitors) for which it has not yet been possible to define clinically meaningful biomarkers beyond the specific diseases for which they have been approved. Identification and validation of appropriate biomarkers for specific agents continue to be essential areas of study.

Modeling approaches, including computer simulations, can be helpful in both improving drug design for enhanced efficacy and identifying potential toxicities of agents prior to clinical testing (17). As knowledge of the important factors that determine both efficacy and toxicity improves, models can be more precise in helping to decide which agents to carry forward into clinical trials.

Another major area of research aims to prevent or overcome development of resistance by cancers to targeted agents. Many mechanisms leading to either primary or secondary development of resistance to targeted agents have been defined, as discussed above. Pharmacokinetic sanctuary sites (such as the brain) continue to be a problem for most new drugs (16, 18). Acquired genetic mutations of a target are detectable through tumor biopsies taken at the time of disease progression, and provide guidance for efforts to develop better drugs and combinations of drugs (19). Mechanisms of drug resistance to antiangiogenic agents, such as bevacizumab resistance in RCC, are poorly understood and thus remain a major challenge. Exploration of strategies to overcome the various mechanisms of resistance is critical for development of new targeted therapies that will be effective in controlling disease for prolonged periods.

Continued improvement in understanding critical processes in cancer development, growth, survival, and metastasis will provide new targets and better drugs, as well as better biomarkers for defining the appropriate patients for specific agents, and a more complete understanding of resistance to targeted agents. Given the complexity and heterogeneity of most cancers, better ways of integrating targeted agents with other anticancer treatment approaches will have to be developed in order to achieve successful long-term control of various cancers.

REFERENCES

1. Hanahan D, Weinberg RA. Hallmarks of cancer: the next generation. *Cell.* 2011; 144: 646-74.

2. Scott AM, Wolchok JD, Old LJ. Antibody therapy of cancer. *Nat Rev Cancer.* 2012; 12: 278-287.

3. Yauch RL, Settleman J. Recent advances in pathway-targeted cancer drug therapies emerging from cancer genome analysis. *Curr Opin Genet Dev.* 2012; 22: 45-49.

4. Sheppard K, Kinross KM, Solomon B, et al. Targeting PI3 inase/AKT/mTOR signalling in cancer. *Crit Rev Oncog.* 2012; 17: 69-95.

5. Lujambio A, Lowe SW. The microcosmos of cancer. *Nature.* 2012; 482: 347-355.

6. Dhomen NS, Mariadason J, Tebbutt N, et al. Therapeutic targeting of the epidermal growth factor receptor in human cancer. *Crit Rev Oncog.* 2012; 17: 31-50.

7. Waldner MJ, Neurath MF. Targeting the VEGF signalling pathway in cancer therapy. *Expert Opin Ther Targets.* 2012; 16: 5-13.

8. Copyright © 2012 PDR Network, LLC, Montvale, NJ 07645.

9. Chabner BA. Early accelerated approval for highly targeted cancer drugs. *N Engl J Med.* 2011; 364: 1087-1089.

10. Wang Z, Rao DD, Senzer N, Nemunaitis J. RNA interference and cancer therapy. *Pharm Res.* 2011: 2983-2995.

11. Flaherty KT, Robert C, Hersey P, et al. Improved survival with MEK inhibition in BRAF-mutated melanoma. *N Engl J Med.* 2012; 367: 107-114.

12. Xu Y, He K, Goldkorn A. Telomerase targeted therapy in cancer and cancer stem cells. *Clin Adv Hematol Oncol.* 2011; 9: 442-455.

13. Muñoz-Pinedo C, El Mjiyad N, Ricci JE. Cancer metabolism: current perspectives and future directions. *Cell Death Dis.* 2012; 3: e248.

14. Gerlinger M, Rowan AJ, Horswell S, et al. Intratumor heterogeneity and branched evolution revealed by multiregion sequencing. *N Engl J Med.* 2012; 366: 883-892.

15. Flaherty K, Infante JR, Falchook GS, et al. Phase I/II study of BRAFi GSK2118436 + MEKi GSK1120212 in patients with BRAF mutant metastatic melanoma who progressed on a prior BRAFi. *Pigment Cell Melanoma Res.* 2011; 25: E1-E11.

16. Katayama R, Shaw AT, Khan TM, et al. Mechanisms of acquired crizotinib resistance in ALK-rearranged lung cancers. *Sci Transl Med.* 2012 4: 120ra17.

17. Lounkine E, Keiser MJ, Whitebread S, et al. Large-scale prediction and testing of drug activity on side-effect targets. *Nature.* 2012; 486: 361-367.

18. Turner NC, Reis-Filho JS. Genetic heterogeneity and cancer drug resistance. *Lancet Oncol.* 2012; 13: e178-e185.

19. Kobayashi S, Boggon T, Dayaram T, et al. Mutation and resistance of non–small-cell lung cancer to gefitinib. *N Engl J Med.* 2005; 352: 786-792.

CHAPTER 11
Antiestrogens

Tanja Badovinac Crnjevic, Paul E. Goss

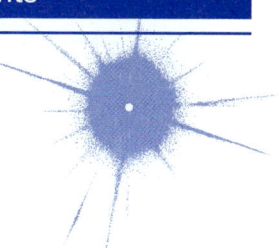

ANTIESTROGENS

Antiestrogen hormonal therapy is the cornerstone of endocrine treatment of hormone-receptor positive breast cancer.

Current antiestrogen treatment options for hormone-receptor positive breast cancer include selective estrogen-receptor modulators (SERMs), selective estrogen-receptor downregulators (SERDs), and aromatase inhibitors (AIs).

■ SELECTIVE ESTROGEN-RECEPTOR MODULATORS

The SERMs are chemically diverse compounds that lack the steroid structure of estrogen but possess a tertiary structure that allows them to bind to estrogen receptors. Depending on the specific end-organ, they exert selective agonist and/or antagonist effects (1).

There are three currently approved SERMS: raloxifene, toremifene, and tamoxifen (**Figure 11-1**). The most widely used SERM for treatment of ER positive breast cancer is tamoxifen.

Tamoxifen

Mechanism of action.   Tamoxifen is a competitive inhibitor of estradiol binding to the ER. In addition to its estrogen antagonist effects on the breast and breast cancer, tamoxifen exerts estrogenic effects on non-breast tissues which influence its overall therapeutic index. Tamoxifen exerts agonist or antagonist effects in part related to ambient estrogen levels. For example on bone metabolism it exerts a partial agonist action in postmenopausal women whereas in premenopausal women its effect on bone is antagonistic (1).

Clinically in women with ER positive disease, 5 years of post-operative adjuvant tamoxifen reduces the annual odds of recurrence of breast cancer by 39% and the annual odds of death by 31%, with comparable effects regardless of age as well as menopausal and nodal status (2).

Absorption, fate, and excretion.   Tamoxifen is readily absorbed following oral administration, with peak concentrations measurable after 3–7 h and steady-state levels being reached at 4–6 weeks. It is a prodrug with little affinity for the estrogen receptor and requires metabolization into its active form endoxifen (4-hydroxy N-desmethyltamoxifen) by the sequential action of CYP2D6 and CYP3A4. A second metabolite, N-desmethyltamoxifen, also has strong antiestrogenic activity. Some selective serotonin reuptake inhibitors (SSRIs) like fluoxetine, paroxetine, and sertraline are potent inhibitors of CYP2D6, and may impair tamoxifen's activation.

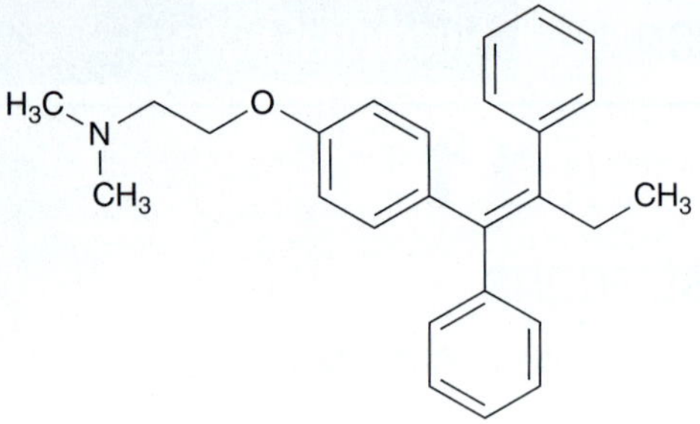

Tamoxifen

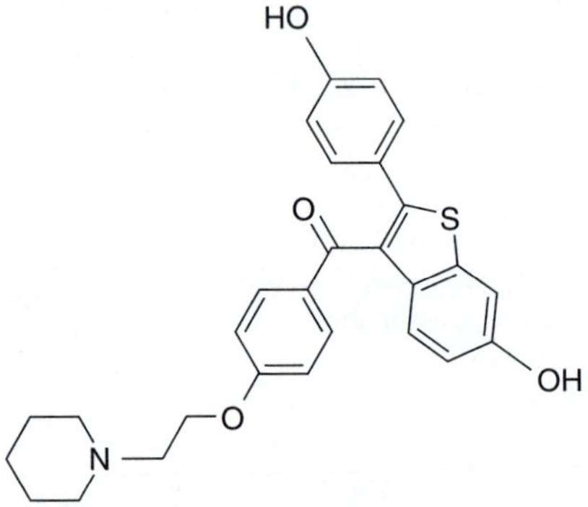

Raloxifene hydrochloride

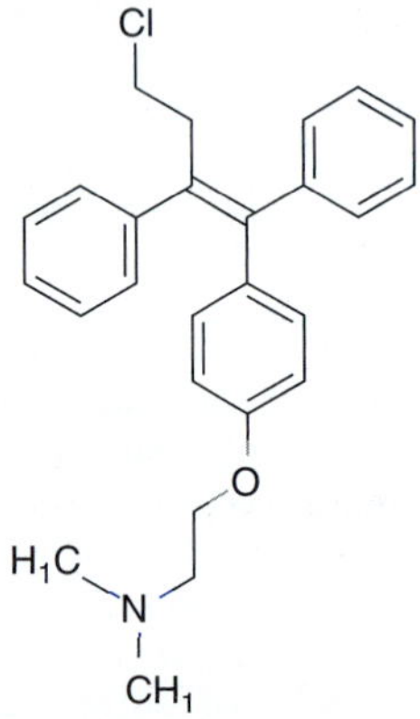

Toremifene

FIGURE 11-1 Chemical structure of selective estrogen receptor modulators: tamoxifen, raloxifene, and toremifene.

It is hypothesized that certain CYP2D6 genotypes and phenotypes are associated with lower endoxifen concentrations and worse breast cancer outcome. However, two published retrospective studies with the largest sample size thus far found no statistically significant association between the presence of poor or intermediate metabolizer phenotype and breast cancer outcome (3, 4). Given the limited and conflicting data, CYP2D6 testing is not recommended as a tool to define the optimal endocrine strategy.

The half-lives of N-desmethyltamoxifen and endoxifen are 14 days or longer. After enterohepatic circulation, glucuronides and other metabolites are excreted in the stool; excretion in the urine is minimal (1).

Therapeutic uses. Tamoxifen citrate (Nolvadex®) is marketed for oral administration. The usual dose prescribed is 20 mg daily.

Tamoxifen is used for (5):

- treatment of ER positive metastatic breast cancer until disease progression.
- adjuvant endocrine treatment of ER positive premenopausal breast cancer alone or in combination with ovarian ablation for 5 years.

- adjuvant endocrine treatment of ER positive postmenopausal breast cancer for 2–3 or 5 years prior to administration of an AI.
- prevention of breast cancer in women at increased risk.

Clinical toxicity. Tamoxifen is generally well tolerated. Side effects are rarely sufficiently severe to require discontinuation of therapy as overall quality of life (QoL) appears not to be impaired (1).

The most common side effects (occurring in greater than 30%) are:

- vasomotor symptoms (hot flashes)
- vaginal discharge
- fluid retention
- loss of libido

Less common side effects (occurring in about 10%–30%) are:

- nausea
- menstrual irregularities
- vaginal bleeding
- mood changes
- increased risk of cataracts, retinal deposits, and decreased visual acuity

Rare but serious side effects include:

- two- to threefold increased risk of endometrial cancer, particularly in postmenopausal women over 60 years taking tamoxifen for ≥2 years; monitoring of abnormal vaginal bleeding with prompt gynecological evaluation is recommended.
- doubling of the rate of deep vein thrombosis and pulmonary embolism; it is recommended to discontinue tamoxifen before elective surgery.

■ SELECTIVE ESTROGEN-RECEPTOR DOWNREGULATORS

SERDs (also termed "pure antiestrogens") bind ER with high affinity, without activating any of the normal transcriptional hormonal responses, and are consequently devoid of any estrogen agonist activity. The lead compound of this class currently approved for the treatment of advanced breast cancer is fulvestrant (Figure 11-2).

Fulvestrant

Mechanism of action. Fulvestrant is a steroidal antiestrogen that binds to the ER with an affinity over 100 times that of tamoxifen, inhibits its dimerization, and increases its degradation. In contrast to tamoxifen, which increases the level of ER expression, fulvestrant is associated with a reduction in the number of detectable ER molecules in cells (6).

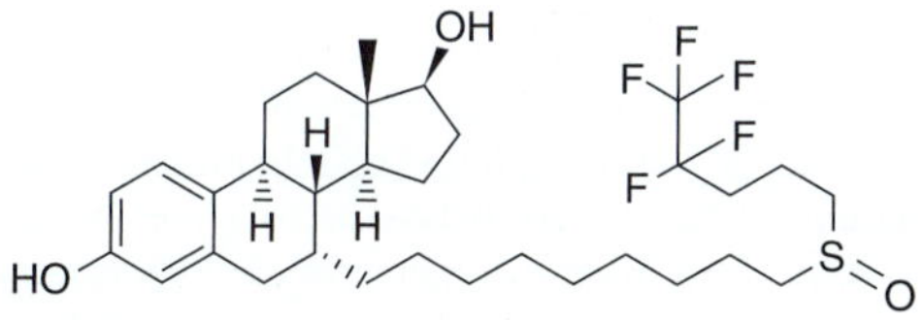

FIGURE 11-2 Chemical structure of fulvestrant.

Absorption, fate, and excretion.   Fulvestrant is administered intramuscularly (i.m.) once monthly. Maximum plasma concentrations are reached at about 7 days after i.m. administration and are maintained over a period of 1 month. The plasma half-life is approximately 40 days. Steady state is achieved in 1 month with a loading dose (500 mg on day 0, 250 mg on day 14, 250 mg on day 28 and q4 weeks thereafter) compared to 4–6 months with the approved dose (250 mg q4 weeks).

There is extensive and rapid distribution of the drug, predominantly to the extravascular compartment.

Various pathways similar to those responsible for endogenous steroid metabolism extensively metabolize fulvestrant. The putative metabolites possess no estrogenic activity and only the 17-keto compound demonstrates a level of antiestrogenic activity about one-fifth than that of fulvestrant. Less than 1% is excreted in the urine (6).

Therapeutic uses.   Fulvestrant (Faslodex®) is available as a long-acting 50 mg/ml solution. It is typically administered as a 250-mg i.m. injection at monthly intervals, but recent data suggest that a high-dose regimen (500 mg) has greater efficacy compared to the approved 250-mg dose. After many years of clinical trials and development, fulvestrant has been approved at a higher dose of 500 mg by the FDA but is still used at the 250 mg dose in some countries (7).

Fulvestrant is used for (5):

- treatment of postmenopausal women with hormone-receptor positive metastatic breast cancer.

Clinical toxicity.   Fulvestrant is generally well tolerated, and QoL outcome measures are maintained over time (8).

Clinical side effects of fulvestrant include:

- nausea
- asthenia
- pain
- vasodilatation (hot flushes)
- headache
- injection site reactions

■ AROMATASE INHIBITORS

In premenopausal women estrogens are synthesized primarily in the ovaries. Following menopause, estrogen is produced by aromatization of circulating androgens in extra-ovarian peripheral tissues, including liver, muscles, skin fat, and connective tissue, and circulates at low levels. Peripheral aromatization depends on androgenic precursors of adrenal origin to generate estradiol and estrone. Aromatase is the enzyme complex responsible for converting androgens (androstenedione and testosterone) to estrogens (estrone [E_1] and estradiol [E_2]). In postmenopausal patients, where only baseline levels of aromatase activity are present, aromatase inhibitors (AIs) effectively lower estrogen levels by 90% to nearly undetectable levels.

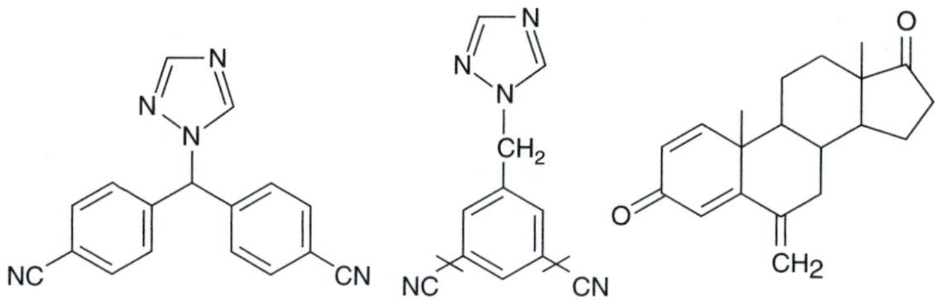

FIGURE 11-3 Chemical structures of aromatase inhibitors.

AIs are not appropriate monotherapy for premenopausal patients, as residual ovarian function can lead to reflex stimulation of FSH, enhanced ovulation, and increased production of estrogen thereby overcoming the effects of the AI.

AIs are classified as type 1 (steroidal aromatase inactivator) or type 2 (nonsteroidal AI) inhibitors according to their structure and mechanism of action (**Figure 11-3**). Type 1 inhibitors are steroidal analogues of androstenedione and bind to the same site on the aromatase molecule, but unlike androstenedione bind irreversibly because of their conversion to reactive intermediates by aromatase. Thus they are commonly known as aromatase inactivators or suicide inhibitors. Type 2 inhibitors are nonsteroidal and bind reversibly to the heme group of the enzyme by way of a basic nitrogen atom (9).

The recently developed AIs, now in common clinical use, include the type 1 steroidal agent, exemestane, and the type 2 nonsteroidal imidazoles anastrozole and letrozole.

Therapeutic use. Several large randomised trials and meta-analyses have shown that AIs are superior to tamoxifen in the treatment of postmenopausal women with ER positive tumors in the metastatic, adjuvant, and neoadjuvant settings. Currently AIs are used for treatment of ER positive metastatic breast cancer and also as adjuvant therapy for early ER positive breast cancer. In the adjuvant setting they can be used as initial adjuvant therapy, as sequential therapy following 2–3 years of tamoxifen (i.e., switching), or as extended therapy following 4.5–6 years of tamoxifen. They have also been tested in the neoadjuvant setting and in chemoprevention of breast cancer in postmenopausal women at high risk for breast cancer (9).

Clinical toxicity. Tamoxifen and AIs have distinct toxicity profiles. Compared to tamoxifen, AIs cause significantly fewer hot flushes, less vaginal discharge or bleeding, and no evidence for uterine carcinoma. While thromboembolism has been associated with AI use in metastatic advanced breast cancer, it is possible that these events have been related to cancer burden rather than therapy and an excess of thrombotic events has not been confirmed in the adjuvant setting with any of the AIs. However, AIs are associated with an increased incidence of musculoskeletal adverse events such as arthralgia, myalgia, and carpal tunnel syndrome. AIs are associated with hypercholesterolemia, and with a higher incidence of cardiovascular events but only in comparison to tamoxifen, which lowers these events. The cardiovascular event rate for subjects taking an AI is not different than the rate for subjects taking a placebo (10).

Due to profound estrogen depletion and accelerated bone resorption, AIs are associated with increased risk of bone loss, osteoporosis, and bone fracture. Currently, most guidelines for postmenopausal patients taking AIs recommend regular monitoring of BMD, supplemental vitamin D and calcium, and initiation of bisphosphonates only after BMD declines to a high risk threshold (e.g., T score 2.5) or if a clinical fracture occurs (11).

Anastrozole

Mechanism of action.   Anastrozole, like letrozole, binds competitively and specifically to the heme of the cytochrome p450 subunit of the aromatase enzyme. Anastrozole 1 mg administered once daily for 28 days reduces androgen aromatization by 96.7%. In addition, anastrozole reduces in situ aromatization in large, ER+ breast tumors. Anastrozole has no clinically significant effect on rates of adrenal glucocorticoid synthesis in postmenopausal women, or on plasma concentrations of luteinising hormone or follicle-stimulating hormone and thyroid hormone.

Absorption, fate, and excretion.   Anastrozole is absorbed rapidly after oral administration with maximal plasma concentrations occurring after 2 h. A high-fat meal increases absorption. Repeated dosing increases plasma concentrations of anastrozole and steady state is attained after 7 days. It has a plasma half-life of 39–62 h. Anastrozole is slowly metabolized by hepatic N-dealkylation, hydroxylation, and glucuronidation. The main metabolite is an inactive triazole. Less than 10% of the drug is excreted as the unmetabolized parent compound (12).

Therapeutic uses.   Anastrozole (Arimidex®) 1 mg is administered once daily orally. Anastrozole is used for (5):

- treatment of postmenopausal women with advanced, hormone-receptor positive breast cancer until disease progression.
- adjuvant treatment of postmenopausal breast cancer: as initial adjuvant therapy for 5 years or as sequential therapy, following 2–3 years of tamoxifen.

Letrozole

Mechanism of action.   In postmenopausal women, letrozole inhibits aromatization throughout the body and reduces in situ aromatization within breast cancers. The drug has no significant effect on the synthesis of adrenal corticoids, aldosterone, or thyroid hormone, and does not alter levels of a range of other hormones.

Absorption, fate, and excretion.   Letrozole is rapidly absorbed after oral administration, and the maximum plasma levels are reached about 1 h after ingestion. Steady-state plasma concentrations of letrozole are reached after 2–6 weeks on treatment. Following metabolism by CYP2A6, and CYP3A4, letrozole is eliminated as an inactive carbinol metabolite in the urine. The elimination half-life is about 40–42 h (13).

Therapeutic uses. Letrozole (Femara®) 2.5 mg is administered orally once daily. Letrozole is used for (5):

- treatment of postmenopausal women with advanced, hormone-receptor positive breast cancer until disease progression.
- adjuvant treatment of postmenopausal breast cancer for 5 years or for 2–3 years following 2–3 years of tamoxifen.
- adjuvant treatment of postmenopausal breast cancer for 5 years following 4.5–6 years of tamoxifen.

Exemestane

Mechanism of action. Exemestane is a potent, orally administered analog of the natural substrate androstenedione. In contrast to the reversible competitive inhibitors, anastrozole, and letrozole, exemestane irreversibly inactivates the enzyme complex (a suicide substrate). Doses of 25 mg per day inhibit aromatase activity by 98% and lower estrone and estradiol levels in plasma by about 90%.

Absorption, fate, and excretion. Exemestane is rapidly absorbed from the gastrointestinal tract reaching maximum plasma levels after 2 h. Its absorption is increased by 40% after a high fat meal. Exemestane has a terminal half-life of approximately 24 h. It is extensively converted in the liver to metabolites inactive against aromatase. A key metabolite, 17-hydroxyexemestane, has weak androgenic activity, which might contribute to antitumor activity and androgenic end-organ effects. Excretion is distributed almost equally between the urine and feces. Since significant quantities of active metabolites are excreted in the urine, doses of exemestane should be adjusted in patients with renal dysfunction (14).

Therapeutic uses. Exemestane 25 mg is administered orally once daily. Exemestane is used for (5):

- treatment of postmenopausal women with advanced, hormone-receptor positive breast cancer until disease progression.
- treatment of postmenopausal women with advanced, hormone-receptor positive breast cancer after failure of a nonsteroidal inhibitor.
- adjuvant treatment of postmenopausal breast cancer: as sequential therapy, following 2–3 years of tamoxifen or as initial adjuvant therapy for 5 years.
- prevention of breast cancer for high-risk postmenopausal women (15), although the drug is not yet approved for this indication.

GnRH agonist

Mechanism of action. Ovarian ablation (OA) is an effective therapy for premenopausal women with ER+ breast cancer. In premenopausal women, where ovaries are the predominant source of estrogen, OA can be accomplished by oophorecotmy or ovarian irradiation. More recently, chemical suppression of ovarian estrogene production with the gonadotropin-releasing hormone (GnRH) analogues is being used. The majority of breast cancer patients are treated with goserelin or leuprolid (16).

For more details on GnRH agonist mechanisms of action, please refer to the Chapter 12 on antiandrogen therapy.

Absorption, fate, and excretion.   Following subcutaneous administration of goserelin, the absorption is rapid and the peak blood concentration occurs between 0.5 and 1.0 h after dosing. Goserelin is released from the depot at a much slower rate initially for the first 8 days, and then there is more rapid and continuous release for the remainder of the 28-day dosing period.

Clearance is very rapid and occurs via a combination of hepatic metabolism and urinary excretion. More than 90% of goserelin is excreted in urine. No dose adjustment is necessary for patients with renal of hepatic impairment (16).

Clinical toxicity.   The most common side effects of GnRH are hot flashes, vaginal dryness, increased sweating, decreased sexual interest, headaches, and mood changes. The use of GnRH agnostic may cause a reduction in BMD and osteoporosis.

Due to tumor flare, transient worsening of symptoms of breast cancer may develop during the first few weeks of treatment (16).

Therapeutic uses (5).   GnRH analogues are usually administered subcutaneously into the anterior abdominal wall below the navel line. Goserelin 3.6 mg is administered every 28 days. Leuprolide is available at various doses and schedules (leuprolide 3.75 mg monthly, leuprolide 11.5 mg every 3 month).

GnRH analogues are used for treatment of premenopausal women with ER+ breast cancer. Their role in protection of the ovaries of women with cancer who are undergoing chemotherapy is being investigated.

In the metastatic setting, GnRH analogues can be used as monotherapy or in combination with antiestrogens (tamoxifen or aromatase inhibitors). The combination of LHRH agonist with tamoxifen appears to be more effective than GnRH alone (17).

In the adjuvant setting, GnRH analogues have been tested alone or in combination with antiestrogens or with chemotherapy. The currently published clinical trials have shown clinical benefit of GnRH. However, comparisons against current clinical standards of care (anthracycline- and/or taxane-based chemotherapy, aromatase inhibitors) are needed before GnRH analogues can be routinely used in the adjuvant treatment of premenopausal women with ER+ early breast cancer (18).

Endocrine resistance.   Although antagonizing estrogen is among the most effective breast cancer treatment, a significant proportion of patients experience disease progression due to either de novo (no response to treatment) or acquired (initial response followed by progression during treatment) resistance to endocrine therapy. Endocrine resistance may occur through multiple mechanisms due to "escape" pathways.

Current concepts and approaches to overcoming endocrine resistance are described below (19).

1. Loss or inactivation of ER or ER pathway

    Downregulation or complete loss of ER occurs in approximately 20% of patients treated with endocrine therapy, and such tumors are no longer driven by estrogens.

Changes in the proteins that form the transcription initiation complexes with the ER can influence effectiveness of endocrine therapy. For example, overexpression of ER coactivator AIB1 (also called SRC3), downregulation of corepressor NCoR, or increased activity of transcriptional factors (AP-1, SP-1, and NF-κB) are associated with endocrine resistance.

2. Alteration of cell cycle and apoptosis regulators

   Preclinical data show that alteration of cell cycle and apoptosis regulators may impact sensitivity to endocrine treatment. In some cases upregulation of positive regulators of the cell cycle and/or downregulation of negative regulators lead to hormonal therapy resistance (19).

3. Dysregulation of membrane tyrosine kinase receptors

   The ER signaling pathway is also regulated by membrane tyrosine kinase receptors. Dysregulation of tyrosine kinase receptors (RKTs) and their downstream signaling pathways can confer resistance to hormonal therapy. For example, overexpression and/or amplification of RKTs such as epidermal growth factor (EGFR), HER2, and insulin-like growth factor (IGF1-R) result in phosphorylation of ER and its coregulators leading to activation of ER in the absence of estrogen. In other cases, deregulation of intracellular signaling elements, such as activating alterations in the PI3 kinase pathway, including mutation of phosphatidylinositol 3-kinase itself, loss of heterozygosity or methylation of the tumor suppressor PTEN gene, and activation of AKT, promotes oncogenic transformation.

In recent years many targeted drugs that inhibit specific pathways have been developed in order to overcome endocrine resistance.

Some clinical trials investigating the combination of endocrine therapy with agents targeting EGFR (gefitinib, erlotinib), HER2 (trastuzumab), or both EGFR and HER2 (lapatinib) receptors have yielded inconclusive results. More promising results come from clinical studies that have focused on novel agents, targeting downstream signaling pathways, such as mTOR. Two randomized trials (BOLERO-2 and TAMRAD) evaluating everolimus with or without endocrine therapy in a selected subgroup of HR-positive metastatic breast cancer patients have demonstrated significant improvement in progression-free survival for the combination. Everolimus was recently approved for treatment of hormone-receptor positive metastatic breast cancer in combination with exemestane in patients progressing on either letrozole or anastrozole (20).

Animal models have illustrated that resistance to endocrine therapy can be induced by chronic endocrine therapy, and preliminary data in humans have suggested that AI withdrawal or intermittent AI therapy may produce clinical advantage (21).

REFERENCES

1. Lawrence BR, Lynn C, Hartmann LC. Selective estrogen receptor modulators–mechanism of action and application to clinical practice. *N Engl J Med.* 2003; 348: 618–629.

2. EBCTCG. Effects of chemotherapy and hormonal therapy for early breast cancer on recurrence and 15-year survival: an overview of the randomised trials. *Lancet.* 2005; 365: 1687–1717.

3. Regan MM, Leyland-Jones B, Bouzyk M, et al. *CYP2D6* genotype and tamoxifen response in postmenopausal women with estrogen-responsive early breast cancer: the Breast International Group 1–98 Trial. *J Natl Cancer Inst.* 2012; 104: 441–451.

4. Rae JM, Drury S, Hayes DF, et al. *CYP2D6* and *UGT2B7* genotype and risk of recurrence in tamoxifen-treated breast cancer patients. *J Natl Cancer Inst.* 2012; 104: 452–460.

5. http://www.nccn.org/professionals/physician_gls/pdf/breast.pdf

6. McCormack P, Sapunar F. Pharmacokinetic profile of the fulvestrant (Faslodex) loading-dose regimen in postmenopausal women with hormone receptor-positive advanced breast cancer. *Breast Cancer Res Treat.* 2007; 106 (Suppl 1): S116.

7. Di Leo A, Jerusalem G, Petruzelka L, et al. Results of the CONFIRM phase III study comparing fulvestrant 250 mg with fulvestrant 500 mg in postmenopausal women with estrogen receptor-positive advanced breast cancer. *J Clin Oncol.* 2010; 28: 4594–4600.

8. Vergote I, Robertson JF. Fulvestrant is an effective and well-tolerated endocrine therapy for postmenopausal women with advanced breast cancer: results from clinical trials. *Br J Cancer.* 2004; 90 (Suppl 1): S11–S14.

9. Strasser-Weippl K, Goss PE. Advances in adjuvant hormonal therapy for postmenopausal women. *J Clin Oncol.* 2005; 23: 1751–1759.

10. Amir E, Seruga B, Niraula S, et al. Toxicity of adjuvant endocrine therapy in postmenopausual breast cancer patients: a systematic review and meta-analysis. *J Natl Cancer Inst.* 2001; 103: 1–11.

11. Reid DM, Doughty J, Eastell R et al. Guidance for management of breast cancer treatment-induced bone loss: a consensus position statement from a UK Expert Group. *Cancer Treat Rev.* 2008; 34: 3–18.

12. Koberle D, Thurlimann B. Anastrozole: pharmacological and clinical profile in postmenopausal women with breast cancer. *Expert Rev Anticancer Ther.* 2001; 1: 169–176.

13. Lonning PE, Geisler J, Bhatnager A. Development of aromatase inhibitors and their pharmacologic profile. *Am J Clin Oncol.* 2003; 26: S3–S8.

14. Lonning PE. Pharmacology and clinical experience with exemestane. *Expert Opin Invest Drugs.* 2000; 9: 1897–1905.

15. Goss PE, Ingle JN, Alés-Martines JE, et al. Exemestane for breast cancer prevention in postmenopausal women. *N Engl J Med.* 2011; 364: 2381–2391.

16. Kiesel LA, Rody A, Greb RR, Szilagyi A. Clinical use of GnRH analogues. *Clin Endocrinol (Oxf).* 2002; 56: 677–687.

17. Prowell TM, Davidson NE. What is the role of ovarian ablation in the management of primary and metastatic breast cancer today? *The Oncologist.* 2004; 9: 507–517.

18. Goel S, Sharma R, Hamilton A, Beith J. LHRH agonists for adjuvant therapy of early breast cancer in premenopausal women. *Cochrane Database Syst Rev.* 2009; 7: CD004562.

19. Giuliano M, Schiff R, Osborne CK, Trivedi MV. Biological mechanisms and clinical implications of endocrine resistance in breast cancer. *Breast.* 2011; 20: 42–49.

20. Baselga J, Campone M, Piccart M, et al. Everolimus in postmenopausal hormone-receptor-positive advanced breast cancer. *N Engl J Med.* 2012; 366: 520–529.

21. Howell A, Dodwell DJ, Anderson H, et al. Response after withdrawal of tamoxifen and progestogens in advanced breast cancer. *Ann Oncol.* 1992; 3: 611–617.

CHAPTER **12**
Antiandrogen Therapy

Bruce A. Chabner

The initial attempt at treating cancer with hormone ablation was implemented by Charles Huggins at the University of Chicago in 1941, when he hypothesized that the prostate depended on testosterone (and, ultimately, its metabolite dihydrotestosterone) for its growth (1). Orchiectomy of patients with advanced prostate cancer reduced serum testosterone to barely detectable levels (less than 50 ng/dl) and produced dramatic relief of bone pain in 90% of such patients. The median duration of response was about 1 year, and hormone-independent tumor emerged in most cases. Huggins was awarded a Nobel Prize for his work.

Since that time, androgen ablation has not changed in concept, but drugs have largely taken the place of orchiectomy. Three basic classes of drugs are used: (i) gonadotrophin releasing hormone (GnRH) agonists, a family of small peptides that promote release, and exhaustion of GnRH from the hypothalamus, thus lowering Gn levels in plasma and blocking androgen release from the testes (medical castration); (ii) small-molecular-weight androgen analogs that inhibit androgen interaction with its receptor in normal and tumor cells; and (iii) drugs that inhibit androgen synthesis in the adrenals and other peripheral, non-gonadal tissues (2).

GnRH AGONISTS

Two GnRH agonists approved for clinical use in the United States are leuprolide and goserelin. These drugs are given by intermittent, monthly to 4-monthly subcutaneous injection, and produce a flair response of testosterone release for several days to weeks, followed by a rapid decline in serum testosterone levels. The flair may induce an increase in bone pain, and in the presence of significant vertebral metastases, symptoms of spinal cord compression may result. In such patients a GnRH antagonist, abarelix, is available to ablate the flair response and offers protection from the short-term progression of disease (3), but is only occasionally used. A more important consideration in the use of GnRH agonists is their lack of effect on adrenal androgen, which makes a small contribution to serum androgen activity and theoretically could be sufficient to maintain or promote tumor growth in the absence of testicular androgen. However, clinical trials of complete androgen blockade with a GnRH agonist and an inhibitor of androgen receptor binding have not yielded conclusively positive results (4), as compared to GnRH agonists alone.

Side effects of GnRH agonists are those of acute androgen deprivation, including vasomotor instability (flushing and sweating), loss of libido, gynecomastia, acute and dramatic bone and muscle loss with an increase in hip fracture rates, truncal obesity, diabetes, and an increased risk of myocardial infarction and sudden cardiac death (5). A "metabolic syndrome" of insulin resistance, increased body fat mass, and changes in plasma lipids can be detected within weeks of initiation of GnRH therapy (6). Bone preservation with bisphosphonates is recommended for patients on long-term GnRH agonist therapy (7).

The GnRH analogs are cleared by both renal excretion and by hepatic metabolism, with an elimination half-life of 3–7 h. Depending on their formulation and dose, plasma concentrations of analog are sufficient to suppress testosterone levels for 1–4 months.

ANDROGEN RECEPTOR INHIBITORS

Four receptor antagonists and one androgen synthesis inhibitor (Table 12-1 and Figure 12-1) have been approved for treatment of prostate cancer. The older compounds (flutamide, bicalutamide, nilutamide) are commonly used with GnRH agonists to block the temporary surge in adrenogens released in response to GnRH agonists and to inhibit the residual effects of adrenal androgens. The newest receptor antagonist, enzalutamide is approved for treatment of advanced, castration resistant prostate cancer after progression on docetaxel (8). As single agents, flutamide, nilutamide, and bicalutamide are not as effective as the GnRH agonists, but their side effect profile is somewhat advantageous. They elevate testosterone levels as a result of inhibition of androgen receptors in the hypothalamus and increased GnRH secretion; thus as single agents they cause less loss of libido

TABLE 12-1　CLINICAL PHARMACOLOGY OF ANTIANDROGENS

Compound	Elimination Half-Life (h)	Daily Dose (mg)
Bicalutamide	140	50
Flutamide (active metabolite)	8	250 every 8 h
Nilutamide	50	300 for 30 d, 150 thereafter
Enzalutamide	42	160
Abiraterone	12	1000 (without food)
		(250 for subjects with Child-Pugh class B hepatic impairment)

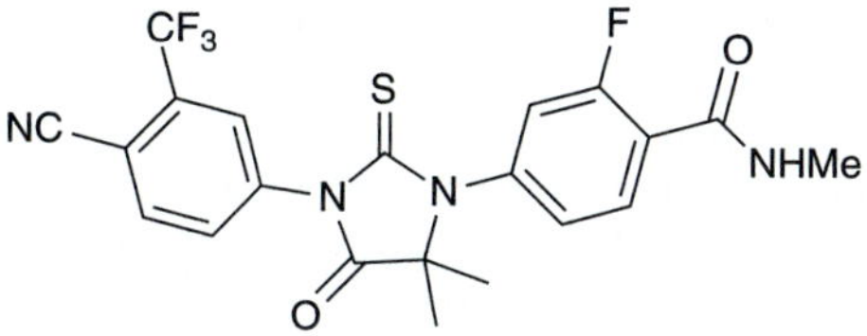

A. Enzalutamide

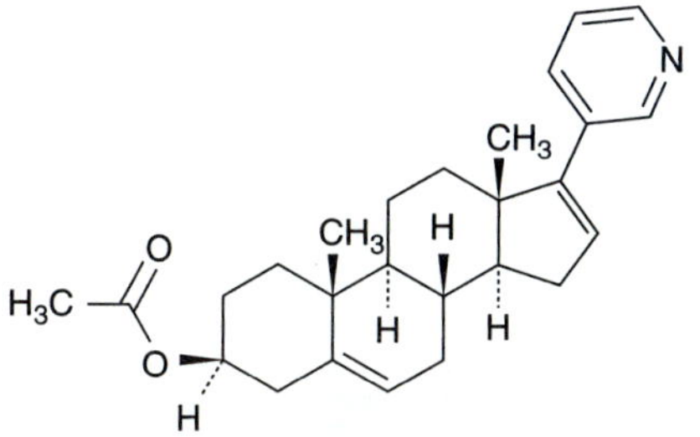

B. Abiraterone

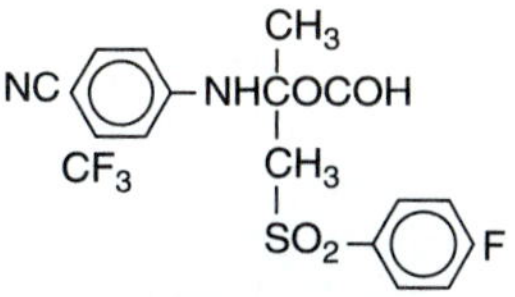

C. Bicalutamide

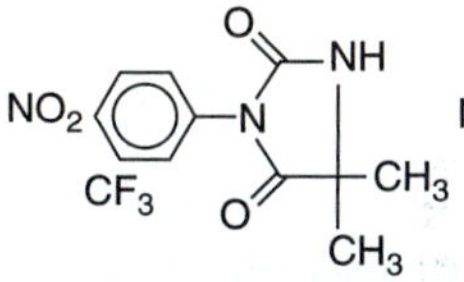

D. Nilutamide

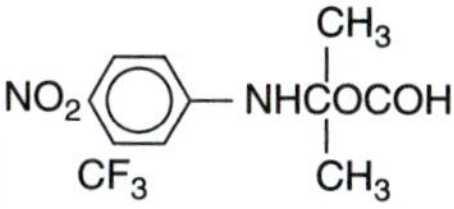

E. Hydroxyflutamide

FIGURE 12-1 Structures of androgen receptor antagonist and degrader, enzalutamide (A), the androgen synthesis inhibitor, abiraterone (B), and the androgen receptor antagonists bicalutamide (C), nilutamide (D), and flutamide (E).

and gynecomastia, and have little effect on bone and muscle mass. However, all three drugs cause rare cases of severe hepatic injury, flutamide causes diarrhea, and nilutamide causes interstitial pneumonitis and visual disturbances (dark adaptation). All are eliminated by hepatic metabolism, and may inhibit the clearance of coumadin, phenytoin, and other agents cleared by hepatic cytochrome-dependent enzymes. Flutamide is rapidly converted to its active alpha-hydroxy metabolite after oral administration. The doses and pharmacokinetics of these antiandrogens are given in Table 12-1. Enzalutamide causes hot flashes, fatigue, and diarrhea as its major side effects; it causes seizures in suprapharmacological doses in animals, and this side effect has been reported in human subjects on this drug.

The newest antiandrogen, enzalutamide, is a potent androgen receptor blocker that promotes degradation of the receptor and uncouples receptor and its coactivators, leading to antitumor responses. It extends survival in patients that have progressed on chemotherapy and prior antiandrogens. Its pharmacokinetic characteristics are shown in Table 12-1. A second new drug, abiraterone, has a unique mechanism of action, blocking the enzyme, 17-alpha hyroxylase/17-20lyase (CYP 17), which converts early steroid molecules to glucocorticoids and androgens in the adrenal glands and in prostate cancer cells. The drug prolongs progression-free survival in patients who have progressed on prior hormonal therapy, although in some patients, the bone scan may "flare" early in the treatment course. Pharmacokinetic features of abiraterone are shown in Table 12-1. Abiraterone's major toxicity is related to depletion of glucocorticoids. Thus replacement doses of prednisone (5 mg twice per day) are required to prevent excess mineralocorticoid, hyperkalemia, fluid retention, and hypertension.

The mechanisms of resistance to GnRH agonists and to receptor inhibitors are not clearly delineated. Resistant cells may develop androgen receptor mutations that allow the small molecule receptor inhibitors, particularly calutamide, nilutamide, and flutamide, to act as agonists (9). In other instances, activation of the phosphoinositol-3 kinase pathway may activate the androgen/receptor complex independent of receptor occupancy (10, 11). Androgen receptor splice variants that activate the receptor complex constitutively, independent of ligand, may also confer resistance (11).

REFERENCES

1. Huggins C, Hodges CV. Studies on prostate cancer. I. The effects of castration, of estrogen, and of androgen injection on serum phosphatases in metastatic carcinoma of the prostate. *Cancer Res.* 1941; 1: 293–297.

2. Sharifi N, Gulley JL, Dahut WL. Androgen deprivation therapy for prostate cancer. *J Am Med Assoc.* 2005; 294: 238–244.

3. Weckermann D, Harzmann R. Hormone therapy in prostate cancer LHRH antagonists versus LHRH analogues. *Eur Urol.* 2004; 46: 279–284.

4. Prostate Cancer Trialists' Collaborative Group. Maximum androgen blockade in advanced prostate cancer: an overview of randomized trials. *Lancet.* 2000; 355: 1491–1498.

5. Keating NL, O'Malley AJ, Smith MR. Diabetes and cardiovascular disease during androgen deprivation therapy for prostate cancer. *J Clin Oncol.* 2006; 24: 4448–4456.

6. Smith MR, Finkelstein JS, McGovern FJ, et al. Changes in body composition during androgen deprivation therapy for prostate cancer. *J Clin Endocrinol Metab.* 2002; 87: 599–603.

7. Shahinian VB, Kuo YF, Freeman JL, Goodwin JS. Risk of fracture after androgen deprivation for prostate cancer. *N Engl J Med.* 2005; 352: 154–164.

8. Scher, H, Fizazi K, Saad F, et al. Increased survival with enzalutamide in prostate cancer after chemotherapy. *N Engl J Med.* 2012; 367: 1187–1197.

9. Taplin ME, Balk SP. Androgen receptor: a key molecule in the progression of prostate cancer to hormone independence. *J Cell Biochem.* 2004; 91: 483–490.

10. Majumder PK, Sellers WR. Akt-regulated pathways in prostate cancer. *Oncogene.* 2005; 24: 7465–7474.

11. Ferrakdeschi R, Pezaro C, Karavasilis V, and de Bono J. Abiraterone and novel antiandrogens: overcoming castration resistance in prostate cancer. *Annu Rev Med.* 2013; 64: 8.1–8.13.

CHAPTER **13**

Interferons

Dan L. Longo

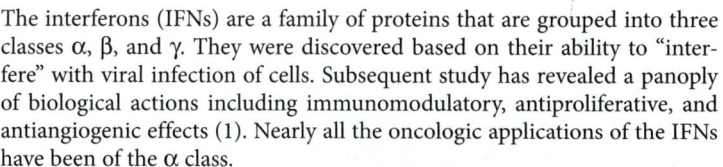

The interferons (IFNs) are a family of proteins that are grouped into three classes α, β, and γ. They were discovered based on their ability to "interfere" with viral infection of cells. Subsequent study has revealed a panoply of biological actions including immunomodulatory, antiproliferative, and antiangiogenic effects (1). Nearly all the oncologic applications of the IFNs have been of the α class.

The α and β IFNs are encoded by a series of genes on chromosome 9p. At least 12 varieties of α IFN exist. A product composed of several species of α IFN produced by stimulated lymphoblasts exists (Wellferon, Burroughs Wellcome), but the predominant forms of IFN in clinical use are recombinant molecules of a single species of α, specifically α2. IFN-α2 is 165 amino acids in length with a molecular weight of about 23 kD. IFN-α2a (Hoffmann-La Roche) differs from IFN-α2b (Schering-Plough) by a single amino acid; IFN-α2a has a lysine at position 23, and IFN-α2b has an arginine. IFN-β has no established role in cancer treatment but is widely used to suppress relapses in multiple sclerosis.

IFN-γ maps to chromosome 12, is 143 amino acids in length, and has minimal sequence homology with IFNs α and β. Its cellular receptor is distinct from the receptor for IFNs α and β, but both types of receptors are widely expressed on all nucleated cells and tissues. Each cell expresses 100–2000 receptors, and the binding constants (K_d) are between 10^{-11} and 10^{-9} M. The α receptor has two chains, one of which is associated with Tyk2 tyrosine kinase and one with JAK1 kinase (2). The genes for the α receptor map to chromosome 21q22.1. The γ receptor also has two chains, one of which is associated with JAK1 kinase and one with JAK2 kinase. The γ receptor genes are on chromosome 6q. Figure 13-1 shows the two forms of receptor for the three classes of IFNs.

IFNs have been approved for use in seven types of cancer, several viral diseases, an autoimmune disease (multiple sclerosis; IFN-β), and an immune deficiency disease (chronic granulomatous disease; IFN-γ) (Table 13-1). In addition to the tumors listed in Table 13-1, IFN-α also has antitumor activity in cutaneous T-cell lymphoma. However, for most of these cancers, IFN is a second- or third-line alternative.

MECHANISM OF ACTION

The wide range of biologic effects of the IFNs has made it difficult to determine a single central mechanism of action. The fact that responses appear to correlate roughly with dose suggests that direct antitumor mechanisms

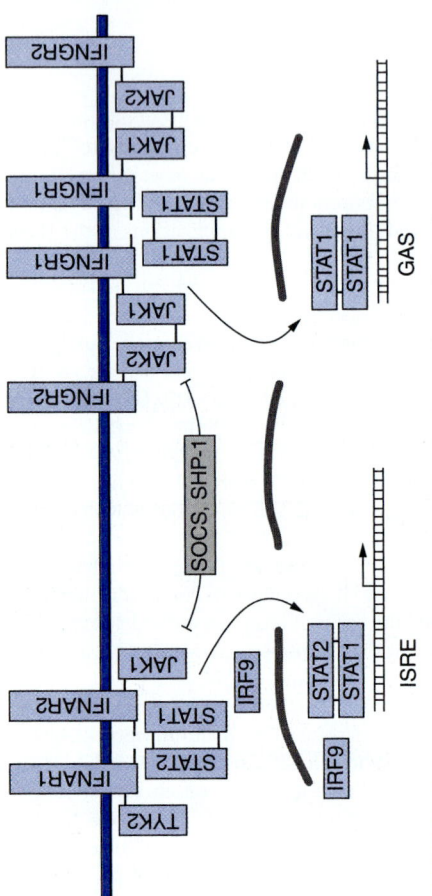

FIGURE 13-1 Components of the interferon (IFN) signaling pathways. The major components responsible for relaying IFN-mediated signals from the cell surface to the regulatory elements of IFN-stimulated genes are represented. GAS, IFN-γ activated site; IFNAR, IFN-α receptor; IFNGR, IFN-γ receptor; ISRE, IFN-stimulated response element; JAK, Janus kinase; SHP, src-homology 2 domain-containing protein tyrosine phosphatase; SOCS, suppressor of cytokine signaling; STAT, signal transducer and activator of transcription; Tyk, JAK family kinase. Small black bars represent tyrosine residues that become phosphorylated and induce complex formation.

TABLE 13-1 USES FOR INTERFERON

Cancers
    Hairy cell leukemia
    Follicular lymphoma
    Myeloma
    Chronic myeloid leukemia
    Kaposi's sarcoma
    Renal cell carcinoma
    Melanoma

Viruses
    Hepatitis C
    Hepatitis B
    Herpes keratitis
    Papillomavirus infections
        Genital warts
        Laryngeal warts

Myeloproliferative syndromes
    Essential thrombocytosis

predominate. IFN-α and IFN-β may exert direct antitumor effects and are capable of boosting mainly innate host defenses. IFN-γ appears to have minimal direct effects on tumor cells but is a potent mediator of effects on immune cells. As a cytokine produced by CD4+ Th1 cells, IFN-γ promotes cytolytic activity from CD8+ cytotoxic T cells. Cells exposed to IFNs are induced to express literally hundreds of new gene products (see http://www.lerner.ccf.org/labs/williams/der.html). They induce cyclin-dependent kinase inhibitors to cause cell cycle arrest and induce FAS and caspases, components of apoptosis pathways (3). IFNs also induce alterations in host defenses. They increase CD8+ cytotoxic T-cell activity, increase NK activity, and stimulate macrophages and dendritic cells. They induce an upregulation of class I MHC molecules in tumors, which could result in more effective recognition of target cells by cytotoxic T cells. In addition, IFNs induce the expression of some known tumor-associated antigens. Many cell effects of IFNs are mediated through the action of a family of proteins called IFN regulatory factors (IRFs) (4). IFNs also inhibit the expression of basic fibroblast growth factor and vascular endothelial growth factor, cytokines involved in tumor angiogenesis.

The in vivo mechanisms of action have not been defined. When biological effects of IFN are measured in man, the assays usually test levels of neopterin (produced by IFN-stimulated monocytes) or β2-microglobulin (shed by IFN-stimulated cells) in the serum or measure the induction of the IFN-inducible 2–5 oligo A synthetase in mononuclear cells.

PHARMACOLOGY

IFN-α is generally administered intramuscularly or subcutaneously. About 80% of an injected dose is absorbed. It is absorbed with a $t_{1/2}$ of 2–2½ h and eliminated with a $t_{1/2}$ of 3–8 h. An intramuscular dose of 72 million units usually produces peak serum levels of 300–500 U/ml (5). The intravenous administration of 20 million units/m^2 produces peak serum levels of about 2500 U/ml. The maximum tolerated dose of IFN-α depends on the route of administration, the frequency of dosing, the duration of treatment, and the patient's willingness to accept toxicities (see below). Most people can tolerate 3–5 million units 3 times a week on a continuous basis.

Efforts to alter the pharmacokinetics of the molecule have been made by attaching polymers of polyethylene glycol (PEG) to the parent molecule (6). Hoffmann-La Roche attached a 40-kD branched chain molecule of PEG to its IFN-α2a and Schering-Plough attached a 25-kD linear chain of PEG to its IFN-α2b. PEG-IFN-α2a has an absorption half-life of 50 h, an elimination half-life of 65 h, and time to maximum serum concentration of 48–80 h. The maximum tolerated dose for PEG-IFN-α2a is 450 µg per week. PEG-IFN-α2b has an absorption half-life of 4–5 h, an elimination half-life of about 40 h, and a time to maximum serum concentration of 15–44 h. The maximum tolerated dose for PEG-IFN-α2b is around 6 µg/kg per week. These pegylated forms sustain measurable blood levels of IFN over a longer period of time. Pegylation may improve the antiviral efficacy of IFN in hepatitis C treatment, but comparisons of efficacy between native and pegylated IFN preparations have been limited in cancer indications. Unpegylated and pegylated IFN appear to be comparably active in chronic myeloid leukemia (7).

TOXICITIES

IFN induces severe flu-like symptoms including fever, chills, rigors, myalgias, arthralgias, malaise, and somnolence in the initial stages of treatment (Table 13-2). If treatment continues, over time these symptoms abate as a reflection of tachyphylaxis. If the course of therapy is interrupted for even short periods, the flu-like symptoms may return upon restarting IFN treatment. With chronic administration, patients often develop severe fatigue, depression, anorexia, and weight loss. These are the major symptoms that may cause an interruption in the course of therapy. Aside from the systemic and nervous system toxicities, myelosuppression and hepatic toxicity are the major organ toxicities. Hypertriglyceridemia is common. Rare patients, particularly those with T-cell tumors, can develop nephrotic syndrome and acute renal failure. Some patients develop autoimmune disorders such as thyroiditis, and some with preexisting autoimmune disease experience an exacerbation of symptoms on IFN.

Myelotoxicity and hepatic toxicity are generally addressed by lowering the dose. Mood changes may be affected by addition of paroxetine. Hypertriglyceridemia can be managed with gemfibrosil. Mechanisms of the toxicity are actively being investigated (8). A surprising level of tolerance for the fatigue and weakness develops among patients chronically receiving IFN. Many patients report not realizing how tired they were until they stopped the drug. For this reason, patient self-evaluation of toxicity often underestimates the level of functional decline associated with IFN administration.

TABLE 13-2 TOXICITIES ASSOCIATED WITH INTERFERON

Acute
    Fever
    Chills and rigors
    Malaise
    Somnolence
    Myalgias
    Arthralgias
    Neutropenia
    Thrombocytopenia
    Anemia
Chronic
    Fatigue
    Depression
    Exhaustion
    Anorexia
    Weight loss
    Sleep disturbances
    Transaminase elevations
    Hypertriglyceridemia
    Nephrotic syndrome
    Development of or exacerbation of preexisting autoimmune disease

INTERFERON RESISTANCE

Resistance to IFN has not been extensively studied. Cellular resistance can be mediated by defects in STAT1 signaling, downregulation of IFN receptors, increased expression of SOCS or SHP1 proteins (these alter IFN signaling), and increased expression of antiapoptotic proteins such as BCL-2. Viruses have adopted a number of mechanisms to resist IFN effects. For example, EBNA-2 of the Epstein-Barr virus and E1A of adenovirus can both inhibit the cellular response to IFN. However, the mechanisms that make most human cancers IFN resistant are not defined.

The development of resistance to IFN in a patient who was responding to it can signal the development of neutralizing anti-IFN antibodies (9). In one study, 16 of 51 patients chronically receiving IFN developed neutralizing antibodies and 6 of the 16 with antibodies acquired IFN resistance. Every patient who had initially responded to IFN and then stopped responding had neutralizing antibodies.

Aggregated forms of IFN are believed to be responsible for the development of antibodies.

REFERENCES

1. Pestka S, Krause CD, Walter MR. Interferons, interferon-like cytokines, and their receptors. *Immunol Rev.* 2004; 202: 8–32.

2. Darnell JE, Jr, Kerr IM, Stark GR. Jak-STAT pathways and transcriptional activation in response to IFNs and other extracellular signaling proteins. *Science.* 1994; 264: 1415–1421.

3. Stark GR, Kerr IM, Williams BR, et al. How cells respond to interferons. *Annu Rev Biochem.* 1998; 67: 227–264.

4. Taniguchi T, Ogasawara K, Takaoka A, Tanaka N. IRF family of transcription factors as regulators of host defense. *Annu Rev Immunol.* 2001; 19: 623–655.

5. Koon HB, McDermott DF. Cytokine therapy for cancer. In BA Chabner, DL Longo (eds.), "Cancer Chemotherapy and Biotherapy: Principles and Practice," 5th edition, Lippincott Williams and Wilkins, Philadelphia, 2011, pp. 579–604.

6. Zeuzem S, Welsch C, Herrmann E. Pharmacokinetics of peginterferons. *Semin Liver Dis.* 2003; 23(Suppl 1): 23–28.

7. Michallet M, Maloisel F, Delain M, et al. Pegylated recombinant interferon alpha-2b vs recombinant interferon alpha-2b for the initial treatment of chronic-phase chronic myelogenous leukemia: a phase III study. *Leukemia.* 2004; 18: 309–315.

8. Kirkwood JM, Bender C, Agarwala S, et al. Mechanisms and management of toxicities associated with high-dose interferon alfa-2b therapy. *J Clin Oncol.* 2002; 20: 3703–3718.

9. Steis RG, Smith JW II, Urba WJ, et al. Resistance to recombinant interferon alfa-2a in hairy-cell leukemia associated with neutralizing anti-interferon antibodies. *N Engl J Med.* 1988; 318: 1409–1413.

CHAPTER **14**

Cytokines, Growth Factors, and Immune-Based Interventions

Dan L. Longo

Cytokines are soluble proteins or glycoproteins that exert trophic effects on a variety of targets based on the expression of particular ligand-specific receptors on the target. All of the cytokines have not yet been identified; but at this time, more than 80 different molecules have been defined. The same cytokine can exert different effects on different cells and tissues. However, the biochemical consequences within the cell of ligand binding to its cellular receptor are similar among all the targets. A number of cytokines have been evaluated for their antitumor effects including the interferons, interleukin-1 (IL1), tumor necrosis factor, IL4, IL12, and others. The rationale for testing these agents as antitumor agents is twofold. First, many of these agents stimulate cells of the immune system, an effect that could promote the immunological killing of the tumor cells. Second, many neoplastic cells retain the cytokine receptors of their normal counterparts; thus, direct biological and potentially antitumor effects are theoretically possible.

Currently, only interferon-α (Chapter 13) and IL2 are approved for use as anticancer agents. Most other tested cytokines have either had little or no antitumor effect or were too toxic when administered systemically as a pharmacologic agent. In general, cytokines work physiologically as paracrine signals coordinating cellular responses in a localized area of release. It has been estimated that in the course of trying to develop IL2 as a therapeutic agent, we administered more of the agent to a few hundred patients than had been produced physiologically in the courses of their entire lives by every man and woman who ever lived.

INTERLEUKIN-2

Interleukin-2 (IL2) is a glycoprotein composed of 133 amino acids and has a molecular weight of 15 kD. It is structurally related to IL4, IL15, and granulocyte-macrophage colony-stimulating factor (GM-CSF). It is normally produced by stimulated T cells and NK cells and acts to promote the proliferation of activated T cells. Resting T cells do not express IL2 receptors and do not respond to the cytokine.

The IL2 receptor has three components: an α-chain, a 55-kD component, also known as CD25, that has only 13 amino acids located intracellularly and functions mainly in binding to IL2; a β-chain, a 75 kD component with a large intracellular component involved in signaling; and the common γ-chain, a 64-kD component called "common" because it is also a shared signaling component of receptors for IL4, IL7, IL9, IL15, and IL21. IL2 binds to the three-component high-affinity receptor with a Kd of 10 pmol/l; in the absence of the α-chain, IL2 binding is termed intermediate and is about 100-fold reduced. High-affinity receptors are mainly expressed on activated T cells; intermediate affinity receptors are expressed on monocytes and NK cells.

Biologic activity. IL2 stimulates the proliferation of activated T cells and promotes the secretion of cytokines from monocytes and NK cells. The main biologic consequence of IL2 stimulation is an increase in cytotoxicity in both T cells and NK cells. IL2 also has a negative regulatory effect on T cells to prevent them from overexpanding or attacking self as IL2 knockout mice have lymphadenopathy and autoimmunity.

Pharmacology. The serum half-life of IL2 after intravenous administration has an α-phase of about 13 min and a more prolonged β-phase of about 90 min. Peak serum levels vary with the dose; 6×10^6 IU/m^2 by IV bolus produces serum levels near 2000 IU/ml. IL2 has been conjugated to polyethylene glycol to prolong its half-life (α 3 h; β 12½ h), but this form is not FDA approved. It is mainly excreted as an inactive metabolite in the urine. When 6×10^6 IU/m^2 IL2 is administered by continuous infusion, it reaches steady-state levels within 2 h at 123 IU/ml and levels fall rapidly after the infusion is stopped. When 6×10^6 IU/m^2 IL2 is administered subcutaneously, peak serum levels of 32–42 IU/ml are reached within 2–6 h.

Method of administration. Chiron IL2 (aldesleukin) is the only form of IL2 currently FDA approved. It is administered in one of three ways. High-dose IL2 is 600,000 or 720,000 IU/kg administered by IV bolus every 8 h until dose-limiting toxicity is reached or a maximum of 15 doses. Low-dose IL2 is 60,000 or 72,000 IU/kg administered by IV bolus every 8 h for 15 doses. A third regimen is for more chronic administration: 250,000 IU/kg subcutaneously daily for 5 days, then 125,000 IU/kg daily for 6 weeks. Considerable data exist on high-dose and low-dose schedules. Much less information is available on the activity of the subcutaneous regimen. Treatment is generally repeated at least once in responding patients.

Because of its life-threatening toxicities (see below), patients must be carefully screened before embarking on a course of IL2 treatment. Patients should undergo cardiac stress testing, pulmonary function tests, brain MRI, and a thorough physical examination and laboratory testing before treatment. They should have a good performance status (0.1 on ECOG scale), no active infections, and normal renal, hepatic, and thyroid function.

Clinical effects. IL2 was approved for use in metastatic renal cell cancer in 1992 and in metastatic melanoma in 1998 (1, 2). High-dose IL2 produces an overall response rate of about 19% in patients with renal cell cancer; however, 8% of patients get complete responses. Both complete and partial responses appear to be quite durable with median response durations of 8–9 years. Thus, median survival is not affected appreciably, but a subset of patients receives substantial benefit from the therapy. Unfortunately, it is not possible to distinguish in advance patients more likely to respond.

High-dose IL2 produces an overall response rate of 16% in metastatic melanoma and 6% of patients achieve complete responses, many of which are long lasting. Median response duration is about 5 years.

The role of high-dose therapy versus low-dose therapy is controversial. Many argue that response rates are the same with the two regimens. However, response durations do not seem to be as durable when low-dose IL2 is used, at least in some studies. Other groups have not seen dramatic differences in efficacy between high- and low-dose regimens, but all groups have noted dramatic differences in toxicities. The mechanism of action of IL2 against these cancers is undefined.

A novel use for IL2 has been developed as more information has emerged about T-cell subsets and their function. A subset of CD4+ T cells known as regulatory T cells (Tregs) are CD25+ and express the FoxoP3 transcription factor. These cells function to suppress T-cell mediated immune responses. Daily administration of IL2 at a dose of 10^6 IU/m^2 is effective in some autoimmune diseases such as chronic graft-vs-host disease and hepatitis C-induced vasculitis (3).

Toxicities. The toxicities from IL2 are life-threatening and are dominated by the capillary leak syndrome (4). Intravascular fluid leaks into the extravascular space, tissues, and alveoli of the lungs. As a consequence, patients develop hypotension, edema, respiratory difficulties, confusion, tachycardia, oliguric renal failure, and electrolyte abnormalities including hypokalemia, hypomagnesemia, hypocalcemia, and hypophosphatemia.

Patients may also experience nausea and vomiting, fever, chills, malaise, and thrombocytopenia. Diarrhea, abnormal liver functions, and neutropenia may occur. Patients often develop a pruritic skin rash over most of the body. Hypothyroidism may also occur. Arrhythmias are a rare complication.

Despite the severity and widespread distribution of the toxic effects of IL2, nearly all the toxicities are reversible within 24–48 h of stopping the drug.

DENILEUKIN DIFTITOX (IL2-DIPHTHERIA HYBRID TOXIN)

Mechanism of action. The fusion protein delivers a potent cellular toxin (diphtheria) to CD25-expressing malignant cells inhibiting cellular protein synthesis and leading to cell death.

Pharmacology. Following the first dose, the agent has a distribution phase half-life of 2–5 minutes and a terminal phase half-life of 70–80 minutes. The development of neutralizing antibodies enhances clearance with subsequent courses.

Administration. Because of infusion reactions, patients are usually premedicated with an antihistamine and acetaminophen before infusion. The drug is given at a dose of 9 or 18 μg/kg/day by IV infusion over 30–60 minutes on 5 consecutive days every 21 days for a total of 8 cycles. The drug is not given if serum albumin levels are less than 3 g/dl.

Toxicity. Hypersensitivity reactions (although most are controllable/preventable by slowing the rate or temporarily interrupting the infusion and treating with antihistamines, acetaminophen, and possibly glucocorticoids, they can be severe or life-threatening); respiratory (dyspnea); gastrointestinal; constitutional (flulike); vascular leak syndrome; rash; elevations of hepatic enzymes (not usually accompanied by other liver abnormalities); renal insufficiency; anemia; thrombocytopenia; hemolysis; proteinuria; and increased risk of infections. Most patients develop antibodies against the toxin/IL2, and these may impact on clearance rates that tend to be two to three times more rapid by the third course. Patients may also lose visual acuity and color vision; thus, these should be monitored during treatment.

Clinical effectiveness. Approved for treatment of persistent or recurrent cutaneous T-cell lymphomas (CTCL) expressing the CD25 antigen (5).

COLONY-STIMULATING FACTORS

The relatively disappointing antitumor efficacy of cytokines has been counterbalanced by the more effective use of a group of cytokines in supportive care of the cancer patient. The lesson learned from these development efforts is that cytokines are more effectively applied to people when they are used to influence their known physiologic targets. Thus, colony-stimulating factors are capable of increasing the production of the cells they normally regulate. However, here, too, we have learned the physiologic limitations of the hematopoietic system. Generally, when we make a patient anemic or granulocytopenic or thrombocytopenic with chemotherapy or radiation therapy, the problem is not that the physiologic response to the cytopenia is limited by poor production of the relevant colony-stimulating factor. Instead the limitation is the number of surviving marrow precursors and the obligate time period for their differentiation into end-stage cells. Thus, even when a cytokine is used to perform its physiologically relevant task, it does not act as a cure-all that erases the prior damage of disease and therapy. Nevertheless, colony-stimulating factors have made a modest contribution to more rapid recovery of blood counts after treatment.

Unfortunately, the magnitude of the effect of colony-stimulating factors has not been sufficient to influence the maximally tolerated doses of myelotoxic agents, a result that was hoped for when these agents were first introduced. However, clinical experience has defined settings in which their use can be beneficial, and guidelines for clinical use have been developed.

■ GRANULOCYTE-COLONY-STIMULATING FACTOR

Granulocyte-colony-stimulating factor (G-CSF) is a 174-amino acid glycoprotein (MW 19,600) encoded by a gene on chromosome 17q11-12 that acts late in myeloid cell differentiation to promote the development of granulocytes. Not only is granulocyte production increased by G-CSF, but the generation of reactive oxygen species by granulocytes is also augmented. Over time additional functions have been uncovered, and its use is now being evaluated in cardiac disease and stroke. It may have a role in suppressing immune reactions.

G-CSF production is usually induced by inflammatory cytokines, and it is produced by fibroblasts, macrophages, and endothelial cells. The receptor for G-CSF is in the cytokine type I receptor family and signals through Janus-like kinase (JAK)/signal transducer and activator of transcription (STAT) pathways.

Biologic activity. When added to bone marrow cell cultures, G-CSF mainly stimulates the development of neutrophils, in contrast to GM-CSF, which induces neutrophil, eosinophil, basophil, monocyte, and dendritic cell development. In addition to increasing neutrophils in the marrow, G-CSF promotes the early release of these cells into the peripheral blood and promotes their ability to phagocytose and kill bacteria. Through the release of metalloproteinases, they also promote the mobilization of hematopoietic stem cells into the peripheral blood.

Pharmacology. Intravenous administration of G-CSF (filgrastim) shows an α-phase half-life of about 8 min and a β-phase half-life of about 2 h. When given subcutaneously, the half-life is 2.5–5.8 h. To prolong the half-life, a 20-kD polyethylene glycol molecule was covalently attached to the N-terminal methionine of filgrastim to produce pegfilgrastim. The half-life of subcutaneously administered pegfilgrastim is 27–47 h.

Method of administration. Filgrastim is generally administered at a dose of 5 µg/kg subcutaneously daily. When given to promote granulocyte recovery, the daily dose is continued until the neutrophil count has increased above 10,000/µl. Pegfilgrastim is usually administered only once at a dose of 100 µg/kg or a total dose of 6 mg subcutaneously. A single dose of pegfilgrastim appears comparable in efficacy to a 10–14 day course of filgrastim. For mobilization of stem cells, the usual dose of filgrastim is 10 µg/kg/day or 5–8 µg/kg twice daily.

Clinical effect. Based on expert opinion and analysis of the world's literature on G-CSF use (6, 7), guidelines have been developed to aid in decision making on who should and who should not receive G-CSF during chemotherapy (Table 14-1). In general, G-CSF is overused in clinical practice.

TABLE 14-1 CLINICAL INDICATIONS FOR NEUTROPHIL
GROWTH FACTORS

Medically necessary

The use of colony-stimulating factors (CSFs) is considered *medically necessary* for patients with cancer with *any* of the following indications:

1. *Primary prophylaxis.* For the prevention of febrile neutropenia (FN) in patients who have a risk of FN of 20% or greater when there are no equally effective regimens not requiring CSFs available. Patients are at high risk based on:
   - Age
   - Medical history
   - Disease characteristics
   - Myelotoxicity of the chemotherapy regimen

2. *For the prevention of FN even when the risk of developing FN is less than 20%* in patients who have other risk factors for FN including any of the following:
   a. Patient age greater than 65 years; or
   b. Poor performance status; or
   c. Previous episodes of FN; or
   d. Extensive prior treatment including large radiation ports; or
   e. After completion of combined chemoradiotherapy; or
   f. Bone marrow involvement by tumor producing cytopenias; or
   g. Poor nutritional status; or
   h. The presence of open wounds or active infections; or
   i. More advanced cancer; or
   j. Other serious comorbidities.

3. *Secondary prophylaxis* with CSFs is recommended for patients who experienced a neutropenic complication from a prior cycle of chemotherapy (for which primary prophylaxis was not received), in which a reduced dose may compromise disease-free or overall survival or treatment outcome. In many clinical situations, dose reduction or delay may be a reasonable alternative.

4. *Use in febrile neutropenic patients.* Adjunctive use with antibiotics in *high-risk, febrile, neutropenic* patients who are at high risk for infection *high-risk, febrile, neutropenic* patients who are at high risk for infection associated complications or have *any of the following* prognostic factors predictive of clinical deterioration:
   a. Expected prolonged (greater than 10 days) and profound (less than $0.1 \times 10^9/l$) neutropenia; or
   b. Age greater than 65 years; or
   c. Uncontrolled primary disease; or
   d. Pneumonia; or
   e. Hypotension and multi organ dysfunction (sepsis syndrome); or
   f. Invasive fungal infection; or
   g. Hospitalized at the time of the development of fever.

(*continued*)

TABLE 14-1 CLINICAL INDICATIONS FOR NEUTROPHIL GROWTH FACTORS (CONTINUED)

5. *Use for dose-dense therapy.* Dose-dense regimens (treatment given more frequently, such as every 2 weeks instead of every 3 weeks) should only be used within an appropriately designed clinical trial or if supported by convincing efficacy data. (For "dose-dense" regimens CSFs are required and recommended by the American Society of Clinical Oncology (ASCO) specifically in the treatment of node positive breast cancer, small cell lung cancer, and diffuse aggressive non-Hodgkin lymphoma.)

6. *Use as adjunct to progenitor cell transplantation.* Administration of CSFs to mobilize peripheral blood progenitor cells (PBPC) often in conjunction with chemotherapy and their administration after autologous, but *not* allogeneic, PBPC transplant.

7. *Use for patients with leukemia or myelodysplastic syndromes.*
    a. *Initial or repeat induction chemotherapy (acute myeloid leukemia [AML]) and consolidation chemotherapy).* For administration shortly after the completion of induction chemotherapy of *AML with patients over* 55 years of age most likely to benefit *or* for patients of any age, after the completion of consolidation chemotherapy for AML. Use of pegylated products for consolidation chemotherapy has not been studied and is not recommended outside clinical trials.
    b. Acute *lymphocytic leukemia (ALL).* In ALL, for administration after completion of the first few days of chemotherapy of the initial induction or first postremission course.
    c. *Myelodysplastic syndromes (MDS).* Intermittent administration of CSF may be considered in a subset of MDS patients with severe neutropenia and recurrent infection.

8. *Use in patients receiving radiation therapy.*

    Radiotherapy. In the absence of chemotherapy, therapeutic use of CSFs may be considered in patients receiving radiation therapy alone if prolonged delays secondary to neutropenia are expected.

9. *Use in older patients.* Prophylactic CSF for patients with diffuse aggressive lymphoma aged 65 years and older treated with curative chemotherapy (CHOP or more aggressive regimens) should be given to reduce the incidence of febrile neutropenia (FN) and infections. (Note. Aside from data available in patients with lymphoma, there is insufficient evidence to support the use of prophylactic CSF in patients solely based on age.)

10. *Use in the pediatric population.*
    a. Will almost always be guided by clinical protocols.
    b. Primary prophylaxis of pediatric patients with a likelihood of FN.
    c. Secondary prophylaxis or therapeutic CSF administration should be limited to high-risk patients. (*Note.* The potential risk for secondary myeloid leukemia or MDS associated with CSF is a concern in children with ALL whose prognosis is otherwise excellent. For these reasons, use of CSF in children with ALL should be with caution.)

TABLE 14-1 CLINICAL INDICATIONS FOR NEUTROPHIL
GROWTH FACTORS (CONTINUED)

11. *Use for radiation injury.* Current ASCO recommendations for the management of patients exposed to lethal doses of total body radiotherapy or accidental total body radiation include the administration of CSF or pegylated G-CSF. This recommendation is based on observation of cases in the Radiation Emergency Assistance Center Training Site in the Radiation Accident Registry Center (REAC/TS registry).

12. *Special comments by ASCO on comparative clinical activity of G-CSF and GM-CSF.* According to ASCO, no guideline recommendation can be made regarding the equivalency of the two colony-stimulating agents, G-CSF and GM-CSF. Further trials are recommended to study the comparative clinical activity, toxicity, and cost effectiveness of G-CSF and GM-CSF.

In addition to the ASCO Guidelines above, CSF agents have other FDA approval or compendia listed indications or orphan drug status including:

1. Chronic administration to reduce the incidence and duration of sequelae of neutropenia (e.g., fever, infections, oropharyngeal ulcers) in symptomatic patients with *congenital neutropenia, cyclic neutropenia, or idiopathic neutropenia.* (FDA approved for Neupogen and included in USPDI for Leukine.)

2. Designated an orphan drug by FDA for the treatment of HIV-infected patients who, in addition, are afflicted with cytomegalovirus retinitis and are being treated with myelosuppressive antiretroviral medication (e.g., ganciclovir; see chart below for off-label compendia).

3. Treatment of moderate to severe aplastic anemia (see chart below for off-label compendia).

4. Treatment for neutropenia associated with HIV infection and antiretroviral therapy (see chart below for off-label compendia).

5. Treatment of drug induced neutropenia (see chart below for off-label compendia).

FDA-Approved Indications for CSFs (Package Labeling, 2002–2005)

Indication	Neulasta (filgrastim)	Neulasta (pegfilgrastim)	Leukine (sargramostim)
Use following induction chemotherapy in AML	×		×
Use in mobilization and following transplantation of autologous PBPC	×		×
Use in myeloid reconstitution after autologous or allogeneic (allogeneic not recommended by ASCO) bone marrow transplantation	×		×
Use in bone marrow transplantation failure or engraftment delay			×

(*continued*)

TABLE 14-1 CLINICAL INDICATIONS FOR NEUTROPHIL GROWTH FACTORS (CONTINUED)

FDA-Approved Indications for CSFs (Package Labeling, 2002–2005)

Indication	Neulasta (filgrastim)	Neulasta (pegfilgrastim)	Leukine (sargramostim)
To decrease incidence of febrile neutropenia in pts with non-myeloid malignancies receiving myelosuppressive chemotherapy associated with a clinically significant incidence of febrile neutropenia	×	×	
For chronic administration to reduce the incidence and duration of sequelae of neutropenia in symptomatic pts with congenital neutropenia, cyclic neutropenia, or idiopathic neutropenia	× ×		
Orphan drug status. AIDS patients with cytomegalovirus retinitis being treated with ganciclovir	×		

Off-label uses listed in compendia (AHFS Online Database, 2005; USPDI Online Database, 2005)

Drug	Indication	Listed in compendia (USPDI or AHFS)
Sargramostim	Chemotherapy-induced neutropenia	USPDI AHFS
Filgrastim	Myeloid engraftment following BMT failure or delay	USPDI
Filgrastim	Myeloid engraftment following hematopoietic stem cell transplant	USPDI
Filgrastim and sargramostim	Neutropenia associated with AIDS	USPDI AHFS
Filgrastim and sargramostim	Myelodysplastic syndromes	USPDI AHFS
Filgrastim and sargramostim	Moderate to severe aplastic anemia	AHFS
Sargramostim	Severe chronic neutropenia (congenital, cyclic, or idiopathic)	USPDI
Filgrastim and sargramostim	Drug-induced neutropenia	USPDI AHFS

TABLE 14-1 CLINICAL INDICATIONS FOR NEUTROPHIL
GROWTH FACTORS (CONTINUED)

Not medically necessary

The use of CSFs is considered *not medically necessary for any of the following*:

1. Routine use in most chemotherapy regimens as prophylaxis; or
2. Receipt of chemotherapy with a risk of febrile neutropenia less than 20% and no significant high risk for complications; or
3. Neutropenic patients who are *afebrile*; or
4. Use as adjunctive therapy to antibiotics in patients with uncomplicated febrile neutropenia, defined as fever less than 10 day duration, no evidence of pneumonia, cellulitis, abscess, sinusitis, hypotension, multiorgan dysfunction, or invasive fungal infection; and no uncontrolled malignancies; or
5. Administration prior to or concurrent with chemotherapy for AML; or
6. Use in relapsed or refractory myeloid leukemia; or
7. Chemo sensitization of myeloid leukemias; or
8. Use to increase the dose intensity of cytotoxic chemotherapy beyond established dosage range for these regimens; or
9. Use in patients receiving concomitant chemotherapy and radiation therapy; particularly involving the mediastinum; or
10. Use either before and/or concurrently with chemotherapy for "priming" effects; or
11. Continued use if no response is seen within 28–42 days (patients who have failed to respond within this time frame are considered nonresponders); or
12. Use in nonchemotherapy-induced infection; or
13. Administration of CSFs to mobilize PBPC after allogeneic PBPC transplant.

Dosage and administration/monitoring

The currently available agents differ in their pharmacokinetic properties. Both sargramostim (Leukine®) and filgrastim (Neupogen®) can be administered intravenously (IV) or subcutaneously (SC), whereas pegfilgrastim (Neulasta®) is administered only SC. Pegfilgrastim is a pegylated form of filgrastim developed to allow for less frequent dosing.

Neulasta® is not labeled for use in leukemias, myelodysplasia, and lymphomas as it has not been studied for this indication. The possibility that pegfilgrastim can act as a growth factor for any tumor type cannot be excluded.

No data support preferential use of filgrastim or pegfilgrastim in the treatment of febrile neutropenia. Similarly, no data support preferential use of filgrastim or sargramostim in the treatment of AML, mobilization of progenitor cells, or following autologous or allogeneic bone marrow transplant. According to the ASCO, no guideline recommendation can be made regarding the equivalency of the two colony-stimulating agents, G-CSF and GM-CSF (Smith, 2006).

Usual doses: filgrastim 5 µg/kg/day; pegfilgrastim 6 mg once; sargramostim 250 µg/m^2/day.

The guidelines suggest that it be used with regimens that have a greater than 20% likelihood of inducing febrile neutropenia. Only a small fraction of frequently used regimens are in this category. Risk of developing febrile neutropenia is reduced by about 50%. In the setting of febrile neutropenia, G-CSF may speed neutrophil recovery by 2 or 3 days. However, its use has not permitted dose escalation of hemotherapy. G-CSF is extremely effective in mobilizing hematopoietic stem cells into the peripheral blood. It is so effective that bone marrow harvest has become unnecessary in the vast majority of stem cell donors. Not only are peripheral blood stem cells easier to collect from the donor, but G-CSF-mobilized cells are also more efficient at reestablishing normal hematopoiesis than bone marrow-derived cells and are associated with shorter periods of neutropenia and thrombocytopenia.

Toxicities. The acute toxicity associated with G-CSF use is minor. A few patients may experience bone pain. In normal individuals receiving G-CSF to mobilize hematopoietic stem cells, rapid splenic enlargement is possible and rare splenic rupture has occurred. Thus, these patients need to be monitored for abdominal or shoulder pain.

More serious concerns are emerging about long-term effects. First, animal studies have shown that the amount of damage to hematopoietic stem cells by cyclic chemotherapy is increased with the use of colony-stimulating factor support to hasten recovery (8). In addition, at least three studies have reported an increase in the incidence of acute leukemia and myelodysplasia when cancer therapy was supported with G-CSF use compared to the incidence with chemotherapy alone (9–11). The precise mechanism of the G-CSF effect is unclear. Possibly, through its antiapoptotic effects, it keeps damaged cells alive that would normally die. Regardless of mechanism, the twofold increased leukemia/myelodysplasia risk is sufficient to motivate clinicians to use the agent more sparingly and only when indicated, especially when cure is the goal.

GRANULOCYTE-MACROPHAGE COLONY-STIMULATING FACTOR

Granulocyte-macrophage colony-stimulating factor (GM-CSF) is a 127-amino acid glycoprotein (MW 22 kD) encoded by a gene on chromosome 5q31 that acts early and late in myeloid cell development. The GM-CSF receptor has a unique α-chain called CSF2R and shares a β-chain with the IL3 and IL5 receptors. It stimulates the common myeloid progenitor to differentiate toward the granulocyte/monocyte progenitor rather than the erthroid/megakaryocyte progenitor, and it stimulates an increase in all the progeny of the granulocte/monocyte progenitor. It also activates granulocytes, monocytes, and macrophages and promotes the antigen-presenting function of dendritic cells. Like G-CSF, it is produced by macrophages, fibroblasts, and endothelial cells, but unlike G-CSF, GM-CSF is also produced by T cells.

Biologic activity. GM-CSF stimulates the production of all three granulocyte types, neutrophils, eosinophils, and basophils. It increases the number of peripheral blood monocytes and supports the differentiation of monocytes into professional antigen-presenting cells called dendritic cells, an activity that has stimulated its testing as a vaccine adjuvant. GM-CSF also improves target killing by antibody-dependent cellular cytotoxicity.

GM-CSF is usually not detectable in the peripheral blood under normal conditions or after the induction of neutropenia. The consequences of its deletion in knockout mice were minor, only a decrease in alveolar macrophages. Thus, GM-CSF is not viewed as a major physiologic regulator of myelopoiesis. Certainly, in its absence, other cytokines are able to stand in for any essential functions it has.

Pharmacology. An intravenously administered dose of GM-CSF (sargramostim) has an α-phase of 5–20 min and a β-phase of 1.1–2.4 h. A subcutaneously administered dose has a half-life of 1.6–5.8 h. A pegylated version of GM-CSF has been generated, but the agent is not approved for use.

Method of administration. Sargramostim is generally given subcutaneously at a dose of 250 $\mu g/m^2$/day for all its indications.

Clinical effect. The clinical effects of GM-CSF mimic those of G-CSF to a large degree. Unfortunately, the agents have not been compared head-to-head. However, in general, the magnitude of the beneficial effects seen with GM-CSF and G-CSF are comparable in magnitude (12). No data suggest that the use of either factor improves the response rate, response duration, or overall survival. GM-CSF has also been used as a vaccine adjuvant and appears to be capable of stimulating both antibody and cellular responses to mildly immunogenic proteins such as idiotypic determinants on immunoglobulin molecules (13).

Toxicities. GM-CSF shares the property of G-CSF to induce bone pain in some patients. In general, GM-CSF is associated with more systemic symptoms than G-CSF including more fevers, muscle aches, and fluid retention. Because of their similar effects on neutrophil counts, G-CSF is used more commonly because of the perception that it produces fewer side effects.

ERYTHROPOIETIN

Erythropoietin (EPO) is a 166-amino acid glycoprotein (MW 21 kD) encoded by a gene on chromosome 7q21 that regulates erythropoiesis. It is produced mainly in the kidney, which senses the level of tissue oxygenation. When levels fall below a certain threshold, hypoxia-inducible factor is produced and acts as a stimulus to produce more EPO. EPO is a hormone that is released by the kidney into the peripheral blood. It binds to the EPO receptor, a 66-kD single-chain molecule expressed on bone marrow erythroid progenitors.

Biologic activity. EPO acts both early and late in red cell production (14). In addition to its effects on the committed erythroid progenitor, it may also exert effects on the early multipotent progenitor cells. EPO suppresses apoptosis and improves the efficiency of red cell production. Additional studies have found that EPO is also produced in neurons and may be involved in protecting hypoxic neurons from cell death (15). Furthermore, EPO appears to exert protective effects on myocardium that has been rendered hypoxic by experimental coronary artery ligation (16). These findings led to clinical trials to evaluate the capacity of EPO to protect hypoxic brain and heart that have thus far been negative (17, 18).

Pharmacology. An intravenously administered dose of EPO in the form of epoetin has a serum half-life of 4–11 h. Subcutaneous administration leads to a more prolonged and more variable kinetics with a half-life of 9–38 h.

Glycosylation can affect the pharmacokinetics greatly. Site-directed mutagenesis was performed to add two N-glycosylation sites producing the product darbepoetin. Its molecular weight is 23% greater than epoetin, but the serum half-life is prolonged about threefold. An intravenous injection has a half-life of 18–25 h; a subcutaneous injection has a half-life of 33–49 h.

Method of administration. The usual dose of epoetin in patients with cancer is 100–150 U/kg administered subcutaneously 3 times weekly. The usual dose of darbepoetin is 200 μg administered once every 2 weeks. No specific level of hemoglobin is used to trigger the intervention. Many physicians intervene when the hemoglobin level falls to 8 g/dl. In the face of cormorbid lung disease or heart disease, a threshold of 10 g/dl may be more appropriate.

Clinical effect. The patients who respond best to EPO have low levels of circulating endogenous EPO and adequate supplies of iron, B_{12}, and folate. In the setting of renal failure, EPO has been very effective at reducing transfusion requirements and improving quality of life. However, in cancer patients, the slow response to EPO has made it difficult to show any influence on the usual efficacy endpoints of response rates, response durations, and survival. Instead, its FDA approval was based on softer quality-of-life data (19, 20). In the absence of complicating factors, a typical patient may get a 1–2 gm/dl increase in hemoglobin over 6–8 weeks of EPO administration. However, an increasing body of data suggests that EPO administration adversely affects the efficacy of concomitantly administered chemotherapy and protects the tumor from chemotherapy-induced killing. Randomized studies in patients with head and neck cancer, lung cancer, and breast cancer have demonstrated poorer response rates and shorter periods of remission in the group of patients receiving chemotherapy or chemotherapy plus radiotherapy together with EPO than in the group of patients receiving the same antitumor treatment without EPO (21). Accordingly, it appears that EPO use should be confined to the palliative care setting and should not be used in patients in whom the goal of therapy is to cure the disease.

Toxicities. EPO is relatively free of toxic symptoms. When the hemoglobin level gets as high as 12 gm/dl, EPO should be stopped because continued use in the setting of hemoglobin levels of 12 gm/dl or above can be associated with hypertension, polycythemia, and thromboembolic disease.

INTERLEUKIN-11

Interleukin-11 (IL11) is a 178-amino acid nonglycosylated protein (MW 23 kD) encoded by a gene on chromosome 19q13 that stimulates thrombopoiesis. Its receptor is a double-chain molecule with a unique α-chain and a second chain called gp130 that it shares with IL6 and leukemia inhibitory factor (LIF). It is produced by bone marrow-derived stromal cells, fibroblasts, and epithelial cells. It plays a critical role in placental and fetal development as IL11 receptor knockout mice fail to develop. IL11 appears to be involved in implantation of the embryo into the endometrium.

Biologic activity. IL11 causes the proliferation of hematopoietic stem cells and megakaryocyte precursors and promotes platelet development independent of thrombopoietin. Some evidence suggests that it may also be a growth factor for hybridomas in vitro. IL11 has also been an agent of interest in inflammatory bowel disease because of its therapeutic effects to minimize bowel inflammation probably through inhibitory effects on the production of proinflammatory cytokines, particularly by monocytes/ macrophages (22, 23).

Pharmacology. Oprelvekin is administered subcutaneously and has a half-life of about 7 h.

Method of administration. Oprelvekin is administered at a dose of 50 µg/ kg/day beginning the day after chemotherapy in a setting where throm-bocytopenia is an expected toxicity. The agent is given daily for periods of 10–21 days until the platelet count reaches 50,000/µl. Treatment should be discontinued at least 2 days before the start of the next treatment cycle.

Clinical effect. The administration of oprelvekin to women with breast cancer who had experienced thrombocytopenia in a prior cycle reduced the requirement for platelet transfusion by about 25%. Of the 96% of women who experienced thrombocytopenia with the drugs alone, the need for platelet transfusion was noted in 70% of those who had received oprelvekin (24). A much more exciting possibility for IL11 is its application to inflam-matory bowel disease where early clinical testing documented a response rate of over 40% (25).

Toxicities. Oprevelkin may produce fatigue, myalgias, arthralgias, and fluid retention with weight gain. The majority of treated patients have fluid retention. Rare patients develop atrial arrhythmias or syncope.

ELTROMBOPAG

Eltrombopag is a biphenyl hydrazine (MW 565) that interacts with the transmembrane domain of the thrombopoietin receptor (cMpl). It is orally bioavailable and stimulates platelet production. The number of megakaryo-cytes and their production of platelets are both enhanced by the promotion of signaling through cMpl.

Pharmacology. After oral administration, the drug achieves a peak concentration in plasma in 2–6 h. Administration with antacids or other sources of divalent cations (e.g., calcium in dairy products) decreases absorption. It is eliminated by the fecal route and metabolized by oxidation and glucuronidation. The metabolism is slower in people of Asian descent.

Method of administration. Eltrombopag is given at a starting dose of 50 mg/day on an empty stomach. If the platelet count is still less than $50K/mm^3$ at 2 weeks, the dose may be increased to 75 mg/day, but not higher. If no response is seen after 4 weeks of treatment, the drug should be discon-tinued. If the platelet count increases above $200K/mm^3$, but less than $400K/mm^3$, the dose may be reduced to 25 mg/day and the platelets rechecked in 2 weeks. If the platelet count exceeds $400K/mm^3$, stop the drug and monitor the platelet count twice a week until the count decreases below $200K/mm^3$ and then restart at a dose 25 mg lower.

Clinical effect. The majority of patients treated with eltrombopag experi-ence an increase in their platelet count within 2 weeks. If the drug is given in support of chemotherapy, it should be stopped 2 or 3 days before the next cycle. No published randomized clinical trials demonstrate efficacy in this setting (the drug has been applied mainly to treat immune thrombo-cytopenia), but clinical experience has suggested that platelet nadirs from chemotherapy can be shortened.

Toxicities. Eltrombopag may cause hepatotoxicity; liver function tests should be carefully monitored. The drug is discontinued of the transaminase level exceeds three times the upper limits of normal. Eltrombopag inhibits the OATP1B1 transporter and may result in increased levels of agents that use this transporter, such as statins.

ROMIPLOSTIM

Romiplostim is an Fc peptide fusion protein (peptibody) produced in *Escherichia coli*; it has two identical single-chain subunits, each of which contains a human IgG1 Fc domain linked at its C-terminus to a peptide comprising two thrombopoietin receptor binding domains. The molecule has no amino acid homology with thrombopoietin, thereby reducing the risk of the development of anti-thrombopoietin neutralizing antibodies, a problem that limited the use of authentic thrombopoietin in patients.

Pharmacology. The pharmacology of the agent is variable. It is administered subcutaneously and achieves peak serum concentrations a median of 14 h later (range 7–50 h) with a half-life of 3.5 days (range 1–34 days). Serum concentrations are not correlated with dose. The agent is cleared faster when the platelet count increases because it binds to the Mpl receptor on platelets.

Method of administration. The drug is administered subcutaneously at a dose of 1 µg/kg once a week and adjusted in 1 µg/kg per week increments up to a maximum dose of 10 µg/kg per week. The drug is not given if the platelet count exceeds 400K/mm^3.

Clinical effect. The drug is active in immune thrombocytopenia. Clinical trials in support of the platelet count in the setting of cancer chemotherapy are ongoing. Most patients respond to the drug with higher platelet production.

Toxicities. Chronic use has led to an increase in reticulin deposition in the marrow, but overt myelofibrosis has not been reported. When the agent is stopped, platelet counts may fall. Platelet counts may increase to a level that promotes thromboembolic complications. Decreasing responses may be due to development of neutralizing antibodies.

Other hematopoietic growth factors are being explored for clinical application, including stem cell factor and FLT-3 ligand. These agents are not currently approved for clinical use.

GROWTH FACTORS

Aside from colony-stimulating factors, most therapeutic strategies that focus on growth factors and their receptors are aimed at blocking the effects of the growth factors. However, growth factors with certain selective properties may be useful in protecting against damage from cancer treatments or in promoting tissue restoration after therapy. A prototype agent is palifermin, keratinocyte growth factor.

■ PALIFERMIN

Palifermin is a 140-amino acid protein (MW 16.3 kD) that differs from endogenous human keratinocyte growth factor by the removal of the first 23 N-terminal amino acids, which improves the stability of the protein. It is a member of the fibroblast growth factor family (FGF7) and binds to keratinocyte growth factor receptor, one of four receptors in the fibroblast growth factor receptor family. The receptor is expressed on epithelial cells of many tissues including the gastrointestinal tract, breast, genitourinary tract, and skin. It is not expressed on hematopoietic cells. It may have trophic effects on involuted thymi.

Biologic activity. Palifermin is produced by mesenchymal cells in response to epithelial injury. When administered to experimental animals, palifermin increases tissue thickness of the tongue, buccal mucosa, and gastrointestinal tract. When given to mice before and after chemotherapy or radiation, palifermin minimized fatalities and reduced weight loss. Palifermin is capable of enhancing the growth of epithelial-derived tumor cell lines in vitro at concentrations >10 µg/ml (generally more than a log higher than levels achieved clinically).

Pharmacology. The elimination half-life of intravenously administered palifermin is about 4.5 h. Levels do not accumulate with three consecutive daily doses. At least a threefold increase in epithelial cell proliferation was detected in healthy subjects who received 40 µg/kg/day for 3 days.

Method of administration. Palifermin is given intravenously on three consecutive days before exposure to the toxic regimen (chemotherapy, radiation therapy, or both) and on 3 consecutive days after treatment at a dose of 60 µg/kg/day. Treatment is given on 6 days.

Clinical effect. Summaries of pivotal clinical trial results are included in the FDA-approved product label (26). Among patients undergoing high-dose therapy and bone marrow transplantation, palifermin reduced duration of grade 3/4 mucositis from 9 to 3 days, reduced incidence of grade IV mucositis from 62% to 20%, and reduced requirement for pain medication by 60% (27). Furthermore, despite the concern about potential adverse effects on growth of carcinomas, palifermin has been applied to the supportive care of patients with colorectal cancer undergoing fluorouracil-based chemotherapy (28). Oral mucositis was dramatically reduced by the use of palifermin, and dose modifications were required in only 14% of the group receiving palifermin compared to 31% of placebo controls. A number of useful supportive measures can further ameliorate the unpleasant consequences of mucositis in patients undergoing cancer treatment (29).

Toxicities. The main toxic effects were grade 3 skin rashes in 3% of patients. Some patients also noted some discoloration of the tongue or mild dysesthesia. Rare patients complained of altered taste. No permanent or life-threatening toxicities were noted.

APPROACHES TO CANCER TREATMENT AND PREVENTION BASED ON ELICITING ANTIGEN-SPECIFIC IMMUNITY

A major goal of oncologists has been to find methods of activating host defenses in the effort to eliminate cancer. The awesome destructive power of the immune system is undeniable, given the consequences of its overactivity in conditions like severe rheumatoid arthritis or multiple sclerosis. We also see the antitumor effects of the immune system in graft-vs-tumor effects that are seen in patients undergoing allogeneic bone marrow transplantation. Those positive effects can be boosted and renewed in some patients with donor lymphocyte infusions. However, despite substantial efforts, not many tumor antigen-specific approaches to cancer therapy are active components of our therapeutic armamentarium. We shall briefly review some promising strategies.

INFECTIOUS DISEASE VACCINES

A number of cancers are known to be caused by infectious agents. Epstein-Barr virus causes lymphomas and nasal lymphoepitheliomas. HTLV-I causes adult T-cell leukemia. *Helicobacter pylori* causes gastric lymphoma and probably some gastric adenocarcinomas. The list of potential targets for vaccine development is quite large. The power of this approach is substantial. Liver cancer from hepatitis B is a major health hazard, particularly in Asia. The institution of a mandatory hepatitis B vaccination program in Taiwan in the 1990s reduced the prevalence of chronic hepatitis B infection in children by over 90% (30).

The newest vaccine that should have cancer preventive activity is the quadrivalent vaccine against the human papillomavirus (HPV) called Gardasil. The vaccine is composed of virus-like particles that express the major capsid protein L1 from four HPV types: 16 and 18 that account for about 70% of cases of cervical cancer and 6 and 11 that account for about 90% of venereal warts (31). An aggressive vaccination campaign should eliminate these types from the population. The question then is whether this would translate into fewer cases of cervical cancer and venereal warts or whether other virus types would emerge to take the place of the eliminated ones.

Additional targets for vaccine approaches to cancer prevention that would make a major impact on cancer incidence worldwide should include hepatitis C, Epstein-Barr virus, and *H. pylori*.

CANCER VACCINES

While cancer prevention by targeting infectious etiologic agents is a clever use of the immune system, the capacity to elicit antitumor immunity in a tumor-bearing host is a challenge we have not yet mastered. The problems are daunting. First, tumor cells are not dramatically different from normal cells; thus, finding a way to attack them uniquely is difficult. One might find a way to activate the immune system that does not distinguish between tumor cells and normal cells. Second, the tumors have undergone several adaptations to protect themselves against host immune attack. They sometimes fail to express major histocompatibility determinants, the molecules through which T cells recognize a target. They erect barriers to penetration by developing high levels of interstitial pressure. Thus, a T cell trying to get into a tumor has to navigate the various natural membrane barriers plus push against a pressure gradient that can be as high as or higher than systolic blood pressure. If the cell manages to overcome those odds, tumors can express Fas ligand, which will kill the T cell where it stands. In addition to these serious local barriers to the immune system, tumors make soluble factors that interfere with the antigen-presenting function of dendritic cells, polarize T cells to the less helpful Th2 phenotype (for making antibody) and away from the more helpful Th1 phenotype (for making cytotoxic cells), and alter the signal transduction machinery making the T cells difficult to activate. In short, efforts at activating the immune system of a tumor-bearing host are like whipping a dead horse.

Nevertheless, if we can define the barriers, we may be able to design strategies to overcome them. Many clever approaches are being tested.

Given the apparent success of allogeneic bone marrow transplantation, one idea has been to vaccinate the normal donor against the tumor and adoptively transfer an immune system that may have an even more powerful and specific antitumor effect. Anecdotal reports have been promising (32), but a systematic evaluation of the strategy is needed.

Another strategy to boost the immune response is to perform the immunization during a period of lymphopenia. Several experimental models have documented that vaccine responses are more robust in animals undergoing homeostasis-driven lymphocyte expansion after a lympholytic stimulus (33). Additional data suggest that it would be wise to selectively deplete CD4+ CD25+ regulatory T cells to boost a vaccine response.

Many investigators are focusing more on the composition of the vaccine than on the immunologic environment into which it will be introduced. Accordingly different investigators favor proteins or peptides as antigens; some use DNA that encode the antigenic determinant; some use DNA encoding both the antigen and an adjuvant molecule such as a chemokine; some pulse dendritic cells with peptides, and some augment the dendritic cells by introducing genes (e.g., GM-CSF) aimed to improve their function. In general, immunologic monitoring of such vaccinations generally shows that tumor-specific T-cell immunity is augmented; but little in the way of an antitumor effect has been seen in cancer-bearing people as a consequence of vaccination strategies.

An exception to this generalization is the work of Bendandi, first at the National Cancer Institute and later at the University of Navarre in Spain (11, 34). In one study, idiotype vaccination of patients rendered disease-free by combination chemotherapy was associated with an immune response, as expected; however, in addition, minimal residual disease detected as persistent cells bearing the t(14;18) translocation disappeared from the blood after vaccination. In a second study of follicular lymphoma patients in relapse, multiple vaccinations following conventional chemotherapy produced longer second remissions than first remissions obtained from either similar or the same chemotherapy. These data suggest that idiotype protein given with GM-CSF not only elicits idiotype-specific T cells, but also those T cells are capable of mediating antitumor effects. This is not the same as seeing a tumor mass shrink under the influence of a vaccine. However, additional evidence for an antitumor effect of the cells comes from an analysis of a relapsed patient. The idiotype of the relapsed tumor was altered; thus, the tumor appeared to have escaped the immune surveillance established by the vaccine.

These results point out an additional problem we will have to face down the line; the emergence of tumor variants that evade detection by altering the antigen that we designed our therapy to attack. The implication of this finding is that we should consider multivalent vaccines that are aimed at more than one tumor antigen, if possible.

A cancer vaccine has been approved for use in the setting of advanced prostate cancer. The vaccine is called sipuleucel T (35) and involves taking antigen-presenting cells from the patient and pulsing them with a fusion protein is composed of prostatic acid phosphatase linked to GM-CSF. These antigen pulsed antigen-presenting cells are then given back to the patient; the pheresis procedure, pulsing, and readministration occurs 3 times 2 weeks apart. Despite the fact that no tumor assessment revealed evidence of a tumor response (size of lesions, PSA level, time to progression), patients receiving the vaccine experienced a median improvement in survival of 4 months. The basis for this improvement is unclear. The study lacked appropriate controls including the administration of antigen-presenting cells pulsed only with GM-CSF.

An additional novel strategy to boost immune effects against tumors is to block the negative regulatory pathways that are designed to prevent the immune system from overreacting to any stimulus. At least two such pathways exist, the CTLA4 regulatory pathway and the PD-1 regulatory pathway. CTLA4 is a homologue of CD28 that is upregulated on activated T cells. It binds to costimulatory molecules CD80 and CD86 on dendritic cells 100 times more efficiently than the physiologic ligand CD28 and the effect of its action is to stop the interaction between the T cell and the antigen-presenting cell and turn off the immune response. Two blocking antibodies to CTLA4 are in clinical trial, ipilimumab (IgG1) and ticilimumab (IgG2). They produce a 15% response rate in metastatic malignant melanoma including complete responses and improve overall survival in metastatic melanoma by 4 months. In addition, responses are sometimes delayed and follow a period of transient tumor expansion as host T cells infiltrate the tumors (36). However, the toxicity profile suggests a breaking of self-tolerance (37). Toxicities include dermatitis, colitis, uveitis, hepatitis, hypophysitis, arthritis, nephritis, and hyperthyroidism. Additional studies are underway using these antibodies to boost vaccine responses and combine them with other targeted therapies.

A second negative regulatory pathway operates in activated T cells. A receptor on T cells called PD-1 (programmed death-1) binds to B7-H1 (also called PD-1 ligand-1 or PD-L1) or to B7-DC (PD-L2) on antigen-presenting cells to inhibit T cell proliferation and function. Antibodies to either PD-1 (nivolumab) (38) or the PD-L1 molecule (39) appear to activate antitumor immune responses and have produced responses in tumor types that are generally refractory to immune therapy, including lung cancer. These studies appear to suggest a reversal of immunologic tolerance to tumors by these agents. Studies are underway to develop combination immunotherapies and to combine these treatments with chemotherapy and targeted agents.

We have chosen not to go into more detail about the specialized studies on adoptive cellular therapies. None is ready to become treatments we need to learn how to give in the office, and the field has been associated with claims that have not withstood efforts at repetition. Suffice it to say that adoptive cellular therapy is an active area of investigation, and based on the successes of allogeneic hematopoietic stem cell transplantation, it seems likely that some adoptive therapy approach will show efficacy as we learn more about the determinants of response. One promising approach worth mentioning is the adoptive transfer of T-cell bearing chimeric antigen receptors. Recombinant receptors containing an antibody molecule and activation domains of molecules involved in T-cell signalling are introduced into T cells and administered in vivo. Responses in a few patients with acute and chronic lymphoid leukemia have been dramatic (40) and point to a novel approach to cancer treatment.

REFERENCES

1. Rosenberg SA. Interleukin 2 and the development of immunotherapy for the treatment of patients with cancer. *Cancer J Sci Am.* 2000; 6 (Suppl 1): S2–S7.

2. McDermott DF. Update on the application of interleukin-2 in the treatment of renal cell carcinoma. *Clin Cancer Res.* 2007; 13: 716s–720s.

3. Koreth J, Matsuoka K, Kim HT, et al. Interleukin-2 and regulatory T cells in graft-vs-host disease. *N Engl J Med.* 2011; 365: 2055–2066.

4. Schwartz RN, Stover L, Dutcher J. Managing toxicities of high-dose interleukin 2. *Oncology.* 2002; 16 (Suppl 13): 11–20.

5. Lansigan F, Stearns DM, Foss F. Role of denileukin diftitox in the treatment of persistent of recurrent cutaneous T-cell lymphoma. *Cancer Manag Res.* 2010; 2: 53–59.

6. Smith TJ, Khatcheressian J, Lyman GH, et al. 2006 update of recommendations for the use of white blood cell growth factors: an evidence-based clinical practice guideline. *J Clin Oncol.* 2006; 24: 3187–3205.

7. Aapro MS, Cameron DA, Pettengell R, et al. EORTC guidelines for the use of granulocyte-colony stimulating factor to reduce the incidence of chemotherapy-induced febrile neutropenia in adult patients with lymphomas and solid tumors. *Eur J Cancer.* 2006; 42: 2433–2453.

8. Hornung RL, Longo DL. Hematopoietic stem cell depletion by restorative growth factor regimens during repeated high-dose cyclophosphamide therapy. *Blood.* 1992; 80: 77–83.

9. Relling MV, Boyett JM, Blanco JG, et al. Granulocyte colony-stimulating factor and the risk of secondary myeloid malignancy after etoposide treatment. *Blood.* 2003; 101: 3862–3867.

10. Smith RE, Bryant J, Decillis A, et al. Acute myeloid leukemia and myelodysplastic syndrome after doxorubicin-cyclophosphamide adjuvant therapy for operable breast cancer: the National Surgical Adjuvant Breast and Bowel Project Experience. *J Clin Oncol.* 2003; 21: 1195–1204.

11. Hershman D, Neugut AI, Jacopson JS, et al. Acute myeloid leukemia or myelodysplastic syndrome following use of granulocyte colony-stimulating factors during breast cancer adjuvant chemotherapy. *J Natl Cancer Inst.* 2007; 99: 196–205.

12. Bohlius J, Reiser M, Schwarzer G, Engert A. Granulopoiesis-stimulating factors to prevent adverse effects in the treatment of malignant lymphoma. *Cochrane Database Syst Rev.* 2004; 1: CD003189.

13. Bendandi M, Gocke CD, Koprin CB, et al. Complete molecular remission induced by patient-specific vaccination plus granulocyte-monocyte

colony-stimulating factor against lymphoma. *Nat Med.* 1999; 5: 1171–1177.

14. Kranz SB. Erythropoietin. *Blood.* 1991; 77: 419–434.

15. Brines ML, Ghezzi P, Keenan S, et al. Erythropoietin crosses the blood brain barrier to protect against experimental brain injury. *Proc Natl Acad Sci USA.* 2000; 97: 10526–10531.

16. Moon C, Krawczyk M, Ahn D, et al. Erythropoietin reduce myocardial infarction and left ventricular functional decline after coronary artery ligation in rats. *Proc Natl Acad Sci USA.* 2003; 100: 11612–11617.

17. Ehrenreich H, Weissenborn K, Prange H, et al. Recombinant human erythropoietin in the treatment of acute ischemic stroke. *Stroke.* 2009; 40: e647–e656.

18. Najjar SS, Rao SV, Melloni C, et al. Intravenous erythropoietin in patients with ST-segment elevation myocardial infarction: REVEAL: a randomized controlled trial. *JAMA.* 2011; 305: 1863–1872.

19. Case DC Jr, Bukowski RM, Carey RW, et al. Recombinant erythropoietin therapy for anemic cancer patients on combination chemotherapy. *J Natl Cancer Inst.* 1993; 85: 801–806.

20. Crawford J, Cella D, Cleeland CS, et al. Relationship between changes in hemoglobin level and quality of life during chemotherapy in anemic cancer patients receiving epoetin alfa therapy. *Cancer.* 2002; 95: 888–895.

21. http://www.fda.gov/cder/drug/infopage/RHE/default.htm

22. Du X, Williams DA. Interleukin 11: review of molecular, cell biology and clinical use. *Blood.* 1997; 89: 3897–3908.

23. Williams DA. Inflammatory cytokines and mucosal injury. *J Natl Cancer Inst Monogr.* 2001; 29: 26–30.

24. Isaacs C, Robert NJ, Bailey FA, et al. Randomized placebo-controlled study of recombinant human interleukin-11 to prevent chemotherapy-induced thrombocytopenia in patients with breast cancer receiving dose-intensive cyclophosphamide and doxorubicin. *J Clin Oncol.* 1997; 15: 3368–3377.

25. Sands BE, Bank S, Sninsky CA, et al. Preliminary evaluation of safety and activity of recombinant human interleukin 11 in patients with active Crohn's disease. *Gastroenterology.* 1999; 117: 58–64.

26. http://www.fda.gov/cder/foi/label/2004/125103lbl.pdf

27. Spielberger R, Stiff P, Bensinger W, et al. Palifermin for oral mucositis after intensive chemotherapy for hematologic cancers. *N Engl J Med.* 2004; 351: 2590–2598.

28. Rosen LS, Abdi E, Davis ID, et al. Palifermin reduces the incidence of oral mucositis in patients with metastatic colorectal cancer treated with fluorouracil-based chemotherapy. *J Clin Oncol.* 2006; 24: 5183–5200.

29. http://www.nci.nih.gov/cancertopics/pdq/supportivecare/oralcomplications/HealthProfessional/page5

30. Shepard CW, Simard EP, Finelli L, et al. Hepatitis B virus infection: epidemiology and vaccination. *Epidemiol Rev.* 2006; 28: 112.

31. Lowy DR, Schiller JT. Prophylactic human papillomavirus vaccines. *J Clin Invest.* 2006; 116: 1167.

32. Kwak LW, Taub DD, Duffey PL, et al. Transfer of myeloma idiotype-specific immunity from an actively immunized marrow donor. *Lancet.* 1995; 345: 1016.

33. Hu HM, Poehlein CH, Urba WJ, Fox BA. Development of antitumor immune responses in reconstituted lymphopenic hosts. *Cancer Res.* 2002; 62: 2914.

34. Inoges S, Rodriguez-Calvillo M, Zabalegui N, et al. Clinical benefit associated with idiotypic vaccination in patients with follicular lymphoma. *J Natl Cancer Inst.* 2006; 98: 1292.

35. Kantoff PW, Higano CS, Shore ND, et al. Sipuleucel-T immunotherapy for castration-resistant prostate cancer. *N Engl J Med.* 2010; 363: 411.

36. Hodi FS, O'Day SJ, McDermott DF, et al. Improved survival with ipilimumab in patients with metastatic melanoma. *N Engl J Med.* 2010; 363: 711.

37. Korman A, Yellin M, Keler T. Tumor immunotherapy: preclinical and clinical activity of anti-CTLA4 antibodies. *Curr Opin Invest Drugs.* 2005; 6: 592.

38. Topalian SL, Hodi, FS, Brahmer JR, et al. Safety, activity and immune correlates of anti-PD-1 antibody in cancer. *N Engl J Med.* 2012; 366: 2443.

39. Brahmer JR, Tykodi SS, Chow LQ, et al. Safety and activity of anti-PD-L1 antibody in patients with advanced cancer. *N Engl J Med.* 2012; 366: 2455.

40. Porter DL, Levine BL, Kalos M, et al. Chimeric antigen receptor-modified T cells in chronic lymphoid leukemia. *N Engl J Med.* 2011; 365: 725.

CHAPTER **15**
Monoclonal Antibodies in Cancer Treatment

Dan L. Longo

Monoclonal antibodies are used in five different ways in the treatment of human conditions. First, antibodies have a variety of effector mechanisms that focus an array of immunologic agents (complement, various effector cells) on the target to which they bind. Second, antibodies can serve as targeting moieties to specifically deliver diverse killing or inhibitory molecules to a specific site. Third, antibodies can be directed at soluble protein or proteoglycan hormones or cytokines or their receptors to antagonize a particular function such as cell growth, invasion, or migration. Fourth, antibodies can be used as antigens to elicit antitumor responses against immunoglobulin-expressing tumors. Fifth, antibodies can be used to alter the pharmacologic behavior of other substances to either increase or decrease their half-life or alter their distribution (e.g., antibodies to digoxin used to treat digoxin toxicity).

Monoclonal antibody technology was developed in 1975 and has been widely applied in biological sciences since then. The first clinical trial of a monoclonal antibody was performed in 1980 and the first FDA approval of a monoclonal antibody for a cancer indication occurred in 1997. Currently 14 monoclonal antibody-based drugs are FDA-approved for therapeutic use; one monoclonal antibody, nofetumomab (NR-LU10, anti-CD56) labeled with technetium-99m is approved for use as an imaging agent in the staging of small-cell lung cancer (it will not be discussed here). Both the list of agents and their approved uses are likely to expand.

ANTIBODY STRUCTURE AND FUNCTION

Antibody structure was initially elucidated by using antibodies as probes of other antibodies. Three sets of determinants were defined. *Isotypes* are determinants that distinguish among the main classes of antibodies of a particular species and are defined by antibodies made in different species. Humans have five main heavy chain isotypes (M, G, A, D, E) and two light chain isotypes (κ, λ). *Allotypes* are small sequence differences or allelic differences between immunoglobulins of the same isotype in different individuals within a species and are defined by antibodies made in the same species. *Idiotypes* are antigenic determinants formed by the antigen-combining site of an antibody that distinguish each clonal B-cell product.

Antibodies are generally composed of four chains, two identical heavy chains (MW ~50,000 Daltons) and two identical light chains (MW ~22–25,000 Daltons). Each chain has a portion with limited sequence variability called the constant region and a portion with extensive sequence variability called the variable region. The heavy and light chains are linked by disulfide bonds and aligned such that the variable regions of the light and heavy chain are adjacent to each other (**Figure 15-1**). A specific antigen is bound by the antibody in the pocket formed by the heavy and light chains. The contact regions between the antigen and the antibody are usually defined by two or three regions of hypervariability within the variable regions. These are called complementarity-determining regions (CDRs).

It is possible to generate an antibody of defined specificity that can bind to nearly any biological molecule by immunizing mice and isolating and immortalizing the B cell that produces the desired antibody. The B cell is then fused to an immunoglobulin nonproducing B-cell line, yielding the monoclonal murine-derived antibodies first used in clinical trials. The efficacy of murine antibodies was found to be limited by several factors. First, murine antibodies cooperate with human effector mechanisms poorly such that important mechanisms like complement fixation and antibody-dependent cellular cytotoxicity were activated weakly or not at all. Second, the human host has developed sophisticated methods to remove animal proteins rapidly from the blood. Therefore, the biological half-life of murine antibodies is short, indeed, much shorter than the biological half-life of human IgG antibodies (~23 days). Third, murine antibodies are themselves

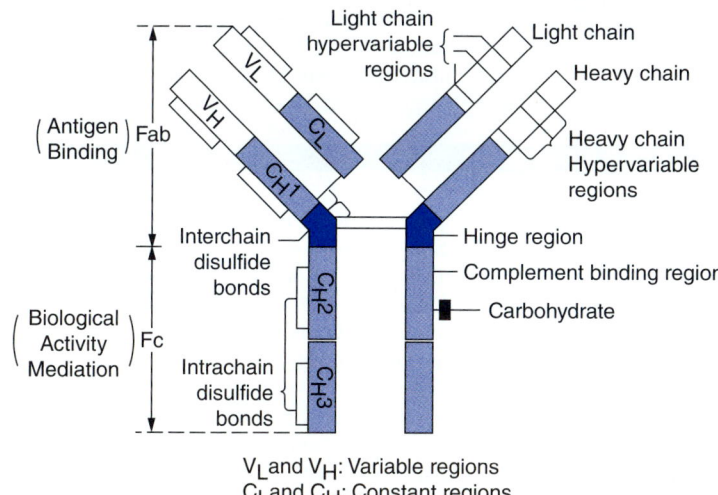

VL and VH: Variable regions
CL and CH: Constant regions

FIGURE 15-1 A schematic depiction of antibody structure and function relationships. (From Wasserman RL, Capra, JD. Immunoglobulins. In MI Horowitz, W Pigman (eds.), *The Glycoconjugates,* Academic Press, New York, 1977, p. 323.)

immunogenic. Thus, human antimouse antibodies to the therapeutic agent result in even more rapid clearance on repeat administration. Other factors that compromised efficacy of early antibody trials were tumor related. Targets were picked that were suboptimal. The target molecule could be shed into the serum and distract the antibody from reaching the cell producing the target. In some cases, target molecules were downregulated such that resistance to the therapeutic antibody emerged.

Many of these problems were addressed in a single technical development; the recombinant production of chimeric antibodies that contained the framework and constant regions of human immunoglobulins with the murine-derived antigen binding portion of the molecule (the variable or hypervariable regions). The first of these chimeric antibodies to gain FDA approval and to become widely used clinically was rituximab, an anti-CD20 antibody. The success of rituximab against lymphoid malignancies derived in large measure from the persistence of the company that owned the rights to it. Based on the rather minor antitumor activity of the murine anti-CD20 antibody, a peer-review process would likely have terminated its clinical development. However, the industrial sponsor took the development a step further and generated a chimeric antibody. That final step corrected nearly all of the defects of the murine antibody and pointed the way to other effective antibodies for clinical use.

The 14 monoclonal antibodies approved for use in patients with cancer are directed at 8 different targets, CD20 (rituximab, ofatumumab, tositumomab, ibritumomab tiuxetan), epidermal growth factor (EGF) receptor (cetuximab, panitumumab), HER2/neu (trastuzumab, pertuzumab, trastuzumab emtansine), CD33 (gemtuzumab ogomycin), vascular endothelial growth factor (bevacizumab), CD52 (alemtuzumab), CD30 (brentuximab vedotin), and CTLA4 (ipilimumab) (**Table 15-1**). Antibodies aimed at dozens of potential targets are in development.

RITUXIMAB (RITUXAN)

CD20, the target of rituximab, is expressed mainly on normal and neoplastic B cells. CD20 is a hydrophobic transmembrane protein of molecular weight 35 kD. CD20 is not expressed on hematopoietic stem cells, pro-B cells or plasma cells, or nonlymphoid tissues. The function of CD20 is unclear; some data have suggested that it functions as a calcium channel. It is not shed or internalized upon antibody binding.

Rituximab is a chimeric IgG1, κ antibody with human constant regions and murine variable regions. Its molecular weight is about 145 kD and it binds CD20 with an affinity of 8 nM. Its antitumor effects are thought to be related to its activation of complement and antibody-dependent cellular cytotoxicity. In addition, signaling through CD20 may activate apoptosis mechanisms. Anti-CD20 improves the antitumor effects of chemotherapeutic agents.

The pharmacokinetics of the agent are influenced by a variety of factors including the tumor burden. Early doses tend to achieve lower serum levels because the tumor and normal B cells bind a larger fraction of an administered dose. The empirically derived treatment schedule is weekly doses of 375 mg/m^2 IV. After the fourth weekly dose, the half-life averages 205 h with a maximum serum concentration of 486 μg/ml. Levels continue to increase with additional weekly administrations. Delivery of rituximab with chemotherapy does not alter its pharmacology. A maximum tolerated dose has not been defined. Doses as high as 500 mg/m^2 are well tolerated. Because of toxicity problems (mainly related to activation of immune effector mechanisms), the drug should be infused at an initial rate of about 50 mg/h.

Toxicities from rituximab are mainly related to the initial infusion. Symptoms generally develop within 30–120 min of starting infusion. In most cases, the symptom complex includes one or more of the following: fever and chills, nausea, pruritis, angioedema, asthenia, headache, bronchospasm, throat irritation, rhinitis, urticaria, myalgia, dizziness, or hypertension. The reactions resolve entirely with either slowing the infusion or temporarily interrupting it. The infusion-related symptoms generally decrease in incidence with each administration from nearly 80% incidence with the first to around 14% with the eighth. Diphenhydramine, acetaminophen, and intravenous fluids are often required to suppress the symptoms. Once symptoms resolve, the administration of rituximab can be reinitiated at about half the rate of the initial infusion. This symptom complex is thought to be largely due to complement activation. The most severe cases can rarely develop adult respiratory distress syndrome, myocardial infarction, ventricular fibrillation, or cardiogenic shock.

Other uncommon problems include the development of tumor lysis syndrome from rapid killing of tumor cells and occasional Stevens-Johnson syndrome with severe mucocutaneous inflammation. When rituximab is administered with chemotherapy, some patients have experienced reactivation

TABLE 15-1 FDA-APPROVED ANTIBODIES FOR CANCER TREATMENT INDICATIONS

Antibody	Target	FDA-Approved indication	Mechanism of action
Trastuzumab (Herceptin®) humanized IgG1	HER2 (ErbB2)	HER2-positive breast cancer, as single agent or in combination with chemotherapy for (i) adjuvant or (ii) palliative treatment; HER2-positive gastric or gastroesophageal junction carcinoma, as first-line treatment in combination with cisplatin and capecitabine/5-FU	Inhibition of HER2 signaling; ADCC
Bevacizumab (Avastin®) humanized IgG1	VEGF	For the palliative treatment of colorectal cancer, non-squamous non-small cell lung cancer, glioblastoma, or renal cell carcinoma	Inhibition of VEGF signaling
Cetuximab (Erbitux®)* chimeric human/murine IgG1	EGFR (ErbB1)	In combination with radiation therapy for the initial treatment of locally or regionally advanced squamous cell cancer of the head and neck (SCCHN); As a single agent for SCCHN patients with whom prior platinum-based therapy has failed; Palliative treatment of pre-treated metastatic EGFR-positive colorectal cancer	Inhibition of EGFR signaling; ADCC
Panitumumab (Vectibix®)* human IaG2	EGFR (ErbB1)	As a single agent for the treatment of pre-treated EGFR-expressing, metastatic colorectal carcinoma	Inhibition of EGFR signaling
Ipilimumab (Yervoy®) IgG1	CTLA-4	For the treatment of unresectable or metastatic melanoma	Inhibition of CTLA-4 signaling
Rituximab (Rituxan® and Mabthera®) chimeric human/murine IgG1	CD20	For the treatment of CD20-positive B cell non-Hodgkin lymphoma (NHL) and chronic lymphocytic leukemia (CLL), and for maintenance therapy for untreated follicular CD20-positive NHL	ADCC; direct induction of apoptosis; CDC
Alemtuzumab (Campath®) humanized IgG1	CD52	As a single agent for the treatment of B cell CLL	Direct induction of apoptosis; CDC

(continued)

177

TABLE 15-1 FDA-APPROVED ANTIBODIES FOR CANCER TREATMENT INDICATIONS (CONTINUED)

Antibody	Target	FDA-Approved indication	Mechanism of action
Ofatumumab (Arzerra®) human IgG1	CD20	Treatment of patients with CLL refractory to fludarabine and alemtuzumab	ADCC; CDC
Gemtuzumab ozogamicin (Mylotarg®) humanized IgG4	CD33	For the treatment of patients with CD33-positive acute myeloid leukemia in first relapse who are 60 years of age or older and who are not considered candidates for other cytotoxic chemotherapy (withdrawn from use in June 2010)	Delivery of toxic payload, calicheamicin toxin
Brentuximab vedotin (Adcetris®) chimeric IgG1	CD30	For the treatment of relapsed or refractory Hodgkin lymphoma and systemic anaplastic lymphoma	Delivery of toxic payload, auristatin toxin
^{90}Y-Ibritumomab Tiuxetan (Zevalin®) murine IgG1	CD20	Treatment of relapsed or refractory, low-grade, or follicular B cell NHL; Previously untreated follicular NHL in patients who achieve a partial or complete response to first-line chemotherapy	Delivery of the radio-isotope yttrium-90
^{131}I-Tositumomab (Bexxar®) murine IgG2	CO20	Treatment of patients with CD20 antigen-expressing relapsed or refractory low-grade, follicular, or transformed NHL	Delivery of the radio-isotope iodine-131; ADCC; direct induction of apoptosis

*Not recommended in colorectal cancer patients whose tumors express mutated KRas of hepatitis B. In general, rituximab is very well tolerated. It only rarely elicits a host antibody response (~1% of patients). The suppression of normal B cells by rituximab is variable in duration depending on the age of the patient and the length of treatment, but most patients recover normal B-cell function within a year of stopping rituximab. No late effects of B-cell suppression have been reported.

Rituximab is effective in nearly all B-cell-derived malignancies that express CD20. It is particularly active when used in combination chemotherapy and has become a component of standard therapy for diffuse large B-cell lymphoma (see the chapter on non-Hodgkin lymphomas). In addition to its standard use in patients with diffuse large B-cell lymphoma, it is also active in follicular lymphoma, mantle cell lymphoma, chronic lymphoid leukemia, and hairy cell leukemia. It is also being used increasingly to treat autoimmune diseases in which autoreactive antibodies play a pathogenetic role (1). These include idiopathic thrombocytopenic purpura, thrombotic thrombocytopenic purpura, autoimmune hemolytic anemia, and some cases of pure red cell aplasia.

OFATUMUMAB (ARZERRA)

Ofatumumab is an IgG1 κ fully human (i.e., not chimeric) monoclonal antibody with specificity for CD20, although it binds an epitope distinct from rituximab. It is approved for use in chronic lymphoid leukemia but is expected to have the same spectrum of antitumor activity as rituximab, given that it attacks the same target. It is thought to kill target cells through complement fixation and activation of antibody-dependent cell-mediated cytotoxicity. Some evidence suggests that it is better at fixing complement and poorer at mediating cellular cytotoxicity than rituximab.

Toxicities include infusion reactions (reduced by premedication with glucocorticoids, acetaminophen, and an antihistamine), neutropenia and thrombocytopenia, infections (especially pneumonia and upper respiratory tract infections), fever, cough, nausea, and diarrhea. The immunosuppression it produces may lead to progressive multifocal leukoencephalopathy or reactivation of hepatitis B.

The agent is cleared mainly by binding to its target. As CD20-bearing cells decrease, its half-life increases. Pharmacokinetics are highly variable, but no adjustments are made based on body weight, age, sex, or creatinine clearance. The antibody is administered as follows: 1. An initial dose of 300 mg; 2. One week later, begin 7 weekly doses of 2000 mg; 3. Four weeks after the seventh weekly dose, give 2000 mg every 4 weeks for 4 doses.

Approval was based on a response rate of 42% among a group of patients with chronic lymphoid leukemia resistant to fludarabine and alemtuzumab (2).

ALEMTUZUMAB (CAMPATH)

CD52, the target of alemtuzumab, is a 21–28 kD cell surface glycoprotein expressed on normal and malignant B and T cells, NK cells, monocytes, macrophages, a subpopulation of granulocytes, as well as a subpopulation of CD34+ bone marrow cells, and on epididymis, sperm, and seminal vesicle, but not on spermatogonia. Its function is unknown. CD52 does not shed or internalize. Alemtuzumab is an IgG1, κ chimeric antibody with human constant and variable framework regions and rat CDRs. It binds to CD52 with a nanomolar affinity and is thought to act through antibody-dependent cellular cytotoxicity.

Alemtuzumab clearance is nonlinear. Its plasma half-life is much shorter for early doses (11 h) than late doses (6 days) presumably because of the depletion of CD52-bearing cells over time. After 12 weeks of doses, the mean AUC is sevenfold higher than the mean AUC after the first dose. No dosage adjustments are required based on age or sex.

Because of infusion-related toxicity, doses are begun at 3 mg/d administered as a 2-h infusion. When infusion-related toxicities are less than or equal to grade 2, the daily dose is escalated to 10 mg. Once that dose is tolerated, one can advance the dose to 30 mg/d. The usual maintenance dose is 30 mg/d 3 times a week, usually a Monday-Wednesday-Friday schedule. Weekly doses exceeding 90 mg total are not recommended because of an increased risk of pancytopenia. Dose escalation from 3 to 30 mg doses can generally be accomplished in a week.

Like rituximab, alemtuzumab is associated with significant infusion-related toxicity with the first dose, decreasing with subsequent administration (3). The symptoms include fever, chills, hypotension, shortness of breath, bronchospasm, and rashes. Rarely the symptoms may progress to adult respiratory distress syndrome, cardiac arrhythmias, myocardial infarction, and heart failure. Routine premedication with diphenhydramine 50 mg and acetaminophen 650 mg 30 min before the infusion is recommended.

The next most common serious toxicity of alemtuzumab is immunosuppression. Because of the widespread expression of CD52 on cells involved in host defenses, patients receiving alemtuzumab become severely immunosuppressed and are susceptible to opportunistic infections such as *Pneumocystic carinii*, aspergillosis and other fungal infections, and intracellular pathogens like *Listeria monocytogenes*. The antibody produces profound lymphopenia. CD4+ T-cell counts do not recover above 200/µl for at least 2 months after stopping treatment and full recovery may take more than 1 year. Antiherpes (acyclovir) and anti-infective (bactrim) prophylaxis is recommended and should be continued until lymphocyte recovery. Opportunistic infections may be seen despite prophylaxis. Because of the immune suppression, patients on alemtuzumab who receive blood products should have those products irradiated to prevent graft-vs-host disease. Patients on alemtuzumab should not receive any live vaccines.

The third serious toxicity associated with alemtuzumab is myelosuppression. Neutropenia, anemia, and thrombocytopenia are common, and rarely patients have developed prolonged and occasionally fatal pancytopenia. The mechanism of the cytopenia may be either direct cytotoxicity or autoimmune; idiopathic thrombocytopenic purpura and autoimmune hemolytic anemia have both been documented. Grade 3 or 4 myelosuppression is noted in 50%–70% of patients.

Nearly 2% of patients receiving alemtuzumab generate antibodies to it, but no adverse effects on toxicity or response have been documented.

The main clinical use for alemtuzumab has been as a salvage therapy for chronic lymphocytic leukemia that is unresponsive to alkylating agents and nucleosides. It is being tested as salvage therapy for other lymphomas and is particularly promising in the treatment of T-cell lymphomas. It is being tested as an immunosuppressive agent in graft-vs-host disease and other conditions of immune hyperreactivity and eosinophilia. It is effective at depleting marrow and peripheral blood collections of T cells in vitro before reinfusing the cells in the setting of allogeneic hematopoietic stem cell transplantation.

BEVACIZUMAB (AVASTIN)

Bevacizumab is an IgG1 recombinant humanized monoclonal antibody that binds to vascular endothelial growth factor (VEGF). The efficacy of the antibody is surprising. Because VEGF is generally secreted locally and acts locally, it would not be expected that a systemically administered antibody to the growth factor itself would achieve relevant concentrations at the sites of production in tissues. The antibody should circulate and be cleared without ever encountering the physiologically relevant VEGF. In general, growth factor receptors make better targets than growth factors themselves because blocking the effects of the ligand at its binding site should be more efficient than attempting to sop up the ligand like a sponge. The proposed mechanism of action of bevacizumab is to prevent the interaction of VEGF with its receptors, Flt-1 and KDR, on the surface of endothelial cells. This should inhibit endothelial cell proliferation and new blood vessel formation and decrease the tumor blood supply. Antiangiogenic drugs also decrease blood vessel permeability, decrease tumor interstitial pressure, and improve delivery of chemotherapy to the tumor.

The half-life of bevacizumab varies according to body weight, sex, and tumor burden; however, the median half-life is around 20 days. The usual dose is 10 mg/kg every 2 weeks. Steady-state serum levels are generally reached by 100 days. It is unknown whether doses need to be adjusted in the setting of renal or hepatic impairment.

Toxicities are overall mild in degree if certain features are monitored and certain clinical situations avoided. Bevacizumab can impair wound healing and has led to wound dehiscences and/or perforations and abscesses in 2%–4% of patients. If possible, the interval between surgery and initiation of therapy should be 4 weeks. After bevacizumab is administered, elective surgery should be delayed at least 4 weeks, if possible, given the 20-day half-life. A second major side effect is bleeding. Mild bleeding in the form of epistaxis occurs in some patients. However, of greater concern is the risk for major pulmonary or gastrointestinal hemorrhage, which has occurred in up to 20% of patients. Active bleeding from the GI tract and hemoptysis are contraindications to bevacizumab use. It should not be used in lung cancer patients with tumor masses that involve the central bronchial airway because of the risk of fatal bronchial hemorrhage. Severe hypertension may also be seen in 7%–10% of patients. The drug should be discontinued if the hypertension cannot be readily controlled. Bevacizumab is also associated with proteinuria in up to 20% of patients, but less than 1% develop nephrotic syndrome. Bevacizumab may also worsen congestive heart failure, particularly in patients who have received antracyclines or radiation therapy involving the heart. Infusion reactions are uncommon and antibodies to bevacizumab have not been documented.

Bevacizumab improves outcome in patients with colorectal cancer and is being tested in a large number of other malignancies (4). Because of the critical and universal role of angiogenesis in cancer biology, bevacizumab is expected to be a useful adjunct to treatment for many types of cancer. Given the success of bevacizumab, antibodies to the VEGF receptor(s) or small-molecular-weight receptor inhibitors may be equally or even more effective therapies.

TRASTUZUMAB (HERCEPTIN)

Trastuzumab is a humanized IgG1 κ antibody that binds to the extracellular domain of HER2/neu, a transmembrane tyrosine kinase growth factor receptor in the EGF receptor family. The target is a 185-kD protein expressed on the surface of about 25% of breast cancers. Tumors with amplification of HER2/neu are generally more refractory to therapy and more aggressive in their rate of progression than HER2/neu-negative tumors. Trastuzumab binding affinity for its target is about 5 nM; it appears to act both by direct tumor growth inhibition and by the activation of antibody-dependent cellular cytotoxicity.

The usual method of administration is to give a loading dose of 4 mg/kg intravenously by 90-min infusion followed by a maintenance dose of 2 mg/kg weekly by 30-min infusion. The mean serum half-life is about 6 days. Steady-state concentrations are achieved between 16 and 32 weeks of therapy with mean trough levels of 79 μg/ml and peak levels of 123 μg/ml. Some patients with HER2/neu-positive breast cancers have detectable levels of soluble receptor in the serum; the presence of circulating target delays the achievement of steady-state levels by a week or two. The disposition of the antibody is not affected by age or renal function. Coadministration with taxanes results in higher trough levels of the antibody (about 50% higher); other chemotherapeutic agents commonly used in breast cancer do not alter trastuzumab clearance.

Trastuzumab produces a 14% response rate when used as a single agent in metastatic HER2/neu-positive (at least 2+ by immunohistology) breast cancer. Responses are more common in patients with higher levels of expression. In combination with chemotherapeutic agents, trastuzumab improves response rates and survival in patients with metastatic disease and improves disease-free and overall survival in the adjuvant setting. In early breast cancer, addition of trastuzumab to adjuvant chemotherapy reduces recurrence rate by 50% and reduces mortality by 30%. In the setting of metastatic disease, addition of trastuzumab to chemotherapy increases response rates by 18%–27%, prolongs disease-free survival by 3–5 months, and improves overall survival by 5–9 months (5).

Adverse reactions from trastuzumab are generally rare. The usual initial infusion reaction from human antibodies occurs in 40% of patients receiving trastuzumab for the first time. The incidence of diarrhea in patients taking trastuzumab alone is about 25%. Use of trastuzumab with myelotoxic chemotherapy may result in an increase in myelosuppression. The most significant toxicity from trastuzumab is heart failure. It occurs in about 4% of patients and affects up to 20% of patients in the setting of past or concurrent treatment with anthracyclines. Patients may present with the usual symptoms and signs of heart failure including dyspnea, peripheral edema, and an S3 gallop. Patients being considered for trastuzumab therapy should undergo thorough baseline evaluation of cardiac function including history, physical exam, electrocardiogram, and an assessment of ejection fraction by echocardiogram or MUGA scan. Advanced age and preexisting cardiac disease increase the risk. Some patients progress to intractable heart failure, but most can be effectively managed by discontinuing the trastuzumab and treating the heart failure. Most of these patients experience gradual improvement in cardiac function with time off therapy. In general, trastuzumab is not withheld in patients with mild decreases in ejection fraction who are asymptomatic. Immunogenicity is low; generally <5% of patients make antibodies to trastuzumab.

Small-molecular-weight inhibitors of HER2/EGFR are in late stages of clinical development and appear to have activity in trastuzumab-resistant patients.

PERTUZUMAB (PERJETA)

Pertuzumab is a recombinant humanized monoclonal antibody that recognizes the extracellular dimerization domain of HER2 and blocks ligand-mediated receptor dimerization with other members of the EGF receptor family. It kills cells by blocking signal transduction through the growth and survival supporting pathways, mitogen-activated (MAP) kinase and phosphoinositidyl-3-kinase (PI3K) pathways. It also mediates antibody-mediated cellular cytotoxicity. This mechanism is distinct from that of trastuzumab, and the combination of pertuzumab plus trastuzumab appears to be more active than trastuzumab alone.

Pharmacokinetics of pertuzumab are linear in the clinically used dose range and the half-life is about 18 days. No dose adjustments are made for body weight or creatinine clearance. Some clinical data suggest that Asian populations may experience more febrile neutropenia with pertuzumab.

Pertuzumab is administered as an intravenous infusion; the first dose is 840 mg given over 60 min. Subsequently, 420 mg is given over 30–60 min every 3 weeks until disease progression. In addition to hypersensitivity to the infusion, toxicities include diarrhea, neutropenia, nausea, fatigue, rash, and peripheral neuropathy. Cardiac effects are rare.

Pertuzumab has single agent activity against HER2+ tumors, but it was approved based on its activity in combination with trastuzumab and docetaxel in metastatic HER2+ breast cancer (6). The combination with pertuzumab increased response rates from 70% to 80% and improved response duration from 12 to 20 months.

TRASTUZUMAB EMTANSINE (KADCYLA)

Trastuzumab emtansine (or ado-trastuzumab emtansine) is an immuno-conjugate between trastuzumab and the maytansine analogue, emtansine, a microtubule inhibitor. It gains access to the cell by binding HER2 and is internalized; the linkage between the antibody and the drug is enzymatically broken down and the free drug penetrates to the cytoplasm. There it binds and disrupts the assembly of microtubules. In addition to its cellular effects, the agent blocks receptor signaling, mediates antibody-dependent cellular cytotoxicity, and prevents the shedding of HER2 from the cell surface.

Pharmacokinetics of trastuzumab emtansine are linear and the half-life is about 4 days. Clearance is not significantly influenced by body weight, tumor burden, albumin levels, or circulating levels of HER2. No adjustments in dose are made by age or race. The emtansine moiety is metabolized by CYP3A4/5 but does not induce or inhibit the cytochrome c enzymes. About 5% of patients develop neutralizing antibodies.

The drug is administered as an infusion at a dose of 3.6 mg/kg every 3 weeks until disease progression. Toxicities include infusion reactions, hepatic toxicity, left ventricular dysfunction, interstitial pneumonitis, thrombocytopenia, and sensory neurotoxicity. It also produces fatigue, nausea, musculoskeletal pain, and headache. The rate of adverse events of grade 3 or greater is about 40%.

In a phase III study comparing trastuzumab emtansine to the combination of lapatinib and capecitabine, the response rate to trastuzumab emtansine (44%) was superior to lapatinib plus capecitabine (31%), and median progression-free survival was improved from 6.4 to 9.4 months and median overall survival from 25 to 31 months (7).

CETUXIMAB (ERBITUX)

Cetuximab is a chimeric human/mouse monoclonal antibody with constant regions of human IgG1 κ origin with murine variable regions that recognize the extracellular domain of the human EGF receptor. The antibody is thought to work mainly by blocking the EGF receptor and starving the tumor of a needed growth factor. This hypothesis is undermined somewhat by data suggesting that some responding patients have tumors that do not express EGF receptors. EGF receptors are overexpressed in most epithelial malignancies.

The usual method of administration is to give a test dose of 20 mg. Patients then receive a loading dose of 400 mg/m^2 by 2-h infusion followed by weekly administration of 250 mg/m^2 by 1-h infusion. Using this regimen, steady-state levels are usually achieved by week 3 with mean peak serum levels being about 200 μg/ml and mean trough serum levels being about 63 μg/ml. Women have about 25% lower clearance rate than men. The half-life is about 5 days (114 h).

Cetuximab was approved for use based on results obtained in patients with metastatic colorectal cancer. In a randomized trial of patients who had previously progressed on irinotecan, cetuximab plus irinotecan produced a 23% overall response rate compared to about 11% for cetuximab alone (8). Median response duration was about 6 months for cetuximab plus irinotecan. Other single-arm cetuximab trials showed response rates of 9%–14% in patients with metastatic colorectal cancer that had progressed following an irinotecan-containing regimen. Although patients were required to have immunohistochemical evidence of EGF receptor expression to be enrolled on these early studies, response did not correlate with either the percentage of positive cells or the intensity of the expression. In a number of other epithelial malignancies, encouraging activity is seen in combination with radiation therapy or chemotherapy in head and neck cancer, non-small cell lung cancer, and pancreatic cancer. Investigations are ongoing to assess the role of antibodies to the EGF receptor versus the small molecule inhibitors of EGF receptor signaling such as gefitinib and erlotinib and whether various combinations or sequences of agents may boost response rates.

Upon first exposure, cetuximab produces the same syndrome associated with other humanized monoclonal antibodies including hives, bronchospasm, and hypotension. Severe reactions are encountered in about 3% of treated patients. Slowing the administration rate and use of antihistamines controls most such reactions. Patients with preexisting interstitial lung disease may have a worsening of symptoms with cetuximab. This problem generally emerges between the 4th and 11th doses of antibody. The antibody causes an acneiform rash in nearly 90% of patients, but is severe in grade in about 10%. The lesions can progress to abscesses requiring incision and drainage, and sepsis can be a complication. Other mucosal surfaces may also be affected by the antibody including nasal, oral, esophageal, and gastrointestinal. Patients on cetuximab also experience malaise (48%), nausea (29%), fever (27%), constipation or diarrhea (25% each), abdominal pain (26%), and headache (26%). Patients should be followed for the development of hypomagnesemia throughout the course of treatment. Low magnesium levels are detected in about half of treated patients and can progress to dangerous levels with attendant hypocalcemia and hypokalemia if not monitored carefully. Antibodies to cetuximab develop in <5% of patients and do not influence response rates.

PANITUMUMAB (VECTIBIX)

Panitumumab, a second antibody to EGF receptor, is a human IgG2 κ antibody with CDRs of murine origin. Overall it contains a smaller proportion of murine sequences than does cetuximab. Like cetuximab, it acts to block the binding of EGF to its receptor and its antitumor effects are thought to be related to loss of EGF receptor signaling (9).

The recommended regimen is 6 mg/kg given once every 2 weeks by 1-h infusion. Steady-state levels are usually reached by the third dose and mean peak concentrations are 213 μg/ml and mean trough concentrations are 39 μg/ml. The elimination half-life is about 7.5 days. Age, sex, race, renal dysfunction, hepatic dysfunction, and level of EGF receptor staining on tumor cells make no noticeable impact on the pharmacokinetics of panitumomab.

Panitumumab was approved based on an 8% response rate in patients with metastatic colorectal cancer whose tumors expressed EGF receptor and whose disease had progressed on or following treatment containing 5-fluorouracil, oxaliplatin, and irinotecan. The median duration of responses was about 4 months. No relationship was found between level of expression of EGF receptors and response rate or duration.

The toxicity profile is nearly identical to cetuximab and includes the initial infusion reaction, skin toxicity, diarrhea, hypomagnesemia, and a 1% risk of pulmonary fibrosis. Its use together with irinotecan is not recommended because it may increase the incidence of severe diarrhea (58% grades 3–4 in one study). Sunlight exposure may worsen the skin reaction to panitumumab. Antibodies are elicited to panitumumab in <4% of patients and are not associated with any alteration in activity or pharmacokinetics.

As the most recently approved antibody for a cancer indication, its activity profile is still actively being defined. There is no reason to suspect that its activity will be substantially different from that of cetuximab.

GEMTUZUMAB OGOMICIN (MYLOTARG)

Gemtuzumab ogomicin is an antibody conjugate. The antibody portion of the molecule is a humanized IgG4 κ antibody that binds to CD33, an adhesion glycoprotein expressed on cells of the myelocytic lineage (but not on pluripotent hematopoietic stem cells or nonhematopoietic cells) and on acute myeloid leukemia cells. The antibody is mainly composed of human sequences with murine CDRs. The antibody is conjugated to calicheamicin, a potent antitumor antibiotic isolated from the bacterium, *Micromonospora echinospora calichensis*. Once the conjugate binds to CD33, it is internalized. The calicheamycin is cleaved away from the antibody and released from the lysosomes intracellularly, and binds DNA in the minor groove to initiate double-strand breaks and cell death.

Gemtuzumab ogomicin is usually administered at a dose of 9 mg/m^2 by 2-h infusion followed by a second dose of 9 mg/m^2 2 weeks later. The elimination half-lives of total and unconjugated calicheamicin are about 45 h and 4 days, respectively, after the first dose and the half-life increases about 50% with the second dose. Clearance is not affected by age, sex, weight, or body surface area.

Gemtuzumab ogomicin is used as a salvage agent in the treatment of acute myeloid leukemia. It was approved for use by the U.S. Food and Drug Administration based on achieving a 26% response rate (13% complete responses) in patients with relapsed acute myeloid leukemia. Response rate and duration of response correlate with the duration of the initial remission. Response rates are 11% for those whose first remission was 6 months or less, 22% for those whose initial remission was 6–12 months, and 35% for those whose first remission was a year or longer. Responding patients survive a median of 1 year following treatment. Response is not influenced by patient age or cytogenetic abnormalities. Because of the many options for younger patients, gemtuzumab ogomicin is often used in patients older than 60 years (10). It is being assessed for its role in postremission therapy as an alternative to bone marrow transplantation in patients who are not candidates or who lack a suitable donor. It is almost always used as a single agent. Data on combination of gemtuzumab ogomicin with other chemotherapy are limited. The dose is usually reduced to 3 mg/m^2 when it is used together with other chemotherapeutic agents. CD33 is also expressed on the malignant cells of acute promyelocytic leukemia; gemtuzumab ogomicin has been used with all-trans retinoic acid with promising results in pilot studies.

In addition to infusion reactions, gemtuzumab ogomicin causes severe myelosuppression. Delayed recovery of platelet counts is often observed in patients who enter complete remission. Patients with peripheral WBC counts above 30,000/μl are susceptible to serious pulmonary dysfunction from cells blocking the pulmonary vessels. Fever, chills, dyspnea, pulmonary infiltrates, pleural effusions, pulmonary edema, and acute respiratory distress syndrome may occur. The WBC count should be reduced below 30,000/μl (with leukapheresis or hydroxyurea) before starting gemtuzumab ogomicin. The antibody conjugate also increases the risk of developing veno-occlusive disease of the liver. Patients undergoing subsequent hematopoietic stem cell transplantation are at higher risk (15%) than patients not undergoing transplantation (1%). Although rare, the syndrome (rapid weight gain, right upper quandrant pain, hepatomegaly, ascites, hyperbilirubinemia, elevated liver enzymes) can progress to death. Another serious complication of gemtuzumab ogomicin therapy is rapid tumor lysis. Patients with large tumor burdens should receive prophylaxis for tumor lysis syndrome. Like other myelotoxic agents, mucositis, bleeding, and febrile neutropenia may complicate its use. The development of antibodies to gemtuzumab ogomicin is very rare and does not affect the treatment course.

Because a randomized Southwest Oncology group study adding gemtuzumab to standard anthracycline plus cytarabine found an increase in day 30 mortality that was not compensated by improved complete response rate, disease-free or overall survival, the manufacturer withdrew the drug from the market in June 2010. Subsequent publications of randomized trial results have suggested some benefit from adding gemtuzumab to the treatment program. Given the genetic heterogeneity of acute myeloid leukemia, it remains possible that gemtuzumab has important efficacy in at least some subsets of patients.

BRENTUXIMAB VEDOTIN (ADCETRIS)

Brentuximab vedotin comprises a chimeric IgG1 antibody specific for human CD30 covalently linked to a protease-sensitive dipeptide linker that binds to monomethyl auristatin E, a microtubule inhibitor. When the immunoconjugate binds to its cell-bound ligand, it is internalized, the linker is broken by lysosomal peptidase activity and the drug portion of the molecule taken into the cytoplasm where it disrupts the microtubule system. It is active in CD30+ tumors including Hodgkin's disease and anaplastic large cell lymphoma (11).

The drug is administered by intravenous infusion at a dose of 1.3 mg/kg over 30 min every 3 weeks. Its serum half-life is 4–6 days. Steady-state levels of the agent are achieved within 21 days, consistent with the q3week schedule of administration. Sex, age, and race do not influence the pharmacology. Some metabolism of the drug is mediated by CYP3A; thus inhibitors of that enzyme might enhance toxicity.

The major toxicities of brentuximab vedotin are peripheral neuropathy (as noted with other microtubule inhibitors), neutropenia, fatigue, nausea, anemia, upper respiratory tract infection, fever, and thrombocytopenia. Cumulative lung toxicity makes combination with bleomycin risky, but patients who have received bleomycin in the past do not seem to be made worse by brentuximab treatment. Rare but serious complications include progressive multifocal leukoencephalopathy and Stevens-Johnson syndrome.

Brentuximab vedotin is highly active in patients with relapsed Hodgkin's disease and anaplastic large cell lymphoma. The overall response rate in a group of treatment refractory patients with Hodgkin's disease, many of whom had progressed after bone marrow transplantation, was 73% with 32% complete responses lasting a median of nearly 2 years. The overall response rate in patients with anaplastic large cell lymphoma was 86% with

57% complete responders lasting more than 1 year. Studies are now being conducted to assess responses to combination therapies in various settings (including primary treatment) of CD30+ tumors.

TOSITUMOMAB AND I-131 TOSITUMOMAB (BEXXAR)

Tositumomab is a murine IgG2a λ monoclonal antibody that binds to human CD20 antigen on normal and malignant B cells (see rituximab above). I-131 tositumomab is the same antibody conjugated to I-131, a beta- and gamma-emitting isotope. The physical half-life of the isotope is 8 days. I-131 tositumomab is targeted to CD20, and it kills cells to which it binds and also kills neighboring cells in the vicinity of the cell to which it binds by delivering radiation.

The use of tositumomab and I-131 tositumomab is divided into two stages; the first step is for dosimetry, and the second for therapy. Each step involves the sequential administration of tositumomab followed by I-131 tositumomab. The first injection of unconjugated anti-CD20 antibody was demonstrated to saturate the spleen and improve the tumor specificity of the subsequently delivered radiopharmaceutical. In the dosimetry phase, 450 mg of tositumomab is given intravenously over 1 h on day 0. Then a dose of I-131 tositumomab containing 5 mCi of I-131 and 35 mg of tositumomab is infused over 20 min. Dosimetry (by external counting of I-131 radioactivity) and biodistribution measurements are then made within 1 h of infusion, on days 2, 3, or 4 and again on days 6 or 7. Certain criteria are then applied to the biodistribution calculation, and if the biodistribution is acceptable, a therapeutic dose of I-131 tositumomab is calculated. Then sometime between day 7 and day 14, the therapeutic step is begun with an infusion of 450 mg tositumomab over 1 h followed by the calculated dose of I-131 tositumomab to deliver 75 cGy of total body radiation. The dosimetry and therapeutic steps together are a course of therapy and patients do not ever receive more than one course (12).

The activity of labeled and unlabeled tositumomab was defined mainly in patients with follicular lymphoma. Overall response rates in patients with relapsed follicular lymphoma were 63%–68% with 29%–33% of the responses defined as complete. Median response duration is about 12–18 months. Some complete remissions appear to be durable.

The main toxicity of unlabeled plus labeled tositumomab is myelosuppression, which can be severe. Platelets decrease to less than 50,000/μl in 53% of patients. Neutrophil counts fall below 1000/μl in 63% of patients. Hemoglobin levels fall below 8 g/dl in 29% of patients. The myelotoxicity is particularly common in the setting of significant marrow involvement with lymphoma; thus, this regimen is not indicated if tumor occupies 25% of more of the marrow space. Febrile neutropenia and other infections were noted in 45% of treated patients. In addition, although patients are pretreated with 3 doses of supersaturated potassium iodide solution, the uptake of radioactive iodine by the thyroid can produce hypothyroidism early on and increase the risk of thyroid cancer years later. The risk of hypothyroidism is about 15% at 4 years. Second malignancies are a problem with this therapy. About 10% of patients develop secondary acute leukemia or myelodysplastic syndrome by 4 years after treatment. In addition, skin, breast, lung, and head and neck cancers may be increased. Other grade 3–4 toxicities are rare. Normal B cells are depleted but this does not lead to hypogammaglobulinemia. About 10% of patients develop human antimurine antibodies, but this is of minor consequence in this group of patients who are unlikely to be exposed to other murine antibodies.

IBRITUMOMAB TIUXETAN (ZEVALIN)

Ibritumomab tiuxetan is a murine IgG1 κ antibody chelated to yttrium-90, a beta-emitting isotope. Ibritumomab binds to human CD20 with an affinity of about 14–18 nM. Tiuxetan is the chelating agent that attaches yttrium-90 to exposed amino groups in lysines and arginines in the antibody sequence. Ibritumomab tiuxetan is used as a salvage regimen for the treatment of CD20-expressing B-cell malignancies.

Like I-131 tositumomab, the ibritumomab tiuxetan therapeutic regimen consists of two steps: dosimetry followed by therapy. Dosimetry is performed by injecting unlabeled rituximab (250 mg/m^2) followed by 5 mCi of indium-111-labeled ibritumomab tiuxetan (containing 1.6 mg of antibody) over 10 min to assess biodistribution of the label. If the biodistribution shows too much lung, renal, or bowel uptake, the therapeutic dose is not given. However, if the biodistribution of the In-111 compound is acceptable, 7–9 days after dosimetry dose, the patient receives a therapeutic dose of 250 mg/m^2 rituximab followed by 0.4 mCi/kg of ibrituximab tiuxetin labeled with Y-90 over 10 min (13). The physical half-life of the isotope is just under 3 days and the mean half-life of Y-90 activity in the blood is 30 h.

The efficacy of ibritumomab tiuxetan appears similar to that of I-131 tositumomab.

Patients who have impaired bone marrow reserve (prior hematopoietic stem cell transplantation, radiation to more than 25% of marrow, current low platelet or neutrophil counts) have been treated with ibritumomab tiuxetan at a lower specific activity (0.3 mCi/kg) with response rates of 67% and median response durations of 12 months.

The most common toxicity of ibritumomab tiuxetan therapy is myelosuppression. In initial studies, platelet counts less than 50,000/μl were noted in 61% of patients and neutrophil counts less than 1000/μl were seen in 57% of patients. The risk of severe thrombocytopenia and neutropenia increased to 75% in patients whose platelet counts were between 100K and 150K at the start of treatment. Median time to nadir is 7–9 weeks and median duration of cytopenias is 3–5 weeks. The duration of the myelosuppression complicates subsequent therapeutic decisions. As would be expected, myeloid malignancies and myelodysplasias have been noted in patients surviving more than a year. Gastrointestinal symptoms (nausea, vomiting, abdominal pain, diarrhea) occur in 10% of patients. Human antimouse antibodies or human antichimeric protein antibodies develop in about 4% of cases. Normal B cells are eliminated but recover after 12–16 weeks. Hypogammaglobulinemia is not a clinically significant sequela. A general problem with the radiopharmaceuticals (both I-131 and Y-90) is the long-term compromise of marrow function. Patients who receive these therapies are not easily treated with subsequent courses of myelotoxic drugs because of the long-term loss of physiologic reserve in the hematopoietic system.

IPILIMUMAB (YERVOY)

CTLA4 is a molecule on the surface of T cells that interacts with CD80 and CD86 on antigen-presenting cells to tamp down an immune response and inhibit T-cell activation. Cancers exploit this pathway by signaling through CTLA4 to suppress the host response. Ipilimumab is a recombinant human IgG1 κ antibody that blocks the interaction between CTLA4 and CD80 or CD86. As a consequence, T cells develop the capacity to be activated. It also exerts effects at the population level tending to reduce the level of inhibitory T regulatory cells and enhancing effector cells. Thus, like bevacizumab, ipilimumab does not act by directly recognizing and killing tumor cells. It acts to alter the tumor host environment to favor the host's resistance to tumor growth and spread through T-cell activation.

Ipilimumab is usually given by 90-min infusion intravenously at a dose of 3 mg/kg, and the treatment is repeated every 3 weeks for a total of four doses. The half-life is 15–16 days and it is not associated with the induction of neutralizing antibodies. This agent behaves in a distinctive fashion from other cancer treatments. While acute toxicities are certainly noted, including fatigue, diarrhea, nausea, decreased appetite, vomiting, constipation, and fever, many of its most significant toxicities are delayed in onset, as are tumor responses. Indeed, the antibody can induce a wide variety of autoimmune diseases as it seems to allow a breach of self-tolerance. Autoimmunity can mediate enterocolitis, hepatitis, dermatitis, neuropathies, and endocrinopathies (including pituitary dysfunction, thyroiditis, Cushing's syndrome, adrenal insufficiency, and hypogonadism). Particular attention must be paid to symptoms that develop as they can be life threatening. Hormone deficiencies can be managed by hormone replacement and autoimmune disorders of particular organ systems like the bowel and liver can be treated with glucocorticoids.

Similarly, the usual time frame of tumor assessment is altered in patients treated with ipilimumab. In some patients, the tumor masses slowly expand occasionally reaching RECIST criteria for progressive disease. However, in contrast to most treatments, a substantial fraction of these tumors are enlarging because of infiltration of the tumor with T cells that will ultimately mediate the destruction of the tumor. Responses may be seen in 15%–20% of patients with melanoma, and median survival is increased from about 6 to about 10 months (14). Considerable efforts are underway to integrate this immunomodulatory therapy into combination regimens that include agents that exert direct antitumor effects.

CONCLUSION

An excellent review article (15) provides more detailed information about the approved antibodies and those in development. Antibodies to PD1 and its ligand, similar to ipilimumab, appear active in blocking the inhibiting effects of cancer on the immune system (16, 17). Monoclonal antibody therapy is burgeoning as a consequence of progress in overcoming the limitations to efficacy discovered in early studies (18).

REFERENCES

1. Rastetter W, Molina A, White CA. Rituximab: expanding role in therapy for lymphomas and autoimmune diseases. *Annu Rev Med.* 2004; 55: 477–503.

2. Wierda WG, Kipps TJ, Mayer J, et al. Ofatumumab as single-agent CD20 immunotherapy in fludarabine-refractory chronic lymphocytic leukemia. *J Clin Oncol.* 2010; 28: 1749–1755.

3. Ravandi F, O'Brien S. Alemtuzumab. *Expert Rev Anticancer Ther.* 2005; 5: 39–51.

4. Gordon MS, Cunningham D. Managing patients treated with bevacizumab combination therapy. *Oncology.* 2005; 69(Suppl 3): 25–33.

5. Plosker GL, Keam SJ. Trastuzumab: a review of its use in the management of HER2-positive metastatic and early-stage breast cancer. *Drugs.* 2006; 66: 449–475.

6. Baselga J, Cortes J, Kim SB, et al. Pertuzumab plus trastuzumab plus docetaxel for metastatic breast cancer. *N Engl J Med.* 2012; 366: 109-119.

7. Verma S, Miles D, Gianni L, et al. Trastuzumab emtansine for HER2-positive advanced breast cancer. *N Engl J Med.* 2012; 367: 1783–1791.

8. Chong G, Cunningham D. The role of cetuximab in the therapy of previously treated advanced colorectal cancer. *Semin Oncol.* 2006; 32(Suppl 9): S55–S58.

9. Saif MW, Cohenuram M. Role of panitumumab in the management of metastatic colorectal cancer. *Clin Colorectal Cancer.* 2006; 6: 118–124.

10. Fenton C, Perry CM. Gemtuzumab ozogomicin: a review of its use in acute myeloid leukaemia. *Drugs.* 2005; 65: 2405–2427.

11. Younes A, Bartlett NL, Leonard JP, et al. Brentuximab vedotin (SGN-35) for relapsed CD30 positive lymphomas. *N Engl J Med.* 2011; 363: 1812–1821.

12. Friedberg JW, Fisher RI. Iodine-131 tositumomab (Bexxar): radioimmunoconjugate therapy for indolent and transformed B-cell non-Hodgkin's lymphoma. *Expert Rev Anticancer Ther.* 2004; 4: 18–26.

13. Gordon LI. Practical considerations and radiation safety in radioimmunotherapy with yttrium-90 ibritumomab tiuxetan (Zevalin). *Semin Oncol.* 2003; 30(Suppl 17): 23–28.

14. Hodi FS, O'Day SJ, McDermott DF, et al. Improved survival with ipilimumab in patients with metastatic melanoma. *N Engl J Med.* 2010; 363: 711–723.

15. Scott AM, Allison JP, Wolchok JD. Monoclonal antibodies in cancer therapy. *Cancer Immunity.* 2012; 12: 14–22.

16. Topalian SL, Hodi FS, Brahmer JR, et al. Safety, activity, and immune correlates of anti-PD1 antibody in cancer. *N Engl J Med.* 2012; 366: 2443–2454.

17. Brahmer JR, Tykodi SS, Chow LQ, et al. Safety and activity of anti-PD-L1 antibody in patients with advanced cancer. *N Engl J Med.* 2012; 366: 2455–2465.

18. Nadler LM, Stashenko P, Hardy R, et al. Serotherapy of a patient with a monoclonal antibody directed against a human lymphoma-associated antigen. *Cancer Res.* 1980; 40: 3147–3154.

CHAPTER 16
Osteoclast-Targeted Therapy: Bisphosphonates and Denosumab
Matthew R. Smith

INTRODUCTION

Bone metastases are a major cause of morbidity in patients with a variety of malignancies including multiple myeloma, breast cancer, and prostate cancer (1). Bone metastases are often described as osteoblastic or osteolytic based on their radiographic appearance. Osteoblastic and osteolytic bone disease represent two extremes of a spectrum, however, and osteoclast number and activity are increased in most bone metastases, including typical osteoblastic metastases from prostate cancer. Pathological activation of osteoclasts appears to play a central role in disease-related skeletal complications.

Osteoclast inhibition by treatment with either a bisphosphonate or a denosumab is a standard part of supportive care for many patients with bone metastases (**Table 16-1**). Bisphosphonates, including pamidronate disodium (Aredia®) and zoledronic acid (Zometa®), are potent inhibitors of osteoclast-mediated bone resorption. Pamidronate disodium and zoledronic acid are approved for the prevention of skeletal-related events (fractures, spinal cord compression, or need for surgery or radiation to bone) in patients with bone metastases from solid tumors or multiple myeloma. Pamidronate disodium and zoledronic acid are also approved for the treatment of hypercalcemia of malignancy. Denosumab (Xgeva®) is a human monoclonal antibody that binds and inactivates receptor activator of nuclear factor-κB ligand (RANKL), a key mediator of osteoclast formation, function, and survival. Denosumab is approved for the prevention of skeletal-related events in patients with bone metastases from solid tumors.

PHARMACOLOGY

■ BISPHOSPHONATES

Bisphosphonates are synthetic analogs of pyrophosphate characterized by a phosphorus-carbon-phosphorus backbone that renders them resistant to hydrolysis (**Figure 16-1**). The R_1 and R_2 carbon side chains determine their pharmacology. Most bisphosphonates contain a hydroxyl group at the R_1 position that confers high-affinity binding to calcium phosphate. The R_2 side chain determines antiresorptive potency. Bisphosphonates with a secondary or tertiary amino group at R_2 (including zoledronic acid) are among the most potent bisphosphonates, with approximately 10,000-fold greater in vitro potency than etidronate, a first-generation bisphosphonate.

TABLE 16-1 OSTEOCLAST-TARGETED THERAPY FOR BONE METASTASES

Generic Name	Trade Name	Dose and Schedule	FDA-Approved Uses in Oncology
Pamidronate disodium	Aredia®	90 mg intravenously (over 2–4 h) every 3–4 wk	• Hypercalcemia of malignancy • SRE prevention in multiple myeloma • SRE prevention in breast cancer
Zoledronic acid	Zometa®	4 mg intravenously (over 15 min) every 3–4 wk	• Hypercalcemia of malignancy • SRE prevention in multiple myeloma • SRE prevention for any solid tumor
Denosumab	Xgeva®	120 mg subcutaneously every 4 wk	• SRE prevention for any solid tumor

Bisphosphonates are adsorbed to calcium phosphate (hydroxyapatite) crystals in bone. Approximately one-half of an intravenously administered dose accumulates in the skeleton. Bisphosphonates preferentially bind to sites of active bone remodeling. Bisphosphonates are not metabolized and are eliminated by renal excretion. Potent nitrogen-containing bisphosphonates (including pamidronate disodium and zoledronic acid) inhibit farnesyl diphosphate synthase, a key enzyme in the mevalonate pathway, and decrease prenylation of essential GTP-binding proteins.

The most common adverse effect of pamidronate disodium and zoledronic acid is an acute phase reaction, a transient flu-like syndrome of fever, arthralgias, and myalgias starting within 24 h after intravenous treatment. Hypocalcemia is also common, but is rarely associated with symptoms. Supplemental calcium (500–1000 mg daily) and vitamin D (at least 400 IU daily) are recommended to reduce the risk of symptomatic hypocalcemia.

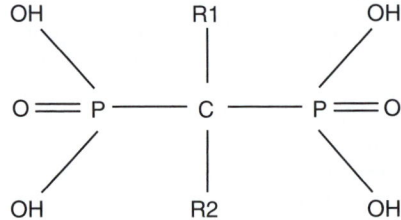

FIGURE 16-1 The molecular structure of bisphosphonates.

Pamidronate disodium and zoledronic acid have potential renal toxicity related to total drug dose and rate of intravenous administration. Treatment is not recommended for patients with creatinine clearance less than 30 ml/min. Dose reductions are recommended for patients with estimated creatinine clearance between 30 and 60 mL/min. Serum creatinine should be monitored before each treatment.

Zoledronic acid and other bisphosphonates are also associated with increased risk of osteonecrosis of the jaw. Most but not all patients who develop osteonecrosis of the jaw have preexisting dental problems. Excellent oral hygiene, baseline dental evaluation for high-risk individuals, and avoidance of invasive dental surgery during therapy are recommended to reduce risk of osteonecrosis of the jaw.

■ DENOSUMAB

Denosumab is a fully human IgG2 monoclonal antibody that binds human RANKL with high affinity, exhibiting a dissociation equilibrium binding constant of 3 pM (2). Denosumab binds to both soluble and membrane-bound primate RANKL. Denosumab does not bind to other tumor necrosis factor family members including TRAIL, CD40 ligand, TNFα, or TNFβ. Denosumab has a long circulatory half-life (>30 days). In contrast to bisphosphonates, denosumab does not accumulate in bone. Denosumab is administered by subcutaneous injection and cleared by metabolism.

Denosumab shares some adverse effects with bisphosphonates. Osteoclast inhibition with denosumab is associated with hypocalcemia. Denosumab is also associated with osteonecrosis of the jaw. In contrast to bisphosphonates, denosumab is not associated with renal toxicity and does not require renal function monitoring or dose adjustments for renal impairment. Denosumab administration is not associated with acute-phase reactions.

CLINICAL USES IN ONCOLOGY

■ HYPERCALCEMIA

Hypercalcemia of malignancy results primarily from increased release of calcium from bone. In the presence of bone metastases, calcium is released from the skeleton by local osteoclast-mediated bone destruction. Hypercalcemia of malignancy may also result from tumor secretion of parathyroid hormone-related protein (PTHrP). PTHrP causes hypercalcemia by osteoclast activation and decreased renal calcium excretion. Many malignancies produce PTHrP, including breast cancer, squamous cell carcinoma, renal cell carcinoma, multiple myeloma, and some types of lymphoma. In addition, 1,25-dihydroxyvitamin D lymphoma syndrome and ectopic hyperpararthyroidism are rare causes of hypercalcemia of malignancy.

Intravenous bisphosphonates are the treatment of choice for mild to severe hypercalcemia of malignancy. Most patients have normal serum calcium levels within several days after treatment with pamidronate disodium or zoledronic acid, and most responses last for 1–4 weeks. In randomized controlled trials, intravenous zoledronic acid achieves higher rates and duration of normocalcemia than pamidronate disodium.

■ PREVENTION OF SKELETAL-RELATED EVENTS

Pamidronate disodium and zoledronic acid decrease skeletal-related events in patients with multiple myeloma or metastatic breast cancer (3, 4). Zoledronic acid also decreases the risk of skeletal complications in patients with bone metastases from prostate cancer, lung cancer, and other solid tumors (5, 6). The optimal timing, schedule, and duration of bisphosphonates for prevention of skeletal-related events are undefined.

Denosumab decreases the risk of skeletal-related events in patients with bone metastases from solid tumors. In randomized controlled trials, denosumab was superior to zoledronic acid for the prevention of skeletal-related events in patients with breast cancer or prostate cancer (7, 8). In another randomized controlled trial, denosumab was similar to zoledronic acid for the prevention of skeletal events in patients with bone metastases for malignancies other than breast cancer or prostate cancer (9). Denosumab is not approved for the treatment of patients with multiple myeloma.

■ PREVENTION OF BONE METASTASES

The establishment of bone metastases involves reciprocal interactions between tumor cells and metabolically active bone (10). Development and progression of bone metastases involve tumor cell adhesion to bone, invasion, new blood vessel formation, and proliferation. Preclinical studies suggest that bisphosphonates and denosumab interfere with several of these steps.

Osteoclast inhibition is associated with delay or prevention of bone metastases in patients with high-risk breast and prostate cancer. In two of three randomized controlled trials of women with high-risk primary breast cancer, clodronate significantly reduced the incidence of new bone metastases (11). In a large randomized controlled trial of men with castration-resistant nonmetastatic prostate cancer, denosumab significantly increased bone metastasis-free survival and time to first bone metastasis (12). Notably, osteoclast-targeted therapies are not currently approved for the prevention of bone metastases.

REFERENCES

1. Roodman GD. Mechanisms of bone metastasis. *N Engl J Med.* 2004; 350: 1655–1664.

2. Lacey DL, Boyle WJ, Simonet WS, et al. Bench to bedside: elucidation of the OPG-RANK-RANKL pathway and the development of denosumab. *Nat Rev Drug Discov.* 2012; 11: 401–419.

3. Van Poznak CH, Von Roenn JH, Temin S. American Society of Clinical Oncology clinical practice guideline update: recommendations on the role of bone-modifying agents in metastatic breast cancer. *J Oncol Pract.* 2011; 7: 117–121.

4. Kyle RA, Yee GC, Somerfield MR, et al. American Society of Clinical Oncology 2007 clinical practice guideline update on the role of bisphosphonates in multiple myeloma. *J Clin Oncol.* 2007; 25: 2464–2472.

5. Rosen LS, Gordon D, Tchekmedyian S, et al. Zoledronic acid versus placebo in the treatment of skeletal metastases in patients with lung

cancer and other solid tumors: a phase III, double-blind, randomized trial—The Zoledronic Acid Lung Cancer and Other Solid Tumors Study Group. *J Clin Oncol.* 2003; 21: 3150–3157.

6. Saad F, Gleason DM, Murray R, et al. Long-term efficacy of zoledronic acid for the prevention of skeletal complications in patients with metastatic hormone-refractory prostate cancer. *J Natl Cancer Inst.* 2004; 96: 879–882.

7. Stopeck AT, Lipton A, Body JJ, et al. Denosumab compared with zoledronic acid for the treatment of bone metastases in patients with advanced breast cancer: a randomized, double-blind study. *J Clin Oncol.* 2010; 28: 5132–5139.

8. Fizazi K, Carducci M, Smith M, et al. Denosumab versus zoledronic acid for treatment of bone metastases in men with castration-resistant prostate cancer: a randomised, double-blind study. *Lancet.* 2011; 377: 813–822.

9. Henry DH, Costa L, Goldwasser F, et al. Randomized, double-blind study of denosumab versus zoledronic acid in the treatment of bone metastases in patients with advanced cancer (excluding breast and prostate cancer) or multiple myeloma. *J Clin Oncol.* 2011; 29: 1125–1132.

10. Mundy GR. Metastasis to bone: causes, consequences and therapeutic opportunities. *Nat Rev Cancer.* 2002; 2: 584–593

11. Dando TM, Wiseman LR. Clodronate: a review of its use in the prevention of bone metastases and the management of skeletal complications associated with bone metastases in patients with breast cancer. *Drugs Aging.* 2004; 21: 949–962.

12. Smith MR, Saad F, Coleman R, et al. Denosumab and bone-metastasis-free survival in men with castration-resistant prostate cancer: results of a phase 3, randomised, placebo-controlled trial. *Lancet.* 2012; 379: 39–46.

CHAPTER **17**
Febrile Neutropenia

Stephen M. Carpenter, Fabrizio Vianello, Mark C. Poznansky

INTRODUCTION

Immune-compromised state refers to a change of the host defense systems that confer an increased susceptibility to infection. Neutropenia remains the major defect of the defense systems predisposing to severe infections. Fever in a neutropenic patient should be considered a medical emergency as it has been demonstrated that a delay in specific therapy is associated with up to a 70% mortality rate (1). In this chapter, we present the medical approach to fever in neutropenic patients by analyzing the predisposing factors, pathogenesis, diagnosis, and treatment.

DEFINITION

Fever in a neutropenic patient is usually defined as a single temperature of >38.3°C (101.3°F), or a sustained temperature >38°C (100.4°F) for more than 1 h. It has to be considered that neutropenic patients may experience clinical deterioration in the absence of fever and that concomitant steroid treatment may also conceal a fever.

Among neutropenic patients, two factors are associated with the increased risk of infection:

- Neutrophil count. The risk increases when the neutrophil count is below $1 \times 10^9/l$. The risk of infection increases further in patients with neutrophil counts of less than $0.1 \times 10^9/l$ neutrophils.
- Duration of neutropenia. A low-neutrophil count and a protracted neutropenia ($0.5 \times 10^9/l$ for 10 days) are major risk factors for infection. A duration of neutropenia of more than 5 weeks is associated with an incidence of infection close to 100%.

Despite this, neutropenic patients remain a heterogeneous population that needs additional parameters that help to define the real risk of infection and tailor a more specific approach for each patient in this category. The risk factors for infection associated with neutropenia include advanced age, poor performance or nutritional status, low baseline and first-cycle nadir blood cell counts, and high-dose chemotherapy. Significant predictors for death, bacteremia, and length of hospital stay include advanced age, hematologic malignancies, disease burden, high fever, and low blood pressure on admission, pneumonia, and single or multiorgan dysfunction.

PATHOGENESIS

A number of predisposing factors other than neutropenia play a role in increasing the risk of infections in neutropenic patients with fever:

- Chemotherapy
- Intravenous or implanted devices
- Hypogammaglobulinemia (i.e., chronic lymphocytic leukemia, multiple myeloma, splenectomy)
- Defects in cell-mediated immunity (ALL, NHL, HD, therapy with fludarabine or alemtuzumab)
- Glucocorticoid therapy
- Disruption of normal anatomic structures

Chemotherapy not only affects the number of neutrophils but also impairs chemotaxis and phagocytosis. Either chemotherapy or radiotherapy-associated mucositis may affect the normal mucosal barrier, predisposing to bacteremia.

The existence of an impairment in neutrophil function preceding chemotherapy as in patients with myelodysplastic syndromes or in the presence of bone marrow failure due to tumor cell invasion predisposes to severe infection or death after chemotherapy (2).

Indwelling catheters and implanted devices pose a significant risk as they can allow access of skin flora directly into blood or subcutaneous tissues or represent a foreign body that bacteria can successfully colonize and infect. Immune defects associated with specific primary cancers may further impair the defense system as in hypogammaglobulinemia associated with CLL or multiple myeloma. Splenectomy predisposes to infection with encapsulated organisms such as *Pneumococcus* or *Meningococcus*.

An increased risk of infection has been observed in patients with Hodgkin's disease as the result of a defect in cell-mediated immunity. Patients with ALL, patients with central nervous system tumors, and patients treated with glucocorticoids are also at increased risk of infections.

ETIOLOGY OF INFECTIONS IN FEBRILE NEUTROPENIA ASSOCIATED PATHOGENS

■ BACTERIA

About 65% of neutropenic patients with fever have infection (Table 17-1). In this group of patients, aerobic gram-negative bacilli represented the most frequent isolates (3). In the past *Pseudomonas aeruginosa* was the most frequent isolate responsible for septic shock and severe pneumonia, and empirical therapy regimens were designed to include antipseudomonal antibiotics. Since the 1980s, gram-positive bacteria have become the most frequent pathogens isolated from patients with febrile neutropenia. More aggressive chemotherapeutic regimens, widespread use of indwelling catheters, and antibiotic prophylaxis have contributed to the trend toward gram-positive infections (4). Coagulase-negative staphylococci are the most common isolates (2), although drug-resistant gram-negative bacteria are causing an increasing number of infections (3).

TABLE 17-1 FACTORS THAT FAVOR A LOW RISK FOR SEVERE INFECTION AMONG PATIENTS WITH NEUTROPENIA

- Absolute neutrophil count of ≥100 cells/mm^3
- Absolute monocyte count of ≥100 cells/mm^3
- Normal findings on a chest radiograph
- Nearly normal results of hepatic and renal function tests
- Duration of neutropenia of <7 days
- Resolution of neutropenia expected in <10 days
- No intravenous catheter-site infection
- Early evidence of bone marrow recovery
- Malignancy in remission
- Peak temperature of < 39°C
- No neurological or mental changes
- No appearance of illness
- No abdominal pain
- No shock, hypoxia, pneumonia or other deep-organ infection, vomiting, or diarrhea

■ FUNGI

It has been demonstrated that up to 20% of patients with neutropenia may experience an invasive mycosis, and this risk is further increased in patients with hematologic malignancies (3) (Table 17-1). Fungi are rarely the cause of fever early during neutropenia, but invasive fungal disease is usually encountered after prolonged neutropenia while on emperic antibiotics.

Risk factors for fungal superinfection include:

- greater than 7 days of profound neutropenia.
- use of quinolones as antibacterial prophylaxis.
- presence of a central venous catheter.
- persistence of fever after 3 days of antibiotic therapy (5).

Superficial and invasive candidiasis and invasive aspergillosis represent the most common infections. *Candida albicans* represents the most common fungal isolate in neutropenic patients followed by *C. tropicalis, C. glabrata,* and *C. parapsilosis.* The use of fluconazole as prophylactic therapy has been associated with an increased frequency of *C. krusei.*

Invasive aspergillosis may be due to *Aspergillus fumigatus, A. terreus, A. flavus,* and *A. niger.* Invasive aspergillosis is associated with a mortality rate approaching 80% in bone marrow transplantation patients with febrile neutropenia (6). The two most common sites of invasive disease are the lungs and the sinuses. Prolonged fever and nodular pulmonary infiltrates resistant to antibiotic therapy often represent the only clues to the diagnosis of invasive aspergillosis. A finding of nodular lesions surrounded by a low-attenuation area ("halo sign") may be evident at a chest CT scan. Isolation from culture or histological detection of *Aspergillus* establishes the definitive diagnosis.

Fusariosis, Trichosporon beigelii, Blastoschizomyces capitatus, Saccharomyces cerevisiae, and *Malassenzia furfur* represent other emerging fungi.

EVALUATION

The initial evaluation of a febrile and neutropenic patient should include a detailed history and physical examination. Symptoms and signs of inflammation may be minimal or even absent in patients with severe neutropenia. A thorough physical examination should be performed, with particular attention to the skin, mucus membranes, sinuses, oropharynx, lung, abdomen, perirectal area, surgical sites, and intravenous lines. In the neutropenic patient, the response to bacterial infection may be misleading, with only minimal erythema and rash, and often without signs associated with cellulitis or abscess formation. All indwelling catheters should be carefully inspected. Lines should also be assessed for any malfunction as poor flow may be a sign of an infected clot.

The examination should include inspection of the perianal area. A digital rectal examination (and rectal temperatures) should generally be avoided. Stool softeners should also be given to patients to avoid hard stools or impaction. Patients should be reassessed daily as new sites of infection can become apparent even 72 h after the initial therapy. In addition, as the neutrophil count rebounds, symptoms and signs of an infection may become evident.

LABORATORY STUDIES

A basic evaluation should include a complete blood cell count with differential measurement of serum levels of creatinine, urea nitrogen, SGOT, SGPT, bilirubin, and electrolytes. Specimens should be obtained immediately for the microbiology laboratory, including two or more blood cultures from the device lumen and from a peripheral vein. Blood cultures should be repeated for persistent fevers.

A sample of sputum may be included in the microbiologic evaluation if the patient can produce it. Culture of urine samples is indicated if signs of symptoms of urinary tract infection do exist, in the presence of urinary catheter or if urinalysis is abnormal.

Lumbar puncture is not recommended as a routine procedure but should be considered if symptoms suggest a CNS infection.

Chest radiographs should be performed even in the absence of pulmonary infection. Even more likely to yield a diagnosis of pneumonia in the neutropenic patient is the high-resolution CT scan, as it frequently reveals pneumonia even in the presence of a normal chest radiography.

If localizing signs or symptoms are present, other tests should be considered, such as skin aspiration or biopsy for culture, stool for culture, and imaging of the CNS, sinuses, and abdomen.

TREATMENT

Treatment for patients with febrile neutropenia include antimicrobial agents and granulocyte-colony stimulating factor (G-CSF). Antibiotics are always administered empirically, ideally within 2 h of recognition (7), and should include appropriate coverage for suspected or known infections (**Figure 17-1**).

■ EMPIRICAL THERAPY

Initial management requires evaluation of the patient to define low or high risk of severe infections (**Table 17-2**). In high-risk patients, several antibiotic regimens have been proposed as initial empirical therapy in febrile neutropenia, but none has demonstrated a clear superiority (8). All regimens have been designed to provide coverage against gram-negative bacilli, especially *P. aeruginosa*.

SINGLE-DRUG THERAPY

- Extended-spectrum cephalosporins: ceftazidime or cefepime
- Antipseudomonal penicillin/beta-lactamase combination: pipericillin-tazobactam
- Carbapenem: imipenem or meropenem

TWO-DRUG THERAPY

- Antipseudomonal penicillin plus an aminoglycoside: piperacillin or ticarcillin or mezlocillin plus gentamycin or tobramycin or amikacin
- Antipseudomonal penicillin plus a fluoroquinolone: piperacillin or ticarcillin or mezlocillin plus ciprofloxacin

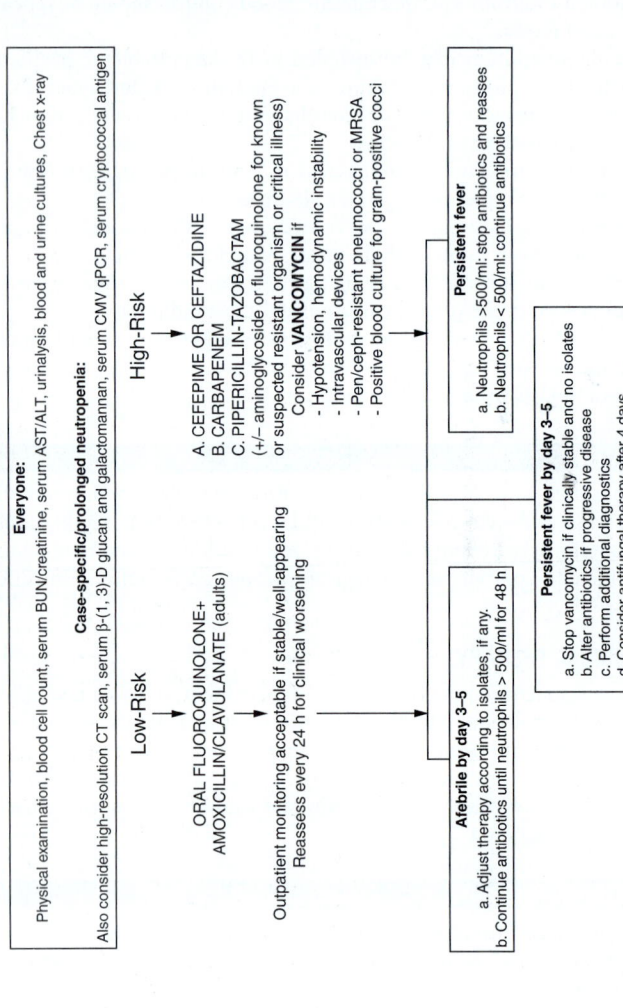

Fever and neutropenia

Everyone:
Physical examination, blood cell count, serum BUN/creatinine, serum AST/ALT, urinalysis, blood and urine cultures, Chest x-ray

Case-specific/prolonged neutropenia:
Also consider high-resolution CT scan, serum β-(1, 3)-D glucan and galactomannan, serum CMV qPCR, serum cryptococcal antigen

Low-Risk

ORAL FLUOROQUINOLONE+
AMOXICILLIN/CLAVULANATE (adults)

Outpatient monitoring acceptable if stable/well-appearing
Reassess every 24 h for clinical worsening

High-Risk

A. CEFEPIME OR CEFTAZIDINE
B. CARBAPENEM
C. PIPERICILLIN-TAZOBACTAM
(+/– aminoglycoside or fluoroquinolone for known
or suspected resistant organism or critical illness)
Consider **VANCOMYCIN** if
- Hypotension, hemodynamic instability
- Intravascular devices
- Pen/ceph-resistant pneumococci or MRSA
- Positive blood culture for gram-positive cocci

Afebrile by day 3–5
a. Adjust therapy according to isolates, if any.
b. Continue antibiotics until neutrophils > 500/ml for 48 h

Persistent fever by day 3–5
a. Stop vancomycin if clinically stable and no isolates
b. Alter antibiotics if progressive disease
c. Perform additional diagnostics
d. Consider antifungal therapy after 4 days

Persistent fever
a. Neutrophils >500/ml: stop antibiotics and reasses
b. Neutrophils < 500/ml: continue antibiotics

FIGURE 17-1 Practical approach to fever and neutropenia.

TABLE 17-2 SCORING INDEX FOR IDENTIFICATION OF LOW-RISK FEBRILE NEUTROPENIC PATIENTS AT TIME OF PRESENTATION WITH FEVER

Characteristic	Score
Extent of illness[a]	
No symptoms	5
Mild symptoms	5
Moderate symptoms	3
No hypotension	5
No chronic obstructive pulmonary disease	4
Solid tumor or no fungal infection	4
No dehydration	3
Outpatient at onset of fever	3
Age <60 y[b]	2

Note: Highest theoretical score is 26. A risk index score of 21 indicates that the patient is likely to be at low risk for complications and morbidity. The scoring system is derived from Reference 50.

[a]Choose 1 item only.

[b]Does not apply to patients 16 y of age. Initial monocyte count of 100 cells/mm^3, no comorbidity, and normal chest radiograph findings indicate children at low risk for significant bacterial infections.

Source: Reference 21.

TWO-DRUG THERAPY (ABOVE) PLUS GLYCOPEPTIDES

- Vancomycin, in selected patients:
  - Catheter-related infections
  - Colonization with penicillin and cephalosporin-resistant pneumococci or MRSA
  - Growth of gram-positive cocci pending final identification
  - Hemodynamic instability

Linezolid or daptomycin should be considered for select resistant gram-positive infections or if vancomycin is not indicated.

A large number of clinical trials performed over the past 30 years have failed to prove the superiority of one antibiotic regimen over others in the management of febrile neutropenia. A patient's risk factors and history, clinical evaluation, the hypothetical source of infection, and the local frequency of specific pathogens should drive the decision.

The antibiotic regimen should still provide broad empirical coverage for the possibility of other pathogens unlike the treatment strategy in most immunocompetent hosts.

Aminoglycosides such as gentamicin and antipseudomonal penicillins represented the conventional therapy for neutropenic patients prior to the advent of fluoroquinolones and third-generation cephalosporins. The advantages of dual therapy over single-drug treatment include synergy against aerobic gram-negative bacilli and reduced risk of resistant strain selection. Nephrotoxicity and ototoxicity associated with aminoglycoside therapy represent the major concern. Toxicity can be minimized by careful monitoring of serum levels and by administering aminoglycoside once a day.

Quinolone-based combinations with beta-lactams represent an option for empirical therapy in patients not treated prophylactically with quinolones (8). However, as low-risk outpatients are being treated empirically with regimens that include fluoroquinolones, resistance is rising, precluding their use in many high-risk inpatients with fever and neutropenia (9).

The next stage corresponds to the development of third- and fourth-generation cephalosporins. In particular, antipseudomonal cephalosporins including ceftazidime and cefepime have potent activity against aerobic gram-negative bacilli including *P. aeruginosa*, and have activity against gram-positive cocci. The effectiveness of ceftazidime led to the introduction of a modified monotherapy in which an aminoglycoside was given for the first 72 h and then discontinued if cultures were negative for aerobic gram-negative bacilli (10).

Monotherapy with a carbamenem is particularly effective in febrile neutropenia of unknown origin in patients who had received prophylactic antibiotics (7, 8). In subgroup analyses, meropenem also appeared to be superior to ceftazidime in patients with severe neutropenia (ANC 100 cells/µl) and in bone marrow transplant recipients (11).

One concern about monotherapy is the possibility that an alarming increase in the frequency of antibiotic-resistant pathogens would be predicted to occur and may eventually reduce the efficacy of this strategy (12).

■ VANCOMYCIN IN EMPIRICAL THERAPY

There is no clear evidence that addition of vancomycin to empirical therapy affects morbidity or mortality. Addition of vancomycin should be considered in patients suffering from hypotension, mucositis, skin or catheter site infection, or have a history of MRSA colonization, or have recent quinolone prophylaxis (Figure 17-1) (13, 14). When vancomycin is added to empirical therapy at the initiation of treatment, subsequent discontinuation of the antibiotic should be considered in the presence of negative blood cultures. The risk of acquiring VRE is cited as another reason for avoiding empirical vancomycin use.

■ THERAPY IN LOW-RISK PATIENTS WITH NEUTROPENIA

Prospective studies have identified patients with fever and neutropenia at low risk for medical complications. These patients have solid tumors, no underlying immunocompromise, and an expected short duration of neutropenia of 5 days or less: in these patients it appears safe to use an oral rather than parenteral therapy (15) (Table 17-2). Comparison of the oral regimen consisting of ciprofloxacin and amoxicillin-clavulanate against intravenous ceftriaxone plus amikacin demonstrated equal efficacy in patients with microbiologically documented infections (16). Oral antibiotic therapy requires very accurate selection of neutropenic patients with a low-risk profile.

■ EMPIRICAL ANTIFUNGAL THERAPY IN FEBRILE NEUTROPENIA

In view of the finding that up to one-third of patients with fever and neutropenia persisting for more than 7 days develop systemic *Candida* or *Aspergillus* infection, empirical treatment with an antifungal drug can be considered, in particular when neutropenia is not expected to resolve within a few days. Diagnostic steps, including fungal isolator blood cultures, fungal cell wall markers including serum β-(1, 3)-D glucan and galactomannan assays, as well as chest CT, should precede the commencement of antifungal therapy.

Antifungal therapeutic options include amphotericin B, lipid formulations of amphotericin B, fluconazole, itraconazole, voriconazole, and the echinocandins: micafungin, caspofungin, or anidulafungin. Amphotericin B has historically been the standard of antifungal therapy in febrile neutropenia with the broadest spectrum of antifungal activity.

When used as lipid formulation, amphotericin causes a lesser incidence of infusion-related fever, chills or rigors, and nephrotoxicity (17). Among azoles, fluconazole has limited activity against *Aspergillus* species and some nonalbicans *Candida* species, and it is generally not recommended for empirical therapy. Intravenous followed by oral itraconazole was found to be as effective as amphotericin B in febrile neutropenic patients (18). Itraconazole should not be used in patients with an estimated creatinine clearance below 30 ml/min and this azole should not be administered for more than 14 days.

Results of three clinical trials assessing the activity of voriconazole and caspofungin have demonstrated their efficacy in the treatment of invasive fungal infections. In one study, voriconazole was superior to liposomal amphotericin B only with respect to documented breakthrough fungal infections, infusion-related toxicity, and nephrotoxicity (19). In another trial, the efficacy of caspofungin in the prevention of breakthrough infections and resolution of fever was superior to liposomal amphotericin B (20). Caspofungin also cured more documented baseline fungal infections than did liposomal amphotericin B. Considering the available evidence, voriconazole and caspofungin both appear to be suitable, and perhaps preferable, alternatives to conventional liposomal amphotericin B as empirical antifungal therapy in patients with persistent fever and neutropenia.

■ HEMATOPOIETIC GROWTH FACTOR (HGF)

Both the Infectious Diseases Society of America and the American Society of Clinical Oncology do not support the routine use of growth factors in febrile neutropenic patients. G-CSF has been reported to decrease the duration of neutropenia, fever, and hospitalization but without significant impact on mortality (21). These agents can be considered in high-risk patients whose risk of fever and neutropenia exceeds 20%. Therapy with G-CSF may be considered to be appropriate in critically ill patients with prolonged neutropenia.

■ ANTIBACTERIAL AND ANTIFUNGAL PROPHYLAXIS

There is no consensus to recommend antimicrobial prophylaxis for all afebrile neutropenic patients. A prophylactic strategy should diminish the attack rate and delay the time to the onset of an infectious complication, but it does not eliminate the risk of infection. The goal would be to provide protection during the period of neutropenia and mucositis. In general, the use of prophylactic antibiotic therapy is not routinely recommended for cancer patients undergoing chemotherapy, although fluoroquinolones can be considered in patients with expected prolonged durations of profound neutropenia. Prophylaxis against *Candida* infection should be considered in patients with a substantial risk of invasive disease, such as stem cell transplants and intensive induction or salvage chemotherapy regimens (21). Vigorous infection-control practices and careful monitoring for the emergence of resistant organisms should accompany any prophylactic program.

REFERENCES

1. Rubin RH, Ferraro MJ. Understanding and diagnosing infectious complications in the immunocompromised host. Current issues and trends. *Hematol Oncol Clin North Am.* 1993; 7: 795–812.

2. Bodey G, Bueltmann B, Duguid W, et al. Fungal infections in cancer patients: an international autopsy survey. *Eur J Clin Microbiol Infect Dis.* 1992; 11: 99–109.

3. Ramphal R. Changes in the etiology of bacteremia in febrile neutropenic patients and the susceptibilities of the currently isolated pathogens. *Clin Infect Dis.* 2004; 39: S25–S31.

4. Cattaneo C, Quaresmini G, Casari S, et al. Recent changes in bacterial epidemiology and the emergence of fluoroquinolone-resistant Escherichia coli among patients with haematological malignancies: results of a prospective study on 823 patients at a single institution. *J Antimicrob Chemother.* 2008; 61:721–728.

5. Nucci M, Colombo AL, Spector N, et al. Breakthrough candidemia in neutropenic patients. *Clin Infect Dis.* 1997; 24: 275–276.

6. Marr KA, Patterson T, Denning D. Aspergillosis. Pathogenesis, clinical manifestations, and therapy. *Infect Dis Clin North Am.* 2002; 16: 875–894, vi.

7. Zuckermann J, Moreira LB, Stoll P, et al. Compliance with a critical pathway for the management of febrile neutropenia and impact on clinical outcomes. *Ann Hematol.* 2008; 87:139–145.

8. Bliziotis IA, Michalopoulos A, Kasiakou SK, et al. Ciprofloxacin vs an aminoglycoside in combination with a beta–lactam for the treatment of febrile neutropenia: a meta–analysis of randomized controlled trials. *Mayo Clin Proc.* 2005; 80: 1146–1156.

9. Bow EJ. Fluoroquinolones, antimicrobial resistance and neutropenic cancer patients. *Curr Opin Infect Dis.* 2011; 24, 545–553.

10. Donowitz GR, Maki DG, Crnich CJ, et al. Infections in the neutropenic patient—new views of an old problem. *Hematology (Am Soc Hematol Educ Program).* 2001; 113–139.

11. Freifeld AG, Walsh T, Marshall D, et al. Monotherapy for fever and neutropenia in cancer patients: a randomized comparison of ceftazidime versus imipenem. *J Clin Oncol.* 1995; 13: 165–176.

12. Raad, II, Escalante C, Hachem RY, et al. Treatment of febrile neutropenic patients with cancer who require hospitalization: a prospective randomized study comparing imipenem and cefepime. *Cancer.* 2003; 98: 1039–1047.

13. Paul M, Borok S, Fraser A, Vidal L, Leibovici L. Empirical antibiotics against gram-positive infections for febrile neutropenia: systematic review and meta-analysis of randomized controlled trials. *J Antimicrob Chemother.* 2005; 55: 436–444.

14. Vardakas KZ, Samonis G, Chrysanthopoulou SA, et al. Role of glycopeptides as part of initial empirical treatment of febrile neutropenic patients: a meta-analysis of randomised controlled trials. *Lancet Infect Dis.* 2005; 5: 431–439.

15. Koh A, Pizzo PA. Empirical oral antibiotic therapy for low risk febrile cancer patients with neutropenia. *Cancer Invest.* 2002; 20: 420–433.

16. Kern WV, Cometta A, De Bock R, et al. Oral versus intravenous empirical antimicrobial therapy for fever in patients with granulocytopenia who are receiving cancer chemotherapy. International Antimicrobial Therapy Cooperative Group of the European Organization for Research and Treatment of Cancer. *N Engl J Med.* 1999; 341: 312–318.

17. Walsh TJ, Finberg RW, Arndt C, et al. Liposomal amphotericin B for empirical therapy in patients with persistent fever and neutropenia. National Institute of Allergy and Infectious Diseases Mycoses Study Group. *N Engl J Med.* 1999; 340: 764–771.

18. Boogaerts M, Winston DJ, Bow EJ, et al. Intravenous and oral itraconazole versus intravenous amphotericin B deoxycholate as empirical antifungal therapy for persistent fever in neutropenic patients with cancer who are receiving broad-spectrum antibacterial therapy. A randomized, controlled trial. *Ann Intern Med.* 2001; 135: 412–422.

19. Walsh TJ, Pappas P, Winston DJ, et al. Voriconazole compared with liposomal amphotericin B for empirical antifungal therapy in patients with neutropenia and persistent fever. *N Engl J Med.* 2002; 346: 225–234.

20. Walsh TJ, Teppler H, Donowitz GR, et al. Caspofungin versus liposomal amphotericin B for empirical antifungal therapy in patients with persistent fever and neutropenia. *N Engl J Med.* 2004; 351: 1391–1402.

21. Freifeld AG, Bow EJ, Sepkowitz KA, et al. Clinical practice guideline for the use of antimicrobial agents in neutropenic patients with cancer: 2010 Update by the Infectious Diseases Society of America. *Clin Infect Dis.* 2011; 52: 427–431.

CHAPTER **18**

Anemia

Zuzana Tothova, James Bradner

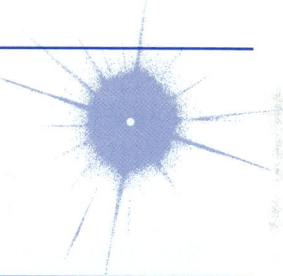

INTRODUCTION

Anemia is defined as a decrease in the red blood cell mass circulating in the bloodstream, and derives from an imbalance in the production and loss of erythrocytes. Symptoms and signs associated with anemia result from impaired oxygen delivery to the tissues. Common symptoms include fatigue, malaise, weakness, dyspnea on exertion, palpitations, and chest pressure. Patients may manifest additional overt signs such as pallor, tachycardia, impaired mentation, high-output congestive heart failure, shock, and death. The 1968 World Health Organization (WHO) criteria define anemia as hemoglobin less than 12 g/dl in women and hemoglobin less than 13 g/dl in men. The current working definition of anemia is a hemoglobin level that is two standard deviations below the mean hemoglobin level for a given sex and age.

TABLE 18-1 NCI GRADING SYSTEM FOR ANEMIA

Grade	Severity	Hemoglobin (g/dl)
0	Normal	12.0–16.0 (women)
		14.0–18.0 (men)
1	Mild	10.0–lower limit of normal
2	Moderate	8.0–<10.0
3	Severe	6.5–<8
4	Life threatening	Life threatening
5	Death	Death

Among patients with cancer, anemia is a prevalent complication of both the disease and its treatment. Nearly 50% of patients have laboratory evidence of anemia at the time of diagnosis with cancer, although it may be initially quite subtle and insidious in onset. With hematologic malignancies, anemia is coincident in as many as 70% of patients. Cancer patients with a particularly increased risk for anemia are those with a low hemoglobin before the diagnosis of cancer, those with lung or gynecologic cancers, and those receiving platinum-based therapy, and female sex (1). Due to the prevalence of anemia with cytotoxic chemotherapy, grading systems have been established to standardize reporting of myelosuppression in clinical studies and to guide clinical decision-making. The grading system offered by the National Cancer Institute is presented in Table 18-1 (2).

Anemia has been shown to decrease quality of life in cancer patients (3). The correlation between fatigue and hemoglobin level is particularly strong, establishing fatigue as a modifiable risk factor for clinical trials of transfusion or erythropoietins (EPOs). A negative impact of anemia on cancer patient prognosis and survival has been reported in both solid and hematologic malignancies (4). Because anemia in the cancer patient is frequently multifactorial, the appropriate diagnostic evaluation and therapeutic interventions must be individualized to fit the cause, the severity of anemia, and the clinical setting. The mainstay of treatment is treating the underlying cause or supportive care with packed red blood cell transfusions and EPO with or without iron supplementation.

ERYTHROPOIESIS

Hematopoiesis and the size of each compartment within its developmental hierarchy, including red blood cell production, are tightly controlled by a dynamic balance of hematopoietic stem cell (HSC) self-renewal and differentiation through subsequent compartments to mature effector cells. HSCs give rise to the common myeloid progenitor (CMP) and subsequently megakaryocyte/erythroid progenitor (MEP) in response to growth factor and cytokine stimulation, as well as instruction by the bone marrow niche. MEP eventually gives rise to red blood cells under the influence of EPO hormone. After nuclear extrusion in the marrow, immature red cells called reticulocytes are released into the circulation. The reticulocytes retain some ribosomes and mRNA that are generally destroyed after the first day in the circulation. The resulting cell is a mature red blood cell. The marrow produces more than a million erythrocytes per second, compensating for the normal 1% daily loss. EPO, a glycoprotein hormone secreted by the kidney (and to a lesser extent by the liver) in response to hypoxia, is primarily responsible for the pace of red cell production, provided that the HSC is normal and adequate supplies of iron are available.

Dietary iron is absorbed in the duodenum and proximal jejunum by apical transporters on enterocytes. The recommended daily allowance (RDA) of iron for adults is 18 mg/day. Absorbed iron then passes across the gut basement membrane into the circulation where it binds transferrin and enters the liver, the primary storage site. Particularly relevant in patients with cancer and systemic inflammatory diseases is the production of hepcidin by the liver and other cells, which impairs iron reutilization by increasing duodenal crypt cell and macrophage iron retention and downregulating iron transporters (5). Elevated hepcidin levels in patients with cancer may impair erythropoiesis. Transferrin receptors on erythrocytic precursors mediate iron uptake.

Red cell production, like other processes that require DNA synthesis, also requires adequate vitamin B_{12} and folate. Dietary folate derives from leafy vegetables and animal products. The RDA of folate for adults is 50 mg/day. Dietary folate, mainly in the form of 5-methyltetrahydrofolate, is absorbed in the jejunum, exhibits significant enterohepatic recirculation, and ultimately enters HSCs by the reduced folate receptor. It is stored in the liver and other tissues as a polyglutamated derivative, and released as needed into the circulation. Dietary cobalamin is derived from animal products. The RDA of cobalamin is 2 μg/day. The first step in cobalamin absorption requires splitting the dietary vitamin from binding proteins in food through the action of acid and pepsin in the stomach. This step is followed by additional proteolysis by pancreatic enzymes, binding of the free cobalamin to intrinsic factor (a glycoprotein secreted by the stomach), and receptor-mediated internalization in the ileum. Medications that impair gastric acid secretion and atrophic gastritis can impair the essential process of splitting vitamin B_{12} from food binders and interfere with intrinsic factor production.

Under normal circumstances, an erythrocyte circulates for 120 days. Thereafter, red cells are removed from circulation by tissue macrophages of the reticuloendothelial system (RES). Heme-bound iron is recycled and stored as ferritin and hemosiderin in the liver, spleen, and bone marrow. Iron stores may be mobilized by release into the plasma and oxidation by ceruloplasmin. Important additional tissues contribute to red cell homeostasis, such as endothelial and serum control of hemostasis and cardiorenal maintenance of plasma volume.

DIAGNOSTIC EVALUATION

The diagnostic evaluation of anemia aims to identify etiologies upon which treatment can be based. A detailed history provides important insights into the pace of development of anemia, and informs the interpretation of laboratory studies. The evaluation of anemia requires a detailed family history, as well as consideration of the family's ethnic, racial, and geographic origins, which may suggest parasites, sickle cell inheritance or thalassemia, or pernicious anemia as causes of anemia. As patients with cancer are frequently treated with agents that cause oxidative stress, glucose-6-phosphate dehydrogenase deficiency with drug-induced hemolysis may become a relevant diagnostic consideration, particularly in patients of Mediterranean and African American origin.

Laboratory evaluation serves to quantify the degree of anemia and the immediate risk posed by the red cell deficit. The hemoglobin concentration in whole blood is routinely used to define anemia. The physiologic reserve of the patient may play a dominant role in the level of symptoms associated with a particular hemoglobin level. The time frame over which the anemia developed and the presence of concurrent illness all influence the degree of symptoms for a particular level of hemoglobin.

Laboratory evaluation of peripheral blood and, if necessary, bone marrow usually yields the cause of anemia. A careful review of the blood smear may reveal morphologic clues useful in confirming the underlying etiology (see below). A complete blood count with differential is obtained to determine if additional hematopoietic lineages are affected. Measurement of the serum creatinine is used to rule out renal failure as a contributing cause or complication. The red cell indices, such as mean corpuscular volume and mean corpuscular hemoglobin, differentiate microcytic anemia from megaloblastic anemia. Among microcytic anemias, the red cell distribution width (RDW) distinguishes between iron deficiency (wide RDW) and thalassemia (narrow RDW). Iron studies (iron, ferritin, and total iron binding capacity) are useful to differentiate iron-deficiency anemia from the anemia of chronic disease. Examination of the stool for occult blood is essential to rule out chronic gastrointestinal bleeding.

Additional studies may diagnose specific etiologies. Reticulocytosis, elevation of serum lactate dehydrogenase and indirect bilirubin, and depressed serum haptoglobin suggest hemolysis. Serum free hemoglobin or urinary hemosiderin reflects intravascular hemolysis. A positive direct antiglobulin (Coombs) test confirms autoimmune hemolytic anemia. In patients with macrocytic anemia, measurement of red blood cell folate levels and plasma homocysteine indicate the presence of folate deficiency, while serum methylmalonic acid and cobalamin are measured to establish B_{12}-deficiency anemias. Low-serum levels of thyroxine or testosterone may also contribute to anemia. In patients with multilineage cytopenias, refractory anemia, or malignancies commonly metastatic to bone, a bone marrow aspirate and biopsy and cytogenetics may establish tumor replacement (myelophthisis) or treatment-related myelodysplasia as the cause.

CLASSIFICATION OF ANEMIA IN PATIENTS WITH CANCER

Anemia can be classified as either relative or absolute. Relative anemia occurs with increases in plasma cell volume, such as with volume overload or pregnancy. Absolute anemia reflects a true decrease in the red cell mass. Causes of anemia in the cancer patient may be ascribed to three fundamental processes:

■ DECREASED RED CELL PRODUCTION (THE DOMINANT FACTOR IN ANEMIA IN CANCER PATIENTS)

- Myelosuppression due to chemotherapy or radiation therapy is the most common etiology of anemia in the cancer patient. Multiagent, dose-intense or dose-dense regimens of nonselective cytotoxins are the most likely causes. Regimens employing cisplatin, taxanes, or alkylating agents are often implicated. Cycles of common regimens lead to progressive anemia, with incomplete recovery between cycles. The anemia is typically normocytic or macrocytic with a low-reticulocyte index.

- Replacement of the normal bone marrow elements by malignancies such as lymphoma, multiple myeloma, or leukemia and less commonly by solid tumors such as metastatic prostate or breast cancer may lead to anemia. In such patients, progressive, normocytic anemia is accompanied by a low-reticulocyte index. Rarely, in such cases, the peripheral blood smear contains early precursors of both the myeloid and erythroid lineages (a leukoerythroblastic response).

- Abnormal stem cell function or impairment in maturation can cause an anemia of underproduction of red cells, as with aplastic anemia, pure red cell aplasia, myelodysplastic syndrome, or acute leukemia. Myelodysplasia is an infrequent sequel of chronic alkylating agent therapy or combined modality therapy with radiation therapy and chemotherapy. A macrocytic anemia with a low-reticulocyte index may be present. The bone marrow examination typically demonstrates dysplastic, immature myeloid, and erythroid forms, and abnormal cytogenetics.

- Due to compromised nutritional status, malabsorption, treatment-related anorexia, and the hypermetabolic demands of the neoplastic process, cancer patients may manifest folate and/or vitamin B_{12}-deficiency anemia. For example, there are reports of cases of pernicious anemia in gastric cancer patients. In the absence of concurrent iron deficiency, both folate and vitamin B_{12} deficiency will result in a macrocytic or megaloblastic anemia with depressed reticulocyte index and elevated plasma homocysteine. Iron-deficiency anemia is prevalent in up to 30%–60% of cancer patients and includes functional iron deficiency, which may result from blood loss or prolonged EPO use, requiring oral or intravenous supplementation. RCTs have shown superior efficacy of iv iron supplementation over oral iron or no iron supplementation in reducing blood transfusion requirement, raising hemoglobin level, and improving quality of life in anemic cancer patients treated with an erythrocyte stimulating agent (ESA) (6).

- Reduced endogenous EPO levels are reported in cancer patients with anemia in the absence of other obvious causes (7). A normocytic anemia with low reticulocytes is seen on the peripheral smear. Renal impairment may contribute to decreased EPO production as a consequence of the malignancy (i.e., multiple myeloma) or therapy (i.e., cisplatin). Serum EPO level may confirm the diagnosis, but is rarely needed to guide the therapeutic intervention.

- Inflammatory cytokines, such as tumor necrosis factor alpha, interleukin-1, interleukin-6, and interferon gamma, may be increased in cancer patients as a consequence of tissue destruction, inflammation, or tumor secretion, and may suppress erythropoiesis by inhibiting survival and differentiation of erythroid progenitor cells.

■ INCREASED RED CELL DESTRUCTION (RARE IN CANCER PATIENTS)

- Autoimmune hemolytic anemia is observed occasionally in B-cell lymphoproliferative disorders, such as chronic lymphocytic leukemia and non-Hodgkin lymphoma. Fludarabine or allogeneic stem cell transplantation may unveil or exacerbate autoimmune anemias. A Coombs test will usually identify a warm agglutinin; other findings are an elevated LDH and depressed haptoglobin. Brisk hemolysis may result in an elevated indirect bilirubin and critically low hemoglobin. The extent of marrow involvement and timing of myelosuppressive therapy will affect the degree of reticulocytosis. Here, effective treatment should include supportive measures, immunosuppressive therapy (i.e., glucocorticoids, intravenous immunoglobulin, or rituximab), and agents targeting the underlying disease.
- Microangiopathic hemolytic anemia occasionally accompanies gastrointestinal malignancies, immunosuppression with cyclosporine or tacrolimus, or exposure to chemotherapeutic agents such as gemcitabine and mitomycin C. Chronic disseminated intravascular coagulopathy can manifest as a mild to moderate anemia.
- Hypersplenism, characterized by increased red cell destruction in the absence of a positive Coombs test, may accompany hematologic malignancies, especially lymphomas. Portal hypertension may lead to a normocytic anemia due to splenic pooling. Patients with significant, refractory hypersplenism may respond well to splenectomy.

■ BLOOD LOSS

- Acute and chronic blood loss is a frequently presenting problem in patients with gastrointestinal and genitourinary malignancies. Disease or chemotherapy-related thrombocytopenia may contribute to the risk of bleeding. Brisk hemorrhage due to tumor erosion into medium and large blood vessels may be life threatening, as observed in locally advanced head and neck or pancreatic cancer. Acute intratumoral hemorrhage is uncommon, but described in hepatocellular carcinoma, sarcoma, metastatic melanoma, and other rapidly proliferative, bulky solid tumors. Unusual causes of life-threatening tumor hemorrhage include bleeding from cavernous hemangioma, splenic hemangiosarcoma, and tumors metastatic to the ovary. Bevacizumab is associated with hemorrhage occasionally, particularly in patients with lung cancer.
- Chronic hemorrhage is a frequent complication of gastrointestinal tumors and gynecologic tumors, in particular endometrial cancer. Often, blood loss is surreptitious and manifests as an iron-deficiency anemia.

INTERVENTION

The adverse consequences of cancer-related anemia warrant intervention appropriate to symptoms and comorbidities. The variable causes of anemia in the cancer patient require specific, directed therapies. Rapid identification of the cause(s) of anemia should prompt the appropriate intervention to correct causes of blood loss, hemolysis, clotting defects, or other reversible processes. Most often, however, no specific and reversible cause is identified other than therapy and the anemia of chronic illness. To replenish red cell mass, two interventions are most often considered: red blood cell transfusion and recombinant EPO with or without iron supplementation.

Transfusion of red blood cells acutely alleviates the symptoms of anemia. However, transfusion is not without risk. Although extremely rare, complications of blood transfusion include volume overload, infection (bacterial, HIV, CMV, HBV, HCV, HTLV), acute transfusion reactions, iron overload, transfusion-related acute lung injury, and allo-immunization. Unless the donor cells are irradiated, there is a risk that donor lymphocytes could induce fatal graft-vs-host disease. Nonetheless, with acute or severe anemia, transfusion may prove life-saving. Under less emergent conditions, the decision to restore red cell mass through transfusion or the use of EPO requires clinical judgment. Evidence-based guidelines for transfusion have been published by a number of organizations, and their conclusions are consistent with a large study that compared restrictive versus liberal transfusion in the critically ill (8). For reasons that remain largely undefined, efforts to keep hemoglobin levels near normal in patients with acute illness are actually associated with poorer overall survival. Without evidence of severe cardiac disease, it is appropriate to restrict transfusion to those patients with a hemoglobin less than 7 g/dl, maintaining levels between 7 and 9 g/dl. The rate of transfusion depends on the severity of symptoms related to hypoxia (dyspnea, fatigue, changes in mental status, tachycardia, angina), taking care to avoid acute fluid overload. A recent Cochrane review analyzed the benefit of blood transfusions in patients with advanced cancer. Although there were no randomized controlled trials (RTCs) available at the time of analysis, meta-analysis of available data pooled from 12 different studies showed a subjective response rate of 31%–70% posttransfusion with effects waning by day 14. However, there was a high 14-day mortality associated with transfusions, and additional studies will be required to shed light on causality versus inappropriate use of transfusions in dying patients (9).

Initially marketed for anemia in advanced renal disease, recombinant EPO was approved by the US FDA for the treatment of cancer-related anemia in 1993 based on quality-of-life endpoints. The two commercially available preparations of recombinant EPO in the United States are epoetin alpha (Epogen, Amgen; Procrit, Ortho Biotech) and the second-generation erythrocyte stimulating agent (ESA) with a longer half-life, darbepoetin alpha (Aranesp, Amgen). Recombinant epoetin alpha is almost identical to the endogenous human glycoprotein, EPO, differing importantly in glycosylation of key residues that prolong half-life. Darbepoetin alpha differs from endogenous EPO at five amino acid residues, allowing for hypoglycosylation and an even more prolonged serum half-life.

Modest clinical efficacy of epoetin alpha and darbepoetin alpha has been established in pivotal, placebo-controlled, registration studies of patients with solid and hematologic malignancies (10–12). Epoetin alpha and darbepoetin alpha demonstrate comparable efficacy in cancer-related anemia. Epoetin alpha was initially studied as a three-time weekly formulation in FDA registration studies. Subsequent clinical trials have established the safety and activity of weekly, high-dose treatment. Weekly epoetin alpha (40,000 units, adjusted in subsequent doses according to the increase in hemoglobin) and darbepoetin alpha every 2 weeks (200 mcg, adjusted) are equally effective (13).

In these and subsequent studies, a consistent, small positive effect has been observed in hemoglobin levels, diminished transfusion requirement and quality of life, though the response develops slowly over several weeks. Evidence-based guidelines have been established and, in general, a consensus has been reached that EPO can produce a symptomatic benefit, but various guideline-developing groups differ in their target hemoglobin. Quality-of-life data support an upper boundary hemoglobin of 12 g/dl (14). However, data have begun to raise the question of whether EPO might protect tumors against therapeutic interventions like radiation therapy and chemotherapy.

An increased risk of adverse complications such as hypertension, venous thromboembolism, and cardiovascular events is reported with recombinant EPO. An international placebo-controlled study of epoetin alpha in patients with metastatic breast cancer was terminated early due to an unexpected, increased recurrence rate and mortality in the treatment arm (15). A study of epoetin beta (NeoRecormon, Roche), approved in Europe for cancer-related anemia, illustrated increased thrombotic and cardiovascular events among treated patients (16). At least eight clinical studies to date have generated data suggesting that EPO is associated with increased risk of cancer recurrence, cancer progression, or death (reviewed in [17]).

For example, the Danish Head and Neck Cancer Study Group trial (DAHANCA 10) compared radiotherapy-to-radiotherapy plus darbepoetin alpha (target hemoglobin 14.0–15.5 g/dl) in the treatment of advanced head and neck cancer. Three-year locoregional control and overall survival were both worse in patients treated with darbepoetin alpha (http://conman.au.dk/dahanca). A double-blind study of 989 patients treated with darbepoetin alpha (target hemoglobin 12 g/dl) or placebo failed to demonstrate a favorable effect of darbepoetin on red cell transfusion requirements. However, patients treated with darbepoetin demonstrated an increase in mortality. A similar study of weekly epoetin alpha (40,000 IU; target hemoglobin 12–14 g/dl) in anemic patients with lung cancer was closed prematurely due to increased mortality in treated patients. Median time to death was 68 days with ESA versus 131 days with placebo. Accordingly the FDA has issued a boxed warning for EPO products (http://www.fda.gov/cder/drug/infopage/RHE/default.htm).

In the most recent Cochrane review of 91 RCTs on managing anemia in cancer patients using ESA, the use of ESAs significantly reduced the need for red blood cell transfusions (RR 0.65), and was associated with a better hematologic response, as well as suggestion of improved quality of life. However, there was strong evidence that ESAs increase mortality (HR 1.17), and less strong evidence that they decrease overall survival (HR 1.05). There was a significantly increased risk of thromboembolic complications (RR 1.52), as well as hypertension (RR 1.30) and inconclusive evidence regarding tumor response (18). As a result of these studies, the American Society of Hematology and the American Society of Clinical Oncology published practice guidelines on the use of ESAs in adult patients with cancer (19), which are outlined in Table 18-2. In summary, EPOs are not FDA approved for use in cancer patients not receiving myelosuppressive chemotherapy with the exception of patients with low-risk myelodysplastic syndromes (MDS) to avoid transfusions, and they are not recommended for patients with hemoglobin >10. EPO is being evaluated clinically for

TABLE 18-2 ASH/ASCO CLINICAL PRACTICE GUIDELINES ON ESA USE IN ADULT CANCER PATIENTS

Undergoing myelosuppressive chemotherapy?	Yes AND Hb <10 g/dl	Consider ESA use after discussing potential harms and benefits
	No	ESA not recommended, except patients with lower risk MDS to avoid transfusions
Recommended length of treatment	Responders	Discontinue when Hb >12, discontinue if Hb rise >1 g/dl in any 2-week period, discontinue with chemotherapy completion
	Non-responders (no diminution in transfusions; Hb rise <1–2 g/dl)	Discontinue after 6–8 weeks
Treatment goal	Curative	ESA not recommended
	Non-curative	ESA may be considered as above
Starting dose	Epoetin	150 U/kg 3 times a week sc OR 40,000 U weekly sc
	Darbepoetin	2.25 μg/kg weekly sc OR 500 μg every 3 weeks sc
Target		Lowest possible Hb level to avoid transfusion

its capacity to limit the size of strokes and myocardial infarcts through its action to protection of hypoxic cells from cell death. It is possible that this protective effect on dying cells will be beneficial in some settings, but all evidence thus far suggests that it is detrimental in patients with cancer. Until the issue is better defined, the use of EPO might wisely be confined to those settings where it is a component of palliative care. Its use as a component of curative regimens is undefined and potentially harmful.

New therapeutic options for treatment of anemia of chronic inflammation (ACI), including that of anemia associated with malignancy, are being actively pursued. Since the iron regulatory hormone hepicidin has been identified as a pathogenic factor in development of ACI, a number of preclinical studies are currently underway investigating the use of hepcidin inhibitors in treatment of ACI (20).

REFERENCES

1. Barrett-Lee PJ, Ludwig H, Birgegard G, et al. Independent risk factors for anemia in cancer patients receiving chemotherapy: results from the European Cancer Anaemia Survey. *Oncology*. 2006; 70: 34–48.

2. Groopman JE, Itri LM. Chemotherapy-induced anemia in adults: incidence and treatment. *J Natl Cancer Inst*. 1999; 91: 1616–1634.

3. Cella D. The Functional Assessment of Cancer Therapy-Anemia (FACT-An) Scale: a new tool for the assessment of outcomes in cancer anemia and fatigue. *Semin Hematol.* 1997; 34(Suppl 2): 13–19.

4. Caro JJ, Salas M, Ward A, et al. Anemia as an independent prognostic factor for survival in patients with cancer: a systemic, quantitative review. *Cancer.* 2001; 91: 2214–2221.

5. Nemeth E, Ganz T. Regulation of iron metabolism by hepcidin. *Annu Rev Nutr.* 2006; 26: 323–342.

6. Aapro M, Osterborg A, Gascon P, et al. Prevalence and management of cancer-related anaemia, iron deficiency and the specific role of i.v. iron. *Ann Oncol.* 2012; 23: 1954–1962.

7. Miller CB, Jones RJ, Piantadosi S, et al. Decreased erythropoietin response in patients with the anemia of cancer. *N Engl J Med.* 1990; 322: 1689–1692.

8. Hebert PC, Wells G, Blajchman MA, et al. A multicenter, randomized, controlled clinical trial of transfusion requirements in critical care. Transfusion Requirements in Critical Care Investigators, Canadian Critical Care Trials Group. *N Engl J Med.* 1999; 340: 409–417.

9. Preston NJ, Hurlow A, Brine J, Bennett MI. Blood transfusions for anaemia in patients with advanced cancer. *Cochrane Database Syst Rev.* 2012; 2: CD009007.

10. Case DC, Jr., Bukowski RM, Carey RW, et al. Recombinant human erythropoietin therapy for anemic cancer patients on combination chemotherapy. *J Natl Cancer Inst.* 1993; 85: 801–806.

11. Hedenus M, Adriansson M, San Miguel J, et al. Efficacy and safety of darbepoetin alfa in anaemic patients with lymphoproliferative malignancies: a randomized, double-blind, placebo-controlled study. *Br J Haematol.* 2003; 122: 394–403.

12. Vansteenkiste J, Pirker R, Massuti B, et al. Double-blind, placebo-controlled, randomized phase III trial of darbepoetin alfa in lung cancer patients receiving chemotherapy. *J Natl Cancer Inst.* 2002; 94: 1211–1220.

13. Glaspy J, Vadhan-Raj S, Patel R, et al. Randomized comparison of every-2-week darbepoetin alfa and weekly epoetin alfa for the treatment of chemotherapy-induced anemia: the 20030125 Study Group Trial. *J Clin Oncol.* 2006; 24: 2290–2297.

14. Crawford J, Cella D, Cleeland CS, et al. Relationship between changes in hemoglobin level and quality of life during chemotherapy in anemic cancer patients receiving epoetin alfa therapy. *Cancer.* 2002; 95: 888–895.

15. Leyland-Jones B. Breast cancer trial with erythropoietin terminated unexpectedly. *Lancet Oncol.* 2003; 4: 459–460.

16. Henke M, Laszig R, Rube C, et al. Erythropoietin to treat head and neck cancer patients with anaemia undergoing radiotherapy: randomised, double-blind, placebo-controlled trial. *Lancet.* 2003; 362: 1255–1260.

17. Oster HS, Neumann D, Hoffman M, et al. Erythropoietin: the swinging pendulum. *Leuk Res.* 2012; 36: 939–944.

18. Tonia T, Mettler A, Robert N, et al. Erythropoietin or darbepoetin for patients with cancer. *Cochrane Database Syst Rev*. 2012; 12: CD003407.

19. Rizzo JD, Brouwers M, Hurley P, et al. American Society of Hematology/ American Society of Clinical Oncology clinical practice guideline update on the use of epoetin and darbepoetin in adult patients with cancer. *Blood*. 2010; 116: 4045–4059.

20. Fung E, Sugianto P, Hsu J, Damoiseaux R, et al. High-throughput screening of small molecules identifies hepcidin antagonists. *Mol Pharmacol*. 2013; 83: 681–690.

CHAPTER **19**

Cancer and Coagulopathy

Rachel P.G. Rosovsky

INTRODUCTION

The association between cancer and thrombosis was first proposed by Armand Trousseau (**Figure 19-1**) when he recognized the condition of *thrombophlebitis migrans*, as a forewarning of occult malignancy (1). In 1865, he remarked, "Should you, when in doubt as to the nature of an affection of the stomach, should you when hesitating between chronic gastritis, simple ulcer, and cancer, observe a vein become infected in the arm or leg, you may dispel your doubt, and pronounce in a positive manner that there is a cancer . . ." (1). Although the association of hemostatic disorders and cancer has been studied extensively over the past 100 years, venous thromboembolism (VTE), defined herein as pulmonary embolus (PE) or deep vein thrombosis (DVT), remains a major cause of morbidity and mortality in cancer patients.

This chapter will explore the pathogenesis of thrombosis in cancer as well as the epidemiology and risk factors. The chapter will also focus on novel risk assessment models and the emergence of new biomarkers to classify patients at high risk of developing VTE. Current diagnostic and management strategies for VTE in cancer patients and the challenges of antithrombotic therapy in this population will be examined. This update will evaluate the results of several randomized controlled trials aimed at assessing the clinical benefit of antithrombotic prophylaxis in cancer outpatients. Finally, new therapeutic developments in this area will be addressed.

PATHOGENESIS

The pathophysiological mechanisms of thrombosis in cancer patients are complex and involve multiple clinical and biological factors including tumor cells, the hemostatic system, inherited and acquired thrombophilia, and exogenous contributors such as chemotherapy and radiotherapy (2).

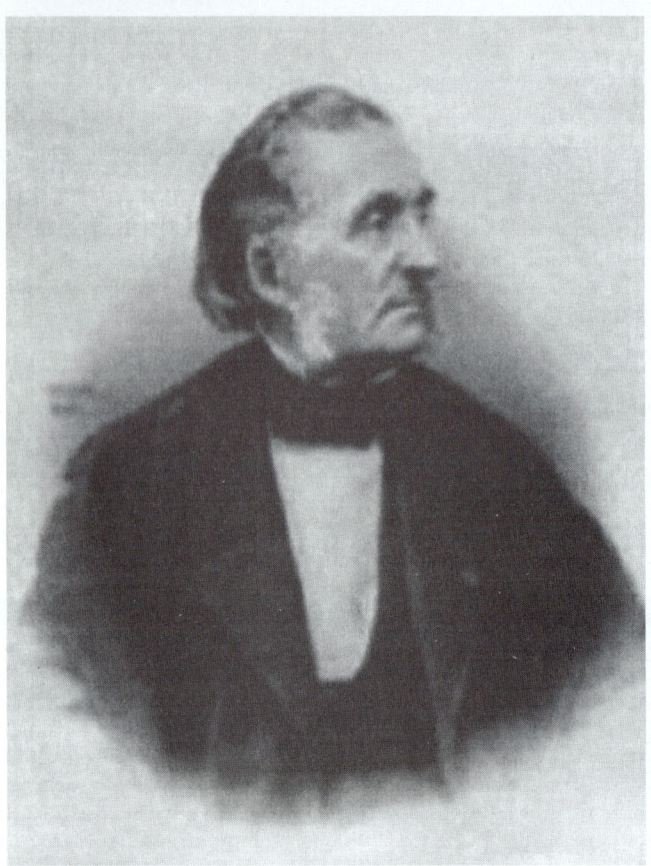

FIGURE 19-1 Armand Trousseau.

Tumors contribute to thrombosis through the expression of procoagulant factors including tissue factor, cancer procoagulant, and adhesion molecules. Recent experimental models of human cancers have shown that an integral feature of neoplastic transformation from cancer cells is through activation of clotting proteins (3–6). The role of tissue factor-bearing microparticles (MP) contributing to thrombin generation has also been explored in vitro and in vivo studies. Zwicker et al. found that VTE developed in 34.8% of cancer patients with elevated levels of MP compared to 0% in those without detectable levels (7). Tumor cells can also induce platelet activation and aggregation through secretion of proteases. Tumor-related release of various cytokines, growth factors, and proteases including tumor necrosis factor α (TNFα), interleukin 1β, and vascular endothelial growth factor (VEGF) contribute not only to angiogenesis and inflammation but also to the activation of the hemostatic system. Furthermore, tumor cells interact directly with the host blood vessels, endothelial cells, leukocytes, and monocytes leading to host cell inflammatory responses (2). These many and varied interactions lead to both a direct and an indirect activation of the clotting system, an increase in thrombin generation, and ultimately a hypercoagulable state.

EPIDEMIOLOGY

Venous thrombosis is a common complication in patients with cancer. Although the exact incidence of VTE in cancer patients is unknown, it occurs in approximately 15%, with reports ranging from 4% to 30% (8, 9). These numbers likely underestimate the problem as VTE often causes no symptoms. In a recent study, clinically unsuspected PE was present in up to 4.4% of oncology patients undergoing CT scans for other indications (10). If symptoms are present, they are often nonspecific or attributed to a patient's underlying malignancy.

Certain malignancies exhibit high rates of VTE, such as hematological malignancies and neoplasms, especially if high grade, of the pancreas, gastrointestinal tract, ovary, brain, colon, kidney, lung, and prostate (11–15). However, it is unclear if the high rates are due to the underlying properties of particular cancers or merely reflect the high prevalence of certain cancers. Nevertheless, it is well documented that cancers diagnosed at the same time as an episode of VTE are more likely to have distant metastases and lower survival rates (16, 17). One study showed that cancer patients with VTE had a 1-year survival of 12% as compared to 36% in cancer patients without VTE (17). Similarly, patients who develop VTE within a year after a cancer diagnosis are more likely to have advanced stage and poorer prognosis when compared to analogous cancer patients without VTE (17). A study of over 235,000 cancer patients showed that after adjusting for age, race, and stage of disease, VTE at the time of or within 1 year of cancer diagnosis was a significant predictor of death within that year (16). VTE is the second leading cause of death in cancer patients, with cancer progression being number one (18). It also appears that cancer patients with VTE are two to three times more likely to have recurrent VTE and two to six times more likely to experience hemorrhagic complications from anticoagulant therapy than noncancer patients with VTE (19, 20). These findings clearly indicate that VTE may be more aggressive and difficult to treat in cancer patients than in noncancer patients.

The association between cancer and thrombosis is further supported by many studies, suggesting that an idiopathic VTE is often associated with occult cancer. Approximately 10% of patients who present with an idiopathic or unprovoked VTE are diagnosed with cancer within the next 1–2 years (21). These provocative findings raise the unanswered question as to whether all patients with idiopathic VTE should undergo extensive cancer screening. The SOMIT study attempted to address this matter (22). Patients with an idiopathic VTE were randomized to either extensive or nonextensive cancer screening and followed for 24 months. Subjects in the extensive screening arm seemed to have a shorter delay in the diagnosis of cancer, their cancers were detected at earlier stages, and they had a lower cancer-related mortality (22). Unfortunately, this trial was stopped prematurely due to recruitment issues leaving these conclusions unsubstantiated.

In a more recent prospective cohort study of 630 patients with a first episode of idiopathic VTE, extensive screening, which included abdominal and chest CT and mammogram, detected six additional cancers (2.0%; 95% CI, 0.74–4.3), compared to limited screening (23). At the 2.5 years of follow-up, cancer was diagnosed in 3.7% in extensive screening group and 5.0% in limited and there was no significant difference in death rates. Thus, this study concluded that the low yield of extensive screening and lack of survival benefit did not support routine screening for cancer in patients with an idiopathic VTE.

A recent systematic review of this question found that an extensive screening strategy employing an abdominal and pelvic CT statistically significantly increased the number of undiagnosed cancer from 49.4% to 67% in patients with an unprovoked VTE (24). However, this review could not address the complication rates, cost-effectiveness, or morbidity and mortality difference associated with an extensive screening approach. The use of PET-CT was recently investigated to screen for occult malignancy in 40 patients who presented with an unprovoked VTE (25). Twenty-five patients (62.5%) had abnormal findings requiring additional evaluations and of these, only one occult malignancy was discovered. This malignancy, however, was detected in a patient with unexplained abdominal pain and unintentional weight loss of 40 pounds, which are symptoms concerning for a malignancy. Hence, larger studies are needed to evaluate the cost-effectiveness of PET-CT in this population.

Current recommendations are to provide age appropriate cancer screening for patients who present with idiopathic VTE, and any additional testing should be driven by what is discovered in a thorough history and physical examination. Given the SOMIT observations, albeit underpowered, future studies evaluating extensive cancer screening for patients with idiopathic VTE are warranted.

RISK FACTORS

Many inherited and acquired risk factors are associated with the development of VTE and are listed in Table 19-1. Cancer patients may have additional risk factors related to their malignancy, including surgery, immobilization, chemotherapy, some forms of hormone therapy, and the presence of indwelling central venous catheters (CVCs). Without appropriate prophylaxis, cancer patients have twice the risk of developing postoperative DVT and three times the risk of developing a fatal PE than patients without cancer (26). Long-term immobilization, often due to lengthy hospital stays, also increases the risk of developing VTE. Furthermore, comorbid conditions, distant metastases, advanced age, obesity, prior history of VTE and elevated platelet count are associated with increased VTE risk (12, 13, 27, 28).

In addition to patient-related risks, there are treatment-related risks. Tamoxifen, estrogen, thalidomide, L-asparaginase, cisplatin, and VEGF inhibitors are a few of the cancer therapies associated with high rates of thromboembolic complications, especially when used in combination with other chemotherapeutic agents. In a trial involving over 2600 women with early stage breast cancer, the incidence of developing VTE was 0.2% with placebo and 0.9% with tamoxifen (29). Another trial involving

TABLE 19-1 RISK FACTORS FOR VENOUS THROMBOEMBOLISM (VTE)*

- Inherited
  - Antithrombin deficiency
  - Protein C deficiency
  - Protein S deficiency
  - Factor V Leiden
  - Prothrombin G20210A
  - Dysfibrinogenemias
- Environmental
  - Smoking
  - Prolonged air travel
- Treatment-related
  - Hormonal (estrogens, tamoxifen)
  - Chemotherapy (bevacizumab, thalidomide)
  - Central venous catheterization
  - Surgery
  - Heparin-induced thrombocytopenia
  - Immobilization
- Comorbid states and diseases
  - Malignancy
  - Advanced age
  - Prior thrombotic event
  - Prolonged immobilization, paresis
  - Pregnancy and the postpartum period
  - Obesity
  - Major trauma
  - Congestive heart failure
  - Antiphospholipid antibody syndrome
  - Myeloproliferative disorders (e.g., essential thrombocytosis, polycythemia vera)
  - Inflammatory bowel disease
  - Paroxysmal nocturnal hemoglobinuria
  - Nephrotic syndrome

*Applies to cancer and noncancer patients.

women with advanced stage breast cancer showed that the incidence of VTE was 2.6% with tamoxifen alone versus 13.6% with tamoxifen plus chemotherapy (30). Similarly, in studies involving multiple myeloma, treatment with thalidomide alone had a risk of 2%. The risk increased to 33% with the addition of chemotherapy (31). Cancer patients who receive either cytotoxic or immunosuppressive therapy have a 6.5-fold increased risk of developing a VTE when compared to noncancer patients, and a twofold increased risk compared to cancer patients not receiving chemotherapy (32). In a recent systematic review of 8216 cancer patients, those receiving cisplatin-based chemotherapy had a significantly increased rate of VTE compared to patients who did not (RR, 1.67l 95% CI, 1.25 – 2.23; p = 0.01) (33). Furthermore, venous thrombosis, and in particular, cortical sinus thrombosis, is a frequent complication of L-asparaginase treatment, and it is related to inhibition of the synthesis of anticoagulant factors, protein C and protein S.

Erythropoiesis-stimulating agents (ESAs) are often given to patients with chemotherapy induced anemia. However, recent studies show that ESAs administered to patients with cancer increase not only risk of VTE but also risk of mortality (13, 34, 35). As such, the FDA label now limits the use of ESA to patients receiving chemotherapy for palliative intent. ESAs are no longer indicated for patients receiving chemotherapy for curative intent.

Many new antiangiogenic agents are under investigation and used in practice to treat a variety of cancers. In a systematic review of 15 RCT, patients receiving bevacizumab, the recombinant humanized monoclonal antibody to VEGF, had an increased risk of VTE compared to controls (RR 1.3; 95% CI, 1.13–1.56; p<0.001) (36). Similarly in a meta-analysis of anti-epidermal growth factor receptor (EGFR) agents, the associated RR of VTEs was 1.32 (95% CI 1.07–1.63; p = 0.01) in patients who received anti-EGFRs versus controls (37). The risk was highest with the use of cetuximab and panitumumab (13).

CVCs are another common risk factor for VTE. These devices are commonplace among cancer patients who require long-term chemotherapy. The reported incidence of catheter-related thrombosis ranges from 5% to 75%, and this wide range likely reflects the distinct types of malignancy, the kind of catheter used, and the duration of its implantation (38). In addition, the complications associated with CVC-related thrombosis can result in loss of catheter function, postphlebitic syndrome of the upper extremity, PE, and even mortality. There have been major efforts to identify disease management approaches to decrease the risk of VTE with CVC, and these mechanisms are discussed in the Prevention section of this chapter.

RISK PREDICTIVE MODELS

Trying to predict the risk of VTE in cancer patients is a major clinical challenge. Patients at high risk of developing VTE may benefit from prophylactic anticoagulation, whereas patients at low risk may have unnecessary and unfavorable consequences from this practice, such as bleeding. Therefore, the development of risk assessment tools and predictive biomarkers to identify high-risk patients is clinically relevant and important.

One novel and promising tool is the Khorana score, which uses baseline clinical and laboratory variables to predict the risk of chemotherapy-associated VTE (39). The score assigns points to cancer site (2 points for very high-risk sites such as pancreatic or gastric and 1 point for high-risk sites such as lung, ovarian, or bladder), platelet count $\geq 350 \times 10^9$/l (1 point), hemoglobin ≤ 10 g/dl or the use of erythropoietin-stimulating agents (1 point), leukocyte count $\geq 11 \times 10^9$/l (1 point), and body mass index ≥ 35 kg/m^2 (1 point). A score of ≥ 3 is considered high risk and correlates with a rate of symptomatic VTE in 6.7% of patients undergoing chemotherapy. This model was recently modified in another study to include platinum or gemcitabine-based chemotherapies (40).

The Ottawa score is another clinical prediction rule aimed at identifying recurrent VTE risk in patients with cancer-associated VTE (41). The independent variables include sex, primary tumor site, tumor-node-metastasis

(TNM) stage, and prior VTE. High-risk predictors include female, lung cancer, and history of VTE and are given 1 point each. Low-risk predictors include breast cancer and stage 1 cancer of any origins and are given −1 and −2 points, respectively. A score of ≤0 correlates with a low clinical probability of recurrent VTE (≤4.5%), whereas a score of ≥1 correlates with a high clinical probability of recurrent VTE (≥19%). Future prospective trials are warranted to demonstrate the reproducibility, generalizability, and safety of the Khorana and Ottawa scores as well as to determine their effectiveness as a tool for treating cancer patients at risk of VTE.

BIOMARKERS

Identifying biomarkers to help predict the risk of VTE in cancer patients is one of the largest growing areas of research. Data from the prospective Vienna Cancer and Thrombosis Study (CATS) demonstrated that elevated levels of P-selectin were predictive of VTE in cancer patients (42). The probability of developing VTE at 6 months was 11.9% in patients with high levels of P-selectin compared to 3.7% in patients with low levels. This group also found that patients with elevated D-dimer and high prothrombin fragment 1+2 (F 1+2) compared to patients with nonelevated levels were associated with an increased risk of VTE (15.5% vs 5%) (43). Thrombin generation is another potential biomarker studied by the Vienna CATS group (44). Elevated peak thrombin levels conferred an 11% risk of developing VTE compared to 4% in patients with lower levels. An expansion of the original Khorana score to include D-dimer and P-selectin appears to improve the VTE risk prediction tool (45). There was a 26-fold higher probability of developing VTE in patients with a high score compared to patients with a low score. However, this expanded risk score requires further validation studies but may be limited by the lack of widely available P-selectin assays.

In the last few years, the role of tissue factor-bearing MP in connection with cancer progression and thrombosis has been investigated. In an immunohistochemical study, high levels versus low levels of MP in pancreatic cancer patients correlated with the development of VTE (26.3% vs 4.5%) (46). Similarly, Zwicker et al. found that VTE developed in 34.8% cancer patients with detectable levels of MP compared to 0% in patients with undetectable levels (7).

Biomarkers may improve the stratification of cancer patients with regard to their risk of VTE. The efficacy and safety of prophylactic anticoagulation in patients with these elevated biomarkers needs to be addressed in well-designed RCTs.

CLINICAL MANIFESTATIONS

Cancer patients can present with a wide range of thromboembolic events. The two most commonly recognized are DVT and pulmonary embolism (PE). However, symptoms and signs may result from migratory thrombophlebitis, nonbacterial thrombotic endocarditis, disseminated intravascular coagulopathy (DIC), thrombotic microangiography, and arterial thrombosis. Cancer patients may also present with multiple clinical sequelae as was originally reported in 1977 by Sack et al. in a review of 182 cases of neoplasia associated with alterations in blood coagulation (47). **Figure 19-2** is an

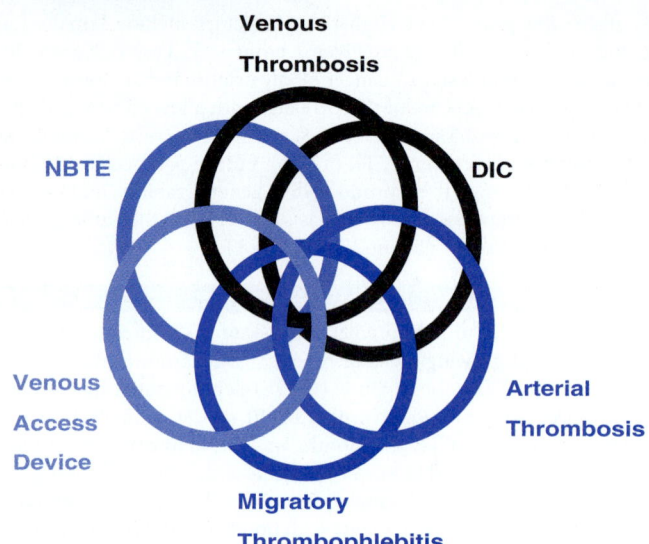

FIGURE 19-2 Venn diagram of relationships between clinical signs.

expansion of the original Venn diagram created by Sack et al. which represents the interrelations between the various clinical phenomena. Discussion of all these clinical presentations is beyond the scope of this chapter and, therefore, only DVT and PE will be presented in detail.

Patients with DVT may experience complaints of leg pain, swelling, tenderness, discoloration, venous distension, or a palpable cord. Nonspecific symptoms of PE include dyspnea, tachypnea, tachycardia, pleuritic chest pain, cough, and wheeze. Signs may include hemoptysis, hypotension, syncope, coma, pleural effusion, or pulmonary infiltrates. Each of these clinical features can be a manifestation of other cardiac or pulmonary processes, such as pneumonia or heart failure, making the diagnosis of PE difficult.

Data from the MASTER registry in Italy demonstrated that the clinical presentation of acute VTE in cancer patients is different and more extensive than in patients without cancer (48). The incidence of bilateral DVT and rates of iliocaval thrombosis were higher in the cancer patients. The management of VTE in the cancer patients was also more problematic with a higher incidence of hemorrhage and need for inferior vena cava (IVC) filters.

Other consequences of DVT and PE include acute morbidity or even death. Some of the short- and long-term complications due to thrombotic events consist of extension of the clot, embolization, postthrombotic syndrome, pulmonary hypertension, and recurrent VTE. Furthermore, there may be significant morbidity associated with long-term anticoagulation or with placement of an IVC filter. The psychological stress and fear that patients face when suffering from a thromboembolic event must also be appreciated. Moreover, the presence of VTE or its complications may cause delays in chemotherapy or other treatments, which may have considerable consequences for the patient. In one of the largest outcome studies of DVT in cancer patients, the most common complication was bleeding, which occurred in 13% of patients (49). PE, death from DVT, and death from anti-coagulation were also observed. The mean length of stay was 11 days with a mean cost of hospitalization of $20,065. VTE as the cause of death was also shown in an autopsy-based study where one out of every seven cancer deaths in the hospital was due to PE (50). Over 60% of those who died of a PE had either limited metastatic or local disease indicating a reasonable chance of prolonged survival if not for the fatal PE (50).

DIAGNOSIS OF VTE

Diagnosing VTE in cancer patients, as in other patients, may be difficult. The signs and symptoms of VTE are often variable and nonspecific, and available diagnostic tests have varying sensitivities and specificities. Moreover, commonly employed models for predicting the probability of VTE have limited value in cancer patients because of the significant additional risk factors at play. Ultimately, a diagnosis requires a combination of modalities.

If VTE is clinically suspected, a common first test is the D-dimer, which reflects the degradation product of cross-linked fibrin. This test is highly sensitive but not specific (51). Because it is elevated in a variety of situations including malignancy, acute VTE, underlying lung abnormalities, recent surgery, hospitalization, and aging, the primary value of the D-dimer test is a negative result, which constitutes strong evidence against significant thrombosis (51). Two recent studies demonstrated that the combination of a normal D-dimer and a low clinical pretest probability was useful in excluding the diagnosis of DVT in cancer patients (52, 53). If the D-dimer test is positive, however, additional diagnostic tests should be performed.

Duplex venous ultrasound (US) imaging, the most widely available modality for diagnosing DVT, is highly sensitive for detecting proximal vein thrombosis but less so for detecting calf vein clots. Therefore, if a patient presents with symptoms suggestive of a calf vein thrombosis but has a negative US test, a repeat test at 3–5 days may be warranted, especially if symptoms persist and no alternative diagnosis has been established. If the US is inconclusive, magnetic resonance imaging (MRI) of the lower extremities is usually definitive.

If PE is suspected, a variety of imaging tests may aid in making the diagnosis, including lung radionuclide scans (VQ), spiral computed tomography (CT), pulmonary angiography, MRI, and magnetic resonance angiography (MRA). Although pulmonary angiography has been the gold standard, it is invasive and often unavailable or impractical and, therefore, has been replaced by CT angiography.

VQ scans, formerly a frequently used diagnostic tool, are now employed only when there is a contraindication to CT scans with contrast, such as renal failure or iodine allergy. VQ scans are helpful when they are either positive or negative, but their results are often inconclusive or confounded by underlying lung abnormalities.

The spiral CT or computerized tomographic angiography (CTA) is highly sensitive for large emboli. Multidetector scanners are able to visualize the subsegmental arteries effectively. Simultaneous imaging of the lower extremities, which is helpful in identifying an associated DVT, can further increase the diagnostic sensitivity of CTA. Moreover, the spiral CT may help identify alternative etiologies for a patient's symptoms if a PE is not identified.

One of the newest diagnostic tools to diagnose PE, MRI/MRA of the chest, has been incompletely evaluated and standardized. Currently studies are underway to assess its accuracy and safety.

TREATMENT

The management of VTE in cancer patients is a challenge due to the frequent presence of a hypercoagulable state, physical obstructions to blood flow, patient immobility, and the general impression that these patients are relatively resistant to anticoagulant therapy. The goals of treatment are to prevent fatal PE, recurrent VTE, and long-term VTE complications. This section will outline current treatment recommendations for both the acute and long-term treatment of VTE in cancer patients based on the seventh American College of Chest Physicians (ACCP) Conference guidelines and Journal of National Comprehensive Cancer Network (JNCCN) (54, 55).

■ ACUTE TREATMENT

The initial treatment for DVT and PE are similar. There are three options for anticoagulation: unfractionated heparin (UFH), low-molecular-weight heparin (LMWH), and fondaparinux sodium. The use of newer anticoagulants to treat VTE in cancer patients is discussed under the section of New Developments.

LMWH is a fragment of UFH and exerts its anticoagulant effect through antifactor Xa and antithrombin activities. It is cleared from plasma by metabolism in the liver, and a small portion is excreted in the urine. LMWH has largely replaced the use of UFH as the initial treatment for VTE because of its similar efficacy, superior safety profile, and pharmacokinetic advantages that allow for once or twice daily subcutaneous administration without laboratory monitoring, lower risk of complications such as heparin-induced thrombocytopenia (HIT) or heparin-induced osteoporosis, and potential for outpatient treatment. LMWH, a weight-based therapy, may need to be episodically monitored in two particular situations: in patients who are at the extremes of body weight or in those suffering from renal failure, the latter situation because of LMWH clearance by renal excretion. This monitoring involves measuring the antifactor Xa activity 3–4 h after subcutaneous injection with a therapeutic goal of 0.5–1.3 U/ml.

If a patient requires a short-acting initial anticoagulant or one that needs to be carefully monitored, is anticipating an invasive procedure, or has a contraindication to LMWH such as severe renal failure, UFH is the favored treatment. UFH, a glycosaminoglycan, exerts its anticoagulant effect at several steps in the formation of fibrin clots. Specifically, when combined with antithrombin III, it inactivates activated factor X and inhibits the conversion of prothrombin to thrombin. UFH is metabolized in the liver and can be reversed with the antidote, protamine sulfate, if necessary. However, unlike LMWH, UFH is usually given intravenously and needs to be monitored frequently, and the dose must be adjusted with the use of nomograms to maintain an activated partial thromboplastin time (aPPT) of 1.5–2.5 times the normal.

A third anticoagulant option is the synthetic pentasaccharide, fondaparinux sodium, which works by indirectly inhibiting factor Xa. It has similar efficacy and safety for the initial treatment of PE and DVT as UFH or LMWH. It is an attractive medication because of its once daily subcutaneous administration and linear pharmacokinetic profile. In addition, it does not cause a syndrome akin to HIT to date. However, it cannot be reversed and its 17-h half-life makes it an unreasonable option in patients who require a short-acting therapy. In addition, because fondaparinux is excreted unchanged in the urine, monitoring is essential in patients with mild or moderate renal insufficiency, and the medication is contraindicated in patients with severe renal failure. The efficacy of fondaparinux for the initial VTE treatment in cancer patients is limited. Results from a post-hoc analysis of the MATISSE trials suggest that fondaparinux may be more efficacious than UFH but less efficacious than LMWH (56).

Other options for the initial treatment of DVT and PE that are not anticoagulants include thrombolytic therapy, thromboendarterectomy, and IVC filters. The use of thrombolytics is controversial in DVT and currently should be considered only for patients with massive iliofemoral thrombosis and at risk for limb gangrene (54, 57). A meta-analysis has helped clarify the use of thrombolytics for the initial treatment of PE (58). While there was no overall benefit of thrombolytics in terms of recurrent PE or death, patients who were hemodynamically unstable (systolic blood pressure <90–100 mmHg) had a significantly lower rate of recurrent PE and death, but a significantly higher rate of major bleeding (58). The use of thrombolytics has also been considered in patients who are hemodynamically stable but exhibit evidence of severe right ventricular dysfunction. Results thus far are not definitive.

Thrombolytic drugs in current use include tissue-type plasminogen activator (t-PA), urokinase, and streptokinase. T-PA, the most commonly used of the group, is given as a 100-mg infusion over 2 h, followed by heparin. In patients refractory to t-PA, one should consider the presence of a saddle embolus, which might require thromboendarterectomy.

IVC filters are another option for the initial treatment of VTE. They are primarily used in patients with recurrent DVT or PE on anticoagulation, or in patients at high risk of bleeding on anticoagulation. There is little published evidence to document an improvement in outcome after their use. Moreover, if necessary, removable filters are preferred.

■ LONG-TERM TREATMENT

Similar to the initial treatment for VTE, the long-term treatment for VTE in cancer patients can be complicated by the concomitant need for chemotherapy, hormone therapy, invasive procedures, or CVCs. In addition, cancer patients have higher rates of recurrent VTE and bleeding with traditional anticoagulant therapy than noncancer patients, which adds a further challenge to their management. For many years, the long-term treatment recommendation for VTE in cancer patients was similar to that of the general population, the vitamin K antagonist (VKA), warfarin (Coumadin).

After the initiation of UFH, LMWH or fondaparinux, warfarin is started on day 1 and adjusted to maintain an INR of 2–3. Given the slow onset of action, there needs to be a 5- to 7-day overlap between the two medications.

Although warfarin has the advantage of being an oral medication, it has significant disadvantages. It requires regular laboratory monitoring, has significant drug interactions because of its cyp 3A4–dependent metabolism, and is influenced by nutritional status. Fortunately, several trials have shown that LMWH is an attractive alternative.

A randomized controlled trial (RCT) demonstrated a clear benefit to LMWH compared with warfarin in cancer patients for long-term treatment or secondary prophylaxis after VTE (59). After 6 months of therapy, cancer patients who received LMWH had a significantly lower rate of recurrent VTE (9%) than those who received warfarin (17%), with no difference in the rates of bleeding (Figure 19-3). In addition, a post-hoc analysis of the patients with nonmetastatic solid tumors revealed a survival advantage in the LMWH group. Twelve-month cumulative mortality in this population was 20% in the LMWH group versus 36% in the warfarin group (60).

The mechanism by which anticoagulants may decrease cancer mortality is not clear. However, in the past decade, multiple trials have suggested a survival advantage in cancer patients receiving LMWH as compared to UFH or warfarin for treatment or prevention of VTE (59). Interestingly, the survival advantages were not solely attributable to decreases in the rate

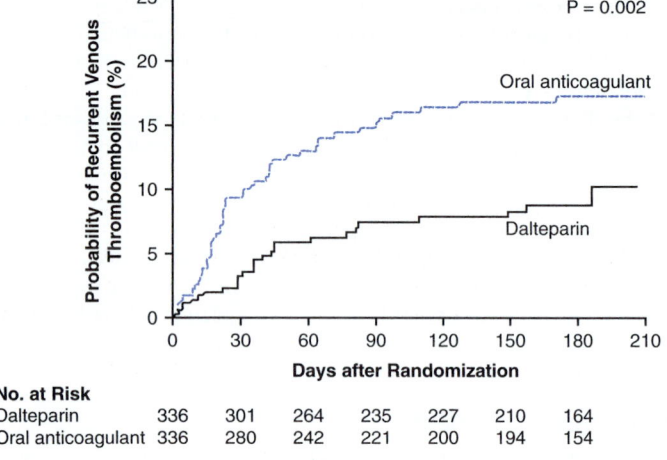

FIGURE 19-3 Recurrent VTE. Kaplan-Meier estimates of the probability of symptomatic recurrent VTE among cancer patients who were randomized to secondary prophylaxis with dalteparin vs warfarin treatment for acute VTE (22). (From Lee AY, Levine MN, Baker RI, et al. Low-molecular-weight heparin versus a coumarin for the prevention of recurrent venous thromboembolism in patients with cancer. *N Engl J Med.* 2003; 349: 146–53. Copyright © 2003. Massachusetts Medical Society. All rights reserved.)

of fatal pulmonary emboli. Three trials studying the value of LMWH in patients without VTE found a significant survival advantage in patients who received LMWH versus placebo (61–63). A recent systematic review and meta-analysis of 4 studies enrolling 898 patients randomized to LMWH versus placebo suggested that LMWH may improve overall survival in cancer patients (64). However, two newer studies did not find a survival benefit with the use of LMWH (23, 65). Furthermore, a number of trials investigating the use of LMWH for thromboprophylaxis in cancer patients receiving chemotherapy have failed to show any survival benefit (66–69). Several ongoing studies are underway to further evaluate this question and to possibly define the tumor types, disease stages, and dosing schedules most likely to have a survival benefit.

LMWHs are thus the most attractive antithrombotic choice for the long-term treatment or secondary prophylaxis in cancer patients. Osteoporosis is a potential complication of LMWH and if no contraindications, these patients should be placed on calcium and vitamin D. Appropriately, the ACCP and JNCCN guidelines recommend LMWH for the first 3–6 months of long-term anticoagulant therapy for cancer patients with VTE (54, 55).

The duration of long-term treatment of acute VTE in cancer patients has not been clearly established. For noncancer patients, in whom the inciting factor has been removed, the recommendation is to treat for 3–6 months. However, in patients with idiopathic VTE, where the inciting factor is unknown and may still exist, two trials have demonstrated decreased recurrence with prolonged anticoagulation beyond 3 months (62, 70). Patients with active cancer are similar to patients with idiopathic VTEs. Thus, current ACCP and JNCCN guidelines recommend anticoagulant therapy as long as there is evidence of active cancer and cancer therapy, whichever is longer (54, 55). Indefinite therapy is recommended for patients with known metastases because their risk of recurrent VTE remains high. It is prudent, however, to re-evaluate patients frequently to re-assess the risk-benefit ratio of continuing anticoagulation.

■ RECURRENT VTE

Recurrent thrombosis is not uncommon in cancer patients with a reported incidence of up to 17% (19, 20, 59). Cancer patients who develop recurrent VTE also have decreased survival (59). In patients who develop a recurrent VTE, one should first determine medication compliance and, if on heparin, rule out HIT. If the patient is on VKA, the recommendation is to switch to LMWH. In patients who develop recurrent VTE while on LMWH, there is evidence to support dose escalation (71). In a small retrospective cohort study of cancer patients who developed a recurrent VTE while on LMWH, increasing the dose by 20%–25% was effective in preventing additional recurrences. In these patients, it may also be useful to check an anti-Xa level at 3–4 h after injection to determine peak plasma concentrations. If the patient is on daily LMWH dosing and develops a recurrent VTE, switching to twice daily dosing is also reasonable. Changing to another anticoagulant such as fondaparinux is an attractive alternative option. There is not enough data on the newer anticoagulation to make a recommendation regarding their use in this setting.

The use of IVC filters in cancer patients with recurrent VTE is controversial. There is no definitive evidence to support this practice and in retrospective series, the risk of recurrent DVT after IVC insertion is as high as 32% (49). Furthermore, these recurrence are associated with significant morbidity and decreased quality of life. These findings are not surprising as filters have no ability to dampen the activated coagulation system in these patients.

■ COMPLICATIONS OF TREATMENT

The treatment of VTE in cancer patients is not without morbidity. Potential complications include bleeding, HIT, heparin-induced osteoporosis, or warfarin or heparin-induced skin necrosis. In two trials involving the use of warfarin, patients with cancer had a clinically and statistically significant increase in the overall incidence of major bleeding compared with noncancer patients: 12.4% and 13.3 per 100 patient-years in patients with cancer versus 4.9% and 2.1 per 100 patient-years in patients without cancer (19, 20). Importantly, the use of LMWH has not been associated with an increased risk of bleeding when compared to warfarin, and some evidence even suggests a decreased risk (59). Similarly, treatment doses of fondaparinux have the same bleeding episodes as compared to LMWH or UFH (56, 72).

In addition to bleeding, there is a 3% risk of HIT with UFH and 1% risk with LMWH (73). Skin necrosis due to heparins or warfarin is another infrequent but serious complication. Skin necrosis presents first with erythema then purpura and hemorrhage, and eventually necrosis (**Figure 19-4**). Specific complications are associated with therapeutic devices, including an increased risk of DVT with IVC filters, and an increased risk of infection with CVCs.

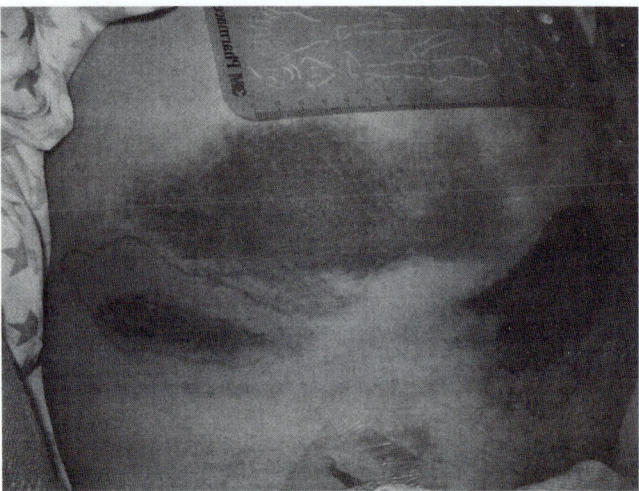

FIGURE 19-4 Low-molecular-weight heparin (LMWH) induced skin necrosis. The ecchymosis seen superiorly and the adjacent indurated, erythematous plaques with central purpura and necrosis are abdominal sites of LMWH injection. (Photo courtesy of Dr. David Kuter, MD, DPhil, MGH.)

PREVENTION

Because of the high rate of VTE in cancer patients, primary prophylaxis has become a major area of interest. This section will briefly discuss preventive strategies associated with surgery, hospitalization, chemotherapy, and CVC.

■ SURGERY

Cancer patients have a twofold higher risk of developing a postoperative DVT and threefold higher risk of fatal PE than noncancer patients undergoing similar procedures (26, 74, 75). Advanced stage of disease, increased duration of anesthesia, prolonged postoperative immobilization, and prior VTE all increase the risk of VTE in the postoperative setting. Trials have led to the conclusion that antithrombotic therapy can reduce the rate of postoperative PE and clinical DVT when comparing LMWH or UFH with no treatment.

Additional studies have shown a significant reduction in postoperative VTE in cancer patients who receive prophylaxis beyond their hospitalization. The ENOXACAN II trial found a 60% reduction in the rate of VTE in cancer patients who received extended LMWH prophylaxis (up to 30 days) after their abdominal or pelvic surgery versus those who received prophylaxis only during their hospital stay (approximately 6–10 days) (76). A recent meta-analysis compared the safety and efficacy of extended use of LMWH (for 3–4 weeks after surgery) to conventional in-hospital prophylaxis and found that the administration of extended LMWH prophylaxis significantly reduced the incidence of VTE (5.93% vs 13.6%, RR 0.44 [CI 95% 0.28 – 0.7]), with no significant difference in major or minor bleeding (77).

Other anticoagulants have also been investigated in this setting. The PEGASUS trial compared fondaparinux to LMWH and found no difference in the rates of postoperative VTE or bleeding in the general population (78). However, in a post-hoc analysis of cancer patients, there was a statistically significant reduction in VTE in the fondaparinux group (4.7%) but not the LMWH group (7.7%) (78). Further studies are needed to confirm this finding. However, it is likely that anticoagulant therapy reduces the postoperative risk of VTE in cancer.

Occasionally, cancer patients may have a contraindication to anticoagulant therapy. In these situations, mechanical forms of prevention can be employed, such as intermittent pneumatic compression devices or compression stockings. However, the efficacy of these measures has not been established by rigorous trials.

Detailed and specific recommendations for prophylactic anticoagulation in cancer patients undergoing surgical procedures can be found in the ACCP guidelines (26, 79).

■ HOSPITALIZATIONS

Cancer patients who are immobile or bedridden with an acute medical illness or because of cancer-related morbidity are at increased risk of developing VTE. In a study in which the vast majority of patients had cancer, the risk of VTE was reduced by 41% in the patients whose physicians received a computer-generated alert reminding them to provide VTE prophylaxis (80). The ACCP and JNCCN recommend that these "high-risk" immobilized and hospitalized cancer patients receive VTE prophylaxis, either a LMWH such as dalteparin (5000 U subcutaneously [sc] everyday [qd]), enoxaparin (40 mg sc qd), or tinzaparin (4500 U sc qd); or UFH (5000 U sc 3 times daily); or fondaparinux (2.5 mg sc qd) (26, 55, 81, 82). For patients with a contraindication to anticoagulant prophylactic therapy, graduated compression stockings or pneumatic compression devices can be used as alternatives.

■ CHEMOTHERAPY

High rates of VTE are associated with the use of chemotherapy. Therefore, the value of thromboprophylaxis has emerged as important research topic. In one of the earliest studies, over 300 women with metastatic breast cancer were randomized to chemotherapy plus or minus warfarin. There was an 85% relative risk reduction of VTE (4.4% vs 0.66%) in the warfarin group with no difference in bleeding rates (83). Despite these significant findings, thromboprophylaxis was not adopted as standard practice at that time.

In the last few years, there has been a surge of trials focusing on the potential benefit of primary thrombosis prophylaxis in ambulatory cancer patients. TOPIC I and TOPIC II investigated the use of the LMWH, certoparin, versus placebo in patients with breast and lung cancer, respectively. In the breast cancer patients, there was no difference in the rates of VTE (4% in both groups); however, there was an increase in major bleeding complications in the LMWH arm (1.7% vs 0%) (84). In the lung cancer patients, there was a nonsignificant trend toward decreased VTE in the LMWH arm compared to placebo (4.5% vs 8.3%, p = 0.07) (84). Another thromboprophylaxis study, PROTECHT (Prophylaxis of Thromboembolism During Chemotherapy) randomized ambulatory patients receiving chemotherapy for advanced cancers to nadroparin or placebo and showed a noteworthy 50% reduction in the rates of symptomatic VTE (2.0% vs 3.9%; p = 0.02) with no difference in bleeding (67). A recent combined analysis of data from PROTECHT and TOPIC II in metastatic or locally advanced lung cancer patients found that LMWHs compared to placebo significantly decreased the rate of VTE (3.2% vs 6.4%) with no difference in major bleeding (85).

Another approach in evaluating the role of prophylactic anticoagulation is to focus on a single site of cancer known to be at high risk of VTE. Two recent prospective studies concentrated on multiple myeloma (MM). In one study, newly diagnosed MM patients receiving a thalidomide-containing regimen were randomized to aspirin (ASA), VKA, or enoxaparin. The incidence of VTE revealed 7.3% in the ASA group, 9.5% in the VKA group, and 4.6% in the LMWH. Historical rates of VTE in this population are reported to be as high as 35% (31). A comparable study randomized newly diagnosed MM patients receiving lenalidomide plus dexamethasone to ASA or enoxaparin and found similar rates of VTE (2.27% ASA and 1.20% enoxaparin) (86). Based on these and other trials, current guidelines recommend outpatient VTE prophylaxis in the form of LMWH or VKA for cancer patients receiving highly thrombogenic thalidomide or lenalidomide-based combination chemotherapy regimens (55, 87, 88).

Given the increased risk of VTE in glioma patients, the PRODIGE study evaluated the use of dalteparin versus placebo in patients with malignant gliomas. Although the trial was closed early due to expiration of study medication, the investigators noted a trend toward reduced rates of VTE and an increased rate of intracranial hemorrhage in the LMWH group (5.1% vs 1.2%) (69). High rates of VTE are also associated with pancreatic cancers, and two recent trials evaluated the use of LMWH exclusively in this population. In CONKO-04, advanced pancreatic cancer patients randomized to enoxaparin had a major reduction in VTE rates at 1 year compared to patients randomized to placebo (5% vs 15.3%; p = <0.01) (89). Similarly, the FRAGEM study demonstrated that pancreatic patients receiving gemcitabine plus nadroparin compared to gemcitabine alone had a 58% risk reduction in VTE (12% vs 28%; p = 0.002) with no difference in bleeding (68). Of note, lethal VTE occurred in 8.3% of the control arm and 0% in the LMWH arm.

The largest study of thromboprophylaxis in ambulatory patients receiving chemotherapy, SAVE-ONCO, randomized 3212 patients with metastatic or locally advanced solid tumors to semuloparin or placebo (66). With a median treatment duration of 3.5 months, semuloparin proved superior to placebo in reducing the risk of VTE (1.2% vs 3.4%; p = <0.001) with no apparent increase in major bleeding.

Two recent meta-analyses were performed to assess the efficacy and safety of LMWH in cancer patients without VTE. The first one, a Cochrane review, included 9 trials (none after 2009) enrolling 2857 patients and found that the effect of heparin therapy on mortality was not statistically significant at 12 months (risk ratio [RR] 0.93; 95% CI 0.85–1.02); however, heparin therapy was associated with a statistically and clinically important reduction in venous thromboembolism (RR 0.55; 95% CI 0.37–0.82) with no significant effect on bleeding (90). The second analysis included over 7000 patients from 11 studies and showed a significant increase in bleeding (RR: 1.32; 95% CI 1.08–1.62) but a decrease in VTE (RR: 0.53; 95% CI 0.42–0.64) in cancer patients who received LMWH compared to placebo or no anticoagulation (91). There was no difference in 1-year mortality rate or major bleeding.

The numerous thromboprophylaxis studies demonstrate that outpatient prophylactic anticoagulation is feasible, safe, and effective. However, it is important to note that these studies do not show a statistically significant reduction in fatal VTE or improvement in overall survival. Furthermore, current guidelines (ACCP, ASCO, NCCN, ESMO) recommend against primary thromboprophylaxis for most ambulatory cancer patients (55, 81, 87, 88). Moreover, the FDA recently voted against approving semuloparin for primary prophylaxis in cancer patients and emphasized the need to create clinically useful tools to better risk stratify patients for thromboprophylaxis.

■ CENTRAL VENOUS CATHETERS

There have been major efforts to decrease catheter-related clotting and its complications with prophylactic anticoagulation. Although the initial studies of CVC thromboprophylaxis demonstrated effectiveness in preventing CVC-related thrombosis, subsequent RCTs showed no benefit (37, 38). Moreover, a recent Cochrane review of 12 RCTs examined the safety and efficacy of VTE prophylaxis in cancer patients with CVC and found no statistically significant effect of UFH, LMWH or VKA on death, DVT, bleeding, infection, or thrombocytopenia (92). Current guidelines state that low-dose warfarin or LMWH to prevent thrombosis related to long-term indwelling CVCs in cancer patients is not warranted (55, 81, 88).

NEW DEVELOPMENTS

■ NOVEL ANTICOAGULANTS

In view of the limitations and side effects associated with the current antithrombotic therapies, better treatments are needed for cancer patients who have unique risks and comorbidities. There is a particular need for longer acting, oral agents that have few drug interactions, do not depend on nutritional status, and do not require monitoring. Thus, there is great interest in the new oral anticoagulants that target the active site of factor Xa or thrombin and their potential role in cancer patients.

These new oral anticoagulants have a highly predictable pharmacological profile that allows them to be taken in fixed doses without laboratory monitoring. Although they have few drug and food interactions, there is little information in how they interact with chemotherapeutic agents. Another limitation is the lack of a reversible agent or an assay to measure their anticoagulant effect. There is also a dearth of experience in how to adjust these medications in patients with thrombocytopenia, which can be common in cancer patients undergoing chemotherapy. Thus, the use of these new agents needs to be rigorously investigated in cancer patients.

The only new agent specifically evaluated in cancer patients is apixaban, a factor Xa inhibitor. A recent pilot study examined the role of apixaban for primary thromboprophylaxis in patients receiving chemotherapy for metastatic or locally advanced solid tumors (93). Patients randomized to apixaban (5 mg, 10 mg, or 20 mg daily) had lower rates of VTE compared to placebo (0% vs 10.3%) with no significant difference in bleeding. This study confirms that apixaban is safe and feasible to use as outpatient prophylaxis. However, its effectiveness for the prevention of VTE in cancer patients needs to be addressed in larger RCTs.

In all the other trials involving novel anticoagulants, cancer patients represent only a small percentage of the patients. Two factor Xa inhibitors, rivaroxaban and apixaban, have been recently tested in large phase III trials for VTE prophylaxis in acutely ill medical patients. The ADOPT trial, which compared extended duration prophylaxis of apixaban to a shorter course of enoxaparin in medically ill patients, found that apixaban was not superior to a shorter course with enoxaparin but was associated with significantly more major bleeding than enoxaparin (94). This trial included only 10% cancer patients, and the authors mentioned no significant difference in these patients with respect to the primary safety endpoint. In a similar design, the MAGELLAN trial, an extended duration of rivaroxaban was compared to a standard course of enoxaparin and was associated with an increased risk of bleeding (95). There were 7.3% active cancer patients in this trial and in a post-hoc analysis, rivaroxaban showed a nonsignificant trend to less efficacy than enoxaparin in this population (RR 1.34; 95% CI 0.71–2.54) (96).

Novel anticoagulants have also been evaluated in the treatment of VTE. In the EINSTEIN-acute DVT and the EINSTEIN-PE trial, rivaroxaban was noninferior when compared to enoxaparin followed by VKA in terms of

VTE and bleeding rates (97, 98). Cancer patients accounted for 9%–12% patients in these trials, and the primary efficacy and safety outcomes were no different in this group as compared to the total group of patients. In the RECOVER trials, dabigatran, a direct thrombin inhibitor, was compared to VKA and the rates of VTE and bleeding were similar in both groups (99). Cancer patients made up 10% of the population, and there was no mention of any difference in outcomes or safety in this group.

■ NOVEL USES OF BIOMARKERS

Several trials have demonstrated the efficacy of LMWH in preventing VTE in cancer patients. However, studies focusing on identifying which patients and which cancers are at greatest risk of VTE and for whom prophylaxis may benefit are needed. Zwicker et al. reported on the first RCT evaluating a novel biomarker-based anticoagulation strategy for thromboprophylaxis (100). Patients with metastatic or locally advanced pancreatic, lung, or colorectal cancers were evaluated based on levels of tissue factor MP. Patients with low levels of MP were observed and patients with elevated levels of MP were randomized to prophylactic enoxaparin versus observation. The incidence of VTE at 2 months was 7.2% in patients with low levels of MP, 5.6% in patients with high levels of MP in the enoxaparin arm, and 27.3% in patients with high levels of MP in the observation arm. Future studies are underway to confirm these encouraging findings.

■ FUTURE DIRECTIONS

Many questions regarding the prevention and treatment of VTE in cancer patients remain unanswered. The evidence linking the use of LMWH to increases in cancer survival in both patients with and without VTE is compelling and is presently being explored. Future investigations will need to address the ideal type and duration of treatment in cancer patients with VTE. Due to the unique challenges in cancer patients, the antithrombotic impact of the new anticoagulants needs to be evaluated specifically in this population. The role of thromboprophylaxis should be investigated with the use of risk stratification approaches combining biomarkers with risk assessment tools. The decision to initiate anticoagulation therapy must not only balance the benefits and risks but also integrate the patient's values and preferences. Lastly, quality-of-life measures should be included in future studies.

CONCLUSION

VTE in cancer patients is a challenging clinical problem. The pathogenesis is complex and multifactorial, and the additional risk factors for cancer patients are often unavoidable. Identifying biomarkers to help predict which patients are at risk of developing VTE are underway and preliminary results are promising. Diagnosing VTE has become more successful and easier with newer noninvasive modalities. The practice of providing extensive screening to identify occult malignancies in patients who present with an idiopathic VTE is intriguing and needs to be explored further. The treatment for VTE can often be difficult and risky, especially given the unique risk factors such as chemotherapy, hormonal therapy, and CVCs, and the comorbidities that are often associated with cancer patients. Moreover, the complications that are related to both VTE and their therapy can cause significant morbidity and even mortality in cancer patients.

LMWH has become a valuable tool for preventing and treating VTE and may have independent beneficial effects on the progression of cancer. Novel agents are an attractive alternative, but their efficacy and safety in cancer patients needs to be investigated. Thromboprophylaxis in patients undergoing surgery or hospitalization appears safe and effective in lowering the risk of VTE. Additional studies employing risk stratification models and measurement of biomarkers are needed to determine the benefit of targeted thromboprophylaxis for primary prevention of VTE in cancer patients.

Given all the limitations and challenges associated with cancer patients and the current available therapies, it is clear that better, safer, and easier treatments are urgently needed. In order to discover these much needed novel treatments, well-designed prospective RCTs specifically for cancer patients are required.

REFERENCES

1. Trousseau A. Phlegmasia alba dolens. *Clinique Medicale de l'Hotel-Dieu de Paris.* 1865; 3: 654–712.
2. Falanga A, Marchetti M, Vignoli A. Coagulation and cancer: biological and clinical aspects. *J Thromb Haemost.* 2013; 11: 223–233.
3. Boccaccio C, Comoglio PM. Genetic link between cancer and thrombosis. *J Clin Oncol.* 2009; 27: 4827–4833.
4. Boccaccio C, Sabatino G, Medico E, et al. The MET oncogene drives a genetic programme linking cancer to haemostasis. *Nature.* 2005; 434: 396–400.
5. Garnier D, Magnus N, D'Asti E, et al. Genetic pathways linking hemostasis and cancer. *Thromb Res.* 2012; 129 (Suppl 1): S22–S29.
6. Rong Y, Post DE, Pieper RO, et al. PTEN and hypoxia regulate tissue factor expression and plasma coagulation by glioblastoma. *Cancer Res.* 2005; 65: 1406–1413.
7. Zwicker JI, Liebman HA, Neuberg D, et al. Tumor-derived tissue factor-bearing microparticles are associated with venous thromboembolic events in malignancy. *Clin Cancer Res.* 2009; 15: 6830–6840.
8. Deitcher SR. Cancer-related deep venous thrombosis: clinical importance, treatment challenges, and management strategies. *Semin Thromb Hemost.* 2003; 29: 247–258.
9. Falanga A, Rickles FR. Pathophysiology of the thrombophilic state in the cancer patient. *Semin Thromb Hemost.* 1999; 25: 173–182.
10. Browne AM, Cronin CG, English C, et al. Unsuspected pulmonary emboli in oncology patients undergoing routine computed tomography imaging. *J Thorac Oncol.* 2010; 5: 798–803.
11. Ahlbrecht J, Dickmann B, Ay C, et al. Tumor grade is associated with venous thromboembolism in patients with cancer: results from the Vienna Cancer and Thrombosis Study. *J Clin Oncol.* 2012; 30: 3870–3875.
12. Blom JW, Doggen CJ, Osanto S, et al. Malignancies, prothrombotic mutations, and the risk of venous thrombosis. *JAMA.* 2005; 293: 715–722.

13. Khorana AA, Dalal M, Lin J, et al. Incidence and predictors of venous thromboembolism (VTE) among ambulatory high-risk cancer patients undergoing chemotherapy in the United States. *Cancer.* 2012; 119: 648–655.

14. Khorana AA, Francis CW, Culakova E, et al. Frequency, risk factors, and trends for venous thromboembolism among hospitalized cancer patients. *Cancer.* 2007; 110: 2339–2346.

15. Paneesha S, McManus A, Arya R, et al. Frequency, demographics and risk (according to tumour type or site) of cancer-associated thrombosis among patients seen at outpatient DVT clinics. *Thromb Haemost.* 2008; 103: 338–343.

16. Chew HK, Wun T, Harvey D, et al. Incidence of venous thromboembolism and its effect on survival among patients with common cancers. *Arch Intern Med.* 2006; 166: 458–464.

17. Sorensen HT, Mellemkjaer L, Olsen JH, et al. Prognosis of cancers associated with venous thromboembolism. *N Engl J Med.* 2000; 343: 1846–1850.

18. Khorana AA. Venous thromboembolism and prognosis in cancer. *Thromb Res.* 2010; 125: 490–493.

19. Hutten BA, Prins MH, Gent M, et al. Incidence of recurrent thromboembolic and bleeding complications among patients with venous thromboembolism in relation to both malignancy and achieved international normalized ratio: a retrospective analysis. *J Clin Oncol.* 2000; 18: 3078–3083.

20. Prandoni P, Lensing AW, Piccioli A, et al. Recurrent venous thromboembolism and bleeding complications during anticoagulant treatment in patients with cancer and venous thrombosis. *Blood.* 2002; 100: 3484–3488.

21. Prandoni P, Lensing AW, Buller HR, et al. Deep-vein thrombosis and the incidence of subsequent symptomatic cancer. *N Engl J Med.* 1992; 327: 1128–1133.

22. Piccioli A, Lensing AW, Prins MH, et al. Extensive screening for occult malignant disease in idiopathic venous thromboembolism: a prospective randomized clinical trial. *J Thromb Haemost.* 2004; 2: 884–889.

23. Van Doormaal FF, Terpstra W, Van Der Griend R, et al. Is extensive screening for cancer in idiopathic venous thromboembolism warranted? *J Thromb Haemost.* 2011; 9: 79–84.

24. Carrier M, Le Gal G, Wells PS, et al. Systematic review: the Trousseau syndrome revisited: should we screen extensively for cancer in patients with venous thromboembolism? *Ann Intern Med.* 2008; 149: 323–333.

25. Rondina MT, Wanner N, Pendleton RC, et al. A pilot study utilizing whole body 18 F-FDG-PET/CT as a comprehensive screening strategy for occult malignancy in patients with unprovoked venous thromboembolism. *Thromb Res.* 2012; 129: 22–27.

26. Geerts WH, Pineo GF, Heit JA, et al. Prevention of venous thromboembolism: the Seventh ACCP Conference on Antithrombotic and Thrombolytic Therapy. *Chest.* 2004; 126 (3 Suppl): 338S–400S.

27. Khorana AA, Francis CW, Culakova E, et al. Thromboembolism in hospitalized neutropenic cancer patients. *J Clin Oncol.* 2006; 24: 484–490.

28. Khorana AA, Francis CW, Culakova E, et al. Risk factors for chemotherapy-associated venous thromboembolism in a prospective observational study. *Cancer.* 2005; 104: 2822–2829.

29. Fisher B, Costantino J, Redmond C, et al. A randomized clinical trial evaluating tamoxifen in the treatment of patients with node-negative breast cancer who have estrogen-receptor-positive tumors. *N Engl J Med.* 1989; 320: 479–484.

30. Pritchard KI, Paterson AH, Paul NA, et al. Increased thromboembolic complications with concurrent tamoxifen and chemotherapy in a randomized trial of adjuvant therapy for women with breast cancer. National Cancer Institute of Canada Clinical Trials Group Breast Cancer Site Group. *J Clin Oncol.* 1996; 14: 2731–2737.

31. Zangari M, Barlogie B, Anaissie E, et al. Deep vein thrombosis in patients with multiple myeloma treated with thalidomide and chemotherapy: effects of prophylactic and therapeutic anticoagulation. *Br J Haematol.* 2004; 126: 715–721.

32. Heit JA, Silverstein MD, Mohr DN, et al. Risk factors for deep vein thrombosis and pulmonary embolism: a population-based case-control study. *Arch Intern Med.* 2000; 160: 809–815.

33. Seng S, Liu Z, Chiu SK, et al. Risk of venous thromboembolism in patients with cancer treated with Cisplatin: a systematic review and meta-analysis. *J Clin Oncol.* 2012; 30: 4416–4426.

34. Bennett CL, Silver SM, Djulbegovic B, et al. Venous thromboembolism and mortality associated with recombinant erythropoietin and darbepoetin administration for the treatment of cancer-associated anemia. *JAMA.* 2008; 299: 914–924.

35. Bohlius J, Wilson J, Seidenfeld J, et al. Recombinant human erythropoietins and cancer patients: updated meta-analysis of 57 studies including 9353 patients. *J Natl Cancer Inst.* 2006; 98: 708–714.

36. Nalluri SR, Chu D, Keresztes R, Zhu X, Wu S. Risk of venous thromboembolism with the angiogenesis inhibitor bevacizumab in cancer patients: a meta-analysis. *JAMA.* 2008; 300: 2277–2285.

37. Petrelli F, Cabiddu M, Borgonovo K, et al. Risk of venous and arterial thromboembolic events associated with anti-EGFR agents: a meta-analysis of randomized clinical trials. *Ann Oncol.* 2012; 23: 1672–1679.

38. Rosovsky RP, Kuter DJ. Catheter-related thrombosis in cancer patients: pathophysiology, diagnosis, and management. *Hematol Oncol Clin North Am.* 2005; 19: 183–202, vii.

39. Khorana AA, Kuderer NM, Culakova E, et al. Development and validation of a predictive model for chemotherapy-associated thrombosis. *Blood.* 2008; 111: 4902–4907.

40. Verso M, Agnelli G, Barni S, et al. A modified Khorana risk assessment score for venous thromboembolism in cancer patients receiving chemotherapy: the Protecht score. *Intern Emerg Med.* 2012; 7: 291–292.

41. Louzada ML, Carrier M, Lazo-Langner A, et al. Development of a clinical prediction rule for risk stratification of recurrent venous thromboembolism in patients with cancer-associated venous thromboembolism. *Circulation.* 2012; 126: 448–454.

42. Ay C, Simanek R, Vormittag R, et al. High plasma levels of soluble P-selectin are predictive of venous thromboembolism in cancer patients: results from the Vienna Cancer and Thrombosis Study (CATS). *Blood.* 2008; 112: 2703–2708.

43. Ay C, Vormittag R, Dunkler D, et al. D-dimer and prothrombin fragment 1 + 2 predict venous thromboembolism in patients with cancer: results from the Vienna Cancer and Thrombosis Study. *J Clin Oncol.* 2009; 27: 4124–4129.

44. Ay C, Dunkler D, Simanek R, et al. Prediction of venous thromboembolism in patients with cancer by measuring thrombin generation: results from the Vienna Cancer and Thrombosis Study. *J Clin Oncol.* 2011; 29: 2099–2103.

45. Ay C, Dunkler D, Marosi C, et al. Prediction of venous thromboembolism in cancer patients. *Blood.* 2010; 116: 5377–5382.

46. Khorana AA, Ahrendt SA, Ryan CK, et al. Tissue factor expression, angiogenesis, and thrombosis in pancreatic cancer. *Clin Cancer Res.* 2007; 13: 2870–2875.

47. Sack GH, Jr., Levin J, Bell WR. Trousseau's syndrome and other manifestations of chronic disseminated coagulopathy in patients with neoplasms: clinical, pathophysiologic, and therapeutic features. *Medicine (Baltimore).* 1977; 56: 1–37.

48. Imberti D, Agnelli G, Ageno W, et al. Clinical characteristics and management of cancer-associated acute venous thromboembolism: findings from the MASTER Registry. *Haematologica.* 2008; 93: 273–278.

49. Elting LS, Escalante CP, Cooksley C, et al. Outcomes and cost of deep venous thrombosis among patients with cancer. *Arch Intern Med.* 2004; 164: 1653–1661.

50. Shen VS, Pollak EW. Fatal pulmonary embolism in cancer patients: is heparin prophylaxis justified? *South Med J.* 1980; 73: 841–843.

51. Stein PD, Hull RD, Patel KC, et al. D-dimer for the exclusion of acute venous thrombosis and pulmonary embolism: a systematic review. *Ann Intern Med.* 2004; 140: 589–602.

52. Carrier M, Le Gal G, Bates SM, Anderson DR, Wells PS. D-dimer testing is useful to exclude deep vein thrombosis in elderly outpatients. *J Thromb Haemost.* 2008; 6: 1072–1076.

53. Di Nisio M, Rutjes AW, Buller HR. Combined use of clinical pretest probability and D-dimer test in cancer patients with clinically suspected deep venous thrombosis. *J Thromb Haemost.* 2006; 4: 52–57.

54. Kearon C, Akl EA, Comerota AJ, et al. Antithrombotic therapy for VTE disease: Antithrombotic Therapy and Prevention of Thrombosis, 9th ed: American College of Chest Physicians Evidence-Based Clinical Practice Guidelines. *Chest.* 2012; 141 (2 Suppl): e419S-e494S.

55. Streiff MB. The National Comprehensive Cancer Center Network (NCCN) guidelines on the management of venous thromboembolism in cancer patients. *Thromb Res.* 2010; 125 (Suppl 2): S128–S133.

56. van Doormaal FF, Raskob GE, Davidson BL, et al. Treatment of venous thromboembolism in patients with cancer: subgroup analysis of the Matisse clinical trials. *Thromb Haemost.* 2009; 101(4): 762–769.

57. Buller HR, Agnelli G, Hull RD, et al. Antithrombotic therapy for venous thromboembolic disease: the Seventh ACCP Conference on Antithrombotic and Thrombolytic Therapy. *Chest.* 2004; 126 (3 Suppl): 401S–428S.

58. Wan S, Quinlan DJ, Agnelli G, et al. Thrombolysis compared with heparin for the initial treatment of pulmonary embolism: a meta-analysis of the randomized controlled trials. *Circulation.* 2004; 110: 744–749.

59. Lee AY, Levine MN, Baker RI, et al. Low-molecular-weight heparin versus a coumarin for the prevention of recurrent venous thromboembolism in patients with cancer. *N Engl J Med.* 2003; 349: 146–153.

60. Lee AY, Rickles FR, Julian JA, et al. Randomized comparison of low molecular weight heparin and coumarin derivatives on the survival of patients with cancer and venous thromboembolism. *J Clin Oncol.* 2005; 23: 2123–2129.

61. Altinbas M, Coskun HS, Er O, et al. A randomized clinical trial of combination chemotherapy with and without low-molecular-weight heparin in small cell lung cancer. *J Thromb Haemost.* 2004; 2: 1266–1271.

62. Kearon C, Ginsberg JS, Kovacs MJ, et al. Comparison of low-intensity warfarin therapy with conventional-intensity warfarin therapy for long-term prevention of recurrent venous thromboembolism. *N Engl J Med.* 2003; 349: 631–639.

63. Klerk CP, Smorenburg SM, Otten HM, et al. The effect of low molecular weight heparin on survival in patients with advanced malignancy. *J Clin Oncol.* 2005; 23: 2130–2135.

64. Lazo-Langner A, Goss GD, Spaans JN, et al. The effect of low-molecular-weight heparin on cancer survival. A systematic review and meta-analysis of randomized trials. *J Thromb Haemost.* 2007; 5: 729–737.

65. Sideras K, Schaefer PL, Okuno SH, et al. Low-molecular-weight heparin in patients with advanced cancer: a phase 3 clinical trial. *Mayo Clin Proc.* 2006; 81: 758–767.

66. Agnelli G, George DJ, Kakkar AK, et al. Semuloparin for thromboprophylaxis in patients receiving chemotherapy for cancer. *N Engl J Med.* 2012; 366: 601–609.

67. Agnelli G, Gussoni G, Bianchini C, et al. Nadroparin for the prevention of thromboembolic events in ambulatory patients with metastatic or locally advanced solid cancer receiving chemotherapy: a randomised, placebo-controlled, double-blind study. *Lancet Oncol.* 2009; 10: 943–949.

68. Maraveyas A, Waters J, Roy R, et al. Gemcitabine versus gemcitabine plus dalteparin thromboprophylaxis in pancreatic cancer. *Eur J Cancer.* 2012; 48: 1283–1292.

69. Perry JR, Julian JA, Laperriere NJ, et al. PRODIGE: a randomized placebo-controlled trial of dalteparin low-molecular-weight heparin thromboprophylaxis in patients with newly diagnosed malignant glioma. *J Thromb Haemost.* 2010; 8: 1959–1965.

70. Ridker PM, Goldhaber SZ, Danielson E, et al. Long-term, low-intensity warfarin therapy for the prevention of recurrent venous thromboembolism. *N Engl J Med.* 2003; 348: 1425–1434.

71. Carrier M, Le Gal G, Cho R, Tierney S, Rodger M, Lee AY. Dose escalation of low molecular weight heparin to manage recurrent venous thromboembolic events despite systemic anticoagulation in cancer patients. *J Thromb Haemost.* 2009; 7: 760–765.

72. Buller HR, Davidson BL, Decousus H, et al. Fondaparinux or enoxaparin for the initial treatment of symptomatic deep venous thrombosis: a randomized trial. *Ann Intern Med.* 2004; 140: 867–873.

73. Warkentin TE. Heparin-induced thrombocytopenia: pathogenesis and management. *Br J Haematol.* 2003; 121: 535–555.

74. Huber O, Bounameaux H, Borst F, et al. Postoperative pulmonary embolism after hospital discharge. An underestimated risk. *Arch Surg.* 1992; 127: 310–313.

75. White RH, Zhou H, Romano PS. Incidence of symptomatic venous thromboembolism after different elective or urgent surgical procedures. *Thromb Haemost.* 2003; 90: 446–455.

76. Bergqvist D, Agnelli G, Cohen AT, et al. Duration of prophylaxis against venous thromboembolism with enoxaparin after surgery for cancer. *N Engl J Med.* 2002; 346: 975–980.

77. Bottaro FJ, Elizondo MC, Doti C, et al. Efficacy of extended thromboprophylaxis in major abdominal surgery: what does the evidence show? A meta-analysis. *Thromb Haemost.* 2008; 99: 1104–1111.

78. Agnelli G, Bergqvist D, Cohen AT, et al. Randomized clinical trial of postoperative fondaparinux versus perioperative dalteparin for prevention of venous thromboembolism in high-risk abdominal surgery. *Br J Surg.* 2005; 92: 1212–1220.

79. Gould MK, Garcia DA, Wren SM, et al. Prevention of VTE in non-orthopedic surgical patients: antithrombotic therapy and prevention of thrombosis, 9th ed: American College of Chest Physicians Evidence-Based Clinical Practice Guidelines. *Chest.* 2012; 141 (2 Suppl): e227S–277S.

80. Kucher N, Koo S, Quiroz R, et al. Electronic alerts to prevent venous thromboembolism among hospitalized patients. *N Engl J Med.* 2005; 352: 969–977.

81. Kahn SR, Lim W, Dunn AS, et al. Prevention of VTE in nonsurgical patients: antithrombotic therapy and prevention of thrombosis, 9th ed: American College of Chest Physicians Evidence-Based Clinical Practice Guidelines. *Chest.* 2012; 141 (2 Suppl): e195S–226S.

82. Wagman LD, Baird MF, Bennett CL, et al. Venous thromboembolic disease. Clinical practice guidelines in oncology. *J Natl Compr Canc Netw*. 2006; 4: 838–869.

83. Levine M, Hirsh J, Gent M, et al. Double-blind randomised trial of a very-low-dose warfarin for prevention of thromboembolism in stage IV breast cancer. *Lancet*. 1994; 343: 886–889.

84. Haas SK, Freund M, Heigener D, et al. Low-molecular-weight heparin versus placebo for the prevention of venous thromboembolism in metastatic breast cancer or stage III/IV lung cancer. *Clin Appl Thromb Hemost*. 2012; 18: 159–165.

85. Verso M, Gussoni G, Agnelli G. Prevention of venous thromboembolism in patients with advanced lung cancer receiving chemotherapy: a combined analysis of the PROTECHT and TOPIC-2 studies. *J Thromb Haemost*. 2010; 8: 1649–1651.

86. Larocca A, Cavallo F, Bringhen S, et al. Aspirin or enoxaparin thromboprophylaxis for patients with newly diagnosed multiple myeloma treated with lenalidomide. *Blood*. 2012; 119: 933–939; quiz 1093.

87. Lyman GH, Kuderer NM. Prevention and treatment of venous thromboembolism among patients with cancer: the American Society of Clinical Oncology Guidelines. *Thromb Res*. 2010; 125 Suppl 2: S120–S127.

88. Mandala M, Falanga A, Roila F. Management of venous thromboembolism (VTE) in cancer patients: ESMO Clinical Practice Guidelines. *Ann Oncol*. 2011; 22 Suppl 6: vi85–vi92.

89. Riess H, Pelzer U, Opitz B, et al. A prospective, randomized trial of simultaneous pancreatic cancer treatment with enoxaparin and chemotherapy: final results of the CONKO-004 trial. *J Clin Oncol*. 2010; 28 (15 Suppl): 4033.

90. Akl EA GS, Barba M, Yosuico VED, et al. Parenteral anticoagulation in patients with cancer who have no therapeutic or prophylactic indication for anticoagulation (Review). The Cochrane Collaboration and published in *The Cochrane Library*. 2013; (1): 1–58.

91. Che DH, Cao JY, Shang LH, et al. The efficacy and safety of low-molecular-weight heparin use for cancer treatment: a meta-analysis. *Eur J Intern Med*. 2013.

92. Akl EA VS, Gunukula S, Yosuico VED, et al. Anticoagulation for patients with cancer and central venous catheters (Review). The Cochrane Collaboration and published in *The Cochrane Library*. 2011(4).

93. Levine MN, Gu C, Liebman HA, et al. A randomized phase II trial of apixaban for the prevention of thromboembolism in patients with metastatic cancer. *J Thromb Haemost*. 2012; 10: 807–814.

94. Goldhaber SZ, Leizorovicz A, Kakkar AK, et al. Apixaban versus enoxaparin for thromboprophylaxis in medically ill patients. *N Engl J Med*. 2011; 365: 2167–2177.

95. Cohen AT, Spiro TE, Buller HR, et al. Rivaroxaban for thromboprophylaxis in acutely ill medical patients. *N Engl J Med*. 2013; 368: 513–523.

96. Cohen AT, Büller HR, Haskell L, et al. Rivaroxaban vs. enoxaparin for the prevention of venous thromboembolism in acutely ill medical patients: Magellan subgroup analyses. *J Thromb Haemost* (International Society on Thrombosis and Haemostasis). 2011; 9 (Suppl 2): 20 (O-MO-034).

97. Bauersachs R, Berkowitz SD, Brenner B, et al. Oral rivaroxaban for symptomatic venous thromboembolism. *N Engl J Med*. 2010; 363: 2499–2510.

98. Buller HR, Prins MH, Lensin AW, et al. Oral rivaroxaban for the treatment of symptomatic pulmonary embolism. *N Engl J Med*. 2012; 366: 1287–1297.

99. Schulman S, Kearon C, Kakkar AK, et al. Dabigatran versus warfarin in the treatment of acute venous thromboembolism. *N Engl J Med*. 2009; 361: 2342–2352.

100. Zwicker JI, Liebman HA, Bauer KA, et al. Prediction and prevention of thromboembolic events with enoxaparin in cancer patients with elevated tissue factor-bearing microparticles: a randomized-controlled phase II trial (the Microtec study). *Br J Haematol*. 2012; 160: 530–537.

CHAPTER **20**
Metabolic Emergencies in Oncology

Ephraim Paul Hochberg

INTRODUCTION

Metabolic emergencies represent rare events in the care of cancer patients. In contrast to the measured pace of most of oncology, these scenarios demand prompt identification and intervention. This chapter reviews tumor lysis syndrome, hyponatremia, and hypercalcemia.

TUMOR LYSIS SYNDROME

■ DEFINITION

Tumor lysis syndrome is a collection of metabolic derangements secondary to the release of tumor cell contents into the extracellular space (Table 20-1). The rapid development of hyperphosphatemia, hyperuricemia, and hyperkalemia can cause devastating renal and cardiac complications. Hypocalcemia occurs secondarily as a consequence of hyperphosphatemia.

Tumor lysis syndrome occurs most frequently in rapidly growing hematologic malignancies such as acute leukemias and Burkitt's lymphoma. In these diseases, it can occur either spontaneously or more commonly 6–72 h following initiation of antitumor therapy. There are case reports of even more rapid onset with the use of targeted therapies. The syndrome is most frequently associated with cytoxic chemotherapy but can occur after

TABLE 20-1 FEATURES OF TUMOR LYSIS SYNDROME

- Hyperkalemia
- Hyperuricemia
- Hyperphosphatemia
- Hypocalcemia
- Metabolic acidosis and renal failure

embolization, radiation, or glucocorticoids. The Cairo-Bishop definitions and grading system for laboratory and clinical tumor lysis syndrome are not widely used in clinical practice (Table 20-2) (1). The National Cancer Institute Common Toxicity Criteria 4.0 system grade TLS by its presence (grade 3), life threatening consequences (grade 4), or death (grade 5).

INCIDENCE AND RISK FACTORS

There are both tumor-related risk factors for tumor lysis syndrome, as well as patient-specific risks. Tumor-specific risks include a large burden of disease, a high-proliferative rate, or a highly treatment-sensitive tumor. Clinically significant tumor lysis syndrome is estimated to occur in up to 30% of patients with Burkitt's lymphoma/B-ALL and 15% of patients with acute myeloid leukemia, although laboratory evidence of tumor lysis syndrome can be present in a larger proportion of patients. There is a significant but lower risk in diffuse large B-cell lymphoma, and rarer reports in chronic lymphocytic leukemia, and multiple myeloma. The use of the monoclonal antibody rituximab has been associated with the development of tumor lysis syndrome in patients with increased numbers of circulating tumor cells ($\geq$25,000) or a large tumor burden. Tumor lysis syndrome is rare in solid tumors, with breast cancer and small cell lung cancer comprising the most common reports. There are case reports of tumor lysis syndrome with a number of targeted therapies (Table 20-3).

Patient comorbidities increase the risk of tumor lysis syndrome. Decreased urinary flow or dehydration, chronic renal insufficiency or frank renal failure, acidic urine, or preexisting hyperuricemia are all risk factors for tumor lysis syndrome development.

MECHANISMS

Purine Catabolism

The major contributing element in the pathophysiology of tumor lysis syndrome is hyperuricemia caused by the release of nucleic acids (purines), which are catabolized to uric acid, leading to elevated plasma urate levels (Figure 20-1). Elevated uric acid levels overwhelm the excretory capacity of the renal tubules particularly in the presence of an acidic pH and low urine flow. Crystalline obstruction of the renal tubules, uric acid nephropathy, renal failure, and uremia may result. Renal failure may also occur due to volume depletion and changes in autoregulation within the kidney.

Intracellular Ion Release

Other intracellular ions are released, including potassium and phosphorus. Hyperkalemia-induced cardiac arrhythmias exacerbated by renal failure are the most life-threatening complication of tumor lysis syndrome.

TABLE 20-2 CAIRO AND BISHOP DEFINITION AND GRADING CLASSIFICATION OF TUMOR LYSIS SYNDROME

	Laboratory TLS*	Grade 0	Grade I	Grade II	Grade III	Grade IV	Grade V
Uric acid	≥476 mmol/l or 25% IFB	LTLS −	LTLS +	LTLS +	LTLS +	LTLS +	LTLS +
Potassium	≥6.0 mmol/l or 25% IFB						
Phosphorous	≥2.1 mmol/l in children or ≥1.45 mmol/l in adults or 25% IFB						
Calcium	≤1.75 mmol/l or 25% DFB						
Creatinine	Not defined	≤1.5 ULN	1.5 × ULN	>1.5–3.0 × ULN	>3.0–6.0 × ULN	>6.0 × ULN	Death
Cardiac arrhythmia/ sudden death	None	None	No intervention indicated	Nonurgent intervention indicated	Symptomatic and incompletely or device controlled	Life threatening	Death
Seizure	None	None	None	One seizure or well controlled by anticonvulsants or infrequent focal motor seizures not interfering with ADL	Seizure with altered consciousness, poorly controlled or generalized seizure despite intervention	Prolonged, repetitive, or difficult to control seizures	Death

*LTLS or laboratory tumor lysis syndrome is alterations in the above values on two different measurements within 3 d before or 7 d after initiation of cytotoxic therapy and assumes a patient has or will receive adequate hydration and a hypouricemic agent.

IFB: Increase from baseline.

DFB: Decrease from baseline.

ULN: Upper limit of normal (all creatinine values are assumed to be age and gender specific).

TABLE 20-3 RISK FACTORS FOR TUMOR LYSIS SYNDROME

	Low Risk	Intermediate Risk	High Risk
Tumor type	Breast, small cell lung cancer	CML, Hodgkin's	High grade lymphoma, Burkitt's, ALL, AML
Tumor burden			
WBC count			>50 × 10 9/l, high blast count
LDH	<200 U/l		>400 U/l
Other			Extensive bone marrow involvement Bulky disease
Treatment intensity			Cisplatin, etoposide, rituximab ionizing radiation, fludarabine, IT MTX, paclitaxel, interferon alpha
Tumor treatment sensitivity	Low		High
Baseline renal function	Normal	Renal insufficiency	Renal failure
Other			Renal infiltration by disease
Baseline serum uric acid	<10 mg/dl		
Other			
Hydration	Euvolemic	Euvolemic	Dehydrated
Serum pH			Acidic
Urine pH	Alkaline		Acidic
Urine output	High		Low
Calcium-phosphorus product			>70

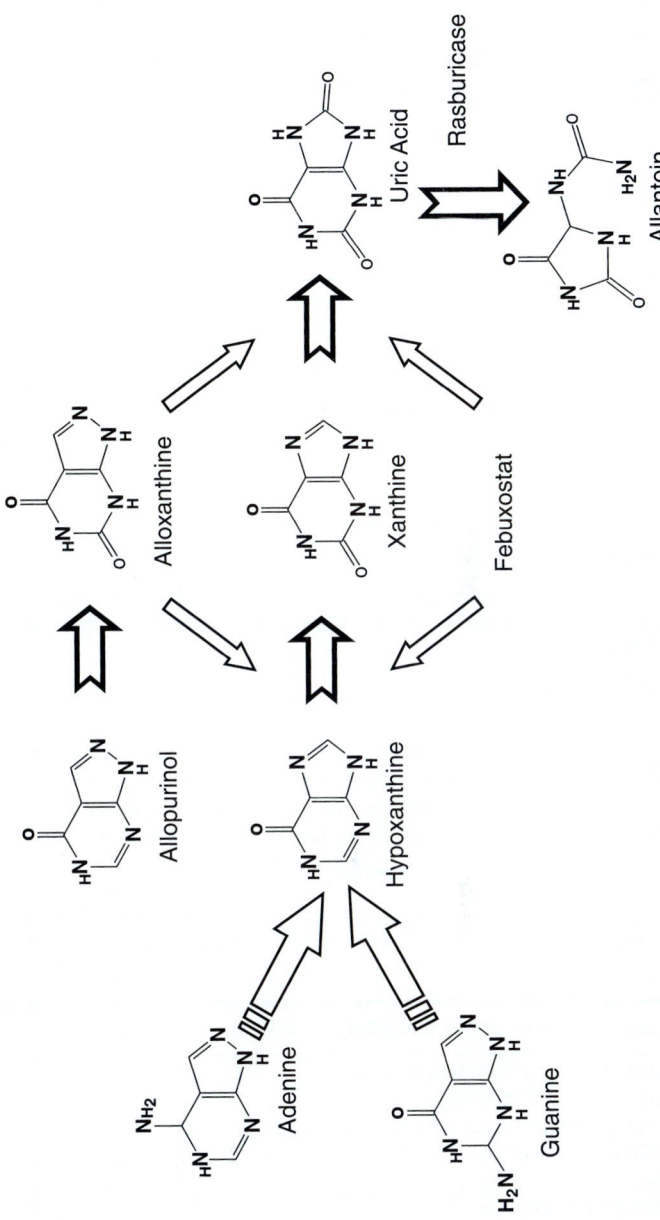

FIGURE 20-1 Uric acid formation via purine catabolism and the mechanism of action of allopurinol, rasburicase, and febuxostat.

TABLE 20-4 CLINICAL SIGNS AND SYMPTOMS OF TUMOR LYSIS SYNDROME

- Nausea, vomiting, diarrhea, lethargy
- Edema and fluid overload, including congestive heart failure and pulmonary edema
- Muscle cramps, paresthesias, tetany
- Acute renal failure or uremia
- Hematuria, flank pain, hypertension, acidosis, oliguria
- Cardiac arrhythmia, hypotension, syncope
- Confusion, hallucinations, seizures
- Death

Intracellular phosphorous, which may be overproduced in malignant cells, is also released, renally excreted, and may precipitate as calcium phosphate in the renal tubules, leading to hypocalcemia, metastatic calcification, intrarenal calcification, nephrocalcinosis, nephrolithiasis, and obstructive uropathy.

Hypocalcemia is generally due to precipitation of calcium phosphate in the soft tissues and kidneys during periods of hyperphosphatemia and inappropriately low levels of 1, 25-dihydroxyvitamin D_3. This can be clinically associated with tetany and cardiac arrhythmias.

■ CLINICAL PRESENTATION

The clinical presentation of tumor lysis syndrome is characterized by the symptoms of the individual electrolyte imbalances and resultant renal failure (Table 20-4).

■ DIFFERENTIAL DIAGNOSIS

The differential diagnosis of tumor lysis syndrome is limited. Injuries to large structures such as ischemic limb or rhabdomyolysis can replicate the varied clinical and laboratory presentations of tumor lysis syndrome but should be clinically apparent. The other laboratory abnormalities may be present to some extent in patients with renal insufficiency from any cause (Table 20-5).

■ THERAPEUTIC AGENTS, MONITORING

See Tables 20-3 and 20-6 for an overview of the following discussion. Patient- and tumor-specific factors are combined in a stratification schema

TABLE 20-5 DIFFERENTIAL DIAGNOSIS OF TUMOR LYSIS SYNDROME

- Tumor infiltration of kidneys or ureters
- Drug associated renal toxicity
- Acute renal failure secondary to other causes
- Acute tubular necrosis
- Sepsis
- Keto or lactic acidosis
- Parathyroid or thyroid disease
- Hemolysis, rhabdomyolysis, crush injuries, or ischemic limb

TABLE 20-6 OVERVIEW OF TUMOR LYSIS PROPHYLAXIS AND TREATMENT

	Prophylaxis	Treatment	
		Moderate or Asymptomatic	Severe or Symptomatic
Hyperkalemia	• Avoid potassium supplements, including dietary sources • Avoid drugs that increase serum potassium	• Sodium polystyrene sulphonate (15 g orally 1–4 ×/d or as a retention enema, 30–50 g rectally every 6 h)	• Insulin (0.1 u/kg) and D5W IV • Sodium bicarbonate (1 mEq/kg) • Loop diuretics • Inhaled beta-agonist • Calcium gluconate 10% (500 mg–2 g) • Hemodialysis or hemofiltration

Hyperuricemia	• Stop drugs that inhibit uric acid excretion
	 • Hydration 2–3 d prior to treatment
	   Allopurinol
	   Febuxostat
		• Hydration (3–6 l/m²) and diuresis
		 ± Alkalinize urine
			• Allopurinol (2/m²/d or 600–800 mg/d orally or 200–400 mg/m²/d IV maximum dose 600 mg/d in adults)
			 • Rasburicase (0.15 or 0.2 mg/kg/d IV over 30 min for 1–7 d)
			 • Hemodialysis or hemofiltration

Renal failure	• Stop nephrotoxic drugs • Hydration	• Renally dose medications • Monitor fluid status • Aggressive fluid and electrolyte management • Aggressive uric acid and phosphate management	• Hemodialysis or hemofiltration
Hyperphosphatemia	• Avoid phosphate and calcium supplements including dietary sources	• Aluminum hydroxide or carbonate (500–1800 mg, 3–6 ×/d between meals) or aluminum carbonate (2 cap/tabs or 12 ml suspension 3–4 ×/d with meals)	• Insulin and dextrose as above • Hemodialysis or hemofiltration
Hypocalcemia		• None	• *Calcium gluconate 50–100 mg/kg IV

* Not recommended.

249

that divides patients into high, intermediate, and low-risk cohorts. High-risk patients include all patients with Burkitt's lymphoma, lymphoblastic lymphoma, or B-cell ALL as well as patients with ALL with a WBC ≥100,000, AML with WBC ≥50,000, or monoblastic subtype. Intermediate-risk patients include all diffuse large B-cell lymphoma, ALL with WBC 50–100,000, AML with WBC 10–50,000, and CLL with WBC ≥10,000 treated with fludarabine as well as all other rapidly proliferating malignancies with an expected rapid response to therapy. Low-risk patients include all indolent lymphomas as well as ALL with a WBC ≤50,000, AML and CLL with WBC ≤10,000 (2).

In patients at high risk of developing tumor lysis syndrome, the decision to delay therapy must be weighed against the risks of tumor lysis syndrome, but in any case prophylactic measures should be instituted. Drugs that contribute to electrolyte abnormalities are nephrotoxic, or block uric acid, or potassium excretion should be stopped.

Hydration and Diuresis

The mainstay of prevention is aggressive hydration and diuresis, with individuals receiving 2–4 times usual maintenance fluids or 3–6 l/m^2/day. These fluids should not initially include potassium, calcium, or phosphate. If the patient is not hypovolemic but is oligo or anuric, diuretics such as furosemide (or mannitol, particularly if furosemide fails) may be used to maintain an appropriate urine output with the following as goals: urine specific gravity should be <1.010 and urine output >150–250 ml/h. Furosemide diuresis may also decrease serum potassium levels. Dosing of diuretics is patient dependent and may be intermittent or continuous.

Traditionally, recommendations have also suggested alkalinization of urine with sodium bicarbonate. However, this is not recommended in the era of recombinant urate oxidase due to the increased risk of urinary xanthine and calcium phosphate deposition, fluid overload, and metabolic alkalosis (3).

Allopurinol

Allopurinol, a xanthine analog that is converted to alloxanthine and acts as a competitive inhibitor of xanthine oxidase, reduces the production of uric acid and the incidence of related obstructive uropathy (Figure 20-1). It does not reduce levels of uric acid already present and leads to lower urate levels over days. Allopurinol may also result in xanthine nephropathy and calculi due to accumulation of xanthine and hypoxanthine, which are renally excreted.

Usual dosing of allopurinol is 2 mg/m^2/day or 600–800 mg/day orally, 12 h to 3 days prior to initiation of chemotherapy (or 200–400 mg/m^2/day IV, 24–48 h before initiation of chemotherapy; maximum dose 600 mg/day if unable to take orally). Allopurinol should be renally dosed in appropriate patients. The intravenous and oral forms have equivalent efficacy.

Allopurinol also reduces the degradation of other purines including 6-mercaptopurine (6-MP) and azothioprine, and therefore, these drugs should be dose-reduced when used with allopurinol.

Rasburicase

Rasburicase (Elitek) is a recombinant urate oxidase that converts uric acid to allantoin, a more soluble compound, which is then renally excreted (Figure 20-1). Usual dosing is 0.20 mg/kg IV over 30 min for 1–5 days and does not require renal dosing. Side effects include anaphylaxis or hypersensitivity reactions (bronchospasm, hypoxemia) in 5% of those who receive this drug. In addition, patients may form antibodies to this drug, the significance of which is currently unknown. Rasburicase should not be used in patients with G-6PD deficiency as hemolytic anemia and methemoglobinemia may occur. In the majority of patients, a single dose is sufficient to control hyperuricemia.

A randomized trial comparing rasburicase, allopurinol, and the combination of the two agents in adult and pediatric patients at high risk for tumor lysis syndrome demonstrated more rapid control of uric acid in a higher percentage of patients in the group treated with rasburicase alone.

Febuxostat

Febuxostat is a nonpurine selective inhibitor of xanthine oxidase used for prevention of gout. A phase 3 trial for tumor lysis syndrome prevention is currently ongoing.

Monitoring

Monitoring for tumor lysis involves twice daily serum electrolytes (more frequently if the patient is at high risk or clinically unstable), and at least daily urinary pH and spot uric acid to creatinine ratio (value should be >1.0), evaluation of volume status (including daily weights, blood pressure, and examination looking for edema, pleural effusions, and ascites), and serum WBC count, LDH, ionized or corrected calcium, and calcium phosphorus product.

ECG changes associated with hyperkalemia include widening of the QRS complex (late manifestations include a sine wave appearance, ventricular arrhythmias, or asystole) and peaked T waves, while hypocalcemia is associated with a long QT secondary to a prolonged ST segment.

■ TREATMENT

Hyperkalemia

Hyperkalemia treatment can be divided into treatment for moderate or asymptomatic hyperkalemia and those for severe or symptomatic hyperkalemia (Table 20-6).

For asymptomatic or moderate hyperkalemia, oral sodium polystyrene sulphonate (Kayexalate), an exchange resin, is the primary treatment (15 g orally 1–4 times daily as a slurry in water or 70% sorbitol or as a retention enema, 30–50 g rectally every 6 h as a warm emulsion in 100 ml aqueous vehicle (sorbitol or D20W), retained for 30–60 min in adults).

For severe cases, Kayexalate in addition to insulin and dextrose, sodium bicarbonate (1 mEq/kg, repeated as needed based on blood gas values), loop diuretics, inhaled beta-agonists, and, in extreme examples, calcium gluconate or chloride is appropriate. For calcium gluconate, the dosage is

2–4 mg/kg of a 10% solution, repeated at 10-min intervals as necessary. Calcium chloride is reserved for emergency situations. Hemodialyis or hemofiltration should also be considered.

Hyperuricemia And Renal Failure

Hyperuricemia should be treated with rasburicase. Hemodialysis or hemofiltration may be necessary.

Renal failure requires aggressive fluid, electrolyte, and uric acid management along with close monitoring for indications requiring hemodialysis or hemofiltration. Hemodialysis indications may include fluid overload, metabolic acidosis, electrolyte disturbances that are recalcitrant to the treatments outlined above, uremia, and hypertension.

Hyperphosphatemia

Hyperphosphatemia is treated with oral aluminum hydroxide (adult dosing: 500–1800 mg, 3–6 times daily between meals) or aluminum carbonate (2 capsules or tablets or 12 ml suspension 3–4 times daily with meals). Insulin and dextrose as administered in hyperkalemia can also be given. Severe or symptomatic cases should receive hemodialysis or hemofiltration.

Hypocalcemia

Moderate or asymptomatic hypocalcemia usually does not require treatment, and the risks of treatment may outweigh the benefits. In severe cases, calcium gluconate 500 mg to 2 g (10% solution) IV in adults at a rate not to exceed 1.5 ml/min can be used but may lead to calcium phosphate precipitation resulting obstructive uropathy or metastatic calcification. In an emergency situation, calcium chloride should be used for hyperkalemia or hypocalcemia at 2–4 mg/kg of a 10% solution, repeated at 10-min intervals as necessary.

HYPONATREMIA

■ INCIDENCE AND RISK FACTORS

Hyponatremia is a common electrolyte abnormality, occurring in many elderly and/or hospitalized patients. In cancer patients, hyponatremia may be due to primary or metastatic disease, cancer-related medical interventions or complications, usually via the syndrome of inappropriate antidiuretic hormone (SIADH), as well as other causes. This section will focus primarily on the diagnosis and treatment of SIADH-related hyponatremia in the setting of malignancy (4).

Malignancy-related hyponatremia is most commonly seen in lung carcinomas, particularly the small cell variant. However, head and neck cancers, leukemia, and mediastinal cancers have also been implicated, along with limited reports in a number of other cancers. Hyponatremia can also be therapy related and has been reported after stem cell transplantation.

■ MECHANISMS

Hyponatremia can be characterized by varying levels of osmolality (Table 20-7). Hypotonic hyponatremia, the most common form, is caused

TABLE 20-7 TYPES OF HYPONATREMIA WITH MECHANISM AND REPRESENTATIVE CAUSES

Hypotonic hyponatremia
Extracellular fluid may be decreased (hypovolemic), euvolemic (dilutional), or increased
    May be hypoosmolar or not depending upon etiology
Isotonic hyponatremia
Shift of water to an isotonic extracellular space Mannitol
Hypertonic hyponatremia
Shift of water to a hypertonic extracellular space Solutes other than sodium, e.g., hyperglycemia
Pseudohyponatremia
Presence of other osmoles in the extracellular space
    Hypertriglyceridemia
    Paraproteinemia

by abnormal retention of water with varying amounts of fluid intake (Table 20-8). Retention of water occurs because the ability of the kidneys to excrete fluid has been impaired or overwhelmed. Edema of the central nervous system is the most concerning consequence of hyponatremia.

Other uncommon causes of hypotonic hyponatremia, not included in Table 20-7, include excessive water intake either orally (as in polydipsia) or via absorption of sodium-free fluids (irrigant solutions, enemas) or reset osmostat syndrome; the latter is a subset of SIADH.

Mechanism Of Siadh

SIADH occurs because of paraneoplastic or ectopic production of antidiuretic hormone (ADH) or arginine vasopressin (AVP). AVP binds to the V2 vasopressin receptor (V2R), a G protein-coupled receptor, in the collecting duct and the ascending limb of the loop of Henle. This leads to increases in intracellular cyclic AMP (c-AMP) that in turn leads to increased water permeability, inappropriate water retention, and, therefore, hyponatremia and hypo-osmolality. Patients with SIADH may exhibit inappropriate thirst (5).

Normally, AVP or V2 vasopressin is produced in the supraoptic and paraventricular nuclei of the hypothalamus and transported down the neurohypophysis, or posterior lobe of the pituitary gland, where it is released into the blood stream when cardiovascular baro- and osmoreceptors signal that blood pressure or plasma volume are too low or plasma osmolality is too high. AVP then acts on the kidney as described above, to retain water and concentrate urine, and may have a direct, pressor effect on arteries and arterioles.

However, the etiology of malignancy-associated hyponatremia may not be due only to ectopic production of AVP (Tables 20-7, 20-8, and 20-9). Consideration should be given to other causes of hyponatremia or SIADH, as this will affect treatment.

TABLE 20-8 CAUSES AND TREATMENT OF HYPOTONIC HYPONATREMIA BY EXTRACELLULAR FLUID VOLUME, TOTAL BODY WATER, AND SODIUM STORES

Decreased Extracellular Fluid	Normal Extracellular Fluid	Increased Extracellular Fluid

Renal sodium losses
  Diuretics
  Osmotic diuretics
  Adrenal disease
  Salt-wasting
  Tubular or keto
  acidosis
	Thyroid or adrenal disease
	SIADH
	  Cancer-related CNS
	  Pulmonary disease
	  Mechanical
	  ventilation
		Cirrhosis
		Congestive heart failure
		Renal failure
		Nephrotic syndrome
		Pregnancy

Other sodium losses
 	
  GI losses
  Bleeding
  Insensible and third
  space losses
	Drugs
	
	  SSRIs, tricyclics
	  Carbamazepine
	  ACE inhibitors
	  Thiazide, loop and
	  osmotic diuretics
	  Morphine, NSAIDs
	Other
	  Pain, nausea, HIV
	  Decreased solutes
	Postoperative state	

Treatment		
• Sodium stores are decreased	• Sodium stores are normal	• Sodium stores are increased
• Total body water is decreased (hypovolemic)	• Total body water may be slightly increased	• Total body water is increased (hypervolemic)
• Volume and sodium deficit must be corrected	• Treat the underlying condition/etiology. May include fluid restriction and/or hypertonic saline	• Treat the underlying condition. May include loss of water

■ DIAGNOSIS

Variable definitions for hyponatremia are used and make comparison of cases difficult. In this chapter, hyponatremia is defined as serum sodium concentration below 135 mmol/l (this is consistent with our institutional range, 135–145 mmol/l, of serum sodium). Diagnostic testing is based upon the hypothesized cause of hyponatremia. For SIADH, the diagnosis should also be based on the criteria in Tables 20-10 and 20-11. AVP level need not be checked. The clinical signs of hyponatremia are listed in Table 20-12.

TABLE 20-9 DIFFERENTIAL DIAGNOSIS OF MALIGNANCY-ASSOCIATED HYPONATREMIA

- Primary or metastatic disease causing:
  - Adrenal insufficiency and steroid withdrawal
  - Thyroid disease
  - Hepatic dysfunction and ascites
  - CNS involvement (stroke, mass, meningitis)
  - Pulmonary disease (including infection) and positive pressure ventilation
  - Renal disease and obstructive uropathy
- Chemotherapeutic agents
  - Vincristine, vinblastine, cyclophosphamide, and cisplatin are most common
  - Nephrotoxicity
- Fluids and parenteral nutrition
- Pain (and drugs used to treat pain—opiates, acetaminophen), nausea and vomiting, diarrhea, bleeding

---

■ PROPHYLAXIS AND MONITORING

There is no prophylaxis for hyponatremia other than to anticipate electrolyte abnormalities, actively replete electrolyte losses, and avoid drugs that induce hyponatremia.

■ TREATMENT

General Comments

Treatment of the underlying disease is the most important therapy. For SIADH tumor response is correlated with resolution of hyponatremia. If other factors, such as drugs, diet, or free water consumption, are worsening the condition, appropriate adjustments should be made.

Hypokalemia is often present with hyponatremia, and correction of hypokalemia will increase serum sodium either via osmotic shifts of sodium and free water or urinary losses. Administration of potassium therefore must be taken into account (see the formula below). Hyperkalemia, without obvious cause, in the presence of hyponatremia warrants consideration of adrenal insufficiency.

Treatment of hypotonic hyponatremia is dependent upon the cause, severity, chronicity, and presence or absence of symptoms. In general, correction of hyponatremia, regardless of etiology, should not exceed 0.5 mM/h or more than 10–15 mEq/l in 24 h unless severe symptoms are present (seizures, coma). In severe cases with acute onset of hyponatremia, rates of correction of 1–3 mM/h have been recommended for short periods. Central pontine myelinolysis can complicate rapid correction (see below).

■ TREATMENT OF SIADH

The initial approach to mild, asymptomatic hyponatremia is fluid restriction to 800 ml/day or a negative water balance.

Symptomatic or moderate to severe hyponatremia will likely require hypertonic saline administration. Isotonic saline should not be used in SIADH.

TABLE 20-10 CLINICAL FEATURES AND RESPONSE TO CLINICAL CHALLENGES BY TYPE OF HYPONATREMIA

	Primary Polydipsia	Hypovolemic	Reset Osmostat	SIADH
Urine osmolality	<100 mOsm/kg	>100 mOsm/kg	100 mOsm/kg	>100 mOsm/kg
Urine sodium	≤20–40 mmol/l	≤20–40 mmol/l	20–40 mmol/l	≥20–40 mmol/l
FE Na	>1%	<1%	>1%	>1%
Water excretion	Normal	Impaired	Normal	Impaired
ADH level	Low	High	Low, normal	High
Serum urea and urate levels	Decreased	Increased	Normal	Decreased
Response to 0.9% saline administration				
Serum Na		>5 mmol/l increase	Depends on osmostat level	No change
FE Na		<0.5% increase	Can concentrate urine if above	>0.5% increase
Following normalization of hyponatremia				
Serum urate				Normalizes
Urine urate				Normalizes
Response to water loading			Able to dilute urine	Unable to dilute urine

*Hyponatremia is not necessary for a diagnosis of cerebral salt wasting, although they often present together.

TABLE 20-11 DIAGNOSTIC FACTORS SUGGESTING SYNDROME OF INAPPROPRIATE ANTIDIURETIC HORMONE (SIADH)

- Serum sodium <134 mmol/l
- Serum osmolality <275 mOsm/kg
- Urine osmolality >300 mOsm/kg or greater than serum pecific gravity may also be elevated
- Urine sodium >40 mmol/l (although not necessarily)
- Serum glucose and albumin should be normal
- Serum creatinine and BUN as well as urine urate are generally low

---

The formula below can assist in determining the expected rise in serum sodium to a given quantity of fluid repletion.

$$\text{Change in serum sodium} = ([\text{Fluid sodium} + \text{fluid potassium}] - \text{serum sodium}) / (\text{total body water} + 1)$$

See Table 20-13. Total body water (TBW) is 0.6 in men and children, and 0.5 for women. These values are slightly lower for older individuals. Based on the goal rate of change, the rate of fluid administration can be calculated.

Another method to determine the amount of saline necessary is to calculate the patient's sodium deficit and then the amount and rate of fluid administration needed to correct this deficit using the formula below:

$$\text{Sodium deficit} = \text{TBW} \times \text{weight (in kg)} \times (\text{desired serum sodium} - \text{current serum sodium})$$

The desired serum sodium is generally 120–125 mmol/l as correction to strictly normal levels of serum sodium via hypertonic saline is generally not necessary or desirable.

Diuresis (with furosemide) may be used to maintain appropriate volume status and to inhibit sodium chloride reabsorption in the kidney and thereby aid in sodium correction, but should be used cautiously to avoid overly rapid correction. Serum sodium should be monitored every 2 h initially and adjustments made accordingly.

Salt supplementation (high-salt diet, salt tablets), loop diuretics, and water restriction are employed in the long-term management for SIADH once severe hyponatremia has been corrected.

TABLE 20-12 CLINICAL SIGNS AND SYMPTOMS OF HYPONATREMIA

- Difficulty concentrating, headache, confusion, personality changes, lethargy
- Anorexia, impaired taste, nausea, vomiting, diarrhea
- Muscle cramps, weakness, fatigue
- Incontinence and oliguria
- Depressed deep tendon reflexes, seizure, coma, cerebral edema/uncal herniation and death

TABLE 20-13 FLUID CHOICE FOR CORRECTION OF HYPONATREMIA

Fluid	mmol/l of Sodium	Extracellular Fluid Distribution (%)
3% NaCl	513	100
0.9% NaCl	154	100
Ringer's lactate	130	97
0.45% NaCl	77	73

Drug Therapies

The vasopressin receptor antagonists produce water diuresis without effecting sodium excretion. Tolvaptan (po) and conivaptan (IV) are currently available in the United States. These agents are limited by the risk of over-rapid correction of serum sodium but can be highly effective in treating hyponatremia. Demeclocycline, a tetracycline antibiotic that can block AVP activation of renal c-AMP, induces a state of nephrogenic diabetes insipidus. It can be given as 600–1200 mg/day in 2–3 divided doses if the above methods fail or cannot be tolerated. Demeclocycline dose should be adjusted for renal and hepatic dysfunction. Photosensitivity, nausea, and nephrotoxicity may occur and it may take days to see a response. Lithium, urea, and fludrocortisone are other medications that have been used in refractory cases.

■ TREATMENT OF OTHER CAUSES OF HYPONATREMIA

Initial techniques for mild, hypervolemic hyponatremia include both fluid and salt restriction. Further treatment must be based on the underlying etiology of the hyponatremia.

Patients who have hypovolemic hyponatremia with sodium loss may benefit from larger volumes of 0.9% sodium chloride initially, especially if blood pressure is low. However, these patients must be monitored closely as they approach euvolemia, as they tend to excrete water more rapidly than sodium as the impetus for ADH release declines, leading to more rapid sodium correction.

Reset osmostat, which is a special case of SIADH, presents as a mild, stable hyponatremia that generally does not require correction and is best treated by treating the underlying condition.

Treatment of hypertonic hyponatremia should be directed at the underlying cause.

■ TREATMENT COMPLICATIONS

A feared complication of overrapid sodium repletion is cerebral myelinolysis. This condition has been described most in the pons where it presents as a rapidly progressive weakness of limbs combined with dysarthria, dysphagia, seizures, and death occurring 2–6 days after correction, with CT and MRI evidence developing 6–10 days after clinical symptoms.

HYPERCALCEMIA

■ INCIDENCE AND RISK FACTORS

Normal values for serum calcium levels are population, laboratory, and laboratory machinery specific. However, one author defined moderate hypercalcemia as total serum calcium (adjusted for albumin) greater than 12 mg/dl and severe as greater than 14 mg/dl. At our institution, normal values for serum calcium are 8.5–10.5 mg/dl and for ionized calcium are 1.14–1.30 mmol/l.

Hypercalcemia may occur in as many as 30% of cancer cases. Among solid tumors, breast cancer, non-small cell lung cancer, squamous cell cancers, head and neck cancer, and renal cancers are highest risk; while among hematologic malignancies, multiple myeloma and lymphoma patients are at the highest risk. Hypercalcemia is uncommonly seen in other solid malignancies, such as colon, prostate, and small cell lung cancer.

The risk for hypercalcemia is determined by the histology and location of the cancer, the duration of illness, and the site of metastases. Risk of death is reported to be higher in individuals with malignancy-associated hypercalcemia.

■ MECHANISMS

Normally PTH and vitamin D act on bone, kidney, and gut to maintain serum calcium levels. Hypercalcemia occurs when either intestinal absorption of calcium increases, bone resorption increases, renal reabsorption increases, or release of tumor-related humoral factors leads to increased serum calcium levels that exceed renal excretion. The two most common causes of malignancy-associated hypercalcemia are local, osteolytic activity of tumor cells and humoral hypercalcemia of malignancy. These two etiologies represent a continuum of malignancy-related pathology (6).

Osteolytic Hypercalcemia

Osteolytic hypercalcemia comprises 20% of cases and is commonly due to breast cancer, myeloma, and lymphoma with substantial bone involvement. Release of osteoclast activating factors including lymphotoxin, IL-1 alpha, TGF alpha and beta, TNF alpha, and IL-6 have been identified, among others. In osteolytic hypercalcemia, phosphate is usually normal, while $1, 25(OH)_2$ vitamin D_3, intestinal reabsorption of calcium and PTH are low, and renal clearance of calcium is increased.

Humoral Hypercalcemia of Malignancy

The other 80% of hypercalcemia cases are due to humoral hypercalcemia via parathyroid hormone related protein (PTHrP) and are usually associated with squamous cell cancers; renal, breast, ovarian, or endometrial cancers; and HTLV-associated ATLL (Acute T cell leukemia/lymphoma). Release of PTHrP appears to contribute to osteolysis locally and systemically by increasing osteoclast activity and therefore bone resorption. Due to close homology with PTH, PTHrP mimics the effect of PTH on renal and skeletal calcium homeostasis.

TABLE 20-14 RARE CAUSES OF HYPERCALCEMIA IN MALIGNANCY

1, 25-dihydroxyvitamin D (calcitriol) secreting cancers
- Rare, usually lymphomas, with extrarenal production
- Tumor cells increase the conversion of $25(OH)D_3$ to $1, 25(OH)_2D_3$, causing increased osteoclastic bone resorption and intestinal absorption of calcium
- PTH and urinary c-AMP are low, with increased urinary calcium excretion and GI absorption

Primary hyperparathyroidism
- Can coexist with PTHrP, in which case, both PTH and PTHrP are elevated. Incidence of copresentation may be 15% and occur most in breast, colon and lymphoma
- In addition, there are rare ectopic PTH secreting tumors
- Leads to increased renal tubular, GI calcium reabsorption, osteoblastic activity, and metabolic acidosis
- In isolated primary hyperparathyroidism, $1, 25(OH)_2$ vitamin D_3 is high

Drugs
- Administration of estrogen or antiestrogens (such as tamoxifen) in the presence of bone metastases has been associated with hypercalcemia

Humoral hypercalcemia should be considered when PTH levels are low, when metastases are absent, and when metabolic alkalosis with low chloride and high bicarbonate concentrations are present. In addition, $1, 25(OH)_2$ vitamin D_3 and phosphorus levels are generally low, while urinary c-AMP concentrations and renal calcium clearance are high.

Other Mechanisms of Hypercalcemia

There are further rare causes of malignancy-associated hypercalcemia that represent a small fraction of cases. These are included in Table 20-14.

■ CLINICAL PRESENTATION

The symptoms of hypercalcemia can be remarkably protean with effects on numerous organ systems (Table 20-15). The presence or absence of

TABLE 20-15 CLINICAL SIGNS AND SYMPTOMS OF HYPERCALCEMIA

• Neurologic	Anxiety, depression, confusion, psychosis and hallucinations, somnolence and coma, hyporeflexia
• Cardiac	QT interval shortening, bradycardia, prolonged PR intervals, widened T waves, arrhythmia
• Gastointestinal	Nausea and vomiting, constipation, anorexia, pancreatitis, peptic ulcer disease
• Renal	Polyuria and dypsia, acute and chronic renal insufficiency, with chronic hypercalcemia: distal renal tubular acidosis, nephrolithiasis, nephrogenic diabetes insipidus
• Musculoskeletal	Weakness or fatigue

TABLE 20-16 DIFFERENTIAL DIAGNOSIS FOR HYPERCALCEMIA

- Primary or tertiary hyperparathyroidism, thyrotoxicosis
- Hypervitaminosis D or A, increased calcium intake (milk alkali), total parenteral nutrition
- Drugs: lithium, thiazide diuretics, theophylline toxicity
- Granulomatous diseases including sarcoidosis, Paget's, acromegaly
- Acute renal failure
- Rhabdomyolysis, immobilization
- Pheochromocytoma, adrenal insufficiency
- Familial hypocalciuric hypercalcemia

symptoms is dependent upon individual patient factors such as severity, chronicity, preexisting mental status, age, concomitant sedatives, or narcotics.

◼ DIFFERENTIAL DIAGNOSIS

The most frequent causes of hypercalcemia are cancer, primary hyperparathyroidism, and vitamin D intoxication (Table 20-16).

◼ DIAGNOSIS

Ideally ionized calcium would be drawn, given variations in calcium level by albumin level and the presence of calcium-binding immunoglobulins. If total serum calcium levels are used, correct for albumin level via the following formula:

$$\text{Corrected Ca} = \text{measured Ca} + 0.8 \times (4.0 - \text{measured albumin})$$

In addition to calcium, serum electrolytes, phosphorus, BUN and creatinine, PTH, and PTHrP (as well as SPEP, UPEP, free serum kappa and lambda light chains, and Bence Jones proteins if myeloma is suspected) are often measured in malignancy-associated hypercalcemia. The presence of bone metastases on radionuclide imaging may also help confirm the diagnosis. Distinguishing between rare causes of malignancy-related hypercalcemia and other causes usually requires further testing, such as vitamin D levels, thyroid function tests, fasting calcium to creatinine urine ratio, chest x-ray, and serum ACE levels.

◼ PROPHYLAXIS AND MONITORING

There are no clear guidelines for the frequency of calcium monitoring. However, it should be based, at least in part, on the expected length of efficacy of any treatment rendered. For instance, for bisphosphonates, the treatment effect generally lasts a month or less. Measurement of serum or ionized calcium, urea and other electrolytes, albumin, volume status including urine output, and mental status are typical.

◼ TREATMENT

The primary treatment of malignancy-associated hypercalcemia is directed toward the underlying cancer. However, Table 20-17 summarizes treatments frequently used as temporizing measures.

TABLE 20-17 TREATMENT FOR MALIGNANCY-RELATED HYPERCALCEMIA

First Line	Dose	Side Effects	Second Line	Dose	Side Effects
Hydration	200–500 ml/h IV normal saline	Volume overload, electrolyte abnormalities	Calcitonin	4–8 IU/kg/d IM or SQ in divided doses Q6–12 h, may need to be given with steroids to avoid side effects	Nausea, flushing, tachyphylaxis, hypersensitivity
Diuresis	Dose by volume status and prior exposure to diuretics				
Bisphosphonates	Pamidronate 30 mg mild HC, 60–90 mg severe HC IV over 2 h in saline or D5W	Renal failure, leucopenia	Gallium nitrate	100–200 mg/m^2 IV over 24 h for 5 d	Nephrotoxicity, pleural effusion and pulmonary infiltrates, optic neuritis
	Zoledronate 4 mg IV over 15 min in saline or D5W 8 mg dosing for relapsed or refractory HC	Renal failure, osteonecrosis			
Dialysis		Hypotension	Plicamycin	25 µg/kg per dose given over 4–6 h in saline. A second dose may be given in 2 d	Renal insufficiency, hepatitis, thrombocytopenia, nausea and vomiting, coagulopathy
			Glucocorticoids*	1 mg/kg/d or 40–60 mg/d prednisone for no more than 10 d	Hyperglycemia, GI bleeding, myopathy, infections, confusion, hypertension

*For vitamin D secreting lymphomas.

First-Line Treatments

Hydration and Diuresis   Mild hypercalcemia can be treated with saline hydration, and, when appropriate, diuresis. Most patients with hypercalcemia are severely dehydrated due to calcium's effect on the kidney's ability to concentrate urine (as in nephrogenic diabetes insipidus) and decreased intake. Isotonic saline is used to improve renal blood flow and encourage calcium excretion via exchange for sodium in the renal distal tubule and is the mainstay of treatment. Attention must be paid to volume overload and electrolyte abnormalities. Loop diuretics (furosemide) may be used to help block renal calcium reabsorption while the patient remains volume replete.

Bisphosphonates   Most cases of hypercalcemia will require further treatment to decrease bone resorption, specifically bisphosphonates. Bisphosphonates are pyrophosphate analogs that inhibit bone resorption via osteoclasts but do not affect renal tubular absorption. Their effect generally occurs within 36–72 h and lasts from 20–30 days. Osteonecrosis of the jaw is a concerning but rare side effect. More common adverse events include bone pain and therapeutic hypocalcemia.

Typical dosing for pamidronate is 30 mg IV for mild and 60–90 mg IV for severe hypercalcemia infused over 2 h in 50–200 ml of saline or D5W. Pamidronate can be used synergistically with calcitonin. Zoledronate dosing is 4 mg IV over 15 min in 50 ml saline or D5W for most cases of hypercalcemia. Zoledronate should be used with caution in patients with renal insufficiency.

Dialysis   Dialysis is available for severe hypercalcemia with acute or chronic renal failure when other treatments cannot be used or are ineffective. However, initiation of dialysis is best reserved for cases in which there are effective treatments for the underlying malignancy.

Supportive Measures and Follow-Up   All patients with hypercalcemia should have efforts made toward removal of exogenous calcium (including TPN, supplements, diet), discontinuation of medications that decrease calcium excretion or reduce renal blood flow (like thiazide diuretics, NSAIDs), and increased mobilization or physical activity.

In patients with hypercalcemia, oral phosphate administration can be used to limit oral calcium bioavailability and can make correction of hypercalcemia easier. Usual dosing is 1–2 g/day orally after meals in divided doses but must be monitored in patients with preexisting renal dysfunction or high serum phosphorus levels. Due to potential side effects, intravenous phosphorus is not recommended.

In cases in which no further cancer treatment can be offered, thought should be given to withholding or withdrawing treatment for hypercalcemia. If neurological depression predominates and other symptoms are not significant (anxiety, gastrointestinal distress), withholding treatment may be preferable and should be discussed with the patient and/or the patient's health-care proxy and family.

Follow-up for hypercalcemia usually includes periodic calcium measurement and bisphosphonate administration.

Second-Line Treatments

Second-line treatments include calcitonin and glucocorticoids. Calcitonin also acts by increasing urinary calcium and can be used synergistically with bisphophonates. Glucocorticoids likely decrease intestinal calcium absorption and inhibit osteoclast-mediated bone resorption and are best used in cases of increased 1, 25(OH)$_2$ vitamin D$_3$ or if the malignancy is responsive to glucocorticoids as a treatment as well (such as lymphoma), given the attendant side effects.

RANK-L (receptor of nuclear factor kappa-B ligand) Agents Denosumab is a fully human monoclonal antibody that targets the RANK ligand. The ligand normally activates pre-osteoclasts into mature osteoclasts and also activates mature osteoclasts. Ongoing clinical trials are testing the efficacy of this agent in hypercalcemia of malignancy.

REFERENCES

1. Cairo M, Bishop M. Tumor lysis syndrome: new therapeutic strategies and classification. *Br J Haematol.* 2004; 127: 3–11.

2. Howard SC, Jones DP, Pui CH. The tumor lysis syndrome. *N Engl J Med.* 2011; 364: 1844–1854.

3. Coiffier B, Altman A. Guidelines for the management of pediatric and adult tumor lysis syndrome: an evidence-based review. *J Clin Oncol.* 2008: 26; 2767–2778.

4. Adrogue HJ, Madias NE. Hyponatremia. *N Engl J Med.* 2000; 342: 1581–1589.

5. Baylis P. The syndrome of inappropriate antidiuretic hormone secretion. *Int J Biochem Cell Biol.* 2003; 35: 1495–1499.

6. Stewart A. Hypercalcemia associated with cancer. *N Engl J Med.* 2005; 352: 373–379.

CHAPTER **21**

Pain Management

Juliet Jacobsen, Vicki Jackson

INTRODUCTION

Cancer causes pain. Although studies give varying results, even the most conservative studies report that at least 20% of patients have pain at diagnosis or in the advanced stages of their illness. Numerous studies show that clinicians often undertreat cancer pain and that undertreated pain causes undue burdens on patients and their families. Clinicians may underestimate how much pain patients feel, or not be facile in pain management techniques that have the potential to greatly improve a patient's quality of life. Patients' misconceptions about pain medications also contribute to inadequate pain management. Patients may be reluctant to take pain medications for fear of addiction or worry that requiring pain medication indicates that death is imminent. Patients at particular risk for undertreatment include women, minorities, the poor, and the old (1).

PAIN ASSESSMENT

With simple treatments, more than 80% of patients can have their pain controlled (2). The first step in devising a pain management plan requires the patient to characterize the pain. It is helpful to distinguish neuropathic pain, which patients will characterize as burning, sharp, or shooting, from visceral and somatic pains, which are dull and aching. In a cancer patient, pain is usually caused by chemotherapy, radiation therapy, or tumor recurrence (3). Understanding the origin of the pain aids in the development of the appropriate pain management plan. Pain from bony metastases, for example, may require an NSAID or radiation, whereas pain from a local recurrence outside of the bone may require only opioids.

The next step is to assess the baseline level of pain using simple, validated methods such as visual analog scales, numerical scales (e.g., from 1 to 10), or pictoral scales (faces, circles of different colors). Many clinicians are unaware that patients with chronic pain will often lack physiologic signs that may indicate pain. Patients with chronic pain rarely show signs of sympathetic arousal such as tachycardia or hypertension. Patient self-report is the gold standard of pain assessment.

A patient's experience of pain is not limited to physical sensation. Depression, anxiety, and existential distress can all exacerbate a patient's perception of and ability to cope with pain. Because psychosocial and spiritual factors play such a large role in a clinician's ability to treat pain, it is critical to include assessment of these factors when developing a comprehensive pain management plan. The comprehensive clinical assessment should therefore include the following:

- Psychological, social, financial, and spiritual sources of coping and of distress
- An assessment of mood disorders: screen for and treat depression and anxiety
- Evaluating how the patient and family are coping with the illness

TREATMENT

The goal of treatment is to adequately manage the pain while trying to minimize toxicity. For moderate pain or pain that persists despite NSAIDs or acetaminophen, it is appropriate to initiate short-acting opioids in conjunction with NSAIDs or acetaminophen (3, 4). Short-acting opioids such as morphine, oxycodone, or hydromorphone have an onset of action of 15–30 min, reach peak effect in about 60 min, and have a duration of action of approximately 4 h. Consider the patient's preferences and experience when choosing an opioid, and avoid codeine except in a patient who has used it with success. Short-acting opioids are dosed every 3–4 h and delivered via the least invasive route that works, preferably oral.

■ STARTING LONG-ACTING OPIOIDS

For a patient with intermittent pain, short-acting opioids may suffice. However, patients with continuous pain or with a combination of continuous and intermittent worsening pain will need to begin long-acting opioids. Long-acting opioids such as sustained-release oxycodone (Oxycontin) or sustained-release morphine (MS Contin) have an onset of action of about 1 h, reach peak effect in 3–4 h, and have a duration of action of 8–12 h.

Choosing the appropriate long-acting opioid dose requires multiple steps. First, determine the total daily dose of short-acting opioid required to provide adequate analgesia. Second, choose the long-acting preparation. Finally, convert the short-acting opioid into the appropriate dose of the long-acting preparation. Commonly morphine or oxycodone is used in a short-acting preparation, and both have long-acting preparations that are inexpensive and well tolerated. When using morphine or oxycodone, the total daily dose of short-acting opioid can be directly converted to long-acting opioid. For example, a patient requiring 5 mg of oxycodone every 3 h is taking a total of 40 mg of oxycodone in a 24-h period. This patient may be started on 20 mg of long-acting oxycodone every 12 h. Alternatively, if the patient requires a different long-acting opioid, it is possible to determine the correct dose using equianalgesic tables (Table 21-1). When converting a patient from one opioid to another, it is important to account for incomplete cross-tolerance by decreasing the dose of the new opioid by 25%–50%.

■ CASE EXAMPLE

A 45-year-old woman with breast cancer metastatic to her ribs presents to clinic and describes aching pleuritic chest pain that is worse with movement. For pain she takes 4 mg of oral hydromorphone (Dilaudid) every 6 h around the clock. She complains that her pain medication wears off, and she is frequently in pain. What are the problems with her pain management? How do you convert her to a long-acting opioid and what breakthrough dose do you give?

Her first problem is that she is not taking an adjuvant that would minimize the toxicity of the opioid. Start an adjuvant medication such as acetaminophen or an NSAID. An NSAID would be a good choice in this patient because NSAIDs are particularly effective for bone metastases. Overall, no NSAID works better than any other. However, individual patients may do best with a particular NSAID. If this works, she could take less opioid.

TABLE 21-1 OPIOID EQUIANALGESIC TABLE (mg)

Hydromorphone (Dilauded)		Morphine		Oxycodone	
IV	Oral	IV	Oral	Oral	IV
1.5	7.5	10	30	20	N/A

Fentanyl transdermal patch 25 mcg/h = 50 mg oral morphine.
Source: Reference 5.

Her second problem is that with her persistent pain, her current dosing interval of 6 h is too long: the short-acting opioid has worn off in 4 h. She could take it more frequently, but every 4-h dosing is cumbersome and interrupts sleep. She needs a long-acting opioid. Since hydromorphone has no long-acting formulation, switch her medication to sustained-release oxycodone (Oxycontin), sustained-release morphine (MS Contin), or transdermal fentanyl. Of these choices, transdermal fentanyl is more difficult to titrate in a patient who is requiring multiple changes in dosing. Oxycodone and morphine, in their respective doses, are similarly effective and easy to titrate. Here is the procedure for changing her medication from oral hydromorphone to long-acting oral morphine:

1. Calculate her 24-h short-acting opioid dose:

$$4 \text{ mg hydromorphone} \times 4 \text{ doses/24 h} = 16 \text{ mg/24 h}$$

2. Look up the equianalgesic conversion from oral hydromorphone to oral morphine:

$$\text{hydromorphone 7.5 mg oral} = \text{morphine 30 mg oral}$$

3. Set up an equation to convert the dose:

$$\frac{7.5 \text{ mg}}{30 \text{ mg}} = \frac{16 \text{ mg}}{X}.$$

Solve for X:

$$X = 64 \text{ mg morphine in 24 h}$$

4. Reduce this dose by 25%–50% due to incomplete cross-tolerance between the old and new opioids. Choosing the lower reduction of only 25%, the final dose is computed as follows:

$$0.25 \times 64 \text{ mg} = 16 \text{ mg reduction}$$
$$64 \text{ mg} - 16 \text{ mg} = 48 \text{ mg oral morphine in 24 h}$$

5. Divide the 24 h total into divided doses. Long-acting morphine can be given q8 or q12. Note: these medications should *not* be dosed tid, but rather q8h to ensure adequate analgesia and to decrease sedation. For this example, the q8h dosing is 48 mg/3 = roughly 15 mg long-acting morphine every 8 h.

■ BREAKTHROUGH DOSING

All long-acting opioids must be paired with an appropriate dose of short-acting medication in the event that the patient experiences breakthrough pain. The usual dose for breakthrough pain is 10%–20% of the total 24-h dose. Opioids prescribed for breakthrough pain may be safely dosed as often as every 1–2 h. Short-acting opioids that are orally dosed reach peak analgesic effect at 1 h and last no more than 4 h. In this example, the patient is taking 45 mg of oral long-acting morphine per day. An appropriate dose for breakthrough pain would be 10%–20% of the total daily long-acting dose or 5–10 mg every 3–4 h as needed.

Taking excessive doses of breakthrough medication can be a symptom of poorly controlled pain. Ideally a patient would not need more than

2–3 breakthrough doses over 24 h. If a patient requires more frequent dosing, the long-acting dose may be too low. To calculate the increase in the long-acting dose, add up the total amount of breakthrough medication taken in 24 h and convert it to the appropriate amount of the long-acting formulation that the patient is already taking. In this example, if your patient consistently took 5 mg of morphine every 4 h for breakthrough pain, the 24-h total (30 mg) should be given instead as long-acting morphine. Her previous dose of morphine 15 mg q8h could be increased to 30 mg in the morning and evening and 15 mg in the afternoon.

SIDE EFFECTS

Common side effects of opioids include nausea, vomiting, sedation, and constipation. Nausea and sedation usually resolve within 1 week. In most cases no psychoimpairment remains 2 weeks after the change in the opioid dose. Constipation, unlike other side effects, does not attenuate with long-term use. Therefore, all patients on opioids require a bowel regimen that includes a stimulant laxative (e.g., senna 2 tab po bid) and stool softener (e.g., docusate [Colace] 100 mg po bid).

■ SAFETY

Care must be taken when dosing opioids in elderly patients or in those with hepatic or renal insufficiency as they will be more sensitive to the medication and experience side effects such as sedation at lower doses. Start at a low dose and increase slowly. The key to safe and competent pain management is assessment and frequent reassessment. Also, watch for delirium and sedation in patients taking concomitant benzodiazepines. Delirium can sometimes improve with a slight reduction in the opioid.

■ OVERSEDATION

Opioid respiratory depression is due to generalized CNS depression. Therefore, when respiratory depression is due to an overdose of opioids, it is always preceded by somnolence. Respiratory depression due to opioids does not commonly occur in patients on a stable dose of opioids unless the patient is experiencing alterations in metabolism or excretion of the drug, has been given another sedating medication such as benzodiazepines, or has developed a new medical complication such as infection. Therefore, if sedation does occur, it is important to do a full medical evaluation. In the sedated but clinically stable patient, initial management includes discontinuation of the opioid, supplemental oxygen, and efforts to arouse the patient. For significant respiratory depression, dilute 0.4 mg naloxone into 10 cc of normal saline and administer 1 cc every 1–2 min until the respiratory rate is satisfactory. The clinical goal is to reverse the respiratory depression without reversing the analgesic effect of the opioid. Beware that too rapid infusion of naloxone may precipitate a pain crisis in a patient on chronic opioids.

DIFFICULT-TO-CONTROL PAIN

Even with standard pain control, some patients still suffer. Patients with severe pain may need rapid titration of opioid medications; for protocols, see the NCCN guidelines on adult cancer pain (www.nccn.org). When pain is difficult to control, consider the following etiologies: neuropathic pain, incident pain, tolerance, addiction, somatization, and (the most frequent) undermedication.

- *Neuropathic pain.* Treat with effective adjuvants such as gabapentin (start 300 mg PO qhs and increase gradually to 300–600 mg po tid, max 3600 mg/day) or tricyclic antidepressants (nortriptyline 10 mg PO qhs and increase to therapeutic dose). Methadone, which blocks opioid and NMDA receptors, may also be helpful.
- *Incident pain* (such as before dressing changes or planned activity). Provide quick-onset, short-acting analgesia with an extra dose of short-acting opioid (use the breakthrough dose, 10%–20% of the daily opioid dose). For incident pain due to bony metastases, consider adjuvants such as NSAIDs (ibuprofen 600–800 mg po tid) or radiation treatment.
- *Tolerance.* Consider increasing the opioid dose or changing the opioid.
- *Psychological addiction.* It is rare in cancer patients treated with opioids (6), but patients who have a history of substance abuse have a higher risk (7).
- *Somatization.* Consult the psychiatry, pain, or palliative-care services.

FENTANYL PREPARATIONS

Transdermal fentanyl, a long-acting fentanyl preparation available in a patch, is changed every 48–72 h (7). It is ideal for patients who have trouble taking oral medication, due to nausea, difficulty swallowing, or gastrointestinal tract dysfunction. Fentanyl, a lipophile, diffuses into the fat of the skin and then into the bloodstream, so place the patch over an area of the body with subcutaneous fat such as the abdomen, upper arm, or buttocks. The patch is not an effective initial treatment for severe pain because at least 12 h are required to build enough drug in the fat reservoir to establish adequate blood levels. Frequent rescue dosing is needed for the first 12–24 h until the fentanyl accumulates. Because the patches need a reservoir of subcutaneous fat, they are not recommended for patients who weigh less than 110 lb or for older cachectic patients. In contrast, febrile patients may have increased absorption and suffer possible toxicity.

Transmucosal immediate release fentanyl (TIRF) products such as Actiq and Fentora have an FDA black box warning and should be used with caution. Because life-threatening hypoventilation could occur at any dose in patients not taking chronic opioids, TIRF is indicated for breakthrough cancer pain only in patients who are already receiving and who are tolerant to opioid therapy. Patients considered opioid tolerant are those who are taking at least 60 mg morphine/day, or an equianalgesic dose of another opioid, for a week or longer. In addition, TIRF products are not interchangeable and converting from one TIRF product to another must be done according to labeled dosing instructions.

METHADONE

Rotation to methadone is complex because methadone has a long half-life and accumulates in the fat stores, and its potency increases when a patient is taking another opioid. Methadone can be up to 10 times more powerful in patients on high doses of opioids than in patients who are opioid naive or on lower doses (Table 21-2). Contact a pain or palliative-care specialist for assistance when converting to methadone.

TABLE 21-2 GUIDELINES FOR IMMEDIATE DISCONTINUATION OF OPIOID AND ROTATION TO METHADONE

Morphine Dose	Ratio to Convert to Methadone
<100 mg/24 h	1 mg of methadone for every 4 mg of morphine (1:4)
101–300 mg/24 h	1:8
301–600 mg/24 h	1:10
601–800 mg/24 h	1:12
801–1000 mg/24 h	1:15
>1000 mg/24 h	1:20

Source: Reference 8.

CONCLUSION

Effective management of cancer pain requires a systematic approach that includes assessment of symptoms, aggressive pharmacologic and nonpharmacologic treatment (relaxation exercises, massage, cognitive-behavioral therapy, and exercise), and education of the patient and family about how to achieve optimal pain control. Involve specialty services when your patient does not respond to standard treatments.

REFERENCES

1. American Pain Society. Guideline for the Management of Cancer Pain in Adults and Children. American Pain Society, Glenview, IL, 2005.

2. Zech DF, Groud S, Lynch J, et al. Validation of World Health Organization guidelines for cancer pain relief: a 10-year prospective study. *Pain.* 1995; 63: 65–76.

3. Portney RK, Lesage P. Management of cancer pain. *Lancet.* 1999; 353: 1695–1700.

4. WHO Expert Committee on Cancer Pain Relief and Active Supportive Care. Cancer Pain Relief and Palliative Care: Report of a WHO Expert Committee. World Health Organization, Geneva, 1990.

5. American Pain Society. Principles of Analgesic Use in the Treatment of Acute Pain and Cancer Pain. American Pain Society, Glenview, IL, 2003.

6. Schug SA, Zech D, Grond S, et al. A long-term survey of morphine in cancer pain patients. *J Pain Symptom Manage.* 1992; 7: 259–266.

7. Passik SD, Kirsh KL, Donaghy KB, et al. Pain and aberrant drug-related behaviors in medically ill patients with and without histories of substance abuse. *Clin J Pain.* 2006; 22: 173–181.

8. Ayonrinde OT, Bridge DT. The rediscovery of methodone for cancer pain management. *Med J Aust.* 2000; 173: 536–540.

CHAPTER **22**
Comprehensive End-of-Life Care
Jennifer Shin, Jennifer Temel

INTRODUCTION

Comprehensive end-of-life (EOL) care is an essential component of oncology. While we aim to cure as many patients as possible, many of them ultimately die of their disease. Our role as clinicians includes guiding patients and their families through the EOL. Comprehensive EOL care encompasses pain and symptom management, psychosocial and spiritual support, caregiver/family support, and discussions about goals of care and advance care planning. This requires skills in communication and symptom management, as well as knowledge of the services available in the community. A multidisciplinary approach is often helpful in providing comprehensive EOL care, and the team may include physicians, nurses, social workers, chaplains, palliative care, and/or hospice.

END-OF-LIFE CARE COMMUNICATION
■ APPROACH TO DIFFICULT CONVERSATIONS

Patients and families consider communication to be one of the most important aspects of EOL care (1). Discussions about goals of care, treatment preferences, and advance care planning can be difficult for clinicians, as well as for patients and families. In order to lead patients and families through these discussions, clinicians should be proficient in communicating about EOL care. Similar to other components of medical care, these communication skills can be learned and practiced (2).

A clinician can approach a difficult conversation using a series of communication steps that may be remembered by using the mnemonic SPIKES (**Table 22-1**) (3, 4). The first step in EOL care communication is to prepare for the discussion by asking the patient who he/she would like present in the discussion and by arranging a quiet, private setting with sitting room for all participants (**S**etup). The clinician should be well prepared for the meeting and know the basic information about the patient's disease, prognosis, and treatment options. The conversation should begin with the clinician establishing what the patient and family know about the illness (**P**erception) and what specific information they would like to know (**I**nvitation). The clinician can then build on the patient's illness understanding by clarifying realistic goals and addressing unrealistic expectations (**K**nowledge). In discussions regarding EOL care, patients and families may express a range of emotions, and it is important to allow them to express these feelings and to recognize and respond to them (**E**mpathize). Finally, it is helpful for the clinician to summarize what was discussed, assess the patient and family's understanding, and make a clear plan about the next steps (**S**ummarize and **S**trategize). These steps can be used in various difficult conversations,

TABLE 22-1 APPROACH TO DIFFICULT CONVERSATIONS

S = SETUP the discussion	• Ask the patient who usually helps to make important decisions and request that they come to the next visit. • Choose a space and time when you are least likely to be interrupted. • Prior to the meeting, review the patient's clinical information and discuss the plan with other providers if necessary.
P = Assess the patient's **PERCEPTION**	• "Can you share with me what you think is happening with your cancer and how you feel the treatments are going?"
I = INVITE the patient to tell you how much information he/she wants to know	• "What things would be helpful for you to know about your disease/treatment?" • "May I share with you some details about your disease/treatment?"
K = Share **KNOWLEDGE**	• Avoid jargon. • Give information in small chunks. • Give a warning that bad news is coming: "Unfortunately, I have some serious news to share with you."
E = EMPATHIZE with emotion	• Allow the patient time to express his/her feelings. • Avoid immediate reassurance or rebuttal. • Acknowledge what the patient is feeling: "I can see how difficult this has been for you and your family."
S = SUMMARIZE and **STRATEGIZE** next steps	• Summarize and check understanding. • Make a clear plan for follow-up.

Source: References 3 and 4.

including communicating bad news, discussing advanced care planning, and shifting from disease-directed therapy to palliative care (4–6).

■ **DISCUSSING PROGNOSIS, MAINTAINING HOPE, AND SETTING REALISTIC GOALS**

Patients facing serious illnesses value being able to prepare for their death (7). Physicians can augment the time that patients have to plan for the last phase of their lives by having honest discussions about prognosis and goals of care.

A patient's understanding of his/her prognosis may directly impact his/her decision-making at the EOL. Cancer patients tend to overestimate their chance of survival, which can lead them to choose life-prolonging therapies or invasive procedures rather than supportive care (8). Additionally, patients must have a clear understanding of the potential impact of therapies on their life expectancy and quality of life in order to make individualized decisions about their care (9).

TABLE 22-2 IDENTIFYING AND REFRAMING GOALS

Identifying Goals	• "What are your hopes for the coming weeks/months?" • "What are you worried about now? In the future?" • "Given the severity of your cancer, what is most important to you now?"
Reframing Goals ("Wish" statements)	• "I wish that there was a chemotherapy that would cure your cancer. Even though cure is not possible, we can meet some of your other goals like staying at home and spending time with your family."

Source: References 4 and 10.

One of the most difficult tasks in oncology is maintaining hope while preparing for inevitable death. Clinicians can address unrealistic hopes (e.g., cure) in an empathic fashion using "wish" statements ("I wish things were different") (10), allowing clinicians to empathize with patients and support their hopes, while acknowledging the realities of their prognosis. "Wish" statements may also help clinicians reframe unrealistic goals and encourage patients to think about new individualized goals (Table 22-2). Although cure may no longer be a possible goal, other realistic goals should be identified (Table 22-2) and may include but are certainly not limited to prolonging life, relief of distressing symptoms, finding personal meaning, and maintaining independence. Clinicians may also encourage their patients to hope for quality time with their loved ones, closure to their lives, and a peaceful death.

In all stages of cancer, patients and families look to their oncologist for guidance. As the focus of care shifts from a disease-directed to a palliative one, oncologists have an ongoing duty to help patients make decisions that are concordant with their goals. A clinician should make recommendations for care aligned with a patient's goals, including the management of symptoms and/or the recommendation of hospice. Although clinicians may be concerned about the impact that EOL discussions may have on patients and caregivers, such discussions have not been associated with higher rates of depression or worry (11). EOL discussions are associated with less aggressive care, including lower rates of ventilation, resuscitation, intensive care unit admission, and earlier hospice enrollment. In contrast, aggressive care is associated with worse patient quality of life and worse caregiver bereavement adjustment (11). The section "Approach to Difficult Conversations" provides a framework for ongoing discussions about goals of care. As these goals evolve, it is important for clinicians to provide individualized recommendations to help patients and families navigate the EOL.

ADVANCE CARE PLANNING

Advance care planning (ACP) is the process by which patients describe their preferences for future care in the event that they become incapable of making medical decisions. It is an important step to ensure that patients' wishes are clearly documented if they are unable to express these wishes themselves. ACP is essential for any patient with a life-limiting illness and is ideally completed prior to a medical crisis or the very EOL. It is important for physicians to systematically introduce the topic of ACP with their patients, as some patients may have already specified their wishes and others may be waiting for their physicians to bring up the topic before creating an advance care plan.

Written advance directives are the basis of ACP and serve two main roles. First, they provide guidance regarding the aggressiveness of care a patient would desire at the time of a life-threatening event (living will). Second, they identify a health-care proxy (durable power of attorney for health care) to communicate a patient's wishes if he/she is unable to do so himself/herself. The designated health-care proxy (or proxies if an alternate proxy is also assigned) should understand that his/her role is to provide decisions based on what the patient would want in that particular situation, not what the proxy would choose for himself/herself.

Advance directives (both living wills and health-care proxies) go into effect only when patients are unable to directly participate in decision-making about their care. There are certain state-specific documents that may be used (Table 22-3). The patient and proxy should have copies of these documents, and a copy should also be placed in the patient's medical record.

Many of the terms used in a living will are ambiguous and require interpretation in the context of the current medical situation. Even when a patient specifies situation-specific instructions in his/her living will, it is impossible to include all of the possible scenarios that a patient may face at the EOL. However, the living will can serve as a catalyst for discussions about goals of care. It may be helpful to meet with the patient, family, and proxy to help guide these discussions with specific mention of some scenarios that patients may face (e.g., life-sustaining treatments in the ICU, artificial nutrition and hydration). Through this process, the patient can consider his/her preferences and make them known to his/her proxy, family, and care team.

TABLE 22-3 USEFUL RESOURCES IN ACP

www.caringinfo.org *A program of the National Hospice and Palliative Care Organization (NHPCO)*	• Download state-specific advance directives • Resources and information for patients about ACP and EOL planning • Resources and information for caregivers • Help with choosing a hospice
http://www.ohsu.edu/polst	• Information about the POLST program for providers, patients, and families • State-specific POLST forms
www.agingwithdignity.org	• Order online and print versions of *Five Wishes*, a living will written in everyday language and a useful tool to initiate and structure conversations about EOL care (available in numerous languages)

A living will documents a patient's preferences regarding medical care, but is not a medical order. A Do Not Resuscitate (DNR) order is written by a clinician to formalize the patient's preference about resuscitation status. This order is usually written when a patient is hospitalized, although a physician may also sign an out-of-hospital DNR order form that a patient can take home (sometimes called a Comfort Care form). This instructs emergency medical personnel on the patient's DNR status. The Physician Orders for Life Sustaining Treatment (POLST) is a form that translates patient goals and preferences into a more comprehensive set of medical orders. The POLST includes orders regarding cardiopulmonary resuscitation (CPR) but also extends to specific medical interventions (e.g., options for comfort measures only, limited interventions including hospitalization, and full treatment) and artificial nutrition/hydration. The POLST may guide discussions and formalize a patient's preferences beyond resuscitation status. POLST programs exist or are in development in 34 states (12).

Initial conversations about treatment preferences and formalizing these discussions into ACP documents and orders should begin early in the course of disease in patients with advanced cancer. As patients decline, it can be difficult for them to think clearly about EOL care preferences. It is also challenging for family members to be objective about a patient's goals when the patient is ill or hospitalized. By beginning this dialogue early in the illness and revisiting it periodically, discussions about EOL care preferences are normalized (13).

PALLIATIVE CARE, HOSPICE, AND BRIDGE PROGRAMS

■ PALLIATIVE CARE

Palliative care is patient- and family-centered care with the goal of anticipating, preventing, and reducing suffering and optimizing the quality of life for patients and families at all stages of a serious illness. It encompasses the management of pain and other distressing symptoms, while incorporating psychosocial and spiritual care tailored to the patient and family's needs. Palliative care can be initiated by the primary oncology team and augmented by consulting and collaborating with an interdisciplinary team of palliative care experts (14), including specially trained physicians, nurses, and often social workers, chaplains, and pharmacists. Palliative care teams can assist the oncology team with symptom management, psychosocial and spiritual support for patients and families, and advance care planning. Specialized palliative care can be administered in a variety of settings (e.g., inpatient and outpatient hospital settings, long-term care facilities, home, hospice), although there is great regional variability in the availability of these services. An important distinction should be made between palliative care and hospice: palliative care is appropriate for any patient facing a serious illness and can be provided concurrently with life-prolonging treatments, while hospice provides palliative care for patients with a prognosis of less than 6 months and who have agreed to focus on comfort as their goal.

In a randomized trial of patients with newly diagnosed metastatic non-small cell lung cancer, patients who were followed by palliative care specialists early in their illness received less aggressive EOL care and had a longer median survival than patients receiving usual care (15). This study and others have demonstrated that palliative care, when combined with standard cancer care or as the main focus of care, leads to better patient and caregiver outcomes (16–18). The National Comprehensive Cancer Network's guidelines recommend that palliative care begin at diagnosis and be administered concurrently with disease-directed, life-prolonging therapies, with a shift to palliative care as the primary goal when these therapies are no longer effective or desired (14). The American Society of Clinical Oncology recently published a provisional clinical opinion suggesting combined oncology and palliative care early in the course of patients with metastatic cancer and/or high symptom burden (19).

■ HOSPICE

Hospice is an essential resource for patients with metastatic cancer as they approach the EOL. Hospice provides comprehensive and compassionate care to patients and their families through an interdisciplinary team (Table 22-4) (20). Most hospice care takes place in the patient's home,

TABLE 22-4 HOSPICE SERVICES AND TEAM MEMBERS

Services
Pain and symptom management
24-h telephone access to a clinician
Assistance with personal care needs
Help with errands (e.g., shopping) and light housework
Spiritual support
Companionship for the patient and family
Patient and family education and counseling
Case management and coordination
Advance care planning
Medications and supplies (pertaining to the hospice diagnosis)
Durable medical equipment
Continuous home care only during brief periods of crisis
Respite services (up to 5 d of inpatient care to allow caregivers a break, no limit to the number of respite care episodes)
Inpatient hospice (for treatment of severe symptoms that cannot be managed at home)
Bereavement counseling

Team Members
Physician (hospice physician, patient's personal physician may also be included)
Nurse
Social worker
Home health aide
Clergy
Bereavement counselor
Speech, physical, and occupational therapists (if needed)
Trained volunteers

Source: From Reference 20.

TABLE 22-5 TRIGGERS FOR EARLY HOSPICE DISCUSSIONS

Change in clinical status
Decline in performance status
Progressive disease
Complication of treatment
Hospitalization
Patient's goals reflect a desire to focus on palliation

although there are nursing facilities that offer hospice care as well as inpatient hospice facilities. Patients are considered eligible for hospice if the referring physician and the hospice medical director certify that they have a life-limiting illness with an estimated life expectancy of less than 6 months. Additionally, the patient must accept a philosophy of comfort care, forgoing disease-directed therapies unless they provide a specific palliative benefit. A DNR order does not need to be signed at the time of enrollment into hospice. Hospice is reimbursed through the Medicare Hospice Benefit, the Medicaid Hospice Benefit, and the majority of private insurers (20).

Families report high levels of satisfaction with hospice (21), and longer hospice stays are associated with better quality of life in patients and less depression in bereaved family members (11, 22). Despite this, only about 42% of people in the United States die while receiving hospice care, and many patients enroll very late in the course of illness with a median length of stay of less than 3 weeks (20). Although this is likely multifactorial in origin, data suggest that patients may enroll in hospice later if their physicians do not discuss hospice, or if these discussions take place in the last few weeks of a patient's life (23, 24). Therefore, it is important for the clinician to initiate a hospice discussion with patients who may benefit from such services. This may be loosely defined by the eligibility criteria, but it may be more helpful to consider specific triggers for earlier hospice discussions (Table 22-5) (6, 25, 26).

■ BRIDGE PROGRAMS

Bridge programs provide many of the services offered by hospice, but eligibility is not limited by a prognosis of less than 6 months or an agreement to forgo life-prolonging therapies. It is important to note that patients do have to meet the criteria for home health care (i.e., homebound with a skilled need), which may be a significant barrier to enrollment in a bridge program. Patients who are receiving bridge program services benefit from a team that is specialized in providing palliative home care, while also undergoing disease-directed therapy. These programs also provide a smooth transition to hospice if the patient chooses to defer additional life-prolonging therapies.

ACKNOWLEDGMENT

This work was supported by R25CA092203 from the National Cancer Institute at the National Institutes of Health.

REFERENCES

1. Wenrich MD, Curtis JR, Shannon SE, et al. Communicating with dying patients within the spectrum of medical care from terminal diagnosis to death. *Arch Intern Med*. 2001; 161: 868–874.

2. Back AL, Arnold RM, Baile WF, et al. Efficacy of communication skills training for giving bad news and discussing transitions to palliative care. *Arch Intern Med*. 2007; 167: 453–460.

3. Baile WF, Buckman R, Lenzi R, et al. SPIKES—a six-step protocol for delivering bad news: application to the patient with cancer. *The Oncologist*. 2000; 5: 302–311.

4. Back AL, Arnold RM, Baile WF, et al. Approaching difficult communication tasks in oncology. *CA Cancer J Clin*. 2005; 55: 164–177.

5. Morrison RS, Meier DE. Clinical practice. Palliative care. *N Engl J Med*. 2004; 350: 2582–2590.

6. Shin J, Casarett D. Facilitating hospice discussions: a six-step roadmap. *J Support Oncol*. 2011; 9: 97–102.

7. Steinhauser KE, Christakis NA, Clipp EC, et al. Factors considered important at the end of life by patients, family, physicians, and other care providers. *JAMA*. 2000; 284: 2476–2482.

8. Weeks JC, Cook EF, O'Day SJ, et al. Relationship between cancer patients' predictions of prognosis and their treatment preferences. *JAMA*. 1998; 279: 1709–1714.

9. Fried TR, Bradley EH, Towle VR, Allore H. Understanding the treatment preferences of seriously ill patients. *N Engl J Med*. 2002. 346: 1061–1066.

10. Quill TE, Arnold RM, Platt F. "I wish things were different": expressing wishes in response to loss, futility, and unrealistic hopes. *Ann Intern Med*. 2001; 135: 551–555.

11. Wright AA, Zhang B, Ray A, et al. Associations between end-of-life discussions, patient mental health, medical care near death, and caregiver bereavement adjustment. *JAMA*. 2008; 300: 1665–1673.

12. Fromme EK, Zive D, Schmidt TA, et al. POLST Registry do-not-resuscitate orders and other patient treatment preferences. *JAMA*. 2012; 307: 34–35.

13. Back AL, Arnold RM, Quill TE. Hope for the best, and prepare for the worst. *Ann Intern Med*. 2003. 138: 439–443.

14. Palliative Care. NCCN Clinical Practice Guidelines in Oncology 2012; Version 2.2012: Available from: www.nccn.org.

15. Temel JS, Greer JA, Muzikansky A, et al. Early palliative care for patients with metastatic non-small-cell lung cancer. *N Engl J Med*. 2010; 363: 733–742.

16. Bakitas M, Lyons KD, Hegel MT, et al. Effects of a palliative care intervention on clinical outcomes in patients with advanced cancer: the Project ENABLE II randomized controlled trial. *JAMA*. 2009; 302: 741–749.

17. Zimmermann C, Riechelmann R, Krzyzanowska M, et al. Effectiveness of specialized palliative care: a systematic review. *JAMA*. 2008; 299: 1698–1709.

18. El-Jawahri A, Greer JA, Temel JS. Does palliative care improve outcomes for patients with incurable illness? A review of the evidence. *J Support Oncol.* 2011; 9: 87–94.

19. Smith TJ, Temin S, Alesi ER, et al. American Society of Clinical Oncology provisional clinical opinion: the integration of palliative care into standard oncology care. *J Clin Oncol.* 2012; 30: 880–887.

20. National Hospice and Palliative Care Organization. Facts and Figures: Hospice Care in America. 2011; Available from: http://www.nhpco.org/files/public/Statistics_Research/2011_Facts_Figures.pdf.

21. Teno JM, Clarridge BR, Casey V, et al. Family perspectives on end-of-life care at the last place of care. *JAMA.* 2004; 291: 88–93.

22. Bradley EH, Prigerson H, Carlson MD, et al. Depression among surviving caregivers: does length of hospice enrollment matter? *Am J Psychiatry.* 2004; 161: 2257–2262.

23. Cherlin E, Fried T, Prigerson HG, et al. Communication between physicians and family caregivers about care at the end of life: when do discussions occur and what is said? *J Palliat Med.* 2005; 8: 1176–1185.

24. Casarett DJ, Quill TE. "I'm not ready for hospice": strategies for timely and effective hospice discussions. *Ann Intern Med.* 2007; 146: 443–449.

25. Conill C, Verger E, Salamero M. Performance status assessment in cancer patients. *Cancer.* 1990; 65: 1864–1866.

26. Mor V, Laliberte L, Morris JN, Wiemann M. The Karnofsky Performance Status Scale. An examination of its reliability and validity in a research setting. *Cancer.* 1984; 53: 2002–2007.

CHAPTER **23**
Depression, Anxiety, and Fatigue

Carlos G. Fernandez-Robles, William F. Pirl

INTRODUCTION

Depression, anxiety, and fatigue are frequent complications of cancer and cancer treatment. Although fatigue can be caused by depression and anxiety, it is a separate symptom that often does not have psychological origins.

An estimated one-third of all people with cancer experience psychosocial distress. Psychosocial distress encompasses both psychiatric disorders as well as emotional states that do not meet full criteria for psychiatric illnesses. Depression, anxiety disorders, and adjustment disorders are the most common psychiatric disorders in cancer patients. Delirium, however, may be more prevalent in hospitalized cancer patients, affecting almost 25%.

REACTION TO DIAGNOSIS OF CANCER

A diagnosis of cancer can elicit a variety of emotions, including sadness, anxiety, anger, and fear. People may have difficulty sleeping, loss of appetite, anxious thoughts about their cancer, poor concentration, and low mood. These symptoms can persist for 3 weeks after diagnosis. Usually by 4 weeks after diagnosis, people have their coping mechanisms in place and the depressive and anxiety symptoms have resolved. Unless the psychological symptoms are severe or are markedly impairing functioning, the diagnosis of a psychiatric disorder is usually reserved during the first 4 weeks after diagnosis, while people are coping with learning they have cancer.

DEPRESSION

Depression can be used to describe a symptom, feeling sad, as well as a serious illness, major depressive disorder (MDD). MDD is associated with poor quality of life, worse adherence to treatment, longer hospital stays, greater desire for death, suicide, and, possibly, increased mortality (1).

■ PREVALENCE

In a recent meta-analysis the prevalence of depression in individuals with cancer by DSM or ICD criteria was 16.3% (13.4–19.5) and for DSM-defined major depression it was 14.9% (12.2–17.7); similarly the prevalence of clinical levels of depressive symptoms, not necessarily MDD, was 19.2% (9.1–31.9) (2).

■ DIAGNOSIS

The diagnosis of MDD is made by using a set of diagnostic criteria that include having a persistently low mood and 5 of the following symptoms for at least 2 weeks: sleep disturbance; loss of interest or anhedonia (inability to experience pleasure); feelings of hopelessness, helplessness, or guilt; low energy; poor concentration; appetite disturbance; psychomotor retardation/agitation; and suicidal ideation. Because many of these symptoms overlap with cancer and cancer treatments, substitutive criteria have been proposed, such as the Endicott criteria. However, the different sets of criteria may not yield markedly different results and in clinical practice physical symptoms that could be related to cancer or cancer treatment are included in making the diagnosis of MDD (3).

■ DIFFERENTIAL DIAGNOSIS

It is important to evaluate possible medical contributions to low mood and to consider the differential diagnosis. Untreated pain, hypothyroidism, and medications such as glucocorticoids and certain chemotherapies (alpha interferon, pemetrexed, and procarbazine) may contribute to MDD. The differential diagnosis includes:

- Adjustment disorder: Low mood has been present for less than 2 weeks or there are less than 5 of the symptoms needed for the diagnosis of MDD. Adjustment disorders are usually in response to a negative event. Treatment usually focuses on symptoms such as sleep disturbance, and antidepressants are usually not prescribed unless the symptoms persist or there is significant impairment in functioning.

- Delirium: Defined as a transient disturbance consciousness with reduced attention and generalized impairment of cognition, can present with waxing and waning severity of symptoms, and be accompanied by sleep-wake disturbance, language impairment, and psychotic symptoms, especially visual hallucinations and paranoid delusions. Agitation does not need to be present and in fact, one subtype of delirium, hypoactive delirium, presents with social withdrawal and inactivity, which is often mistaken for MDD. Addressing the underlying cause and the use of antipsychotics, not antidepressants, are the treatment for delirium.

- Fatigue: Although difficult to tease apart from MDD, because of overlapping symptoms, attention to clinical symptoms can facilitate its diagnosis. Anhedonia (markedly diminished interest or pleasure in activities) may be the best distinguishing factor for MDD. Depressed patients usually complain of fatigue early in the day, whereas energy levels in cancer-related fatigue are at its best at this time of the day. Severe hopelessness and suicidal ideation are usually less frequent in fatigue.

- Anxiety: Tearfulness and depressed mood can occur in anticipation of negative events, like disease progression or cancer recurrence. In this case the low mood is not persistent and is usually triggered by the anxious thoughts. However, anxiety and MDD often occur together.

- Personality disorders: Can present with depressed mood, but the mood symptoms are not usually constant and persistent. Mood changes are usually triggered by a perceived injury or threat of abandonment. People with personality disorders can have difficulties maintaining stable social support and a history of self-harmful behavior like cutting. Although antidepressants and other psychotropic medications may be useful in managing specific symptoms, the treatment of personality disorders is primarily behavioral.

- Apathy: A neurological symptom that can also look like MDD and it is associated with a lesion in the frontal or temporal lobes. There is little spontaneous action or speech; responses are delayed, short, slowed, or absent; and it is usually associated with cognitive impairment and older age. Stimulants and dopaminergic medications may be helpful.

■ TREATMENT

Treatment for MDD consists of antidepressants and/or psychotherapy. Severe cases of MDD, especially those that endanger a patient's life, may be treated with electroconvulsive therapy. Although complementary treatments such as herbal preparations, acupuncture, and massage are available, there is currently little data on their efficacy for treating MDD in cancer patients. Suicidal ideation should be assessed and, if present, a referral to a mental health professional should be made.

Antidepressants

Antidepressants are commonly used to treat MDD comorbid with cancer (Table 23-1). Overall, limited evidence from three randomized trials and two trials comparing active treatments suggest that cancer patients may benefit from pharmacological treatments of depression (4). Antidepressants should be selected with potential side effects in mind. Side effects can

TABLE 23-1 SELECTED ANTIDEPRESSANTS COMMONLY USED IN CANCER PATIENTS

Medication	Beneficial for These Comorbid Symptoms	Potential for Drug Interactions	Side Effects	Starting Dose	Dose Range
Selective Serotonin Reuptake Inhibitors (SSRIs)					
Escitalopram (Lexapro)	Anxiety, hot flashes	Low	Nausea, anxiety, insomnia, headache, sexual dysfunction	10 mg qd	10–20 mg qd
Citalopram (Celexa)	Same as above, also available as liquids			20 mg qd	20–40 mg qd
Sertraline (Zoloft)			Same as above but more GI side effects	25–50 mg qd	50–200 mg qd
Serotonin-Norepinephrine Reuptake Inhibitors (SNRIs)					
Venlafaxine (Effexor)	Neuropathic pain, hot flashes	Low	Nausea, constipation, sedation, insomnia, increased blood pressure	25 mg bid-tid; 37.5–75 mg qd of extended release capsule (XR)	75–300 mg per day
Duloxetine (Cymbalta)	Neuropathic pain, hot flashes	Moderate: substrate for CYP 1A2 + 2D6; inhibitor of CYP 2D6	Nausea, anorexia, constipation, sedation, insomnia	20 mg bid	20–30 mg bid
Desvenlafaxine (Pristiq)	Neuropathic pain Hot flashes	Low	Nausea, dizziness, dry mouth, diarrhea, sweating	50 mg	No additional benefit is demonstrated with dose >50 mg/d

Tricyclics

Nortriptyline (Pamelor)	Inexpensive, diarrhea, sleep problems; neuropathic pain	Moderate: Substrate for CYP 1A2 + 2D6	Constipation, orthostatic hypotension, sedation, dry mouth, cardiac conduction, confusion	10–25 mg qhs	25–150 mg qhs (dosed by serum level)

Newer Generation Antidepressants

Mirtazapine (Remeron)	Least GI side effects, sleep problems, anorexia, available in dissolving tablet	Low	Sedation, weight gain	15 mg qhs	15–45 mg qhs
Buproprion (Wellbutrin, Zyban)	Fatigue, least sexual side effects	Moderate: Inhibitor of CYP 2D6	Tremor, insomnia, restlessness, lowers seizure threshold	100 mg bid	200–450 mg/d

impact tolerability, but also be helpful with accompanying symptoms such as sleep disturbance and poor appetite. Some of the selective serotonin reuptake inhibitors (SSRIs) (fluoxetine, fluvoxamine, and paroxetine) and buproprion may interfere with the metabolism of commonly used medications in oncology because of their effects on cytochrome p450 2D6 system (5). Additionally, the FDA recently warned of higher doses of citalopram leading to QT prolongation and arrhythmias, especially when used with medications altering its metabolism (6). Antidepressants usually take about 4 weeks to see full benefit, but some patients may show signs of improvement earlier. Antidepressants should be continued for 9–12 months after remission of depressive symptoms if this has been the person's first episode. Patients with recurrent MDD should continue the medication longer in order to lessen the chances of recurrence.

Stimulant medications may be beneficial for MDD in medically ill patients, but the evidence to supporting this practice is derived from case series and no trials have been reported in cancer patients. Stimulants, such as methylphenidate and dextroamphetamine, may lift mood, increase appetite, and improve fatigue. Effects of stimulants are usually seen within 1 week.

Psychotherapy

Psychotherapy often needs to take a flexible approach because of medical morbidity and the demands of cancer treatment. Referrals should be made to trained therapists with experience in working with medically ill patients, if possible. Because issues around coping with cancer are often the focus, certain short-term therapies that target current life stresses and strengthen coping skills, such as cognitive-behavioral therapy, may be beneficial. Similar to antidepressants, these short-term therapies may still take weeks to see improvement.

ANXIETY

Anxiety can also be used to describe an emotional experience, feeling nervous, and also to refer to set of psychiatric disorders. Anxiety becomes a psychiatric disorder when it leads to functional impairment. Several kinds of anxiety disorders are seen in people with cancer, such as phobias, panic disorder, generalized anxiety disorder, and post-traumatic stress disorder (PTSD), as well as some presentations of anxiety that do not fit into the current diagnostic system, like persistent anxiety around cancer recurrence.

■ PREVALENCE

In a large-scale study of adult outpatients at a tertiary cancer center, clinical levels of anxiety were present in 34% of patients (7). A meta-analysis of 70 studies found that actual anxiety disorders were present in 10.3% of patients, whereas 19.4% patients meet criteria for adjustment disorders (2).

■ DIAGNOSIS

- Phobia: extreme anxiety about a specific thing that leads to avoidance. Common phobias in medical settings include needles, blood, and confined spaces. Although the use of anxiolytic medication, like lorazepam, before entering into a phobic situation may be helpful, the primary treatment is behavioral therapy.

- Panic: a constellation of physical symptoms (shortness of breath, palpitations, chest pain, abdominal discomfort, nausea, headache, and numbness/tingling) along with anxious cognitions, such as "I am dying" or "I need to get out of here immediately." Panic attacks are recurrent, unexpected, and usually last less than 30 min. Panic usually first presents in early adulthood and onset late in life is unusual. Pulmonary emboli, which can have similar symptoms, can be misdiagnosed as a panic attack.
- Generalized anxiety disorder: unrealistic and excessive worry for at least 6 months that is accompanied by motor tension, autonomic hyperactivity, or excessive vigilance.
- PTSD: a constellation of symptoms that persist months after a traumatic event. Symptoms include nightmares, flashbacks, avoidance behaviors related to the trauma, and hypervigilance. Although having cancer can be thought of as "traumatic," the specific event is usually a particular point in time, such as waking up intubated and restrained in an intensive care unit.

■ TREATMENT

Similar to MDD, anxiety is treated with medications, psychotherapy, or both.

Medications

Because anxiety symptoms in cancer patients are often time limited or episodic, quick onset of action makes benzodiazepines particularly useful. These agents should be selected on the basis of their half-lives and duration of action. Short- or intermediate-acting lorazepam may be useful for situational anxiety around receiving a MRI, while longer acting clonazepam may be useful for preventing panic attacks throughout the day. In patients with impaired hepatic function, lorazepam, oxazepam, and temazepam are preferred because they undergo glucuronide conjugation. Side effects include sedation, ataxia, disinhibition, and confusion, especially in the elderly. Benzodiazepines can cause dependence and withdrawal, which is more likely with the shorter acting ones, like alprazolam.

Low-dose atypical antipsychotic medications, such as olanzapine and quetiapine, can also be useful for the immediate treatment of anxiety. They may be used for anxiety resistant to benzodiazepines or in people in whom benzodiazepines should be avoided, such as someone who developed confusion from a benzodiazepine or someone with serious substance abuse.

Antidepressants are effective for the treatment of anxiety disorders, but do not provide immediate relief. Higher doses and longer duration of treatment may be required compared to the treatment of MDD. Additional medications, like benzodiazepines, may be needed for more immediate relief while waiting at least 4 weeks for effects. Other agents such as buspirone, anticonvulsants (gabapentin and pregabalin), hydroxyzine, propanolol, and clonidine are sometimes used in the clinical practice of managing anxiety;

these agents do not have US Food and Drug Administration indications for anxiety treatment and have not been systematically studied in anxiety treatment trials in cancer.

Psychotherapy

Short-term targeted therapies that include increasing distress tolerance and strengthening coping skills; identifying cognitive distortions and catastrophizing; and systematic desensitization may be particularly beneficial. Other techniques such as distraction, relaxation exercises, and visualization are also helpful.

FATIGUE

Cancer-related fatigue (CRF) is the most commonly reported symptom in people with cancer and it is the symptom that causes the most functional impairment (8). CRF may be the presenting symptom at the time of cancer diagnosis, occur during treatment, and persist into survivorship in some people. Often CRF will have identifiable causes that can be treated. Although psychiatric disorders, especially MDD and anxiety, can contribute to CFR, they are often not present.

■ REVALENCE

Reports on the rate of CFR in people affected by cancer vary widely because of differing measures of fatigue and heterogeneous populations. It is estimated that 60%–90% of patients have fatigue (9, 10).

■ DIAGNOSIS

CFR is characterized by a pervasive and persistent sense of tiredness not relieved by sleep or rest. Its diagnosis is largely clinical. The National Comprehensive Cancer Network (NCCN) recommends screening for fatigue at visits with a one-item, 0–10 scale, similar to screening for pain, with "0" being "no fatigue," and "10" being "the most severe fatigue." Scores of 4 or greater are recommended to have further evaluation.

Evaluation should consist of identifying any possibly modifiable causes of fatigue such as anemia, pain, sleep disturbance (insomnia, difficulty staying asleep, and sleep apnea), emotional distress (major depressive disorder and anxiety), poor nutrition, inactivity/deconditioning, medications and chemotherapies that cause fatigue (e.g., gemcitabine, glucocorticoids, narcotics, antiemetics, and beta-blockers), and other medical conditions such as hypothyroidism, hypogonadism, adrenal insufficiency, hypercalcemia, hepatic failure, and cardiovascular or pulmonary compromise. Fatigue can also be a side effect of radiation therapy. The time course of the onset of fatigue is important in trying to identify possible causes as well as detecting preexisting fatigue in people with fibromyalgia and chronic fatigue syndrome.

■ TREATMENT

NCCN guidelines suggest initially treating any underlying reversible cause of fatigue as described above. Persistent fatigue may be treated with stimulants, exercise, and behavioral interventions.

Medications

A recent Cochrane Review of drug treatment of CFR (11), after combining five randomized controlled studies, concluded that current evidence supports the use of psychostimulants for this condition. NCCN guidelines recommend the use of methylphenidate after other non-pharmacological approaches have failed. Other agents, such as dextroamphetamine and modafinil, have also been commonly used in the clinical treatment of CRF. Stimulants may raise blood pressure and heart rate and should be used with caution in patients with cardiac disease. Multiple studies have found a recognizable reduction in fatigue with erythropoietin; however, new safety concerns suggest that any seen benefit is outweighed by the increase risk of harm from these drugs in patients with mild anemia (12). Additional studies with selective serotonin reuptake inhibitors and glucocorticoids have failed to demonstrate any superiority over placebo for these classes of drugs.

Exercise

Several studies have demonstrated the benefit of exercise for fatigue in people with cancer (12). A physical therapist can design an exercise program, containing both strength training and cardiovascular, that is appropriate for a person with physical limitations from cancer or cancer treatments. For medically complicated patients, exercise might best be done in a cardiovascular or pulmonary rehabilitation center.

Behavioral Interventions

Behavioral interventions have focused on energy conservation; prioritizing activities and delegating if possible; problem solving around difficulties caused by the fatigue; improving organizational skills; and trying to maximize functioning through careful observation of symptoms and planning activities around them.

REFERENCES

1. Richardson J, Sheldon D, Krailo M, et al. The effect of compliance with treatment on survival among patients with hematologic malignancies. *J Clin Oncol.* 1990; 8: 356–364.

2. Mitchell AJ, Chan M, Bhatti H, et al. Prevalence of depression, anxiety, and adjustment disorder in oncological, haematological, and palliative-care settings: a meta-analysis of 94 interview-based studies. *Lancet Oncol.* 2011; 12: 160–174.

3. Kathol RG, Mutgi A, Williams J, et al. Diagnosis of major depression in cancer patients according to four sets of criteria. *Am J Psychiatry.* 1990; 147: 1021–1024.

4. Williams S, Dale J. The effectiveness of treatment for depression/depressive symptoms in adults with cancer: a systematic review. *Br J Cancer.* 2006; 94: 372–390.

5. Kalash GR. Psychotropic drug metabolism in the cancer patient: clinical aspects of management of potential drug interactions. *Psycho-oncology.* 1998; 7: 307–320.

6. US Food and Drug Administration. FDA drug safety communication: abnormal heart rhythms associated with high doses of Celexa (citalopram hydrobromide). http://www.fda.gov/Drugs/DrugSafety/ucm269086.htm

7. Brintzenhofe-Szoc KM, Levin TT, Li Y, et al. Mixed anxiety/depression symptoms in a large cancer cohort: Prevalence by cancer type. *Psychosomatics.* 2009; 50: 383–391.

8. Curt CA, Breitbart W, Cella D, et al. Impact of cancer-related fatigue on the lives of patients: new findings from the fatigue coalition. *The Oncologist.* 2000; 5: 353–360.

9. Vainio A. Prevalence of symptoms among patients with advanced cancer: an international collaborative study. Symptom Prevalence Group. *J Pain Symptom Manage.* 1996; 12: 3–10.

10. Lawrence DP, Kupelmick B, Miller K, et al. Evidence report on the occurrence, assessment, and treatment of fatigue in cancer patients. *JNCI Monograph.* 2004; 32: 40–50.

11. Minton O, Richardson A, Sharpe M, et al. Drug therapy for the management of cancer-related fatigue. *Cochrane Database Syst Rev.* 2010; (7): CD006704.

12. Ahlberg K, Ekman T, Gaston-Johansson F, et al. Assessment and management of cancer-related fatigue in adults. *Lancet.* 2003; 362: 640–650.

CHAPTER **24**
Acute Myeloid Leukemia

Amir T. Fathi

ETIOLOGY AND EPIDEMIOLOGY

Acute myeloid leukemia (AML) is an aggressive and frequently lethal hematologic malignancy, with a median age of presentation beyond the sixth decade. Approximately 12,000 new cases of AML are diagnosed in the United States each year, and most cases are idiopathic. However, AML is increasingly seen in survivors of other cancers who were previously exposed to chemotherapy and radiotherapy. Alkylating agents, such as melphalan and chlorambucil, can give rise to therapy-related AML, with a median time of onset of 5–10 years, and associated abnormalities in chromosomes 5 and 7. Inhibitors of topoisomerase, such as etoposide and anthracyclines, can also cause a therapy-related AML, with a median time of onset of 2–3 years. These cases of AML are often associated with balanced chromosomal translocations at 11q23 and involve alterations of the mixed lineage leukemia (MLL) protein. Myelodysplastic syndrome and myeloproliferative disorders, such as polycythemia vera and myelofibrosis, can also progress to AML. The "secondary" leukemias that derive from previous therapy or other myeloid diseases have significantly worse outcomes than the "de novo" cases of AML. Of note, the risk of leukemia is 20-fold higher in patients with Down's syndrome (1). Common mutations with prognostic value in AML include the *FLT3*-internal tandem duplication (ITD) mutation and the *NPM1* (nucleophosmin) mutation. The *FLT3-ITD* mutation, identified in approximately a quarter of patients, leads to the production of an abnormal, constitutively active FLT3 receptor tyrosine kinase on the surface of leukemic cells. This in turn leads to uncontrolled proliferation of undifferentiated blasts and a higher propensity for relapse and poor outcomes (2, 3). The *NPM1* mutation, on the other hand, is associated with a better prognosis if present as an isolated lesion, and affects a larger proportion of patients with AML. This mutation leads to the aberrant sequestration of altered nucleophosmin proteins in the cytoplasm, and disruption of regulated cell cycling in malignant cells (4, 5).

- Most cases of AML are idiopathic.
- AML may arise secondary to prior chemotherapy or radiotherapy, or from underlying myelodysplastic/myeloproliferative processes.

◼ PATHOPHYSIOLOGY

Acute leukemia is a clonal disease derived from leukemic stem cells. DNA mutations render myeloid precursor cells incapable of normal differentiation and maturation and promote unchecked proliferation, leading to the acute leukemic phenotype. The myeloblasts proliferate in the bone marrow compartments, resulting in hematopoietic insufficiency and progressive cytopenias. When myeloblasts expand outside of the bone marrow, severe peripheral leukocytosis may result, leading to additional sequelae, such as leukostasis and significant tumor lysis. Rarely extravascular solid tumors, known as chloromas or granulocytic sarcomas, may arise in tissue.

■ DIAGNOSIS

AML can be subtle in its presentation with some patients presenting with days to weeks of nonspecific symptoms, such as fatigue, shortness of breath, and bleeding. A complete blood count, examination of the peripheral blood smear, and bone marrow aspirate and biopsy are essential in establishing the diagnosis of acute leukemia. The myeloblasts classically have distinct nucleoli, fine chromatin, scant cytoplasm, and azurophilic granules. The characteristic Auer rods are formed by azurophilic granules within lysosomes, although they are not essential for diagnosis. Histochemical stains can be helpful; for example, acute monocytic leukemia can be differentiated using a nonspecific esterase stain. Immunophenotyping by flow cytometry helps to establish a definitive diagnosis and distinguish AML from acute lymphoblastic leukemia (ALL). As examples, CD33 is positive in approximately 75% of patients with AML, CD13 is positive in approximately 70% of patients with AML, and CD14 is positive in more than 50% of the monocytic and myelomonocytic subtypes. The most widely used classification system for AML is that developed by the World Health Organization (WHO), and organizes this malignancy according to morphologic, karyotypic, and molecular features (6) (Table 24-1).

- History and exam may reveal fatigue, shortness of breath, pallor, petechiae, fever, night sweats, and occasionally splenomegaly. Skin, gum, and CNS lesions can be seen, but are more frequent in monocytic variants.
- On laboratory examination, the white blood cell count may be normal, high, or low. Anemia and thrombocytopenia are frequent. Examination of the peripheral blood smear is essential and often reveals myeloblasts and other early progenitor cells, and occasionally a myelophthisic picture.
- Diagnostic evaluation includes a bone marrow aspirate and biopsy with flow cytometry, histochemical stains, cytogenetics, and molecular evaluation (e.g., fms-like tyrosine kinase [*FLT3*] and nucleophosmin [*NPM1*]). Definition of AML: >20% myeloblasts in peripheral blood or bone marrow.

■ TREATMENT

Treatment of AML traditionally involves remission induction chemotherapy, followed by post-remission therapy (consolidation). The most commonly used form of induction chemotherapy is the so-called "7+3" regimen, consisting of 3 days of an anthracycline, such as idarubicin 12 mg/m^2/day, and 7 days of infusional cytarabine at a dose ranging from 100 to 200 mg/m^2 (7). Experimental trials are underway to assess the addition of novel agents such as the proteosome inhibitor bortezomib or

TABLE 24-1 2008 WHO CLASSIFICATION OF ACUTE MYELOID LEUKEMIA (AML) AND RELATED NEOPLASMS

Acute myeloid leukemia with recurrent genetic abnormalities

-AML with t(8;21)(q22;q22); *RUNX1-RUNX1T1*

-AML with inv(16)(p13.1;q22) or t(16;16)(p13.1;q22); *CBFB-MYH11*

-APL with t(15;17)(q22;q12); *PML-RARA*

-AML with t(9;11)(p22;q23); *MLLT3-MLL*

-AML with t(6;9)(p23;q34); *DEK-NUP214*

-AML with inv(3)(q21;q26.2) or t(3;3)(q21;q26.2); *RPN1-EVI1*

-AML (megakaryoblastic) with t(1;22)(p13;q13); *RBM15-MKL1*

-AML with mutated NPM1

-AML with mutated CEBPA

Acute myeloid leukemia with myelodysplasia-related changes

Therapy-related myeloid neoplasms

Acute myeloid leukemia, not otherwise specified

-AML with minimal differentiation

-AML without maturation

-AML with maturation

-Acute myelomonocytic leukemia

-Acute monoblastic/monocytic leukemia

-Acute erythroid leukemia: pure erythroid leukemia or erythroleukemia, erythroid/myeloid

-Acute megakaryoblastic leukemia

-Acute basophilic leukemia

-Acute panmyelosis with myelofibrosis

Myeloid sarcoma

Myeloid proliferations related to Down syndrome

-Transient abnormal myelopoiesis

-Myeloid leukemia associated with Down syndrome

Blastic plasmacytoid dendritic cell neoplasm

(Adapted from Reference 6.)

oral antagonists to the FLT3 tyrosine kinase, which is altered in a sizeable percentage of patients (8). The addition of the anti-CD33 humanized antibody-drug conjugate gemtuzumab ozogamicin to induction chemotherapy led to an improvement in overall survival in AML patients aged 50–70 years old in one study (9). This agent is not available for use in the United States, but may become an important adjunct to therapy in the future, based on these results.

For patients with so-called "favorable-risk" disease, such as those with the karyotypic abnormalities inversion 16 or translocation 8;21 or those harboring isolated NPM1 alterations, consolidation chemotherapy is given for 2–4 months following achievement of remission, usually with high doses of cytarabine, in doses of 3 g/m^2/bid on days 1, 3, and 5 of therapy for 3–4 cycles. Consolidation chemotherapy with high-dose cytarabine can also be considered for those patients without favorable- or poor-risk features, who thus fall into an "intermediate-risk" category. The landmark study performed by the Cancer and Leukemia Group B (CALGB) showed superior survival to the high dose ara-c regimen compared to lower doses (7, 10). As yet, there is no established role for maintenance therapy for patients with AML (11).

Patients with a high risk of relapse, considered "high-risk," including those with complex cytogenetic abnormalities or secondary AML, should be considered for allogeneic stem cell transplantation in first remission. Long-term disease-free survival rates for patients with AML in first remission receiving an allogeneic transplant from a fully matched sibling donor are 60%–70% with a transplant-related mortality of 10%–15%. Results are significantly worse for patients in second or subsequent remission.

Elderly patients or patients with significant comorbidity may not tolerate induction chemotherapy well. Elderly patients are more likely to have poor risk cytogenetics and a history of myelodysplasia. Patients under the age of 70 years with a good performance status should be considered for induction chemotherapy (12, 13). Some older and frailer patients may be considered for treatment with DNA methyltransferase inhibitors (DMNTIs) such as 5-azacitidine or decitabine. A phase III randomized study of 5-azacitidine in myeloid malignancies included a large number of AML patients and demonstrated a survival benefit for this agent (14). Because DNMTI therapy can be given on an outpatient basis and is not as intensive and morbid as induction chemotherapy, it is now increasingly used in older patients with advanced myelodysplastic syndromes and AML. Older patients may also be treated with supportive or palliative approaches including the use of the cytoreductive agent hydroxyurea (13) or lower doses of cytarabine (13, 15). The palliative benefit of such therapy is undefined.

The majority of patients with AML relapse, but the optimal treatment of relapsed disease has not been defined. Relapsed AML is not curable with standard chemotherapy alone. Patients who relapse more than 1 year after their initial therapy can be treated with idarubicin and cytosine arabinoside again. Patients who relapse within 1 year after their first induction are treated with combinations that include other agents such as mitoxantrone and etoposide. If a second remission is achieved, these patients should be considered for allogeneic stem cell transplantation as a curative attempt.

- Induction chemotherapy with an anthracycline and infusional cytarabine is the traditional approach to initial management of AML.
- Consolidation chemotherapy with high-dose cytarabine following achievement of first remission can lead to cure in a subset of patients with favorable- or intermediate-risk AML.
- Allogeneic stem cell transplantation is advised for patients at high risk of relapse or for patients in second complete remission.

■ COMPLICATIONS

Both AML and its treatment can pose several life-threatening complications. The death rate from complications of induction therapy is approximately 5%–10%. Leukostasis is more common with a blast count >100,000 and can be characterized by pulmonary infiltrates, visual changes, and CNS bleeding. The treatment consists of intravenous fluids, hydroxyurea to lower the white blood count, or leukapheresis.

Infection is the most common cause of death in patients with AML. Patients are functionally neutropenic even if their neutrophil count is not suppressed. Gram-positive infections, such as those caused by *Staphylococcus* and *Streptococcus*, have become the most common bacterial infections; gram-negative infections, however, may be more immediately life threatening. The use of quinolones for prophylaxis has created the emergence of resistant gram-negative organisms. *Candida* and *Aspergillus* are the most common fungal infections. *Aspergillus* should be considered in patients with nodular or cavitary pneumonias. All febrile patients with AML should be presumed to have an infection and treated with broad spectrum gram-negative antibiotics, such as cefepime or cefotaxime. Broad gram-positive coverage with vancomycin should be initiated if there is suspicion of skin infection, intravenous line involvement, or documented gram-positive infection.

Tumor lysis syndrome occurs because of the rapid destruction of tumor cells with release of intracellular electrolytes and uric acid (see Chapter 20). The syndrome can progress to severe electrolyte imbalance, acute renal failure, and life-threatening cardiac arrhythmias. Intravenous fluids and allopurinol should be started before the start of chemotherapy. The recombinant urate oxidase rasburicase abruptly lowers the uric acid level and should be employed in patients at high risk of or experiencing tumor lysis (16). Laboratory parameters for electrolytes, uric acid, and LDH should be followed closely, every few hours, in newly diagnosed patients and those recently started on therapy.

Bleeding is usually related to thrombocytopenia, and patients should receive prophylactic platelet transfusions for platelet counts below 10×10^9/l. Disseminated intravascular coagulation (DIC) is most commonly seen with acute promyelocytic leukemia (APL, see below) but can also be seen with other variants of AML, particularly the monocytic variants. Treatment involves replacement of clotting factors with fresh frozen plasma and repletion of fibrinogen with cryoprecipitate.

Leukemic meningitis occurs in less than 10% of adult AML patients at the time of diagnosis, more frequently in patients with the monocytic variants of AML. Leukemic meningitis is treated with intrathecal therapy with methotrexate or cytarabine given via lumbar puncture twice weekly until the CNS is cleared of involvement.

- Management of leukostasis includes aggressive cytoreduction with an agent such as hydroxyurea, prompt start of induction therapy, and leukapheresis. Red blood cell transfusions can increase leukostasis acutely and should be avoided unless absolutely necessary.
- Platelet, fresh frozen plasma, and cryoprecipitate transfusions can be employed to decrease risk of bleeding or complications from DIC.

- Fevers on presentation are broadly covered with antibiotics.
- For suspicion of tumor lysis syndrome, preventive measures with allopurinol and IV hydration are employed. Rasburicase can be used to effectively decrease uric acid in patients at risk for or experiencing severe tumor lysis.

■ **PROGNOSIS**

The overall 5-year survival for patients with AML is 25%, 40% for patients under age 60 years, and 10% for patients over age 60 years. Remission is achieved in the majority of patients, but relapse is common, particularly in older patients. Older age, complex cytogenetic abnormalities, and secondary AML are poor prognostic factors (Table 24-2). Cytogenetics can help define prognostic categories and determine who should receive more aggressive post-remission therapy, such as bone marrow transplantation (Table 24-3). Patients with the karyotypic abnormalities, translocation (8;21) or inversion 16, have a more favorable prognosis. Patients with abnormalities of chromosomes 5 or 7 or complex (>3) cytogenetic abnormalities have a worse prognosis. Approximately 40% of adult AML patients have normal cytogenetics at diagnosis and, thus, have an "intermediate-risk" prognosis. Molecular markers are also important in delineating prognosis in this group of patients. *FLT3-ITD* (internal tandem mutation) alterations connote a poor prognosis, and isolated *NPM1* (nucleophosmin) gene mutations carry a more favorable prognosis, with the recommended approach being stem cell transplantation after obtaining remission for the population of patients carrying isolated *FLT3-ITD* mutations and chemotherapy-based consolidation for those carrying isolated *NPM1* mutations (5, 17).

TABLE 24-2 ACUTE MYELOID LEUKEMIA (AML)—PROGNOSTIC FEATURES

Poor-Risk Prognostic Features

-Age over 65 y

-Presence of a FLT3-ITD mutation

-Poor-risk cytogenetics (e.g., -7, -7q, -5, or complex [> 3 chromosomal abnormalities])

-AML arising from preceding myelodysplasia or chronic myeloproliferative states

-Therapy-related disease (AML secondary to prior chemotherapy or radiation exposure)

-Presence of granulocytic sarcoma (extramedullary disease)

-Acute bilineal or biphenotypic leukemia

Better-Risk Prognostic Features

-Presence of an NPM1 mutation (without concurrent FLT3-ITD mutation)

-Presence of a CEBPα mutation

-"Good" risk cytogenetics (e.g., t(15;17), inv(16), t(16;16), t(8;21))

TABLE 24-3 CYTOGENETIC ABNORMALITIES IN THE ACUTE MYELOID LEUKEMIAS

Cytogenetics	Disease	Molecular Marker	Prognosis
T(8;21)	AML		Good
T(15;17)	APML	PML-RAR-alpha	Good
Inversion 16	AML		Good
Normal	AML		Intermediate
-5	AML		Poor
-7	AML		Poor
11q23	AML	MLL	Poor

ACUTE PROMYELOCYTIC LEUKEMIA

ETIOLOGY AND EPIDEMIOLOGY

Acute promyelocytic leukemia (APL) is a rare form of acute myeloid leukemia, accounting for only 10%–15% of all AMLs diagnosed in the United States.

PATHOPHYSIOLOGY

The breakpoint on chromosome 15 in APL occurs at the PML transcription unit and on chromosome 17, at the retinoic acid receptor alpha gene. A chimeric PML-RAR-alpha gene product is created. This PML-RAR-alpha transcript renders the aberrant promyelocytes sensitive to the differentiating effects of therapy with all trans-retinoic acid (ATRA) and arsenic trioxide.

DIAGNOSIS

It is critical to make the diagnosis of APL quickly since treatment is different than for other subtypes of AML and since patients are at acute risk of mortality due to complications related to DIC. Characteristic morphology (Figure 24-1) is the presence of promyelocytes with intense azurophilic (red) granules. However, in the microgranular variant of APL, the granules can be very small and difficult to visualize on Wright stain. The diagnosis of APL can be made by cytogenetics revealing the classic t(15;17) translocation. Molecular diagnostics by PCR analysis can confirm the presence of PML-RAR-alpha. The white blood cell count is frequently lower in patients with APL than in the other subtypes of AML, and a higher white blood cell count at presentation portends a worse prognosis.

- Initial assessment of APL involves a detailed history and physical exam, with careful attention to bleeding and thrombosis, possible signs of ongoing DIC.
- Laboratory evaluation should include CBC, chemistry panel, uric acid, LDH, PT, PTT, and a full DIC screen. Bone marrow biopsy with collection of specimens for cytogenetics and molecular diagnostic studies for PML-RAR-alpha are essential diagnostic steps.

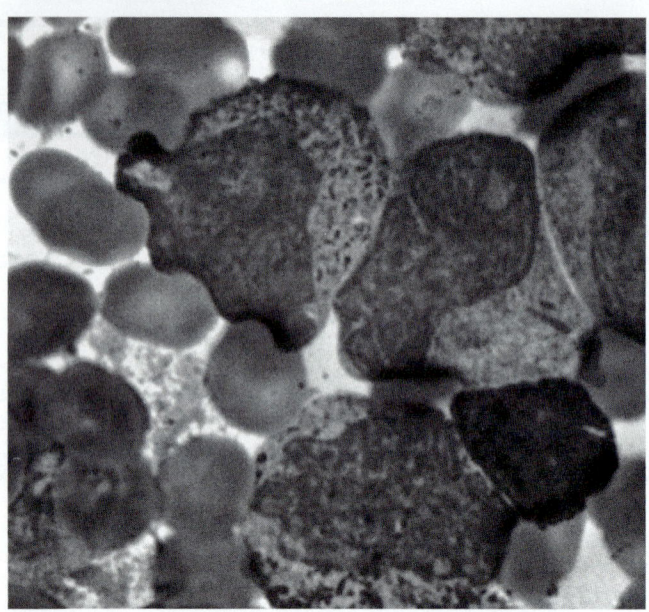

FIGURE 24-1 Aberrant promyelocytes of acute promyelocytic leukemia (APL), with prominent azurophilic granules seen within the cytoplasm. Also seen are Auer rods, needle-shaped inclusion bodies containing clumps of azurophilic granules, which are found in the cytoplasm of malignant cells in various forms of AML, including APL.

■ TREATMENT

It is important to start therapy for APL promptly; up to 17% of patients with APL die before or at the time of diagnosis (18). If the diagnosis of APL is suspected, treatment should be started with all-trans retinoic acid (ATRA) (19). Initial induction therapy for APL begins with ATRA given orally; cytotoxic chemotherapy, such as daunorubicin 50 mg/m²/day for 4 days and cytarabine 100 mg/m²/day for 7 days, begins 3–4 days after ATRA. The French APL trial reported a complete remission rate of 92% and a relapse rate of 6% with the ATRA plus chemotherapy approach. ATRA rapidly corrects the coagulation defects in APL-associated DIC. Consolidation following induction chemotherapy consists of a combination of ATRA with anthracyclines and arsenic trioxide, although consolidation approaches can vary. The role of maintenance therapy is controversial (20). The incorporation of arsenic trioxide into therapy for APL has led to recent improvements in outcomes. Arsenic trioxide is the most active agent in APL and is thought to act by direct degradation of the PML-RAR-alpha transcript, allowing transcription of target genes and normal differentiation (21). The combination of ATRA and arsenic trioxide is highly active and becoming the initial treatment of choice.

Elderly patients can be treated with ATRA alone or ATRA in combination with arsenic. Arsenic trioxide is often included in the treatment of relapsed APML. Electrolyte replacement and frequent EKG monitoring for prolonged QTc are part of routine monitoring during arsenic therapy. For relapsed patients, a regimen of arsenic trioxide to achieve a second remission followed by autologous stem cell transplant for PCR-negative patients will cure an additional 60% of relapsed patients (21–24).

- With suspicion for APL, start ATRA promptly
- Upon confirmation of the diagnosis, continue ATRA followed by anthracycline-based chemotherapy.
- Consolidation chemotherapy for APL includes cycles of ATRA plus an anthracycline, and of arsenic trioxide.
- Maintenance therapy with ATRA can be considered for some patients.
- For relapsed patients, arsenic trioxide followed by autologous SCT is an effective approach for long-term disease-free survival.

■ COMPLICATIONS

Tumor lysis, infection, bleeding, and leukostasis can occur with APL, as with the other AML variants. DIC and bleeding are often more prominent and lethal features of APL, and although the process of DIC in APL is complex, release of tissue factor and increased production of prothrombin complexes have been demonstrated in the malignant cells of patients (25–27). DIC can present with acute intravascular sequelae such as thrombosis or bleeding, including those involving the central nervous system. Prompt treatment for DIC can include reversal of coagulopathy with infusion of cryoprecipitate, fresh frozen plasma, and platelets as necessary.

APL also has the unique potential complication of ATRA syndrome. This syndrome is related to the infiltration of the lung and other organs with tumor cells that have differentiated into granulocytes under the influence of ATRA, and can occur within the first few days of ATRA administration. It can be associated with a rapid rise in the white blood cell count, and onset of fever, weight gain, and shortness of breath with pulmonary infiltrates. ATRA syndrome can be treated by promptly starting dexamethasone 10 mg twice daily. Severe cases may require temporary discontinuation of ATRA or initiation of cytoreduction with hydroxyurea.

A rare complication of ATRA therapy is pseudotumor cerebri, characterized by increased intracranial pressure, headaches, nausea, and visual changes. This complication is more common in children, and is treated by discontinuation of ATRA and diuretics such as mannitol. It can at times be difficult to distinguish this significant syndrome from severe headaches, which are a common toxicity associated with ATRA (21, 22).

- ATRA syndrome can manifest as weight gain, leukocytosis, and pulmonary infiltrates, and can be initially managed with IV dexamethasone.
- To prevent bleeding due to DIC, transfuse cryoprecipitate to fibrinogen >150, fresh frozen plasma to normalize PT, and platelets to platelet count >50,000 or higher depending on clinical presentation and risks.
- Prompt (<24 h) initiation of ATRA therapy is necessary to avoid potentially fatal complications of DIC and bleeding.

■ PROGNOSIS

APL has the most favorable prognosis of all the acute leukemias in adults. More than 90% of patients will achieve complete molecular remission after induction and consolidation therapy. Marrows performed at 10–14 days after chemotherapy will often be cellular and hard to interpret; therefore, unlike other AML subtypes, the bone marrow should be assessed 4–5 weeks post-chemotherapy, at the time of count recovery. The majority of patients will have molecular evidence of disease after induction therapy, but after consolidation therapy, molecular testing for PML-RAR-alpha by PCR should be negative. Conversion from negative to positive PML-RAR-alpha is a harbinger of hematologic relapse. Over 80% of patients will be long-term survivors (18, 19).

REFERENCES

1. Lowenberg B, Downing JR, Burnett A. Acute myeloid leukemia. *N Engl J Med.* 1999; 341: 1051–1062.

2. Fathi AT, Chabner BA. FLT3 inhibition as therapy in acute myeloid leukemia: a record of trials and tribulations. *The Oncologist.* 2011; 16: 1162–1174.

3. Fathi A, Levis M. FLT3 inhibitors: a story of the old and the new. *Curr Opin Hematol.* 2011; 18: 71–76.

4. Fallini B, Mecucci C, Tiacci E, et al. Cytoplasmic nucelophosmin in acute myelogenous leukemia with a normal karyotype. *N Engl J Med.* 2005; 352: 254–266.

5. Schnittger S, Schoch C, Kern W, et al. Nucleophosmin gene mutations are predictors of favorable prognosis in acute myelogenous leukemia with a normal karyotype. *Blood.* 2005; 106: 3733–3739.

6. Vardiman JW, Thiele J, Arber DA, et al. The 2008 revision of the World Health Organization (WHO) classification of myeloid neoplasms and acute leukemia: rationale and important changes. *Blood.* 2009; 114: 937–951.

7. Farag S, Ruppert AS, Mrozek K, et al. Outcome of induction and postremission therapy in younger adults with acute myeloid leukemia with normal karyotype: a Cancer and Leukemia Group B study. *J Clin Oncol.* 2005; 23: 482–493.

8. Attar E, DeAngelo D, Supko J, et al. Phase I and pharmacokinetic study of bortezomib in combination with idarubicin and cytarabine in patients with AML. *Clinical Cancer Research.* 2008; 14: 1446–1450.

9. Castaigne, S, Pautas C, Terre C, et al. Fractionated doses of gemtuzumab ozogamicin (GO) combined to standard chemotherapy (CT) improve event-free and overall survival in newly-diagnosed *de novo* AML patients aged 50–70 years old: a prospective randomized phase 3 trial from the Acute Leukemia French Association (ALFA). *Blood* (ASH Annual Meeting Abstracts). 2011; 118: 6.

10. National Comprehensive Cancer Network. Acute myeloid leukemia: clinical practice guidelines in oncology. *J Compr Cancer Netw.* 2003; 4: 520–539.

11. Anderson JE, Kopecky KJ, Willman CL, et al. Outcomes after induction chemotherapy for older patients with acute myeloid leukemia is not improved with mitoxantrone and etoposide compared to cytarabine and daunorubicin: a Southwest Oncology Group study. *Blood.* 2002; 100: 3869–3872.

12. Rowe JM, Neuberg D, Friedenberg W, et al. A phase 3 study of three induction regimens and of priming with GM-CSF in older adults with acute myeloid leukemia: a trial by the Eastern Cooperative Oncology Group. *Blood.* 2004; 103: 479–485.

13. Estey EH. How I treat older patients with AML. *Blood*. 2000; 96: 1670–1673.

14. Fenaux P, Mufti G, Hellstrom-Lindberg E, et al. Efficacy of azacitidine compared with that of conventional care regimens in the treatment of higher-risk myelodysplastic syndromes: a randomised, open-label, phase III study. *Lancet Oncology*. 2009; 10: 223–232.

15. Löwenberg B, Suciu S, Archimbaud E, et al. Mitoxantrone versus daunorubicin in induction-consolidation chemotherapy—the value of low-dose cytarabine for maintenance of remission, and an assessment of prognostic factors in acute myeloid leukemia in the elderly: final report. *J Clin Oncol*. 1998; 16: 872–881.

16. Jeha S, Kantarjian H, Irwin D, et al. Efficacy and safety of rasburicase, a recombinant urate oxidase in the management of malignancy-associated hyperuricemia in pediatric and adult patients: final results of multicenter compassionate use trial. *Leukemia*. 2005; 19: 34–38.

17. Schlenk RF, Döhner K, Krauter J, et al. Mutations and treatment outcome in cytogenetically normal acute myeloid leukemia. *N Engl J Med*. 2008; 358: 1909–1918.

18. Park JH, Qiao B, Panageas KS, et al. Early death rate in acute promyelocytic leukemia remains high despite all-trans retinoic acid. *Blood*. 2011; 118; 1248–1254.

19. Sanz MA, Tallman MS, Lo-Coco F. Tricks of the trade for the appropriate management of newly diagnosed acute promyelocytic leukemia. *Blood*. 2005; 105: 3019–3025.

20. Powell BL, Moser BK, Stock W, et al. Adding mercaptopurine and methotrexate to alternate week ATRA maintenance therapy does not improve the outcome for adults with acute promyelocytic leukemia (APL) in first remission: results from North American leukemia intergroup trial C9710. *Blood* (ASH Annual Meeting Abstracts). 2011; 118: 258.

21. Tallman MS and Altman JK. How I treat acute promyelocytic leukemia. *Blood*. 2009; 114: 5126–5135.

22. Lo Coco F, Avvisati G, Vignetti M, et al. Retinoic acid and arsenic trioxide for acute promyelocytic leukemia. *N Engl J Med*. 2013; 369: 111–121.

23. Sanz MA, Martin G, Gonzalez M, et al. Risk-adapted treatment of acute promyelocytic leukemia with all-trans-retinoic acid and anthracycline monotherapy: a multicenter study by the PETHEMA group. *Blood*. 2004; 103: 1237–1243.

24. Tallman MS, Nabhan C, Feusner JH, et al. Acute promyelocytic leukemia: evolving therapeutic strategies. *Blood*. 2001; 99: 3554–3558.

25. Gralnick HR, Abrell E. Studies of the procoagulant and fibrinolytic activity of promyelocytes in acute promyelocytic leukaemia. *Br J Haematol*. 1973; 24: 89–99.

26. Andoh K, Kubota T, Takada M, et al. Tissue factor activity in leukemia cells. Special reference to disseminated intravascular coagulation. *Cancer*. 1987; 59: 748–754.

27. Bauer KA, Rosenberg RD. Thrombin generation in acute promyelocytic leukemia. *Blood*. 1984; 64: 791–796.

CHAPTER **25**
Myelodysplastic Syndromes
Eyal C. Attar

INTRODUCTION

Myelodysplastic syndromes (MDS) represent premalignant entities that share many characteristics with acute myeloid leukemia (AML). These clonal hematopoietic stem cell (HSC) disorders are characterized by pancytopenia resulting from failure of normal hematopoiesis. The bone marrow shows hypercellularity, arrested maturation in one or more cellular lineages, and an increase in bone marrow myeloid precursors. Clinical symptoms result from cytopenias. Approximately one-third of patients ultimately progress to AML. Treatment involves supportive care and the use of agents capable of ameliorating cytopenias and delaying development of AML. However, hematopoietic stem cell transplantation (HCT) represents the only potentially curative treatment for MDS.

KEY FEATURES

- One or more peripheral blood cytopenias.
- Hematopoietic cell dysplasia.
- Bone marrow hypercellularity.
- Ringed sideroblasts in a subset of patients.
- Less than 20% bone marrow and peripheral blood myeloblasts.
- Abnormal cytogenetics are observed in approximately 50% of patients. Approximately 20% of patients have characteristic, interstitial deletions within the long arm of chromosome 5, which are associated with clinical response to immunomodulatory drugs (IMIDs).
- MDS may be related to prior chemotherapy and/or radiation for another medical condition (therapy-related MDS or T-MDS).
- Approximately 30% of patients with MDS develop AML.

EPIDEMIOLOGY

Approximately 15,000–30,000 new cases of MDS are diagnosed in the United States each year. MDS is three to four times more prevalent than AML and follows a more indolent course. MDS is likely underdiagnosed. MDS is one cause of anemia in the elderly.

ETIOLOGY

The exact cause of MDS is unknown in most patients. However, intrinsic defects in hematopoietic cells and extrinsic defects associated with the bone marrow microenvironment are involved in the pathogenesis of this disorder.

While most patients with MDS have spontaneously arising, de novo, disease, a portion of patients has therapy-related MDS (T-MDS). Such patients have received chemotherapy and/or radiation in the past, possibly for another malignancy or autoimmune disorder. T-MDS develops within a period of 3–10 years following chemotherapy and is associated with complex chromosomal abnormalities, often involving alterations of chromosomes 5 and/or 7. In addition, T-MDS is associated with a more aggressive clinical course and poorer prognosis in comparison to de novo MDS.

CLINICAL CHARACTERISTICS

- Median age is approximately 70 years.
- Slightly more common in males than in females.
- Prevalence is 50,000–100,000 cases in the United States.
- May be associated with prior chemotherapy, radiation, or environmental exposures to genotoxic agents.

CLASSIFICATION OF MDS

The World Health Organization (WHO) classification system includes refractory anemia (RA), RA with ringed sideroblasts (RARS), refractory cytopenia with multilineage dysplasia (RCMD), and MDS with isolated deletion of 5q for patients harboring a distinct interstitial deletion within the long arm of chromosome 5 (1). Patients with elevated bone marrow blasts of 5%–9% have RA with excess blasts I (RAEB-I) and patients with 10%–19% blasts have RAEB-II. Individuals with 20% or greater myeloblasts in the marrow or peripheral blood have AML.

PROGNOSIS

The most commonly used system to assess a patient's prognosis is the International Prognostic Scoring System (IPSS) (2). This system assigns a score at diagnosis within each of three categories: the percentage of bone marrow blasts, cytogenetics, and the number and degrees of cytopenias (Table 25-1). The scores are added to yield the IPSS category (Low, Int-1, Int-2, and High). The median survival for patients with Low-, Int-1-, Int-2-, and High-risk disease is 5.7, 3.5, 1.2, and 0.4 years, respectively. Importantly, this system applies only to patients with de novo MDS and was not developed using information from patients with T-MDS, who uniformly have a worse prognosis.

Additional staging systems have emerged. The WPSS system incorporates the WHO category and whether a patient requires transfusions (3). This system may be used dynamically throughout a patient's illness to assess prognosis. Another system stratifies patients within IPSS categories using five refined cytogenetic subgroups (4). Indeed, a revised IPSS (IPSS-R) has been developed which incorporates these five subgroups along with blast percentage, hemoglobin, platelet count, and ANC (Greenberg P., et al., American Society of Hematology Meeting, December, 2011).

Other factors affect prognosis. The presence of abnormally localized immature progenitors (ALIPS) within the bone marrow is associated with worse prognosis. These collections of immature, CD34 positive cells are displaced from their customary paratrabecular location to the central marrow space and are associated with decreased survival and increased risk of transformation to AML, even within IPSS subgroups. Dependence upon blood transfusions and elevated ferritin levels are also associated with worse prognosis.

TABLE 25-1 THE INTERNATIONAL PROGNOSTIC SCORING SYSTEM (IPSS)

(a) COMPONENTS OF THE IPSS

	Score				
	0	0.5	1.0	1.5	2.0
Percentage of BM blasts	<5	5–10	–	11–20	21–30
Karyotype	Good (NL, Y-, 5q-, 20q-)	Intermediate (all others)	Poor (complex, Chr 7)	–	–
Cytopenias	0/1	2/3	–	–	–

RBC ≡ HgB <10

WBC ≡ ANC <1800

Plt ≡ <100K

(b) RELATIONSHIP OF THE IPSS TO MEDIAN OVERALL SURVIVAL AND TIME TO 25% OF PATIENTS TRANSFORMING TO AML

	Score	Overall Median Survival (year)	Time to 25% of Patients Transforming to AML (Year)
Low	0	5.7	9.4
Int-1	0.5–1.0	3.5	3.3
Int-2	1.5–2.0	1.2	1.1
High	2.5–3.5	0.4	0.2

KEY ELEMENTS OF PROGNOSIS

- IPSS scoring system (Table 25-1):
  - Percentage of bone marrow blasts
  - Cytogenetics
  - Number and degrees of cytopenias
- Additional parameters important when assessing prognosis:
  - ALIPS
  - Requirement for blood product transfusions
  - Therapy-related MDS
  - Elevated ferritin

PATHOPHYSIOLOGY

MDS involvement of multiple hematopoietic lineages suggests the disease arises in a primitive hematopoietic cell, or HSC. However, the microenvironment, too, contributes significantly to disease pathogenesis.

■ MDS IS A CLONAL STEM CELL DISORDER

The hypercellular bone marrow in MDS is clonal in origin and the clonal genetic lesion resides within a primitive HSC. MDS arises from a primitive, multipotent HSC capable of homing and engraftment.

■ GENOMIC INSTABILITY

Genomic instability within hematopoietic cells further indicates the presence of a cell-intrinsic defect. Clonal genetic abnormalities are observed in the bone marrow of 50% of patients with de novo MDS and 80% of patients with secondary MDS. The majority of abnormalities are nonrandom. The presence of genetic alterations, in most cases, is associated with inferior prognosis. However, one particular genetic alteration, interstitial deletion within the long arm of chromosome 5, paradoxically confers a favorable prognosis.

T-MDS is an example of the contribution of genomic instability to MDS pathogenesis. T-MDS occurs in younger patients than de novo MDS and is more often associated with chromosomal abnormalities. Karyotypic abnormalities include deletion of large portions of, or entire, chromosomes (-5, -7, 7q-, 13q-, 17p-, and -18) (5).

Clinically, T-MDS follows exposure to agents that cause DNA damage and accounts for approximately 10%–20% of MDS/AML. Affected individuals have been previously treated for lung cancer, breast cancer, childhood acute lymphoblastic leukemia, rheumatoid arthritis, and other oncologic and autoimmune disorders requiring chemotherapy and/or irradiation. T-MDS is associated with a poorer prognosis than de novo MDS, with a median survival of approximately 9 months. Injury associated with topoisomerase inhibitor chemotherapy, such as etoposide, has the earliest onset, often within 2–3 years of exposure. Typical mutations involve core binding factor on chromosomes 16 or 21 and the mixed-lineage leukemia (MLL) gene on 11q. In contrast, alkylating agents such as chlorambucil and cyclophosphamide result in a more latent T-MDS, arising 4–7 years following exposure. Alkylator-associated T-MDS is often associated with abnormalities of chromosomes 5 and/or 7. Exposure to radiation may result in delayed onset of T-MDS, even 10 years or longer following exposure. This category of injury is associated with mutations in the AML1 gene. Genotoxic insult from occupational solvents, such as benzene, is clearly associated with development of MDS/AML. Bone marrow disorders associated with stem cell defects such as paroxysmal nocturnal hemoglobinuria (PNH) and aplastic anemia (AA) may evolve into MDS.

■ 5Q- INTERSTITIAL DELETION

Approximately 5%–20% of patients with MDS harbor an interstitial deletion within the long arm of chromosome 5, with or without additional cytogenetic abnormalities. This represents the most common single cytogenetic abnormality in MDS (6).

These patients differ from those with T-MDS, who have losses of large regions of 5q or the entire chromosome 5 and have a distinctly inferior prognosis. Instead, interstitial deletion of genomic DNA between bands q13 and q34 is prognostically favorable compared to other types of MDS. Most importantly, patients with 5q- are exquisitely responsive to the class of agents known as immunomodulators (IMIDs). Patients harboring the 5q- interstitial deletion but carrying additional cytogenetic abnormalities are also responsive to IMIDs, although they have a worse prognosis when compared to patients with isolated interstitial deletion of 5q.

Approximately half of patients with 5q- have isolated deletion of 5q- and clinical features comprising the "5q- syndrome": RA, mild leukopenia, atypical megakaryocytes, normal or increased platelets, transfusion dependence, and extended survival with low risk of transformation to AML. 5q- syndrome is twice as common in women as men and has a median age of 68 years. The pathogenesis and clinical features of the 5q- syndrome may be related to haploinsufficiency of the RPS14 gene and to loss of miR-145, both on chromosome 5q (7, 8).

GENETIC MUTATIONS WITH NORMAL KARYOTYPE

About 50% of patients have somatic mutations in one or more of at least 18 genes. Mutations in RUNX1, TP53, and NRAS are associated with severe thrombocytopenia and a higher percentage of blast cells in the bone marrow (9). Mutations in TP53, EZH2, and ETV6 are associated with a greater than twofold increased risk of death.

ABNORMAL DIFFERENTIATION

A major clinicopathologic feature of MDS is altered differentiation on cytologic examination of the bone marrow aspirate and biopsy, which displays arrested differentiation and dysplasias affecting one or more lineages. In vitro differentiation of MDS bone marrow is diverted toward nonerythroid lineages, explaining the clinical anemia observed in these patients. MDS marrow contains lower levels of erythroid progenitors and requires several-fold higher concentrations of erythropoietin (Epo) to support in vitro erythroid colony growth. This is clinically relevant, as patients with MDS are often resistant to exogenous Epo or require higher doses to support erythropoiesis than required for other diseases.

■ INCREASED PROLIFERATION AND APOPTOSIS

Cell cycle analyses have demonstrated increased cellular proliferation in MDS marrow, particularly in the myeloid lineage. However, this is accompanied by an increase in cellular apoptosis. The net balance is a hypercellular bone marrow but ineffective hematopoiesis.

Proliferation and apoptosis have been specifically studied in primitive CD34+ cells from MDS. In early stages of disease such as RA and RARS, apoptosis is greatest and exceeds proliferation. In progressive stages of disease, the ratio of apoptosis to proliferation equalizes. Progression is associated with reductions in both proliferation and apoptosis (10).

■ MICROENVIRONMENT

Several abnormalities of the environment in which hematologic progenitors proliferate contribute to the pathogenesis of MDS. The most notable example of the potential role of the microenvironment is evidenced in a murine model where mice lacking expression of Dicer1 strictly within osteoprogenitors develop MDS and, in some case, AML (11).

Another potential contributor to MDS pathogenesis is increased secretion of pro-apoptotic cytokines by bone marrow fibroblasts and macrophages, resulting in increased hematopoietic cell apoptosis. Cells and stroma from MDS patients secrete increased levels of TNF-α, interleukin-6, and IFN-γ relative to normal controls. Agents such as IMIDs inhibit TNF-α and IL-6 secretion and reduce bone marrow angiogenesis.

T-lymphocytes are hypothesized to provide immune surveillance in MDS and undergo activation and proliferation in an attempt to eradicate the malignant clone. Indeed, use of immunosuppressive medications such as cyclosporine and eliminating activated T cells using antithymocyte globulin (ATG) can improve cytopenias, particularly in patients with hypoplastic MDS (12).

CLINICAL PRESENTATION

The clinical presentation of MDS relates to the number and degree of cytopenias. Anemia, the most common cytopenia in MDS and seen in 80%–90% of patients, may manifest as a sensation of light headedness, fatigue, chest pain, dyspnea, palpitations, and depression. Leukopenia is the second most common cytopenia in MDS, present in 50% of affected individuals. Manifestations include recurrent lung, sinus, and skin infections. Thrombocytopenia is present in 25% of patients and may result in easy bruising, epistaxis, petechiae, gastrointestinal bleeding, and hematuria. In addition, qualitative defects in hematopoietic cell function may result in clinical signs and symptoms, even in the presence of adequate blood counts. For example, neutrophil dysfunction may contribute to infection, while platelet dysfunction may result in hemorrhage even if the blood counts are within the normal range.

1. *Anemia.* Light headedness, fatigue, chest pain, dyspnea, palpitations, and depression.
2. *Leukopenia.* Lung, sinus, and skin infections.
3. *Thrombocytopenia.* Easy bruising, epistaxis, petechiae, gastrointestinal bleeding, and hematuria.

DIAGNOSTIC STUDIES

The initial evaluation of uni- or multilineage cytopenias begins with careful history taking. Medications, such as antibiotics and chemotherapeutic agents, are common causes. Also, infections caused by parvovirus, HBV, HCV, EBV, CMV, and HIV suppress hematopoiesis, and their presence may be discerned by history, physical examination, and laboratory studies.

When MDS is suspected, a complete blood count with differential is necessary to identify the number and severity of cytopenias. An elevated erythroid mean corpuscular volume (MCV) is often, although not always, present in MDS. Evaluation of iron levels by assessing the iron (Fe), total iron binding capacity (TIBC), and ferritin levels is necessary to assess baseline iron stores, to determine whether iron supplementation is required to enhance hematopoiesis, or identify situations of Fe overload. The B_{12} and folate levels should also be assessed to ensure adequate substrates for hematopoiesis. An Epo level is helpful in deciding whether exogenous erythroid growth factor administration will be likely to help patients with anemia. Levels of copper and ceruloplasmin should be checked, particularly in patients with ringed sideroblasts within the bone marrow.

A bone marrow aspiration and core biopsy is essential for the diagnosis of MDS. The percentage of bone marrow cellularity is assessed on the core biopsy, while the myeloblast percentage is calculated using the aspirate. Morphologic assessment of myeloid and erythroid dysplasia is made using the aspirate, while megakaryocyte dysplasia is most easily assessed on the core. Flow cytometry is utilized to identify monotypic populations of lymphoid and myeloid cells. Cytogenetic analysis is performed on the aspirate. If cytogenetic information cannot be obtained, FISH may be used to disclose critical genetic deletions.

Bone marrow studies may reveal alternative causes for cytopenias, such as other hematologic malignancies including AML and non-Hodgkin lymphomas, and solid tumors metastatic to the bone. Hypoplastic MDS, hypoplastic anemia, and aplastic anemia may be determined on the bone marrow core. PNH may be detected by flow cytometric assessment of the glycosylphosphatidylinositol (GPI) linked proteins CD55 and CD59.

Laboratory studies used to diagnose MDS:

- Peripheral blood
  - CBC with differential, MCV
  - Fe, TIBC, ferritin, copper, ceruloplasmin
  - B_{12}, folate
  - Epo level
- Bone marrow aspiration and biopsy
  - Morphologic analysis of dysplasia using the aspirate and core biopsy
  - Quantitation of myeloblasts using the bone marrow aspirate
  - Flow cytometry to identify monoclonal populations of lymphoid and myeloid cells, PNH, and T-cell large granular lymphocytes
  - Cytogenetics to identify chromosomal alterations (FISH is used when cytogenetic information cannot be obtained)

THERAPIES FOR MDS

A broad range of management options exists for MDS including amelioration of hematologic deficits with blood product support and administration of growth factors, the use of novel agents aimed at restoring normal hematopoiesis and reducing the malignant clone (Table 25-2), and HCT for patients with high-risk disease for whom a donor can be identified.

■ SUPPORTIVE CARE

The goal of supportive care is to reduce morbidity and improve quality of life (QoL). Supportive care for MDS consists of cytokine growth factors capable of stimulating myelo- and erythropoiesis, transfusion of red blood cells (RBCs) and platelets, and antibiotics. Anemia has been clearly linked to diminished QoL that can be improved by increasing the hemoglobin (HgB). Age, comorbidities, and lifestyle determine the optimal target HgB level for each patient. However, most patients derive clinical benefit by maintaining an HgB of at least 9 g/dl and HCT of at least 27%, although lower transfusion thresholds are required for patients with symptoms of anemia and with other comorbidities, such as cardiopulmonary disease.

Initial treatment of anemia may be achieved by periodic administration of erythroid growth factors such as epoetin alfa, Procrit, or darbepoetin alfa, Aranesp. Responses to epoetin alfa and darbepoetin alfa are 20%–70% depending on the patient population. Epoetin alfa may be initiated at

TABLE 25-2 FDA-APPROVED THERAPEUTIC AGENTS FOR MDS

Name	Class	FDA Indication
5-Azacitidine (Vidaza)	Cytidine analog, DNA methyltransferase inhibitor	All FAB subtypes of MDS: • RA and RARS (if accompanied by neutropenia or thrombocytopenia or requiring transfusions) • RAEB • RAEB-T • CMMoL
Decitabine (Dacogen)	Cytidine analog, DNA methyltransferase inhibitor	• All FAB subtypes • All IPSS subtypes of MDS excluding Low- risk patients
Lenalidomide (Revlimid)	Immunomodulatory drug (IMID)	Patients with transfusion-dependent anemia due to Low and Int-1 IPSS MDS associated with deletion of 5q cytogenetic abnormality, with or without additional cytogenetic abnormalities

40,000–60,000 units weekly, while darbepoetin is given at 200–300 mcg every 1–2 weeks. However, dose adjustments will be required to achieve the desired laboratory and clinical benefit. HgB rises of 1–4 g/dl may be achieved. Both agents appear to have similar efficacy in MDS (13). There may be potential synergy achieved by adding G-CSF (filgrastim, Neupogen), which should be considered if there is no response to epoetin or darbepoetin alone after a period of 6 weeks (14). Patients with elevated endogenous Epo levels (>500 mU/ml) and those requiring RBC transfusions are unlikely to respond to erythroid growth factors alone.

Patients who fail to respond to growth factors require RBC supplementation via periodic transfusions. Individuals with advanced MDS by IPSS score are more likely to require RBC transfusions than those with lower risk disease. Leukodepleted products are recommended to decrease alloimmunization, prevent nonhemolytic febrile transfusion reactions, and reduce the transmission of cytomegalovirus (CMV). Other complications include iron and volume overload, infections, and graft-versus-host disease. Blood products should be irradiated to prevent potentially fatal graft-versus-host disease.

Infections are treated with antibiotics. Myeloid growth factors are not routinely used for prophylaxis of uninfected individuals, even if neutropenic. However, they may be added for resistant or recurrent infections, particularly in patients with an ANC <500/μL. Platelet transfusions are used to treat patients with thrombocytopenia. Prophylactic transfusions are typically used when the platelet count is <10,000/μL. However, transfusions may be required at higher levels such as 20,000 or 30,000 if accompanied by signs of bleeding or petechiae.

■ IRON-CHELATION THERAPY

Both increased intestinal absorption and transfusional overload account for elevated iron in MDS. While total body iron stores are normally between 3 and 5 g, tissue overload with subsequent dysfunction occurs when the total body iron load is 15–20 g. A serum ferritin of 1000 ng/ml corresponds with a total body iron load of approximately 5 g. Current guidelines are to consider iron-chelation therapy in patients who have received more than 20–25 units of packed RBCs or who have a serum ferritin exceeding approximately 2500 ng/ml. Chelation may be achieved by use of the parenteral agent deferoxamine (Desferal), or one of the two oral chelators, deferiprone (not approved in the United States) and deferasirox (Exjade). Consideration must be given toward balancing the cost and convenience of chelation therapy with the potential benefit. In general, chelation therapy should be considered in young patients with Low/Int-1 IPSS scores who have low levels of bone marrow myeloblasts and iron overload.

Although the relationship of iron-chelation therapy to overall survival has not been prospectively assessed, one retrospective study found that transfusional iron overload, defined as a ferritin level exceeding 1000 ng/ml, was associated with inferior survival in patients with RA and RARS receiving pRBC transfusions compared to patients whose ferritin levels remained below <1000 ng/ml. Retrospective analyses have demonstrated that heavily transfused patients with Low- and Int-1-risk MDS have improved survival, but prospective studies are needed (15, 16).

■ HYPOMETHYLATING AGENTS

Epigenetic DNA hypermethylation is common in MDS. Hypermethylation results in transcriptional silencing and may contribute to the pathogenesis of MDS by decreasing expression of tumor suppressor genes, genes involved in differentiation, and cyclin-dependent kinase inhibitors (CDKIs). DNA methyltransferase inhibitors (DMTIs) promote hypomethylation via their incorporation into DNA and inhibition of DNA methyltransferases. Like histone deacetylase inhibitors (HDACs), DMTIs have the capacity to promote cellular differentiation in vitro. Such approaches are of obvious relevance to patients with MDS, in which the bone marrow often shows hypercellularity and a block in differentiation.

The DMTI 5-azacitidine (Vidaza), a cytidine analog, was the first agent to receive approval by the FDA for the treatment of MDS. Azacitidine is approved for all FAB subtypes of MDS, including RA and RARS with neutropenia or thrombocytopenia or requiring transfusional support. Azacitidine's activity was established in a study of 191 patients with MDS randomized to receive azacitidine versus best supportive care (17). Complete and partial responses were observed in 7% and 10% of patients, respectively, treated with azacitidine compared to none in the control arm. Overall improvement was observed in 37% of patients with azacitidine versus 5% with best supportive care. Time to leukemia or death was significantly increased from 13 to 21 months in the azacitidine group. In addition, QoL in the categories of fatigue, dyspnea, physical functioning, positive effect, and psychologic distress was improved in the treatment arm. The effect of azacitidine on improving overall survival (OS) in patients with Int-2- and High-risk MDS was established in the AZA-001 study, where 358 patients were randomized to receive azacitidine versus a conventional care regimen consisting of low-dose cytarabine, induction chemotherapy, or best supportive care alone (18). Patients treated with azacitidine had a median 9-month improvement in OS compared to the CCR arm. In addition, the complete remission (CR) rate and the hematologic response rate in patients receiving azacitidine were 17% and 49%, compared to 8% and 29% in those treated with CCR.

Decitabine (5-deoxyazacitidine, Dacogen) is a deoxycytidine analog that inhibits DNA methylation. Decitabine's activity was established in a study of 170 patients with MDS randomized to receive either decitabine at a dose of 15 mg/m² given intravenously over 3 h every 8 h for 3 days (at a dose of 135 mg/m² per course) and repeated every 6 weeks, or best supportive care (19). Patients treated with decitabine achieved an overall response rate of 17%, including 9% complete responses. In comparison, no responses were seen in the supportive care group. In addition, patients treated with decitabine had a trend toward a longer median time to progression to AML or death compared with patients who received supportive care alone (all patients, 12.1 months versus 7.8 months [$P = 0.16$]), although improvement was statistically significant in patients with IPSS Int-2- and High-risk disease (12.0 months versus 6.8 months [$P = 0.03$]) and in those with de novo disease (12.6 months versus 9.4 months [$P = 0.04$]). In a subsequent randomized study of 233 patients with intermediate- and high-risk MDS treated with decitabine versus best supportive care, a significant survival benefit was not observed in the decitabine arm (20).

■ IMMUNOMODULATORS (IMIDs)

IMIDs are oral agents that suppress secretion of inflammatory cytokines but also modulate the immune response and inhibit angiogenesis. Thalidomide (Thalomid), the first member of this family to show activity in MDS, is highly teratogenic and is associated with significant side effects including neuropathies, constipation, drowsiness, and fatigue, and has been superseded by lenalidomide (Revlimid), the second agent to gain FDA approval for the treatment of MDS. Lenalidomide is approved for patients with Low- or Int-1-risk MDS who are transfusion dependent and who have a deletion in chromosome 5q. Lenalidomide has fewer side effects than thalidomide.

The efficacy of lenalidomide in MDS was initially observed in a phase II study of 43 patients. Erythroid and cytogenetic responses were most prominent in patients with the 5q- interstitial deletion. In a phase II study of 148 patients with Low- and Int-1-risk MDS who were transfusion dependent, transfusion independence was achieved in 67% of patients while an additional 9% had minor erythroid responses (21). The median duration of response exceeded 104 weeks. Also, 45% of patients had complete cytogenetic remissions, while another 28% had minor cytogenetic responses.

In a similarly designed study, 214 patients with Low- and Int-1-risk MDS who were transfusion dependent and lacked a deletion in 5q were treated with lenalidomide (22). The majority of patients (78%) had a normal karyotype. Transfusion independence was achieved in 26% of patients, while an additional 17% had minor erythroid responses. Of the 47 (22%) patients with abnormal cytogenetics, 9 (19%) achieved a cytogenetic response of which 4 were complete. The median duration of transfusion independence was 41 weeks. The most common toxicities of lenalidomide include neutropenia and thrombocytopenia, which appear to be more common in patients with the 5q- interstitial deletion than in other patients.

■ IMMUNE SUPPRESSION

Some patients with MDS demonstrate elevated levels of inflammatory cytokines within the blood and/or abnormal lymphoid collections within the bone marrow. These findings suggest that immune dysregulation is operative in MDS pathogenesis and raises the possibility that immune suppression may result in clinical benefit. In a study of 61 patients with primarily low-risk MDS by FAB treated with equine ATG, responses were seen in all three hematopoietic lineages (12). Of these, 21 of 61 patients became transfusion independent, with a median duration of 36 months, 10 of 21 with severe thrombocytopenia achieved sustained responses, and 6 of 11 patients with severe neutropenia had significant improvements. Other studies have shown activity of ATG in MDS, particularly in patients with RA and RARS. Variables noted to predict response to therapy include young age (<60 years), expression of the HLA-DR15 antigen, and shorter duration of RBC transfusion dependence.

■ ADDITIONAL AGENTS UNDER INVESTIGATION

Like DNA methyltransferases, histone deacetylases suppress gene transcription and are active in patients with MDS. Thus, the role of histone deacetylase inhibitors (HDACs) is under investigation in MDS. A trial of the orally bioavailable HDAC, vorinostat (suberoylanilide hydroxamic acid, SAHA), has shown activity. The Ras/Raf kinase signaling pathway is activated in a variety of malignancies including MDS and AML. Agents capable of inhibiting this pathway include arsenic trioxide (AsO_3, Trisenox), farnesyl-transferase inhibitors (FTIs), which block necessary steps required for Ras activation, and direct pathway inhibitors, such as the Raf kinase inhibitor Bay 43-9006 (Sorafenib).

The proteasome, a catalytic, multisubunit protease involved in protein degradation, is an antineoplastic target inhibited by bortezomib (Velcade). This agent, capable of suppressing levels of the master transcription factor, nuclear factor-kappa B (NF-κB), is approved for use in multiple myeloma. Elevated levels of nuclear NF-κB have been identified in primitive leukemia cells from patients with leukemia in addition to CD34+ bone marrow cells from patients with high-risk MDS, suggesting a role for the inhibitor in myeloid malignancies.

■ STEM CELL TRANSPLANTATION

Care of those with advanced disease presents a considerable clinical challenge. Intensive chemotherapy regimens have not provided improvements in long-term outcomes. However, HCT is an important consideration offering potential cure.

Allogeneic stem cell transplantation remains the only potential cure for MDS, although long-term survival is only approximately 30%. An estimated

10%–15% of patients are eligible for HCT, which is generally performed in patients with adequate performance status and for whom a suitable donor is identified. HCT may be performed until age 75 years using reduced-intensity conditioning approaches. A retrospective study of 836 MDS patients transplanted with stem cells from HLA-identical sibling donors revealed comparable overall survival in patients receiving either myeloablative or reduced intensity conditioning (23). Autologous HCT remains an option for individuals without suitable allogeneic candidates, although the majority of patients relapse within 2 years (24).

Optimal timing of allogeneic HCT represents a balance between maximizing chances of long-term survival while decreasing transplant-related morbidity and mortality. A decision-model analysis was conducted to determine the relationship between IPSS score and timing of HCT (25). This model concluded that for patients <60 years receiving myeloablative conditioning, early HCT increased overall survival for patients with Int-2- or High-risk disease. In contrast, HCT could be delayed for a brief period of time for those with Low- or Int-1-risk disease, provided the HCT is done before leukemic transformation. A similar analysis in adults aged 60–70 years found a life-expectancy and quality-adjusted survival benefit for early transplantation of individuals with Int-2- and High-risk disease. These strategies maximize overall survival for low-risk patients while decreasing the early morbidity and mortality of transplantation.

PRINCIPLES OF THERAPY

Treatment of MDS requires consideration of patient age, treatment preference, IPSS score, performance status, presence of antecedent hematologic disorder (AHD), and availability of an HLA-matched stem cell donor. A treatment schema is provided in **Figure 25-1**. Patients with secondary MDS have a worse prognosis relative to those with de novo MDS. If the patient is a candidate for intensive therapy, an allogeneic donor must be sought and preparations made for allogeneic SCT. If the patient is deemed unsuitable or an appropriate donor cannot be identified, therapies consisting of supportive care, azacitidine, decitabine, and/or clinical trial should be considered.

For patients with Low- or Int-1-risk MDS and anemia, cytogenetic status influences the starting therapy. Initial treatment for patients with the 5q-interstitial deletion, with or without additional cytogenetic abnormalities, is with lenalidomide. If an adequate response is not achieved after a period of approximately 3 months, attention is turned toward azacitidine, decitabine, or clinical trials in addition to supportive care. For Low/Int-1-risk patients lacking the 5q- cytogenetic deletion, initial treatment is based upon the serum Epo level and transfusion status. Patients with elevated serum Epo levels and/or those dependent upon RBC transfusions are unlikely to respond to exogenous erythropoietic growth factors and, therefore, treatment commences with supportive care, azacitidine, decitabine, and/or clinical trials. Lenalidomide may be effective in improving anemia, even in patients lacking the 5q- interstitial deletion. Antilymphocyte therapy consisting of ATG may be effective in patients who are HLA-DR15 positive, who harbor trisomy 8, or who have a hypocellular MDS.

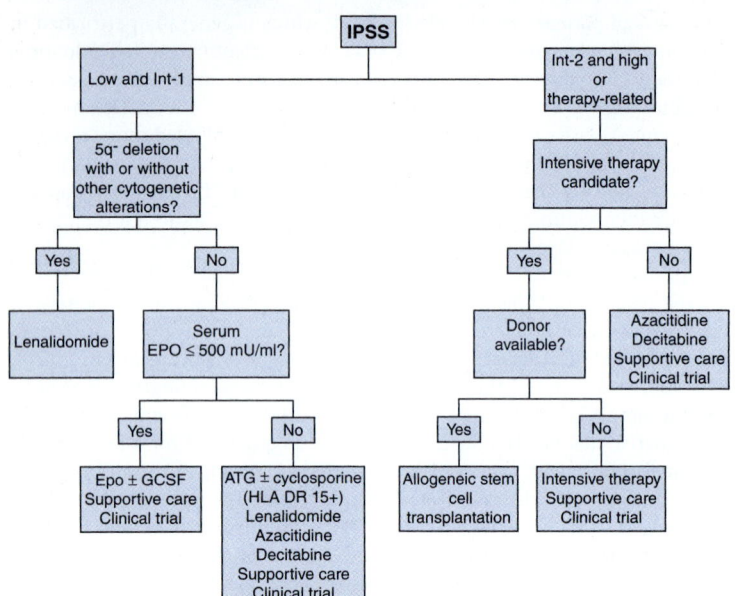

FIGURE 25-1 Treatment schema for patients with MDS.

Patients with neutropenia and infections require myeloid growth factors and antibiotics. Patients with clinically significant thrombocytopenia should receive platelet transfusions and/or antifibrinolytic agents (aminocaproic acid). Azacitidine, decitabine, or clinical trials may be beneficial for individuals with thrombocytopenia and/or neutropenia.

For Int-2- and High-risk patients, HCT represents the best initial therapy for young patients with HLA-matched donors. If a donor cannot be identified or if the patient is not a candidate for HCT, azacitidine, decitabine, chemotherapy agents, and/or supportive care are reasonable choices.

REFERENCES

1. Swerdlow S, Campo E, Harris N, et al. *WHO Classification of Tumours of Haematopoietic and Lymphoid Tissues.* Lyon: International Agency for Research on Cancer (IARC); 2008.

2. Greenberg P, Cox C, LeBeau MM, et al. International scoring system for evaluating prognosis in myelodysplastic syndromes. *Blood.* 1997; 89: 2079–2088.

3. Malcovati L, Germing U, Kuendgen A, et al. Time-dependent prognostic scoring system for predicting survival and leukemic evolution in myelodysplastic syndromes. *J Clin Oncol.* 2007; 25: 3503–3510.

4. Schanz J, Tuchler H, Sole F, et al. New comprehensive cytogenetic scoring system for primary myelodysplastic syndromes (MDS) and oligoblastic acute myeloid leukemia after MDS derived from an international database merge. *J Clin Oncol.* 2012; 30: 820–829.

5. Mauritzson N, Albin M, Rylander L, et al. Pooled analysis of clinical and cytogenetic features in treatment-related and de novo adult acute myeloid leukemia and myelodysplastic syndromes based on a consecutive series of 761 patients analyzed 1976–1993 and on 5098 unselected cases reported in the literature 1974–2001. *Leukemia*. 2002; 16: 2366–2378.

6. Nimer SD. Clinical management of myelodysplastic syndromes with interstitial deletion of chromosome 5q. *J Clin Oncol*. 2006; 24: 2576–2582.

7. Ebert BL, Lee MM, Pretz JL, et al. An RNA interference model of RPS19 deficiency in Diamond-Blackfan anemia recapitulates defective hematopoiesis and rescue by dexamethasone: identification of dexamethasone-responsive genes by microarray. *Blood*. 2005; 105: 4620–4626.

8. Kumar MS, Narla A, Nonami A, et al. Coordinate loss of a microRNA and protein-coding gene cooperate in the pathogenesis of 5q-syndrome. *Blood*. 2011; 118: 4666–4673.

9. Bejar R, Stevenson K, Abdel-Wahab O, et al. Clinical effect of point mutations in myelodysplastic syndromes. *N Engl J Med*. 2011; 364: 2496–2506.

10. Parker JE, Mufti GJ, Rasool F, et al. The role of apoptosis, proliferation, and the Bcl-2-related proteins in the myelodysplastic syndromes and acute myeloid leukemia secondary to MDS. *Blood*. 2000; 96: 3932–3938.

11. Raaijmakers MH, Mukherjee S, Guo S, et al. Bone progenitor dysfunction induces myelodysplasia and secondary leukaemia. *Nature*. 2010; 464: 852–857.

12. Molldrem JJ, Leifer E, Bahceci E, et al. Antithymocyte globulin for treatment of the bone marrow failure associated with myelodysplastic syndromes. *Ann Intern Med*. 2002; 137: 156–163.

13. Mannone L, Gardin C, Quarre MC, et al. High dose darbopoetin alfa the treatment of lower risk MDS: results of a phase II study. *Br J Haematol*. 2006; 133: 513–519.

14. Hellstrom-Lindberg E, Gulbrandsen N, Lindberg G, et al. A validated decision model for treating the anaemia of myelodysplastic syndromes with erythropoietin + granulocyte colony-stimulating factor: significant effects on quality of life. *Br J Haematol*. 2003; 120: 1037–1046.

15. Rose C, Brechignac S, Vassilief D, et al. Does iron chelation therapy improve survival in regularly transfused lower risk MDS patients? A multicenter study by the GFM (Groupe Francophone des Myelodysplasies). *Leuk Res*. 2010; 34: 864–870.

16. Guariglia R, Martorelli MC, Villani O, et al. Positive effects on hematopoiesis in patients with myelodysplastic syndrome receiving deferasirox as oral iron chelation therapy: a brief review. *Leuk Res*. 2011; 35: 566–570.

17. Silverman LR, Demakos EP, Peterson BL, et al. Randomized controlled trial of azacitidine in patients with the myelodysplastic syndrome: a study of the cancer and leukemia group B. *J Clin Oncol*. 2002; 20: 2429–2440.

18. Fenaux P, Mufti GJ, Hellstrom-Lindberg E, et al. Efficacy of azacitidine compared with that of conventional care regimens in the treatment of higher-risk myelodysplastic syndromes: a randomised, open-label, phase III study. *Lancet Oncol*. 2009; 10: 223–232.

19. Kantarjian H, Issa JP, Rosenfeld CS, et al. Decitabine improves patient outcomes in myelodysplastic syndromes: results of a phase III randomized study. *Cancer.* 2006; 106: 1794–1803.

20. Lubbert M, Suciu S, Baila L, et al. Low-dose decitabine versus best supportive care in elderly patients with intermediate- or high-risk myelodysplastic syndrome (MDS) ineligible for intensive chemotherapy: final results of the randomized phase III study of the European Organisation for Research and Treatment of Cancer Leukemia Group and the German MDS Study Group. *J Clin Oncol.* 2011; 29: 1987–1996.

21. List A, Dewald G, Bennett J, et al. Lenalidomide in the myelodysplastic syndrome with chromosome 5q deletion. *N Engl J Med.* 2006; 355: 1456–1465.

22. Raza A, Reeves JA, Feldman EJ, et al. Phase 2 study of lenalidomide in transfusion-dependent, low-risk, and intermediate-1 risk myelodysplastic syndromes with karyotypes other than deletion 5q. *Blood.* 2008; 111: 86–93.

23. Martino R, Iacobelli S, Brand R, et al. Retrospective comparison of reduced intensity conditioning and conventional high dose conditioning for allogeneic hematopoietic stem cell transplantation using HLA identical sibling donors in myelodysplastic syndromes. *Blood.* 2006; 108: 836–846.

24. Ducastelle S, Ades L, Gardin C, et al. Long-term follow-up of autologous stem cell transplantation after intensive chemotherapy in patients with myelodysplastic syndrome or secondary acute myeloid leukemia. *Haematologica.* 2006; 91: 373–376.

25. Cutler CS, Lee SJ, Greenberg P, et al. A decision analysis of allogeneic bone marrow transplantation for the myelodysplastic syndromes: delayed transplantation for low-risk myelodysplasia is associated with improved outcome. *Blood.* 2004; 104: 579–585.

CHAPTER **26**

Myeloproliferative Neoplasms

Jerry L. Spivak

POLYCYTHEMIA VERA

■ INTRODUCTION

Polycythemia vera (PV) is a clonal disorder of a multipotent hematopoietic stem cell in which overproduction of morphologically normal red cells, white cells, and platelets occurs in the absence of an apparent cause. The commonest of the chronic myeloproliferative disorders, PV, is uncommon, occurring at an average frequency of 2/100,000, but with increasing age, rates as high as 18/100,000 have been observed. Females predominate, particularly below age 40 years.

PATHOGENESIS

The etiology of PV is unknown. Abnormalities of chromosomes 1, 8, 9, 13, and 20 have been identified in up to 30% of PV patients, but they are neither specific for the disorder nor necessary for its pathogenesis; in many instances they appear to occur as secondary events and their expression can be enhanced by exposure to chemotherapeutic agents (1). Erythropoietin-independent in vitro erythroid colony formation is a characteristic feature of PV, although not specific for it, since this behavior has also been observed in primary myelofibrosis (PMF) and essential thrombocytosis. Constitutive activation of JAK2 (2), which is the cognate tyrosine kinase for type 1 hematopoietic growth factor receptors such as the erythropoietin, thrombopoietin, and granulocyte colony-stimulating factor receptors, has been identified to be the molecular basis for such growth factor independence in PV and its companion myeloproliferative disorders PMF and essential thrombocytosis.

The mechanism for constitutive JAK2 activation in the chronic myeloproliferative disorders is an acquired point mutation in the autoinhibitory JH2 domain of the JAK2 gene, replacing valine with phenylalanine (V617F). JAK2 is located on the short arm of chromosome 9 and loss of heterozygosity for 9p is a common cytogenetic lesion in PV, leading to homozygosity for the JAK2 V617F mutation; in some patients, there is also reduplication of chromosome 9. In PV, approximately 90% of patients express the JAK2 V617F mutation, of which approximately 35% are homozygous for it. Approximately 5% have a JAK2 exon 12 activating mutation. No clinical differences have been identified between heterozygotes and those homozygous for JAK2 V617F, nor are there any clinical differences between PV patients expressing JAK2 V617F and those who do not. Thus, although the JAK2 V617F mutation provides an explanation for the hematopoietic growth factor independence of PV hematopoietic cells in vitro, their apoptosis resistance and their uncontrolled growth in vivo, the absence of the mutation in some patients with classical PV, and its expression in PMF and essential thrombocytosis patients strongly suggest that other as yet unidentified molecular lesions are involved in the pathogenesis of these disorders.

CLINICAL FEATURES

PV is extremely variable in its presenting manifestations as well as its clinical features, which also change over the course of the disorder. Because its onset can be insidious, an abnormal blood count is often the first sign of the disease. In approximately 40% of patients, there will be an increase in red cells, white cells, and platelets. In approximately 15% of patients, erythrocytosis will be the sole presenting manifestation. In approximately 5%–10% of patients, an elevated platelet count may be the first manifestation of the disease, while in the rest, erythrocytosis and thrombocytosis or leukocytosis are the presenting blood abnormalities. Extramedullary hematopoiesis as manifested by palpable splenomegaly occurs in approximately 40% of patients at the time of diagnosis; rarely, myelofibrosis can be the initial manifestation of PV with erythrocytosis becoming evident later on. Since PV is a hypercoagulable state, arterial or venous thrombosis may also be the first manifestation of the disease. Classically, in young women, the thrombosis most commonly involves the hepatic veins, often as the presenting manifestation and often with an apparently normal hematocrit due to concomitant plasma volume expansion. Pruritus, usually aquagenic, is also not uncommon as a presenting manifestation, but PV is often not initially recognized as its cause. Erythromelalgia, in which the extremities become warm, red, and painful; migraine headaches; or other neurologic disturbances such as vertigo or visual disturbances are also characteristic symptoms that indicate the presence of an elevated red cell mass or thrombocytosis.

■ LABORATORY ABNORMALITIES

In addition to increases in the red cell, granulocyte, and platelet counts, the MCV can be low if red cell mass expansion or gastrointestinal blood loss depletes body iron stores. An elevated leukocyte alkaline phosphatase and serum vitamin B_{12} and vitamin B_{12} binding capacity due to increased release of granulocyte transcobalamin III reflect neutrophil activation, presumably due to JAK2 V617F, which is also responsible for the increased expression of granulocyte PRV-1 mRNA (CD177). When the platelet or leukocyte counts are elevated, spurious hyperkalemia may be observed, as can hypoglycemia and a low pO_2 if blood samples are not collected on ice and in the presence of sodium azide. Elevation of the serum alkaline phosphatase occurs with extramedullary hematopoiesis and becomes more marked after splenectomy.

Abnormalities of coagulation in PV are largely limited to platelet function. These include defective platelet aggregation to ADP, epinephrine, or collagen alone or in combination and loss of alpha granules and dense bodies. When the platelet count exceeds 1,000,000/ml, higher molecular weight von Willebrand multimers will be absorbed by the platelets and degraded, leading to a reduction in ristocetin cofactor activity and an acquired form of von Willebrand's disease, although spontaneous bleeding due to this is uncommon.

■ DIAGNOSIS

Elevation of the red cell mass is the sine qua non of PV, the only feature that distinguishes it from its companion myeloproliferative disorders, PMF and essential thrombocytosis, and the feature of the disease that is responsible for its most frequent serious consequences, thrombosis and hemorrhage. Unfortunately, erythrocytosis is not unique to PV, and in recent years the very means for identifying the presence of erythrocytosis, direct determination of the red cell mass by isotope dilution, has become unavailable in many medical centers. Attempts to resolve this issue by the use of surrogate markers for direct red cell mass determination have not proved to be useful (3). For example, specific hematocrit or hemoglobin levels are woefully inadequate as indicators of the red cell mass unless the hematocrit is >60% (hemoglobin >20 g/dl) in a man, or >52% in a woman (hemoglobin >17 g/dl). The reasons for this are a consequence of blood rheology and the unique pathophysiology of PV with respect to blood volume regulation.

For example, when erythrocytosis occurs as a consequence of hypoxia, there is a simultaneous reduction in the plasma volume as the body attempts to maintain a normal total blood volume. This contributes to the observed increase in hematocrit. In PV, however, particularly in women, as the red cell mass rises, the plasma volume either rises or fails to decrease. Furthermore, with splenomegaly, there is a compensatory increase in plasma volume. Both of these situations lead to hematocrit values that are spuriously low with respect to the actual red cell mass (4). As a corollary, a decrease in the plasma volume alone can lead to a falsely elevated hematocrit, when in fact the red cell mass is normal.

The recent discovery of the JAK2 V617F mutation has greatly simplified the evaluation of a high hematocrit and the diagnosis of PV. This is because first, benign disorders causing erythrocytosis are more common than PV (Table 26-1) and second, because surrogate markers for the latter lack sensitivity and specificity. For example, while the serum erythropoietin level

---

TABLE 26-1 CAUSES OF ERYTHROCYTOSIS

Relative erythrocytosis
   Hemoconcentration secondary to dehydration, androgens, or tobacco abuse
Absolute erythrocytosis
   Hypoxia
      Carbon monoxide intoxication
      High-affinity hemoglobin
      High altitude
      Pulmonary disease
      Right to left shunts
      Sleep apnea syndrome
      Neurologic disease
   Renal disease
      Renal artery stenosis
      Focal sclerosing or membranous glomerulonephritis
      Renal transplantation
   Tumors
      Hypernephroma
      Hepatoma
      Cerebellar hemangioblastoma
      Uterine fibroma
      Adrenal tumors
      Meningioma
      Pheochromcytoma
   Drugs
      Androgens
      Recombinant erythropoietin
   Familial (with normal hemoglobin function erythropoietin receptor mutations)
   Polycythemia vera

is lower in PV than in other disorders causing erythrocytosis, the serum erythropoietin level can also be normal in PV as well as in secondary forms of erythrocytosis. Similarly, the bone marrow examination can be normal in PV or even mimic that of PMF or essential thrombocytosis. Cytogenetic abnormalities are present in only 30% of PV patients and are not pathognomonic for the disease, while other markers such as elevation of the leukocyte alkaline phosphatase and endogenous erythroid colony formation are merely consequences of the constitutively active JAK2.

Figure 26-1 illustrates an algorithm for the evaluation of the patient with a high hematocrit. When red cell mass and plasma volume determinations are not available, it is reasonable to start with an assay for JAK2 V617F with the knowledge that a positive assay only indicates the presence of a myeloproliferative disorder, while a negative assay does not exclude such a disorder. In the absence of a red cell mass determination, a positive JAK2 V617F assay in a patient with a high hematocrit obligates the physician to phlebotomize the patient to the normal hematocrit for gender as discussed below.

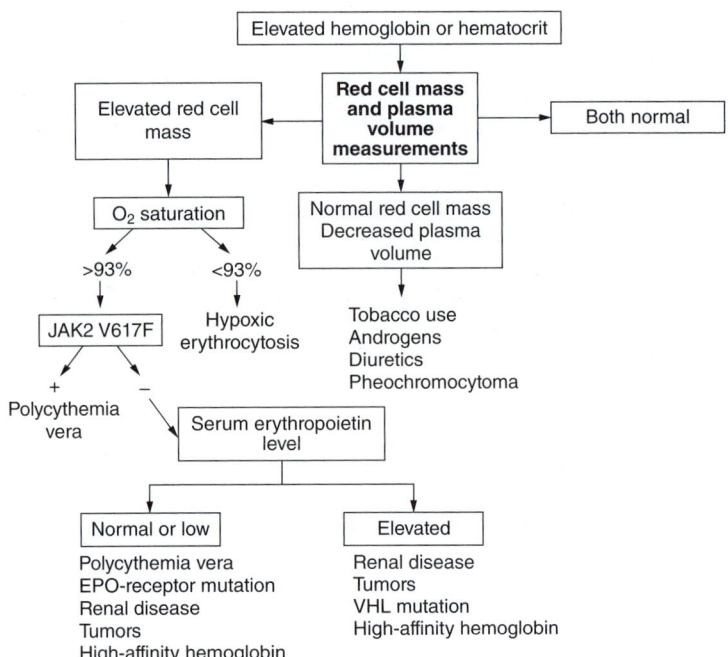

FIGURE 26-1 Algorithm for the diagnosis of polycythemia vera. The first requirement is to establish the basis for an elevated hemoglobin or hematocrit. If it is determined that there is an elevated red cell mass, an assay for JAK2 V617F will establish the diagnosis in over 90% of patients with polycythemia vera. A negative JAK2 V617F assay does not, however, exclude a myeloproliferative etiology and in the absence of splenomegaly, leukocytosis, or thrombocytosis; further studies will be required.

■ NATURAL HISTORY

Most classical hematology textbooks suggest that the natural history of PV follows an inevitable course from erythrocytosis through myelofibrosis and myeloid metaplasia to acute leukemia if the patient does not die first from some other complication or comorbidity. This depiction ignores the clinical heterogeneity of the disease, its modification by improved therapies, and the earlier stages at which PV is now usually recognized. In this regard, prognosis does not appear to be influenced by the presence or the absence of JAK2 V617F or whether this mutation is expressed homozygously or heterozygously.

The complications of PV are listed in Table 26-2. Erythrocytosis, not thrombocytosis, is responsible for the major thrombotic complications of PV; minor transient thrombotic or ischemic complications such as erythromelalgia, ocular migraine, or digital infarction do involve the platelets but are exacerbated by erythrocytosis, which promotes platelet activation, platelet-leukocyte interactions, as well as endothelial cell activation and damage, all of which enhance thrombogenesis. Erythrocytosis can also cause hypertension, splenomegaly, and exacerbate aquagenic pruritus. Acid-peptic disease leading to gastrointestinal hemorrhage and iron deficiency occur at a higher frequency in PV patients than in the general population; the roles of vascular stasis, excess histamine, or other cytokine production are unknown, but the frequency of *Helicobacter* infection is increased in PV.

Over time, there will be a gradual increase in the leukocyte and platelet counts, but the leukocytosis is not usually progressive unless there is disease acceleration, while asymptomatic thrombocytosis requires no therapy. The development of excessive extramedullary hematopoiesis with massive splenomegaly and hepatomegaly is a serious complication of PV, occurring in about 10%–15% of patients. These patients are at a higher risk of subsequent leukemic transformation (5).

Splenomegaly can lead to mechanical discomfort, easy satiety, portal hypertension, and cachexia. Marrow fibrosis is another expected event

TABLE 26-2 THE COMPLICATIONS OF POLYCYTHEMIA VERA

Complication	Cause
• Thrombosis, hemorrhage, hypertension	• Elevated red cell mass, decreased vWF multimers
• Organomegaly	• Extramedullary hematopoiesis or elevated red cell mass
• Pruritus, acid-peptic disease	• Inflammatory mediators
• Erythromelalgia	• Thrombocytosis
• Hyperuricemia, gout, renal stones	• Increased cell turnover
• Myelofibrosis	• Reaction to the neoplastic clone
• Acute leukemia	• Therapy-induced or clonal evolution

in the natural history of PV. It is essential to distinguish between the development of increased marrow reticulin as a consequence of marrow cell hyperplasia and the hematopoietic stem cell disorder, PMF. There is no evidence that myelofibrosis in PV represents a bad prognostic sign or that it impairs marrow function in the absence of exposure to agents that damage the bone marrow; it is stem cell failure that is the problem. Rarely, pulmonary hypertension has developed with long-standing disease; in some patients this may be due to extramedullary hematopoiesis, while in others there may be pulmonary fibrosis.

Spontaneous acute leukemia develops in PV at an incidence of approximately 1.5%–2.5%; this usually occurs within the first 8 years of the disease and most commonly in patients older than 60 years. Chemotherapy or radiation-induced acute leukemia occurs at rates as high as 10% when these patients are exposed to ^{32}P or alkylating agents. The role of hydroxyurea as a leukemogen has been a matter of debate, but in one randomized prospective clinical trial (6, 7), hydroxyurea was associated with a 10% incidence of acute leukemia after 10 years; hydroxyurea is also a proven tumor promoter when used in conjunction with ^{32}P or an alkylating agent or with UV light exposure.

■ TREATMENT

PV is generally an indolent disease in which survival is measured in decades in the majority of patients. Most estimates of disease survival have failed to take into account the toxic forms of therapy that have been generally employed, the inadequate use of phlebotomy, and the later stages at which the disease was previously recognized clinically. Furthermore, it is now apparent that PV is a heterogenous disorder with both indolent and aggressive forms and that aggressive chemotherapy has not improved survival (8). There is currently no curative therapy for PV with the possible exception of allogeneic bone marrow transplantation, a therapy not suitable for the older patients who most commonly develop this disorder (9). Thus, treatment should be tailored to disease manifestations. Unfortunately, in contrast to PMF, prognostic risk stratification according to laboratory features has not yet been possible with the exception that a prior history of thrombosis is an adverse risk factor for recurrent thrombotic events.

Erythrocytosis is the greatest initial threat to health because of the adverse effects of hyperviscosity (thrombosis, hemorrhage, hypertension, headache, and impaired cognitive function). Therefore, the red cell mass should be lowered by phlebotomy to achieve a hematocrit of ≤42% (hemoglobin ≤12 g%) in women and ≤45% (hemoglobin ≤14 g%) in men (8). This can be done quickly in all but the frailest because phlebotomy stimulates rapid plasma volume expansion. Repeated phlebotomies will be necessary to maintain the hematocrit at a normal level and to induce iron deficiency, but once this is achieved, the need for phlebotomy will diminish. Phlebotomy therapy actually improves platelet function, does not contribute significantly to thrombocytosis, and does not lead to myelofibrosis, and it must be remembered that the higher the hematocrit, the greater the extent of tissue damage with thrombosis (8). Pruritus, usually aquagenic, is a distressing symptom in approximately 30% of patients. There is no single effective remedy. Phlebotomy, antihistamines, PUVA light therapy, interferon alpha, and hydroxyurea have all been effective but none uniformly. Hyperuricemia (uric acid >10 mg/dL) responds well to allopurinol.

Platelet-related microvascular complications include migraine, visual auras, transient ischemic attacks, erythromelalgia, and digital infarction. Aspirin is a specific remedy for erythromelalgia but with migraine, it may be necessary to lower the platelet count as well to achieve relief using conventional remedies. Symptomatic thrombocytosis causing acquired von Willebrand's disease will also require platelet count reduction. Asymptomatic thrombocytosis without a significant reduction in ristocetin cofactor activity (<30%) requires no treatment in the absence of a thrombotic risk factor. In this regard, it is important to emphasize that there is no correlation between the platelet count and thrombosis, and no study to date has demonstrated that in the absence of hematocrit control, platelet count reduction prevents arterial or venous thrombosis. Hydroxyurea does appear to be more effective than anagrelide in the prevention of transient ischemic attacks but not venous or arterial thrombosis. The use of prophylactic low dose aspirin therapy is no substitute for adequate control of the red cell mass and has not been demonstrated to have clinical efficacy in asymptomatic PV patients who are adequately phlebotomized.

Control of extramedullary hematopoiesis involving the spleen and liver is the most challenging therapeutic problem in PV but fortunately not one that involves every patient. Interferon alpha, and its pegylated congener in particular, is the drug of choice for this because it lacks the potential for bone marrow damage (10). A recent study demonstrated that durable molecular remissions could be achieved with pegylated interferon (11). Since interferon's side effects can be significant with chronic use, in the absence of a complete molecular remission, intermittent use is a prudent strategy. In some patients, splenomegaly may be refractory to interferon and chemotherapy, and mechanical discomfort, cachexia, and portal hypertension will demand treatment. If bone marrow transplantation is not an option, the newly approved nonspecific JAK2 inhibitor, ruxolitinib, is the drug of choice in this situation (see the primary myelofibrosis chapter). Low-dose thalidomide is another option worth considering with surgery as the choice of last resort because of the high complication rate associated with it. The postoperative complications of splenectomy include wound dehiscence, hernias, bleeding, portal or mesenteric vein thrombosis, exuberant hepatic extramedullary hematopoiesis, and extreme leukocytosis and thrombocytosis, all of which can be very difficult to control. Splenic irradiation is only a temporary solution and not advisable unless surgery is not an option (12).

■ PREGNANCY

The opportunity for pregnancy should not be denied to women with PV who have no medical contraindications and prior thrombosis is not one of these. The major threat to a successful outcome is failure to maintain the red cell mass at a safe level. Since there is an expansion of the plasma volume with pregnancy normally, there will be masking of the expanded red cell mass. A normal hematocrit in a pregnant woman is never normal and this is doubly true in PV. It is essential to phlebotomize these patients to a hematocrit of <33% and avoid iron supplements; folic acid supplementation is mandatory. Thrombocytosis and splenomegaly may mandate the use of interferon alpha. Given the elevation of von Willebrand factor that occurs during pregnancy, aspirin therapy may be prudent but this is unproved.

PRIMARY MYELOFIBROSIS

■ INTRODUCTION

Primary myelofibrosis (PMF) is the least common and most enigmatic of the chronic myeloproliferative disorders. Most frequent after age 60 years, PMF has an incidence of approximately 1/100,000 with male predominance. Previously known as agnogenic myeloid metaplasia, idiopathic myelofibrosis, primary osteomyelofibrosis, or myelofibrosis with myeloid metaplasia, it is important to note that both the first and last appellations actually describe a pathologic process that is not restricted to the disease PMF but can be caused by a variety of benign and malignant processes (Table 26-3). Like its companion myeloproliferative disorders, PV and essential thrombocytosis, PMF is a clonal hematopoietic stem cell disorder, but in contrast to them, it is associated not only with overproduction of blood cells without an obvious cause but also, in many patients, with anemia, leucopenia, or thrombocytopenia.

■ PATHOGENESIS

The etiology of PMF is unknown. Although irradiation and exposure to organic chemicals such as toluene and benzene can cause marrow fibrosis,

TABLE 26-3 DISORDERS CAUSING MYELOFIBROSIS

Malignant
Acute leukemia (lymphocytic, myelogenous, megakaryocytic)
Chronic myelogenous leukemia
Hairy cell leukemia
Hodgkin disease
Idiopathic myelofibrosis
Lymphoma
Multiple myeloma
Myelodysplasia
Metastatic carcinoma
Polycythemia vera
Systemic mastocytosis
Nonmalignant
HIV infection
Hyperparathyroidism
Renal osteodystrophy
Systemic lupus erythematosus
Tuberculosis
Vitamin D deficiency
Thorium dioxide exposure
Gray platelet syndrome

no other consistent environmental risk factors have been identified for PMF and familial transmission is rare. Cytogenetic abnormalities occur in more than 50% of patients but generally involve the same chromosomes as in PV and essential thrombocytosis, and none appear to be involved in its pathogenesis. Myelofibrosis is the hallmark of the disorder, but there is good retrospective histologic evidence that a premyelofibrotic phase of the disease exists (13), supporting other evidence that the fibrosis is a consequence of the disease, not its cause.

Normally, hematopoiesis is extravascular, and hematopoietic progenitor cell proliferation and differentiation in the marrow are supported by accessory cells such as macrophages, adipocytes, reticulum cells, fibroblasts, and endothelial cells, all of which are embedded in an extracellular matrix of collagens. PMF represents the deposition of additional collagen fibrils that are thicker and contiguous. The earliest phase of marrow fibrosis is the deposition of reticulin, which represents collagen fibrils coated with matrix substances such as hyaluronic acid that are argyrophilic and stain with silver. As the quantity of collagen increases relative to matrix substances, the fibrils eventually become reactive with the classical histological collagen stains.

Osteosclerosis in PMF represents only the deposition of minerals on the marrow trabeculae as opposed to the combined osteoblastic and osteoclastic activity that characterizes metabolic bone disease, and is thought to be due to overproduction of osteoprotegerin, which is an osteoclast inhibitor. With advancing myelofibrosis, there is also a reduction in the number of hematopoietic cells in the marrow with the exception of the megakaryocytes. Disease duration, spleen size, and prognosis do not correlate with the degree of myelofibrosis or the type of collagen staining pattern.

The stimulus for the marrow fibrosis and osteosclerosis that are central features of PMF are not entirely understood, but both megakaryocytes and monocytes appear to be involved through the elaboration of the fibrogenic cytokines, particularly TGF-β and thrombopoietin. Animal models of myelofibrosis and osteosclerosis, which have been created by overexpression of thrombopoietin, impaired expression of the hematopoietic transcription factor GATA-1, or transplantation of hematopoietic cells overexpressing JAK2 V617F, further implicate megakaryocytes and other hematopoietic progenitor cells in these processes.

Importantly, a variety of techniques have been employed to definitively demonstrate that the fibroblastic component of PMF is not monoclonal but rather reactive, in contrast to the hematopoietic cells in this disorder, which are clonal and primary. The latter exhibit the hematopoietic growth factor hypersensitivity and growth factor-independent in vitro colony-forming activity that is characteristic of all three chronic myeloproliferative disorders. Bone marrow neoangiogenesis is another characteristic feature of PMF that is thought to be due to increased VEGF production.

■ CLINICAL FEATURES

As with the other chronic myeloproliferative disorders, PMF may first be recognized during a routine health maintenance evaluation due to abnormal blood counts or a palpable spleen. However, in contrast to the other chronic myeloproliferative disorders, PMF can present with significant constitutional symptoms such as fever, night sweats, anorexia, pruritus, weakness, fatigue, and weight loss. In some patients, particularly men, thrombocytosis alone may be the first manifestation of the disease and, less commonly, isolated leukocytosis. In general, the cases of so-called essential thrombocytosis take approximately 4–7 years to develop the complete myelofibrosis phenotype, but in these patients, bone marrow examination may initially reveal changes inconsistent with the diagnosis of essential thrombocytosis. This situation has been designated as the cellular or premyelofibrotic phase of PMF (13).

Palpable splenomegaly, which can be modest or extreme, is the most common clinical finding, but occasionally patients are encountered before palpable splenomegaly has developed, putting them in a diagnostic limbo. Hepatomegaly is less common and not seen in the absence of splenomegaly. Lymphadenopathy is very uncommon and, when localized, should suggest another diagnosis.

■ LABORATORY ABNORMALITIES

Any combination of blood count abnormalities can be encountered in PMF. Anemia is the most common abnormality, and a normal hematocrit in a patient with splenomegaly should suggest the presence of PV; indeed, retrospectively approximately 10% of patients in most published series of PMF actually had PV. The anemia is usually normochromic and normocytic and a hemolytic component is rare. Folic acid deficiency, however, can complicate the disorder due to an increased turnover of marrow cells. Leukocytosis is common but not usually to the degree found in chronic myelogenous leukemia. The platelet count is usually normal or elevated, but modest thrombocytopenia can be seen in approximately 25% of patients. Nucleated red blood cells, myelocytes, promyelocytes, and even blast cells may be present in the blood, creating the classical leukoerythroblastic blood picture. Tear drop-shaped red cells reflect the presence of splenomegaly. The leukocyte alkaline phosphatase can be low, normal, or high. With hepatic extramedullary hematopoiesis, the serum alkaline phosphatase will be increased. The JAK2 V617F mutation occurs in approximately 50% of PMF patients and is often homozygous in its expression, but this abnormality does not correlate with disease activity. The more important abnormality, which does correlate with disease phenotype, is clonal dominance by the malignant clone. Platelet function abnormalities in PMF parallel those in the other chronic myeloproliferative disorders, but PMF patients are particularly prone to bleeding (14).

Bone marrow is inaspirable when there is marrow fibrosis, necessitating a biopsy. The bone marrow biopsy in PMF may reveal a hypercellular marrow with myeloid hyperplasia, an increase in large dysplastic megakaryocytes occurring in clusters and, in some patients, widening of the bony trabecula. An increase in collagen and osteoid deposition, sinusoidal dilatation, neoangiogenesis with extramedullary hematopoiesis, and a reduction in cellularity with erythroid islands and megakaryocyte sparing may also be encountered. The reticulin stain will show a dense pattern of argyrophilic fibers in a contiguous pattern with sinusoidal accentuation. If collagen deposition is extensive, the trichrome stain will be positive. It is important to remember, however, that marrow histology is not uniform with respect to biopsy sampling, and marrow histology cannot be relied on to stage this disorder.

■ **RADIOLOGIC ABNORMALITIES**

Osteosclerosis but not myelofibrosis can be detected radiologically, most commonly as an increase in medullary bone density in the proximal long bones. Rib and vertebral involvement are also common and even the skull can be affected. The presence of radiologically evident osteosclerosis suggests involvement of at least 40% of the marrow cavity and is related to the extent of the myelofibrosis and splenomegaly but not disease duration or prognosis. Hypertrophic osteoarthropathy with painful periostitis and onion skinning of the tibiae is an uncommon complication of PMF and could be another consequence of the neoangiogenesis that characterizes this disorder.

■ **CYTOGENETIC ABNORMALITIES**

Cytogenetic abnormalities are more common in PMF than in its companion myeloproliferative disorders, but they are mostly nonspecific. They include 20q-, 13q-, trisomy 8, trisomy 9, partial trisomy 1q, 5q-, -5, 7q-, -7, 12p-, i(17q), and 9p reduplication. In contrast to its companion myeloproliferative disorders, however, trisomy 8 and 12p- as well as certain complex chromosomal abnormalities appear to confer a poor prognosis in PMF (15).

■ **DIAGNOSIS**

Given the inability to aspirate bone marrow when myelofibrosis is present, distinguishing PMF from the many other disorders that cause myelofibrosis (Table 26-3) is a difficult task. Clinical criteria have been formulated to facilitate this (Table 26-4), but they are either inadequate or uncritical.

TABLE 26-4 DIAGNOSTIC CRITERIA FOR MYELOFIBROSIS WITH MYELOID METAPLASIA

Necessary criteria

1) Diffuse bone marrow fibrosis
2) Absence of the Philadelphia chromosome or BCR-ABL rearrangement in peripheral blood cells

Optional criteria

1) Splenomegaly of any grade
2) Anisopoikilocytosis with teardrop erythrocytes
3) Presence of circulating immature myeloid cells
4) Presence of circulating erythroblasts
5) Presence of clusters of megakaryocytes and anomalous megakaryocytes in bone marrow biopsy sections
6) Myeloid metaplasia
   A diagnosis of MMM is acceptable if the following combinations are present: the two necessary criteria plus any other two optional criteria when splenomegaly is present; the two necessary criteria plus any four optional criteria when splenomegaly is absent

---

(From Italian consensus conference on diagnostic criteria for myelofibrosis with myeloid metaplasia. *Br J Haematol.* 1999; 104: 730–737.)

TABLE 26-5 CAUSES OF EXTRAMEDULLARY HEMATOPOIESIS AND A LEUKOERYTHROBLASTIC REACTION

Carcinoma metastatic to the bone marrow
Lymphoma involving the bone marrow
Idiopathic myelofibrosis
Polycythemia vera
Chronic myelogenous leukemia
Myelodysplasia
Acute hepatic injury
Hemolytic anemia

For example, the presence of extramedullary hematopoiesis as defined by circulating nucleated red cells and myelocytes is a feature of many disorders other than PMF (Table 26-5). Although splenomegaly has been considered an optional diagnostic criterion in one classification, splenomegaly is present in over 90% of patients at the time of diagnosis. Thus, at a minimum, in the absence of splenomegaly, it is probably not possible to distinguish PMF clinically from the many disorders that mimic it.

The most important disorders with respect to differential diagnosis are chronic myelogenous leukemia, PV, acute myelofibrosis, myelodysplasia, hairy cell leukemia, primary bone marrow lymphomas, multiple myeloma, metastatic carcinoma, and systemic mastocytosis. The most difficult of this group to identify are acute myelofibrosis and myelodysplasia with myelofibrosis. The former is a rapidly progressive form of acute leukemia, which can have extramedullary hematopoiesis without palpable splenomegaly; the latter is somewhat more indolent but carries an equally poor prognosis. In either instance, an increase in marrow blast cells, micromegakaryocytes, specific chromosome abnormalities, and an increase in marrow CD34+ cells favor an acute myeloid malignancy or myelodysplasia rather than PMF, in which there is an increase in circulating CD34+ cells (16).

The JAK2 V617F mutation can be used to distinguish PMF from chronic myelogenous leukemia and nonmyeloid hematopoietic malignancies in approximately 50% of cases; absence of the mutation, however, is not helpful. From a diagnostic perspective, bone marrow aspiration and biopsy with cytogenetics, flow cytometry using peripheral blood, marrow immunohistochemistry with respect to CD34+ cells, and a JAK2 V617F assay should suffice to differentiate PMF from the other disorders that mimic it.

■ NATURAL HISTORY

The natural history of PMF is highly variable. In its most aggressive form, there is progressive bone marrow failure with expanding extramedullary hematopoiesis. The consequences of this include splenic and hepatic enlargement, portal hypertension, anemia, thrombocytopenia, leukocytosis or leukopenia, hyperuricemia, cachexia, and in some patients, pulmonary hypertension or transformation to acute leukemia. The actuarial frequency of transformation in one series was 21% at 8 years, a frequency much higher than in PV or essential thrombocytosis. No organ or body cavity is immune

TABLE 26-6 INTERNATIONAL PROGNOSTIC SCORING SYSTEM FOR PMF

Staging Risk Factors

Age >65 y

Constitutional symptoms

Hemoglobin <10 g%

WBC >25,000/µl

Circulating blast cells ≥1%

Scoring System

Risk Group	Risk Score	Median Survival (Months)
Low	0	135
Intermediate-1	1	95
Intermediate-2	2	48
High	3	27

(From Reference 18.)

to the development of extramedullary hematopoiesis, which can invade the lymph nodes, kidneys, adrenals, ovaries, dura, spinal canal, skin, mediastinum, mesentery, pulmonary parenchyma, and the pleural, peritoneal, and retroperitoneal spaces (17). Progressive, disseminated extramedullary hematopoiesis can also be a harbinger of leukemic transformation. Fortunately, however, this scenario is not the fate of every patient.

Although previous estimates of survival indicated that life expectancy in this disorder was distinctly inferior to its companion myeloproliferative disorders, subsequent studies have indicated that PMF is not a monolithic illness and, with risk stratification, it has been possible to identify patients whose disease is indolent rather than progressive. For this purpose, two useful risk stratification schemes have recently been proposed: the first for risk stratification at diagnosis (the International Prognostic Scoring System [IPSS]) (18) (Table 26-6), and the second during the course of the disease (the Dynamic IPSS plus [DIPPS plus]) (15). Age >65 years, anemia (hemoglobin <10 g/dL), leukocyte count (>25,000/ml), circulating blast cell count (≥1%), and constitutional symptoms are the criteria for IPSS risk stratification, a scoring system similar to that employed for risk stratification in myelodysplasia. The DIPSS plus adds thrombocytopenia (platelets <100,000/ml), transfusion dependence, and unfavorable cytogenetics. JAK2 V617F expression correlated only with older age at diagnosis and a history of thrombosis or pruritus but not prognosis, while the impact on prognosis of newly described but low frequency mutations in PMF has not yet been assessed.

■ TREATMENT

There is no specific therapy for PMF and allogeneic bone marrow transplantation is the only potentially curative therapy. Unfortunately, this approach has been most effective in patients under age 45 years with good prognosis disease, and when viewed with the context of the DIPSS plus, survival correlated with the scoring stage with the low-risk patients faring better than all other groups. Transplant-related mortality was high at 28%; relapse-free survival was 100% at 5 years in low-risk patients, but was 51%, 54%, and 30% for int-1, int-2, and high-risk patients, respectively, which was not better or even worse than their intrinsic natural history (19). Recently, reduced intensity conditioning was found to decrease transplant-related mortality and achieve remission rates of greater than 70% (20). However, prospective studies will be required to establish the most effective conditioning regimen (21). Splenomegaly and myelofibrosis per se did not appear to impact negatively on engraftment.

Bone marrow failure and progressive splenomegaly are the two most pressing problems in the management of PMF. Anemia is the most common problem and can be multifarious with respect to etiology, which can include hemodilution, blood loss, hemolysis, and folic acid or vitamin B_6 deficiency. In patients with constitutional symptoms, prednisone therapy may be effective in alleviating anemia as well as the constitutional symptoms since a cytokine storm of varying extent is a feature of PMF. If the serum erythropoietin level is less than 125 mU/ml, a trial of recombinant erythropoietin is worthwhile with the caveat that this could increase spleen or liver size. Impeded androgens such as danazol have been tried in this situation with modest success, but these agents have side effects that make their long-term use unattractive and much of their benefit may actually be virtual since these agents also contract the plasma volume.

Progressive splenomegaly with or without hepatomegaly is a difficult therapeutic problem in PMF since it gives rise to mechanical problems such as early satiety, diarrhea, abdominal discomfort, sequestration of leukocytes and platelets, splenic infarction, portal hypertension, and esophageal varices. Cachexia is an inevitable complication. A number of therapies have been tried in this situation, including low-dose alkylating agents, hydroxyurea, interferon alpha, imatinib mesylate, and thalidomide. Alkylating agents such as busulfan and melphalan at doses of 2–4 mg/day have proved effective but have the potential for substantial hematologic and nonhematologic toxicity and are also leukemogenic; their use should be reserved for specific situations where other remedies have not been effective. Hydroxyurea is effective in controlling leukocytosis and thrombocytosis but can exacerbate anemia. Neither interferon nor imatinib has proved effective in advanced PMF, but the former may be effective in the early stages of the disorder. However, both appear to have substantial toxicity in this group of patients. Thalidomide at low doses in combination with prednisone has proved to be effective in ameliorating anemia as well as thrombocytopenia in PMF patients and also reducing spleen size in approximately 20% (22). Lenolidamide has also been used in PMF with minimal success but has the disadvantage of being myelotoxic in contrast to thalidomide. Low-dose alkylating agents have also been used but are myelotoxic and genotoxic, particularly if used with hydroxyurea.

The most important therapeutic advance for PMF patients is the recent development of nonspecific JAK2 inhibitors, the first of which, ruxolitinib (Jakafi), has been FDA approved for patients with advanced disease, regardless of the presence of a JAK2 mutation (23, 24). Given orally with a recommended starting dose of 15 mg bid, ruxolitinib has proved effective in reducing splenomegaly by approximately 35% in at least 50% of patients and alleviating constitutional symptoms by suppressing inflammatory cytokine production with improvement in exercise tolerance and weight gain in up to 50% of patients. Symptomatic improvement and reduction in spleen size can be seen within 12 weeks with a durable effect as long as the drug is continued. Ruxolitinib's major toxicity is marrow suppression with the exacerbation or induction of anemia or thrombocytopenia. Discontinuation of the drug will also lead to the reappearance of constitutional symptoms within 7 days, and thus, the drug should be tapered slowly or the use of glucocorticoids considered should the cytokine rebound be severe. To date, ruxolitinib has had no significant impact on the JAK2 V617F allelic burden or the size of the malignant stem cell pool. Nevertheless, it is an important new therapy, which should reduce the need for splenectomy and improve the lives of PMF patients without the risk of increasing genetic instability in the involved hematopoietic stem cell clone, as may occur with hydroxyurea.

In some patients, splenectomy may be necessary for massive splenomegaly because of the failure of other treatment options. This is a major undertaking with significant postoperative complications including hemorrhage, splenic vein thrombosis, infection, hepatomegaly, exuberant leukocytosis or thrombocytosis, and abdominal hernias. Neither anemia nor thrombocytopenia is significantly improved in most patients. In one series, the incidence of acute leukemia increased postsplenectomy. Splenic irradiation has been employed in patients thought to be unfit for surgery. This is often effective in reducing spleen size and ameliorating symptoms temporarily and can be repeated, although not always with the same result. However, myelosuppression is frequent and the mortality rate as a consequence can be as high as 50%. By contrast, irradiation can be useful in controlling localized soft tissue sites of extramedullary hematopoiesis or periostitis. In summary, lacking specific therapy for PMF, treatment in this disorder must be tailored to the individual patient.

ESSENTIAL THROMBOCYTOSIS

■ INTRODUCTION

Essential thrombocytosis (ET) is the most nebulous of the chronic myeloproliferative disorders, since its only identifying marker, thrombocytosis, is not specific for it. Like PMF and PV, ET is a clonal disorder involving a multipotent hematopoietic stem cell. However, unlike its companion myeloproliferative disorders, hematopoiesis is not globally disturbed, women predominate, and overall life span is superior. The frequency of ET is approximately 2/100,000. The frequency of the disorder increases with age with a mean age at diagnosis of 51 years. In women, the incidence appears to be biphasic with a peak at age 50 years and a second at age 70 years.

■ PATHOGENESIS

The etiology of ET is unknown. Although thrombopoietin is essential for the survival of primitive hematopoietic stem cells, overproduction of thrombopoietin does not recapitulate ET in animal models or in familial thrombocytosis due to mutations in the 5′ UTR of the thrombopoietin gene or the thrombopoietin receptor gene (MPL). In contrast to PV, where the plasma level of erythropoietin is severely reduced due to the expansion of the red cell mass, in ET, the thrombopoietin level is normal or elevated despite expansion of the megakaryocyte mass, preventing its distinction from secondary forms of thrombocytosis on this basis.

A number of epigenetic abnormalities found in PV and PMF, such as increased expression of granulocyte PRV-1 mRNA and reduced expression of the thrombopoietin receptor, Mpl, in megakaryocytes and platelets, are also found in ET. Cytogenetic abnormalities similar to those found in PV and PMF are also present in ET, but at a much lower frequency. The frequency of the JAK2 V617F mutation is also lower in this disorder than in the other chronic myeloproliferative disorders, and homozygosity for the mutation is rarely present. Some investigators have claimed that ET patients expressing JAK2 V617F have a "PV-like" phenotype. However, a consistent failure on the part of these investigators to exclude PV by performing a red cell mass determination renders these claims specious.

■ CLINICAL FEATURES

First recognized in 1920, ET has been known by a variety of names, including hemorrhagic thrombocythemia, idiopathic thrombocytosis, and primary thrombocytosis. This ambivalence reflects the lack of a specific diagnostic marker for ET and the fact that the thrombocytosis can be associated with either thrombosis or hemorrhage. Furthermore, with the advent of electronic particle counters, thrombocytosis is now being recognized in individuals who are asymptomatic. This was most often true in women and did not vary with age. Microvascular occlusive syndromes such as migraine, transient ischemic attacks, visual disturbances, dizziness, or erythromelalgia are the most common presenting complaints but are, of course, not specific for the disease. Hemorrhage, usually involving the mucous membranes and generally mild, has been more common in some series than thrombotic episodes, which could be arterial or, less frequently, venous. Interestingly, hemorrhage was more common with platelet counts greater than $1,000,000/\mu l$, and thrombosis when the platelet count was lower.

The physical examination in ET is usually normal. Splenomegaly is present in less than 30% of reported patients at diagnosis and even then is minimal in extent. Significant splenomegaly, isolated hepatomegaly, or lymphadenopathy should suggest another cause for the thrombocytosis.

■ LABORATORY ABNORMALITIES

Thrombocytosis is the major laboratory abnormality in ET with the platelet count averaging $1,000,000/\mu l$ or greater in most large studies. It is not possible, however, to distinguish reactive thrombocytosis from ET simply on the basis of platelet number. Anemia is uncommon and usually mild, and an elevated hemoglobin or hematocrit level should suggest PV. A mild neutrophilic leukocytosis is common, but when the leukocyte count is greater than $15,000/\mu l$ or there is significant anemia or a leukoerythroblastic reaction, another diagnosis should be considered. Many patients are iron deficient but paradoxically correction of the deficit usually does not influence the platelet count. Pseudohyperkalemia occurs as a consequence of platelet potassium release during blood clotting when the platelet count is elevated. A very high platelet count can also cause pseudohypoglycemia and hypoxemia if blood for glucose and oxygen tension measurements is not collected on ice and in the presence of a metabolic inhibitor. It is of interest that the serum erythropoietin level can be low in ET, making this test not useful for distinguishing between PV and ET.

Coagulation abnormalities in ET are a consequence of intrinsic platelet abnormalities or the platelet count (25). Abnormalities of platelet structure include an increase in mean platelet volume and distribution width, loss of alpha granules and dense bodies, and disorganization of the platelet microtubular and canalicular systems. Surface expression of CD41 and the thrombopoietin receptor, Mpl, are decreased, while the expression of P-selectin and thrombospondin are increased; the intracellular ADP, PF4, and 5-HT content are reduced. The majority of patients have increased platelet aggregation in response to epinephrine, ristocetin, ADP, and collagen. Paradoxically, however, the bleeding time is increased in less than 20% of patients. Thromboxane excretion is frequently increased and suppressible by salicylate therapy, suggesting continuous intravascular platelet activation. However, there is no correlation between the platelet abnormalities and thrombosis in this disorder.

Acquired von Willebrand's disease is an interesting feature of ET as well as the other chronic myeloproliferative disorders (26). As the platelet count increases, generally above $1,000,000/\mu l$, the platelets adsorb and destroy the highest molecular weight plasma von Willebrand multimers, leading to a reduction in ristocetin cofactor activity. Patients with this abnormality are at risk of bleeding, particularly if exposed to salicylates.

■ CYTOGENETIC ABNORMALITIES

Cytogenetic abnormalities are uncommon in ET and none is pathognomonic for the disorder. The common cytogenetic abnormalities include trisomy 1, 8, 9, and 21, 1q-, 13q-, and 20q-. Since both chronic myelogenous leukemia and the 5q- syndrome can present with thrombocytosis, cytogenetic analysis constitutes an important part of the diagnostic evaluation.

■ DIAGNOSIS

Establishing a diagnosis of ET is more difficult than for the other chronic myeloproliferative disorders because ET lacks any unique identifying characteristics or a specific diagnostic marker, and because thrombocytosis can be the initial manifestation of PV or PMF, either of which may not become clinically apparent for many years after the onset of the thrombocytosis (27, 28). Furthermore, there is as yet no agreement as to what platelet count threshold should be used for the diagnosis of ET. A number of diagnostic criteria have been developed, but they rely on the exclusion of other disorders and their complexity emphasizes the difficulties inherent in the diagnosis of this disease. The extent of the problem can be simply visualized from the number of benign and malignant disorders that can cause thrombocytosis (Table 26-7). Furthermore, it is apparent from epidemiologic

TABLE 26-7 CAUSES OF THROMBOCYTOSIS

Tissue inflammation
Collagen vascular disease, inflammatory bowel disease
Malignancy
Infection
Myeloproliferative disorders
Polycythemia vera, idiopathic myelofibrosis, essential thrombocytosis, chronic myelogenous leukemia
Myelodysplastic disorders
5q- syndrome, idiopathic refractory sideroblastic anemia
Postsplenectomy, or hyposplenism
Hemorrhage
Iron deficiency anemia
Surgery
Rebound
Correction of vitamin B_{12} or folate deficiency, post-ethanol abuse
Hemolysis
Familial
Thrombopoietin overproduction, constitutive Mpl activation

studies of JAK2 V617F expression, platelet Mpl expression, and clonality that there is substantial heterogeneity among ET patients with respect to these abnormalities and, except for lack of JAK2 V617F homozygosity, no specificity. Attempts to distinguish the cellular phase of PMF from ET solely on the basis of bone marrow morphology have not been convincing, but a JAK2 V617F allele burden greater than 50%, anemia, significant leukocytosis (>15,000/μl), or a leukoerythroblastic reaction should suggest the presence of a different myeloproliferative disorder (29).

From a prognostic prospective, the most serious illnesses associated with thrombocytosis that need to be excluded are chronic myelogenous leukemia, myelodysplasia (5q- syndrome), sideroblastic anemia, PMF, and PV. It also needs to be emphasized that chronic myelogenous leukemia can present with isolated thrombocytosis alone in the absence of leukocytosis or basophilia. From this perspective, a bone marrow aspirate and biopsy for morphology, flow cytometry, cytogenetics, and peripheral blood FISH for bcr-abl, since this can be positive in the absence of the Philadelphia chromosome, are the essential diagnostic tests. A negative assay for JAK2 V617F does not exclude the diagnosis of ET, nor does its presence have any implications with respect to diagnosis or the clinical course.

■ **NATURAL HISTORY**

Most but not all studies of ET have found that life span was not significantly different from the general population. A recent study of low-risk ET suggests that the most important risk factor for thrombosis in ET is tobacco use, particularly in the presence of cardiovascular risk factors. Otherwise, the traditional risk factors including age ≥60 years, prior thrombosis, and leukocytosis (>15,000/μl) were not predictive (30). Additionally, rates of venous thrombosis were higher in women than men. Importantly, regardless of the type of therapy employed, the risk of thrombosis appeared to reach a plateau after 9 years. A platelet count of 1,000,000/µl or greater is the major risk factor for hemorrhage. Transformation to myelofibrosis or PV occurs in approximately 20% of patients over the first decade after diagnosis (27, 28). Spontaneous leukemic transformation occurs but is uncommon and most instances are a consequence of myelotoxic drug exposure.

■ TREATMENT

The first rule of therapy for ET is accuracy in diagnosis, particularly because life span is generally not reduced in this disease and its treatment differs from the other chronic myeloproliferative disorders it mimics. The second rule of therapy is to do no harm. Stated differently, the treatment cannot be worse than the disease. Thrombosis, either macrovascular or microvascular, is the major impediment to health in ET, but there is no correlation between the height of the platelet count and thrombosis, rendering problematic the formulation of a treatment endpoint on that basis. In general, patients with ET who have had a prior major vessel thrombosis should be treated no differently with respect to anticoagulation and risk factor reduction than their counterparts with a normal platelet count. The most difficult decision then becomes how best to manage the platelet count (31).

Patients with ET under age 60 years, who have no cardiovascular risk factors or a prior thrombosis, are not at a greater risk of thrombosis than their age-matched counterparts with a normal platelet count (30, 32). Treatment in these patients should be directed at the alleviation of microvascular symptoms such as ocular migraine or erythromelalgia. Aspirin is a specific remedy for these and can be given daily or on as needed basis. Ibuprofen can be substituted if a shorter acting agent is required. When the platelet count is greater than 1,000,000/µl, ristocetin cofactor activity should be measured before using either agent in a symptomatic patient and, if reduced, platelet count reduction rather than platelet inactivation will be necessary. In some patients, particularly those with migraine, platelet inactivation may not be sufficient to control symptoms. The safest method to lower the platelet count then becomes the major issue.

Current therapy for controlling the platelet count includes hydroxyurea, anagrelide, interferon alpha, alkylating agents, and ^{32}P. All of these agents are usually effective but each has distinct disadvantages. The most serious of these is myelotoxicity leading to acute leukemia, which has been demonstrated unequivocally for the alkylating agents and ^{32}P. Whether hydroxyurea is leukemogenic has been a matter of debate. It also enhances the leukemogenic effect of the alkylating agents and ^{32}P, whether given before or after them. Since the use of chemotherapeutic agents has not been shown to improve longevity in the chronic myeloproliferative disorders, their use should not be routine but restricted to situations where other forms of therapy have been ineffective.

Two randomized clinical trials provide some guidance to this end. In a study of ET patients older than 60 years, hydroxyurea was not more effective than aspirin in preventing arterial thrombosis (33) and failed to prevent venous thrombosis. In a much larger study of high-risk patients with thrombocytosis taking aspirin, in whom the platelet count was normalized, hydroxyurea was not more effective than anagrelide in preventing arterial thrombosis and was actually less effective in preventing venous thrombosis. Hydroxyurea was, however, more effective in preventing transient ischemic attacks (34) because it is a nitric oxide donor. Therefore, in patients over age 60 years who have risk factors for thrombosis and who are experiencing transient ischemic attacks, hydroxyurea is the drug of choice. Otherwise, a safer alternative such as interferon alpha or anagrelide should be used when there is a clinical indication to lower the platelet count. In the case of both, given the side effects associated with long-term use, their use should be intermittent if possible (35). If long-term use is planned, periodic cardiac monitoring is also indicated. Finally, the combination of aspirin and anagrelide has been associated with an increased incidence of gastrointestinal hemorrhage (34).

Acquired von Willebrand syndrome caused by thrombocytosis requires no treatment unless there is a need for surgery or the patient experiences spontaneous bleeding (26). In this instance, platelet count reduction will be required. In an emergent situation, platelet pheresis can be employed but this is not a particularly efficient approach when there is extreme thrombocytosis. Administration of epsilon aminocaproic acid is an effective remedy for bleeding in this situation.

■ PREGNANCY

Special mention needs to be made about pregnancy since ET is so common in young women. Pregnancy has an ameliorating effect on the thrombocytosis in this disorder and, while first trimester abortions are increased, there is no correlation between platelet count and obstetrical complications. No specific therapeutic intervention has been proved to be uniformly effective, but low-dose aspirin has been recommended as prophylactic therapy and, when there has been prior thrombosis, low-molecular-weight heparin. Interferon alpha can also be given safely during pregnancy if platelet count reduction is necessary. Perhaps the most important recommendation is to be sure that the patient does not actually have PV. Stated differently, a normal hematocrit in a pregnant woman with ET should suggest the presence of PV.

REFERENCES

1. Gangat N, Strand J, Lasho TL, et al. Cytogenetic studies at diagnosis in polycythemia vera: clinical and JAK2V617F allele burden correlates. *Eur J Haematol*. 2008; 80: 197–200.

2. Vainchenker W, Dusa A, Constantinescu SN. JAKs in pathology: role of Janus kinases in hematopoietic malignancies and immunodeficiencies. *Semin Cell Dev Biol*. 2008; 19: 385–393.

3. Johansson PL, Safai-Kutti S, Kutti J. An elevated venous haemoglobin concentration cannot be used as a surrogate marker for absolute erythrocytosis: a study of patients with polycythaemia vera and apparent polycythaemia. *Br J Haematol*. 2005; 129: 701–705.

4. Lamy T, Devillers A, Bernard M, et al. Inapparent polycythemia vera: an unrecognized diagnosis. *Am J Med*. 1997; 102: 14–20.

5. Beer PA, Delhommeau F, Lecouedic JP, et al. Two routes to leukemic transformation following a JAK2 mutation-positive myeloproliferative neoplasm. *Blood.* 2010; 115: 2891–2900.

6. Najean Y, Rain J. Treatment of polycythemia vera: the use of hydroxyurea and pipobroman in 292 patients under the age of 65 years. *Blood.* 1997; 90: 3370–3377.

7. Kiladjian JJ, Chevret S, Dosquet C, et al. Treatment of polycythemia vera with hydroxyurea and pipobroman: final results of a randomized trial initiated in 1980. *J Clin Oncol.* 2011; 29: 3907–3913.

8. Spivak JL. Polycythemia vera myths, mechanisms, and management. *Blood.* 2002; 100: 4272–4290.

9. Ballen KK, Woolfrey AE, Zhu X, et al. Allogeneic hematopoietic cell transplantation for advanced polycythemia vera and essential thrombocythemia. *Biol Blood Marrow Transplant.* 2012; 18: 1446–1454.

10. Silver RT. Treatment of polycythemia vera with recombinant interferon alpha (rifnalpha) or imatinib mesylate. *Curr Hematol Rep.* 2005; 4: 235–237.

11. Kiladjian JJ, Cassinat B, Chevret S, et al. Pegylated interferon-alfa-2a induces complete hematologic and molecular responses with low toxicity in polycythemia vera. *Blood.* 2008; 112: 3065–3072.

12. Elliott MA, Chen MG, Silverstein MN, Tefferi A. Splenic irradiation for symptomatic splenomegaly associated with myelofibrosis with myeloid metaplasia. *Br J Haematol.* 1998; 103: 505–511.

13. Thiele J, Kvasnicka HM, Mullauer L, et al. Essential thrombocythemia versus early primary myelofibrosis: a multicenter study to validate the WHO classification. *Blood.* 2011; 117: 5710–5718.

14. Murphy S, Davis JL, Walsh PN, Gardner FH. Template bleeding time and clinical hemorrhage in myeloproliferative disease. *Arch Intern Med.* 1978; 138: 1251–1253.

15. Gangat N, Caramazza D, Vaidya R, et al. DIPSS Plus: A refined dynamic international prognostic scoring system for primary myelofibrosis that incorporates prognostic information from karyotype, platelet count, and transfusion status. *J Clin Oncol.* 2011; 29: 392–397.

16. Barosi G, Hoffman R. Idiopathic myelofibrosis. *Semin Hematol.* 2005; 42: 248–258.

17. Rumi E, Passamonti F, Boveri E, et al. Dyspnea secondary to pulmonary hematopoiesis as presenting symptom of myelofibrosis with myeloid metaplasia. *Am J Hematol.* 2006; 81: 124–127.

18. Cervantes F, Dupriez B, Pereira A, et al. New prognostic scoring system for primary myelofibrosis based on a study of the International Working Group for Myelofibrosis Research and Treatment. *Blood.* 2009; 113: 2895–2901.

19. Ditschkowski M, Elmaagacli AH, Trenschel R, et al. DIPSS scores, pre-transplant therapy and chronic GVHD determine outcome after allogeneic hematopoietic stem cell transplantation for myelofibrosis. *Haematologica.* 2012; 97:1574–1581.

20. Rondelli D, Barosi G, Bacigalupo A, et al. Allogeneic hematopoietic stem-cell transplantation with reduced-intensity conditioning in intermediate- or high-risk patients with myelofibrosis with myeloid metaplasia. *Blood*. 2005; 105: 4115–4119.

21. Ballen KK, Shrestha S, Sobocinski KA, et al. Outcome of transplantation for myelofibrosis. *Biol Blood Marrow Transplant*. 2010; 16: 358–367.

22. Mesa RA, Steensma DP, Pardanani A, et al. A phase 2 trial of combination low-dose thalidomide and prednisone for the treatment of myelofibrosis with myeloid metaplasia. *Blood*. 2003; 101: 2534–2541.

23. Verstovsek S, Mesa RA, Gotlib J, et al. A double-blind, placebo-controlled trial of ruxolitinib for myelofibrosis. *N Engl J Med*. 2012; 366: 799–807.

24. Harrison C, Kiladjian JJ, Al-Ali HK, et al. JAK inhibition with ruxolitinib versus best available therapy for myelofibrosis. *N Engl J Med*. 2012; 366: 787–798.

25. Wehmeier A, Sudhoff T, Meierkord F. Relation of platelet abnormalities to thrombosis and hemorrhage in chronic myeloproliferative disorders. *Semin Thromb Hemost*. 1997; 23: 391–402.

26. Michiels JJ, Budde U, van der PM, et al. Acquired von Willebrand syndromes: clinical features, aetiology, pathophysiology, classification and management. *Best Pract Res Clin Haematol*. 2001; 14: 401–436.

27. Jantunen R, Juvonen E, Ikkala E, et al. Development of erythrocytosis in the course of essential thrombocythemia. *Ann Hematol*. 1999; 78: 219–222.

28. Cervantes F, Alvarez-Larran A, Talarn C, Gomez M, Montserrat E. Myelofibrosis with myeloid metaplasia following essential thrombocythaemia: actuarial probability, presenting characteristics and evolution in a series of 195 patients. *Br J Haematol*. 2002; 118: 786–790.

29. Barbui T, Thiele J, Passamonti F, et al. Survival and disease progression in essential thrombocythemia are significantly influenced by accurate morphologic diagnosis: an international study. *J Clin Oncol*. 2011; 29: 3179–3184.

30. Alvarez-Larran A, Cervantes F, Pereira A, et al. Observation versus antiplatelet therapy as primary prophylaxis for thrombosis in low-risk essential thrombocythemia. *Blood*. 2010; 166: 1205–1210.

31. Schafer AI. Thrombocytosis. *N Engl J Med*. 2004; 350: 1211–1219.

32. Ruggeri M, Finazzi G, Tosetto A, et al. No treatment for low-risk thrombocythaemia: results from a prospective study. *Br J Haematol*. 1998; 103: 772–777.

33. Cortelazzo S, Finazzi G, Ruggeri M, et al. Hydroxyurea for patients with essential thrombocythemia and a high risk of thrombosis. *N Engl J Med*. 1995; 332: 1132–1136.

34. Harrison CN, Campbell PJ, Buck G, et al. Hydroxyurea compared with anagrelide in high-risk essential thrombocythemia. *N Engl J Med*. 2005; 353: 33–45.

35. Emadi A, Spivak JL. Anagrelide: 20 years later. *Expert Rev Anticancer Ther*. 2009; 9: 37–50.

CHAPTER **27**
Chronic Myeloid Leukemia
Karen Ballen

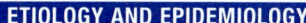

ETIOLOGY AND EPIDEMIOLOGY

Chronic myeloid leukemia (CML) is a clonal disorder of the hematopoietic stem cell affecting every lineage (except T lymphocytes). It affects about 5500 people a year in the United States and has a median age of onset in the sixth decade. The cause of CML is unknown.

PATHOPHYSIOLOGY

CML was one of the first human cancers associated with a chromosomal abnormality, the translocation 9;22, or Philadelphia chromosome. This translocation creates a novel fusion gene, bcr-abl, between the abl gene on chromosome 9 and the bcr gene on chromosome 22. The fusion gene protein product expresses an activated tyrosine kinase. The uncontrolled kinase activity of the bcr-abl takes over the normal functions of the normal ABL enzyme, causing unregulated cellular proliferation and decreased apoptosis.

NATURAL HISTORY

The disease is characterized by a stable phase that may be clinically silent and lasts 3–4 years. Accumulation of genetic damage over that time, particularly mutations in p53, can then lead to disease acceleration and a predominance of myeloblasts in the marrow and peripheral blood. Once disease acceleration occurs, median survival is usually less than 1 year. The development of acute leukemia may be of lymphoid, myeloid, or erythroid differentiation.

DIAGNOSIS

Most patients with CML, particularly in the stable phase (<5% myeloblasts in the bone marrow), are asymptomatic. An elevated WBC may be noted on a routine physical exam. Patients in accelerated phase (5%–20% marrow blasts) may have night sweats, adenopathy, and splenomegaly. The blast crisis (>20% marrow or blood blasts) has similar presentation to acute leukemia. The blood smear and bone marrow in CML will show an abundance of cells in all stages of maturation. (**Figure 27-1**). The definitive diagnosis can be made by the presence of the bcr-abl translocation in the blood or bone marrow, determined by PCR analysis. Variant chromosomes are seen in 5% of patients and do not affect prognosis (1).

- Positive bcr-abl in blood or marrow diagnostic of CML—bone marrow not needed for diagnosis but helpful to rule out more advanced stage of disease.
- Chronic phase: high WBC, often asymptomatic, <5% blasts

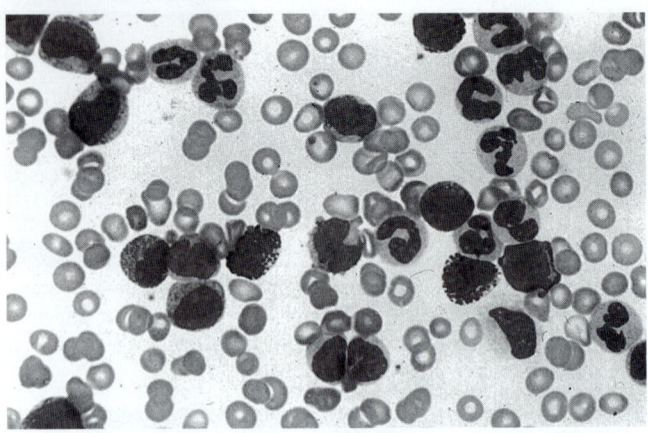

FIGURE 27-1 Chronic myeloid leukemia in stable phase-peripheral blood. Early myeloid cells and basophilia are characteristic.

- Accelerated phase: may be symptomatic, 5%–20% blasts
- Blast crisis: 70% present as a myeloid acute leukemia, 30% lymphoid, and similar to acute leukemia, the diagnosis is based on >20% blasts.

TREATMENT

The treatment for CML has changed dramatically since the approval of imatinib (Gleevec) in 2002 (2). Imatinib is a tyrosine kinase inhibitor that blocks the kinase activity of bcr-abl and inhibits the proliferation of Philadelphia chromosome positive progenitors. Chronic phase disease is treated with imatinib at a dose of 400 mg/day. Approximately 95% of chronic phase patients receiving imatinib will have a complete hematologic response, 87% complete cytogenetic response, and 77% major molecular response (3) (see Table 27-1). After 2 years, CML progresses in 3% of patients with a major cytogenetic response (<35% Philadelphia positive metaphases) and 12% of patients without a major cytogenetic response (4). Side effects of imatinib include nausea, rashes, headache, diarrhea, fluid

TABLE 27-1 DEFINITIONS OF RESPONSE FOR PATIENTS WITH CHRONIC MYELOGENEOUS LEUKEMIA

	Definition
Complete hematologic response	Platelet $<450 \times 10^9$/l White blood count $<10 \times 10^9$/l Nonpalpable spleen
Complete cytogenetic response	No Philadelphia positive metaphases
Complete molecular response	Non-detectable bcr-abl level
Major molecular response	Bcr-abl <0.10r

retention, and cytopenias. Patients who are intolerant of imatinib or who do not have a molecular remission should be switched to the second generation tyrosine kinase inhibitors dasatinib or nilotinib. These drugs induce a quicker molecular remission than imatinib, and may also be used for initial therapy (4). In a randomized trial, nilotinib yielded better progression-free survival, as compared to imatinib. Discontinuation of tyrosine kinase inhibitors in patients with a complete molecular response is controversial (5). Patients in remission should have peripheral blood monitoring for the bcr-abl transcript every 3 months until a major molecular response, and every 6 months thereafter.

Allogeneic stem cell transplantation is now reserved only for very young patients (under age 30 years), for patients who do not attain a molecular remission on imatinib, dasatinib, or nilotinib, for patients with the T315I mutation (who are resistant to tyrosine kinase inhibitors by virtue of steric hindrance of drug binding to the ATP binding site of the kinase), or for patients in accelerated or chronic phase. Cure rates of 70% have been reported with either related or unrelated allogeneic donors. However, the 100-day transplant-related mortality is 10%–15% (see Chapter 37). A significant advance in the transplantation field is the recognition that leukemia control is dependent on an allogeneic graft-versus-leukemia effect, first demonstrated in CML patients. CML patients with graft-versus-host disease have a lower risk of relapse, and patients who relapse after allogeneic transplantation can be cured by donor lymphocyte infusions.

- Initial therapy with imatinib at 400 mg daily.
- Dasatinib or nilotinib for patients who are imatinib intolerant or resistant (these drugs may also be considered for upfront therapy).
- Allogeneic stem cell transplantation for patients with tyrosine kinase inhibitor resistance, the T315I mutation, or accelerated/blast crisis.
- Ponatinib, a new abl kinase inhibitor, was rationally designed to overcome resistance to imatinib and is effective in tumors bearing the T315I mutation (6).

PROGNOSIS

The prognosis for patients with CML has dramatically improved since the introduction of imatinib (7). Patients who achieve a complete cytogenetic remission and a 3-log reduction in bcr-abl transcript have a progression-free survival of 100% at 2 years. Overall survival has improved to about 80% at 10 years (8).

REFERENCES

1. Marzocchi G, Castagnetti F, Luatti S, et al: Variant Philadelphia translocations: molecular-cytogenetic characterization and prognostic influence on frontline imatinib therapy, a GIMEMA Working Party on CML analysis. *Blood.* 2011; 117: 6793–6800.
2. Goldman JM, Melo JV. Chronic myeloid leukemia—advances in biology and new approaches to treatment. *N Engl J Med.* 2003; 349: 1451–1464.
3. Jabbour E, Kantarjian H, O'Brien S, et al. The achievement of an early complete cytogenetic response is a major determinant for outcome in

patients with early chronic phase chronic myeloid leukemia treated with tyrosine kinase inhibitors. *Blood.* 2011; 118: 4541–4546.

4. Saglio G, Kim DW, Issarangrisil S, et al: Nilotinib versus imatinib for newly diagnosed chronic myeloid leukemia. *N Engl J Med.* 2010; 362: 2251–2259.

5. Mahan FX, Rea D, Guilhot F, et al. Discontinuation of imatinib in patients with chronic myeloid leukemia who have maintained complete molecular remission for at least 2 years: the prospective, multicentre Stop Imatinib (STIM) trial. *Lancet Oncology.* 2010; 11: 1029–1035.

6. Cortes JE, Kantarjian H, Shah NP, et al. Phase I trial of ponatinib in refractory Ph+ chromosome leukemias. *N Engl J Med.* 2012; 367: 2075–2088.

7. Kantarjian H, Sawyers C, Hochhaus A, et al. Hematologic and cytogenetic responses to imatinib mesylate in chronic myelogeneous leukemia. *N Engl J Med.* 2002; 346: 645–652.

8. Kantarjian H, O'Brien S, Jabbour E, et al. Improved survival in chronic myeloid leukemia since the introduction of imatinib therapy: a single institute historical experience. *Blood.* 2012; 119: 1981–1987.

CHAPTER **28**

Acute Lymphoblastic Leukemia and Lymphoma

James W. Fraser, Janet E. Murphy, Eyal C. Attar

INTRODUCTION

Acute lymphoblastic leukemia (ALL) is a highly aggressive neoplasm of hematopoietic cells of lymphoid lineage. Collections of abnormal T- or B lymphoblasts may be found in the bone marrow, peripheral blood, and other extramedullary sites. ALL is predominantly a childhood cancer, with two-thirds of new cases diagnosed in children younger than 15 years of age. ALL was uniformly fatal until the 1960 but, due to advances in chemotherapy and supportive care, is now cured in over 80% of children. Adults diagnosed with ALL, in contrast, have a poor overall prognosis. Important factors in assessing prognosis are the age of the patient, type of lymphoid cell involved (T cell vs B cell), and the presence of high-risk cytogenetic markers, such as the t(9;22) (BCR–ABL) translocation. Burkitt's lymphoma, a malignancy of mature B cells, has been historically classified as a B-ALL due to its high-grade leukemia-like features but is both diagnostically and prognostically a separate entity from precursor B-ALL. Burkitt's lymphoma is addressed in the chapter on non-Hodgkin lymphomas.

- ALL is the most common malignancy of childhood.
- Childhood ALL has a much better prognosis than adult ALL.
- Highly aggressive lymphoid malignancy with B-cell (80%) and T-cell (20%) immunophenotypes.
- Certain cytogenetic alterations, such as t(9;22), are associated with inferior prognosis while others, such as t(12;21), are associated with favorable outcomes.

EPIDEMIOLOGY AND ETIOLOGY

Leukemia comprises 32% of malignancies in children younger than 15 years. Of these, the majority are ALL. Each year approximately 2400 children in the United States are diagnosed with ALL. The peak incidence in children is between ages 2 and 5. Leukemia rates are significantly higher in Caucasian children, with a nearly threefold higher incidence over African-American children. ALL is almost 30% more common in males than females. Overall, the incidence of childhood ALL has increased in the past 20 years at a rate of 0.9% per year. Adult ALL is less common, with approximately 1000 new cases diagnosed per year. The incidence of ALL decreases from age 15 until 50; then a second, minor increase in new cases appears. A third peak appears at age 80. The lifetime risk of developing ALL is 0.13%, or approximately 1 in 789 men and women (1).

Several reports have suggested that inadvertent exposure to radiation in utero and postnatal radiation treatment for such conditions as tinea capitis and thymic enlargement increase the risk of ALL (2). A common cytogenetic translocation involving ETV-6 was retrospectively detected in neonatal blood spots of children who were diagnosed with ALL between ages 2 and 5, suggesting that ALL can be initiated by somatic translocation in utero but requires additional molecular events to fully develop (3). Limited and/or inconsistent evidence links ALL to parental smoking, infection, diet, electromagnetic fields, hydrocarbons and, possibly, radiation delivered during the course of diagnostic studies such as CT scans (4).

The following characteristics are associated with ALL:

- Male sex
- Age 2–5
- Caucasian race
- Higher socioeconomic status (SES)
- Hereditary factors (Down syndrome, Bloom syndrome, ataxia telangectasia, neurofibromatosis, Klinefelter syndrome, Shwachman syndrome, and Langerhans cell histiocytosis)
  - Radiation and chemical exposure is controversial but may increase overall risk of ALL both in utero and during childhood
  - Overall likelihood of developing ALL in one's lifetime is 0.13%, or 1 in 789

ALL CLASSIFICATION

Proper characterization of the specific hematopoietic lineage involved in ALL is crucial for assessing risk and for treatment. ALL may be classified according to the presence or absence of various cell surface and intracellular markers.

Both immunohistochemistry and flow cytometry may be used to identify expression of cell surface and cytoplasmic proteins. These techniques use panels of lineage-specific antibodies directed against B-lymphoid and T-lymphoid antigens to stain patient bone marrow and lymph node samples. Common immunophenotypes are presented in Table 28-1.

Both B and T lymphoblasts typically express terminal deoxytransferase (TdT) and/or the primitive hematopoietic cell surface marker CD34. Approximately 80% of adult ALL patients have B-ALL, while 5% have Burkitt's (an aggressive tumor of peripheral follicular B cells) and the remainder are precursor T-cell ALL.

Precursor B-ALL cells express CD19 and at least one other B-lineage marker such as CD20, CD24, CD22, CD21, or CD79. More than 90% also express CD10, a marker known as CALLA, or common ALL antigen. In addition, 25% of patients have cytoplasmic Ig staining.

Precursor T-cell leukemias express CD7, TdT, and cytoplasmic CD3 antigen. Expression of CD1a is highly characteristic of T-ALL. More highly differentiated thymocytes acquire CD2 and CD5 and, later, CD4 and CD8. Mature thymocytes express functional T-cell receptor (TCR) and surface CD3. TCR rearrangement studies may be conducted to establish clonality.

TABLE 28-1 COMMON IMMUNOPHENOTYPE PROFILES OF LYMPHOID AND MYELOID MALIGNANCIES

| | | Primitive | | | B-lymphoid | | | T-lymphoid | | Myeloid | | |
		TdT	CD34	CD1a	CD10 (cALLa)	CD20	sIg	CD4	CD8	CD13	CD33	MPO
B cell	Precursor B-cell ALL	+	+	–	+	–	–	–	–	–	–	–
	Mature B-cell	–	–	–	–	+	+	–	–	–	–	–
T cell	Precursor T-cell ALL	+	–	+	±	–	–	–	–	–	–	–
	Mature T-cell	–	–	–	–	–	–	+	+	–	–	–
Myeloid		–	+	–	–	–	–	–	–	+	+	+

MPO, myeloperoxidase; sIg, surface immunoglobulin.
+ denotes >50% positive.
– denotes <50% positive.
NOTE: This is a general schema, exceptions exist. For example, biphenotypic and multilineage leukemias may coexpress multiple lineage markers.

343

As in adults, approximately 80% of children with ALL too have B-ALL, whereas 2% have mature B-cell (Burkitt's) leukemia/lymphoma and 15% T-ALL.

- ALL may be classified as B- or T-cell origin using intracellular and cell surface markers.
- B-ALL markers most commonly include: CD10, CD19, CD20, CD21, CD22, CD24, and CD34 and TdT. Twenty-five percent of B-ALL will have cytoplasmic Ig staining.
- T-ALL markers include CD7, TdT, CD1a, and cytoplasmic CD3. More differentiated leukemia markers of T-cell origin include CD2, CD5, and CD4 or CD8.

DIAGNOSIS OF ALL

■ CLINICAL PRESENTATION

Children with ALL may have an insidious or explosive course before diagnosis, whereas adults present more uniformly with rapid-onset disease. Physical signs and symptoms are the result of marrow failure from leukemia cell proliferation.

Patients commonly present with signs and symptoms of anemia, such as pallor, fatigue, lethargy, and, in adults, cardiac angina. Thrombocytopenia, another common sign, manifests as easy bruising, bleeding, and petechiae. Underproduction of normal neutrophils predisposes patients to infections, such as pneumonias, tooth infections, and sinusitis.

Leukemia cell expansion within the marrow may lead to bone pain and, in young children, resistance to walking. Extramedullary deposition leads to lymphadenopathy, hepatosplenomegaly with abdominal tenderness to palpation, and testicular enlargement, while involvement of the CNS leads to headaches, nausea, vomiting, and cranial nerve palsies. A mediastinal mass, which may be seen in T-cell ALL, may result in chest discomfort, shortness of breath, dyspnea on exertion, and superior vena cava syndrome.

Rapidly proliferating disease may result in spontaneous tumor lysis with renal failure and electrolyte imbalances. Many patients present with fevers without infectious etiologies.

A summary of clinical features is presented in Table 28-2.

■ DIAGNOSTIC STUDIES

The WHO classification describes three distinct entities of ALL: B-ALL with recurrent genetic abnormalities, B-ALL not otherwise specified (cytogenetically normal), and T-ALL. To classify a hematologic malignancy as ALL, there must be at least 25% involvement of precursor lymphoblasts committed to the B-cell or T-cell lineage present in the bone marrow and blood. This diagnostic criterion contrasts with AML, which requires ≥20% myeloblasts in the bone marrow or blood for diagnosis. Burkitt's lymphoma is classified as a "mature" B-ALL and is the exception to this rule. Burkitt's cells are negative for both myeloperoxidase (MPO) and TdT but stain positively for B-cell markers and, often, have light chain restriction.

The diagnostic workup consists of blood tests, imaging, bone marrow aspiration and biopsy, and lumbar puncture (LP) (Table 28-3). The CBC

TABLE 28-2 CLINICAL MANIFESTATIONS OF ALL

Marrow failure
- Anemia: pallor, fatigue, lethargy, angina
- Thrombocytopenia: bruising, petechiae
- Neutropenia: infection

Clonal expansion
- Bone pain, resistance to walking in children
- Tender lymphadenopathy
- Hepatosplenomegaly
- Fever
- Mediastinal mass
- Testicular mass

CNS infiltration
- Headache
- Nausea, vomiting
- Cranial nerve palsies

---

and peripheral blood smear may show leukocytosis with lymphoblasts (Figure 28-1) with decreases in normal blood counts. Serum chemistries reflect the degree of tumor burden and cell lysis; patients with tumor lysis exhibit hyperuricemia, hypocalcemia, hyperphosphatemia, hyperkalemia, and elevated LDH. Bone marrow aspiration reveals hypercellularity with increased lymphoblasts. CNS involvement is present in 5%–15% of adults and children alike, and is more frequently associated with the precursor T-cell immunophenotype. LP and subsequent CNS analysis will show blasts by cell count and cytology and may demonstrate an elevated opening pressure and protein and glucose derangements. Evidence exists that a traumatic LP may seed the CNS in unaffected children. Consequently, a traumatic tap as suggested by the presence of red blood cells in the cell analysis represents an indication for intensification of CNS therapy (5). An anterior mediastinal mass may be detected in 5%–10% of children and 15% of adults by chest X-ray, a finding more commonly associated with T-ALL.

RISK STRATIFICATION

■ CLINICAL FACTORS

Treatment of ALL is based on assignment of risk derived from immunophenotype, cytogenetics, and clinical prognostic factors. In children, the Rome/NCI (*National Cancer Institute*) criteria have traditionally assigned children to standard versus high-risk categories for treatment based on age and WBC count at diagnosis. Children ages 1–9 with B-cell ALL who present with WBC count <50,000/μl at diagnosis are considered standard risk, while all others are high risk. Recent trials have employed Children's Oncology Group (COG) criteria for risk assessment, in which age and WBC count

TABLE 28-3 WORKUP AND FINDINGS SEEN IN ALL

CBC and peripheral smear
- Leukocytosis or leukopenia
- Lymphoblasts
- Anemia
- Thrombocytopenia

Serum chemistries
- Hyperuricemia
- Hyperkalemia
- Hypocalcemia
- Hyperphosphatemia
- Elevated LDH reflective of high-tumor burden and cell lysis

Bone marrow
- Homogeneous lymphoblast field with hypercellular marrow (>25% blasts)
- Residual myeloid and erythroid precursors are morphologically normal
- A few/absent megakaryocytes

LP
- CNS blasts
- Elevated opening pressure
- Elevated protein
- Decreased glucose

Radiology
- Anterior mediastinal mass (more often associated with T-cell ALL)
- PET/CT scanning of the neck, chest, abdomen, and pelvis may reveal lymphadenopathy
- Testicular ultrasound for patients with a scrotal mass

determine initial risk; cytogenetics and subsequent response to therapy substratify patients during treatment into a four-category algorithm that maximizes cure rate and minimizes exposure to toxic chemotherapies in low-risk patients.

Factors that influence prognosis in children are summarized in Table 28-4. Overall, mature B cell and precursor T-cell ALL immunophenotypes have poorer prognosis, and children with leukemias of this origin are assigned to the high-risk treatment group regardless of blast count at presentation. Age at presentation is crucial, with the age group 1–9 being most favorable. Children younger than 1 year have an exceptionally poor prognosis, with aggressive disease (higher WBC at presentation, often accompanied by massive hepatosplenomegaly) attributed to a high frequency of the t(4;11) MLL-AF4 translocation, which occurs in 50% of infants. Adolescents (10–20 years) have a poorer prognosis than younger

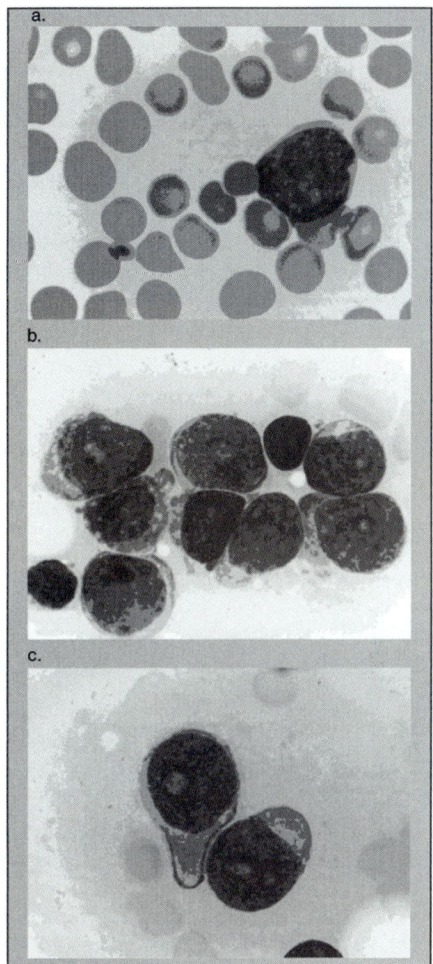

FIGURE 28-1 Morphology of ALL cells. Slides showing: (A) peripheral smear with lymphoblasts, and (B) bone marrow aspirate. Leukemic lymphoblasts are large cells with a high nuclear-to-cytoplasmic ratio and prominent nucleoli. Cells with "hand mirror" contours may be seen in the peripheral blood in ALL. (Courtesy Rob Hasserjian, MGH Cancer Center.)

children, presenting more frequently with T-cell disease and Philadelphia-positive B-cell disease. Interestingly, young adults in their late teens have improved outcomes when treated on pediatric protocols compared to adult protocols. This may relate to increased use of non-myelotoxic drugs and stricter compliance with pediatric treatments—possibly aided by increased parental participation ("the mommy factor") (6).

Patient ethnicity has historically been a factor: African-Americans and Native Americans have generally experienced poorer outcomes, with higher

TABLE 28-4 PROGNOSTIC FACTORS IN CHILDHOOD ALL

Age	Favorable 1–9 Years at Diagnosis	Unfavorable <1, >10 Years at Diagnosis
WBC at presentation	<50,000/µl	>50,000/µl
Immunophenotype	Precursor B-cell type	Mature B-cell type
		Precursor T-cell type and sequelae: mediastinal mass and CNS involvement
Race	Caucasian	Other (though normalizes with equal access to care)
Organ involvement (lymph nodes, spleen, liver, testes)	Absent	Present
CBC	Anemia and thrombocytopenia (implies indolent onset)	Absence of anemia or thrombocytopenia (implies explosive onset)
CNS involvement	Absent	Present
Response to therapy	Clearance of blasts by day 7	Nonclearance of blasts
Cytogenetics	t(12; 21) ETV-6	t(9; 22) BCR–ABL
	Hyperdiploidy >50	t(4; 11) AF4/MLL
	Trisomies 4, 10, 17	t(1; 19) E2A/PBX
		Hypodiploidy

WBC counts, increased prevalence of lymphadenopathy, and mediastinal mass on presentation. However, this difference is reduced when patients are provided equal access to care (7).

Important clinical factors include organ involvement (lymph nodes, spleen, liver, testes), which portends poor prognosis, as does the absence of anemia and thrombocytopenia, which correlates with explosive disease. Likewise, CNS involvement is associated with a lower rate of remission and higher rate of relapse. Finally, clearance of blasts is routinely measured at days 7 and 14 of induction chemotherapy; nonclearance of blasts at these time points is associated with a 2.7-fold relative risk of relapse in children and half to two-thirds less chance of 5-year overall survival in adults (8, 9).

Risk assignment in adults is less succinctly defined. In the absence of consensus guidelines, individual consortia have developed parameters to govern their trials. The Cancer and Leukemia Group B (CALGB) criteria for high-risk patients include:

1. age greater than 30, which is inversely correlated with achievement of complete remission (CR), duration of CR, and overall survival. The linear worsening of prognosis with age in adult ALL makes it difficult to define a threshold of low versus high risk.

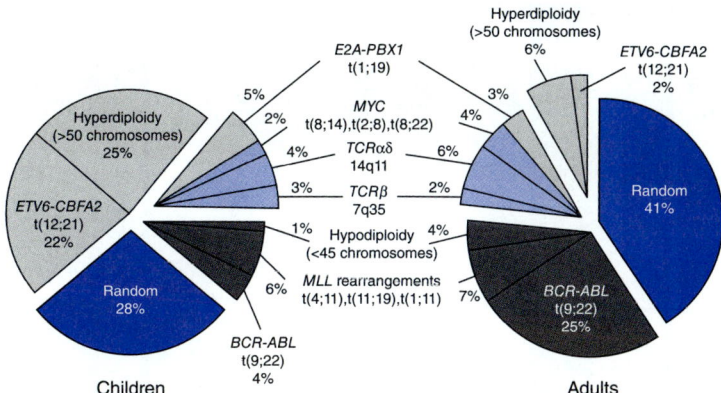

FIGURE 28-2 Estimated frequencies of specific genotypes among children and adults with ALL. (From Pui E. Drug therapy: acute lymphoblastic leukemia. *N Engl J Med.* 1998; 339: 605–615. Copyright © 1998 Massachusetts Medical Society. All rights reserved.)

2. WBC at presentation >30,000/μl
3. Presence of a mediastinal mass

■ CYTOGENETICS

Genetic lesions in ALL are common and correlated with immunophenotype, response to treatment, and disease recurrence (Figure 28-2). The WHO identifies six cytogenetic subcategories associated with prognosis in precursor B-cell ALL, summarized in Table 28-5. In children, classical cytogenetic lesions associated with favorable prognosis in precursor B-cell disease are the t(12;21) (TEL/AML) translocation, found in 15%–25% of children with ALL, and hyperdiploidy, with chromosome counts >50 per cell, found in 30% of children (vs 2% of adults). Trisomies of chromosomes 4, 10, 17, while not a WHO subcategory, also correlate with favorable prognosis in children (10).

Treatment failure in B-ALL is associated with the t(4;11) (MLL-AF4) translocation, commonly found in infantile ALL with high blast counts (11). In both adults and children, the Philadelphia chromosome t(9;22) (BCR–ABL) portends negative prognosis. Prevalence of t(9;22) is striking in older adults, with 50% of patients over 50 exhibiting this mutation. Both the 210-kD gene product, identical to the one found in CML, and a smaller, 190-kD protein are found in Ph+ ALL, with equal prognostic implications (12). Finally, the t(1;19) (E2A-PBX1) translocation is associated with early treatment failure in B-ALL (13).

Prognosis in T-ALL is not as well correlated with specific cytogenetic mutations. The T-cell immunophenotype more often presents with aggressive features, including mediastinal mass and CNS infiltration, but no single karyotype confers this risk. Approximately 50% of precursor T-cell clones have activating mutations of the NOTCH1 gene, but the prognostic significance of this mutation is not yet defined (14). Preclinical studies are currently underway assessing the efficacy of notch inhibitors, such as

TABLE 28-5 WORLD HEALTH ORGANIZATION (WHO) PROGNOSTIC IMPLICATIONS OF GENETIC ALTERATIONS IN PRECURSOR B-LYMPHOBLASTIC LEUKEMIA

Cytogenetic Finding	Genetic Alteration	Function	Frequency (Children)	Frequency (Adults)	Prognosis
t(9;22)(q34;q11.2)	BCR/ABL	Fusion product with constitutive protein tyrosine kinase activity; enhances clone proliferation and survival.	3%–4%	25%	Unfavorable
t(4;11)(q21;q23)	AF4/MLL	Disrupts homeobox genes, which regulate normal transcription of hematopoietic stem cells.	2%–3%, but 50% of infants	5%–6%	Unfavorable
t(1;19)(q23;p13.3)	E2A/PBX	Disrupts the activity of HOX-PBX dimers, which normally regulate hematopoietic differentiation.	6% (25% of pre-B ALL)		Unfavorable
t(12;21)(p13;q22)	ETV-6	Fusion product of two transcription factors, TEL and AML1. Inhibits normal AML1 activity, resulting in altered stem-cell differentiation.	20%–25%		Favorable
Hyperdiploid >50			30%	2%	Favorable
Hypodiploidy			2%	2%	Unfavorable

Adapted and expanded from Brunning RD, Borowitz M, Matutes E, et al. Precursor B lymphoblastic leukaemia/lymphoblastic lymphoma (precursor B-cell acute lymphoblastic leukaemia). In E Jaffe, N Harris, H Stein, J Vardiman (eds). *World Health Organization Classification of Tumors, Pathology and Genetics, Tumors of Haematopoietic and Lymphoid Tissues.* IARC Press, Lyon, 2001, p. 113.

γ-secretase inhibitors, in both B- and T-ALL (15, 16). Translocations involving the TCR genes on chromosomes 7 and 14 are common.

Additional genetic techniques, such as microarray gene expression profiling and comparative genomic hybridization (CGH), are being used to explore novel molecular lesions operative in ALL. These techniques may be used to further substratify patients within cytogenetic groups but are most useful in patients who have normal cytogenetics.

TREATMENT

Chemotherapy is the mainstay of treatment for ALL. The treatment regimen depends upon immunophenotype and clinical and molecular risk category. Table 28-6 provides a global approach to the treatment of patients with ALL.

With standard protocols, children with ALL attain remission in 98% of cases, with 80% surviving at least 5 years from diagnosis (17). In contrast, approximately 85% of adults achieve CR, with a median duration of remission of 15 months and ultimate cure rate of only 25%–40%.

Mature B-cell ALL does not respond well to chemotherapy traditionally used for precursor ALL. However, event-free survival (EFS) rates exceeding 90% have been obtained with treatments designed for Burkitt's lymphoma, which emphasize cyclophosphamide and the rapid rotation of antimetabolites in high dosages (Table 28-7). This strategy differs from therapies for precursor ALL, which involve sequential modules of remission induction, intensification, CNS prophylaxis, and maintenance. Patients with large sites of disease, as in precursor T-cell ALL with a mediastinal mass, often require involved field radiation therapy in addition to systemic chemotherapy. Typical regimens for precursor and mature B-cell ALL are provided in Table 28-7.

Remission induction aims to restore normal blood counts and marrow appearance, reduce the percentage of blasts to <5%, and eliminate extramedullary disease. Standard treatment regimens consist of vincristine, a glucocorticoid (usually prednisone or dexamethasone), L-asparaginase, and, often, an anthracycline such as doxorubicin or daunorubicin. Three to four drugs are used for standard-risk patients, while up to seven drugs may be used in high-risk cases. For adult patients, a five-drug regimen known as "CAVP-L" incorporates the alkylating agent cyclophosphamide with daunorubicin, vincristine, prednisone, and L-asparaginase and is commonly used for induction (18). Another regimen known as "Hyper-CVAD" utilizes hyperfractionated doses of cyclophophamide in induction alternating with cycles of cytarabine and methotrexate. *Intensification* aims to eliminate residual leukemia, prevent relapse, and reduce the possible emergence of drug-resistant cells. In children, high-dose methotrexate with mercaptopurine is commonly used. Reinduction with the initial drug combination often follows after several months.

Maintenance therapy preserves remission. ALL requires 2–3 years of maintenance, significantly longer than other chemoresponsive cancers. Standard maintenance regimens may incorporate daily mercaptopurine, weekly methotrexate, and monthly pulses of vincristine and prednisone.

CNS prophylaxis While the incidence of CNS involvement is relatively rare (5%–15%), the CNS represents a sanctuary site for ALL that may be

TABLE 28-6

Risk		Low-risk ALL	High-risk ALL	Very high risk ALL	Mature B-cell ALL
	B-lineage	WBC <30 K	WBC >30 K	Ph1/ ber-abl* +	
	T-lineage	WBC <100 K	WBC >100 K		
	Time to CR	<4 weeks	>4 weeks Pro B-ALL, Pro T-ALL		
Pretreatment			Consider Vinc/Pred if pretreatment for bulky disease		Cyclophos- phamide/ prednisone for bulky disease
Multiple-agent chemotherapy			Yes		Short, intensive cycles (4–6 depending upon regimen)
CNS prophylaxis			Yes		Yes
Consolidation/ intensification			Yes		
BMT in CRI		Consider allo if MRD available	Allo if MRD available	Allo if MRD available, MUD for younger patients if MRD not available; Auto SCT for all others	No
Maintenance 6- MP/MTX intensification for 2 years		In patients not transplanted	In patients not transplanted	Yes	No

*Patients with t(9;22) should receive a bcr/abl tyrosine kinase inhibitor continuously throughout every phase of treatment.

TABLE 28-7 COMMON ADULT ALL TREATMENT REGIMENS

Precursor acute B-cell lymphoblastic leukemia/lymphoma

- CALGB 19802 (Stock, et al. *Blood*. 2003; 102: 1375a)
- CALGB 9111 (Larson, et al. *Blood*. 1998; 92: 1556)

Precursor acute T-cell lymphoblastic leukemia/lymphoma

- GMALL/MSCMCC (Hoelzer, et al. *Blood*. 2002; 99: 4379)

Mature B-cell leukemia/Burkitt's lymphoma

- GMALL (German Multicenter Study Group for Treatment of Adult ALL) (Hoelzer, Ludwig, et al. *Blood*. 1996; 87: 495.)
- BFM GMALL/NHL 2002(Hoelzer, et al. *Blood*. 2003; 102: 236a)
- BFM 86 (Reiter, et al. *Blood*. 1994; 84: 3122-3133)
- Modified Magrath Regimen (Lacasce, et al. *Leuk Lymphoma*. 2004; 45: 761-767.)
- (R)-HyperCVAD (Thomas et al. *J Clin Oncol*. 1999; 17: 2461-2470, Thomas et al. *Cancer*. 2006; 106: 1569-1580.)

the source of systemic relapse at a later date or site of disease occurrence despite systemic remission. The CNS is routinely prophylaxed using intrathecal (IT) chemotherapy consisting of methotrexate and/or cytarabine. Cranial irradiation, too, is a standard component of prophylaxis.

Supportive care includes administration of white blood cell growth factors, antibiotics for infection prophylaxis and treatment, blood product transfusions, and treatment of electrolyte disturbances.

Response to therapy The efficacy of chemotherapy is evaluated by repeated analysis of peripheral blood and bone marrow samples at regular intervals. Response to therapy is measured in several ways:

1. Time interval to achieve CR with induction chemotherapy. Adults who do not achieve CR by 4 weeks are twice as likely to relapse, and have a negligible 5-year disease-free survival rate.

2. Detection of minimal residual disease. More sensitive techniques such as flow cytometry and PCR can detect one lymphoblast in 10^4 and 10^6 normal cells, respectively. Current research has correlated an MRD $>10^{-4}$ with significantly lower rates of relapse-free survival within the first year, within 5 years (15% vs 71% MRD neg) and higher rates of treatment failure following autologous stem-cell transplant (77% vs 25% MRD neg) in non T-ALL (19). However, an MRD $>10^4$ detected before allogeneic stem-cell transplantation does not appear to have a significant effect on outcome.

Allogeneic hematopoietic cell transplantation has been shown to improve outcomes in high-risk groups such as t(9;22)-positive adults. Indeed, prospective outcome data on 267 unselected adult patients with (9;22) positive ALL showed 5-year OS to be 44% and 36% for patients who received sibling matched allo-HSCT (hematopoietic stem-cell transplantation) or matched unrelated HSCT, respectively, versus 19% who underwent chemotherapy alone (20). Following remission induction, patients undergo conditioning with chemotherapy (and sometimes radiation therapy) and transplantation with allogeneic hematopoietic cells. Transplantation not only provides hematopoietic rescue but also donor lymphocytes, which may mediate a graft versus leukemia/lymphoma effect (21). Recent evidence suggests that even adults with standard risk disease benefit from allo-HSCT over standard consolidation and maintenance chemotherapy if a matched related donor is available.

Nonmyeloablative strategies are currently under investigation for older patients and those unable to receive myeloablative conditioning due to other medical conditions. Current research is evaluating the benefit of purged autologous hematopoietic stem cells, reduced-intensity conditioning regimens, and use of alternative stem cells sources such as cord blood.

Salvage chemotherapy Relapsing patients undergo reinduction with repeated use of induction agents or salvage regimens based on high-dose cytarabine in combination with other agents such as mitoxantrone. Allogeneic transplantation, when possible, frequently follows for such high-risk patients if remission is attained. Despite the benefit of these therapies in the short term, only 7% of patients with relapsed ALL achieve an overall survival >5 years (22). Relapsed patients who undergo allo-HCT have improved survival compared to those who do not.

Novel treatments Advances in survival have outpaced significant alterations in chemotherapy for ALL; survival is attributed to improvements in risk stratification such that patients receive sufficient chemotherapy while toxicities are minimized. Current investigation in pharmacogenomics may result in personalized approaches to chemotherapy types and dosages. For example, discovery of an autosomal recessive polymorphism in the thiopurine methyltransferase (TPMT) gene, responsible for inactivation of 6-mercaptopurine, has altered how chemotherapy is dosed. TPMT-deficient patients achieve toxic levels when standard doses of 6-MP are administered, but their event-free survival has been historically better—a finding with implications for optimal dosing in wild-type patients as well (23). In the future, pharmacogenomics may help to identify polymorphisms and permit dosing to maximal effect in patients.

The targeted ABL kinase inhibitor imatinib mesylate (Gleevec) has shown activity in patients with t(9;22)-positive disease, mainly when administered with standard chemotherapies (24). Second generation tyrosine kinase inhibitors that include dasatinib (Sprycel) and nilotinib (Tasigna) also have activity in Ph+ disease. The novel nucleoside analogue clofarabine is approved in pediatric ALL, while nalarabine (ara-G) is approved in relapsed and refractory T-ALL. Current trials are evaluating the benefit of monoclonal antibodies, such as the anti-CD20 agent rituximab (Rituxan), inotuzumab ozogamicin (a conjugate of calicheamicin with an anti-CD22 antibody), bispecific T-cell engager (BiTEs) antibodies such as blinatumomab (one portion binds T cells and the other CD19 on B-cell tumor cells), the proteasome inhibitor bortezomib, and inhibitors of molecular targets perturbed in ALL, such as NOTCH.

REFERENCES

1. National Cancer Institute. SEER Stat Facts Sheet, Acute Lymphoblastic Leukemia. Available at: http://seer.cancer.gov/statfacts/html/alyl.html.

2. National Cancer Institute. Adult ALL Treatment, Childhood ALL Treatment, SEER Pediatric Monograph. Available at: http://www.cancer.gov/cancertopics/pdq/treatment/adultALL/HealthProfessional ttp://www.cancer.gov/cancertopics/pdq/treatment/childhoodALL/HealthProfessional. Accessed February 17, 2006.

3. Wiemels JL, Cazzaniga G, Daniotti M, et al. Prenatal origin of acute lymphoblastic leukaemia in children. *Lancet.* 1999; 354: 1499–1503.

4. Pearce MS, Salotti JA, Little MP, et al. Radiation exposure from CT scans in childhood and subsequent risk of leukemia and brain tumours: a retrospective study cohort. *Lancet.* 2012; 380: 499–505.

5. Gajjar A, Harrison PL, Sandlund JT, et al. Traumatic lumbar puncture at diagnosis adversely affects outcome in childhood acute lymphoblastic leukemia. *Blood.* 2000; 96: 3381–3384.

6. Boissel N, Auclerc M-F, Lheritier V, et al. Should adolescents with acute lymphoblastic leukemia be treated as old children or young adults? Comparison of the French FRALLE-93 and LALA-94 trials. *J Clin Oncol.* 2003; 21: 774–780.

7. Pui CH, Sandlund JT, Pei D, et al. Results of therapy for acute lymphoblastic leukemia in black and white children. *J Am Med Assoc.* 2003; 290: 2001–2007.

8. Steinherz PG, Gaynon PS, Breneman JC, et al. Cytoreduction and prognosis in acute lymphoblastic leukemia—the importance of early marrow response: report from the Children's Cancer Group. *J Clin Oncol.* 1996; 14: 389–398.

9. Cortes J, Fayad, L, O'Brien S, et al. Persistence of peripheral blood and bone marrow blasts during remission induction in adult acute lymphoblatic leukemia confers a poor prognosis depending on treatment intensity. *Clinical Cancer Research.* 1999; 5: 2491–2497.

10. Brunning RD, Borowitz M, Matutes E, et al. Precursor B lymphoblastic leukaemia/lymphoblastic lymphoma (precursor B-cell acute lymphoblastic leukaemia). In E Jaffe, N Harris, H Stein, J Vardiman (eds.), *World Health Organization Classification of Tumors, Pathology and Genetics, Tumors of Haematopoietic and Lymphoid Tissues* IARC Press, Lyon, 2001, pp. 111–117.

11. Heerema NA, Sather HN, Ge J, et al. Cytogenetic studies of infant acute lymphoblastic leukemia: poor prognosis of infants with t(4;11)—a report of the Children's Cancer Group. *Leukemia.* 1999; 13: 679–686.

12. Secker-Walker L, Craig JM. Prognostic implications of breakpoint and lineage heterogeneity in Philadelphia-positive acute lymphoblastic leukemia: a review. *Leukemia.* 1993; 7: 147–151.

13. Foa R, Vitale A, Mancini M, et al. E2A-PBX1 fusion in adult acute lymphoblastic leukemia: biological and clinical features. *Br J Haematol.* 2003; 120: 484–487.

14. Weng AP, Ferrando AA, Lee W, et al. Activating mutations of NOTCH1 in human T cell acute lymphoblastic leukemia. *Science*. 2004; 306: 269–271.

15. Meng X, Wasowska K, Girodon F, et al. GSI-I (Z-LLN;e-CHO) inhibits γ-secretase and the proteosome to trigger cell death in precursor-B acute lymphoblastic leukemia. *Leukemia*. 2011; 25: 1135–1146.

16. Samon JB, Castillo-Martin M, Hadler M, et al. Preclinical analysis of the γ-secretase inhibitor PF-03084014 in combination with glucocorticoids in t-cell acute lymphoblastic leukemia. *Mol Cancer Ther*. 2012; 11:1565–1575.

17. Maloney KW, Schuster JJ, Murphy S, Pullen J, Camitta BA. Long-term results of treatment studies for childhood acute lymphoblastic leukemia: Pediatric Oncology Group studies from 1986–1994. *Leukemia*. 2000; 14: 2276–2285.

18. Larson RA, Dodge RK, Burns CP, et al. A five-drug remission induction regimen with intensive consolidation for adults with acute lymphoblastic leukemia: cancer and leukemia group B study 8811. *Blood*. 1995; 85: 2025–2037.

19. Patel B, Rai L, Buck G, et al. Minimal residual disease is a significant predictor of treatment failure in non T-lineage adult acute lymphoblastic leukaemia: final results of the international trial UKALL XII/ECOG2993. *Br J Haematol*. 2009; 148: 80–89.

20. Fielding AK, Rowe JM, Richards SM, et al. Prospective outcome data on 267 unselected adult patients with Philadelphia chromosome-positive acute lymphoblastic leukemia confirms superiority of allogeneic transplantation over chemotherapy in the pre-imatinib era: results from the international ALL trial MRCUKALLXII/ECOG2993. *Blood*. 2009; 113: 4489–4496.

21. Dhedin N, Dombret H, Thomas X, et al. Autologous stem cell transplantation in adults with acute lymphoblastic leukemia in first complete remission: analysis of the LALA-85, -87 and -94 trials. *Leukemia*. 2006; 20: 336–344.

22. Fielding AK, Richards SM, Chopra R, et al. Outcome of 609 adults after relapse of acute lymphoblastic leukemia (ALL); an MRC UKALL12/ECOG 2993 study. *Blood*. 2007; 109: 944–950.

23. Stanulla M, Schaeffeler E, Flohr T, et al. Thiopurine methyltransferase (TPMT) genotype and early treatment response to mercaptopurine in childhood acute lymphoblastic leukemia. *J Am Med Assoc*. 2005; 293: 1485–1489.

24. Thomas DA, Faderl S, Cortes J, et al. Treatment of Philadelphia chromosome-positive acute lymphocytic leukemia with hyper-CVAD and imatinib mesylate. *Blood*. 2004; 103: 4396–4407.

CHAPTER **29**
Chronic Lymphocytic Leukemia/ Small Lymphocytic Lymphoma

Philip C. Amrein

INTRODUCTION

Chronic lymphocytic leukemia (CLL) is a neoplastic disease characterized by the accumulation of monoclonal lymphocytes in blood, bone marrow, and lymphoid tissues. These lymphocytes are small, mature-appearing B cells typically expressing CD19, CD5, and CD23. It is generally a disease of older people and prognosis ranges widely from a few years to many years, but it is not considered curable outside of the bone marrow transplant setting. At times these neoplastic cells predominate in lymph nodes leading to the classification as a lymphoma. Hence, the WHO in 2008 has defined this neoplasm as chronic lymphocytic leukemia/small lymphocytic lymphoma (CLL/SLL) (1).

EPIDEMIOLOGY

CLL is the most common form of leukemia among adults of Western societies and accounts for 30% of all leukemias. In the United States, 16,060 new cases or 4.2 per 100,000 persons and 4580 deaths are projected for 2012 (2, 3). The male-to-female ratio is approximately 3:2. CLL accounts for 1% of all cancers, and is a disease of older adults with a median age of 72 years; only 10% of patients are <50 year old. The disease tends to run in families. When multiple members of a family have CLL, a detectable clone of CLL cells can be found by flow cytometry in 13.5% of apparently healthy first-degree relatives of patients. Also, among normal individuals >40 years of age, a clone of B cells consistent with CLL can be found by multiparameter flow cytometry in 3.5% of subjects (4). It is uncertain whether these individuals will progress to clinically significant disease. CLL is uncommon in Asia.

BIOLOGY

■ CAUSE

The cause is unknown. Environmental factors such as exposure to radiation, sunlight, chemical toxins, or viruses are not associated with an increased incidence of the disease. HLA haplotype is not associated with disease susceptibility.

■ MOLECULAR DEFECT

CLL cells are characterized by a defective B-cell receptor (CD79a and CD79b) that does not respond properly to antigen engagement but is associated with constitutive signaling intracellularly through immuno-receptor tyrosine-based activation motifs (ITAMs) to activate a cascade of kinases including Lyn and Syk leading to proliferation, inhibition of apoptosis, or, on occasion, promotion of apoptosis (5, 6). These changes lead to an accumulation of CLL cells in G0. CLL cells derive from antigen-experienced B lymphocytes and have the phenotype of activated cells.

During an immune response, normal B cells encountering antigen will travel to a germinal center and undergo a series of point mutations in the immunoglobulin genes, which result in a more snug fit for the antigen in its binding site. These somatic mutations can be detected by sequencing the immunoglobulin heavy-chain variable-region (IgV_H) genes. Patients with CLL cells that contain somatic mutations in their Ig genes (a little over 50%) will have a much better prognosis than patients with CLL cells containing germline Ig sequences. Two surrogate markers for mutational status are more easily obtainable than mutational analysis: CD38, a cell-surface enzyme involved in regulating B-cell activation, and ZAP-70, the 70-kD zeta-associated protein normally found in T cells and NK cells (5). CD38 levels tend to be high in CLL cells bearing unmutated Ig genes and can be easily assayed by routine flow cytometry. The intracellular protein ZAP-70 can also be assayed by flow cytometry, but it is technically more difficult. Elevated levels of ZAP-70 are also associated with CLL expressing unmutated Ig genes.

CLL cells can develop other cytogenetic abnormalities. Commonly detected clonal evolutions involve DNA deletions at chromosomes 13q14, 11q22-23, 17p13, and 6q21.

■ IMMUNE DYSREGULATION

Patients with CLL frequently demonstrate immune dysregulation ranging from hyperreactivity to external stimuli such as insect bites to frank immunodeficiency with frequent infections. CLL cells elaborate immune suppressive cytokines such as CD27 or transforming growth factor-β, which impede immune activation. CLL cells can also downmodulate CD40 ligand on CD4 T cells, which results in defective function of T cells as well as the initial steps in immunoglobulin production. Paradoxically autoimmunity may develop leading to autoimmune hemolytic anemia, idiopathic thrombocytopenic purpura (ITP), pure red cell aplasia, or autoimmune neutropenia. Usually the pathogenic autoantibodies are not produced by the CLL cells but are produced by normal lymphocytes and plasma cells in response to factors produced by the CLL cells.

CLINICAL PRESENTATION

Most patients with CLL present with mild symptoms of fatigue or malaise. Over 25% will present asymptomatically with incidental lymphocytosis in blood and nearly 80% of patients have nontender lymphadenopathy. Occasionally, patients will present with advanced disease with fever, sweats, weight loss, anemia, thrombocytopenia, or recurrent infections. Although computerized axial tomography (CT) scans are not part of the routine evaluation of CLL, they can on occasion demonstrate massive lymphadenopathy not otherwise appreciated. Rarely, lymphadenopathy in CLL will be responsible for organ dysfunction such as ureteral obstruction with hydronephrosis or biliary obstruction. Splenomegaly is present initially in approximately 50% of patients and may cause discomfort or early satiety. Patients may have anemia or thrombocytopenia. It is of critical importance to assess whether the cause is bone marrow infiltration or destruction by autoantibodies, as the treatment approach may vary according to the mechanism. The examination of the peripheral blood smear will generally show a lymphocytosis of mature-appearing lymphocytes with occasional larger lymphocytes and smudge cells. The smudge cells, which are broken lymphocytes resulting from the technique to prepare the blood smear, are characteristic of CLL. Despite very high lymphocyte counts in some patients with CLL, hyperleukocytosis with pulmonary or cerebral symptoms requiring emergency intervention is rare; patients have generally tolerated lymphocyte counts as high as 800,000/μl without problems of hyperviscosity. Bone marrow biopsies performed at the time of presentation will show infiltrating CLL cells. The pattern of infiltration is said to be prognostic, and four patterns are recognized: interstitial, nodular, mixed, and diffuse (prognosis going from better to worse). A Coombs test is recommended at the time of presentation because approximately 20% of patients will test positive; however, only 8% will have autoimmune hemolytic anemia. Approximately 15% of patients will present with normochromic normocytic anemia that is not associated with anti-RBC antibodies.

DIAGNOSIS

■ SPECIFIC CRITERIA

The diagnostic criteria for CLL have evolved over time, and currently most clinicians follow the criteria outlined in 2008 by the World Health Organization(WHO)(1) and by the International Workshop on Chronic Lymphocytic Leukemia (IWCLL) (7). Accordingly, the diagnosis of CLL requires a lymphocytosis of >5000/μl with cells that are B cells (positive for CD19, CD20, and CD23) and carry the aberrantly expressed T-cell marker CD5. Monoclonality needs to be demonstrated by surface immunoglobulin restriction to either kappa or lambda light chain. The lymphocytosis must also consist of <55% prolymphocytes, otherwise a diagnosis of prolymphocytic leukemia is favored. In the event that fewer than 5000/ul B-lymphocytes are detected in the peripheral blood, a diagnosis of SLL may be made with the presence of lymphadenopathy and/or splenomegaly. With neither lymphadenopathy nor splenomegaly a diagnosis of monoclonal B-lymphocytosis (MBL) may be made with <5000/ul monoclonal B-cells in the peripheral blood. Although approximately 80% of cases will have an abnormal karyotype by fluorescence in-situ hybridization (FISH) analysis, no specific cytogenetic abnormality defines the disease.

■ DIFFERENTIAL DIAGNOSIS (SEE TABLE 29-1)

Benign Lymphocytosis Patients may present with a high lymphocyte count when infected with various organisms such as: viruses, *Bordetella pertussis*, or *Toxoplasma gondii*. Usually, the lymphocytosis is not sustained, however,

TABLE 29-1A IMMUNOPHENOTYPE OF CLL AND SIMILAR NEOPLASMS (WORLD HEALTH ORGANIZATION CRITERIA)

Neoplasms	Surface Ig	CD2	CD3	CD4	CD5	CD7	CD8	CD10	CD11c	CD19	CD20	CD23	CD103
CLL/SLL[1]	dim		-	-	+			-	dim	+	dim	+	
B-PLL[2]	++				+/-					+	+	+/-	
T-PLL[3]		+	+	+/-		+	+/-						
T-LGL[4]	-		+	+/-	-	-	+						
HCL[5]	++							-	++	+	++	-	++
MCL[6]	++				+			-		+	+	-	
SMZL[7]	+				-			-		+	+	-	-
FL[8]	+				-			+		+	+	+/-	

[1]Chronic lymphocytic leukemia/small lymphocytic lymphoma.
[2]B-Prolymphocytic leukemia.
[3]T-Prolymphocytic leukemia.
[4]Large granular lymphocyte leukemia.
[5]Hairy cell leukemia.
[6]Mantle cell leukemia.
[7]Splenic marginal zone lymphoma.
[8]Follicular lymphoma.

TABLE 29-1B IMMUNOPHENOTYPE OF CLL AND SIMILAR NEOPLASMS

Neoplasms	Cyclin D1	Bcl-2	Bcl-6	TCR	Annexin A1	FMC7	TdT
CLL/SLL[1]	−			−	−	−	
B-PLL[2]					−	+	
T-PLL[3]				+			−
T-LGL[4]				+			
HCL[5]	+/−				+	+	
MCL[6]	+	+	−		−	+	
SMZL[7]	−		−		−		
FL[8]		+	+		−		

[1]Chronic lymphocytic leukemia/small lymphocytic lymphoma.
[2]B-Prolymphocytic leukemia.
[3]T-Prolymphocytic leukemia.
[4]T-Large granular lymphocyte leukemia.
[5]Hairy cell leukemia.
[6]Mantle cell leukemia.
[7]Splenic marginal zone lymphoma.
[8]Follicular lymphoma.

flow cytometry will not show monoclonal surface Ig or expression of CD5 on B cells.

Distinguishing Cll from other B-cell leukemias (WHO criteria) CLL is generally easily distinguished from other monoclonal B-cell malignancies that can be associated with lymphocytosis. CLL is surface Ig weak (others are strong), CD5 positive (others are negative), CD23 positive (others are negative), and CD79b/CD22 weak (others are strong). In addition, the antibody FMC7 does not react with CLL cells but does react with other B-cell leukemias.

B-prolymphocytic leukemia When the percentage of prolymphocytes in blood exceeds 55% in a patient who otherwise makes criteria for CLL, a diagnosis of prolymphocytic leukemia is made. It accounts for 1% of lymphoid leukemias. The prolymphocytes are larger cells being 10–15 μm in diameter (vs 7–10 μm for CLL cells), and they have more cytoplasm, frequently have nucleoli, and stain brightly for surface immunoglobulin. Prognosis is worse for prolymphocytic leukemia.

T-prolymphocytic leukemia (T-PLL) In about 2% of cases of small lymphocytic leukemia, the blood contains small- to medium-sized T-lymphoid cells with nongranular basophilic cytoplasm and round or oval nuclei with a nucleolus. Patients often have hepatosplenomegaly and lymphadenopathy and 20% have skin infiltration. The tumor cells are CD2, CD3, and CD7 positive while TdT and CD1a are negative. In 60%, the cells express CD4 but not CD8; in 15% they express CD8 but not CD4; and in 25% they express both CD4 and CD8. The course of disease is rapid with median survival of 1 year.

T-cell large granular lymphocytic leukemia In 2%–3% of cases of small lymphocytic leukemia, the cells in the peripheral blood have abundant cytoplasm that contains azurophilic granules. These patients usually present with neutropenia and minimal lymphocytosis. Flow cytometry shows these cells to be T cells, being positive for CD3, CD8, and the T-cell receptor (TCR). The cells are positive for CD57 in over 80% of cases and usually negative for CD4. The course of disease is often indolent.

Hairy cell leukemia In about 2% of cases of small lymphocytic leukemia, the blood smear will show a minimal lymphocytosis with lymphocytes demonstrating villous projections. Flow cytometry is diagnostic with cells positive for CD19, CD20, CD22, CD25, CD103, CD11c, and annexin A1. Flow cytometry will be negative for CD5 and CD10. Note that some cells may be positive for cyclin D1. Soluble CD25 levels are elevated. Patients present with splenomegaly and pancytopenia; monocytopenia is often noted. Long remissions have been obtained using cladribine or other nucleosides.

Mantle cell lymphoma with blood involvement These cells in blood and lymph nodes may look very much like CLL cells, and flow cytometry is required for a secure diagnosis. The cells are positive for CD5, FMC-7, and cyclin D1, and they have bright surface immunoglobulin, while being negative for CD10, CD23, and BCL6. Aberrant phenotypes exist, so genetic confirmation is desirable by testing for t(11;14)(q13;q32), which is the translocation of IGH with CCND1, the gene for cyclin D1. Prognosis for mantle cell lymphoma is generally much worse than that for CLL.

Splenic marginal zone lymphoma Patients generally present with splenomegaly and lymphocytosis with the lymphoid cells containing villous projections. Flow cytometry distinguishes these cells, since they are positive for CD19, CD20, CD79a, and surface immunoglobulin. Importantly, the cells are negative for CD5, CD10, CD23, annexin A1, and cyclin D1. The disease usually follows an indolent course.

Follicular lymphoma with blood involvement Examination of the blood smear usually shows these cells to have cleaved nuclei, while CLL cells do not. The flow cytometry pattern shows cells positive for CD10, CD19, CD20, CD22, and surface immunoglobulin with a bright pattern. They are positive for BCL2 and BCL6, while being negative for CD5.

EVALUATION OF THE PATIENT

The following evaluation is commonly performed on patients with CLL:

History and physical examination (B symptoms, lymphadenopathy, splenomegaly)

Complete blood count with differential, reticulocyte count, Coombs test, and LDH

Routine chemistries, uric acid, liver function tests including albumin and globulin

Hepatitis B serologies should be done, if treatment with rituximab is likely

Serum protein electrophoresis

Beta-2-microglobulin

Flow cytometry of blood: CD5, CD10, CD19, CD20, CD23, CD38, cyclin D1

Clinical trials may request ZAP-70 and IgVH mutational analysis

Lymph node biopsy: Immunohistochemical panel: CD3, CD5, CD10, CD20, CCD1

Bone marrow biopsy with cytogenetics and FISH analysis: del(11q), trisomy 12, del(13q), del(17p). Consider FISH analysis for t(11;14) when mantle cell lymphoma is suspected

Note that physical examination and peripheral blood examination are usually adequate for initial evaluation of asymptomatic patients, and bone marrow biopsy is usually delayed until treatment is imminent or when indicated to assess the pathophysiologic basis of anemia or thrombocytopenia. Clinical trials may require CT scans to assess response. Note that PET scans are generally not indicated unless Richter's transformation (histologic progression to diffuse large B-cell lymphoma with an accelerated pace of disease) is suspected.

PROGNOSTIC FACTORS

■ STAGING

Using clinical data from the physical examination and the complete blood count with differential, an estimate of prognosis can be obtained. The critical features used to assign clinical stage of disease are the presence of lymphadenopathy, splenomegaly, or hepatomegaly, and the presence of anemia and/or thrombocytopenia. The Rai (8) and Binet (9) staging classifications for CLL are shown in Table 29-2. Prognosis varies from 2 years with advanced stage disease to over 10 years with early stage disease.

■ MUTATIONAL STATUS

In about half of cases of CLL, immunoglobulin V_H genes have undergone somatic mutation, and this event is associated with an improved prognosis compared to patients whose cells express unmutated Ig genes. Determining mutational status of Ig genes is highly specialized and not widely available. The presence of ZAP-70 in the cytoplasm and CD38 on the surface of CLL cells has been found to correlate with the presence of unmutated Ig genes and a poorer prognosis. In one study (Figure 29-1), at approximately 10 years the mutated group and the CD38 negative group both showed 80% survival, while the unmutated group and the CD38 positive group both showed approximately 40% survival (10). Similar results have been seen when CLL patients have been analyzed based on ZAP-70 expression (11).

■ KARYOTYPE

Cytogenetic studies, including analysis by FISH techniques, can also identify patients with distinct prognosis. In one large report, 82% of the cases contained a chromosomal aberration by FISH techniques (12). The five most frequently encountered aberrations were a deletion in 13q, a deletion in 11q, trisomy 12, a deletion in 17p, and a deletion in 6q (Table 29-3). Prognosis varied widely with a median survival of 2.5 years for patients with the 17p deletion compared to 10 years or more for patients with a normal karyotype, trisomy 12, or a 13q deletion (Figure 29-2).

TABLE 29-2 STAGING SYSTEMS FOR CHRONIC LYMPHOCYTIC LEUKEMIA (8, 9)

	Criteria	Median Survival (y)
RAI STAGING SYSTEM		
Stage*		
0 (low-risk)	Lymphocytes > 15 × 10⁹/l Bone marrow >40% lymphocytes	>10
I and II (intermediate-risk)	Blood and bone marrow lymphocytosis, lymphadenopathy liver or spleen enlargement	6
III and IV (high-risk)	Blood and bone marrow lymphocytosis plus anemia (hemoglobin <11 g/dl) or thrombocytopenia (platelets <100 × 10⁹/l)	2
BINET STAGING SYSTEM		
Group*		
A	No anemia or thrombocytopenia, less than three of the following five areas involved: axillary, inguinal, cervical (unilateral or bilateral), liver, spleen	9
B	No anemia or thrombocytopenia; three or more involved areas	5
C	Anemia (hemoglobin <10g/dl) or thrombocytopenia (platelets <100 × 10⁹/l)	2

*Autoimmune hemolytic anemia and thrombocytopenia are independent of stage or group. Reproduced with permission from Handin R, Lux S, Stossel T (eds). *Blood: Principles and Practice of Hematology.* Philadelphia, JB Lippincott, 1995, p. 789.

■ **OTHER FACTORS**

Short doubling time of the lymphocyte count is associated with a poor prognosis; median survival for patients with a doubling time <12 months is about 5 years compared to a survival of 12 years for a longer doubling time. Bone marrow histology for patients with CLL (as noted above) has been studied; those with a diffuse pattern of involvement have been associated with a poorer prognosis and complications with cytopenias. Elevated beta-2-microglobulin is associated with poorer prognosis. Elevated LDH may indicate the presence of Richter transformation, which occurs at some point in 5%–10% of patients with CLL. The transformation marks the conversion to a diffuse large B-cell lymphoma generally resistant to treatment and associated with survival of 3–6 months. Telomerase activity when high has been linked

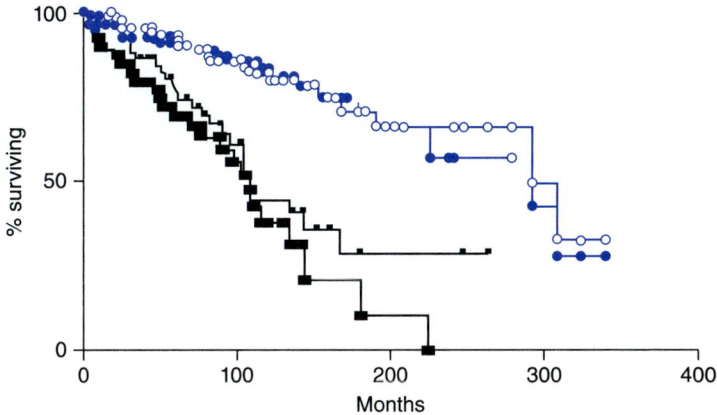

FIGURE 29-1 Survival curves of 145 patients with B-CLL. Comparisons were made of patients whose cells are CD38+ (⊥. N = 60) or CD 38-(●. N = 85) and have mutated (○. N = 95) or unmutated (■. N = 50) IgVH genes from date of diagnosis of CLL. (From Hamblin TJ, Orchard JA, Ibbotson RE, et al. CD38 expression and immunoglobulin variable region mutations are independent prognostic variables in chronic lymphocytic leukemia, but CD38 expression may vary during the course of the disease. *Blood.* 2002; 99: 1023-1029.)

TABLE 29-3 INCIDENCE OF CHROMOSOMAL ABNORMALITIES IN 325 PATIENTS WITH CHRONIC LYMPHOCYTIC LEUKEMIA

Aberration	No. of Patients (%)*
13q deletion	178 (55)
11q deletion	58 (18)
12q trisomy	53 (16)
17p deletion	23 (7)
6q deletion	21 (6)
8q trisomy	16 (5)
t(14q32)	12 (4)
Clonal abnormalities	268 (82)
Normal karyotype	57 (18)

*One hundred seventy five patients had one aberration, 67 had two aberrations, and 26 had more than two aberrations.

From Dohner H, et al. Genomic aberrations and survival in chronic lymphocytic leukemia. *N Engl J Med.* 2000; 343: 1910-1916.

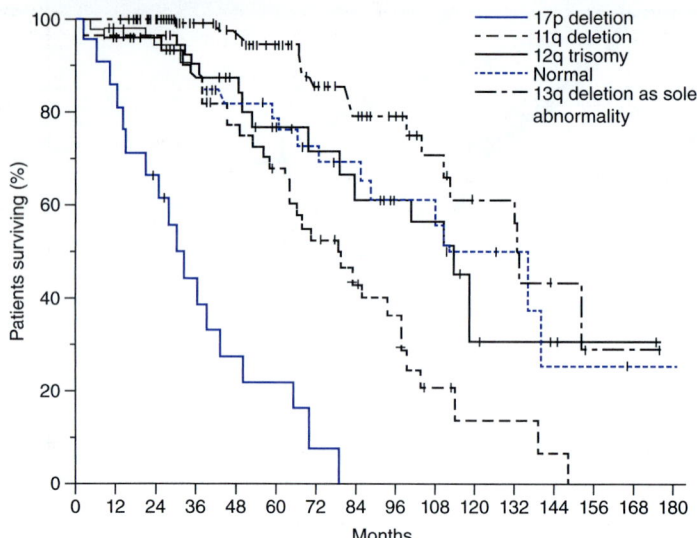

FIGURE 29-2 Probability of survival from the date of diagnosis among the patients in the five genetic categories. The median survival times for the groups with 17p deletion, 11q deletion, 12q trisomy, normal karyotype, and 13q deletion as the sole abnormality were 32, 79, 114, 111, and 133 months, respectively. Twenty-five patients with various other chromosomal abnormalities are not included in the analysis. (From Dohner H, et al. *N Engl J Med*. 2000; 343: 1910-1916.)

to the presence of short telomeres and aggressive histology. The patients with unmutated CLL tend to have high telomerase activity and short survival.

Most of these prognostic factors are not employed in clinical decision-making.

TREATMENT

■ INDICATIONS

The indication to treat a CLL patient is based on the emergence of symptoms caused by the tumor mass (pain, organ compromise, or constitutional symptoms) or the development of anemia and/or thrombocytopenia. It is important to investigate the mechanisms of any cytopenia. The development of an autoimmune cytopenia does not influence overall survival, and these autoimmune cytopenias generally can be controlled by immunosuppressive therapy with glucocorticoids or rituximab or, in some instances, by splenectomy. If expansion of CLL cells in the bone marrow is the basis for the cytopenia, therapy aimed at controlling the tumor is indicated because the patient will not improve significantly without such therapy, and this advanced stage represents a threat to survival. Generally, the indications to treat as outlined by the IWCLL are reasonable guidelines for general practice, and they are provided in Table 29-4 (7).

TABLE 29-4 INDICATIONS FOR TREATMENT OF CLL PATIENTS—IWCLL 2008 (7)

1. Worsening of anemia or thrombocytopenia
2. Splenomegaly with spleen tip >6 cm below the costal margin
3. Symptomatic lymph nodes or any lymph node >10 cm
4. Progressive lymphocytosis with a doubling in blood within 6 mo
5. Autoimmune anemia or thrombocytopenia poorly responsive to glucocorticoids
6. Weight loss of >10% within the past 6 mo
7. Fatigue with ECOG performance status of >2 due to disease
8. Fever with temperature >100.5°F for 2 wk not due to infection
9. Night sweats for >1 mo not due to infection

◼ INTENSITY OF TREATMENT

Once a decision is made to treat a patient, one must consider whether a mild treatment is best or a more intense approach is indicated. The clinical features used to make this decision generally are: age of the patient, performance status, comorbid conditions, ability to monitor the patient closely, and the specific wishes of the patient.

◼ SPECIFIC DRUGS OR REGIMENS

Most patients with CLL are treated with one or a combination of the following drugs: chlorambucil, fludarabine, cyclophosphamide, rituximab, ofatumumab, bendamustine, alemtuzumab, and glucocorticoids. As initial treatment in newly diagnosed patients, single-agent chlorambucil administered in pill form is appropriate for older patients that may not be fit for more aggressive intravenous approaches; however, most patients can tolerate single-agent fludarabine given intravenously, which has been shown to be more active than chlorambucil (Figure 29-3). The randomized trial demonstrating the higher response rate of fludarabine, however, also showed that patients in both groups had a median survival of approximately 5 years (13). Clinical trials have shown that responses improve when cyclophosphamide or rituximab (anti-CD20) is added to fludarabine (Table 29-5). Using the three drugs together as a combination has resulted in further improvement (14), and the "FCR" regimen has become the current standard of treatment for younger more fit patients with CLL. The overall response rate and complete response rate of FCR as reported by Tam was 95% and 72% with an overall survival of 77% at 6 years (15). The high response rate and improved survival was confirmed in a randomized trial reported by Hallek. (16) Trials with bendamustine and/or rituximab have shown similar high response rates with slightly less toxicity and are more widely used in somewhat older patients (17, 18). Doses and schedules of the FCR, BR, and other commonly used regimens are shown in Table 29-6.

The treatment of relapsed and refractory CLL is more challenging, and the choice of therapy is often determined by risk stratification. Patients

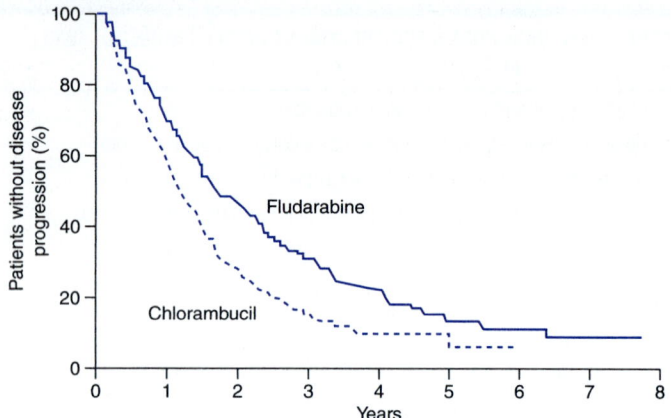

FIGURE 29-3 Proportion of CLL patients without disease progression, according to treatment group. The median time to progression was significantly longer in the fludarabine group than in the chlorambucil group (20 vs 14 months, $P < 0.001$). (From Rai KR, et al. *N Engl J Med.* 2000; 343: 1750-1757.)

who have had a progression-free survival of more than 3 years generally should be treated with the same regimen used to achieve the first remission, and another long remission would be expected. Patients progressing within 3 years of prior treatment should undergo cytogenetic analysis for the presence of del(17p). If present, consideration should be given to using alemtuzumab as a single agent (19) or using high-dose methylprednisolone in combination with either rituximab (20) or with alemtuzumab (21), since further use of alkylating agents has been disappointing in this setting. Clinical trials employing new agents also should be strongly considered for patients progressing within 3 years. Using the FCR regimen in relapsed CLL was reported to result in an overall response rate of 74%, a complete

TABLE 29-5 REPORTED COMPLETE AND OVERALL RESPONSE RATES (CR AND OR) IN VARIOUS CLINICAL TRIALS FOR PREVIOUSLY UNTREATED CHRONIC LYMPHOCYTIC LEUKEMIA (CLL)

Regimen	Patients	CR (%)	OR (%)	Reference
Chlorambucil	181	4	37	(13)
Fludarabine	170	20	63	(13)
Fludarabine + cyclophosphamide	34	35	88	(16)
Fludarabine + rituximab	51	47	90	(39)
Fludarabine, cyclophosphamide, rituximab	300	72	95	(15)

TABLE 29-6 REGIMENS USEFUL IN THE TREATMENT OF CLL

Regimen	Dose and schedule
1. Chlorambucil	10 mg/day PO or 40 mg/m^2 PO day 1 q28d
2. Fludarabine	25 mg/m^2 IV days 1–5 q28d
3. Fludarabine plus Cyclophosphamide	25 mg/m^2 IV days 1–3 q28d 250 mg/m^2 IV days 1–3 q28d
4. Fludarabine plus Rituximab	25 mg/m^2 IV days 1–5 q28d 375 mg/m^2 IV d1 q28d
5. Fludarabine plus Cyclophosphamide plus Rituximab	25 mg/m^2 IV on days 2–4 (or on days 1–3) 250 mg/m^2 IV for 3 days with fludarabine 375 mg/m^2 IV day 1
6. Bendamustine plus Rituximab	70 mg/m2/day on days 1 and 2 375 mg/m2 on day 0 (or on day 1)

response rate of 30%, and an overall survival of 47 months; however, the regimen was not recommended for patients with del(17p) or with fludarabine refractory disease (22). After cytoreductive therapy consideration should be given in younger patients to consolidating the response with an allogeneic stem-cell transplant.

■ BONE MARROW TRANSPLANTATION

Bone marrow transplantation, or hematopoietic stem-cell transplantation (SCT), is appropriate treatment for only a small subset of patients with CLL for several reasons. Many patients with CLL have indolent disease and do not need treatment on presentation or perhaps ever. The median age of patients with CLL is 72 years, and therefore many such patients are elderly and medically unfit to consider the transplant option. Nevertheless, high-dose therapy with hematopoietic stem cell support has been tested extensively over the years in younger patients with relapsed or refractory disease.

Autologous SCT has not been accepted as standard treatment in CLL, but continues to be tested in clinical trials. Initial enthusiasm for this treatment has faded with the recognition that patients seem not to be cured, with no observed plateau on the reported survival curves. In addition, there is the concern regarding the development of secondary malignancies, especially MDS/AML, which occurred in 12% of patients at 5 years in one trial (23). There are three recently reported randomized trials of autologous SCT used as first-line or second-line therapy in CLL. Results showed significant improvement in event-free survival (EFS) in all studies, but no improvement in overall survival (OS) when compared with various non-transplant chemotherapy strategies (24-26). For these reasons, autologous SCT for patients with CLL is currently recommended only in the experimental setting.

Myeloablative SCT similarly has been extensively tested in CLL but has been used successfully only in relatively young and very fit patients. While potentially curative, the high treatment-related mortality in this population has limited its feasibility. Past registry data have indicated a 46% treatment-related mortality for patients with CLL treated with myeloablative SCT (27), and the estimated 5-year overall survival in another study was only 32% (28). With the relative success of reduced-intensity conditioning (RIC) SCT, most centers have been focusing on this form of transplantation for CLL patients.

RIC SCT is better suited for the elderly patients typical of CLL. Lower intensity conditioning has greatly reduced the treatment-related mortality, and the ability of the graft versus leukemia effect to eradicate residual CLL has been gratifying. The results of a recently completed multi-institutional study of RIC SCT in relapsed and refractory CLL has been published (29). In this trial the treatment-related mortality at 5 years was 23%, the EFS was 39%, and the OS was 50%.

The European Group for Blood and Marrow Transplantation (EBMT) has recently set guidelines for the use of SCT in patients with high-risk CLL (30). Autologous SCT is considered only for clinical trials, but allogeneic SCT may be considered for the following high-risk patients with CLL:

- Fludarabine resistant: non-response or early relapse (<12 months) after purine analogue-based therapy.
- Relapse <24 months after purine analogue combinations or auto-SCT (plus high-risk genetics)
- p53 mutation with treatment indication

In conclusion, allo-SCT remains the only truly curative treatment for CLL, but its use is limited to younger, more fit patients with high-risk disease, generally as indicated by the EBMT. The focus in the transplant setting has been with the use of reduced intensity conditioning, which has resulted in acceptable treatment-related mortality, not seen with myeloablative regimens.

FUTURE DIRECTIONS

■ CONSOLIDATION WITH ALEMTUZUMAB

Patients with CLL characterized by deletions of 17p13 have a particularly resistant form of disease, possibly due to alterations in p53. Alemtuzumab is particularly effective in this population of patients leading to the concept of consolidating patients with alemtuzumab treatment after more conventional treatment to eradicate any resistant cells that may be left behind. Results of such studies have shown the emergence of a population of patients without detectable minimal residual disease and prolonged disease-free interval; however, there is also an enhanced risk for opportunistic infections with this approach, which currently limits its use and applicability (31, 32).

■ MINIMAL RESIDUAL DISEASE

As treatment becomes more effective, there is a need to evaluate patients with lower tumor burden than can be detected by clinical measures. Studies using polymerase chain reaction (PCR) techniques for the IgV_H gene can detect 1 CLL cell in 10,000 on a reliable basis, but the procedure is labor intensive. Multiparameter flow cytometry is also capable of detecting 1 CLL cell in 10,000 when certain antibodies are used. One set of antibodies shown to be effective for this is CD5, CD19, CD20, and CD79b. Detection of minimal residual disease (MRD) is clinically useful, as trials now show a survival advantage for those patients who are rendered MRD negative (33). Most future clinical trials will include MRD monitoring for those achieving a clinical complete remission. Additional data are needed to assess whether clinical decisions can be made based on the MRD results.

■ NEW DRUGS

Several new drugs undergoing evaluation in clinical trials are already showing activity in CLL. Although it is unclear at this time how useful they will become, they have stirred the interest of many investigators. A short list of active new agents includes flavopiridol (34), lenalidomide (35), CAL101, an inhibitor of PI3K (36), and ibrutinib, an inhibitor of the Bruton tyrosine kinase (37, 38).

■ SUPPORTIVE CARE

The hypogammaglobulinemia encountered frequently with CLL and as a consequence of using certain drugs (fludarabine, rituximab, alemtuzumab, and glucocorticoids) can lead to an increased risk of serious infections. When a patient experiences his or her second serious infection, monthly intravenous infusions of immunoglobulin are recommended to reduce this infectious risk, but immunoglobulin is expensive and treatments are frequently accompanied by significant infusional reactions. Severe neutropenia is also frequently encountered with the various treatments for CLL and should be treated with growth factor support and, in certain situations, prophylactic oral antibiotics.

CONCLUSIONS

Considerable progress has been made in understanding the biology of CLL and in the development of new and more effective treatments. Because the prognosis of patients with CLL is quite variable, such that some patients may never need treatment while other patients very quickly encounter serious life-threatening complications of progressive disease, the assessment of prognosis for each patient has become a very important exercise. Very long-term remissions are now possible in a subset of patients, and the testing for minimal residual disease by flow cytometry has become routine for patients achieving a clinical complete remission. The outlook for CLL patients has improved, and ongoing research promises further steady progress.

REFERENCES

1. Muller-Hermelink HK, Montserrat E, Catovsky D, et al. Chronic lymphocytic leukemia/small lymphocytic lymphoma. In: Swerdlow SH, Campo E, Harris NL, et al (eds). *WHO Classification of Tumors of Haematopoietic and lymphoid Tissues,* fourth edition, Lyon, WHO Press, 2008; pp 32-37.

2. Siegel R, Naishadham D, Jemal A. Cancer statistics. *CA Cancer J Clin.* 2012; 62:10-29.

3. Howlader N, Noone AM, Krapcho M, et al (eds). SEER Cancer Statistics Review, 1975-2009 (Vintage 2009 Populations), National Cancer Institute. Bethesda, MD, http://seer.cancer.gov/csr/1975_2009_

pops09/, based on November 2011 SEER data submission, posted to the SEER web site, 2012.

4. Rawstron AC, Green MJ, Kuzmicki A, et al. Monoclonal B lymphocytes with the characteristics of "indolent" chronic lymphocytic leukemia are present in 3.5% of adults with normal blood counts. *Blood.* 2002; 100: 635-639.

5. Chiorazzi N, Rai KR, Ferrarini M. Chronic lymphocytic leukemia. *N Engl J Med.* 2005; 352: 804-815.

6. Contri A, Brunati AM, Trentin L, et al. Chronic lymphocytic leukemia B cells contain anomalous Lyn tyrosine kinase, a putative contribution to defective apoptosis. *J Clin Invest.* 2005; 115: 369-378.

7. Hallek M, Cheson, BD, Catovsky D, et al. Guidelines for the diagnosis and treatment of chronic lymphocytic leukemia: a report from the International Workshop on Chronic Lymphocytic Leukemia updating the National Cancer Institute-Working Group 1996 guidelines. *Blood.* 2008; 111: 5446-5456.

8. Rai KR, Sawitsky A, Cronkite EP, et al. Clinical staging of chronic lymphocytic leukemia. *Blood.* 1975; 46: 219-234.

9. Binet JL, Auquier A, Dighiero G, et al. A new prognostic classification of chronic lymphocytic leukemia derived from a multivariate survival analysis. *Cancer.* 1981; 48: 198-206.

10. Hamblin TJ, Orchard JA, Ibbotson RE, et al. CD38 expression and immunoglobulin variable region mutations are independent prognostic variables in chronic lymphocytic leukemia, but CD38 expression may vary during the course of the disease. *Blood.* 2002; 99: 1023-1029.

11. Rassenti LZ, Huynh L, Toy TL, et al. ZAP-70 compared with immunoglobulin heavy-chain gene mutation status as a predictor of disease progression in chronic lymphocytic leukemia. *N Engl J Med.* 2004; 351: 893-901.

12. Dohner H, Stilgenbauer S, Benner A, et al. Genomic aberrations and survival in chronic lymphocytic leukemia. *N Engl J Med.* 2000; 343: 1910-1916.

13. Rai KR, Peterson BL, Appelbaum FR, et al. Fludarabine compared with chlorambucil as primary therapy for chronic lymphocytic leukemia. *N Engl J Med.* 2000; 343: 1750-1757.

14. Keating MJ, O'Brien S, Albitar M, et al. Early results of a chemoimmunotherapy regimen of fludarabine, cyclophosphamide, and rituximab as initial therapy for chronic lymphocytic leukemia. *J Clin Oncol.* 2005; 23: 4079-4088.

15. Tam CS, O'Brien S, Wierda W, et al. Long-term results of the fludarabine, cyclophosphamide, and rituximab regimen as initial therapy of chronic lymphocytic leukemia. *Blood.* 2008; 112: 975-980.

16. Hallek M, Fischer K, Fingerle-Rowson G, et al. Addition of rituximab to fludarabine and cyclophosphamide in patients with chronic lymphocytic leukaemia: a randomised, open-label, phase 3 trial. *Lancet.* 2010; 376: 1164-1174.

17. Knauf WU, Lissichkov T, Aldaoud A, et al. Phase III randomized study of bendamustine compared with chlorambucil in previously untreated patients with chronic lymphocytic leukemia. *J Clin Oncol.* 2009; 27: 4378-4384.

18. Fischer K, Cramer P, Busch R, et al. Bendamustine combined with rituximab in patients with relapsed and/or refractory chronic lymphocytic leukemia: a multicenter phase II trial of the German Chronic Lymphocytic Leukemia Study Group. *J Clin Oncol.* 2011; 29: 3559-3566.

19. Lundin J, Kimby E, Bjorkholm M, et al. Phase II trial of subcutaneous anti-CD52 monoclonal antibody alemtuzumab (Campath-1H) as first-line treatment for patients with B-cell chronic lymphocytic leukemia (B-CLL). *Blood.* 2002; 100: 768-773.

20. Castro JE, Sandoval-Sus JD, Bole J, et al. Rituximab in combination with high-dose methylprednisolone for the treatment of fludarabine refractory high-risk chronic lymphocytic leukemia. *Leukemia.* 2008; 22: 2048-2053.

21. Pettitt AR, Jackson R, Carruthers S, et al. Alemtuzumab in combination with methylprednisolone is a highly effective induction regimen for patients with chronic lymphocytic leukemia and deletion of TP53: final results of the national cancer research institute CLL206 trial. *J Clin Oncol.* 2012; 30: 1647-1655.

22. Badoux XC, Keating MJ, Wang X, et al. Fludarabine, cyclophosphamide, and rituximab chemoimmunotherapy is highly effective treatment for relapsed patients with CLL. *Blood.* 2011; 117: 3016-3024.

23. Milligan DW, Fernandes S, Dasgupta R, et al. Results of the MRC pilot study show autografting for younger patients with chronic lymphocytic leukemia is safe and achieves a high percentage of molecular responses. *Blood.* 2005; 105: 397-404.

24. Michallet M, Dreger P, Sutton L, et al. Autologous hematopoietic stem cell transplantation in chronic lymphocytic leukemia: results of European intergroup randomized trial comparing autografting versus observation. *Blood.* 2011; 117: 1516-1521.

25. Sutton L, Chevret S, Tournilhac O, et al. Autologous stem cell transplantation as a first-line treatment strategy for chronic lymphocytic leukemia: a multicenter, randomized, controlled trial from the SFGM-TC and GFLLC. *Blood.* 2011; 117: 6109-6119.

26. Brion A, Mahe B, Kolb B, et al. Autologous transplantation in CLL patients with B and C Binet stages: final results of the prospective randomized GOELAMS LLC 98 trial. *Bone Marrow Transplant.* 2012; 47: 542-548.

27. Michallet M, Archimbaud E, Bandini G, et al. HLA-identical sibling bone marrow transplantation in younger patients with chronic lymphocytic leukemia. European Group for Blood and Marrow Transplantation and the International Bone Marrow Transplant Registry. *Ann Intern Med.* 1996; 124: 311-315.

28. Sorror ML, Storer BE, Sandmaier BM, et al. Five-year follow-up of patients with advanced chronic lymphocytic leukemia treated with allogeneic hematopoietic cell transplantation after nonmyeloablative conditioning. *J Clin Oncol*. 2008; 26: 4912-4920.

29. Dreger P, Brand R, Hansz J, et al. Treatment-related mortality and graft-versus-leukemia activity after allogeneic stem cell transplantation for chronic lymphocytic leukemia using intensity-reduced conditioning. *Leukemia*. 2003; 17: 841-848.

30. Dreger P, Corradini P, Kimby E, et al. Indications for allogeneic stem cell transplantation in chronic lymphocytic leukemia: the EBMT transplant consensus. *Leukemia*. 2007; 21: 12-17.

31. Moreton P, Kennedy B, Lucas G, et al. Eradication of minimal residual disease in B-cell chronic lymphocytic leukemia after alemtuzumab therapy is associated with prolonged survival. *J Clin Oncol*. 2005; 23: 2971-2979.

32. Lin TS, Donohue KA, Byrd JC, et al. Consolidation therapy with subcutaneous alemtuzumab after fludarabine and rituximab induction therapy for previously untreated chronic lymphocytic leukemia: final analysis of CALGB 10101. *J Clin Oncol*. 2010; 28: 4500-4506.

33. Rawstron AC, Kennedy B, Evans PA, et al. Quantitation of minimal disease levels in chronic lymphocytic leukemia using a sensitive flow cytometric assay improves the prediction of outcome and can be used to optimize therapy. *Blood*. 2001; 98: 29-35.

34. Lin TS, Ruppert AS, Johnson AJ, et al. Phase II study of flavopiridol in relapsed chronic lymphocytic leukemia demonstrating high response rates in genetically high-risk disease. *J Clin Oncol*. 2009; 27: 6012-6018.

35. Chen CI, Bergsagel PL, Paul H, et al. Single-agent lenalidomide in the treatment of previously untreated chronic lymphocytic leukemia. *J Clin Oncol*. 2011; 29: 1175-1181.

36. Furman RR, Byrd JC, Brown JR, et al. CAL-101, An isoform-selective inhibitor of phosphatidylinositol 3-Kinase P110, demonstrates clinical activity and pharmacodynamic effects in patients with relapsed or refractory chronic lymphocytic leukemia (abstract 55). *Proc Am Soc of Hematology*. 2010.

37. de Rooij MF, Kuil A, Geest CR, et al. The clinically active BTK inhibitor PCI-32765 targets B-cell receptor- and chemokine-controlled adhesion and migration in chronic lymphocytic leukemia. *Blood*. 2012; 119: 2590-2594.

38. Byrd JC, Furman RR, Coutre SE, et al. The Bruton's tyrosine kinase (BTK) inhibitor PCI-32765 (P) in treatment-naive (TN) chronic lymphocytic leukemia (CLL) patients (pts): interim results of a phase Ib/II study (abstract 6507). *J Clin Oncol*. 2012; (Suppl).

39. Byrd JC, Peterson BL, Morrison VA, et al. Randomized phase 2 study of fludarabine with concurrent versus sequential treatment with rituximab in symptomatic, untreated patients with B-cell chronic lymphocytic leukemia: results from Cancer and Leukemia Group B 9712 (CALGB 9712). *Blood*. 2003; 101: 6-14.

CHAPTER **30**
Plasma Cell Disorders

Noopur Raje, Dan L. Longo

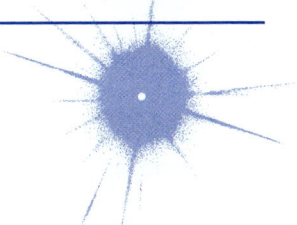

INTRODUCTION

Plasma cell disorders are a group of related diseases arising from a common progenitor belonging to the B-cell lineage. They are characterized by the expansion of plasma cells in the bone marrow (BM) and nearly always accompanied by the presence of a monoclonal immunoglobulin (Ig) or Ig fragment in the serum and/or urine of patients (1). Monoclonal gammopathy of undetermined significance (MGUS), multiple myeloma (MM), Waldenstrom's macroglobulinemia (WM), primary amyloidosis, and heavy chain diseases (HCD) all belong to this group of disorders. Dysproteinemias or plasma cell dyscrasias are some of the other terms used to refer to this unique group of disorders.

Normal B-cell differentiation is characterized by a process of Ig VDJ rearrangement, somatic mutation, and Ig class switching resulting in maturation of antibody-producing plasma cells. Ig variable (VH) gene sequence analysis indicates that myeloma tumor cells are postfollicular, and originate from a memory cell undergoing isotype switch events. Translocations involving switch regions indicate that the final oncogenic molecular event in myeloma occurs late in B-cell ontogeny. Five heavy-chain isotypes (M, G, A, D, E) and two light-chain isotypes (κ and λ) are present and are typically identified by serum or urine protein electrophoresis as a sharp spike in the gamma region. The isotype is further identified and quantitated by immunofixation and is referred to as the monoclonal component, that is, arising from the neoplastic clone. This is a useful biomarker and helps determine responses in patients with plasma cell disorders. More recently an ELISA-based assay is being used to detect light chains in the serum. This is particularly useful in patients with amyloidosis, light chain MM, and nonsecretory MM.

MONOCLONAL GAMMOPATHY OF UNDETERMINED SIGNIFICANCE

Monoclonal gammopathy of undetermined significance (MGUS) is seen in 1% of patients over age 50 and 3% of people over age 70 and is associated with the presence of a monoclonal Ig which is less than 3.5 g/l (2). It is differentiated from MM by fewer than 5% monoclonal BM plasma cells and lack of end organ damage like bone lesions, anemia, hypercalcemia, or renal dysfunction. In a large series of 1384 patients followed longitudinally at the Mayo Clinic, 115 patients progressed to MM (relative risk [RR] 25), IgM lymphoma (RR 2.4), primary amyloidosis (RR 8.4), macroglobulinemia (RR 46), chronic lymphocytic leukemia (RR 0.9), or plasmacytoma (RR 8.5). The risk of progression of MGUS to MM or related disorders is about 1% per year (2); risk factors for progression include high serum monoclonal protein (≥1.5 g/dl), non-IgG MGUS, and abnormal serum free light chain ratio (3). At this time, treatment for MGUS and smoldering MM consists of risk stratification and close observation (2). Clinical trials are however being conducted to target this population.

MULTIPLE MYELOMA

■ EPIDEMIOLOGY

MM is a plasma cell dyscrasia characterized by a clonal proliferation of lymphoid B cells and infiltration of the BM by plasma cells (1, 4). It is the second most common hematologic malignancy, and is responsible for at least 2% of cancer-related deaths. It is estimated that 21,700 new cases of MM and 10,710 deaths from MM will occur in the United States in 2012 (5). African-Americans and Pacific Islanders have a reported high incidence of MM followed by Europeans and North American Caucasians. Low incidence rates have been reported for Asians living in Asia and the United States (6). In addition to MGUS, potential risk factors for the development of MM include exposure to irradiation or petroleum products. Familial cases have also been reported, suggesting a possible genetic predisposition. Myeloma has also been found to occur with somewhat greater frequency in farmers, paper producers, furniture manufacturers, and wood workers.

■ BIOLOGY

Cytokines like interleukin-6 (IL-6) and insulin-like growth factor-1 (IGF-1) confer a growth and survival advantage to MM cells. Regulation of the mitogen-activated protein kinase (MAPK) and phosphatidylinositol 3′-kinase/Akt kinase (p13 kinase/AKT) pathways by these and other cytokines and activation of the survival Janus Kinase/signal transducer and activator of transcription (JAK/STAT) pathway may be involved in the pathogenesis. The role of adhesion molecules and the BM microenvironment is also critical to tumor cell growth and survival. Adhesion molecules mediate both homotypic and heterotypic adhesion of tumor cells to either extracellular matrix (ECM) proteins or bone marrow stromal cells (BMSCs). After class switching in the LN, adhesion molecules, including CD44, VLA-4, VLA-5, LFA-1, CD56, Syndecan-1, and MPC-1, mediate homing of myeloma cells to the BM, and adhesion to BMSCs and ECM. Such binding not only localizes tumor cells to the BM microenvironment, but also stimulates IL-6 transcription and secretion from BMSCs with related paracrine growth of myeloma cells. In addition to homing to the BM, loss of some of these adhesion molecules results in migration at the time of disease progression. The binding of MM cells to BMSCs also regulates cell cycle progression and plays a role in the development of adhesion-mediated drug resistance (4). A variety of chromosomal abnormalities are found in MM. Based on conventional cytogenetic analysis, chromosome 13 deletions were predominant and associated with a poor prognosis. Techniques like spectral karyotyping have identified chromosomal abnormalities in the majority of MM patients and are broadly classified into hyperdiploid (HRD) or nonhyperdiploid (NHRD) tumors. Five recurrent IgH translocations have been seen in MM including MMSET and FGFR3 (15%), cyclin D3 (3%), cyclin D1 (15%), c-maf (5%) genes, and MAFB (2%) accounting for a prevalence of 40%. All MM tumor cells have high levels of cyclin D1, D2, and D3 including

MGUS suggesting a unifying early oncogenic event (7, 8). Dysregulation of cyclin genes renders MM cells more susceptible to proliferative stimuli resulting in selective expansion in response to BMSCs and/or cytokines like IL-6 and IGF-1. On the basis of gene expression profiles, a new molecular classification has been proposed that categorizes patients based on the five major translocations and cyclin D overexpression in MM. Whole genome and whole exome sequencing of 38 MM patients identified mutations in genes involved in protein translation (e.g., mutations in *DIS3* [also known as *RRP44*] and *FAM46C*), histone methylation, blood coagulation, and members of the NF-κB signaling (9). Four percent of patients had activating mutations in the BRAF kinase, suggesting a potential role for BRAF inhibitor-directed therapy.

■ DIAGNOSTIC CRITERIA

The diagnosis of MM is based on the presence of well-defined major and minor criteria (Table 30-1) (10). These criteria help distinguish MM from other plasma cell dyscrasias and B-cell malignancies associated with a

TABLE 30-1 DURIE–SALMON CRITERIA FOR DIAGNOSIS OF MYELOMA

Major criteria

1. Plasmacytomas on tissue biopsy
2. BM plasmacytosis (>30% plasma cells)
3. Monoclonal immunoglobulin spike on serum or urine electrophoresis: IgG >3.5 g/dl or IgA >2.0 g/dl; κ or λ light chain urinary excretion > 1.0g/day

Minor criteria

a. BM plasmacytosis (10%–30% plasma cells)
b. Monoclonal immunoglobulin spike present but at a lower magnitude than above
c. Lytic bone lesions
d. Normal IgM< 500 mg/l, IgA < l g/l, or IgG < 6 g/l

The diagnosis of myeloma requires a minimum of one major and one minor criterion, although (1) + (a) is not sufficient or three minor criteria that must include (a) and (b).

Patients with the above criteria associated with

- absent or limited bone lesions (≥3 lytic lesions), no compression fractures
- stable paraprotein levels IgG < 70 g/l, IgA <50 g/l
- no symptoms and associated disease features including Karnofsky performance status > 70%, hemoglobin > 10 g/l, normal serum calcium, serum creatinine <2 mg/dl, and no infections
- plasma cell labelling index ≤ 0.5% are categorized as those with indolent myeloma and do not require immediate therapy.

Adapted from Durie BG. Staging and kinetics of multiple myeloma. *Semin Oncol.* 1986; 13: 300–309.

paraprotein. They also help differentiate MM from solitary plasmacytoma. Solitary plasmacytomas are collections of monoclonal plasma cells originating in either bone (solitary osseous plasmacytoma, SOP) or soft tissue (extramedullary plasmacytoma, EMP) and are very responsive to local radiation treatment. The mean age of diagnosis of solitary plasmacytomas is usually younger than MM and approximately 70% of EMPs can be cured with local treatment alone. EMPs typically involve the lymphoid tissues of the upper aerodigestive tract. SOPs have a higher rate of progression to MM and therefore patients with plasmacytomas require prolonged follow-up (11).

■ CLINICAL AND LABORATORY FEATURES

The mean age at diagnosis for MM is 62 years for men and 61 years for women. A slight male preponderance has been described. BM infiltration with plasma cells is commonly seen (**Figure 30-1**). Most of the symptoms associated with MM are a result of the end-organ damage caused by either MM tumor cell infiltration and/or the associated paraprotein. Symptoms of bone pain and anemia remain the most common presenting features affecting 80% of the patients. Other features include renal insufficiency, hypercalcemia, and symptoms associated with infection and hyperviscosity (12) (**Table 30-2**).

Bone disease and hypercalcemia MM typically presents with osteolytic bone lesions (**Figure 30-2**). These may be associated with pathologic and compression fractures of the vertebral bodies. Bone scans and serum alkaline phosphatase are usually normal because of the absence of osteoblastic activity. Increased tumor burden results in production of osteoclast-activating factors like lymphotoxin (LT), TNF-α, hepatocyte growth factor (HGF), IL-6, IL-1, metalloproteinases, RANKL, and insulin-like growth factor-binding protein 4 (IGFIV) resulting in increased osteoclastogenesis and increased bone resorption. Bone resorption leads to increased calcium in extracellular fluid.

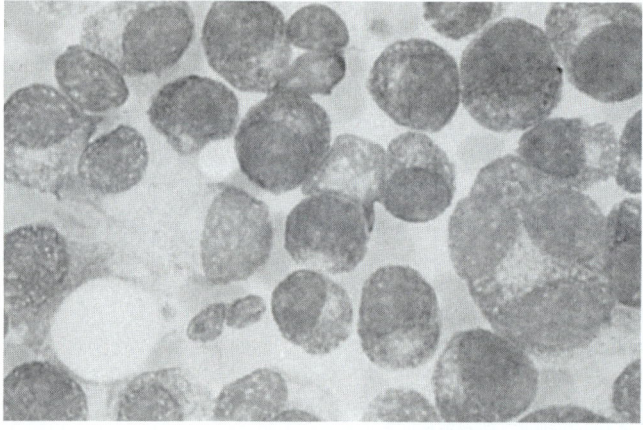

FIGURE 30-1 Photomicrograph of clusters of plasma cells in a bone marrow specimen.

TABLE 30-2 CLINICAL FEATURES OF MULTIPLE MYELOMA

Organ Involvement	Pathogenesis	Signs and Symptoms
Skeletal system	↑osteoclastogenesis ↑OAFs by tumor cells Tumor cell infiltration	Bone pains Osteoporosis Lytic disease Pathologic fractures Hypercalcemia Cord compression
Hematopoietic system	Tumor cell infiltration Inhibitory cytokines ↓Erythropoietin ↑Antibodies Hyperviscosity	Anemia Neutropenia Thrombocytopenia Bleeding
Renal	Light chain disease Myeloma kidney Dehydration Amyloid Urate nephropathy	Renal failure Hypercalcemia
Immune system	Hypogammaglobulinemia ↓ neutrophil migration	Infections
Neurologic	↑ Antibodies Hyperviscosity Tumor infiltration	Neuropathies Strokes Cord compression

A skeletal survey is routinely performed on patients with MM to evaluate for bone disease. MRI is more sensitive and is being increasingly used in patients. In addition to defining bone disease, it can highlight BM infiltration.

Anemia Anemia in MM can be due to a number of factors, including tumor infiltration of the BM, renal impairment, the myelosuppressive effects of tumor products and chemotherapy, and a deficient production of erythropoietin (EPO) relative to the degree of anemia.

Renal failure Renal failure in MM predicts for an adverse outcome. The causes of renal failure in MM are often multifactorial and include hypercalcemia, MM kidney, hyperuricemia, toxicity from intravenous urography, dehydration, plasma cell infiltration, pyelonephritis, medications like nonsteroidal anti-inflammatory drugs, and amyloidosis.

Hyperviscosity Hyperviscosity is characterized clinically by spontaneous bleeding with headache and neurologic and visual disorders.

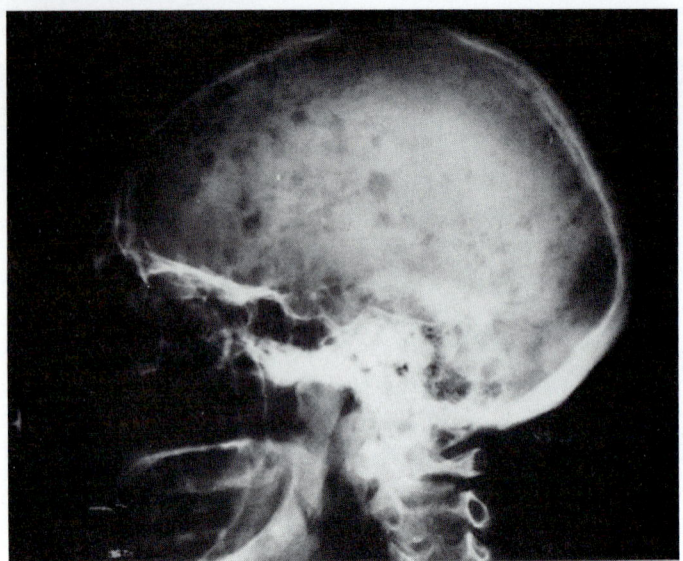

FIGURE 30-2 Radiograph of the head showing lytic lesions in the skull. The lesions have no osteoblastic activity and do not appear on nuclear medicine bone scans. (Photo provided by Dr. Geraldine Schechter.)

Hyperviscosity is commonly seen with IgM paraproteins, although the IgG3 subclass has also been associated with this syndrome.

Recurrent infections Patients with MM are at an increased risk of infections because of the underlying hypogammaglobulinemia. *Streptococcus pneumoniae* and hemophilus infections usually occur early and typically during response to chemotherapy. Gram-negative infections occur in refractory, advancing disease; in the setting of previous antibiotic therapy; instrumentation; immobilization; colonization with hospital flora; and azotemia. Fatal infections may be hospital acquired, emphasizing the need to minimize indwelling foreign bodies such as catheters in patients with MM.

Cardiac failure The median age of patients with MM is more than 60 years; such patients are at an increased risk of cardiovascular disease. Patients are uniquely susceptible to cardiac ischemia and/or congestive heart failure (CHF) due to myocardial infiltration with amyloid, causing dilated or restricted cardiomyopathy, hyperviscosity syndrome, and/or anemia. MM patients are also susceptible to high-output CHF of unclear etiology.

Neuropathies In MM, a symmetric, distal sensory or sensorimotor neuropathy is most common and is associated with axonal degeneration, with or without amyloid deposition. In some cases, neuropathy is associated with monoclonal antibodies directed against peripheral nerve myelin.

Laboratory evaluation identifies a monoclonal Ig in serum and/or urine in the majority of cases. In most series, 50%–60% of patients with myeloma have both serum and urinary monoclonal protein; 20%–30% of patients have serum without urinary protein; 15%–20% patients have monoclonal protein in urine only, and only 1%–2% patients do not secrete monoclonal protein in blood and/or urine but have evidence of BM infiltration with plasma cells. IgG or IgA monoclonal proteins are most common, and IgD or IgE proteins are rare. The natural history of myeloma is a progressive increase in tumor growth. The M protein doubling time, which is reflective of the myeloma growth rate, shortens with each relapse. Eventually marrow failure develops, with sideroblastic anemia, leukopenia, and thrombocytopenia. The median interval from marrow failure to death is 3 (range 1–9) months. Infection (52%) and renal failure (21%) account for the majority of deaths in patients with myeloma.

■ PROGNOSTIC FACTORS

Multiple attempts have been made to define clinical and laboratory parameters which have prognostic significance. The Durie–Salmon staging system has been most commonly utilized (13). Staging in this system correlated with tumor cell mass and was further subdivided into A and B based on renal function. Based on this system, survival duration is 61.2 months for patients with Stage IA disease, 54.5 for Stages IB + IIA + IIB, 30.1 months for Stage IIIA, and 14.7 months for Stage IIIB disease. A newer staging system has been has been validated in over 10,000 MM patients based on presenting serum albumin and β2-microglobulin levels (14). This system classifies patients into three stages with median survivals of 62 months for Stage I, 44 months for Stage II, and 29 months for stage III disease (Table 30-3).

FISH and conventional karyotype may be used to risk-stratify patients (15-17). Gene expression profiling is also used to identify patients with high risk disease, although this does not as yet guide clinical decision making (18).

A quarter of newly-diagnosed patients will have intermediate- to high-risk disease, including patients with deletion 17p (leading to loss of tumor suppressor p53), t(4:14), or t(14;16) by FISH. The majority of patients will have standard risk disease, including patients with hyperdiploid karyotype. Patients with standard risk disease have an expected median survival of over 6–7 years, whereas patients with high-risk disease have a median survival of roughly 3 years (19).

TABLE 30-3 NEW INTERNATIONAL STAGING SYSTEM FOR MULTIPLE MYELOMA

Stage	Serum β2 Microglobulin	Serum Albumin	Median Survival
I	<3.5 mg/l	≥3.5 g/dl	62 mo
II	<3.5 mg/l or 3.5–5.5 mg/l	<3.5 g/dl any level	44 mo
III	≥5.5 mg/l	any level	29 mo

Adapted from Greipp PR, San Miguel J, Durie BG, et al. International staging system for multiple myeloma. *J Clin Oncol.* 2005; 23: 3412-3420. Reprinted with permission from the American Society of Clinical Oncology.

■ TREATMENT

Between 5% and 10% of MM patients have an indolent course (see Table 30-1) and do not require immediate therapy. For the majority of patients, MM treatment is indicated at the time of diagnosis. Treatment is subdivided into specific antitumor therapy and supportive care measures.

SUPPORTIVE CARE MEASURES

Bone disease and hypercalcemia The use of bisphosphonates for the treatment of MM-related bone disease has greatly improved the quality of life of MM patients. Pamidronate has demonstrated efficacy in a prospective randomized trial by reducing skeletal-related events, including pathologic fractures, radiation therapy to bone, and spinal cord compression in patients with Durie–Salmon stage III MM and ≥ one lytic bone lesion (20). More potent bisphosphonates, such as zoledronate, have undergone clinical evaluation and offer the advantage of shorter infusion times compared to pamidronate.

In addition to playing an important supportive role, bisphosphonates may have a direct antitumor effect. The MRC Myeloma IX trial compared zoledronic acid to oral clodronic acid and found that zoledronic acid reduced mortality by 16% and increased median overall survival from 44.5 months to 50 months (21). The benefit of zoledronic acid on skeletal morbidity was also seen in patients without bone lesions at baseline (22). A key concern with bisphosphonates, especially zoledronic acid, is the risk of osteonecrosis of the jaw (ONJ) (23). In the MRC Myeloma IX trial, the rate of ONJ was 4% (21). Attention to dental hygiene and minimizing invasive procedures may reduce the risk of ONJ (24).

Denosumab is a monoclonal antibody to RANK ligand that also inhibits osteoclasts and showed promising activity in MM in a phase II trial (25). While denosumab was superior to zoledronic acid in patients with solid tumors and bone metastases, denosumab was inferior in a subset analysis of MM patients in a phase III trial (26). However, interpretation is limited based on the small numbers in the trial. A larger phase III study (NCT01345019) focusing on patients with MM is ongoing.

Vertebroplasty (injection of methyl methacrylate or bone cement) and kyphoplasty (use of an inflatable balloon followed by instillation of bone cement) are percutaneous procedures for treating compression fractures, and have also been used in the setting of MM (27, 28).

The treatment of hypercalcemia consists of maintaining hydration, treatment of the underlying MM, as well as inhibition of osteoclastic bone resorption with glucocorticoids, calcitonin, mithramycin, and/or bisphosphonates.

Anemia EPO administration is beneficial in managing the anemia of MM if baseline serum EPO levels are not elevated above 50 U/ml. Many physicians begin the use of EPO in patients whose hgb levels fall below 10–11 g/dl. The starting dose is 150 U/kg subcutaneously three times a week. Make sure the patient is not iron deficient before initiating EPO treatment. The dose may be doubled if no response is seen after 8 weeks of treatment.

Renal dysfunction Aggressive hydration and treatment of the underlying MM are the usual measures taken. Decisions about dialysis are affected by the status of the underlying disease.

Hyperviscosity Clinical findings improve with vigorous plasmapheresis, which reduces both MM protein concentration and serum viscosity. Plasmapheresis is more effective when the paraprotein is IgM, because 80% of the IgM remains intravascular. IgG hyperviscosity requires more frequent and complete plasmapheresis.

Infections Patients should be taught to take the onset of fever seriously and seek immediate medical attention. Patients who have survived a serious infection may benefit from monthly infusions of intravenous immunoglobulin, although they are expensive.

■ INITIAL ANTITUMOR TREATMENT

The status of MM therapy is in a period of dynamic change. The past two decades have seen dramatic advances in the treatment of MM, beginning with the publication of a randomized trial investigating the use of high-dose melphalan and autologous stem-cell transplant in 1996 (29), followed by the introduction of immunomodulatory drugs thalidomide(30) and lenalidomide (31) and the proteasome inhibitor bortezomib (32). With these new treatments, the 5-year survival rate has increased in the Surveillance Epidemiology and End Results (SEER) database from 28.8% from the period of 1990-1992 to 34.7% in years 2002-2004 to 40.3% in years 2003-2007 (33, 34). Previously, most of the survival benefit observed was in younger patients, but a more recent analysis showed that older patients over the age of 70 were deriving benefit as well (33, 34).

Oral administration of melphalan and prednisone (MP) has been the standard of care for over five decades in elderly MM patients. This form of therapy produces objective response in 50%–60% of patients. The shortcomings of MP have stimulated investigators to use many combinations of chemotherapeutic agents. Several different combinations have been tested and two large overviews of over 10,000 patients have demonstrated that MP had equivalent efficacy and survival to combination chemotherapy (35, 36). MP therefore still remains a very reasonable treatment strategy for elderly MM patients. A number of developments promise to be improvements over MP. Palumbo and colleagues have incorporated the use of thalidomide in combination with MP in newly diagnosed patients with MM over the age of 65 years (37). The addition of thalidomide resulted in a 76% complete or partial response rate compared to 47% in the MP arm. This translated into a doubling of the 2-year event-free survival (EFS) to 54% versus 27%. Randomized trials with the use of other novel agents like bortezomib (a proteasome inhibitor) and lenalinamide (a thalidomide analogue) with MP have proven benefits. For example, the VISTA trial compared the regimen of bortezomib, melphalan, prednisone (VMP) to melphalan and prednisone (MP) in patients who were not candidates for autologous stem-cell transplant (38). Overall survival was significantly improved in the VMP group versus MP group, with 3-year overall survival of 68.5% versus 54% respectively (39).

Strategies aimed at improving the tolerability of treatment and decreasing risk of adverse events include using a lower dose of dexamethasone (40), decreasing the frequency of bortezomib to weekly (41, 42), and changing the mode of administration from intravenous to subcutaneous (43). These changes have maintained the efficacy of treatment and allowed for longer duration of exposure to therapy.

Patients under the age of 65 years are potential autologous transplant candidates. Historically, beginning in the 1980s, the combination of vincristine, doxorubicin, and dexamethasone (VAD) was used for induction (44). However, highly active regimens using lenalidomide and/or bortezomib have replaced VAD. Examples of modern regimens in use include doublet combinations of bortezomib and dexamethasone (45) and lenalidomide and dexamethasone (40) as well as triplet combinations of lenalidomide, bortezomib, dexamethasone (RVD)(46) and cyclophosphamide, bortezomib, dexamethasone (CyBorD) (47). A quadruplet combination where cyclophosphamide is added to RVD has been studied in the EVOLUTION trial, though no substantial advantage over three-drug combinations was noted in a phase II trial (48). The choice of regimen may vary depending on drug availability from country to country. After four cycles of RVD, 75% of patients in a phase II trial achieved a partial response or better (as defined by a reduction in the monoclonal protein by 50% or more); this increased to 100% with additional cycles (46). Drugs with potential for stem cell toxicity such as melphalan are generally not used during induction (49). The number of cycles of treatment, especially with lenalidomide-containing regimens is limited to roughly four cycles, as additional cycles may compromise the ability to collect stem cells (50, 51).

High-dose therapy The rationale for the administration of high doses of alkylating agents (melphalan) with or without total body irradiation, followed by transplantation of syngeneic, allogeneic, and autologous BM or peripheral blood progenitor cells (PBPCs), is based on the fact that MM is uniformly fatal and MM cells have demonstrated a dose–response curve to chemotherapy with a high proportion of patients achieving complete responses when higher doses of therapy are given.

Allogeneic stem-cell transplantation Experience with allografting has been disappointing in MM largely because of the high transplant-related mortality (TRM). Syngeneic BMT has been done infrequently, but some patients reported from Seattle and the European BM Transplant Group (EBMT) have remained progression-free at long intervals post-BMT. The EBMT and Seattle groups have reported on allografting in MM with similar results demonstrating an overall survival (OS) of 20%–28% associated with a high TRM of 41%–44% (52, 53). Nonetheless, molecular remissions, due in part to a graft-versus-myeloma (GVM) effect, have been noted in allogeneic BMT, and the emphasis now is to develop strategies to achieve and maintain high remission rates while avoiding TRM. The use of nonmyeloablative transplantation is one such alternative strategy which preserves GVM allogeneic immunity while avoiding the toxicity of allografting and is currently under investigation. Early data demonstrate reduced TRM (10%–20%) with improved OS but follow-up remains short (54).

Autologous stem-cell transplantation High-dose chemoradiotherapy followed by transplantation of either autologous BM or PBPCs has achieved high (40%) CR rates, but the median duration of these responses has been only 2–3 years. The Intergroupe Francais du Myelome (IFM 90), a national French study, first demonstrated the efficacy of autologous BMT over conventional chemotherapy in 200 MM patients (29). Several randomized trials and case-controlled studies have been performed and the results have been variable. For example, the MRC randomized study confirmed a 12-month survival benefit for the transplanted arm (55). In contrast, the US Intergroup randomized trial was unable to confirm the benefits of transplantation (56). Despite the use of aggressive approaches like transplantation, few, if any, patients are cured. To improve upon the results of high-dose chemotherapy, the French group have compared single versus double autografts and their data suggest that two sequential transplants may benefit a subset of patients with MM who did not achieve a complete remission after the first transplant (57). Studies are underway addressing the role of autologous transplant in the context of novel drugs.

Maintenance therapy To extend the duration of complete remission following autologous stem-cell transplant, maintenance regimens have been proposed. The increased tolerability and efficacy of newer anti-MM agents has increased the attractiveness and the applicability of this approach; previous attempts at maintenance therapy with older conventional chemotherapy agents such as melphalan or interferon were not beneficial (58).

- *Lenalidomide:* Three randomized trials have explored the use of lenalidomide as maintenance therapy, with two of the trials following autologous stem-cell transplant (59, 60) and one trial after 9 months of melphalan-based therapy in patients ineligible for high-dose treatment (61). In all three trials, there was a near doubling in progression free survival with lenalidomide maintenance, for example, from 27 to 46 months in the CALGB 100104 study (60). Furthermore, the CALGB study showed an overall survival benefit with lenalidomide: 15% of the lenalidomide group had died compared to 23% in the placebo group ($P < 0.03$) and at 3 years, the overall survival was 88% in the lenalidomide group compared to 80% in the placebo group.

Risk of secondary malignancy: However, a significant concern with maintenance therapy with lenalidomide is the risk of secondary malignancy. The risk of second primary cancers was roughly double in the maintenance group, (7%–7.7%) compared to the placebo group, (2.6%–3%). The secondary cancers observed included both hematological malignancies such as acute myelogenous leukemia as well as solid tumors. This increased risk of secondary malignancies and the risk-benefit ratio of maintenance therapy should be considered.

Bortezomib: Bortezomib has also been studied as maintenance therapy. In the HOVON-65/GMMG-HD4 study, bortezomib was given every 2 weeks and was associated with increasing the near CR and CR rate from 31% to 49% (62).

■ REFRACTORY DISEASE

Almost all patients who initially respond to treatment will eventually relapse. Proteosome inhibitors like bortezomib and immunomodulatory drugs like thalidomide and lenalidomide have provided a significant advance in the therapy of relapsed MM. Newer generation carfilzomib and pomalidomide continue to contribute significant benefits to these patients.

■ FUTURE DIRECTIONS

Despite the use of aggressive approaches like transplantation and the use of novel agents like bortezomib, thalidomide, and lenalidomide, MM remains incurable. In order to overcome resistance to current therapies and improve patient outcome, novel biologically based treatment approaches that target mechanisms whereby MM cells grow and survive in the BM are needed. Our understanding of the biology of MM has allowed the development of several promising targeted therapies that can attack the MM cell in its BM microenvironment and, it is hoped, overcome classic drug resistance. These include next generation proteasome inhibitors such as carfilzomib, MLN 9708, and marizomib (63) as well as new immunomodulatory drugs such as pomalidomide (64). Carfilzomib was recently approved by the FDA in July 2012 for patients who have progressive disease after at least two prior therapies, including bortezomib and an immunomodulatory agent.

Newer targets for treatment include CS1, a cell surface glycoprotein that is highly expressed in MM cells. CS1 is neutralized by the monoclonal antibody elotuzumab (65). Another target is B-cell activating factor (BAFF), a growth factor for B cells, and serum levels of BAFF are increased in MM patients (66–68). Tabalumab (LY2127399) is a monoclonal antibody targeting BAFF under clinical development for MM (69). The aggresome, which like the proteasome, also degrades misfolded and unfolded proteins, is also another novel target for anti-MM therapy through inhibition of histone deacetylase 6 (HDAC6) (70, 71). Other agents under development include cyclin dependent kinase (CDK) (72), aurora kinase (73), mTOR (74), and activin inhibitors (75), which have promising activity in vitro and are in early phase clinical trials (76, 77).

WALDENSTROM'S MACROGLOBULINEMIA (WM)

The diagnosis of WM requires an IgM serum level of at least 3.0 g/dl in association with an increase in lymphocytes or plasmacytoid lymphocytes in the marrow. WM corresponds most closely to the lymphoplasmacytic lymphoma (LPA) under the World Health Organization (WHO) classification of lymphoid tumors (LPL/immunocytoma of the Revised European–American (REAL) classification of lymphoma). Like MM, BM involvement is common; however, no lytic bone disease is noted with WM (78). The median age of onset of WM is 61 years. Symptoms are characteristically vague and nonspecific, with the most common being weakness, anorexia, and weight loss. Symptoms due to peripheral neuropathy and Raynaud phenomenon can precede more serious manifestations. Lymphadenopathy, splenomegaly, and/or hepatomegaly are present in 30%–40% of cases, and at least 20%–25% lymphoplasmacytoid cells are usually present in the marrow. Visceral involvement of small bowel and peripheral nerves can cause the clinical sequelae of malabsorption and neuropathy, respectively. Hemorrhagic complications are common, attributable to abnormal bleeding times, decreased platelet adhesiveness, or direct interference by the IgM protein with the release of platelet factor 3 and with coagulation factors. An important part of the differential diagnosis is to exclude the less common entity of IgM MM, which is characterized by lytic bone disease and an absence of organomegaly and/or lymphocytic involvement; rarely, WM can progress to IgM MM. Amyloidosis occurs rarely in WM. Hyperviscosity syndrome, described earlier as a rare complication in MM, occurs more commonly in the setting of excess IgM and is characterized by mucosal bleeding and neurologic, ocular, and cardiovascular abnormalities. Plasmapheresis is more useful to remove excess IgM than it is in the setting of excess IgG monoclonal proteins and related hyperviscosity in MM.

The median survival of patients with WM is approximately 50 months. In contrast to persons with MM, many individuals with WM have indolent disease requiring no therapy for long periods of time, with survivals in excess of 20 years. A high IgM level is not in itself an indication to initiate therapy. A prognostic model has been developed for WM based on an analysis of 585 patients seen at the Mayo Clinic (79). Age greater than 65 years and organomegaly were the major risk factors; absence of both was associated with a median survival of nearly 11 years, while the presence of one or both factors predicted a median survival of 4.2 years.

A consensus panel on WM has developed recommendations for initiation of therapy in WM. Hematocrit of <30, platelet count <100,000, symptoms attributable to WM, hyperviscosity, moderate to severe neuropathies, symptomatic cryoglobulinemia, and cold agglutinin disease are some indicators to start therapy. Low-dose therapy with alkylating agents like chlorambucil has resulted in overall response rates of 50%. However, this is a stem cell toxic agent and acute leukemia has developed in patients with WM. Nucleoside analogs, fludarabine and 2-chlorodeoxyadenosine, have demonstrated efficacy with overall response rates of 30%–70% with more rapid cytoreduction. Monoclonal antibody therapy with rituximab, a chimeric anti-CD20 monoclonal antibody, produces responses in both treated and untreated patients with low-grade lymphoma. Given that the CD20 antigen is typically present in WM, rituximab has been given to WM patients and a clinical response is seen in about one-third of previously treated patients. Ongoing studies are looking at combining rituximab with fludarabine in the treatment of WM. Salvage strategies for treatment of WM have included reuse of the first-line agent, combination chemotherapy like CHOP and CVP, and stem-cell transplantation. Novel agents like thalidomide, lenolinamide, and bortezomib used in MM are also being studied for the treatment of WM.

A MYD88 L265P somatic mutation has been seen in 91% of WM patients with early evidence that this may be targeted by drugs like Bruton's tyrosine kinase inhibitors (80).

HEAVY-CHAIN DISEASES (HCD)

The HCD are rare lymphoplasmacytic malignancies. They are classified based on the heavy-chain isotype (81).

Gamma HCD was originally described by Franklin and coworkers in a patient with malignant lymphoma whose serum and urine contained large amounts of the Fc fragment of IgG. It is characterized by the presence of a portion of the Ig heavy chain in the serum or urine or both. The median age at diagnosis is similar to MM, about 60 years. Most common presenting symptoms are weakness, fatigue, and fever, associated with lymphadenopathy and hepatosplenomegaly. In addition to Ig heavy chain in serum or urine, a lymphoplasmacytic marrow infiltrate is noted in most cases. The clinical course can be fulminant and rapidly progressive; alternatively, the monoclonal heavy chain can persist for years in otherwise asymptomatic patients. Thus, survival is variable, but the median is only 12 months. Treatment options for patients with active disease are similar to those used for lymphoma or MM, whereas patients with indolent disease should be followed expectantly without therapy.

Cases of αHCD, μHCD, and δHCD have also been described. αHCD is typically associated with Mediterranean lymphoma affecting the gastrointestinal tract, beginning with plasma cells that produce a heavy chain and aggregate in the intestinal tract and subsequent transformation into a malignant non-Hodgkin lymphoma of the immunoblastic type. μHCD is extremely rare and may be associated with chronic lymphocytic leukemia. The ideal therapy for HCD is not known because of its rarity, but intensive chemotherapy including intravenous cyclophosphamide, doxorubicin, vincristine, and oral prednisone appears to offer some patients long-term remissions.

AMYLOIDOSIS

Amyloidosis is relatively rare as a clinically significant disease. The amyloid found in most cases of amyloidosis can be assigned to one of two types, according to whether the fibrils consist mainly of the variable region of Ig light chains (AL, or primary amyloidosis) or protein A (AA, or secondary amyloidosis). Protein A is not related to any known immunoglobulin. In AL, amyloid primarily involves the heart, tongue, gastrointestinal tract, and skin, whereas AA primarily results in fibril deposition in liver, kidney, and spleen. A review of 229 patients with AL documented MM in 47 (21%) patients. Initial presenting symptoms were fatigue and weight loss, with pain more common in those who also had MM. Hepatomegaly and macroglossia were present in up to one-third of patients with AL; renal insufficiency was present in half of patients, and proteinuria (defined as albuminuria with immune globulin, seen only in MM) was documented in 82% of patients. Nephrotic syndrome, CHF, orthostatic hypotension, carpal tunnel syndrome, and peripheral neuropathy were all more common in those without MM (30%–70% of patients studied) than in persons with (<20%) MM. Overall median survival was 12 months, 5 months for those with MM in contrast to 13 months for individuals without MM (82).

Treatment for AL is unsatisfactory. Only 18% patients responded to MP, although median survival for responders was prolonged at 89.4 months; only 5% of patients with primary AL survive ≥10 years. Early reports suggest that dose-intensive melphalan with blood stem cell support can achieve CR, with improvement in performance status and clinical remission of organ-specific disease. Attempts to improve outcomes for patients with symptomatic and advanced multisystem disease may require both solid and stem-cell transplantation, as well as the use of less intensive conditioning regimens. Novel drugs with promise in the treatment of MM are also being tested in patients with amyloidosis.

REFERENCES

1. Rajkumar SV, Kyle RA. Multiple myeloma: diagnosis and treatment. *Mayo Clin Proc.* 2005; 80: 1371–1382.

2. Kyle RA, Rajkumar SV. Monoclonal gammopathy of undetermined significance. *Clin Lymphoma Myeloma.* 2005; 6: 102–114.

3. Rajkumar SV, Kyle RA, Therneau TM, et al. Serum free light chain ratio is an independent risk factor for progression in monoclonal gammopathy of undetermined significance. *Blood.* 2005; 106: 812–817.

4. Hideshima T, Bergsagel PL, Kuehl WM, et al. Advances in biology of multiple myeloma: clinical applications. *Blood.* 2004; 104: 607–618.

5. Siegel R, Naishadham D, Jemal A. Cancer statistics, 2012. *CA Cancer J Clin.* 2012; 62: 10–29.

6. Herrinton LJ, Weiss NS, Olshan AF, et al (eds). Myeloma: biology and management. *Epidemiol Myeloma.* 1997: 150.

7. Bergsagel PL, Kuehl WM. Molecular pathogenesis and a consequent classification of multiple myeloma. *J Clin Oncol.* 2005; 23: 6333–6338.

8. Shaughnessy JD, Jr., Barlogie B. Using genomics to identify high-risk myeloma after autologous stem cell transplantation. *Biol Blood Marrow Transplant.* 2006; 12(1 Suppl 1): 77–80.

9. Chapman MA, Lawrence MS, Keats JJ, et al. Initial genome sequencing and analysis of multiple myeloma. *Nature.* 2011; 471: 467–472.

10. Durie BG. Staging and kinetics of multiple myeloma. *Semin Oncol.* 1986; 13: 300–309.

11. Dimopoulos MA, Moulopoulos LA, Maniatis A, et al. Solitary plasmacytoma of bone and asymptomatic multiple myeloma. *Blood.* 2000; 96: 2037–2044.

12. Kyle RA. Multiple myeloma: review of 869 cases. *Mayo Clin Proc.* 1975; 50: 29–40.

13. Durie BG, Salmon SE. A clinical staging system for multiple myeloma. Correlation of measured myeloma cell mass with presenting clinical features, response to treatment, and survival. *Cancer.* 1975; 36: 842–854.

14. Greipp PR, San Miguel J, Durie BG, et al. International staging system for multiple myeloma. *J Clin Oncol.* 2005; 23: 3412–3420.

15. Kumar SK, Mikhael JR, Buadi FK, et al. Management of newly diagnosed symptomatic multiple myeloma: updated Mayo Stratification of Myeloma and Risk-Adapted Therapy (mSMART) consensus guidelines. *Mayo Clin Proc.* 2009; 84: 1095–1110.

16. Fonseca R, Bergsagel PL, Drach J, et al. International Myeloma Working Group molecular classification of multiple myeloma: spotlight review. *Leukemia.* 2009; 23: 2210–2221.

17. Rajkumar SV. Multiple myeloma: 2012 update on diagnosis, risk-stratification, and management. *Am J Hematol.* 2012; 87: 78–88.

18. Zhou Y, Barlogie B, Shaughnessy JD Jr. The molecular characterization and clinical management of multiple myeloma in the post-genome era. *Leukemia.* 2009; 23: 1941–1956.

19. Rajkumar SV. Treatment of multiple myeloma. *Nat Rev Clin Oncol.* 2011; 8: 479–491.

20. Berenson JR, Lichtenstein A, Porter L, et al. Efficacy of pamidronate in reducing skeletal events in patients with advanced multiple myeloma. Myeloma Aredia Study Group. *N Engl J Med.* 1996; 334: 488–493.

21. Morgan GJ, Davies FE, Gregory WM, et al. First-line treatment with zoledronic acid as compared with clodronic acid in multiple myeloma (MRC Myeloma IX): a randomised controlled trial. *Lancet.* 2010; 376: 1989–1999.

22. Morgan GJ, Child JA, Gregory WM, et al. Effects of zoledronic acid versus clodronic acid on skeletal morbidity in patients with newly diagnosed multiple myeloma (MRC Myeloma IX): secondary outcomes from a randomised controlled trial. *Lancet Oncol.* 2011; 12: 743–752.

23. Woo SB, Hellstein JW, Kalmar JR. Narrative [corrected] review: bisphosphonates and osteonecrosis of the jaws. *Ann Intern Med.* 2006; 144: 753–761.

24. Dimopoulos MA, Kastritis E, Bamia C, et al. Reduction of osteonecrosis of the jaw (ONJ) after implementation of preventive measures in patients with multiple myeloma treated with zoledronic acid. *Ann Oncol.* 2009; 20: 117–120.

25. Vij R, Horvath N, Spencer A, et al. An open-label, phase 2 trial of denosumab in the treatment of relapsed or plateau-phase multiple myeloma. *Am J Hematol.* 2009; 84: 650–656.

26. Henry DH, Costa L, Goldwasser F, et al. Randomized, double-blind study of denosumab versus zoledronic acid in the treatment of bone metastases in patients with advanced cancer (excluding breast and prostate cancer) or multiple myeloma. *J Clin Oncol.* 2011; 29: 1125–1132.

27. Dudeney S, Lieberman IH, Reinhardt MK, et al. Kyphoplasty in the treatment of osteolytic vertebral compression fractures as a result of multiple myeloma. *J Clin Oncol.* 2002; 20: 2382–2387.

28. Fourney DR, Schomer DF, Nader R, et al. Percutaneous vertebroplasty and kyphoplasty for painful vertebral body fractures in cancer patients. *J Neurosurg.* 2003; 98(1 Suppl): 21–30.

29. Attal M, Harousseau JL, Stoppa AM, et al. A prospective, randomized trial of autologous bone marrow transplantation and chemotherapy in multiple myeloma. Intergroupe Francais du Myelome. *N Engl J Med.* 1996; 335: 91–97.

30. Singhal S, Mehta J, Desikan R, et al. Antitumor activity of thalidomide in refractory multiple myeloma. *N Engl J Med.* 1999; 341: 1565–1571.

31. Dimopoulos M, Spencer A, Attal M, et al. Lenalidomide plus dexamethasone for relapsed or refractory multiple myeloma. *N Engl J Med.* 2007; 357: 2123–2132.

32. Richardson PG, Barlogie B, Berenson J, et al. A phase 2 study of bortezomib in relapsed, refractory myeloma. *N Engl J Med.* 2003; 348: 2609–2617.

33. Brenner H, Gondos A, Pulte D. Recent major improvement in long-term survival of younger patients with multiple myeloma. *Blood*. 2008; 111: 2521–2526.

34. Pulte D, Gondos A, Brenner H. Improvement in survival of older adults with multiple myeloma: results of an updated period analysis of SEER data. *The Oncologist*. 2011; 16: 1600–1603.

35. Gregory WM, Richards MA, Malpas JS. Combination chemotherapy versus melphalan and prednisolone in the treatment of multiple myeloma: an overview of published trials. *J Clin Oncol*. 1992; 10: 334–342.

36. Combination chemotherapy versus melphalan plus prednisone as treatment for multiple myeloma: an overview of 6,633 patients from 27 randomized trials. Myeloma Trialists' Collaborative Group. *J Clin Oncol*. 1998; 16: 3832–3842.

37. Palumbo A, Bringhen S, Caravita T, et al. Oral melphalan and prednisone chemotherapy plus thalidomide compared with melphalan and prednisone alone in elderly patients with multiple myeloma: randomised controlled trial. *Lancet*. 2006; 367: 825–831.

38. San Miguel JF, Schlag R, Khuageva NK, et al. Bortezomib plus melphalan and prednisone for initial treatment of multiple myeloma. *N Engl J Med*. 2008; 359: 906–917.

39. Mateos MV, Richardson PG, Schlag R, et al. Bortezomib plus melphalan and prednisone compared with melphalan and prednisone in previously untreated multiple myeloma: updated follow-up and impact of subsequent therapy in the phase III VISTA trial. *J Clin Oncol*. 2010; 28: 2259–2266.

40. Rajkumar SV, Jacobus S, Callander NS, et al. Lenalidomide plus high-dose dexamethasone versus lenalidomide plus low-dose dexamethasone as initial therapy for newly diagnosed multiple myeloma: an open-label randomised controlled trial. *Lancet Oncol*. 2010; 11: 29–37.

41. Bringhen S, Larocca A, Rossi D, et al. Efficacy and safety of once-weekly bortezomib in multiple myeloma patients. *Blood*. 2010; 116: 4745–4753.

42. Reeder CB, Reece DE, Kukreti V, et al. Once- versus twice-weekly bortezomib induction therapy with CyBorD in newly diagnosed multiple myeloma. *Blood*. 2010; 115: 3416–3417.

43. Moreau P, Pylypenko H, Grosicki S, et al. Subcutaneous versus intravenous administration of bortezomib in patients with relapsed multiple myeloma: a randomised, phase 3, non-inferiority study. *Lancet Oncol*. 2011; 12: 431–440.

44. Rajkumar S. Multiple myeloma: the death of VAD as initial therapy. *Blood*. 2005; 106: 2–3.

45. Harousseau JL, Attal M, Avet-Loiseau H, et al. Bortezomib plus dexamethasone is superior to vincristine plus doxorubicin plus dexamethasone as induction treatment prior to autologous stem-cell transplantation in newly diagnosed multiple myeloma: results of the IFM 2005-01 phase III trial. *J Clin Oncol*. 2010; 28: 4621–4629.

46. Richardson PG, Weller E, Lonial S, et al. Lenalidomide, bortezomib, and dexamethasone combination therapy in patients with newly diagnosed multiple myeloma. *Blood*. 2010; 116: 679–686.

47. Reeder CB, Reece DE, Kukreti V, et al. Cyclophosphamide, bortezomib and dexamethasone induction for newly diagnosed multiple myeloma: high response rates in a phase II clinical trial. *Leukemia*. 2009 Jul; 23(7): 1337–1341.

48. Kumar S, Flinn I, Richardson PG, et al. Randomized, multicenter, phase 2 study (EVOLUTION) of combinations of bortezomib, dexamethasone, cyclophosphamide, and lenalidomide in previously untreated multiple myeloma. *Blood*. 2012; 119: 4375–4382.

49. Prince HM, Imrie K, Sutherland DR, et al. Peripheral blood progenitor cell collections in multiple myeloma: predictors and management of inadequate collections. *Br J Haematol*. 1996; 93: 142–145.

50. Kumar S, Dispenzieri A, Lacy MQ, et al. Impact of lenalidomide therapy on stem cell mobilization and engraftment post-peripheral blood stem cell transplantation in patients with newly diagnosed myeloma. *Leukemia*. 2007; 21: 2035–2042.

51. Paripati H, Stewart AK, Cabou S, et al. Compromised stem cell mobilization following induction therapy with lenalidomide in myeloma. *Leukemia*. 2008; 22: 1282–1284.

52. Gahrton G, Svensson H, Cavo M, et al. Progress in allogenic bone marrow and peripheral blood stem cell transplantation for multiple myeloma: a comparison between transplants performed 1983–93 and 1994–8 at European Group for Blood and Marrow Transplantation centres. *Br J Haematol*. 2001; 113: 209–216.

53. Bensinger WI, Maloney D, Storb R. Allogeneic hematopoietic cell transplantation for multiple myeloma. *Semin Hematol*. 2001; 38: 243–249.

54. Badros A, Barlogie B, Siegel E, et al. Improved outcome of allogeneic transplantation in high-risk multiple myeloma patients after nonmyeloablative conditioning. *J Clin Oncol*. 2002; 20: 1295–1303.

55. Child JA, Morgan GJ, Davies FE, et al. High-dose chemotherapy with hematopoietic stem-cell rescue for multiple myeloma. *N Engl J Med*. 2003; 348: 1875–1883.

56. Barlogie B, Kyle RA, Anderson KC, et al. Standard chemotherapy compared with high-dose chemoradiotherapy for multiple myeloma: final results of phase III US Intergroup Trial S9321. *J Clin Oncol*. 2006; 24: 929–936.

57. Attal M, Harousseau JL, Facon T, et al. Single versus double autologous stem-cell transplantation for multiple myeloma. *N Engl J Med*. 2003; 349: 2495–2502.

58. Ludwig H, Durie BG, McCarthy P, et al. IMWG consensus on maintenance therapy in multiple myeloma. *Blood*. 2012; 119: 3003–3015.

59. Attal M, Lauwers-Cances V, Marit G, et al. Lenalidomide maintenance after stem-cell transplantation for multiple myeloma. *N Engl J Med*. 2012; 366: 1782–1791.

60. McCarthy PL, Owzar K, Hofmeister CC, et al. Lenalidomide after stem-cell transplantation for multiple myeloma. *N Engl J Med*. 2012; 366: 1770–1781.

61. Palumbo A, Hajek R, Delforge M, et al. Continuous lenalidomide treatment for newly diagnosed multiple myeloma. *N Engl J Med*. 2012; 366: 1759–1769.

62. Sonneveld P, Schmidt-Wolf IG, van der Holt B, et al. Bortezomib induction and maintenance treatment in patients with newly diagnosed multiple myeloma: results of the randomized phase III HOVON-65/GMMG-HD4 trial. *J Clin Oncol*. 2012; 30: 2946–2955.

63. Moreau P, Richardson PG, Cavo M, , et al. Proteasome inhibitors in multiple myeloma: 10 years later. *Blood*. 2012; 120: 947–959.

64. Lacy MQ, Tefferi A. Pomalidomide therapy for multiple myeloma and myelofibrosis: an update. *Leuk Lymphoma*. 2011; 52: 560–566.

65. Lonial S, Vij R, Harousseau JL, Facon T, et al. Elotuzumab in combination with lenalidomide and low-dose dexamethasone in relapsed or refractory multiple myeloma. *J Clin Oncol*. 2012; 30: 1953–1959.

66. Moreaux J, Legouffe E, Jourdan E, et al. BAFF and APRIL protect myeloma cells from apoptosis induced by interleukin 6 deprivation and dexamethasone. *Blood*. 2004; 103: 3148–3157.

67. Neri P, Kumar S, Fulciniti MT, et al. Neutralizing B-cell activating factor antibody improves survival and inhibits osteoclastogenesis in a severe combined immunodeficient human multiple myeloma model. *Clin Cancer Res*. 2007; 13: 5903–5909.

68. Tai YT, Li XF, Breitkreutz I, et al. Role of B-cell-activating factor in adhesion and growth of human multiple myeloma cells in the bone marrow microenvironment. *Cancer Res*. 2006; 66: 6675–6682.

69. Raje N. Phase I study of LY2127399, a human anti-BAFF antibody, and bortezomib in patients with previously treated multiple myeloma. *J Clin Oncol*. 2011; 29: Abstract 8012.

70. Hideshima T, Bradner JE, Wong J, et al. Small-molecule inhibition of proteasome and aggresome function induces synergistic antitumor activity in multiple myeloma. *Proc Natl Acad Sci USA*. 2005; 102: 8567–8572.

71. Santo L, Hideshima T, Kung AL, et al. Preclinical activity, pharmacodynamic, and pharmacokinetic properties of a selective HDAC6 inhibitor, ACY-1215, in combination with bortezomib in multiple myeloma. *Blood*. 2012 Mar 15; 119: 2579–2589.

72. Santo L, Vallet S, Hideshima T, et al. AT7519, A novel small molecule multi-cyclin-dependent kinase inhibitor, induces apoptosis in multiple myeloma via GSK-3beta activation and RNA polymerase II inhibition. *Oncogene*. 2010 Apr 22; 29: 2325–2336.

73. Gorgun G, Calabrese E, Hideshima T, et al. A novel Aurora-A kinase inhibitor MLN8237 induces cytotoxicity and cell-cycle arrest in multiple myeloma. *Blood*. 2010; 115: 5202–5213.

74. Cirstea D, Hideshima T, Rodig S, et al. Dual inhibition of akt/mammalian target of rapamycin pathway by nanoparticle albumin-bound-rapamycin

and perifosine induces antitumor activity in multiple myeloma. *Mol Cancer Ther.* 2010; 9: 963–975.

75. Vallet S, Mukherjee S, Vaghela N, et al. Activin A promotes multiple myeloma-induced osteolysis and is a promising target for myeloma bone disease. *Proc Natl Acad Sci USA.* 2010; 107: 5124–5129.

76. Cirstea D, Vallet S, Raje N. Future novel single agent and combination therapies. *Cancer J.* 2009; 15: 511–518.

77. Mahindra A, Laubach J, Raje N, et al. Latest advances and current challenges in the treatment of multiple myeloma. *Nat Rev Clin Oncol.* 2012; 9: 135–143.

78. Dimopoulos MA, Anagnostopoulos A. Waldenstrom's macroglobulinemia. *Best Pract Res Clin Haematol.* 2005; 18: 747–765.

79. Ghobrial IM, Fonseca R, Gertz MA, et al. Prognostic model for disease-specific and overall mortality in newly diagnosed symptomatic patients with Waldenstrom macroglobulinaemia. *Br J Haematol.* 2006; 133: 158–164.

80. Treon SP, Xu L, Yang G, et al. MYD88 L265P somatic mutation in Waldenstrom's macroglobulinemia. *N Engl J Med.* 2012; 367: 826–833.

81. Witzig TE, Wahner-Roedler DL. Heavy chain disease. *Curr Treat Options Oncol.* 2002; 3: 247–254.

82. Rajkumar SV, Gertz MA. Advances in the treatment of amyloidosis. *N Engl J Med.* 2007; 356: 2413–2415.

CHAPTER **31**
Diffuse Large B-Cell Lymphoma

Jennifer Gao, Ephraim Paul Hochberg

Lymphomas are a malignancy arising from lymphoid cells, with more than 60 distinct variants identified by the World Health Organization (WHO). Lymphomas can originate in B cells, T cells, or natural killer cells, and are broadly categorized into Hodgkin lymphoma (HL) and non-Hodgkin lymphoma (NHL). Within NHL, further differentiation is made based on clinical presentation and histology. About 85% of lymphomas in the United States and Western Europe are of B-cell origin. Diffuse large B-cell lymphoma (DLBCL) is the most common subtype of NHL in North America and the focus of this chapter. The majority of the information in this chapter is applicable to DLBCL-NOS (not otherwise specified). Short discussions of other subtypes of diffuse large B-cell lymphoma and of other lymphomas of large B cells are included at the end of this chapter.

EPIDEMIOLOGY

DLBCL is a B-cell lymphoma characterized by malignant proliferations of lymphocytes at various stages during the normal B-cell maturation process and accounts for 30%-40% of all NHL cases. The annual incidence is approximately 16.5 per 100,000 people per year, with a slightly higher incidence in men compared to women (SEER). Comparing incidence based on race, Caucasians have the highest and American Indians/Alaskan Natives the lowest (SEER). The median age of diagnosis is 67 years old.

In a majority of patients, no clear risk factor can be identified; although the proportion of Epstein-Barr virus associated DLBCL is greater in the elderly, suggesting a possible viral connection. HIV strongly increases the risk of lymphoma, with DLBCL being the most common HIV-associated lymphoid malignancy. The underlying pathophysiology is likely due to chronic antigenic stimulation causing polyclonal B-cell expansion and then subsequent emergence of monoclonal B cells. Autoimmune rheumatologic diseases, such as Sjogren's, lupus, and rheumatoid arthritis have also been associated with the development of DLBCL, especially in patients with detectable autoantibodies and substantial clinical involvement. In these diseases, chronic immune stimulation may promote lymphoma development although the role of immunosuppressive medication regimens is also being studied. Finally, a small number of patients present with histologic progression or transformation to DLBCL after a diagnosis of an indolent NHL, such as follicular lymphoma, or chronic lymphocytic leukemia. Transformation of chronic lymphocytic leukemia into diffuse large B-cell lymphoma is known as Richter's transformation.

PATHOLOGY

Definitive diagnosis is made via excisional biopsy or core needle biopsy (fine needle aspiration is inadequate) with hematopathologic review of slides. Microscopic examination usually demonstrates a diffuse infiltrate of large lymphoid cells completely effacing the normal nodal architecture. The neoplastic cells are large lymphocytes with nuclei greater than twice the size of small lymphocyte nuclei, prominent nucleoli, and amphiphilic to basophilic cytoplasm. Histology can reveal centroblastic and immunoblastic cell types but these distinctions are not highly reproducible and do not have clinical implications. For most DLBCL subtypes, the cells express the pan-B cell markers CD19, CD20, and CD79a. CD5 is expressed in 5%–10% of cases and blastoid mantle cell lymphoma should be excluded in these cases by absence of the t(11;14). Overexpression of BCL6 is common.

CHARACTERISTICS

The WHO divides DLBCL into subtypes based on clinical, morphological, immunological, and genetic features (Table 31-1).

Pathogenic mutations commonly seen in DLBCL-NOS involve BCL-6, BCL-2, c-Myc, as well as genes in the NF-κB pathway.

Gene-expression profiling has divided DLBCL into distinct molecular subtypes: activated B-cell subtype (ABC), germinal-center B-cell subtype (GCB), type 3, and primary mediastinal B-cell lymphoma (PMBL). These subtypes are characterized by distinct clinical presentations, differential gene expression, and likely arise from B cells at varying stages of differentiation. A number of immunohistochemical algorithms have been reported to replicate profiling based subtype classification. Further studies

TABLE 31-1 DIFFUSE LARGE B-CELL LYMPHOMA SUBTYPES

Diffuse large B-cell lymphoma, not otherwise specified (DLBCL-NOS)
    Common morphologic variants
        Centroblastic
        Immunoblastic
        Anaplastic
    Molecular subgroups
        Germinal centre B-cell-like (GCB)
        Activated B-cell-like (ABC)
    Immunohistochemical subgroups
        CD5-positive DLBCL
        Germinal centre B-cell-like (GCB)
        Nongerminal centre B-cell-like (non-GCB)

Diffuse large B-cell lymphoma subtypes
    T-cell/histiocyte-rich large B-cell lymphoma
    Primary DLBCL of the CNS
    Primary cutaneous DLBCL, leg type
    EBV-positive DLBCL of the elderly

Other lymphomas of large B cells
    Primary mediastinal (thymic) large B-cell lymphoma
    Intravascular large B-cell lymphoma
    DLBCL associated with chronic inflammation
    Lymphomatoid granulomatosis
    ALK-positive LBCL
    Plasmablastic lymphoma
    Large B-cell lymphoma arising in HHV8-associated multicentric Castleman disease
    Primary effusion lymphoma

Borderline cases
    B-cell lymphoma, unclassifiable, with features intermediate between diffuse large B-cell lymphoma and Burkitt lymphoma
    B-cell lymphoma, unclassifiable, with features intermediate between diffuse large B-cell lymphoma and classical Hodgkin lymphoma

are underway to determine the impact of these subtypes on therapy choice and outcome, and gene expression profiling is not currently used routinely.

DIAGNOSIS AND STAGING

DLBCL patients may present with symptoms of a rapidly enlarging lymph nodes, commonly in the neck or abdomen, sometimes accompanied by B symptoms of fevers, night sweats, and unintentional weight loss (Table 31-2). Up to 40% of patients will present with extranodal disease.

TABLE 31-2 B SYMPTOMS

Fever >38°C

Drenching sweats, especially at night

Unintentional weight loss >10% of body weight over a period of 6 mo or less

Staging is via the Ann Arbor staging system, which was originally developed for Hodgkin lymphoma (HL) (Table 31-3).

Approximately 27% will presents with stage I disease and 50% with advanced stage disease at diagnosis (SEER).

Initial evaluation of newly diagnosed DLBCL should include (NCCN) (1):

- Thorough history and physical examination with attention to nodal areas and to the liver and spleen
- B symptom inventory
- Performance status assessment
- International Prognostic Index score calculation (see Prognosis below)
- Laboratory studies: CBC with differential, comprehensive metabolic panel, LDH, uric acid, hepatitis B testing
- Imaging: CT of the chest/abdomen/pelvis with attenuation corrected PET or full diagnostic PET-CT
- Cardiac status: assessment of ejection fraction if anthracycline based chemotherapy regimen is planned
- Bone marrow biopsy with or without aspirate
- Pregnancy test

In selected cases, lumbar puncture (in patients with neurologic signs or symptoms or bone marrow involvement), HIV test, CNS imaging, and fertility discussions may also be useful (NCCN).

Functional imaging (FDG-PET) is used at diagnosis to accurately stage patients as well as early during the course of chemotherapy to risk stratify patients and guide treatment. It is nearly 100% sensitive for DLBCL when lymph nodes are above the size detection limit.

TABLE 31-3 ANN ARBOR STAGING SYSTEM (NCCN)

Stage I: single lymph node group

Stage II: two or more lymph node groups on the same side of the diaphragm

Stage III: lymph nodes on both sides of the diaphragm involved, subscript S = splenic involvement

Stage IV: disseminated disease involving extranodal organs (not including spleen, which is considered lymphoid tissue)

For stages I-III subscript E = extralymphatic organ/site involvement

- A = absence of systemic symptoms; B = presence of systemic symptoms
- X = bulky disease (>10-cm nodal mass or >1/3 intrathoracic diameter if mediastinal mass)

TABLE 31-4 REVISED INTERNATIONAL PROGNOSTIC INDEX (IPI)

IPI Score	Risk Group	4-Year PFS (%)	4-Year OS (%)
0	Very good	94	94
1–2	Good	80	79
3–5	Poor	53	55

OS, overall survival; PFS, progression-free survival.
Clinical factors worth 1 point each: age >60, serum LDH above upper value of normal, ECOG performance status 2 or greater, Ann Arbor stage III or IV, two or more extranodal disease sites.

PROGNOSIS

Prognosis is determined based on the International Prognostic Index (IPI) (2), a scoring system prognostic in the setting of rituximab-based chemotherapy regimens for event-free survival, progression-free survival, and overall survival in 2010 (3). It is based on five clinical factors (Table 31-4):

1. Age > 60
2. Serum LDH above upper value of normal
3. ECOG performance status 2 or greater
4. Ann Arbor stage III or IV
5. Two or more extranodal disease sites

The overall survival of patients at 4 years ranges from 94% for zero risk factors, down to 55% for patients with 3–5 risk factors.

Between 5% and 11% of patients with newly diagnosed diffuse large B-cell lymphoma will have concurrent translocations of *myc* and *BCL-2*. These cases are colloquially known as "double hit lymphomas" and have a poor prognosis with standard therapy.

Two recent studies have demonstrated that 20%–30% of newly diagnosed patients will have increased expression of *myc* and *BCL-2* without a translocation. These patients have a response rate, progression-free survival, and overall survival intermediate between standard DLBCL and double hit lymphomas (4). The standard chemotherapy regimen of R-CHOP (Table 31-5) does not appear to provide satisfactory outcomes in this population and the therapeutic standard of care has not yet been established.

TABLE 31-5 R-CHOP CHEMOTHERAPY REGIMEN

Rituximab 375 mg/m^2 IV on day 1

Cyclophosphamide 750 mg/m^2 IV on day 1

Doxorubicin (hydroxydaunorubicin) 50 mg/m^2 IV on day 1

Vincristine (Oncovin) 1.4 mg/m^2 (max 2 mg) IV on day 1

Prednisone 100 mg po daily on days 1–5

Cycles are given every 21 days.

FRONT-LINE CHEMOTHERAPY

The mainstay of DLBCL treatment is combination chemotherapy. The current standard chemotherapy regimen is R-CHOP every 21 days (Table 31-5).

Rituximab is a chimeric monoclonal anti-CD20 IgG1 antibody that has demonstrated an additive effect when combined with CHOP to improve both progression-free and overall survival. One of the earliest reports of this survival benefit was from the Groupe d'Etude des Lymphomas de l'Adulte (GELA), which showed that in DLBCL patients over 60 years of age, regardless of IPI score at diagnosis, the addition of rituximab to CHOP improved complete remission and overall survival rates at 2 years by 10%–15% (5). Since then, several subsequent studies have confirmed this benefit in other DLBCL patient cohorts, affirming R-CHOP as first line treatment in DLBCL. R-CHOP given every 14 days has been compared to R-CHOP at 3-week intervals and is not superior.

■ LIMITED-STAGE DIFFUSE LARGE B-CELL LYMPHOMA: STAGES I AND II

Patients with stage I or II bulky disease, defined as ≥10 cm in size, should receive 6 cycles of R-CHOP. Radiation therapy does not improve outcome over chemotherapy alone.

Patients with nonbulky disease, defined as <10 cm in size, can receive either 3 cycles of R-CHOP with radiation therapy or 6 cycles of R-CHOP without radiation therapy. The use of radiation therapy places the patient at a lifetime increased risk of second malignancy.

The decision to proceed with radiation therapy after chemotherapy completion depends on PET imaging results after completing R-CHOP. Biopsy should be considered in this setting with a positive PET scan:

- If there is a complete response (PET negative), then treatment is complete.
- Patients with a partial response (PET positive) should undergo biopsy. Those with persistent disease have the option of: (1) receiving radiation therapy to the PET positive site, (2) receiving high dose therapy with autologous stem-cell transplant, or (3) enrollment in a clinical trial. Repeat PET imaging is performed after completing the course of treatment with a repeat biopsy needed if scans return yet again positive.
- Patients with no response or progressive disease after the initial chemotherapy should receive treatment for refractory disease (see below).

Advanced-Stage Diffuse Large B-Cell Lymphoma: Stages III And IV

Patients with advanced stage disease should receive 6 cycles of R-CHOP. After the first 2–4 cycles of R-CHOP interim PET scans may sometimes be used to guide treatment; however, this approach has not been validated in prospective clinical trials.

- Those with a complete response (PET negative) should complete 6 cycles of R-CHOP and then have repeat PET scans. If the final scans continue to be negative; observation is indicated. If the final scans are positive, then treatment should be based on the algorithm for refractory disease below (after a biopsy has been obtained).

TABLE 31-6 FIRST-LINE CHEMOTHERAPY IN PATIENTS WITH POOR LEFT VENTRICULAR FUNCTION

RCEPP: rituximab, cyclophosphamide, etoposide, prednisone, procarbazine

RCDOP: rituximab, cyclophosphamide, liposomal doxorubicin, vincristine, prednison

RCNOP: rituximab, cyclophosphamide, mitoxantrone, vincristine, prednisone

DA-EPOCH: etoposide, prednisone, vincristine, cyclophosphamide, doxorubicin + rituximab

RCEOP: rituximab, cyclophosphamide, etoposide, vincristine, prednisone

- Those with an interim partial response (PET positive) should complete 6 cycles of R-CHOP and have a final scan performed. Then the patient is managed as above for those with final scan negative or positive.
- For those without any response on interim restaging, patients should be treated for refractory disease. However, it is very rare that a PET scan is required to detect the failure of chemotherapy to produce a response. Refractory disease is nearly always a clinical diagnosis, often made by the patient.

In cases of poor left ventricular function, standard anthracyclines or anthracenediones cannot be used and alternative chemotherapy regimens and schedules are preferred (Table 31-6) (6).

Rarely, patients will present with central nervous system involvement at initial diagnosis. In patients with CNS parenchymal disease, high-dose systemic methotrexate is incorporated into first-line chemotherapy regimens. In leptomeningeal disease, intrathecal methotrexate and cytarabine or high-dose systemic methotrexate are both options. Limited data suggest that autologous stem-cell transplantation in first remission for these patients may improve outcome.

◼ RELAPSED/REFRACTORY DLBCL

Although R-CHOP has improved outcome in DLBCL patients, approximately a third of patients will either relapse or prove refractory to initial therapy. The majority of relapses occur within 2–3 years of treatment. Late relapses (after 5 years) constitute ~7% of all progressions after R-CHOP.

Autologous stem-cell transplant has been the standard of care for patients with relapsed DLBCL.

In the European PARMA trial, Philip et al. (7) studied 215 patients with relapsed NHL who had received two courses of conventional chemotherapy. Of these, 109 responded to the initial chemotherapy and 54 of these were assigned to receive four more courses of chemotherapy with or without radiation therapy, and 55 were assigned to receive intensive chemotherapy and an autologous bone marrow transplant. They followed the patients for 63 months and found a response rate of 84% in the transplant group and 44% in the nontransplant group. At 5 years, the event-free survival rate was 46% in the transplant group and 12% in the nontransplant group ($P = 0.001$). The overall survival rate was 53% and 32% in the two groups

TABLE 31-7 SECOND-LINE CHEMOTHERAPY BEFORE HD-SCT, ALL USUALLY WITH RITUXIMAB

ICE: ifosfamide, carboplatin, etoposide

DHAP: dexamethasone, high-dose cytarabine/anthracycline, procarbazine

ESHAP: etoposide, methylprednisolone, cytarabine/anthracycline, cisplatin

GDP: gemcitabine, dexamethasone, cisplatin/carboplatin

GemOx: gemcitabine, oxaliplatin

MINE: mesna, ifosfamide, mitoxantrone, etoposide

($P = 0.038$). The PARMA trial was performed before rituximab entered the standard of care for DLBCL.

The CORAL trial (8) included relapsed or refractory patients with CD20+ DLBCL. The majority of patients had been treated with R-CHOP as their initial therapy. These patients were randomized to receive R-DHAP (rituximab, dexamethasone, cytarabine, and cisplatin) versus R-ICE (rituximab, ifosfamide, etoposide, carboplatin). Those who responded to this second treatment then received autologous stem-cell transplant followed by a second randomization to maintenance rituximab or observation. Approximately 200 patients were randomized to the R-ICE and R-DHAP arms, with no difference in overall response rates seen between the groups (63.5% vs 62.8%). Of the 206 patients that went on to receive ASCT, there was no difference noted between the R-ICE and R-DHAP groups when comparing event-free (26% vs 35%, $P = 0.6$) or overall survival (47% vs 51%, $P = 0.5$). Notably the response rate, event-free survival, and overall survival were significantly inferior for patients who had received rituximab in the front-line setting.

Second-line chemotherapy regimens are listed in Table 31-7. Fit patients with complete or partial responses should proceed to HD-SCT. Patients with chemotherapy-resistant relapse should be evaluated for clinical trials or palliative treatment.

For patients not eligible for HD-SCT or with relapse after HD-SCT, several new agents are currently under investigation (Table 31-8).

■ **CENTRAL NERVOUS SYSTEM PROPHYLAXIS**

Central nervous system recurrence in DLBCL is rare, with risk estimates ranging from 3% to 9% in the rituximab era. While rituximab has been shown to have partial protective effects against CNS relapse, patients with advanced disease stage, elevated LDH, IPI 3–5, and involvement of extranodal sites (particularly orbit, sinus/posterior nasal space, breast, testicle, bone, and bone marrow) are still at high risk for CNS relapse (9). Options for prophylaxis of central nervous system relapse include intrathecal methotrexate as well as systemic intravenous methotrexate. Our standard approach is to provide intravenous methotrexate prophylaxis at a dose of 3.5 g/m² with leukovorin rescue on day 15 of R-CHOP cycles 1, 3, and 5 to patients with either bone marrow involvement, testicular disease, or

TABLE 31-8 NOVEL TARGETED THERAPIES

Enzastaurin

BCR-signaling inhibitors

Bortezomib

Lenalidomide

Navitoclax

BCL-6 inhibitors

Bruton's tyrosine kinase inhibitors

Novel unconjugated monoclonal antibodies

Antibody drug conjugates

the combination of an elevated LDH and more than one extranodal site of disease.

■ TUMOR LYSIS SYNDROME

Tumor lysis syndrome is fully discussed in Chapter 20. DLBCL is generally considered to be intermediate risk for tumor lysis syndrome and recommended prophylaxis includes hydration and allopurinol.

■ HEPATITIS B REACTIVATION

Reactivation of the hepatitis B virus has been reported in patients treated with rituximab monotherapy, chemotherapy, or with the combination. This reactivation may result in severe hepatitis including hepatic failure or death. Patients who are HBsAg positive are at a high risk of reactivation but HBsAg-negative HBcAb-positive patients can also reactivate. Antiviral prophylaxis reduces the risk of reactivation substantially, but the optimal duration of prophylaxis after the completion of therapy is unknown. Viral load should be monitored monthly.

■ PROGRESSIVE MULTIFOCAL LEUKOENCEPHALOPATHY (PML)

PML is a fatal central nervous system infection caused by JC virus. It has been reported in patients treated with rituximab for a variety of indications. Diagnosis is usually made by PCR of the virus from the CSF or a brain biopsy.

■ CHEMOTHERAPY SIDE EFFECTS

Common and important serious adverse events seen with R-CHOP include infection in 7%–10%, thrombocytopenia and anemia in less than 1%, nausea and vomiting in 4% (with proper antiemetic prophylaxis), and alopecia in 40% of patients.

While empiric granulocyte colony-stimulating factor (G-CSF) use is not routinely recommended, R-CHOP falls into an intermediate febrile neutropenia risk category. G-CSF should be considered in patients with the following characteristics:

- >65 years old
- Poor performance status

- Bone marrow involvement
- Impaired renal or hepatic function
- Chemotherapy-induced neutropenia severe enough to cause delays in treatment

It is recommended that 24 hours elapse between chemotherapy and G-CSF. Antibiotic prophylaxis, especially against *Pneumocystis jiroveci* pneumonia should be considered in regimens containing glucocorticoids, purine analogs, or high-dose chemotherapy.

Other common chemotherapy side effects include a low risk of cardiotoxicity, therapy-induced myelodysplasia, sensory neuropathy, and infertility.

■ DLBCL SUBTYPES

In this section, we will highlight some key aspects of a few DLBCL subtypes.

Primary Mediastinal Large B-Cell Lymphoma (PMBCL)

PMBCL is a rare subtype accounting for 5% of all DLBCL and is thought to arise from thymic medullary B cells. It is commonly seen in adolescents and young adults, with a median age of diagnosis in the fourth decade of life and a male-female ratio of 1:2. It is sometimes histologically confused with nodular sclerosis classical Hodgkin lymphoma; however, PMBCL has upregulation of the NFkB pathway and usually expresses the pan B-cell markers CD20 and CD 79a. PMBCL typically presents as a rapidly progressive and locally invasive anterior mediastinal mass, frequently causing symptoms of cough, dyspnea, dysphagia, and superior vena-cava syndrome (seen in up to 30%–50% of patients) due to local compressive effects. Regional spread can also cause lung, chest wall, pleural, and pericardial infiltration. PMBCL is diagnosed at stage I or II in 80% of patients. Because of the rarity of this subtype, prospective trials have not fully defined the standard of care. Chemotherapy commonly consists of DA-EPOCH chemotherapy regimen and is associated with a 5-year survival of ~95%. Radiation therapy is not needed when DA-EPOCH chemotherapy is used.

Intravascular Large-B Cell Lymphoma

Intravascular DLBCL is a rare subtype of DLBCL, occurring in less than 1 person per 1 million. Initially described in 1959, it was characterized as an angiotropic large-cell lymphoma. By 2008, the WHO defined this as an extranodal DLBCL, with growth restricted to the lumina of small vessels, particularly capillaries. It primarily affects the elderly population and 91% of patients present at advanced stage. The most common presenting symptoms are caused by occlusion of terminal vascular beds and include cutaneous findings, CNS symptoms (including sensorimotor deficits, paresthesias, aphasias, seizures, visual changes, vertigo, and altered mental status) as well as renal involvement. Fever and B symptoms are relatively common. It frequently also involves the kidneys, lungs, and endocrine glands, although lymph nodes are usually spared. R-CHOP chemotherapy is the mainstay of care although some centers include CNS-directed therapies given the proclivity of this lymphoma for involvement of vascular structures within the brain parenchyma. There may be two distinct subtypes of this disease, a Western form with predominant end-organ manifestations and an Asian form that presents with prominent systemic symptoms, pancytopenia and hemophagocytosis.

EBV-Positive DLBCL of the Elderly

EBV-positive DLBCL was originally described in elderly Japanese patients (Oyama). It is a clonal EBV+ B cell neoplasm seen in patients over the age of 50 without known prior lymphomas or immunodeficiencies. It is an aggressive subtype and frequently has extranodal involvement on presentation, which carries a poor prognosis. There is speculation that this particular DLBCL subset is related to immunosenescence. Many elderly patients who are diagnosed with EBV-positive DLBCL have other medical comorbidities that limit the chemotherapy regimens and number of cycles that can be given.

T-cell/Histiocyte-Rich Large B-cell Lymphoma

T-cell/histiocyte-rich large B-cell lymphoma (THRBCL) is characterized by scattered single neoplastic malignant B cells in a background of reactive T cells and histiocytes. The B cells are never seen in sheets or substantial aggregates. Cases of THRBCL are seen in patients with nodular lymphocyte predominant Hodgkin lymphoma and the interrelationship between these diseases has not been fully defined. Care must be taken to distinguish these two entities as the therapies and outcomes are distinct. Epidemiologically, it is most frequent in middle-aged men. Compared with DLBCL-NOS, THRBCL has a propensity toward involvement of the bone marrow, liver, and spleen. Treatment involves R-CHOP-based chemotherapy regimens, with a response rate similar to that of traditional DLBCL.

Primary DLBCLs of the CNS

Discussed in Central Nervous System Malignancies (see Chapter 62).

Double hit lymphomas Double hit lymphomas are a group of B-cell lymphomas with recurrent chromosomal breakpoints that results in activation of oncogenes. Of these, *BCL2* and *myc* rearrangements are most common; however, rearrangements involving *bcl6* are also seen. These lymphomas are typically highly aggressive and may have clinical features that overlap with Burkitt lymphoma and DLBCL. At presentation, extranodal disease, bone marrow, and CNS involvement are frequently seen. The overall prognosis is poor and as of 2013, no standard therapy has yet been defined.

B-cell lymphoma unclassifiable with features intermediate between diffuse large B-cell lymphoma and Burkitt lymphoma (BclU) Burkitt lymphoma (BL) is an aggressive B-cell non-Hodgkin lymphoma which is characterized by *c-myc* translocations and a high proliferation index. Morphologically, BL has a "starry sky" appearance, with numerous macrophages that have ingested apoptotic debris amidst a background of neoplastic lymphoid cells. Epstein-Barr virus (EBV) is strongly associated with endemic BL, but also occurs in sporadic and HIV-associated cases. BclU are diseases with biological, clinical, and genetic features of both BL and DLBCL. Clinically most patients present with advanced stage disease and extranodal involvement is common. There is substantial overlap between this clinically and morphologically defined entity and DHL which is defined genetically. The optimal therapy of this disease is unknown although many centers use R-EPOCH with high response rates and excellent long-term survival.

B-cell lymphoma unclassifiable with features intermediate between diffuse large B-cell lymphoma and classical Hodgkin lymphoma This disease is defined as a B-cell lymphoma with clinical, morphologic, and immunophentypic features of classical HL and DLBCL, most commonly the primary mediastinal subtype. These lymphomas typically present in younger men in the second and third decade of life with a mediastinal mass. Histologically sheets of tumor cells are seen within fibrous stroma although often the architecture varies in different areas of the same tumor from the appearance of classical HL to that of PMBL. Rare true composite lymphomas of PMBL and cHL have also been reported. These lymphomas are typically CD20 and CD79a while also expressing CD30 and CD15. There is no consensus on the optimal therapy of this rare disease.

REFERENCES

1. National Comprehensive Cancer Network Guidelines. Diffuse Large B-Cell Lymphoma. Version 2. 2012.

2. Shipp MA, Yeap BY, Harrington DP, et al. A predictive model for aggressive non-Hodgkin's lymphoma. *N Engl J Med.* 1993; 329: 987–994.

3. Ziepert M, Hasenclever D, et al. Standard International Prognostic Index remains a valid predictor of outcome for patients with aggressive CD20+ B-cell lymphoma in the rituximab era. *J Clin Oncol.* 2010; 28: 2373-2380.

4. Snuderl M, Kolman OK, et al. B-cell lymphomas with concurrent IGH-BCL2 and MYC rearrangements are aggressive neoplasms with clinical and pathologic features distinct from Burkitt lymphoma and diffuse large B-cell lymphoma. *Am J Surg Pathol.* 2010; 34: 327–340.

5. Coiffer B, Lepage E, et al. CHOP chemotherapy plus rituximab compared with CHOP alone in elderly patients with diffuse large-B-cell lymphoma. *N Engl J Med.* 2002; 346: 235–242.

6. Fields PA, Linch DC. Treatment of the elderly patient with diffuse large B cell lymphoma. *British J Haematol.* 2012; 157: 159–170.

7. Philip T, Guglielmi C, Hagenbeek A, et al. Autologous bone marrow transplantation as compared with salvage chemotherapy in relapses of chemotherapy-sensitive non-Hodgkin's lymphoma. *N Engl J Med.* 1995; 333: 1540–1545.

8. Gisselbrecht C, et al. R-ICE versus R-DHAP in relapsed patients with CD20 diffuse large B-cell lymphoma (DLBCL) followed by autologous stem cell transplantation: CORAL study. *J Clin Oncol.* 2009; 27(15s).

9. Villa D, Connors JM, et al. Incidence and risk factors for central nervous system relapse in patients with diffuse large B-cell lymphoma: the impact of the addition of rituximab to CHOP chemotherapy. *Ann Oncology.* 2010; 21: 1046–1052.

CHAPTER **32**
Hodgkin's Disease

Dan L. Longo

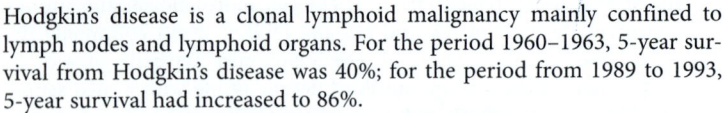

Hodgkin's disease is a clonal lymphoid malignancy mainly confined to lymph nodes and lymphoid organs. For the period 1960–1963, 5-year survival from Hodgkin's disease was 40%; for the period from 1989 to 1993, 5-year survival had increased to 86%.

EPIDEMIOLOGY

About 7500 new cases are diagnosed in the United States each year (roughly 2.9 per 100,000 population) (1). Males are affected somewhat more often than females (M:F 1.4:1). Hodgkin's disease accounts for about 11% of all lymphomas and is about half as common as multiple myeloma. It has a bimodal age distribution with the first peak in the late twenties and a second peak in late life. The etiology is unknown. Farmers, wood workers, and meat workers are at somewhat increased risk. A minor increased risk is associated with an HLA-linkage disequilibrium. Hodgkin's disease can complicate the genetic disease and ataxia telangiectasia, and occurs at increased frequency in patients with AIDS. An identical twin of an affected person is at 99-fold increased risk of developing the disease. Some geographic clusters have been noted and molecular studies have implicated Epstein–Barr virus (EBV) in the pathogenesis of some cases, particularly cases in Central and South America and patients with mixed cellularity histology (2) (see below).

PATHOLOGY

Two major forms of Hodgkin's disease are recognized: classical Hodgkin's disease accounts for 95% of cases and nodular lymphocyte predominant Hodgkin's disease accounts for 5% (3). Classical Hodgkin's disease is divided into four histologic subtypes: nodular sclerosis (70% of cases), mixed cellularity (20% of cases), lymphocyte rich (3%–5% of cases), and lymphocyte depleted (<2% of cases). As diagnostic methods have improved, cases of lymphocyte depleted Hodgkin's disease have declined both because some cases were actually other lymphoma entities and because earlier diagnosis has made the entity more rare.

The malignant cell of Hodgkin's disease is the Reed–Sternberg cell; it has different forms in distinct histologic subtypes. In classical Hodgkin's disease, it is usually derived from a follicular center B cell that has clonally rearranged its immunoglobulin genes but does not transcribe them. Thus, no tumor immunoglobulin molecules are detected. From a clinical perspective, the distinction between classical Hodgkin's disease and nodular lymphocyte predominant Hodgkin's disease is critical because the entities differ in natural history and in standard approach to treatment. The distinction between subsets of classical Hodgkin's disease is not technically difficult, but carries little impact as the natural history and management are not affected by the subset diagnosis.

Hodgkin's Disease CHAPTER 32 407

TABLE 32-1 IMMUNOPHENOTYPE OF MALIGNANT CELLS IN HODGKIN'S DISEASE

	Classical Hodgkin's Disease	Nodular Lymphocyte Predominant Hodgkin's Disease
CD30	+	−
CD15	+	−
EMA	−	+
CD45	−	+
CD20, CD79	±	+
J Chain	−	+

Immunophenotypic studies define differences between classic and nodular lymphocyte predominant Hodgkin's disease (see Table 32-1). All forms of Hodgkin's disease share three histologic features: effacement of the normal lymph node architecture; infiltration with a broad range of normal-appearing cells including reactive T cells, plasma cells, histiocytes, neutrophils, eosinophils, and stromal cells (the malignant cells are usually 3% or less of the total cells in an enlarged node); and presence of the characteristic neoplastic cells.

Nodular sclerosis Hodgkin's disease is the most common form in the United States and is slightly more common in women than men and in the younger age group. The disease grows in nodules separated by bands of collagen fibrosis and the Reed–Sternberg cell is the "lacunar" variant. The name derives from a fixation artifact that causes the cytoplasm to retract leaving a single or multilobed nucleus surrounded by a clear area.

Mixed cellularity Hodgkin's disease grows in a diffuse pattern and has a florid inflammatory cell background. Reed–Sternberg cells are usually binucleated with prominent nucleoli that give the cell an "owl's eyes"-like appearance.

Nodular lymphocyte predominant Hodgkin's disease is characterized by the lymphocyte and histiocyte (L&H) Reed–Sternberg cell variant that is also called a popcorn cell because of a lobulated nuclear contour that resembles popcorn. The cell expresses B-cell markers, surface immunoglobulin, often expresses epithelial membrane antigen (EMA), and cytoplasmic J chains. Unlike the Reed–Sternberg cell in classic Hodgkin's disease, it is CD30 and CD15 negative. The T cells that cluster around the neoplastic cells often express CD57, a natural killer cell marker and the tumor nodules contain a vague meshwork of CD21+ follicular dendritic cells. It is said that the number of infiltrating CD68+ macrophages influences the risk of relapse; more CD68+ cells correlate with shorter remission duration.

GENETICS

Unlike other lymphoid malignancies, Hodgkin's disease does not have a characteristic genetic lesion. The cells are aneuploid; Reed–Sternberg cells contain two–eight copies of individual chromosomes (3). A variety of genetic abnormalities have been noted, but none recurs in different cases at high frequency. Cells may contain mutant p53. Evidence for Epstein–Barr virus is noted in 30%–60% of cases, varying with the technique used to detect it. It is commonly present in a clonal episome; however, the only consistent viral gene expressed in the cells containing the EBV genome is LMP1. Its role in the genesis or maintenance of the malignant cells is undefined.

CLINICAL FEATURES OF CLASSICAL HODGKIN'S DISEASE

Patients usually present with painless adenopathy localized to the neck. The mediastinum is involved in the majority of patients (~2/3), occasionally with large masses. When the mediastinal shadow is greater than 1/3, the greatest chest diameter on PA chest radiograph, the mediastinal involvement is considered massive. B symptoms are present in 20%–25%. The disease tends to start in cervical nodes (left side more commonly than right) and march to contiguous lymph node groups. The first intraabdominal site is most often the spleen. Because the spleen has no afferent lymphatics, spleen involvement implies hematogenous spread. The liver is never involved unless the spleen is involved. Involvement of Waldeyer's ring or epitrochlear nodes is rare. Extranodal involvement is also unusual; when present, bone marrow, liver, lung, pleura, and pericardium are the most commonly involved sites.

In patients with B symptoms, the pattern of the fever may be intermittent. Pel–Ebstein fever describes a pattern in which fever is noted more or less continuously for 1 or 2 weeks followed by afebrile periods of similar duration. However, Pel–Ebstein fevers are unusual. When present, fever tends to occur every evening and breaks while the patient is sleeping giving rise to drenching night sweats.

Pruritis is common, but is not a B symptom. Patients occasionally experience pain in involved lymph nodes upon ingesting alcohol. This is thought to be due to alcohol-induced degranulation of eosinophils. A wide range of symptoms may be noted based on the direct effects of the tumor or paraneoplastic syndromes from tumor products. These symptoms are listed in Table 32-2.

Patients with AIDS who develop Hodgkin's disease are more likely to have mixed cellularity histology and to have extranodal involvement (2/3 of cases).

CLINICAL FEATURES OF NODULAR LYMPHOCYTE PREDOMINANT HODGKIN'S DISEASE

Patients are predominantly male, in the 30–50-year age group, and usually present with localized peripheral adenopathy involving the cervical, axillary, or inguinal nodes. Mediastinal, spleen, or bone marrow involvement is rare.

DIAGNOSIS AND STAGING

The diagnosis depends on an excisional lymph node biopsy. Needle aspiration is an inadequate diagnostic procedure in a patient with undiagnosed lymphadenopathy. Once a diagnosis is made, a variety of tests are performed to define the extent of disease and the presence or absence of factors that affect prognosis (see Table 32-3). As a result of the testing, the patient is assigned a stage of disease based upon the Cotswolds modification of the

TABLE 32-2 CLINICAL MANIFESTATIONS OF HODGKIN'S DISEASE

Findings at presentation
    Adenopathy, most often cervical
    Mediastinal mass
    Splenomegaly (in 25%)

Symptoms
    Fever, unexplained weight loss, night sweats
    Pruritis
    Alcohol-induced pain in enlarged lymph nodes
    Bone pain (rare)
    Pericardial effusion or tamponade (rare)
    Pleural effusion

Laboratory findings
    Granulocytosis
    Thrombocytosis
    Eosinophilia
    Elevated erythrocyte sedimentation rate
    Elevated alkaline phosphatase

Paraneoplastic syndromes
    Dermatologic
    Nodular prurigo
    Ichthyosis
    Psoriaform lesions
    Erythema nodosum
    Dermatomyositis
    Linear IgA bullous dermatosis
    Leukocytoclastic vasculitis
    Toxic epidermal necrolysis

Renal and metabolic
    Nephrotic syndrome
    Hypercalcemia
    Hypoglycemia
    Lactic acidosis

Neurologic
    Brachial plexopathy
    Guillian–Barre syndrome
    Sensory ganglionitis
    Acute cerebellar degeneration
    Stiff-man syndrome
    Ophelia syndrome

Ann Arbor staging classification (see Table 32-4) (4). Because of the orderly progression of Hodgkin's disease from one lymph node-bearing site to the contiguous node-bearing site, the staging system is an anatomic-based system. However, improvements in treatment over the last 30 years have changed the role of staging in patient management. Stage no longer affects prognosis as primary treatment leads to the cure of about 80% or greater of all patients at all stages of disease. Clinical features other than stage of disease may affect prognosis (Table 32-5).

Most patients receive systemic chemotherapy either alone or as part of a combined modality treatment program. Accordingly, the need for precise pathologic staging and exploratory laparotomy has vanished. This change in practice has served to reduce the acute surgical morbidity and mortality risk of the staging laparotomy and to avoid the increased risk of infection associated with splenectomy. Thus, the current state-of-the-art in staging evaluation is to perform clinical staging tests and to include systemic therapy in the management of all patients.

TABLE 32-3 RECOMMENDED STAGING EVALUATION IN PATIENTS WITH HODGKIN'S DISEASE

Mandatory procedures

Excisional biopsy of an involved lymph node

History with attention to B symptoms

Physical examination, record bidimensional dimensions of adenopathy, splenomegaly

Laboratory tests

    CBC, differential count, platelet count

    Chemistry panel, liver and renal function tests

    Erythrocyte sedimentation rate

Radiographic tests

    PA and lateral chest radiograph

    Abdominal and pelvic computed tomography (CT)

    Bipedal lymphogram (not widely available, yet the best test for paraaortic nodes)

    Bilateral bone marrow biopsies and aspirates

    Nuclide imaging

        PET scan or gallium scan

Procedures useful under certain circumstances

    Thoracic computed tomography if chest radiograph abnormal (of minimal value if chest x-ray normal)

    Liver biopsy if there is evidence of splenic or hepatic involvement

    Bone scan if bone pain is present

    Echocardiography if pericardial disease is suspected

TABLE 32-4 STAGING CLASSIFICATION FOR HODGKIN'S DISEASE

Stage	Definition
I	Involvement of a single lymph node region or structure (e.g., spleen)
II	Involvement of two or more lymph node regions on the same side of the diaphragm
III	Involvement of lymph node regions or structures on both sides of the diaphragm
IV	Involvement of extranodal site(s) beyond that designated as "E," more than one extranodal deposit at any location, any involvement of liver or bone marrow
A	No symptoms
B	Unexplained weight loss >10% of body weight in last 6 mo Unexplained fever >38°C in the previous month Recurrent drenching night sweats in the previous month
X	Bulky disease: ≥10 cm maximal diameter of a nodal mass, mediastinal mass >1/3 chest diameter
E	Localized solitary involvement of extralymphatic tissue except liver and bone marrow: if this is the only site of disease, it is stage IE By limited direct extension from a known nodal site Single-discrete site proximal to a regional involved nodal site (IIE)

The most poorly evaluated common site of disease is the paraaortic lymph nodes. Bipedal lymphography is more sensitive and specific than abdominal CT in detecting paraaortic node involvement; however, the skill to perform lymphatic channel cannulation is disappearing from radiology departments and, unfortunately, the test is not widely available. However, the widespread use of systemic treatment has resulted in no apparent cost in survival as a consequence of inaccurate abdominal staging.

TREATMENT

■ PRIMARY TREATMENT OF NODULAR LYMPHOCYTE PREDOMINANT HODGKIN'S DISEASE

Patients with localized disease are often managed with involved-field radiation therapy (5). The disease may have long periods of remission punctuated by intermittent relapses that do not appear to affect overall survival. The natural history is quite prolonged with survival that is generally as good as or better than classical Hodgkin's disease. Patients with advanced stage disease are usually managed like patients with classical Hodgkin's disease (see below). About 3%–5% of patients may undergo histologic progression to diffuse large B-cell lymphoma that is derived from the same malignant clone that gave rise to the Hodgkin's disease. Such lymphomas are usually responsive to combination chemotherapy and patients are often put into long-term complete remission.

TABLE 32-5 PROGNOSTIC FACTORS IN VARIOUS SETTINGS

Early stage disease
    B symptoms
    Massive mediastinal involvement

Advanced stage disease
    Serum albumin <4 g/dl
    Hemoglobin <10.5 g/dl
    Male sex
    Age >45 years
    Stage IV disease
    Leukocytosis >15,000/mm^3
    Lymphcytopenia <600/mm^3 or <8% of total white count

Once treatment has begun
    Disease progression through treatment
    Failure to achieve a complete response
    Persistent PET-positive disease after cycle 2 or 3

After relapse
    Short duration of initial remission
    B symptoms
    Multiple relapses

PRIMARY TREATMENT OF CLASSICAL HODGKIN'S DISEASE

Combination chemotherapy is the cornerstone of Hodgkin's disease treatment. ABVD combination chemotherapy appears to have the best overall efficacy with the least acute and chronic toxicity (6, 7). Clinical staging followed by six cycles of ABVD chemotherapy is certainly a reasonable management approach. Controversy surrounds the use of radiation therapy in the management of Hodgkin's disease. Many have taken the approach that a shorter course of chemotherapy (e.g., 2 cycles of ABVD) together with 20-Gy mantle-field or involved-field radiation therapy (8) should further improve disease control. While combined modality therapy does somewhat lower the risk of relapse in previously involved lymph nodes, combined modality therapy has not been demonstrated to improve overall survival in early stage (9) or advanced stage disease (10). A key component to assess the impact of treatment is to measure both acute and chronic toxicities.

Radiation therapy to the mediastinum is associated with a threefold increased risk of *fatal* myocardial infarction (11) and an increased risk of second malignancies in as many as 30% of patients within 30 years of treatment (12). By contrast, randomized comparisons between ABVD versus ABVD plus radiation therapy have not demonstrated significant differences in outcome (13). In the range of doses used to treat Hodgkin's disease, no convincing evidence has been obtained of a dose-response curve such that lower doses of radiation therapy are less likely to produce late fatal complications.

Thus, it is safest to reserve radiation therapy only for the subset of patients who need it to optimize control of their disease.

Who, then, needs radiation therapy? About 5%–12% of patients treated with six cycles of ABVD chemotherapy will not achieve a complete response. This subset of patients benefits from the use of radiation therapy to convert the partial response to a complete response. Patients with low-volume residual disease have a very high rate of conversion to durable complete response. Patients with larger volume residual disease have about a 50% chance of achieving a durable remission. The small group of patients who have a tumor that grows in the face of chemotherapy have a poor prognosis and should be managed with salvage chemotherapy; see below.

Other patients might also benefit from added radiation therapy. Some data suggest that the persistence of PET-positive disease after two or three cycles of chemotherapy may identify patients at risk of relapse if managed with chemotherapy alone. In one series, 80% of patients had no residual PET-positive disease after two cycles of therapy; among the 20%, who had residual PET positivity, two-thirds of those patients relapsed (14). Other data are persuasive that it is PET negativity at the end of treatment that is the superior predictor of outcome (15). Thus, while prospective trials are being performed, it should be possible to define criteria that permit the use of radiation therapy in the subset of patients who have the greatest need for its therapeutic effects while protecting the 80% or so of patients who do well without exposing them to the late toxicities of radiation therapy. Until prospective clinical trial evidence emerges that mid-cycle PET positivity is sufficiently strong a predictor of outcome that one can base treatment decisions on it, the safest approach is to add radiation therapy only to the subset of patients with positive PET scans at the end of their planned course of chemotherapy.

Other regimens have been advocated including Stanford V (16) and BEACOPP (17). Stanford V is a combined modality regimen that involves administering radiation therapy to 100% of patients. It should be kept in mind that it takes 20–30 years to assess the late complications from radiation therapy. Comments about technical advances that should lower the risks are meaningless until a lower risk is actually demonstrated. No one has demonstrated any therapeutic radiation technique that is not associated with late second malignancies. Furthermore, comparison of Stanford V to ABVD in randomized trials suggested that the regimens were comparable in efficacy (18, 19). BEACOPP is a multidrug alkylating agent-based regimen that is said to be superior to COPP/ABVD based on a randomized clinical trial (20). However, BEACOPP is highly myelotoxic, causes infertility and is likely to have an unacceptable late toxicity profile, including secondary leukemia and myelodysplasia, especially because 75% of the patients also received involved-field radiation therapy. Efforts to improve treatment outcome by combining the active agents into 7-, 8-, or 10-drug regimens have not demonstrated clear superiority over ABVD alone.

■ SALVAGE TREATMENT

High-dose chemotherapy with autologous hematopoietic stem-cell transplantation is the cornerstone of salvage therapy for patients with Hodgkin's disease who relapse or who experience progression during remission induction.

The likelihood of success is related to the initial remission duration (21). Those whose initial remission lasted more than 12 months may have a 75%–80% of achieving a durable second remission. Initial remissions shorter than 12 months identify a group of patients that have about a 40%–50% chance of achieving a second durable remission. Patients with progressive disease during induction chemotherapy generally have a 20% or less chance of attaining durable remission.

Salvage treatment is administered in two phases; first a conventional dose regimen to achieve major reduction in tumor bulk and promote mobilization of hematopoietic stem cells into the peripheral blood followed by high-dose therapy with stem cell support. The choice of the conventional dose regimen is usually based on the original remission duration.

In general, patients who experience long initial remissions remain sensitive to the drugs that induced the first remission. However, alkylating agent-based regimens like MOPP (22) or ChlVPP (23) may offer some advantage over a second course of ABVD in the setting of resistant disease (7) as the mechanisms of resistance to natural products like vinblastine and doxorubicin do not appear to influence alkylating agent-based killing. Patients with initial remissions lasting less than 1 year should receive an alkylating agent-based conventional-dose salvage regimen. Patients who experienced progressive disease on ABVD may respond to MOPP or MOPP-like regimens. However, a newer regimen with novel agents such as ESHAP (etoposide, methylprednisolone, high-dose cytarabine, cisplatin) (24) may be more effective. A novel agent that appears to have substantial activity in the salvage setting is brentuximab vedotin, an antibody-drug immunoconjugate targeting CD30 on the surface of the tumor cells (25). Once the agent binds to CD30, its linker releases the antitubulin drug, monomethyl auristatin E, into the cell and response rates are as high as 70%. One has considerable freedom of choice in selecting the conventional dose regimen. The goal is to achieve as close to a complete response as possible before embarking on the high-dose chemotherapy regimen. Patients entering the high-dose therapy phase with the lowest tumor bulk generally have the highest likelihood of attaining a durable remission.

A number of myeloablative regimens have been employed in the salvage treatment of Hodgkin's disease including BEAM (26), CVB (27), and high-dose melphalan (28) (see Chapter 38). One has not been convincingly shown to be better than the others. It is important that the treating physician has experience using the regimens at these high doses. Doses and schedules of all the regimens are provided in Table 32-6. Low-dose preparative regimens are also being tested.

The consequence of this overall approach to treatment is cure of about 85%–90% of the patients. However, some patients will not obtain a durable remission after high-dose therapy with stem cell support. It is important to keep in mind that it is still possible to provide palliation in such patients with the judicious use of single-agent chemotherapy. For example, weekly low-dose vinblastine (29) is extremely effective at controlling disease progression at doses that are not myelosuppressive. Anecdotes of prolonged survival with such palliative approaches foster a spirit of continuing to explore novel treatment options. Gemcitabine (30) has activity in patients with refractory disease. In addition, new approaches are in development including exploitation of the

TABLE 32-6 TREATMENT PROGRAMS FOR HODGKIN'S DISEASE

Primary treatment programs

ABVD

Doxorubicin 25 mg/m^2 IV days 1, 15

Bleomycin 10 U/m^2 IV days 1, 15

Vinblastine 6 mg/m^2 IV days 1, 15

Dacarbazine 375 mg/m^2 IV days 1, 15

28-day cycle

MOPP

Nitrogen mustard 6 mg/m^2 IV days 1, 8

Vincristine 1.4 mg/m^2 IV days 1, 8 (NO cap at 2 mg; dose reduction for motor, not sensory, neuropathy)

Procarbazine 100 mg/m^2 po days 1–14

Prednisone 40 mg/m^2 po days 1–14

28-day cycle

ChIVPP

Chlorambucil 6 mg/m^2 (10 mg maximum) po days 1–14

Vinblastine 6 mg/m^2 (10 mg maximum) IV days 1, 8

Procarbazine 100 mg/m^2 po days 1–14

Prednisone 40 mg/m^2 po days 1–14

28-day cycle

Stanford V

Nitrogen mustard 6 mg/m^2 IV on weeks 1, 5, and 9

Doxorubicin 25 mg/m^2 IV on weeks 1, 3, 5, 7, 9, and 11

Vinblastine 6 mg/m^2 IV on weeks 1, 3, 5, 7, 9, and 11

Vincristine 1.4 mg/m^2 (capped at 2 mg) IV on weeks 2, 4, 6, 8, 10, and 12

Bleomycin 5 U/m^2 IV on weeks 2, 4, 6, 8, 10, and 12

Etoposide 60 mg/m^2 IV on days 1 and 2 of weeks 3, 7, and 11

Prednisone 40 mg/m^2 po every other day on weeks 1–10

12 weeks of therapy followed by radiation therapy to 36 Gy

BEACOPP

Bleomycin 10 U/m^2 IV day 8

Etoposide 100 mg/m^2 IV days 1–3

Doxorubicin 25 mg/m^2 IV day 1

Cyclophosphamide 650 mg/m^2 IV day 1

Vincristine 1.4 mg/m^2 (2 mg maximum) IV day 8

Procarbazine 100 mg/m^2 po days 1–7

(continued)

TABLE 32-6 TREATMENT PROGRAMS FOR HODGKIN'S DISEASE (CONTINUED)

BEACOPP (Continued)	
	Prednisone 40 mg/m^2 po days 1–14
	21-day cycles
Escalated BEACOPP	
	Bleomycin 10 mg/m^2 IV day 8
	Etoposide 200 mg/m^2 IV days 1–3
	Doxorubicin 35 mg/m^2 IV day 1
	Cyclophosphamide 1250 mg/m^2 IV day 1
	Vincristine 1.4 mg/m^2 IV day 8
	Procarbazine 100 mg/m^2 po days 1–7
	Prednisone 40 mg/m^2 po days 1–14
	G-CSF SC from d8*
	21-day cycles
Conventional-dose salvage programs	
If ABVD was the initial treatment program, MOPP or ChIVPP should be the initial salvage regimen	
If MOPP or ChIVPP was the initial treatment program, ABVD should be the initial salvage regimen	
CR or good PR should be followed by high-dose therapy and autologous hematopoietic stem-cell transplantation	
If disease fails to respond or progresses through the initial salvage regimen	
ASHAP	
	Doxorubicin 10 mg/m^2/day continuous IV infusion days 1–4
	Methylprednisolone 500 mg/day IV days 1–5
	Cisplatin 25 mg/m^2/day continuous IV infusion days 1–4
	Cytosine arabinoside 1.5 g/m^2 IV day 5
	2–3 28-day courses and then high-dose therapy with transplant
Mini-BEAM	
	Carmustine 60 mg/m^2 IV day 1
	Etoposide 75 mg/m^2 IV days 2–5
	Cytarabine 100 mg/m^2 IV q12h days 2–5
	Melphalan 30 mg/m^2 IV day 6
	2–3 28-day cycles and then high-dose therapy with transplant
If patient relapses after high-dose therapy with autologous hematopoietic stem cells, consider allogeneic transplant	
If bone marrow donor is unavailable, useful palliative regimens include single agents	

(continued)

TABLE 32-6 TREATMENT PROGRAMS FOR HODGKIN'S DISEASE (CONTINUED)

Vinblastine 4–6 mg total dose IV weekly

Gemcitabine 1000 mg/m² IV days 1, 8 every 4 weeks

High-dose salvage and marrow ablative preparative programs

CBV

        Carmustine 300 mg/m² IV day–6

        Cyclophosphamide 1500 mg/m²/d IV days–6, –5, –4, –3

        Etoposide 125 mg/m² IV q12h days–6, –5, –4

        Stem cells on day 0

BEAM

        Carmustine 300 mg/m² IV day–6

        Etoposide 200 mg/m² IV days–5, –4, –3, –2

        Cytarabine 200 mg/m² IV q12h days–5, –4, –3, –2

        Melphalan 140 mg/m² IV day–1

        Stem cells on day 0

*Until recovery of WBC to at least 1000/mL on 3 consecutive days.

expression of CD30 on the tumor cells by agonistic antibodies and immunotoxins (25). For the subset of patients with matched sibling donors, allogeneic bone marrow transplantation is also an option and mini-transplants are being evaluated as an experimental approach.

■ LONG-TERM FOLLOW-UP

About half of the patients destined to relapse will do so in the first year after treatment, and nearly all the relapses occur within 5 years of treatment. While it is common to follow patients every few months for the first couple of years gradually extending the interval between visits, there is no evidence that careful surveillance detects relapses sooner or that treatment outcome of those relapses is improved by the careful surveillance. Most relapses are detected by the patients themselves.

The point of routine follow-up of treated patients is not just monitoring for relapse but also monitoring for early and late toxicities of the disease and its treatment (31). Patients treated for Hodgkin's disease have an increased risk of secondary non-Hodgkin lymphoma, often diffuse large B-cell lymphomas involving the gastrointestinal tract. As this complication seems to occur with equal frequency regardless of the treatment approach, it is thought to be a feature of the underlying disease. Patients also remain at infectious disease risk for up to a year after their treatment. This problem has been greatly ameliorated by the omission of splenectomy from staging workups and the decline in the use of splenic radiation therapy. Chemotherapy regimens each have their own special concerns. ABVD treatment must be monitored for bleomycin-related pulmonary dysfunction using diffusion tests, and bleomycin should be withheld if the diffusing capacity declines greater than

25%. The doses of doxorubicin are generally below the level that is associated with cardiac dysfunction, but patients need to be queried regarding exercise tolerance and fatigue. Alkylating agent-based regimens (MOPP, ChlVPP, BEACOPP) induce infertility and, when used together with radiation therapy, increase the risk of developing acute leukemia and/or a myelodysplastic syndrome. The absolute risk is about 3%, and returns to zero if no marrow damage has appeared within 10 years of treatment (32). The alkylating agent-based regimens also induce premature menopause; while this may somewhat reduce the risk of breast cancer, it increases the risk of osteoporosis.

Radiation therapy can produce xerostomia, dental caries, dysgeusia, and hypothyroidism, and can accelerate atherosclerosis with a threefold increased risk of fatal myocardial infarction. It also increases the risk of second malignancies in or adjacent to the treatment fields. The risk of second cancers begins to appear about 5 years after treatment and increases steadily for at least 30 years. A woman treated with mediastinal radiation therapy at age 25 years has a 30% absolute risk of developing breast cancer by age 55 years, compared to a 3% risk for an age-matched control. It is important that patients be informed of the risk and that healthy behaviors be encouraged including frequent surveillance. Women who received chest radiation therapy might benefit from breast cancer chemoprevention with tamoxifen or an aromatase inhibitor, but studies confirming a benefit have not yet been undertaken and many of these cancers are hormone receptor negative. In addition, lung cancers, sarcomas, melanomas, and thyroid cancers also occur with increased frequency after radiation therapy.

REFERENCES

1. Jemal A, Murray T, Ward E, et al. Cancer statistics 2005. *CA Cancer J Clin.* 2005; 55: 10–30.

2. Mueller NC, Grufferman S. Epidemiology of Hodgkin's disease. In P Mauch, JO Armitage, V Diehl (eds). *Hodgkin's Disease,* Lippincott Williams and Wilkins, Philadelphia, 1999, p. 61.

3. Stein H, Delsol G, Pileri S, et al. Hodgkin lymphoma. In ES Jaffe, NL Harris, H Stein, et al (eds). *World Health Organization Classification of Tumors; Pathology and Genetics; Tumours of Haematopoietic and Lymphoid Tissues.* IARC Press, Lyon, 2001, p. 237.

4. Lister TA, Crowther D, Sutcliffe SB, et al. Report of a committee convened to discuss the evaluation and staging of patients with Hodgkin's disease: Cotswolds meeting. *J Clin Oncol.* 1989; 7: 1630–1636.

5. Diehl V, Sextro M, Franklin J, et al. Clinical presentation, course, and prognostic factors in lymphocyte-predominant Hodgkin's disease and lymphocyte-rich classical Hodgkin's disease; report from the European Task Force on Lymphoma Project on Lymphocyte-Predominant Hodgkin's disease. *J Clin Oncol.* 1999; 17: 776–783.

6. Bonadonna G, Zucali R, Monfardini S, et al. Combination chemotherapy of Hodgkin's disease with adreiamycine, bleomycin, vinblastine, and imidazole carboxamide versus MOPP. *Cancer.* 1975; 36: 252–259.

7. Canellos GP, Anderson JR, Propert KJ, et al. Chemotherapy of advanced Hodgkin's disease with MOPP, ABVD, or MOPP alternating with ABVD. *N Engl J Med.* 1992; 327: 1478–1484.

8. Engert A, Plutschow A, Eich HT, et al. Reduced treatment intensity in patients with early-stage Hodgkin's lymphoma. *N Engl J Med.* 2010; 363: 640-652.

9. Specht L, Gray RG, Clarke MJ, Peto R. Influence of more extensive radiotherapy and adjuvant chemotherapy on long-term outcome of early-stage Hodgkin's disease: a meta-analysis of 23 randomized trials involving 3,888 patients. International Hodgkin's Disease Collaboratorive Group. *J Clin Oncol.* 1998; 16: 830–843.

10. Loeffler M, Brosteanu O, Hasenclever D, et al. Meta-analysis of chemotherapy versus combined modality treatment trials in Hodgkin's disease. International Database on Hodgkin's Disease Overview Study Group. *J Clin Oncol.* 1998; 16: 818–829.

11. Hancock SL, Tucker MA, Hoppe RT. Factors affecting late mortality from heart disease after treatment of Hodgkin's disease. *J Am Med Assoc.* 1993; 270: 1949–1955.

12. Travis LB, Hill D, Dores GM, et al. Cumulative absolute breast cancer risk for young women treated for Hodgkin lymphoma. *J Natl Cancer Inst.* 2005; 97: 1428–1437.

13. Straus DJ, Portlock CS, Qin J, et al. Results of a prospective randomized clinical trial of doxorubicin, bleomycin, vinblastine and dacarbazine (ABVD) followed by radiation therapy (RT) versus ABVD alone for stages I, II and IIIA nonbulky Hodgkin disease. *Blood.* 2004; 104: 3483–3489.

14. Hutchings M, Loft A, Hansen M, et al. FDG-PET after two cycles of chemotherapy predicts treatment failure and progression-free survival in Hodgkin lymphoma. *Blood.* 2006; 107: 52–59.

15. Barnes JA, LaCasce AS, Zukotynski K, et al. End-of-treatment but not interim PET scanning predicts outcome in non-bulky limited stage Hodgkin's lymphoma. *Ann Oncol.* 2011; 22: 910-915.

16. Bartlett NL, Rosenberg SA, Hoppe RT, et al. Brief chemotherapy, Stanford-V, and adjuvant radiotherapy for bulky or advanced-stage Hodgkin's disease. *J Clin Oncol.* 1995; 13: 1080–1089.

17. Diehl V, Franklin J, Hasenclever D, et al. BEACOPP, a new dose-escalated accelerated regimen, is at least as effective as COPP/ABVD in patients with advanced-stage Hodgkin's lymphoma: interim report from a trial of the German Hodgkin's Lymphoma Study Group. *J Clin Oncol.* 1998; 16: 3810–3821.

18. Hoskin PJ, Lowry L, Horwich A, et al. Randomized comparison of Stanford V regimen and ABVD in the treatment of advanced Hodgkin's lymphoma: United Kingdom National Research Institute Lymphoma Group Study ISRCTN 64141244. *J Clin Oncol.* 2009; 27: 5390-5396.

19. Gordon LI, Hong F, Fisher RI, et al. Randomized phase III trial of ABVD versus Stanford V with or without radiation therapy in locally

extensive and advanced stage Hodgkin lymphoma: An Intergroup study coordinated by the Eastern Cooperative Oncology Group. *J Clin Oncol.* 2013; 31: 684-691.

20. Engert A, Diehl V, Franklin J, et al. Escalated-dose BEACOPP in the treatment of patients with advanced-stage Hodgkin's lymphoma: 10 years of follow-up of the GHSG HD9 study. *J Clin Oncol.* 2009; 27: 4548-4554.

21. Longo DL, Duffey PL, Young RC, et al. Conventional-dose salvage combination chemotherapy in patients relapsing with Hodgkin's disease after combination chemotherapy: the low probability for cure. *J Clin Oncol.* 1992; 10: 210–218.

22. DeVita VT Jr, Simon RM, Hubbard SM, et al. Curability of advanced Hodgkin's disease with chemotherapy. Long-term follow-up of MOPP-treated patients at the National Cancer Institute. *Ann Intern Med.* 1980; 92: 587–595.

23. Dady PJ, McElwain TJ, Austin DE, et al. Five years' experience with ChlVPP: effective low-toxicity combination chemotherapy for Hodgkin's disease. *Br J Cancer.* 1982; 45: 851–859.

24. Aparicio J, Segura A, Garcera S, et al. ESHAP is an active regimen for relapsing Hodgkin's disease. *Ann Oncol.* 1999; 10: 593–595.

25. Younes A, Bartlett NL, Leonard JP, et al. Brentuximab vedotin (SGN-35) for relapsed CD30-positive lymphomas. *N Engl J Med.* 2010; 363: 1812-1821.

26. Gribben JG, Linch DC, Singer CR, et al. Successful treatment of refractory Hodgkin's disease by high-dose combination chemotherapy and autologous bone marrow transplantation. *Blood.* 1989; 73: 340–344.

27. Jagannath S, Dicke KA, Armitage JO, et al. High-dose cyclophosphamide, carmustine, and etoposide and autologous bone marrow transplantation for relapsed Hodgkin's disease. *Ann Intern Med.* 1986; 104: 163–168.

28. Stewart DA, Guo D, Sutherland JA, et al. Single-agent high-dose melphalan salvage therapy for Hodgkin's disease: cost, safety, and long-term efficacy. *Ann Oncol.* 1997; 8: 1277–1279.

29. Little R, Wittes RE, Longo DL, Wilson WH. Vinblastine for recurrent Hodgkin's disease following autologous bone marrow transplant. *J Clin Oncol.* 1998; 16: 584–588.

30. Santoro A, Bredenfeld H, Devizzi L, et al. Gemcitabine in the treatment of refractory Hodgkin's disease: results of a multicenter phase II study. *J Clin Oncol.* 2000; 18: 2615–2619.

31. Bookman MA, Longo DL. Concomitant illness in patients treated for Hodgkin's disease. *Cancer Treat Rev.* 1986; 13: 77–109.

32. Blayney DW, Longo DL, Young RC, et al. Decreasing risk of leukemia with prolonged follow-up after chemotherapy and radiotherapy for Hodgkin's disease. *N Engl J Med.* 1987; 316: 710–714.

CHAPTER **33**
Follicular Lymphoma
Amy Sievers, Ann LaCasce

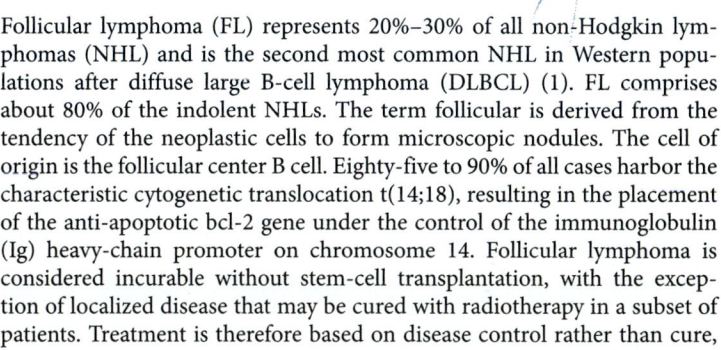

Follicular lymphoma (FL) represents 20%–30% of all non-Hodgkin lymphomas (NHL) and is the second most common NHL in Western populations after diffuse large B-cell lymphoma (DLBCL) (1). FL comprises about 80% of the indolent NHLs. The term follicular is derived from the tendency of the neoplastic cells to form microscopic nodules. The cell of origin is the follicular center B cell. Eighty-five to 90% of all cases harbor the characteristic cytogenetic translocation t(14;18), resulting in the placement of the anti-apoptotic bcl-2 gene under the control of the immunoglobulin (Ig) heavy-chain promoter on chromosome 14. Follicular lymphoma is considered incurable without stem-cell transplantation, with the exception of localized disease that may be cured with radiotherapy in a subset of patients. Treatment is therefore based on disease control rather than cure, and eventual relapse after treatment is the usual natural history of FL (2).

INCIDENCE

The incidence of follicular lymphoma is approximately 2.2–3.2 per 100,000 in the United States and Western Europe (3). Follicular lymphoma is more common in Caucasians than in people of African or Asian descent and typically affects the middle-aged or elderly with an average age at diagnosis of 60 years. The disease occasionally occurs in children or young adults. FL in children is a distinct clinical entity, presenting with localized disease that is often eradicated with initial therapy. In contrast, adults with FL typically present with advanced stage disease and experience recurrence after standard treatment. Although there are no universally accepted risk factors for the development of FL, herbicides and pesticides have been linked with the disease. Familial cases represent a small proportion of total incidence, and there appears to be a slightly increased risk in relatives of patients with FL.

PRESENTATION

Clinically, patients with FL often present with asymptomatic peripheral lymphadenopathy or have enlarged lymph nodes detected incidentally on imaging studies. Although hilar and mediastinal nodes are frequently involved, large mediastinal masses are uncommon. The spleen and bone marrow are commonly involved by disease, but CNS and organ involvement is uncommon. Infiltration of the bone marrow is present in 60%–80% of patients at time of diagnosis. The majority of patients (70%–80%) will present with advanced stage disease, and up to 25% will have B symptoms or an elevated serum LDH level. Although bone marrow involvement is common and sensitive molecular testing frequently identifies circulating lymphoma cells, cytopenias are uncommon at presentation.

In addition to the classic presentation of FL as described above, there are a few distinct clinical variants. Primary intestinal follicular lymphoma is often found incidentally on endoscopy performed for unrelated indications and most often involves the second portion of the duodenum. Pediatric lymphoma is another variant and has distinct features as noted above. Intrafollicular neoplasia, or in situ FL, refers to follicles with high levels of BCL-2 expression but without other features of FL. This condition has relatively low rates of progression to disseminated FL. Rarely, patients will present with diffuse large B-cell lymphoma (DLBCL) with concurrent, previously undiagnosed FL. Prognosis for these patients with transformation is significantly worse than for de novo DLBCL without underlying FL. Of note, DLBCL with t(14;18) translocation does not necessarily imply transformed FL. Histologic features of coexisting FL, most commonly presenting with involvement of the bone marrow with FL, in addition to DLBCL are required for the diagnosis of transformed FL. Histologic transformation most commonly occurs after a variable period of FL, is a natural feature of the disease rather than a side effect of treatment, and when it occurs, it signals an acceleration in the natural history of disease.

DIAGNOSIS

The diagnosis of FL is typically determined by examination of an involved lymph node, ideally by means of an excisional biopsy of a complete node. Fine needle aspirates are not adequate to fully assess the architecture of the disease and establish the grade of the lymphoma. Bone marrow biopsy is an important component of staging but does not allow for disease grading. FL is one of the few lymphomas where morphologic evaluation alone is often sufficient for diagnosis. Distinguishing FL from reactive follicular hyperplasia or other types of lymphomas may be difficult on occasion. FL most commonly appears as tightly packed nodules of varying size and shape consisting of a mixture of small lymphocytes with cleaved nuclei and large lymphocytes with noncleaved nuclei that efface the normal lymphoid architecture. This is in contrast to a normal lymph node, where follicles are more uniform in appearance and interfollicular elements are more prominent. Additionally, FL nodules typically have lower Ki-67 fractions and decreased numbers of phagocytic cells compared with reactive nodes. FL less commonly involves lymph nodes in a diffuse pattern and involved lymph nodes may have both nodular and diffuse areas of disease involvement. Bone marrow involvement typically appears as paratrabecular lymphoid aggregates.

FL grading is based on the relative frequency of large noncleaved cells in the histologic specimen. Of note, grading of FL is notoriously nonconcordant between pathologists and with sequential readings by the same pathologist. Grading criteria are:

- Grade 1: 0–5 large cells per high power field (follicular small cleaved)
- Grade 2: 6–15 large cells per high power field (follicular mixed)
- Grade 3: >15 large cells per high power field (follicular large cell)
  - 3A: small cleaved cells present
  - 3B: small cleaved cells absent, solid sheets of large cells present

Grades 1, 2, and 3A are felt to represent a spectrum of disease, whereas the biology of grade 3B is distinct from the other subsets and cells typically lack CD10 and BCL-2 expression. Immunohistochemistry and flow cytometry demonstrate CD19, CD20, CD21, and CD79 positivity. CD10 is positive in up to 90% of cases. CD5, CD43, and CD11c are negative, and CD23 expression is variable although more commonly negative. The neoplastic cells typically express monoclonal surface immunoglobulin, most commonly IgM or IgG. Cytoplasmic BCL-2 is strongly expressed in most grade 1, 2, and 3A FL, but is less commonly found in grade 3B disease.

Cytogenetic analysis demonstrates a BCL-2 translocation in 85%–90% of cases, typically as the result of a (14;18) translocation between the BCL-2 gene on chromosome 18 and the Ig heavy chain on chromosome 14. This translocation can also be found in up to 30% of cases of de novo DLBCL and occasionally in germinal center B cells in healthy individuals. Translocations between BCL-2 and the kappa light chain on chromosome 2 or lambda light chain on chromosome 22 are less common. All three translocations result in constitutive activity of BCL-2 leading to cellular resistance to apoptosis. BCL-2 translocations may also be identified by FISH and by PCR. The prognostic significance of minimal residual disease following therapy has not been clearly demonstrated. In addition, BCL-6 translocations on chromosome 3 are identifiable in 5%–15% of cases of FL and are more common in grade 3B disease, usually signifying a more aggressive clinical course. BCL-2 and BCL-6 translocations are not mutually exclusive, although FL harboring both mutations is uncommon.

STAGING AND PROGNOSIS

The Ann Arbor staging classification is employed in FL (4, 5):

- Stage 1: Limited to one lymph node region or lymphoid organ, or a single extranodal site (IE).
- Stage II: Limited to two or more lymph node regions on the same side of the diaphragm, or a single extranodal site with associated nodal involvement.
- Stage III: Involvement of lymph node regions or lymphoid organs on both sides of the diaphragm.
- Stage IV: Disseminated involvement of one or more extralymphatic sites, including liver, pleura, CNS, or bone marrow, with or without associated lymph node involvement.

Patients with persistent fevers, drenching night sweats, or a loss of >10% total body weight are considered to have B symptoms. Patients with FL are typically staged with computed tomography (CT) scans of the chest, abdomen, and pelvis as well as a bone marrow biopsy. Additional studies, such as CT scans of the neck, may be indicated based on individual clinical situations. FL is uniformly FDG avid on positron emission tomography (PET), and PET scans may upstage patients with FL compared with CT scan alone. Although a number of recent studies have examined the prognostic role of pretreatment, interim, and end-of-treatment PET scans, no clear guidelines exist on the use of this imaging modality and its use is currently investigational in FL (6, 7).

The best predictors of disease course and outcome are the factors that comprise the Follicular Lymphoma International Prognostic Index (FLIPI) score and disease grade. The FLIPI was developed using a retrospective multivariate analysis of over 4000 patients with follicular lymphoma from 1985 to 1992, before the routine use of rituximab. The prognostic value of the FLIPI has been validated in subsequent clinical trials (8, 9). The FLIPI score is based on the following criteria:

- Age >60
- Ann Arbor stage III of IV
- Hemoglobin <12.0 g/dL
- Involved nodal areas >4
- Serum LDH greater than the upper limit of normal

Five- and 10-year overall survival (OS) rates were determined based on the number of adverse factors present.

- Low risk (0–1 adverse factors): 91% and 71%
- Intermediate risk (2 adverse factors): 78% and 51%
- High risk (≥3 adverse factors): 52% and 36%

The FLIPI2 examined approximately 900 patients receiving therapy from 2003 to 2005 and identified the following criteria as independently prognostic (10):

- Age >60
- Bone marrow involvement
- Hemoglobin <12.0 g/dL
- Largest node >6 cm
- Elevated serum β2 microglobulin

The 3-year progression-free survival (PFS) was 91%, 69%, and 51%, and OS 99%, 96%, and 84% for patients with low (0), intermediate (1–2), and high (3) risk factors, respectively. Of note, only patients who received therapy were included in the analysis and the FLIPI2 prognostic score has not been prospectively validated in clinical trials.

Disease grade is also an important prognostic factor. Grades 1 and 2 disease have a similar clinical course and are treated uniformly. In general, grade 3 disease is more aggressive, though grade 3A disease may behave in a fashion more similar to grades 1 and 2 disease. Grade 3B is felt to represent a distinct entity and behaves more like DLBCL. Pathologic distinction between grades 3A and 3B disease may be difficult even with expert hematopathology consultation.

Finally, emerging data from gene expression profiling studies suggest that the tumor microenvironment and tumor immunology may predict disease behavior. Immune responses enriched with T cells as compared to those with higher percentages of monocytes/macrophages or dendritic cells appear to correlate with more favorable survival and lower rates of transformation to DLBCL (11, 12).

TREATMENT

Given that chemotherapy has not been curative in advanced stage FL and early therapy has not been shown to improve survival, the decision of when to begin treatment and the selection of therapy must balance symptoms from disease and influence of the cancer diagnosis on the patient with both disease- and treatment-related complications. The median survival for FL is in the range of 7–10 years, although extremes on either end occur. Overall survival may be significantly higher since the advent of rituximab. The 15%–20% of patients diagnosed with early-stage disease are potentially curable with local radiotherapy (RT). The mainstay of treatment for the remaining patients is systemic chemotherapy and/or immunotherapy, with a goal of disease control rather than cure. Radioimmunotherapy is another effective approach for some patients. More aggressive and toxic therapies may achieve better initial responses, but do not appear to translate into improved survival. As therapy has become more effective with incorporation of rituximab into combination chemotherapy regimens as well as its use as maintenance therapy, a larger fraction of patients achieve complete remissions and remissions are more durable than the median of 2 years achieved with older treatment regimens. For younger patients with relapsed or refractory disease, stem-cell transplantation may offer the potential for long-term control of the disease, at the expense of higher toxicity.

■ TREATMENT OF EARLY STAGE DISEASE

Involved field radiotherapy (RT) may cure a subset of patients with nonbulky localized FL. RT leads to a 10-year OS of 60%–80% and median survival of 19 years, with some patients achieving cure (13). Larger doses and larger fields of radiation do not appear to improve outcomes, although randomized trials of radiation field are underway. In general, patients receive total doses of 24–30 Gy with additional boosts of up to 6 Gy for bulky or slowly responsive disease. Despite data supporting the use of RT in this setting, only 27%–34% of patients with limited stage FL receive RT according to multiple large studies (14, 15). Often curative RT is not offered to patients because physicians assume that the disease is widespread. Although localized disease accounts for only 15%–20% of patients, the use of RT offers the potential for cure that may be lost if patients are managed by the watch-and-wait approach. All patients should have the disease staged including scans and bone marrow biopsy. RT may be omitted in a subset of patients due to abdominal disease, or stage II disease that is noncontiguous and/or would require large RT fields. While RT is the recommended therapy for most cases of early stage FL, among patients who are not appropriate candidates for RT based on the location and/or bulk or extent of disease, watchful waiting or systemic therapy may be reasonable options. Both combined chemoimmunotherapy and immunotherapy alone are options for systemic therapy of early stage disease, although data are limited as to efficacy in this setting. There are no clear data to suggest combined systemic and radiotherapy improves outcomes in early stage FL. In addition, a recent study analyzing patterns of care in a large number of patients with stage I FL showed excellent outcomes with a number of treatment approaches including RT, chemoimmunotherapy, or immunotherapy alone with or without RT and observation (16).

Although up to 20% of patients are diagnosed with early stage disease based on standard staging procedures with CT scans and unilateral bone marrow biopsy, a subset of patients will have occult higher stage disease. The studies evaluating the role of RT in localized disease predated the use of PET scans. At present, there are no data to suggest that using more sensitive means of detecting occult disease such as PET scans or peripheral blood or bone marrow assessment by PCR translates into better outcomes.

■ TREATMENT OF ADVANCED STAGE DISEASE

Multiple randomized clinical trials have demonstrated no advantage to early therapy versus a "watch and wait" strategy in asymptomatic patients with advanced stage follicular lymphoma. Both the Groupe d'Etude des Lymphomes Folliculaires (GELF) and British National Lymphoma

Investigation developed criteria to determine when treatment of advanced-stage FL is indicated (17, 18). Extracting from both of these guidelines, primary indications for treatment in advanced stage FL include: (1) symptomatic bulky lymphadenopathy or splenomegaly, (2) compromise of organ function from disease, either directly or through nodal compression, (3) significant B symptoms, (4) significant cytopenias, (5) transformation to a more aggressive NHL, (6) presence of symptomatic effusions or other extra-nodal disease, or (7) an increase in the pace of disease. However, the GELF criteria are the most frequently invoked criteria for not treating:

- Maximum diameter of disease <7 cm
- Fewer than 3 nodal sites
- No systemic symptoms
- Spleen <16 cm on CT
- No significant effusions
- No risk of local compressive symptoms
- No circulating lymphoma cells
- No marrow compromise (Hgb <10 g/dL, WBC count <1.5×10^9/L, platelet count <100×10^9/L)

Among patients for whom treatment is indicated, there are a number of potential regimens for the initial treatment FL. For patients with a lower burden of disease who are frail or who have significant comorbidities, rituximab monotherapy is an option. The overall response rates range from 50% to 70% with a median time to progression from 13 to 34 months (19, 20). For the majority of patients requiring therapy, chemoimmunotherapy is the treatment of choice. In general, FL is sensitive to either single-agent chemotherapy such as alkylating agents or purine analogs, or combination regimens such as cyclophosphamide, doxorubicin, vincristine, and prednisone (CHOP) or cyclophosphamide, vincristine, and prednisone (CVP). Overall response rates with rituximab plus chemotherapy are 80%–100%. Multiple randomized studies have demonstrated benefit in PFS with the addition of rituximab in combination with chemotherapy (chemoimmunotherapy) compared to chemotherapy alone. Some of these studies have also shown an OS benefit with the incorporation of rituximab (21, 22). Rituximab in combination with fludarabine has comparable response rates to R-CVP and R-CHOP at the expense of increased toxicity, particularly myelosupression and risk of stem cell damage. More recently the alkylating agent bendamustine, which structurally also has purine analog-like features, has shown promise in terms of both efficacy and tolerability (23). Bendamustine in combination with rituximab is rapidly becoming the standard initial systemic therapy for FL based on preliminary data demonstrating improved complete response (CR) rates and PFS as well as tolerability as compared to R-CHOP (24, 25). OS is similar, though the follow-up is relatively short at this time.

Disease-free intervals can often be prolonged and partial responses (PRs) potentially converted to CRs with the use of maintenance rituximab in both the up-front and relapsed/refractory setting (26). In the PRIMA trial, patients responding to an initial combination regimen were randomized to observation or rituximab every 8 weeks for 2 years (27). Patients in the rituximab group had a 3-year PFS of 75% compared to 57.6% in the observation group. An influence on OS has not yet been demonstrated in the up-front setting. At this time, both maintenance rituximab and retreatment with rituximab at the time of progression remain acceptable options.

Grade 3 FL

Grade 3A follicular lymphoma is typically treated in a manner consistent with grades 1 and 2. Grade 3B disease, however, is often managed as DLBCL with anthracycline-based combination chemotherapy, such as R-CHOP or dose-adjusted EPOCH-R (rituximab, etoposide, prednisone, vincristine, cyclophosphamide, doxorubicin). Studies comparing grades 3A and 3B have not been consistent in terms of response to therapy and prognosis. This may, in part, be due to the lack of diagnostic reproducibility. Some studies have demonstrated that patients with grade 3B disease may experience long-term disease control with initial anthracycline-based chemotherapy (28).

Large Cell Transformation

Patients with FL have a risk—from 3% to 7% annually—of transformation to a more aggressive NHL, most commonly DLBCL. Transformation is often heralded by rapidly enlarging masses, the onset of systemic symptoms, and a rapidly rising LDH. Suspicion of aggressive transformation should prompt immediate biopsy and treatment. Patients with transformed disease are treated with regimens appropriate for aggressive lymphoma such as R-CHOP. More intensive regimens, such as dose-adjusted R-EPOCH are currently being studied. The prognosis for previously treated patients with histologic transformation to DLBCL is generally poor with most series showing a median survival <12 months, though patients who are chemotherapy naive at the time of transformation have a more favorable prognosis. A subset of patients treated with R-CHOP may achieve long-term remissions after consolidation with high-dose chemotherapy and autologous stem cell rescue; 5-year disease-free survivals range from 30% to 60% (29). However, the low-grade follicular component may reemerge after therapy. Rarely, transformation is associated with the acquisition of a MYC translocation or overexpression, a "double hit" lymphoma in the case of both MYC and BCL-2 translocations, which is associated with a particularly poor prognosis (30).

Stem-cell Transplantation

The role of high-dose therapy with autologous stem-cell transplant (ASCT) for patients with FL is controversial. Several prospective trials examining ASCT in previously untreated FL have shown improvements in CR rate and PFS without a benefit in overall survival (31, 32). A small randomized study of relapsed FL in the pre-rituximab era showed that stem-cell transplantation demonstrated improved PFS and OS compared to standard chemotherapy (33). In addition, single institution studies have shown 10-year PFS of 30%–50%. A plateau in PFS after 10 years has been identified in some very mature studies, possibly suggesting that ASCT may be curative in approximately a quarter of patients (34). Earlier studies reported up to 10%–20% transplant-related mortality (TRM) with ASCT, though in the modern era TRM of 4%–5% is more usual. In the era of total body irradiation-containing preparatory regimens, the risk of myelodysplastic syndrome/acute myeloid leukemia (MDS/AML) was greater than 10% in some series. Chemotherapy-only conditioning regimens appear to have a substantially lower risk. In general, ASCT is reserved for patients with aggressive histology transformations or for patients with chemosensitive relapsed or refractory disease and good performance status. The role of maintenance rituximab following ASCT has not been clearly defined but it is widely used.

Allogeneic transplantation, primarily through a graft-versus-lymphoma immune response, offers the best chance of cure in FL. Because of the substantial risk of TRM (up to 30%–40% at 1 year in older studies) and the risk of chronic GHVD, allogeneic SCT has generally been reserved for patients with good performance status whose disease is chemotherapy resistant or has an extremely poor prognosis, such as patients who have relapsed after ASCT. Outcomes are better, however, among patients without transformed disease and who have received fewer previous lines of therapy. Although the risk of toxicity is high, rates of long-term disease-free survival with allogeneic transplant exceed 60% in some series (35, 36). TRM is lower with reduced-intensity conditioning regimens or T-cell-depleted transplants, but the optimal conditioning regimen has not been defined.

Radioimmunotherapy

Radioimmunotherapy (RIT) is another effective therapy in FL. Currently two radiolabeled anti-CD20 monoclonal antibodies are approved by the FDA: Yttrium-90 ibritumomab tiuxetan (Zevalin) and Iodine-131 tositumomab (Bexxar). These agents have not been compared directly in randomized clinical trials. RIT is typically employed in the relapsed/refractory setting, with the majority of patients responding, including those who have received prior rituximab. In addition, responses are often more durable than those obtained from previous treatments. RIT as initial treatment is highly active, though it has not been compared directly to rituximab alone. In addition, consolidation after chemotherapy prolongs progression-free survival, but again this strategy has not been compared to chemoimmunotherapy or to maintenance rituximab (37). In addition, RIT is also being added to conditioning regimens before both autologous and allogeneic transplantation (38). Thus far the toxicities of RIT have been acceptable, with hematologic effects occurring for approximately 4–8 weeks after therapy due to the radiation effects on the bone marrow. This effect on the marrow has been associated with a small risk of prolonged cytopenias and myelodysplastic syndrome. Though published reports claim no permanent marrow damage from RIT, clinical experience suggests that marrow tolerance to subsequent courses of chemotherapy is compromised by RIT.

Refractory or Relapsed Disease

Patients with primary progressive disease or patients who fail to achieve a PR—defined as 50% reduction in the burden of disease—with initial treatment are considered to have refractory disease. In managing patients who display primary refractory or relapsed disease in the setting of a rising serum LDH, disproportionate growth in one area, new development of extranodal disease, or new "B" symptoms, obtaining a repeat biopsy to exclude transformation to DLBCL is indicated. Therapeutic options for patients with relapsed FL are dictated by treatment goals. Additionally, indications for treatment or relapsed/refractory disease are similar to indications for initial treatment. Treatment options include watchful waiting, monotherapy with immunotherapy, combined chemoimmunotherapy, RIT, clinical trials, and stem-cell transplantation. For patients with refractory disease or short durations of remission who respond to subsequent therapy and are appropriate candidates, stem-cell transplantation may be considered. A number of novel agents such as lenalidomide and bortezomib are active and numerous other drugs are in clinical trials, including novel antibodies, antibody drug conjugates, and Bruton's tyrosine kinase (BTK) and BCL-2 inhibitors (39–41).

Monitoring

There are no consensus guidelines on monitoring of FL and the frequency of imaging is highly controversial given the potential risk from radiation exposure related to serial scans. A reasonable approach is clinical examination and laboratory tests including CBC, comprehensive metabolic profile, LDH, and possibly $\beta2$-microglobulin every 3–6 months for the first year after diagnosis or after treatment, and then every 6–12 months thereafter. Relapses are almost always detected by the patient. Imaging is generally performed at time of diagnosis and before initiation of treatment, and then following the completion of treatment. Surveillance imaging is left to the discretion of the treating physician and patient. As noted previously, a proper biopsy is a key component of the initial diagnosis and should be considered at recurrence, particularly if clinical, laboratory, or radiographic findings suggest transformation.

SUMMARY

FL is the most common subtype of indolent lymphoma. A subset of patients with localized disease may achieve long-term disease control with radiotherapy. FL is not usually cured with chemotherapy or chemoimmunotherapy alone. Stem-cell transplant is potentially curative in selected younger and good performance status patients with relapsed or refractory disease. The mainstay of treatment for advanced-stage disease is combination chemoimmunotherapy, often followed by maintenance immunotherapy. There are numerous options for systemic treatment. OS is 13–15 years for most patients, although patients with transformation to more aggressive histologies have a poorer prognosis.

REFERENCES

1. Swerdlow SH, Campo E, Harris NL, et al. *World Health Organization Classification of Tumours of Haematopoietic and Lymphoid Tissues.* 2008; Lyon: IARC Press.
2. NCCN Guidelines v. 1.2013: Non-Hodgkin Lymphomas http://www.nccn.org/professionals/physician_gls/pdf/nhl.pdf%5D.
3. Morton LM, Wang SS, Devesa SS, et al. Lymphoma incidence patterns by WHO subtype in the United States, 1992-2001. *Blood.* 2006; 107: 265–276.
4. Carbone PP. Second Joint Working Conference: National Cancer Institute Chemotherapy Program. Working session report: clinical trials. *Cancer Chemother Rep 3.* 1972; 3: 73–75.

5. Lister TA, Crowther D, Sutcliffe SB, et al. Report of a committee convened to discuss the evaluation and staging of patients with Hodgkin's disease: Cotswolds meeting. *J Clin Oncol.* 1989; 7: 1630–1636.

6. Trotman J, Fournier M, Lamy T, et al. Positron emission tomography-computed tomography (PET-CT) after induction therapy is highly predictive of patient outcome in follicular lymphoma: analysis of PET-CT in a subset of PRIMA trial participants. *J Clin Oncol.* 2011. 29: 3194–3200.

7. Dupuis J, Berriolo-Riedinger A, Julian A, et al. Impact of [18F]fluorodeoxyglucose positron emission tomography response evaluation in patients with high-tumor burden follicular lymphoma treated with immunochemotherapy: a prospective study from the Groupe d'etudes des Lymphomes de l'Adulte and GOELAMS. *J Clin Oncol.* 2012; 30: 4317–4322.

8. Solal-Celigny P, Roy P, Colombat P, et al. Follicular lymphoma international prognostic index. *Blood.* 2004; 104: 1258–1265.

9. Relander T, Johnson NS, Farinha P, et al. Prognostic factors in follicular lymphoma. *J Clin Oncol.* 2010; 28: 2902–2913.

10. Federico M, Bellei M, Marcheselli L, et al. Follicular lymphoma international prognostic index 2: a new prognostic index for follicular lymphoma developed by the international follicular lymphoma prognostic factor project. *J Clin Oncol.* 2009; 27: 4555–4562.

11. Canioni D, Salles G, Mounier N, et al. High numbers of tumor-associated macrophages have an adverse prognostic value that can be circumvented by rituximab in patients with follicular lymphoma enrolled onto the GELA-GOELAMS FL-2000 trial. *J Clin Oncol.* 2008; 26: 440–446.

12. Glas AM, Knoops L, Delahaye L, et al. Gene-expression and immunohistochemical study of specific T-cell subsets and accessory cell types in the transformation and prognosis of follicular lymphoma. *J Clin Oncol.* 2007; 25: 390–398.

13. Guadagnolo BA, Li S, Neuberg D, et al. Long-term outcome and mortality trends in early-stage, Grade 1-2 follicular lymphoma treated with radiation therapy. *Int J Radiat Oncol Biol Phys.* 2006; 64: 928–934.

14. Friedberg JW, Taylor MD, Cerhan JR, et al. Follicular lymphoma in the United States: first report of the national LymphoCare study. *J Clin Oncol.* 2009; 27: 1202–1208.

15. Pugh TJ, Ballonoff A, Newman F, Rabinovitch R. et al. Improved survival in patients with early stage low-grade follicular lymphoma treated with radiation: a Surveillance, Epidemiology, and End Results database analysis. *Cancer.* 2010; 116: 3843–3851.

16. Friedberg JW, Byrtek M, Link BK, et al. Effectiveness of first-line management strategies for stage I follicular lymphoma: analysis of the National LymphoCare Study. *J Clin Oncol.* 2012; 30: 3368–3375.

17. Ardeshna KM, Smith P, Norton A, et al. Long-term effect of a watch and wait policy versus immediate systemic treatment for asymptomatic advanced-stage non-Hodgkin lymphoma: a randomised controlled trial. *Lancet.* 2003; 362: 516–522.

18. Brice P, Bastion Y, Lepage E, et al. Comparison in low-tumor-burden follicular lymphomas between an initial no-treatment policy,

prednimustine, or interferon alfa: a randomized study from the Groupe d'Etude des Lymphomes Folliculaires. Groupe d'Etude des Lymphomes de l'Adulte. *J Clin Oncol.* 1997; 15: 1110–1117.

19. McLaughlin P, Grillo-Lopez AJ, Link BK, et al. Rituximab chimeric anti-CD20 monoclonal antibody therapy for relapsed indolent lymphoma: half of patients respond to a four-dose treatment program. *J Clin Oncol.* 1998; 16: 2825–2833.

20. Colombat P, Salles G, Brousse N, et al. Rituximab (anti-CD20 monoclonal antibody) as single first-line therapy for patients with follicular lymphoma with a low tumor burden: clinical and molecular evaluation. *Blood.* 2001; 97: 101–106.

21. Marcus R, Imrie K, Belch A, et al. CVP chemotherapy plus rituximab compared with CVP as first-line treatment for advanced follicular lymphoma. *Blood.* 2005; 105: 1417–1423.

22. Hiddemann W, Kneba M, Dreyling M, et al. Frontline therapy with rituximab added to the combination of cyclophosphamide, doxorubicin, vincristine, and prednisone (CHOP) significantly improves the outcome for patients with advanced-stage follicular lymphoma compared with therapy with CHOP alone: results of a prospective randomized study of the German Low-Grade Lymphoma Study Group. *Blood.* 2005; 106: 3725–3732.

23. Cheson BD, Rummel MJ. Bendamustine: rebirth of an old drug. *J Clin Oncol.* 2009; 27: 1492–1501.

24. Rummel MJ, Niederle N, Maschmeyer G, et al. Bendamustine plus rituximab versus CHOP plus rituximab as first-line treatment in patients with indolent and mantle cell lymphomas: updated results from the StiL NHL1 study (abstract 3). *J Clin Oncol.* 2012; 30: 6s.

25. Rummel JR, Niederle N, Maschmeyer G, et al. Bendamustine plus rituximab is superior in respect of progression free survival and complete remission rate when compared to CHOP plus rituximab as first-line treatment of patients with advanced follicular, indolent, and mantle cell lymphomas: final results of a randomized phase III study of the StiL (abstract 405). *Blood.* 2009; 114: 405.

26. van Oers MH, Klasa R, Marcus RE, et al. Rituximab maintenance improves clinical outcome of relapsed/resistant follicular non-Hodgkin lymphoma in patients both with and without rituximab during induction: results of a prospective randomized phase 3 intergroup trial. *Blood.* 2006; 108: 3295–3301.

27. Salles G, Seymour JF, Offner F, et al. Rituximab maintenance for 2 years in patients with high tumour burden follicular lymphoma responding to rituximab plus chemotherapy (PRIMA): a phase 3, randomised controlled trial. *Lancet.* 2011; 377: 42–51.

28. Wahlin BE, Yri OE, Kimby E, et al. Clinical significance of the WHO grades of follicular lymphoma in a population-based cohort of 505 patients with long follow-up times. *Br J Haematol.* 2012; 156: 225–233.

29. Oliansky DM, Gordon LI, King J, et al. The role of cytotoxic therapy with hematopoietic stem cell transplantation in the treatment of

follicular lymphoma: an evidence-based review. *Biol Blood Marrow Transplant.* 2010; 16: 443–468.

30. Johnson NA, Savage KJ, Ludkovski O, et al. Lymphomas with concurrent BCL2 and MYC translocations: the critical factors associated with survival. *Blood.* 2009; 114: 2273–2279.

31. Ladetto M, De Marco F, Benedetti F, et al. Prospective, multicenter randomized GITMO/IIL trial comparing intensive (R-HDS) versus conventional (CHOP-R) chemoimmunotherapy in high-risk follicular lymphoma at diagnosis: the superior disease control of R-HDS does not translate into an overall survival advantage. *Blood.* 2008; 111: 4004–4013.

32. Schaaf M, Reiser M, Borchmann P, et al. High-dose therapy with autologous stem cell transplantation versus chemotherapy or immuno-chemotherapy for follicular lymphoma in adults. *Cochrane Database Syst Rev.* 2012; 1: CD007678.

33. Schouten HC, Qian W, Kvaloy S, et al. High-dose therapy improves progression-free survival and survival in relapsed follicular non-Hodgkin's lymphoma: results from the randomized European CUP trial. *J Clin Oncol.* 2003; 21: 3918–3927.

34. Rohatiner AZ, Nadler L, Davies AJ, et al. Myeloablative therapy with autologous bone marrow transplantation for follicular lymphoma at the time of second or subsequent remission: long-term follow-up. *J Clin Oncol.* 2007; 25: 2554–2559.

35. van Besien K, Loberiza FR Jr, Bajorunaite R, et al. Comparison of autologous and allogeneic hematopoietic stem cell transplantation for follicular lymphoma. *Blood.* 2003; 102: 3521–3529.

36. Soiffer RJ, Freedman AS, Neuberg D, et al. CD6+ T cell-depleted allogeneic bone marrow transplantation for non-Hodgkin's lymphoma. *Bone Marrow Transplant.* 1998; 21:1177–1181.

37. Morschhauser F, Radford J, Van Hoof A, et al. Phase III trial of consolidation therapy with yttrium-90-ibritumomab tiuxetan compared with no additional therapy after first remission in advanced follicular lymphoma. *J Clin Oncol.* 2008; 26: 5156–5164.

38. Press OW, Eary JF, Gooley T, et al. A phase I/II trial of iodine-131-tositumomab (anti-CD20), etoposide, cyclophosphamide, and autologous stem cell transplantation for relapsed B-cell lymphomas. *Blood.* 2000; 96: 2934–2942.

39. Witzig TE, Wiernik PH, Moore T, et al. Lenalidomide oral monotherapy produces durable responses in relapsed or refractory indolent non-Hodgkin's Lymphoma. *J Clin Oncol.* 2009; 27: 5404–5409.

40. Fowler N, Kahl BS, Lee P, et al. Bortezomib, bendamustine, and rituximab in patients with relapsed or refractory follicular lymphoma: the phase II VERTICAL study. *J Clin Oncol.* 2011; 29: 3389–3395.

41. Friedberg JW, Vose JM, Kelly JL, et al. The combination of bendamustine, bortezomib, and rituximab for patients with relapsed/refractory indolent and mantle cell non-Hodgkin lymphoma. *Blood.* 2011; 117: 2807–2812.

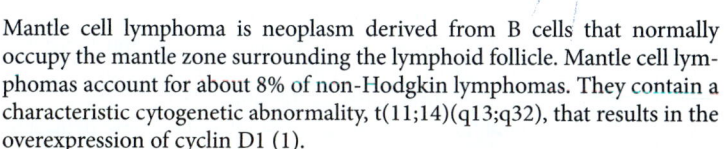

CHAPTER **34**
Mantle Cell Lymphoma

Dan L. Longo

Mantle cell lymphoma is neoplasm derived from B cells that normally occupy the mantle zone surrounding the lymphoid follicle. Mantle cell lymphomas account for about 8% of non-Hodgkin lymphomas. They contain a characteristic cytogenetic abnormality, t(11;14)(q13;q32), that results in the overexpression of cyclin D1 (1).

CLINICAL FEATURES

Patients with mantle cell lymphoma are typically older white men. The disease usually (90%) presents in advanced stage (III or IV) and very often includes extranodal involvement of the bone marrow (80%), gastrointestinal tract (80% histologically involved, 25% symptomatic), and liver, in addition to lymphadenopathy and enlarged spleen and nodal tissue in Waldeyer's ring. The peripheral blood may show lymphocytosis but clonal abnormal cells are detectable by flow cytometry even when lymphocytosis is absent. B symptoms are present in 20%. Cells overexpressing cyclin D1 are detected in asymptomatic normal people rarely (5%–8%), but it is not clear that their presence presages the development of lymphoma. Involvement of the gastrointestinal tract may produce multiple lymphomatous polyposis.

The natural history of the disease is variable. About 15% of patients may have an indolent clinical course. In the extreme, a patient may not manifest progressive disease over many years of follow-up without treatment. However, the majority of patients show disease progression within the first 1 or 2 months of diagnosis. About 10% of patients show extremely rapid disease progression and follow a downhill course in a few months. The usual patient responds to chemotherapy but complete remissions are seldom durable and the median survival is 3–5 years (2).

PATHOLOGY AND GENETIC FEATURES

Mantle cell lymphomas are not graded according the WHO Classification of Lymphoid Tumors but classical variants and highly aggressive variants (blastoid and pleomorphic) are recognized. The classical form involves vaguely nodular sheets of small to intermediate size lymphoid cells often with a notched nuclear contour. The overexpression of cyclin D1 is a hallmark and is usually associated with the characteristic t(11;14)(q13;q32) translocation juxtaposing the cyclin D1 gene with the immunoglobulin heavy chain gene. Rare mantle cell lymphomas do not overexpress cyclin D1; these tend to overexpress cyclin D2 or D3. An unusual translocation of cyclin D2 to the immunoglobulin kappa light-chain gene [t(2:12)(p12;p13)] has been observed in some cases. The pattern of gene expression in these unusual variants mimics the pattern seen in cyclin D1-overexpressing tumors (3).

The malignant cell of mantle cell lymphoma expresses surface immuno-globulin (IgM and IgD) intensely, CD20, and CD5, but not CD10 or BCL6. Cyclin D1 and BCL-2 are expressed in the cytoplasm and are thought to be key to tumorigenesis. Cyclin D1 expression interferes with the G1 checkpoint (controlled by RB, the retinoblastoma protein, p27kip) at which the cell takes inventory and assesses its ability to enter DNA synthesis. BCL-2 prevents the programmed cell death that would normally occur in cells that were not ready for the G1/S transition (4). The cells accumulate genetic damage through defects in DNA repair mechanisms and the molecular profile is marked by overexpression of proliferation-related genes (5). The immunoglobulin variable region genes of the tumor cells are germline in the majority of cases but an important subset of the tumors have hypermutated variable regions suggesting that antigen selection may play a role in some tumors. Tumor cells also express SOX11 but its role is unclear. SOX11 is generally not expressed in other forms of lymphoma.

Many studies also suggest a role for the Ki-67 index in predicting outcome. Ki-67 is expressed in all phases of the cell cycle but is not expressed in resting cells; thus, it is a marker for growth fraction. The index is the fraction of cells in a tumor expressing Ki-67; in general, the higher the index, the more aggressive the tumor. A difficulty in applying the index clinically is the absence of standardization and the absence of wide availability of the test. The study of prognostic factors has not shown that Ki-67 staining adds independent significance to the clinical prognostic factors (6).

STAGING WORKUP

Once an excisional tumor biopsy has documented the diagnosis (needle aspirates are not indicated and only serve to delay definitive diagnosis), essential staging procedures are history inquiring about B symptoms and gastrointestinal tract symptoms, physical examination with careful measurement and documentation of involved lymph nodes, complete blood count with flow cytometry to assess the presence of monoclonal B cells, serum chemistry profile with special attention to lactate dehydrogenase (LDH) levels, bone marrow biopsy with or without an aspirate, and CT scan of the chest, abdomen, and pelvis. The role of positron emission tomography is not established. Sigmoidoscopy/colonoscopy is not necessary in asymptomatic patients but many of these patients will have lower GI tract involvement. Although a large fraction of patients have bone marrow involvement, the disease rarely involves the central nervous system. Sampling of cerebrospinal fluid and central nervous system prophylaxis are not indicated.

Patients can be grouped into low, intermediate, and high risk on the basis of four factors: age, performance status, LDH elevations, and white blood cell count (see Table 34-1). At the moment, therapy for mantle cell lymphoma is not risk-adapted; thus, the main value of the index is to predict outcome rather than guide decision making. An indolent disease subset can be identified by taking a watch-and-wait approach for a short time. Patients with indolent disease often have exclusively extranodal disease, tumor cells expressing hypermutated immunoglobulin variable region genes, and absence of aneuploidy. Most of these features are not readily available to the

TABLE 34–1 MANTLE CELL LYMPHOMA INTERNATIONAL PROGNOSTIC INDEX

Points	Age, y	ECOG	LDH/ULN	WBC, 10^9/L
0	<50	0–1	<0.67	<6.700
1	50–59	0–1	0.67–0.99	6.700–9.999
2	60–69	2–4	1.0–1.49	10.000–14.999
3	70	2–4	>1.50	≥15.000

Points are summed:

Low risk	0–3 points	70% 5-year survival
Intermediate risk	4–5 points	50% 5-year survival
High risk	6–11 points	15% 5-year survival

LDH was weighted according to the ratio to the upper limit of normal (ULN). Thus, for an ULN of 240 U/L, the cutpoints were 180 U/L, 240 U/L, and 360 U/L, for example.
Modified from Hoster E, Dreyling M, Klapper W, et al. A new prognostic index (MIPI) for patients with advanced mantle cell lymphoma. *Blood.* 2008; 111: 558–565.

clinician, and thus the indolent subset is mainly recognized on the basis of absence of progression under clinical observation.

TREATMENT

No consensus exists on a standard therapy for mantle cell lymphoma. A wide variety of chemotherapy programs have been tested and results recently summarized (7, 8). A key first step is to be certain that the patient does not have indolent disease by observing for disease progression over the period of a month or two. Classic mantle cell lymphoma will progress in most cases. For patients who are thought to be medically eligible for high-dose therapy and autologous hematopoietic stem-cell transplantation, the usual initial therapy is R-CHOP (rituximab, cyclophosphamide, doxorubicin, vincristine and prednisone), rituximab with high-dose cytarabine, followed by high-dose therapy and autologous stem cell rescue. Alternative treatment regimens include hyper-CVAD (cyclophosphamide, doxorubicin, vincristine, and dexamethasone) alternated with high-dose methotrexate and cytarabine and bendamustine plus rituximab. Nucleosides like fludarabine and cladribine also have activity but are more often used in salvage therapy.

The use of rituximab as maintenance therapy appears to prolong progression-free survival but it is not clear whether this treatment is keeping active disease out of site without a major impact on overall survival (9). For older, less-fit patients, R-CHOP or rituximab plus bendamustine with rituximab maintenance therapy is often used as primary therapy. Therapy may be expected to induce responses in more than 85% of cases and complete remissions in about 50%–60%. Remissions tend to be more short-lived than those seen with similar therapy in diffuse large B-cell lymphoma; median progression-free survival ranges from 1.5 to 3 years. Maintenance rituximab may extend remission durations.

A variety of novel approaches are being tested. Lenalidomide, vorinostat (a histone deacetylase inhibitor targeting chromatin), bortezomib (proteasome inhibitor), temsirolimus (mTOR inhibitor), ibrutinib (Bruton's tyrosine kinase inhibitor), and a number of immunologic strategies including vaccination, IL-21, and adoptively transferred T cells are all being explored.

REFERENCES

1. Swerdlow SH, Campo E, Seto M, Muller-Hermelink HK. Mantle cell lymphoma. In Swerdlow SH, Campo E, Harris NL, et al (eds). *WHO Classification of Tumours of Haematopoietic and Lymphoid Tissues.* IARC Press, 2008, pp. 229–232.

2. Chandran R, Gardiner SK, Simon M, Spurgeon SE. Survival trends in mantle cell lymphoma in the United States over 16 years, 1992-2007. *Leuk Lymphoma.* 2012; 53: 1488–1493.

3. Fu K, Weisenberger DD, Greiner TC, et al. Cyclin D1-negative mantle cell lymphoma: a clinicopathologic study based on gene expression profiling. *Blood.* 2005; 106: 4315–4321.

4. Jares P, Colomer D, Campo E. Molecular pathogenesis of mantle cell lymphoma. *J Clin Invest.* 2012; 122: 3416–3423.

5. Rosenwald A, Wright G, Wiestner A, et al. The proliferation gene expression signature is a quantitative integrator of oncogenic events that predicts survival in mantle cell lymphoma. *Cancer Cell.* 2003; 3: 185–197.

6. Hoster E, Dreyling M, Klapper W, et al. A new prognostic index (MIPI) for patients with advanced mantle cell lymphoma. *Blood.* 2008; 111: 558–565.

7. Witzens-Harig M, Hess G, Atta J, et al. Current treatment of mantle cell lymphoma: results of a national survey and consensus meeting. *Ann Hematol.* 2012; 91: 1765–1772.

8. Li Z-M, Zucca E, Ghielmini M. Open questions in the management of mantle cell lymphoma. *Cancer Treat Rev.* 2013; 39: 602–609.

9. LaCasce AS, Vandergrift JL, Rodriguez MA, et al. Comparative outcome of initial therapy for younger patients with mantle cell lymphoma: an analysis from the NCCN NHL database. *Blood.* 2012; 119: 2092–2099.

CHAPTER **35**
Peripheral T-cell Lymphomas

Jeffrey A. Barnes, Jeremy S. Abramson

INTRODUCTION

The peripheral T-cell lymphomas are a heterogeneous group of lymphoid malignancies each with a distinct clinical presentation and prognosis. The term "peripheral" denotes mature T-cell neoplasms, differentiating them from the precursor lymphoid diseases T-cell acute lymphoblastic leukemia and lymphoblastic lymphoma. Treatment regimens for peripheral T-cell lymphomas are generally derived from data extrapolated from trials of aggressive non-Hodgkin lymphoma (NHL) before the advent of CD20-directed therapies of which T-cell lymphomas represent approximately 10% of the studied population. While therapies are often overlapping, T-cell lymphomas in general have an inferior prognosis to their B-cell counterparts. Recent advances have been made, however, with development of treatments specifically directed at peripheral T-cell lymphomas.

EPIDEMIOLOGY

In 2012, there were an estimated 70,130 new cases of NHL in the United States with approximately 18,940 deaths (1). T-cell lymphoma is an uncommon subtype of NHL representing just 12% of all cases (2). The T-cell lymphomas have been subdivided by the most recent WHO classification scheme into predominantly leukemic, nodal, and extranodal variants (Table 35-1) (3). The International Peripheral T-cell Lymphoma project

TABLE 35-1 T/NK-CELL NEOPLASMS

Predominantly Leukemic	Predominantly Extranodal
• T-cell prolymphocytic leukemia	• Extranodal NK/T cell lymphoma, nasal type
• T-cell large granular lymphocytic leukemia	• Enteropathy-associated T-cell lymphoma
• Chronic NK-cell lymphoproliferative disorder	• Hepatosplenic T-cell lymphoma
• Aggressive NK-cell leukemia	• Subcutaneous panniculitis-like T-cell lymphoma
• Adult T-cell leukemia/lymphoma	• Hydroa vaccineforme-like lymphoma
• Systemic EBV+ T-cell lymphoproliferative disease of childhood (associated with chronic active EBV infection)	• Mycosis fungoides
	• Sezary syndrome
	• Primary cutaneous anaplastic large-cell lymphoma
	• Primary cutaneous aggressive epidermotropic CD8+ cytotoxic T-cell lymphoma
	• Primary cutaneous gamma-delta T-cell lymphoma
	• Primary cutaneous small/medium CD4+ T-cell lymphoma

Predominantly Nodal

• Peripheral T-cell lymphoma, not otherwise specified

• Angioimmunoblastic T-cell lymphoma

• Anaplastic large-cell lymphoma (ALCL), ALK+/−

Adapted from Reference 3. The WHO classification of tumours of haematopoetic and lymphoid tissue.

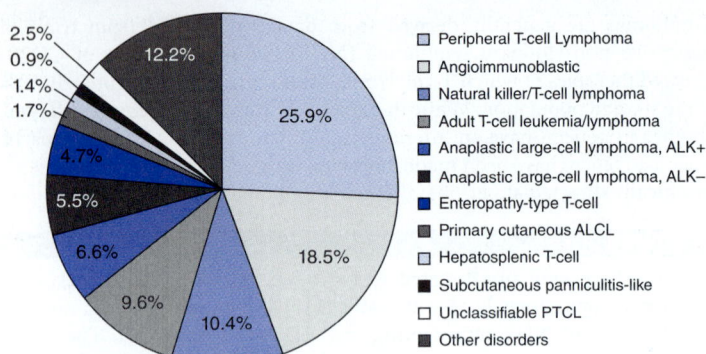

Figure 35-1 International T-cell Lymphoma Study: frequency of subtypes. (From Reference 4.)

determined the relative frequencies and geographic variation of T-cell lymphoma of subtypes with peripheral T-cell lymphoma-not otherwise specified (PTCL-NOS) being the most common, followed by angioimmu-noblastic T-cell lymphoma (AITL), anaplastic large-cell lymphoma(ALCL), and adult T-cell leukemia/lymphoma (ATLL) (Figure 35-1) (4). Notably, there are significant geographic differences in the incidence of these entities with PTCL-NOS being the most common in North America and Europe, whereas extranodal nasal NK T-cell lymphoma (ENKTL) and ATLL are more common in Asia due to the seroprevalence of the EBV virus and HTLV-1 viruses, respectively (Table 35-2).

PERIPHERAL T-CELL LYMPHOMA NOS

DIAGNOSIS

PTCL-NOS is the most common subtype of T-cell lymphoma in the United States representing approximately 35% of all T-cell lymphomas (4%–5% of all lymphomas). PTCL-NOS presents at a median age of 61 years with a male-to-female ratio of approximately 2:1 (5). Typically patients present with advanced stage disease (69%), elevated LDH (49%), B symptoms (35%), and extranodal disease (56%) (6). The diagnosis is optimally made based on excisional lymph node biopsies with final needle aspirates normally inadequate. PTCL can be a heterogeneous disease by morphology with most biopsies demonstrating medium-sized or large cells with irregular, pleomorphic, hyperchromatic, or vesicular nuclei with prominent nucleoli and many mitotic figures (3). Immunophenotypic features include CD4 expression more common than CD8 expression with frequent antigen loss of CD5 and CD7, antigens normally expressed on T cells. The T-cell receptor beta chain is usually expressed allowing differentiation from gamma/delta T-cell lymphomas and NK cell lymphomas. Similar to other lymphomas, PTCL-NOS is staged according to the Ann Arbor staging system (Table 35-3) (37). Initial evaluation should include:

TABLE 35-2 MAJOR LYMPHOMA SUBTYPES BY GEOGRAPHIC REGION

Lymphoma Subtypes	North America (%)	Europe (%)	Asia (%)
PTCL-NOS	34.4	34.3	22.4
Angioimmunoblastic	16.0	28.7	17.9
Anaplastic, ALK+	16.0	6.4	3.2
Anaplastic, ALK−	7.8	9.4	4.3
NK/T-cell	5.1	4.3	22.4
ATLL	2.0	1.0	25.0
Enteropathy type	5.8	9.1	1.9
Hepatosplenic	3.0	2.3	0.2
Primary cutaneous ALCL	5.4	0.8	0.7
Subcutaneous panniculitis-like	1.3	0.5	1.3
Unclassifiable T-cell	2.3	3.3	2.4

PTCL, peripheral T-cell lymphoma; NOS, not otherwise specified; ALCL, anaplastic large-cell lymphoma; NKTCL, natural killer/T-cell lymphoma.
Adapted from Reference 4.

TABLE 35-3 ANN ARBOR STAGING SYSTEM

- Stage I
  - Single nodal region or lymphoid structure (spleen, thymus, Waldeyer's ring) or single limited extralymphatic site (IE)
- Stage II
  - Involvement of two or more nodal regions on the same side of the diaphragm, alone or with involvement of a contiguous limited extralymphatic site (IIE)
- Stage III
  - Involvement of nodal regions or lymphoid structures on both sides of the diaphragm
- Stage IV
  - Diffuse involvement of one or more extralymphatic sites, with or without associated nodal involvement
- A or B is added to denote presence of systemic "B" symptoms: unexplained fever, night sweats, or loss of >10% of body weight over previous 6 months
- X is added to denote bulky disease: >1/3 widening of mediastinum at T-5-6, or nodal mass >10 cm
- S denotes splenic involvement. E denotes extranodal involvement

Adapted from Reference 37.

- Physical examination with attention paid to nodal areas, hepatospleno-megaly, and performance status.
- Laboratory studies including complete blood count with differential, LDH, uric acid, calcium, and liver function tests.
- Bone marrow biopsy in select cases (of prognostic importance)
- Imaging studies including CT scans of the chest, abdomen, and pelvis. The majority of PTCL-NOS will also be PET avid, and so PET/CT may be obtained.
- Evaluation of cardiac function including ejection fraction for those patients receiving an anthracycline.

■ PROGNOSIS

The 5-year overall survival for PTCL-NOS is approximately 32%. The prognostic index for PTCL-NOS (PIT) was developed to risk stratify patients based on four adverse risk factors including age greater than 60, performance status of 2 or higher, elevated LDH, and bone marrow involvement. Patients in group 1 with no adverse factors, group 2 with one factor, group 3 with two factors, and group 4 with three or four factors have a 5-year overall survival of 62%, 52.9%, 33%, and 18% respectively (**Figure 35-2**) (7).

■ TREATMENT

Peripheral T-cell lymphomas are traditionally treated like other aggressive NHLs with combination chemotherapy including CHOP-like regimens (cyclophosphamide, doxorubicin, vincristine, and prednisone). The complete remission rate for patients receiving an anthracycline-containing regimen such as CHOP is approximately 56% compared to 70%–90% for patients with diffuse large B-cell lymphoma receiving R-CHOP (6). The German high-grade NHL study group retrospectively analyzed 343 patients (70 with PTCL-NOS) comparing 6–8 cycles of CHOP to CHOP plus etoposide as

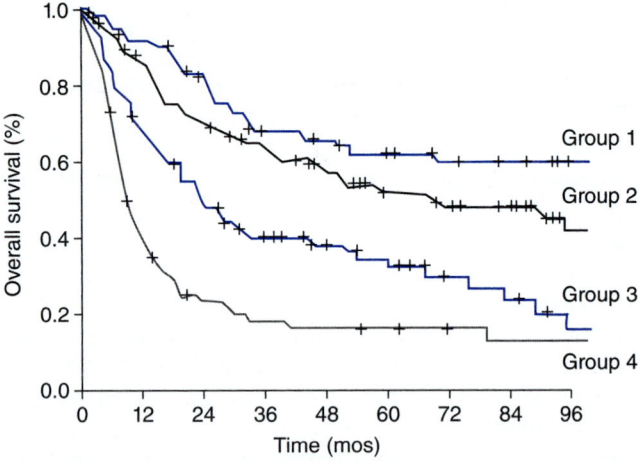

Figure 35-2 Overall survival according to the prognostic index for PTCL-NOS (PIT). (From Reference 7.)

well as 14- versus 21-day treatment intervals. While no difference was seen in CHOP 14 versus CHOP 21, there was a statistically significant improvement in 3-year event-free survival favoring inclusion of etoposide (75.4%) compared to CHOP alone (51.0%) (8).

Given the poor outcomes with standard chemotherapy, consolidation with high-dose chemotherapy and autologous stem-cell transplant (ASCT) has been explored. Retrospective studies have shown an improvement in 5-year overall survival to 68% compared to the predicted 32% (9); however, such analyses are confounded by selection bias of the most favorable patients and inclusion of patients with ALK+ ALCL who have a decidedly more favorable prognosis compared to PTCL-NOS. A prospective trial of up-front ASCT excluding patients with ALK+ ALCL showed a 3-year overall survival of 48% (10). The 3-year overall survival rate was 71% for the two-thirds of patients with chemosensitive disease enrolled on the trial that underwent ASCT versus 11% for the patient who did not undergo ASCT. There are also retrospective data for allogeneic stem-cell transplant for patients with refractory peripheral T-cell lymphomas including PTCL-NOS with 2-year overall survival to 55% but with nonrelapse mortality of 22% (11).

Several novel agents have activity in PTCL-NOS (Table 35-4). The histone deactylase inhibitor romidepsin is approved in the United States for patients with PTCL-NOS having received one prior therapy based on a phase II trial showing a response rate of 25% but with a complete response rate of 15% and a median duration of response of 17 months (12). The main toxicities of romidepsin include cytopenias, GI toxicity, and the potential for arrhythmias. Pralatrexate, a novel antifolate agent, is also approved for patients with relapsed or refractory PTCL-NOS with an overall response rate of 29% and complete response rate of 11% with main toxicities including cytopenias and mucositis (38). Gemcitabine, a nucleoside analog, also has significant activity with overall response rates of approximately 50% (13). There are several other agents that have shown promise in small clinical trials including brentuximab vedotin (for patients with CD30+ disease) (39), alemtuzumab (40), denileukin diftitox (41), and bortezomib (42). Both alemtuzumab and denileukin diftitox have been combined with CHOP-like chemotherapy but early trials were limited due to increased infectious complications. Given the poor predictive outcomes for both up-front and salvage therapy, participation in clinical trials both at diagnosis and relapse are encouraged.

ANAPLASTIC LARGE CELL LYMPHOMA

DIAGNOSIS

Anaplastic large-cell lymphoma (ALCL) represents approximately 12% of the peripheral T-cell lymphomas seen in the United States each year or approximately 2% of all non-Hodgkin lymphomas (4). ALCL can be further subclassified as expressing or lacking expression of the protein anaplastic lymphoma kinase (ALK). ALK-positive tumors have a translocation of chromosome 2 and chromosome 5 with resultant fusion of ALK on chromosome 2 with the nucleophosmin gene on chromosome 5 to produce t(2;5), and tend to present in the first three decades of life with a median age of 34 years. ALK-negative patients present at a median age of 58 (14).

TABLE 35-4 NOVEL AGENTS FOR PERIPHERAL T-CELL LYMPHOMAS

Compound	Mechanism of Action	N	Response Rate	Outcome	Toxicity
Romidepsin (12)	Histone deacetylase inhibitor	131	ORR 25%, CRR 15%	Median DOR 17 mo	Thrombocytopenia, neutropenia, infection
Pralatrexate (38)	Novel antifolate	111	ORR 29%, CRR 11%	Median DOR 10.1 mo	Thrombocytopenia, mucositis, neutropenia, anemia
Gemcitabine (13)	Nucleoside analog	39	ORR 51%, CRR 30%	Median DOR 34 mo for patients in CR	Thrombocytopenia, neutropenia, LFT abnormalities
Brentuximab vedotin (for ALCL only) (39)	Anti-CD30 antibody conjugated to the micro-tubule toxin monomethyl auristatin-E	58 with ALCL	ORR 86 %, CRR 57%	Median DOR 12.6 mo	Neuropathy, neutropenia, thrombocytopenia
Alemtuzumab (40)	Anti-CD52 monoclonal antibody	10	ORR 60%	Not reported	Infection
Denileukin diftitox (41)	Interleukin-2 linked to diphtheria toxin	27	ORR 48%	Median PFS 6 mo	Capillary leak syndrome, infusion reactions
Bortezomib (42)	Proteasome inhibitor	15	ORR 67%	Not reported	Thrombocytopenia, neutropenia, neuropathy

CRR, complete response rate; DOR, duration of response; ORR, overall response rate; PFS, progression-free survival.

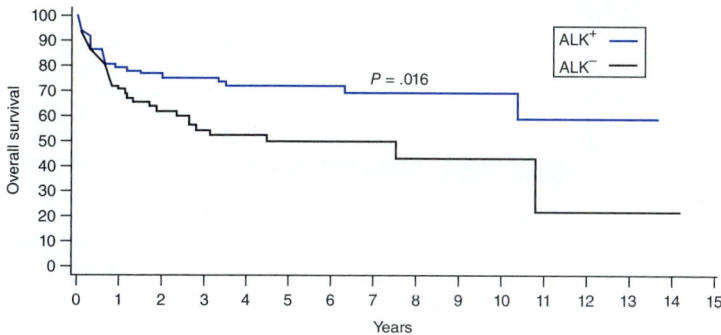

Figure 35-3 Overall survival according to ALK status in ALCL. (From Reference 14.)

Both ALK+ and ALK− ALCL often present at advanced stage (58%–65%) with elevated LDH (37%–46%), extranodal disease ~20%, and B symptoms (60%). As with PTCL-NOS, the diagnosis is made on excisional lymph node biopsies showing effacement of lymph node architecture with large anaplastic cells often with reniform nuclei and are positive for CD30, CD25, and epithelial membrane antigen (EMA). The staging and pretreatment evaluations are similar to those as listed above for PTCL-NOS.

◼ PROGNOSIS

ALCL has an improved prognosis compared to PTCL-NOS, but with a distinct difference between the ALK+ and ALK− variants. ALK+ ALCL has a 5-year overall survival of 70% compared to 49% for ALK− ALCL (**Figure 35-3**) (14). The IPI score typically used for DLBCL is able to effectively risk stratify patients with ALCL regardless of the ALK status.

◼ TREATMENT

Patients with ALCL are treated with anthracycline-containing CHOP-like regimens similar to PTCL-NOS based on extrapolation of data from trials aggressive NHLs including both B- and T-cell lymphomas. As above with PTCL-NOS, retrospective studies evaluating the addition of etoposide to a CHOP-like regimen have shown improvement in both the 3-year event-free survival and overall survival for ALK+ ALCL (75.8% and 89.8%) and ALK− ALCL (45.7% and 62.1%) (8).

Given the excellent prognosis of ALK+ ALCL patients treated with CHOP-like chemotherapy, upfront consolidation with high-dose chemotherapy and autologous stem-cell transplant is not recommended. Patients with ALK− ALCL are much more likely to relapse and go onto salvage therapies including autologous stem-cell transplant resulting in long-term remissions of only 30%–40%. ALCL is uniformly CD30 positive making the CD-30 directed antibody-drug conjugate brentuximab vedotin an appealing agent. A phase II trial of 58 patients (26% of whom had received prior autologous SCT and 62% of whom were refractory to front-line treatment) demonstrated an overall response rate of 86%, complete response rate of 57% with 97% of patients having observed reductions in tumor size (**Figure 35-4**) (15). The median

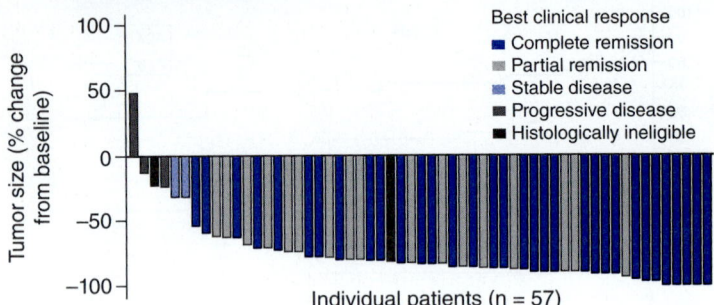

Figure 35-4 Maximum tumor reduction in patients with relapsed refractory ALCL after brentuximab vedotin. (From Reference 15.)

duration of response was 12.6 months with an estimated 12-month overall survival rate of 70%. Given brentuximab vedotin's remarkable single agent activity in relapsed and refractory disease, studies are ongoing with this agent in combination with chemotherapy and earlier in the treatment paradigm. The ALK inhibitor crizotinib (recently approved for non-small cell lung cancer harboring ALK mutations) has been tested in four refractory ALK+ ALCL patients all of whom responded (16); however, its role in this otherwise favorable disease subset is unclear at this time as the majority of patients with ALK+ ALCL will be cured with existing standard therapies.

ANGIOIMMUNOBLASTIC T-CELL LYMPHOMA

■ DIAGNOSIS

Angioimmunoblastic T-cell lymphoma (AITL) represents approximately 19% of all the T-cell lymphoma seen in the United States every year or approximately 1%–2% of all NHLs (4). A majority of patients with AITL present with the relatively abrupt onset of systemic symptoms including fevers, a pruritic skin rash, nonbulky adenopathy, and organomegaly; a unique clinical presentation compared to other non-Hodgkin lymphomas. The median age of onset is 65 years with a slight male predominance (17). The majority of patients present with advanced stage and extranodal disease is present in approximately one-third of patients. As the historical name of angioimmunoblastic lymphadenopathy with dysproteinemia (AILD) suggests, 30% of patients will present with polyclonal hypergammaglobulinemia, or other protein abnormalities including small amounts of paraprotein or positive tests for autoantibodies. Given the constellation of rapid onset fevers, rashes, and nonbulky adenopathy, patients with AITL are often sent for rheumatologic or infectious disease evaluation before their lymphoma diagnosis, leading to a delay in therapy. Positive tests for rheumatoid factor, antinuclear antibody, Lyme, and other conditions contribute to initially incorrect diagnoses. These patients are frequently started on glucocorticoids confounding the diagnosis of lymphoma with a median time to diagnosis over 6 months from the onset of symptoms. Patients may also present with recurrent infections related to immune deficiency secondary to both the neoplastic process and their immunosuppressive treatments. Ten to twenty percent of patients will have concurrent autoimmune cytopenias, immune-mediated thrombocytopenia (ITP), and/or autoimmune hemolytic anemia (AIHA). As with PTCL-NOS and ALCL, the diagnosis is made on excisional lymph node biopsies demonstrating effacement of lymph node architecture with a paracortical polymorphous infiltrate of small- to medium-sized CD4-positive T cells and proliferation of arborizing high endothelial venules. There is also often an associated expansion of EBV-positive B immunoblasts that are polyclonal. The staging and pretreatment evaluations are similar to those as listed above for PTCL-NOS with the addition of testing for circulating paraproteins and autoimmune cytopenias.

■ PROGNOSIS

AITL has a poor prognosis with a 5-year overall survival of 32% and 5-year failure-free survival of 18% (4). The prognostic index score is less valuable in this histology since the majority of patients present with high-risk scores.

■ TREATMENT

As with PTCL-NOS and ALCL, AITL is customarily treated with CHOP-like regimens based on extrapolation from aggressive NHL trials with a complete remission rate for those receiving an anthracycline-containing regimen of approximately 60%. No survival differences have been observed in patients treated with combination chemotherapy that included an anthracycline compared to those receiving an anthracycline-sparing regimen, but definitive conclusions cannot be reached based on this retrospective data (17). Given the poor outcome in the majority of patients treated with standard chemotherapy, autologous stem-cell transplant in first and second remission has been retrospectively evaluated. In 146 patients with a median follow-up of 31 months, there was an estimated 4-year overall survival of 59%, which is improved compared to historical controls (18). As with all retrospective studies, these findings must be interpreted with attention to biases including selecting for patients that are younger with fewer comorbidities making them eligible for transplant and therefore likely to do better than historical controls regardless of the transplant procedure.

EXTRANODAL NK/T-CELL LYMPHOMA, NASAL TYPE

■ DIAGNOSIS

Extranodal NK/T-cell lymphoma, nasal type (ENKTL) is an uncommon T-cell lymphoma in North America and Europe representing around 5% of cases but with a significantly increased incidence in Asia where it represents approximately 22% of new T-cell lymphomas and 9% of all lymphomas (4). Patients present at a median age of 43 years with a slight male predominance and symptoms of nasal obstruction due to the presence of a mass lesion in the upper aerodigestive tract. The majority of patients present with localized disease (76%), with a good performance status, normal LDH (63%), and lack of B symptoms (35%) (19). Diagnostic biopsies show frequent ulceration of the mucosal surfaces by a diffuse lymphomatous infiltrate positive for CD2, CD3, and CD56, and will often demonstrate an angiocentric and angiodestructive growth pattern.

■ PROGNOSIS

ENKTL nasal type has an improved outcome compared to other PTCLs, owing to the more likely presentation at limited stage disease. The estimated 5-year overall survival is about 49%, but is improved in patients with localized disease who have a 5-year overall survival of approximately 76%. Specific prognostic models for ENKTL have been proposed with adverse risk factors including the presence of B symptoms, advanced stage, elevated LDH, and lymph node involvement demonstrating 5-year overall survival of 81%, 64%, 34%, and 7%, for those with 0, 1, 2, and 3 or more risk factors, respectively. (**Figure 35-5**) (19). Local invasion through bone or soft tissues also negatively affects prognosis.

■ TREATMENT

ENKTL nasal type relies heavily upon the use of radiation therapy for curative intent. With doses ranging from 40 to 65Gy (higher than typical radiation doses for other lymphomas), complete remission rates are

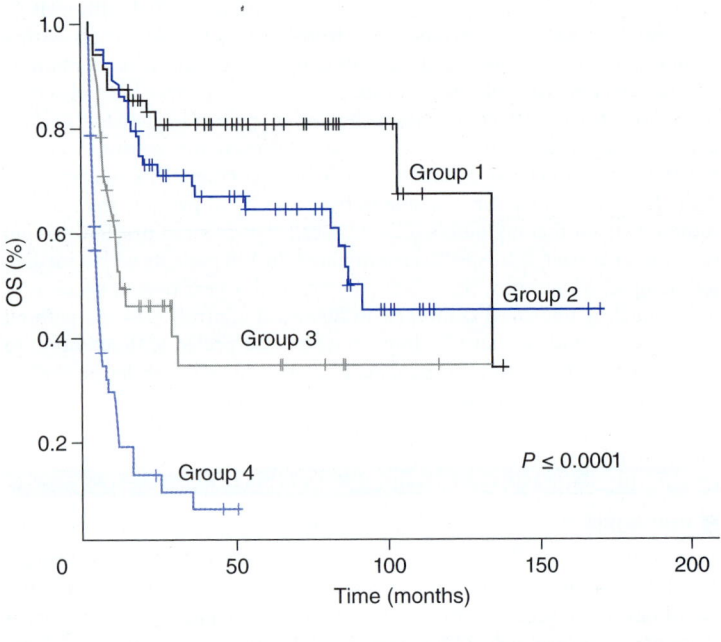

Risk group	No. of factors'	No. of patients	%	% 5-Year OS	SE	RR	95% CI
Group 1	0	60	27	80.9	5.5	1.0	N/A
Group 2	1	68	31	64.2	6.5	1.8	0.9–3.5
Group 3	2	44	20	34.4	9.5	4.1	2.0–8.3
Group 4	3 or 4	47	22	6.6	4.3	13.6	7.0–26.6

Figure 35-5 Overall survival for patients with extranodal NK/T-cell lymphoma. (From Reference 19.)

approximately 87% for radiation therapy alone with a 5-year overall survival of 71% for patients with stage IE and IIE disease (20). Small prospective trials of combined modality therapy with radiation therapy given either with concurrent cisplatin followed by VIPD (etoposide, ifosfamide, cisplatin, and dexamethasone) or DeVIC (dexamethasone, etoposide, ifosfamide, and carboplatin) have shown modestly increased overall survival but with increased toxicity (21, 22). Patients with advanced stage disease are not candidates for curative radiotherapy, and asparaginase-based regimens may perform better than other chemotherapy programs in this disease. The steroid, methotrexate, ifosfamide, L-asparaginase, and etoposide (SMILE) regimen produces an overall response rate of 79% in patients with stage IV disease, with a 1-year overall survival of 55%, though at the cost of significant toxicity (23). The AspaMetDex regimen (L-asparaginase, methotrexate and dexamethasone) is less toxic than SMILE and has shown an encouraging complete remission rate of 61% in patients with refractory disease with median overall survival of 1 year, suggesting that further testing is warranted of L-asparaginase in the up-front treatment of ENKTL (24).

ADULT T-CELL LEUKEMIA/LYMPHOMA

◼ DIAGNOSIS

Adult T-cell leukemia/lymphoma (ATLL) is a rare entity in North America and Europe but has a significantly increased incidence in Asia and in the Caribbean where it is directly linked to the prevalence of human T-cell leukemia virus 1 (HTLV-1) infection. There is often a long latency with most affected individuals exposed to the virus early in life. HTLV-1 is transmitted in breast milk and by exposure to peripheral blood or blood products. There are four clinical variants of ATLL that affect the clinical presentation and prognosis including acute, lymphomatous, chronic, and smoldering types. The acute type is most common and presents with disseminated leukemic and bone marrow involvement, lymphocytosis, skin rash, and generalized lymphadenopathy. Hypercalcemia at presentation is quite common, as are pulmonary infiltrates. The differential diagnosis of the lung infiltrates include leukemic infiltration and opportunistic infection given the uniform immunosuppressive state associated with the disease. The lymphomatous type, as the name implies, presents with adenopathy and/or extranodal masses, but without significant involvement of peripheral blood and bone marrow. The chronic type presents with a lymphocytosis but with mild adenopathy and follows a more indolent course. Finally the smoldering type presents without peripheral blood or marrow involvement and with frequent cutaneous involvement. The median age of onset is 62 years with the majority of patients presenting with stage IV disease (73%) (25). While a broad spectrum of cytologic features may be present, the characteristic finding in the peripheral blood is of CD4+, CD8–, CD25+ T cells with the characteristic flower-shaped nucleus with many nuclear convolutions and lobules (**Figure 35-6**). Unlike the other T-cell lymphomas, the diagnosis often can be made on peripheral blood with correlation with HTLV-I serologies. Unlike other leukemias, bone marrow involvement is often patchy. ATLL is staged according to the Ann Arbor system, with a

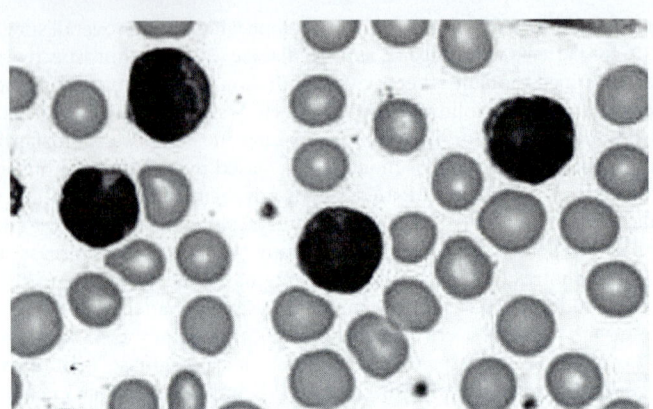

Figure 35-6 Peripheral blood smear from patient with acute ATLL. (Photo courtesy of Dr. Judith Ferry, Massachusetts General Hospital Department of Pathology.)

similar workup as for other T-cell lymphomas, but with staging of the blood with flow cytometry and attention to the risk of hypercalcemia, opportunistic infection, and occasionally spontaneous tumor lysis syndrome.

■ PROGNOSIS

The prognosis for ATLL is dependent on the subtype with the smoldering and chronic variants having significantly better survival compared to the lymphomatous and acute subtypes. The IPI score can be used to stratify patients with the lymphomatous subtype but is not very helpful in the other variants (25). For patients with the acute subtype, the ATL prognostic index is based on five factors including advanced Ann Arbor stage, performance status greater than one, serum albumin less than 3.5 g/dL, age greater than 70, and levels of soluble IL-2 receptors <20,000 U/ml and can separate patients into low- (scores 0–2), intermediate- (scores 3–4), and high-risk groups (score 5) with a 2-year overall survival rates of 37%, 17%, and 2%, respectively (26).

■ TREATMENT

The smoldering and chronic variants of ATLL can follow an indolent course and patients may be followed with observation alone until the disease become symptomatic. The aggressive variants of ATLL including the acute and lymphomatous types carry a poor prognosis when treated with CHOP-like regimens. Given that ATLL presents in a leukemic phase with a significant burden of disease and a high incidence of preexisting hypercalcemia, close attention must be paid to development of treatment-related tumor lysis syndrome. Overall response rates to initial therapy are approximately 70% but the duration of response is frequently short (25). Given the poor prognosis with standard therapies, allogeneic stem-cell transplantation should be considered in eligible ATLL patients with available donors given the evidence for a graft versus leukemia effect and signal of efficacy in small series.

Consideration of novel agents and early enrollment in clinical trials is warranted. Novel treatment approaches including targeting the HTLV-I virus itself may offer additional benefit compared to chemotherapy. Small studies examining the use of antiviral therapy with zidovudine plus interferon produced high response rates approaching 90% but a short median event-free survival of approximately 7 months (27). The addition of zidovudine and interferon to chemotherapy improved overall response rates from 49% to 81% although no difference was seen in progression-free or overall survival (28). For patients with relapsed or refractory disease, treatment with denileukin diftitox, alemtuzumab, pralatrexate, and histone deacetylase inhibitors may be considered based on the PTCL-NOS data, but response rates and duration of response are quite limited based on small amounts of data.

UNCOMMON SUBTYPES

■ CUTANEOUS T-CELL LYMPHOMAS

Mycosis Fungoides, Sézary Syndrome

Cutaneous lymphomas represent less than 2% of all NHLs, 75% of which are cutaneous T-cell lymphomas (CTCL). Mycosis fungoides is the most common type of CTCL, often presenting in older adults with a male-to-female ratio of 2:1. Patients often present with a prolonged indolent course with scaling skin plaques/lesions that wax and wane. Most patients present with limited stage disease confined to the skin alone and are treated with skin directed therapies including topical glucocorticoids, topical nitrogen mustard, topical retinoids, and UV light therapy usually enhanced by psoralen sensitization. For disease that is unresponsive to skin-directed therapies, the oral retinoid bexarotene and low-dose methotrexate can be used. The prognosis for limited stage patients is excellent with a median overall survival in excess of 10 years. Patients with advanced stage disease including disseminated cutaneous disease or visceral involvement have dramatically inferior prognosis. Multiagent chemotherapy, such as CHOP-like regimens, have overall response rates of 60%–80% but significant infectious risks and very brief duration of response; therefore, single-agent approaches are more often employed. Liposomal doxorubicin, gemcitabine, and methotrexate all have significant activity and can be used with palliative intent.

Sézary syndrome (SS) accounts for 5% of all cutaneous T-cell lymphomas, and is defined as the presence of a circulating CTCL count of 1000 cells per microliter of peripheral blood. The disease is often accompanied by widespread skin disease that is called erythroderma. SS is an aggressive disease with an overall survival rate at 5 years of less than 10%. Several targeted agents have been approved for CTCL and but few have been evaluated in patients with Sézary syndrome. Denileukin diftitox has response rates in CTCL of up to 50% with a 10% complete response rate (29). The histone deacetylase inhibitors vorinostat and romidepsin are effective in CTCL with responses seen in up to one-third of patients but no complete responses have been seen (30, 31). The CD52-directed monoclonal antibody alemtuzumab is highly active in patients with SS, where low-dose therapy (10- or 15-mg delivered subcutaneously three times a week) was found to have an overall response rate of 86% and a complete response rate of 21% in one small study (32).

Primary Cutaneous CD30-Positive T-Cell Lymphoproliferative Disorders

Primary cutaneous CD30-positive T-cell lymphoproliferative disorders are the second most common type of CTCL behind mycosis fungoides (33). This group of diseases includes lymphomatoid papulosis (LyP) and primary cutaneous anaplastic large-cell lymphoma. LyP is a chronic, recurrent, self-healing papulonodular skin eruption with histologic features of a CD30-positive CTCL. LyP generally occurs in adults and can be differentiated from primary cutaneous ALCL by the presence of skin lesions at different stages of development that resolve without intervention. LyP in general does not require therapy although in patients with truly persistent painful disease, low-dose methotrexate can be used as suppressive therapy. Primary cutaneous ALCL shares similar histologic features with LyP demonstrating non-epidermotropic infiltrates of large CD30-positive tumor cells (34). Unlike systemic ALCL, most cutaneous ALCLs do not express ALK. While primary cutaneous ALCL exists on a spectrum with LyP, the lesions in ALCL do not spontaneously remit. The major differential diagnosis of primary cutaneous ALCL is systemic ALCL with secondary skin involvement. Patients should be carefully examined for lymphadenopathy or organ involvement. Isolated lesions can be treated with local radiation therapy (electron beam) or surgical excision with chemotherapy rarely indicated. Primary cutaneous ALCL has an excellent prognosis; estimated 10-year survival exceeds 90%.

Subcutaneous Panniculitis-Like T-Cell Lymphoma/Primary Cutaneous Gamma-Delta T-Cell Lymphoma (SPTCL)

SPTCL is a rare T-cell lymphoma representing less than 1% of the T-cell lymphomas seen each year. It is a disease with a female predominance with a median age of 36 years with 20% of patients presenting before age 20 years (35). Historically, it has been divided in two groups based on T-cell receptor expression. Those with alpha/beta T-cell receptors carry a more favorable prognosis and usually present without skin findings and rarely have involvement of other nonsubcutaneous sites. Those with the gamma/delta T-cell receptor have an unfavorable prognosis and may present with ulcerated skin lesions. Patients often will have an associated autoimmune disorder such as SLE or juvenile RA, and presentation with an associated hemophagocytic syndrome may be seen in >20% of cases.

■ T-CELL LARGE GRANULAR LYMPHOCYTIC LEUKEMIA

T-cell large granular lymphocytic leukemia (T-LGL) is a rare lymphoproliferative disorder characterized by a population of clonal LGL cells between 2 and 20 K/ul in the peripheral blood without an identified cause (3). Reactive T-cell LGLs can be seen in response to viral infections, posttransplant T-cell expansions, and connective tissue diseases and should be differentiated from a malignant process. LGL is a rare disease occurring primarily in older adults with a strong association with rheumatoid arthritis. Patients usually present with recurrent infections secondary to neutropenia. Other cytopenias may also be seen including anemia and thrombocytopenia. Up to 14% of patients may present with pancytopenia making the distinction from aplastic anemia difficult. Splenomegaly is usually present, but is not massive as may be seen in other splenic predominant disease such as splenic marginal zone lymphoma or hairy cell leukemia.

Evaluation of the peripheral blood smear typically shows large lymphocytes with moderate to abundant cytoplasm and prominent azurophilic granules. The bone marrow often shows a normocellular or hypocellular marrow. The LGL infiltrate can be variable and difficult to visualize. When present there is usually an interstitial/intrasinusoidal infiltrate of CD3+, CD8+, TCR-alpha/beta+ cytotoxic T cells. Abnormally, decreased or lost expression of CD5 and/or CD7 is common. Most are positive for CD57 and CD16 as well as perforin and granzyme B, typical of cytoxic T cells. TCR PCR for gene rearrangements can be used to confirm clonality, though false positives do occur and should be interpreted in the context of the entire clinicopathologic picture.

The prognosis for LGL is excellent with most cases taking an indolent course. Indications for treatment are cytopenias, particularly neutropenia. Several agents can be employed including low-dose weekly methotrexate with or without prednisone, daily oral cyclosporine or cyclophosphamide, and less commonly chemotherapy agents such as pentostatin.

■ ENTEROPATHY-ASSOCIATED T-CELL LYMPHOMA

Enteropathy associated T-cell lymphoma (EATL) is a rare peripheral T-cell lymphoma representing less than 5% of cases. This disease occurs exclusively in patients with underlying celiac disease, but the celiac disease and lymphoma may be diagnosed concurrently at the time the patient presents with a lymphoma complication. Patients with celiac disease are recommended to maintain a gluten-free diet, which reduces the risk of developing this lymphoma. Patients typically present with abdominal pain, GI bleeding, and occasionally bowel perforation. Patients may have a poor performance status and hypoalbuminemia at diagnosis due to protein wasting. Abdominal masses show ulcerating lesions that invade the wall of the intestine with medium to large lymphoid cells with vesicular nuclei, prominent nucleoli, and moderate pale cytoplasm. Prognosis is quite poor with a 5-year overall survival of 29% (4). As with other T-cell lymphomas patients are often treated with CHOP-like regimens. A novel regimen of ifosfamide, etoposide, epirubicin, and methotrexate followed by autologous stem-cell transplant generated 5-year progression-free and overall survival of 52% and 60%, respectively. These numbers are greatly improved over historical controls; however, this is a small study (36).

■ HEPATOSPLENIC T-CELL LYMPHOMA

Hepatosplenic T-cell lymphoma (HSL) is an extremely rare form of T-cell lymphoma representing less than 2% of all cases of T-cell lymphoma (4). The median age of onset is 34 years with a male predominance. There is preferential involvement of the vascular sinusoids of the liver, spleen, and bone marrow, but adenopathy is generally not present. Patients frequently present with B symptoms organomegaly, and cytopenias. This disease may occur in patients with immune suppression, most commonly after a solid-organ transplantation when it occurs at median of 10 years posttransplant. All patients may initially respond to multiagent chemotherapy, but durations of remission are brief and the 5-year overall survival approaches 0% (4).

CONCLUSIONS

The peripheral T-cell lymphomas are mature T-cell neoplasms each with distinct clinical presentations. Attention to pattern recognition of their unique clinical presentations and close collaboration with expert hematopathologists are needed to make accurate diagnoses. Treatment regimens are extrapolated from trials of aggressive lymphomas of which T-cell lymphomas represent an approximate 10% of the study populations. Aside from ALK+ ALCL, prognosis is generally poor and early consideration for participation in clinical trials is warranted to identify more effective therapies for these uncommon and aggressive diseases.

REFERENCES

1. American Cancer Society. Cancer facts and figures 2012. 2012.

2. Anderson JR, Armitage JO, Weisenburger DD, for the Non-Hodgkin's Lymphoma Classification Project. Epidemiology of the non-Hodgkin's lymphomas: distributions of the major subtypes differ by geographic locations. *Ann Oncol.* 1998; 9: 717–720.

3. Swerdlow S, Campo E, Harris NL, et al (eds). WHO classification of tumours of haematopoetic and lymphoid tissue. Lyon, IARC, 2008.

4. Vose J, Armitage J, Weisenburger D, International T-Cell Lymphoma Project. International peripheral T-cell and natural killer/T-cell lymphoma study: pathology findings and clinical outcomes. *J Clin Oncol.* 2008; 26: 4124–4130.

5. Rüdiger T, Weisenburger DD, Anderson JR, et al. Peripheral T-cell lymphoma (excluding anaplastic large-cell lymphoma): results from the non-Hodgkin's lymphoma classification project. *Ann Oncol.* 2002; 13: 140–149.

6. Weisenburger DD, Savage KJ, Harris NL, et al. Peripheral T-cell lymphoma, not otherwise specified: a report of 340 cases from the international peripheral T-cell lymphoma project. *Blood.* 2011; 117: 3402–3408.

7. Gallamini A, Stelitano C, Calvi R, et al. Peripheral T-cell lymphoma unspecified (PTCL-U): a new prognostic model from a retrospective multicentric clinical study. *Blood.* 2004; 103: 2474–2479.

8. Schmitz N, Trumper L, Ziepert M, et al. Treatment and prognosis of mature T-cell and NK-cell lymphoma: an analysis of patients with T-cell lymphoma treated in studies of the german high-grade non-Hodgkin lymphoma study group. *Blood.* 2010; 116: 3418–3425.

9. Rodriguez J, Conde E, Gutierrez A, et al. The results of consolidation with autologous stem-cell transplantation in patients with peripheral T-cell lymphoma (PTCL) in first complete remission: the spanish lymphoma and autologous transplantation group experience. *Ann Oncol.* 2007; 18: 652–657.

10. Reimer P, Rudiger T, Geissinger E, et al. Autologous stem-cell transplantation as first-line therapy in peripheral T-cell lymphomas: results of a prospective multicenter study. *J Clin Oncol.* 2009; 27: 106–113.

11. Delioukina M, Zain J, Palmer JM, et al. Reduced-intensity allogeneic hematopoietic cell transplantation using fludarabine-melphalan

conditioning for treatment of mature T-cell lymphomas. *Bone Marrow Transplant.* 2012; 47: 65–72.

12. Coiffier B, Pro B, Prince HM, et al. Results from a pivotal, open-label, phase II study of romidepsin in relapsed or refractory peripheral T-cell lymphoma after prior systemic therapy. *J Clin Oncol.* 2012; 30: 631–636.

13. Zinzani PL, Venturini F, Stefoni V, et al. Gemcitabine as single agent in pretreated T-cell lymphoma patients: evaluation of the long-term outcome. *Ann Oncol.* 2010; 21: 860–863.

14. Savage KJ, Harris NL, Vose JM, et al. ALK- anaplastic large-cell lymphoma is clinically and immunophenotypically different from both ALK+ ALCL and peripheral T-cell lymphoma, not otherwise specified: report from the international peripheral T-cell lymphoma project. *Blood.* 2008; 111: 5496–5504.

15. Pro B, Advani R, Brice P, et al. Brentuximab vedotin (SGN-35) in patients with relapsed or refractory systemic anaplastic large-cell lymphoma: results of a phase II study. *J Clin Oncol.* 2012; 30: 2190–2196.

16. Pogliani EM, Dilda I, Villa F, et al. High response rate to crizotinib in advanced, chemoresistant ALK+ lymphoma patients. ASCO Meeting Abstracts. 2011; 29(15_Suppl): e18507.

17. Federico M, Rudiger T, Bellei M, et al. Clinicopathologic characteristics of angioimmunoblastic T-cell lymphoma: analysis of the international peripheral T-cell lymphoma project. *J Clin Oncol.* 2013; 31: 240–246.

18. Kyriakou C, Canals C, Goldstone A, et al. High-dose therapy and autologous stem-cell transplantation in angioimmunoblastic lymphoma: complete remission at transplantation is the major determinant of outcome-lymphoma working party of the European group for blood and marrow transplantation. *J Clin Oncol.* 2008; 26: 218–224.

19. Lee J, Suh C, Park YH, et al. Extranodal natural killer T-cell lymphoma, nasal-type: a prognostic model from a retrospective multicenter study. *J Clin Oncol.* 2006; 24: 612–618.

20. Li Y, Yao B, Jin J, et al. Radiotherapy as primary treatment for stage IE and IIE nasal natural killer/T-cell lymphoma. *J Clin Oncol.* 2006; 24: 181–189.

21. Yamaguchi M, Tobinai K, Oguchi M, et al. Phase I/II study of concurrent chemoradiotherapy for localized nasal natural killer/T-cell lymphoma: Japan clinical oncology group study JCOG0211. *J Clin Oncol.* 2009; 27: 5594–5600.

22. Kim SJ, Kim K, Kim BS, et al. Phase II trial of concurrent radiation and weekly cisplatin followed by VIPD chemotherapy in newly diagnosed, stage IE to IIE, nasal, extranodal NK/T-cell lymphoma: consortium for improving survival of lymphoma study. *J Clin Oncol.* 2009; 27: 6027–6032.

23. Yamaguchi M, Kwong YL, Kim WS, et al. Phase II study of SMILE chemotherapy for newly diagnosed stage IV, relapsed, or refractory extranodal natural killer (NK)/T-cell lymphoma, nasal type: the NK-cell tumor study group study. *J Clin Oncol.* 2011; 29: 4410–4416.

24. Jaccard A, Gachard N, Marin B, et al. Efficacy of L-asparaginase with methotrexate and dexamethasone (AspaMetDex regimen) in patients with refractory or relapsing extranodal NK/T-cell lymphoma, a phase 2 study. *Blood.* 2011; 117: 1834–1839.

25. Suzumiya J, Ohshima K, Tamura K, et al. The international prognostic index predicts outcome in aggressive adult T-cell leukemia/lymphoma: analysis of 126 patients from the international peripheral T-cell lymphoma project. *Ann Oncol.* 2009; 20: 715–721.

26. Katsuya H, Yamanaka T, Ishitsuka K, et al. Prognostic index for acute- and lymphoma-type adult T-cell Leukemia/Lymphoma. *J Clin Oncol.* 2012; 30: 1635–1640.

27. Hermine O, Allard I, Levy V, et al. A prospective phase II clinical trial with the use of zidovudine and interferon-alpha in the acute and lymphoma forms of adult T-cell leukemia/lymphoma. *Hematol J.* 2002; 3: 276–282.

28. Hodson A, Crichton S, Montoto S, et al. Use of zidovudine and interferon alfa with chemotherapy improves survival in both acute and lymphoma subtypes of adult T-cell leukemia/lymphoma. *J Clin Oncol.* 2011; 29: 4696–4701.

29. Prince HM, Duvic M, Martin A, et al. Phase III placebo-controlled trial of denileukin diftitox for patients with cutaneous T-cell lymphoma. *J Clin Oncol.* 2010; 28: 1870–1877.

30. Piekarz RL, Frye R, Turner M, et al. Phase II multi-institutional trial of the histone deacetylase inhibitor romidepsin as monotherapy for patients with cutaneous T-cell lymphoma. *J Clin Oncol.* 2009; 27: 5410–5417.

31. Duvic M, Olsen EA, Breneman D, et al. Evaluation of the long-term tolerability and clinical benefit of vorinostat in patients with advanced cutaneous T-cell lymphoma. *Clin Lymphoma Myeloma.* 2009; 9: 412–416.

32. Bernengo MG, Quaglino P, Comessatti A, et al. Low-dose intermittent alemtuzumab in the treatment of Sezary syndrome: clinical and immunologic findings in 14 patients. *Haematologica.* 2007; 92: 784–794.

33. Willemze R, Jaffe ES, Burg G, et al. WHO-EORTC classification for cutaneous lymphomas. *Blood.* 2005 May 15; 105: 3768–3785.

34. Bekkenk MW, Geelen FA, van Voorst Vader PC, et al. Primary and secondary cutaneous CD30(+) lymphoproliferative disorders: a report from the dutch cutaneous lymphoma group on the long-term follow-up data of 219 patients and guidelines for diagnosis and treatment. *Blood.* 2000 Jun 15; 95: 3653–3661.

35. Willemze R, Jansen PM, Cerroni L, et al. Subcutaneous panniculitis-like T-cell lymphoma: definition, classification, and prognostic factors: an EORTC cutaneous lymphoma group study of 83 cases. *Blood.* 2008; 111: 838–845.

36. Sieniawski M, Angamuthu N, Boyd K, et al. Evaluation of enteropathy-associated T-cell lymphoma comparing standard therapies with a novel regimen including autologous stem cell transplantation. *Blood.* 2010; 115: 3664–3670.

37. Lister TA, Crowther D, Sutcliffe SB, et al. Report of a committee convened to discuss the evaluation and staging of patients with hodgkin's disease: Cotswolds meeting. *J Clin Oncol.* 1989; 7: 1630–1636.

38. O'Connor OA, Pro B, Pinter-Brown L, et al. Pralatrexate in patients with relapsed or refractory peripheral T-cell lymphoma: results from the pivotal PROPEL study. *J Clin Oncol.* 2011; 29: 1182–1189.

39. Pro B, Advani R, Brice P, et al. Brentuximab vedotin (SGN-35) in patients with relapsed or refractory systemic anaplastic large-cell lymphoma: results of a phase II study. *J Clin Oncol.* 2012; 30: 2190–2196.

40. Zinzani P, Alinari L, Tani M, et al. Preliminary observations of a phase II study of reduced-dose alemtuzumab treatment in patients with pretreated T-cell lymphoma. *Haematologica.* 2005; 90: 702–703.

41. Dang NH, Pro B, Hagemeister FB, et al. Phase II trial of denileukin diftitox for relapsed/refractory T-cell non-hodgkin lymphoma. *Br J Haematol.* 2007; 136: 439–447.

42. Zinzani PL, Musuraca G, Tani M, et al. Phase II trial of proteasome inhibitor bortezomib in patients with relapsed or refractory cutaneous T-cell lymphoma. *J Clin Oncol.* 2007; 25: 4293–4297.

CHAPTER **36**

Uncommon B-Cell Lymphomas

Jeremy S. Abramson, Jeffrey A. Barnes

Multiple uncommon B-cell lymphomas each account for only a small percentage of non-Hodgkin lymphomas overall, but should be familiar to clinicians based on their unique clinical and pathologic features, natural histories, and approaches to therapy. These diseases reviewed in this chapter include Burkitt lymphoma, plasmablastic lymphoma, primary effusion lymphoma, lymphomatoid granulomatosis, hairy cell leukemia, and cutaneous B-cell lymphomas.

BURKITT'S LYMPHOMA

■ INTRODUCTION

Burkitt's lymphoma is a highly aggressive mature B-cell lymphoma accounting for approximately 3% of new non-Hodgkin lymphoma (NHL) diagnoses annually in the United States. The disease has endemic, immunodeficiency-associated, and sporadic variants. Endemic Burkitt's lymphoma was the initial entity described as a rapidly progressive tumor most commonly occurring in the jaws of children in equatorial Africa, Brazil, and Papua New Guinea (1). This subtype occurs at a median age of 5–7, and is uniformly positive for Epstein–Barr virus (EBV). Immunodeficiency-associated Burkitt's lymphoma occurs most commonly in HIV-infected individuals, but may also be seen in patients following solid-organ transplantation or other immunodeficient states. These tumors express the EBV virus in approximately one-third of cases. Sporadic Burkitt's lymphoma occurs in healthy adults with a male predominance and a median age of 30–40 (2, 3). EBV is usually negative in immunocompetent patients.

■ DIAGNOSIS AND STAGING

Diagnosis should be made by excisional biopsy. Pathologically, Burkitt's lymphomas are characterized by a diffuse infiltrate of monomorphic medium-sized lymphoid cells with coarse chromatin, basophilic cytoplasm, frequent mitoses, and interspersed tingible-body-macrophages ingesting apoptotic debris and giving the tumor the classic "starry sky" appearance on low-power microscopy (**Figure 36-1**) (4). Immunohistochemical staining shows the cells to express pan B-cell markers (CD19, CD20, and CD79a) and markers of germinal center derivation (CD10 and BCL6). BCL-2 should be negative. Staining for Ki67 demonstrates a proliferation fraction that is usually approaching 100%. The genetic *sine qua non* is the rearrangement of the MYC proto-oncogene on chromosome 8, usually in the t(8;14), or occasionally the variant translocations t(2;8) or t(8;22) where the site of translocation of MYC is to the transcriptionally active immunoglobulin heavy-(chromosome 14) or light-chain genes (kappa on chromosome 2 or lambda on chromosome 22). In endemic Burkitt's lymphoma, the MYC breakpoint is usually upstream of the first coding exon and the immunoglobulin heavy chain breakpoint is in the joining (J) region. In sporadic and HIV-associated Burkitt's lymphoma, the MYC breakpoint is often between exons 1 and 2 and the heavy chain breakpoint is in the switch region. These distinct molecular changes are not always noted. The MYC translocation in Burkitt lymphoma typically occurs in the context of a simple karyotype.

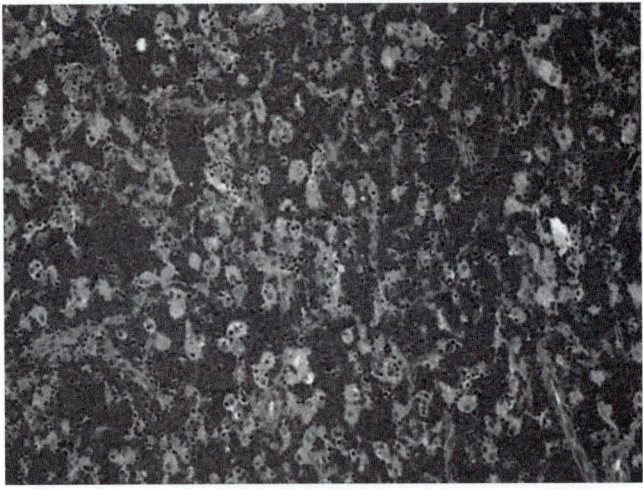

Figure 36-1 Burkitt's lymphoma. Low-power view showing monomorphic medium-sized malignant cells effacing the lymph node architecture with areas of clearing formed by tingible body macrophages ingesting apoptotic debris.

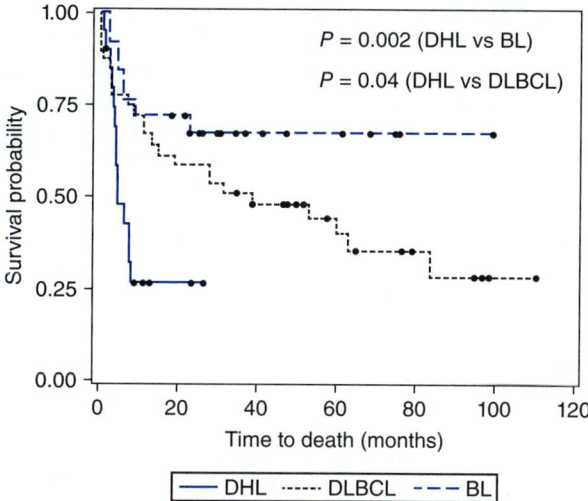

$P = 0.002$ (DHL vs BL)

$P = 0.04$ (DHL vs DLBCL)

— DHL ····· DLBCL - - - BL

Figure 36-2 Overall survival of double hit lymphoma compared to Burkitt's lymphoma and diffuse large B-cell lymphoma. (From Snuderl M, et al. *Am J Surg Pathol.* 2010;34:327–340.)

In settings of atypical morphologic, immunohistochemical, or genetic features, such as BCL-2 expression or a complex karyotype, those cases would generally not be classified as a Burkitt's lymphoma, but rather as B-cell lymphoma unclassifiable with intermediate features between diffuse large B-cell lymphoma and Burkitt lymphoma. Such cases generally occur in older adults and will often be characterized as a "double hit lymphoma" harboring dual translocations of MYC and BCL-2, usually in the setting of a complex karyotype, and carrying a significantly worse prognosis than Burkitt lymphoma of diffuse large B-cell lymphoma (5) (**Figure 36-2**).

Burkitt's lymphoma presents clinically as rapidly progressive nodal and/or extranodal masses. Nonendemic cases of Burkitt's lymphoma have a predilection for abdominal sites, particularly the ileocecal valve, but may present virtually anywhere in the body including any nodal or extranodal region, the head and neck, bone marrow, liver, kidneys, breast, soft tissues, skin, or central nervous system. Systemic "B" symptoms of fever, drenching night sweats, and weight loss may occur. Cases of immunodeficiency-associated Burkitt's lymphoma similarly present at advanced stage, often involving both nodal and extranodal sites. LDH is elevated in the majority of patients with Burkitt's lymphoma, and spontaneous tumor lysis may be present at diagnosis.

Following diagnosis, staging for Burkitt's lymphoma includes full body CT scans, ideally in concert with a full body PET scan given the increased sensitivity of this modality, particularly for extranodal sites of disease. The bone marrow is assessed with a bone marrow aspiration and biopsy, and spinal fluid should be evaluated by cytology and flow cytometry. HIV status should be checked along with viral load and CD4 count. Most

HIV-associated Burkitt's lymphomas occur in patients with a median CD4 count in the 200s (2). Hepatitis B serologies should be checked given risk of HBV reactivation in patients treated with intensive chemotherapy, particularly when rituximab is included. Tumor lysis labs should be checked at baseline. Evaluation of cardiac ejection fraction with echocardiography or multigated acquisition (MUGA) scan is advised in anticipation of anthracycline-containing therapy.

In addition to Ann Arbor staging, Burkitt patients may be classified as either low- or high-risk based on extent of disease and LDH value. Low-risk patients have a completely resected mass or limited disease less than 10 cm, a favorable performance status, and a normal LDH. All other patients are considered high risk.

■ TREATMENT

Treatment has historically been with highly intensive alternating cycles of chemotherapy directed at both the systemic and CNS compartments (6, 7). The anti-CD20 monoclonal antibody rituximab has been included with intensive chemotherapy based on noncomparative data showing encouraging results when added to combination chemotherapy (2, 8). The CODOX-M/IVAC regimen (cyclophosphamide, vincristine, doxorubicin, methotrexate alternating with ifosfamide, etoposide, and cytarabine) with rituximab produces a 3-year overall survival of nearly 80% (Table 36-1) (2). Patients with low-risk disease receive 3 cycles of the R-CODOX-M alone, while patients with high-risk disease receive 4 alternating cycles of R-CODOX-M and R-IVAC. Adverse prognostic factors include advanced age and involvement of the CNS at diagnosis. HIV infection is not an adverse predictor of outcome, but does require increased attention to supportive care including white blood cell growth factor support, prophylactic antibiotics against opportunistic infections, and attention to drug-drug interactions with the HIV-directed antiretroviral therapy. The R-HyperCVAD/MA regimen (rituximab, hyperfractionated cyclophosphamide, vincristine, doxorubicin and dexamethasone alternating with high-dose methotrexate and cytarabine) administered for 8 alternating cycles also produces encouraging results with 3-year overall survival approaching 90% (Table 36-2) (8). Both regimens include intrathecal chemotherapy for prophylaxis of the CNS, with additional intrathecal doses included for patients with an involved CNS at diagnosis. The overall course of therapy with HyperCVAD is twice as long as the complete course of therapy for CODOX-M/IVAC. Both regimens are highly intensive with virtually all patients experiencing grade 4 hematologic toxicity, and so supportive care for all patients is essential, including blood product support as needed, white blood cell growth factor support, antibiotic prophylaxis against *P. jiroveci*, and tumor lysis prophylaxis and monitoring at initiation of therapy. Patients with HIV should receive concurrent combination antiretroviral therapy (cART) in addition to intensive supportive care and infectious prophylaxis. Elderly patients tolerate these intensive regimens poorly, and so less intensive approaches should be considered. The infusional dose-adjusted EPOCH-R regimen (etoposide, prednisone, vincristine, cyclophosphamide, doxorubicin and rituximab) is better tolerated than the highly intensive approaches and has shown superb efficacy in a small study in predominantly younger patients

TABLE 36-1 MODIFIED R-CODOX-M/R-IVAC REGIMEN

R-CODOX-M[a]

Day	1	2	3	4	5	6	7	8	9	10	11	12	13
Rituximab 375 mg/m^2	x[b]												
Cyclophosphamide 800 mg/m^2	x	x											
Vincristine[c] 1.4 mg/m^2	x									x			
Doxorubicin 50 mg/m^2	x												
Methotrexate 3 g/m^2													
Leucovorin rescue										x	x	x	x
IT Cytarabine 50 mg	x		x[d]		x[d]								
IT Methotrexate 12 mg	x												
G-CSF[e]			x	x	x	x						x	x

R-IVAC[a]

Day	1	2	3	4	5	6	7	8	9	10	11	12	13
Ifosfamide 1500 mg/m^2	x	x	x	x	x								
Mesna	x	x	x	x	x								
Etoposide 60 mg/m^2	x	x	x	x	x								

(continued)

TABLE 36-1 MODIFIED R-CODOX-M/R-IVAC REGIMEN (CONTINUED)

Cytarabine 2 g/m² q12h × 4 doses	X	X							
IT methotrexate 12 mg			X						
IT cytarabine 50 mg		X[f]	X[f]						
G-CSF			X	X	X	X	X	X	X

[a]Low-risk patients receive 3 cycles of R-CODOX-M. High-risk patients receive 4 alternating cycles of R-CODOX-M and R-IVAC. Cycles are resumed once ANC is greater than 1000 and platelet count is >75,000. Average cycle length is 21 days.

[b]Rituximab should be administered on day 3 of cycle 1 to reduce tumor lysis risk, and on day 1 of all subsequent cycles.

[c]Vincristine capped at 2 mg.

[d]Only high-risk patients receive IT cytarabine on day 3. For patients with active CNS disease at diagnosis, additional intrathecal cytarabine should be administered on days 3 and 5 of the first cycle of R-CODOX-M.

[e]Neulasta may be substituted for G-CSF on day 2 of each cycle. If ANC <1000 on day 12 of R-CODOX-M, restart G-CSF.

[f]For patients with active CNS disease at diagnosis, intrathecal cytarabine should be administered on days 3 and 5 of the first cycle of R-IVAC.

Adapted from References 2 and 32.

TABLE 36-2 R-HYPERCVAD-MA

R-HyperCVAD[a]

Day	1	2	3	4	5	6	7	8	9	10	11	12	13	14
Rituximab 375mg/m²	x[b]										x			
Cyclophosphamide 300 mg/m² q12h × 6 doses	x	x	x											
Mesna	x	x	x											
Vincristine 2 mg				x							x			
Doxorubicin 50 mg/m² via 24-h continuous infusion				x										
Dexamethasone 40 mg	x	x	x	x							x	x	x	x
IT cytarabine 100 mg							x							
IT methotrexate 12 mg[c]		x												
G-CSF[d]					x	x	x	x	x	x				

R-MA[a]

Day	1	2	3	4	5	6	7	8	9	10	11	12	13	14
Rituximab 375 mg/m²		x[b]						x[b]						

(continued)

461

TABLE 36-2 R-HYPERCVAD-MA (CONTINUED)

Methotrexate 1 g/m² via 24-h continuous infusion	x						
Cytarabine 3 g/m² q12h × 4 doses		x					
Leucovorin rescue		x	x	x			
IT cytarabine 100 mg					x		
IT methotrexate 12 mg[c]		x					
G-CSF[d]			x	x	x	x	x	x

[a]Patients receive 8 alternating courses of R-HyperCVAD and methotrexate/cytarabine. Cycle length is 21 days.
[b]Rituximab administered only with cycles 1–4.
[c]Reduce dose to 6 mg if administering via Ommaya reservoir.
[d]G-CSF continued until WBC reached ≥3 × 10^9/L or bone pain present.
Adapted from Reference 8.

TABLE 36-3 DOSE-ADJUSTED[a] EPOCH-R

Day	1	2	3	4	5	6	7	8	9	10
Rituximab 375mg/m^2	x									
Etoposide[a] 50 mg/m^2/day by continuous infusion	x	x	x	x						
Doxorubicin[a] 10 mg/m^2/day by continuous infusion	x	x	x	x						
Vincristine 0.4 mg/m^2/day by continuous infusion	x	x	x	x						
Cyclophosphamide[a] 750 mg/m^2					x					
Prednisone 60 mg/m^2/BID	x	x	x	x	x					
IT Methotrexate 12 mg[b]	x				x					
G-CSF[c]						x	x	x	x	x

[a]CBC is checked twice weekly for dose adjustment. Cycle length is 21 days.
- If ANC nadir ≥0.5 × 10^9/L, then 20% increase in etoposide, doxorubicin, and cyclophosphamide for next cycle.
- If ANC nadir <0.5 × 10^9/L for 1 or 2 measurements, then maintain dose level.
- If ANC nadir <0.5 × 10^9/L for ≥3 measurements, then 20% decrease in etoposide, doxorubicin, and cyclophosphamide for next cycle.
- If platelet nadir <25 × 10^9/L on any measurement, then 20% decrease in etoposide, doxorubicin, and cyclophosphamide for next cycle.

[b]Intrathecal MTX given on days 1 and 5 of cycles 3–6 for patients without CNS involvement. Patients with CNS involvement receive IT therapy beginning with cycle 1. Treatment for active CNS disease is twice weekly until 2 weeks past negative cytology, then weekly × 6 doses, then monthly × 6 doses. Dose is 6 mg if given via Ommaya reservoir.

[c]G-CSF continued until ANC reached ≥5 × 10^9/L.

Adapted from References 9 and 33.

with Burkitt's lymphoma (Table 36-3) (9). This regimen is currently under study in a broader Burkitt lymphoma population in a phase II clinical trial. If these data are validated in the multicenter study, EPOCH-R may emerge as an appealing alternative to the more intensive regimens currently employed for the majority of patients.

PLASMABLASTIC LYMPHOMA

■ INTRODUCTION

Plasmablastic lymphoma (PBL) is a highly aggressive mature B-cell lymphoma initially described in HIV patients with a predilection for the oral cavity (10). Since the initial report, this disease has also been seen in HIV noninfected patients accounting for close to one-third of PBL cases, and includes patients following solid organ transplantation, as well as immunocompetent adults (11). The majority of patients are men, and the median age is approximately 40 years in HIV-infected patients and 60 years in patients

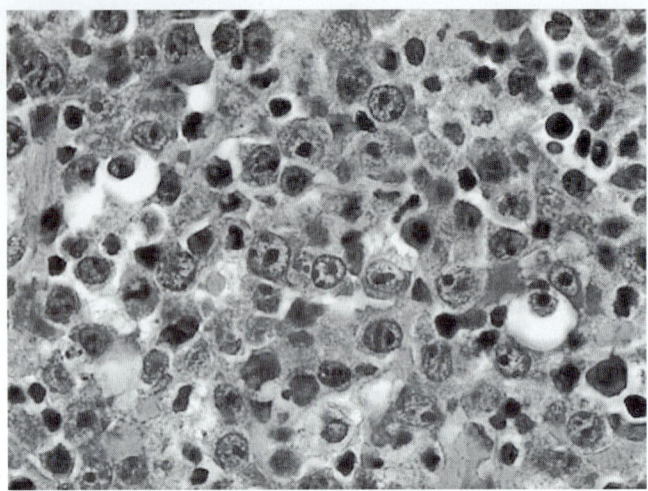

Figure 36-3 Plasmablastic lymphoma. High-power view of large malignant B-cells in PBL with an immunoblastic appearance.

without HIV. Most patients present with advanced stage disease, usually involving extranodal sites, oral cavity and sinuses, orbit, gastrointestinal tract, bone, skin, soft tissues, and central nervous system. LDH is commonly elevated. Among HIV patients, the median CD4 count is 165 cells/mm³ (12).

■ DIAGNOSIS AND STAGING

PBL is characterized histologically by large lymphoid cells that may have either immunoblastic or plasmacyctic differentiation (Figure 36-3) (4). Mitoses are frequent and the Ki67 proliferation fraction is generally close to 100%, reflecting the highly aggressive disease kinetics. By immunohisto-chemistry, the cells are usually negative for CD20 and positive for plasma cell markers CD38 and CD138. EMA and CD30 are commonly expressed, and EBV is detected in the majority of cases by in situ hybridization for EBV RNA. HHV8 is negative, unlike in primary effusion lymphoma. PBL should be evaluated for MYC rearrangements, which have been detected in approximately half of cases (13).

Staging should include a full body PET/CT given the role of functional imaging in high-grade lymphomas and increased sensitivity for extranodal sites. Bone marrow aspiration and biopsy should be performed. Lumbar puncture is recommended, as well as brain MRI for patients with CNS symptoms. All patients should have HIV checked, as well as CD4 count and viral load for HIV-infected patients. Spontaneous tumor lysis syndrome may occur, so tumor lysis labs should be checked at baseline, as well as an echocardiogram if an anthracycline-containing regimen is planned.

■ TREATMENT

PBL is a highly proliferative neoplasm and is rapidly fatal without therapy. The estimated median survival is 14 months, with 31% of patients alive at

5 years (12). Patients presenting with localized disease enjoy a more favorable prognosis. As with other HIV-associated lymphomas, cART should be considered a vital component for therapy in all patients with PBL in the setting of HIV infection, but rapid initiation of chemotherapy is essential. CHOP is associated with a high rate of treatment failure with low survival rate, and is not recommended, and so the more intensive regimens typically used in Burkitt's lymphoma should be considered, including dose-adjusted EPOCH, CODOX-M/IVAC, or HyperCVAD (Tables 36-1 through 36-3). Rituximab should be included only for the small number of cases that express CD20. Patients with localized disease should have radiation therapy included as combined modality therapy given the historic chemoresistance of this disease. All patients receiving intensive chemotherapy should be monitored for tumor lysis syndrome and receive supportive care with G-CSF and antibiotic prophylaxis against *P. jiroveci* and other pathogens as dictated by CD4 count.

The proteosome inhibitor bortezomib is used routinely in the management of the plasmacytic neoplasm multiple myeloma, providing rationale for use in PBL. Presently, only case reports exist to support efficacy, and further data are needed. CD30 is usually expressed in PBL, making the CD30-targeted agent brentuximab vedotin also worthy of investigation in the setting of a clinical trial.

PRIMARY EFFUSION LYPHOMA

■ INTRODUCTION

Primary effusion lymphoma (PEL), also known as body cavity lymphoma, is an uncommon B-cell lymphoma most commonly seen in advanced AIDS. Rare cases have also been observed in the absence of HIV infection, including in patients following solid organ transplantation, or in the setting of chronic hepatitis C or autoimmune diseases. PEL is uniformly associated with HHV-8 infection (also called the Kaposi's sarcoma herpes virus), the same viral pathogen that causes Kaposi's sarcoma and multicentric Castleman's disease. Patients with one HHV-8-associated disease are at increased risk for developing another. Given that most of these patients have advanced AIDS, concurrent opportunistic infections are also common, and must be considered in the differential diagnosis at presentation.

Patients typically present with a pleural effusion, pericardial effusion, or ascites. The leptomeninges are a rare site of involvement. Clinical presentation is related to the site of the effusion such as shortness of breath in pleural or pericardial PEL, and abdominal distention in patients with peritoneal disease.

An uncommon variant of this rare lymphoma may occur as solid tumors, often in extranodal locations, but with the same morphologic and immunohistochemical features and associated HHV8 expression. These cases have been dubbed "extracavitary" or "solid-phase" PEL.

■ DIAGNOSIS

Diagnosis is by aspiration of fluid from the involved body cavity for cytologic evaluation, flow cytometry, and cell block analysis with immunohistochemistry. Any associated solid tumors should also be biopsied. Given that PEL may present with concomitant Castleman's disease or Kaposi's sarcoma, adenopathy and skin lesions should be evaluated and biopsied. Attention should also be paid to possible concomitant opportunistic infections in patients with HIV and low CD4 counts.

The malignant effusion is characterized by large lymphoid cells that usually have plasmacytic differentiation with expression of CD45, CD30, CD38, and CD138, and no CD20 expression. HHV8 infection is a defining pathologic feature and can be detected by staining for viral gene product LANA-1. EBV coinfection is present in the majority of cases and is optimally detected by in situ hybridization for EBV RNA.

Staging should include full body CT scans with consideration of PET imaging as this has improved sensitivity for extranodal sites. Bone marrow biopsy is usually obtained.

■ TREATMENT

Prognosis of PEL is poor, with an estimated median survival of 6 months (14). The lymphoma rarely disseminates outside of body cavities, but the prognosis is driven in large part by the underlying HIV that is present in most patients with this disease resulting in death due to advanced AIDS and opportunistic infections, as well as progressive lymphoma. Adverse predictors of prognosis include poor performance status and absence of prior cART at the time of diagnosis (14).

Initiation of cART is standard as a vital component of treatment, and has been associated with responses in the absence of chemotherapy, and an improved outcome. CHOP (cyclophosphamide, doxorubicin, vincristine, and prednisone) has a reported response rate of 42% but with a short overall survival (15). The dose-adjusted EPOCH regimen (16) has been well studied in other HIV-associated lymphomas and should be considered based on encouraging efficacy in HIV-associated DLBCL and Burkitt lymphoma, but the efficacy specifically in PEL is unknown. Rituximab should not be routinely included given the CD20 negativity in this tumor, but can be added in rare CD20+ cases. A number of novel approaches hold promise as effective therapies as well. Antiviral therapy carries appeal given the HHV-8-mediated pathogenesis, though the cells are lytically infected and thus not sensitive to traditional agents like ganciclovir. Induction of the lytic phase of the virus may sensitize the cells to antiviral therapy, and this is a subject of investigation in clinical trials of HHV-8- and EBV-mediated lymphomas. Intrapleural cidofovir has been reported in case reports to induce responses, and may be considered in patients who are not candidates for systemic chemotherapy (17). The anti-CD30 antibody drug conjugate brentuximab vedotin holds promise as an effective targeted therapy given the superb activity in other CD30+ diseases Hodgkin lymphoma and anaplastic large T-cell lymphoma, and is currently under investigation.

LYMPHOMATOID GRANULOMATOSIS

■ INTRODUCTION

Lymphomatoid granulomatosis (LyG) is a rare EBV-associated angiocentric and angioinvasive lymphoproliferative disease that primarily involves extranodal sites. It generally occurs in patients age 50–70 year old and with a 2:1 male predominance (18). Though the disease may occur in immuno-compromised patients such as HIV patients, organ transplant recipients, or those with congenital immunodeficiency, this disease occurs most commonly in previously immunocompetent individuals. All patients have evidence of impaired immune function at diagnosis (19), raising the question of whether the disease causes the immunodeficiency, or conversely is occurring in the setting of a previously undiagnosed immune-deficient milieu. The lungs are involved in nearly all patients, usually bilaterally, followed by kidneys, skin, central nervous system, and liver. The presenting symptoms are usually cough, dyspnea, and chest discomfort related to pulmonary involvement, often associated with fever and malaise. The subacute onset with fevers and respiratory symptoms will often lead to an initial diagnosis of a respiratory infection. Respiratory symptoms and chest x-ray findings of bilateral lung nodules that predominate in the middle and lower lobes may wax and wane. Skin lesions of LyG are most commonly maculopapular and may ulcerate. Patients may present with symptoms referable to CNS involvement which occurs in approximately one-third of patients and may cause altered mental status, cranial neuropathy, gait disturbance, or seizures (20).

■ DIAGNOSIS

The diagnosis may be difficult to make given the nonspecific clinical presentations that are more suspicious for respiratory infections or primary neurologic diseases. Given the polymorphous nature of the infiltrate, fine needle and core needle biopsies are usually nondiagnostic and so wedge biopsies via video-assisted thoracoscopic surgery are recommended. On biopsy, the lesions are characterized by an angioinvasive polymorphous inflammatory infiltrate of lymphocytes, plasma cells, immunoblasts, and histiocytes (4). A variable number of large atypical EBV+ lymphocytes are present. The disease is graded based on the number of large EBV+ cells in the infiltrate with the cells being infrequent or absent in grade 1 lesions, occasional (5–20 per high power field) in grade 2 lesions, and numerous (>50/ high power field) in grade 3 lesions (4). Grade 3 lesions may contain large aggregates or sheets of the atypical cells, and necrosis may be present. The cells are typically positive for CD20 and variable for CD30. CD15 is absent. The background T cells are more commonly CD4 than CD8. Clonality by immunoglobulin gene rearrangements can be demonstrated in the majority of grade 2 and 3 lesions, but may not be seen in grade 1. Laboratory studies are usually unremarkable, though a polyclonal hypergammaglobulinemia may be seen. CT scans of the chest, abdomen, and pelvis should be performed at diagnosis, and brain MRI if CNS symptomatology is present, though this disease is not traditionally staged using the Ann Arbor system.

■ TREATMENT

Historically, prognosis was poor with a median survival of less than 2 years (20). Some patients, particularly with grades 1 and 2 disease, may have a lengthy waxing and waning natural history, while grade 3 lesions are typically aggressive with a short overall survival without aggressive treatment. For patients with asymptomatic or minimally symptomatic grades 1 and 2 disease, close observation is appropriate as spontaneous remissions may occur. Glucocorticoids have been utilized with little success with most patients doing poorly (21). Interferon has been utilized for patients with grades 1 and 2 disease starting with a dose of 7.5 million units thrice weekly and escalated based on response (18). Sixty percent of patients achieved a complete remission, including the majority of patients with CNS disease, but the median time to response is 9 months. The progression-free survival at 5 years was 56%. Among patients with grade 3 disease, response to interferon is low, but the dose-adjusted EPOCH-R regimen produced a complete response rate of 66% and 40% progression-free survival at 2 years (Table 36-3) (18). Rituximab either alone or in a low-intensity chemoimmunotherapy platform such as R-CVP (rituximab, cyclophosphamide, vincristine, and prednisone) is a reasonable strategy in patients who cannot tolerate intensive combination chemotherapy, but evidence of success is limited to case reports with no prospective clinical trials reported (22, 23). Patients may succumb to infectious complications given the immune-deficiency associated with LyG, or may undergo transformation to high-grade DLBCL. Such patients should be treated with aggressive chemoimmunotherapy regimens such as dose-adjusted EPOCH-R or R-CHOP, or with traditional second-line DLBCL regimens if those regimens have already been employed.

HAIRY CELL LEUKEMIA

■ INTRODUCTION

Hairy cell leukemia (HCL) is a low-grade B-cell lymphoproliferative disease initially described in 1958 as leukemic reticuloendotheliosis (24). HCL occurs at a median age of 50 with a male predominance of approximately 5:1. The name derives from the circulating cells that may be observed in the peripheral blood as medium-large size lymphoid cells with oval nuclei and abundant pale blue cytoplasm with fine circumferential hair-like projections (**Figure 36-4**). Despite the name of "leukemia," most patients present with a very small amount of circulating disease. The dominant disease burden in HCL is found in the bone marrow and spleen (**Figure 36-5**), leading to the most common presentation of symptomatic splenomegaly and pancytopenia. Lymphadenopathy is uncommon. Absolute monocytopenia is observed in the majority of patients. Patients may present with bleeding due to thrombocytopenia or recurrent opportunistic infections.

■ DIAGNOSIS

Diagnosis of HCL is usually by evaluation of blood and bone marrow. In the blood, the typical hairy cells may be observed, but are often few in number and can also difficult to distinguish from other malignant cells such as the villous lymphocytes often seen in splenic marginal zone lymphoma. The characteristic pattern on flow cytometry are cells that are positive for CD20 and negative for CD5, CD10, and CD23 (4). Expression of CD103, CD25, and CD11c are typically seen in HCL, helping to distinguish it from splenic marginal zone lymphoma or lymphoplasmacytic lymphoma. On bone marrow examination, the HCL cells are observed with their abundant cytoplasm,

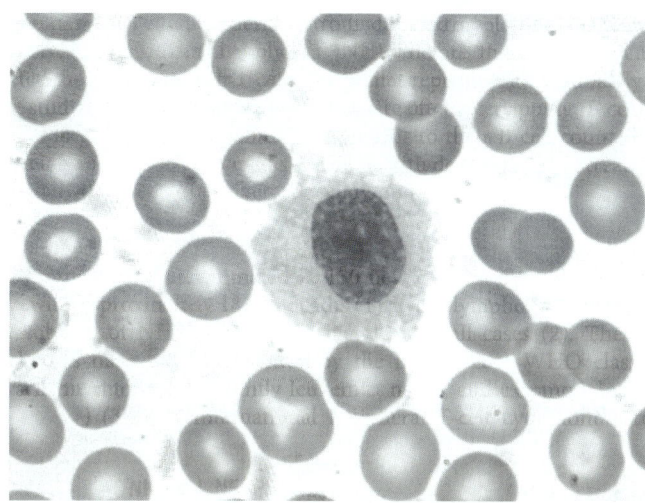

Figure 36-4 Hairy cell leukemia. Peripheral smear showing a typical hairy cell with an oval nucleus, abundant cytoplasm and ruffled indistinct border with circumferential fine hairlike projections.

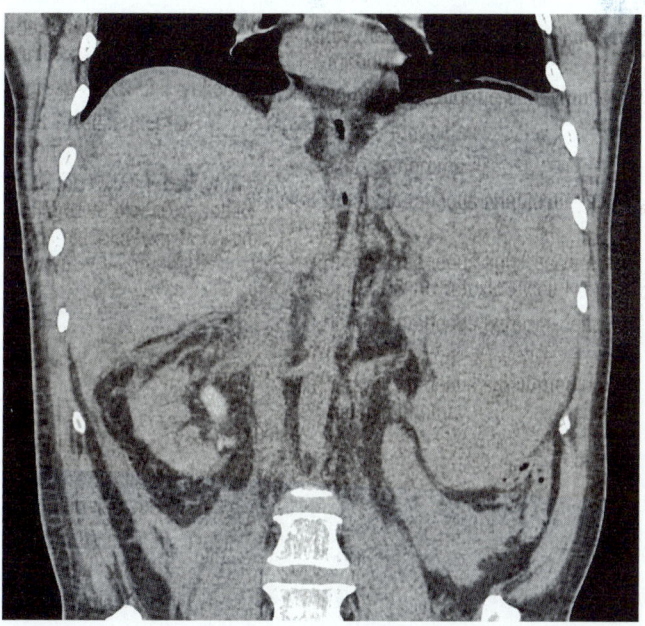

Figure 36-5 Splenomegaly in hairy cell leukemia (HCL). Massive splenomegaly in a patient with HCL seen in this coronal image of a noncontrast enhanced abdominal CT scan.

oval nucleus, and distinct cell borders, giving it a classic "fried-egg" appearance. Reticulin is increased in the bone marrow in HCL, and can impair the ability to draw an aspirate, making a "dry tap" common at diagnosis. The infiltrate in the marrow may be patchy and subtle, so can be overlooked in the absence of careful examination.

■ TREATMENT

HCL is an indolent disease that is exquisitely sensitive to therapy with most patients enjoying an excellent prognosis. Patients may be observed if they have asymptomatic disease without cytopenias, recurrent infections, systemic symptoms, or symptomatic splenomegaly. Initial therapy when indicated is with the nucleoside analogue cladribine or pentostatin (Table 36-4). Cladribine administered for a single cycle as a 7-day continuous infusion (0.1 mg/kg/day) produces a complete response in the vast majority of patients in most series with a median duration of response of approximately 8 years (Figure 36-6) (25). Favorable outcomes have also been reported using a single cycle of a 5-day bolus regimen with a dose of 0.14 mg/kg/day (26), but the continuous infusion is preferred if available given that the preponderance of the data employs infusional therapy. Pentostatin administered at 2–4 mg/m^2 every 14 days until maximal response produces high complete response rates with similarly encouraging disease-free survival rates as observed with cladribine (Figure 36-7), and studies of both agents demonstrate that greater than 90% of patients remain alive a decade following therapy (Table 36-4) (27). Given the prolonged myelosuppression of a single cycle of cladribine, pentostatin is preferred as initial therapy in patients with active infections at the time therapy is to be initiated. At disease progression, nucleoside analogues remain quite active, and so retreatment is preferred. Rituximab has also demonstrated encouraging single agent activity in the setting of relapse (26, 28). More recently, BRAF V600E mutations have been identified as the culprit genetic lesion in nearly all cases of HCL, yielding an appealing target for future therapy (29). The BRAF inhibitor vemurafenib has demonstrated activity in refractory HCL cases in case reports (30), but the role for this therapy in HCL remains undefined given the excellent outcomes achieved already with standard nucleoside analogues. Long-term follow-up of patients with HCL should monitor for recurrence as well as secondary malignancies, which are increased in this patient population.

TABLE 36-4 INITIAL TREATMENT OPTIONS FOR HAIRY CELL LEUKEMIA

Treatment	Dose and Schedule	Duration of Therapy
Cladribine by continuous infusion (25)	0.1 mg/kg per day by continuous IV infusion for 7 days	Single cycle of therapy
Cladribine by bolus (26)	0.14 mg/kg by 2 hour IV bolus per day for 5 days	Single cycle of therapy
Pentostatin by bolus	2–4 mg/m^2 IV every 14 days	Until maximal response, up to 1 year

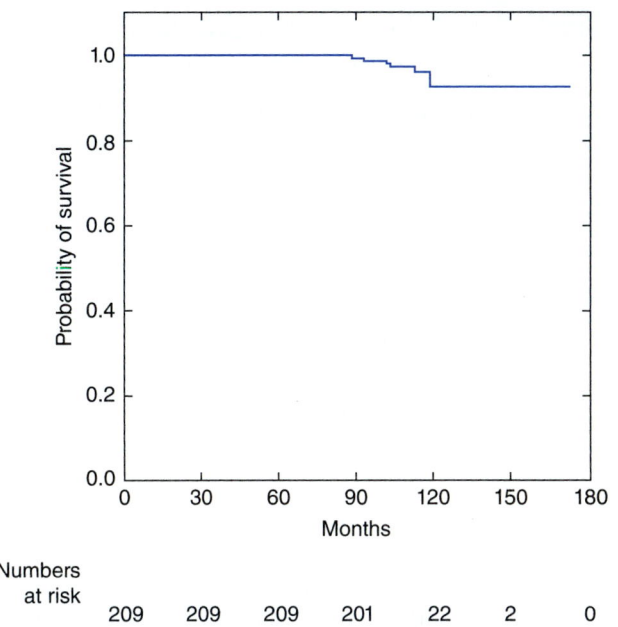

Figure 36-6 Cladribine and for hairy cell leukemia (HCL). Overall survival of 209 patients with HCL treated with cladribine. 97% of patients are alive at 108 months. (From Goodman GR, et al. *J Clin Oncol.* 2003. 21:891–896.)

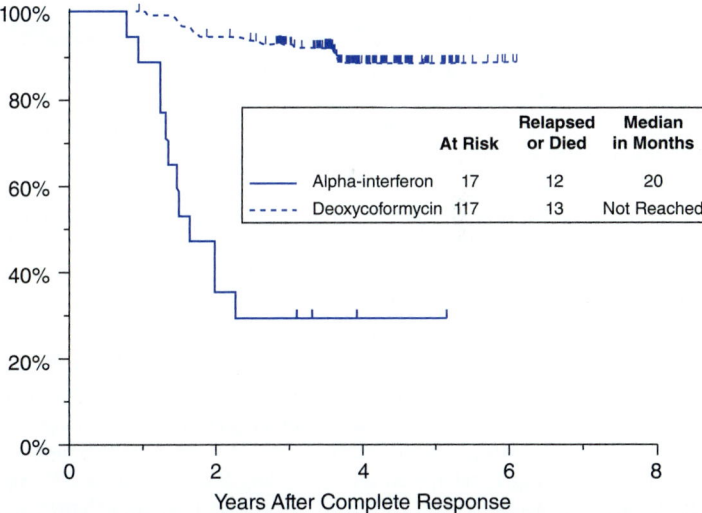

Figure 36-7 Pentostatin for hairy cell leukemia. Superior relapse-free survival for pentostatin compared to alpha-interferon in a randomized trial in untreated HCL. (From Grever M, et al. *J Clin Oncol.* 1995. 13:974–982.)

CUTANEOUS B-CELL LYMPHOMAS

Cutaneous lymphomas without systemic disease are a rare subset of non-Hodgkin lymphomas representing less than 10% of all new cases diagnosed annually, and approximately 25% of all cutaneous lymphomas. The majority of cutaneous lymphomas are from T-cell derivation, with mycosis fungoides being the most common type. Initial evaluation of any cutaneous B-cell lymphoma should include systemic staging with CT scans, as systemic B-cell lymphomas may secondarily involve the skin. The majority of primary cutaneous B-cell lymphomas are primary cutaneous follicle center lymphoma (PCFCL). These are CD20+ and BCL6+ with variable CD10 expression. The majority are BCL-2 negative and strong expression of BCL-2 should prompt suspicion for cutaneous involvement by systemic follicular lymphoma. They behave in an indolent manner and the vast majority can be cured with radiation therapy alone with the complete response rate approaching 100% (31). Primary cutaneous marginal zone lymphoma is another indolent cutaneous lymphoma with a high cure rate with radiation therapy alone.

Primary cutaneous diffuse large B-cell lymphoma, leg type (PCLBCL) is a much more aggressive disease compared to other cutaneous B-cell lymphomas with 5-year overall survival of 40%–60%. It is, as the name suggests, mainly found on the lower extremities, but 10%–15% may be found on the trunk with no findings on the legs. It usually has larger cells that are CD20+, BCL6+, and CD10– with variable expression of BCL-2 and MUM-1. This disease should be approached as other systemic diffuse large B-cell lymphomas and treated with R-CHOP with or without involved field radiotherapy.

REFERENCES

1. Burkitt D. A sarcoma involving the jaws in African children. *Br J Surg.* 1958; 46: 218–223.

2. Barnes JA, Lacasce AS, Feng Y, et al. Evaluation of the addition of rituximab to CODOX-M/IVAC for Burkitt's lymphoma: a retrospective analysis. *Ann Oncol.* 2011; 22: 1859–1864.

3. Mead GM, Barrans SL, Qian W, et al. A prospective clinicopathologic study of dose-modified CODOX-M/IVAC in patients with sporadic Burkitt lymphoma defined using cytogenetic and immunophenotypic criteria (MRC/NCRI LY10 trial). *Blood.* 2008; 112: 2248–2260.

4. Swerdlow SH, Campo E, Harris NL, et al. *WHO Classification of Tumours of Hematopoietic and Lymphoid Tissues.* Lyon, WHO, 2008.

5. Snuderl M, Kolman OK, Chen YB, et al. B-cell lymphomas with concurrent IGH-BCL2 and MYC rearrangements are aggressive neoplasms with clinical and pathologic features distinct from Burkitt lymphoma and diffuse large B-cell lymphoma. *Am J Surg Pathol.* 2010; 34: 327–340.

6. Magrath I, Adde M, Shad A, et al. Adults and children with small non-cleaved-cell lymphoma have a similar excellent outcome when treated with the same chemotherapy regimen. *J Clin Oncol.* 1996; 14: 925–934.

7. Thomas DA, Cortes J, O'Brien S, et al. Hyper-CVAD program in Burkitt's-type adult acute lymphoblastic leukemia. *J Clin Oncol.* 1999; 17: 2461–2470.

8. Thomas DA, Faderl S, O'Brien S, et al. Chemoimmunotherapy with hyper-CVAD plus rituximab for the treatment of adult Burkitt and Burkitt-type lymphoma or acute lymphoblastic leukemia. *Cancer.* 2006; 106: 1569–1580.

9. Dunleavy K, Little RF, Pittaluga S, et al. A prospective study of dose-adjusted (DA) EPOCH with rituximab in adults with newly diagnosed Burkitt Lymphoma: a regimen with high efficacy and low toxicity. *Ann Oncol.* 2008; 19: iv83–iv84.

10. Delecluse HJ, Anagnostopoulos I, Dallenbach F, et al. Plasmablastic lymphomas of the oral cavity: a new entity associated with the human immunodeficiency virus infection. *Blood.* 1997; 89: 1413–1420.

11. Rafaniello Raviele P, Pruneri G, Maiorano E. Plasmablastic lymphoma: a review. *Oral Dis.* 2009; 15: 38–45.

12. Castillo JJ, Winer ES, Stachurski D, et al. Prognostic factors in chemotherapy-treated patients with HIV-associated plasmablastic lymphoma. *The Oncologist.* 2010; 15: 293–299.

13. Valera A, Balague O, Colomo L, et al. IG/MYC rearrangements are the main cytogenetic alteration in plasmablastic lymphomas. *Am J Surg Pathol.* 2010; 34: 1686–1694.

14. Boulanger E, Gerard L, Gabarre J, et al. Prognostic factors and outcome of human herpesvirus 8-associated primary effusion lymphoma in patients with AIDS. *J Clin Oncol.* 2005; 23: 4372–4380.

15. Simonelli C, Spina M, Cinelli R, et al. Clinical features and outcome of primary effusion lymphoma in HIV-infected patients: a single-institution study. *J Clin Oncol.* 2003; 21: 3948–3954.

16. Little RF, Pittaluga S, Grant N, et al. Highly effective treatment of acquired immunodeficiency syndrome-related lymphoma with dose-adjusted EPOCH: impact of antiretroviral therapy suspension and tumor biology. *Blood.* 2003; 101: 4653–4659.

17. Halfdanarson TR, Markovic SN, Kalokhe U, et al. A non-chemotherapy treatment of a primary effusion lymphoma: durable remission after intracavitary cidofovir in HIV negative PEL refractory to chemotherapy. *Ann Oncol.* 2006; 17: 1849–1850.

18. Dunleavy K, Roschewski M, Wilson WH. Lymphomatoid granulomatosis and other epstein-barr virus associated lymphoproliferative processes. *Curr Hematol Malig Rep.* 2012; 7: 208–215.

19. Sordillo PP, Epremian B, Koziner B, et al. Lymphomatoid granulomatosis: an analysis of clinical and immunologic characteristics. *Cancer.* 1982; 49: 2070–2076.

20. Katzenstein AL, Carrington CB, Liebow AA. Lymphomatoid granulomatosis: a clinicopathologic study of 152 cases. *Cancer.* 1979; 43: 360–373.

21. Jaffe ES, Wilson WH. Lymphomatoid granulomatosis: pathogenesis, pathology and clinical implications. *Cancer Surv.* 1997; 30: 233–248.

22. Hu YH, Liu CY, Chiu CH, Hsiao LT. Successful treatment of elderly advanced lymphomatoid granulomatosis with rituximab-CVP combination therapy. *Eur J Haematol.* 2007; 78: 176–177.

23. Zaidi A, Kampalath B, Peltier WL, et al. Successful treatment of systemic and central nervous system lymphomatoid granulomatosis with rituximab. *Leuk Lymphoma.* 2004; 45: 777–780.

24. Bouroncle BA, Wiseman BK, Doan CA. Leukemic reticuloendotheliosis. *Blood.* 1958; 13: 609–630.

25. Goodman GR, Burian C, Koziol JA, et al. Extended follow-up of patients with hairy cell leukemia after treatment with cladribine. *J Clin Oncol.* 2003; 21: 891–896.

26. Robak T, Blasinska-Morawiec M, Krykowski E, et al. 2-chlorodeoxyadenosine (2-CdA) in 2-hour versus 24-hour intravenous infusion in the treatment of patients with hairy cell leukemia. *Leuk Lymphoma.* 1996; 22: 107–111.

27. Else M, Ruchlemer R, Osuji N, et al. Long remissions in hairy cell leukemia with purine analogs: a report of 219 patients with a median follow-up of 12.5 years. *Cancer.* 2005; 104: 2442–2448.

28. Thomas DA, O'Brien S, Bueso-Ramos C, et al. Rituximab in relapsed or refractory hairy cell leukemia. *Blood.* 2003; 102: 3906–3911.

29. Tiacci E, Trifonov V, Schiavoni G, et al. BRAF mutations in hairy-cell leukemia. *N Engl J Med.* 2011; 364: 2305–2315.

30. Dietrich S, Glimm H, Andrulis M, et al. BRAF inhibition in refractory hairy-cell leukemia. *N Engl J Med.* 2012; 366: 2038–2040.

31. Senff NJ, Noordijk EM, Kim YH, et al. European Organization for Research and Treatment of Cancer and International Society for Cutaneous Lymphoma consensus recommendations for the management of cutaneous B-cell lymphomas. *Blood.* 2008; 112: 1600–1609.

32. Lacasce A, Howard O, Lib S, et al. Modified magrath regimens for adults with Burkitt and Burkitt-like lymphomas: preserved efficacy with decreased toxicity. *Leuk Lymphoma.* 2004; 45: 761–767.

CHAPTER **37**

Immunology of Hematopoietic Stem Cell Transplantation

Srinivas Viswanathan, Yi-Bin Chen

Hematopoietic stem cell transplantation (HSCT) has wide applications in the treatment of hematologic malignancies, congenital and acquired disorders of hematopoiesis, and autoimmune disease. Transplanted hematopoietic progenitors can reconstitute the full spectrum of hematopoietic cells in a recipient host, and can also confer immunologic antitumor activity. HSCT is therefore employed for both cellular replacement and for cancer immunotherapy. This chapter reviews the basic immunology of HSCT.

MAJOR CELLULAR TYPES

Following HSCT, donor hematopoietic progenitor cells migrate to the recipient bone marrow and differentiate to generate all cell types of the erythroid, myeloid, and lymphoid lineages. The following hematopoietic cell types are thought to play key physiologic roles:

- $CD34^+$ cells: The population of cells containing the hematopoietic progenitors capable of repopulating the recipient marrow. HSCT grafts are usually quantified based on the $CD34^+$ population. In certain selective cellular depletion protocols, donor hematopoietic cells can be purified for $CD34^+$ cells prior to transplantation. Doses of more than or equal to 2×10^6/kg (recipient weight) CD34-expressing progenitor cells are typically required in autologous or adult allogeneic adult donor products. Requirements are approximately one log lower for umbilical cord products.
- B-cells: Lymphocytes whose chief role is to produce antibodies against specific antigens to mediate humoral immunity. The role of B cells in chronic graft-versus-host disease (cGVHD) has been recognized.
- $CD8^+$ T cells: Cytotoxic T cells that recognize antigenic peptides presented on major histocompatibility (MHC) Class I proteins. In the presence of either a costimulatory signal or stimulatory cytokines (secreted by $CD4^+$ Th and other cells), $CD8^+$ T cells undergo clonal expansion and lyse their targets via the release of perforin and granzyme.
- $CD4^+$ $helper$ T (Th) $cells$: Helper T cells that can develop into either Th1 or Th2 effector T cells. Th1 cells support the cellular immune response by stimulating killing by macrophages and $CD8^+$ T cells. Th2 cells support the antibody response by stimulating B-cell proliferation and

475

antibody production. A third subset of Th cells (Th17 cells) has been identified although its role in HSCT is yet to be defined.

- *Natural killer (NK) cells:* Cytotoxic lymphocytes central to the innate immune response. NK cells kill cells that have lost cell-surface expression of self MHC I in a perforin- and granzyme-dependent manner. NK cells are also key effectors in humoral immunity, mediating antibody-dependent cellular cytotoxicity (ADCC).
- *Regulatory (Treg) cells:* A subset of CD4+ T cells that functions in a regulatory capacity to modulate the immune response and suppress autoimmunity. Ongoing clinical trials are exploring different ways to expand Treg cells to control GVHD.
- *Dendritic cells:* Antigen-presenting cells (APCs) that express high levels of both MHC I and MHC II and efficiently present antigens to T cells. Dendritic cells stimulate naïve T cells within lymphoid tissues. Dendritic cells within the thymus eliminate T cells that are selective for self-antigens through the process of negative selection.

GRAFT-VERSUS-HOST DISEASE

Graft-versus-host disease (GVHD) results from an immunologic response against antigenic disparities between donor hematopoietic cells and host tissues. GVHD comprises a significant proportion of morbidity and mortality associated with HSCT. Historically, GVHD had been classified into acute (traditionally occurring within 100 days of transplant) and chronic (traditionally occurring after 100 days of transplant) phases. However, recent consensus definitions have transitioned to a classification based solely on clinical manifestations, rather than the timing of symptoms after HSCT. There is also an acute-chronic GVHD overlap syndrome which has manifestations of both classic acute and chronic disease (Table 37-1).

Significant acute GVHD (aGVHD) complicates up to half of all HLA-matched stem cell transplants and a higher proportion of mismatched transplants. The most commonly involved sites of aGVHD are the skin, liver, and gastrointestinal tract. Clinical features include a maculopapular rash, liver function test abnormalities (traditionally, elevations in direct bilirubin and alkaline phosphatase), and high-volume diarrhea accompanied by abdominal cramping. Histologic features differ by organ, and it is worth noting that the overall clinical picture, and not pathologic findings, is the gold standard for diagnosis. Skin involvement by aGVHD is characterized histologically by dermal and epidermal lymphocytic infiltration. Liver aGVHD is characterized by lymphocytic infiltration of small bile ducts, leading to bile duct damage and degeneration, and intestinal aGVHD is characterized by crypt cell necrosis, increased apoptosis, and a loss of intestinal epithelium (1, 2).

The pathogenesis of aGVHD is thought to be driven by donor T-cell-mediated damage of host cells as well as by local and systemic release of inflammatory cytokines. This is thought to occur via a multistep process: (1) Damage to host tissues by the conditioning regimen (classically, high doses of chemotherapy and radiation) stimulates the release of proinflammatory cytokines including IL-1, IL-6, TNF-α, and IFN-γ; (2) increased MHC molecule expression on host APCs including dendritic cells in

TABLE 37-1 COMPARISON OF FEATURES OF ACUTE GVHD AND Chronic GVHD

	Acute GVHD	Chronic GVHD
Timing	<100 days posttransplant[a]	>100 days posttransplant[a]
Clinical and pathologic features	Maculopapular rash Abnormal liver function tests Diarrhea	Fibrotic changes in multiple organ systems
Predominant cell types involved	T cells	T cells B cells
Standard prophylaxis	Calcineurin inhibitor + methotrexate +/– ATG Calcineurin inhibitor + MMF	
Alternative Prophylaxis	Post-HSCT high-dose cyclophosphamide T-cell depletion	
First-line treatment	Glucocorticoids	Glucocorticoids
Second-line treatment	MMF Sirolimus IL-2 antagonists TNF-α antagonists Pentostatin Extracorporeal pheresis	MMF Sirolimus Rituximab Calcineurin inhibitors Extracorporeal pheresis Local therapies

ATG = antithymocyte globulin; GVHD = Graft-versus-host disease; MMF = mycophenolate mofetil.

[a]Typical distinction, but clinical features trump timing in definition.

response to cytokines; (3) presentation of alloantigens to donor T cells by activated host APCs triggers T-cell activation, leading to IL-2 and IFN-γ production; (4) CD4$^+$ T cells stimulate expansion of the donor CD8$^+$ T cells that mediate the cytotoxic effects of GVHD; and (5) direct damage by the cytotoxic actions of activated donor CD8$^+$ T-cells and inflammatory cytokines result in the clinical manifestations of acute GVHD (Figure 37-1).

Every allogeneic HSCT requires some form of prophylaxis against GVHD. This can be accomplished through (1) pharmacologic methods (most commonly) or (2) ex vivo T-cell depletion methods. The accepted international standard for pharmacologic prophylaxis against aGVHD involves a calcineurin inhibitor (either cyclosporine or tacrolimus) in combination with several low doses of post-HSCT methotrexate. Calcineurin inhibitors are generally continued at therapeutic levels for several months with gradual tapering to discontinuation if there are no signs of GVHD.

The initial treatment for patients who develop clinical aGVHD despite appropriate prophylaxis involves high-dose systemic glucocorticoids, usually

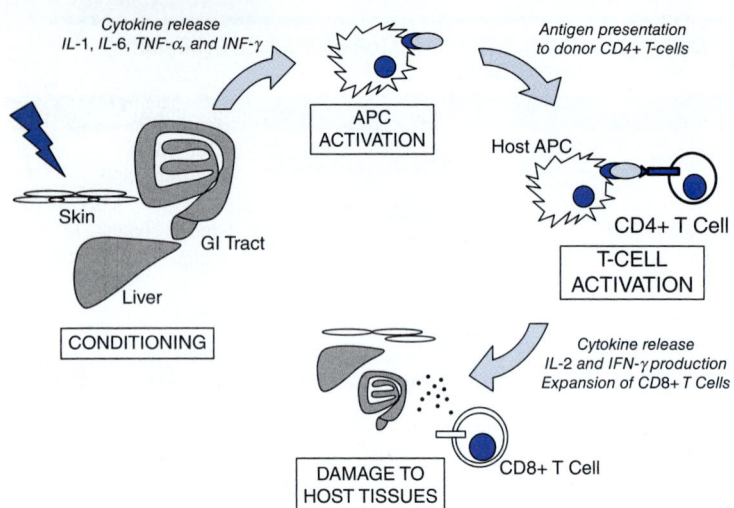

FIGURE 37-1 Schematic of the steps leading to GVHD. In the afferent phase, damage to host tissues by conditioning regimen leads to inflammatory cytokine production and upregulation of MHC on host APCs. Subsequently, recipient and donor APCs activate donor-derived T cells. Cytotoxic (CD8) T cells then cause damage to host tissues.

at doses of 1–2 mg/kg/day of prednisone or its equivalent. Glucocorticoids provide durable remission in only 50% of patients, and those who fail initial therapy have high mortality rates (3, 4). There is no standard second-line therapy and a number of agents have been tried, including mycophenolate mofetil, sirolimus, IL-2 antagonists, TNF-α antagonists, pentostatin, and extracorporeal pheresis.

Chronic GVHD (cGVHD) develops in a subset of patients with acute GVHD, and also arises in the absence of any preceding acute GVHD. The most commonly involved sites are the eyes, skin, respiratory tract, esophagus, and liver. Clinically, chronic GVHD is pleomorphic and heterogeneous, with many features resembling classic autoimmune diseases such as lupus, Sjogren's syndrome, vitiligo, and scleroderma. In contrast to the inflammatory changes that are typically found in aGVHD biopsies, pathologic hallmarks of cGVHD include a dense fibrosis of involved tissues with occasional infiltration of mononuclear cells (5).

Both donor B cells and donor T cells appear to play important roles in the pathophysiology of chronic GVHD. T-cells have been implicated in cGVHD in multiple mouse models, as well as by the fundamental observation that cGVHD incidence is significantly less in patients who undergo transplants from T-cell depleted grafts. The role of B cells has emerged recently from studies showing antibodies specific for proteins coded from the Y chromosome in female donor—male recipient transplants (6). In addition, other studies have also demonstrated that B-cell activating factor (BAFF), a pro-B-cell growth factor, is present at high levels in patients with active chronic GVHD (7).

Many of the same agents used for treatment of aGVHD are also used for the treatment of cGVHD, including systemic glucocorticoids, calcineurin inhibitors, mycophenolate mofetil, sirolimus, and extracorporeal pheresis. Given the recent data implicating the role of B cells in cGVHD, the anti-CD20 antibody rituximab has also been employed with encouraging results (8). Chronic GVHD has emerged as the most important determinant of quality of life in long-term survivors of HSCT (9), and, unfortunately, many trials that have shown some success in reducing acute GVHD have not had a significant effect on preventing chronic GVHD. Therefore, one of the primary focuses of future research in HSCT involves better prevention and treatment of chronic GVHD.

GRAFT-VERSUS-LEUKEMIA

The existence of an immunologic graft-versus-leukemia (GVL) effect has been supported by several observations: (1) with comparable conditioning regimens, allogeneic transplants result in a lower relapse rate than autologous or syngeneic transplants; (2) multiple series have observed that patients who develop acute or chronic GVHD have a lower incidence of disease relapse than those who do not (10); and (3) donor leukocyte infusions (DLI) alone were able to achieve remission for many patients with relapsed chronic myeloid leukemia (CML) after HSCT (11). Although antitumor effects of HSCT have been most widely studied in the setting of leukemia, regression of other hematologic malignancies has also been clearly described following HSCT, leading to the use of the broader term graft-versus-malignancy (GVM). The recognition of the GVM effect has led to the increasing popularity of protocols employing nonmyeloablative and reduced-intensity conditioning regimens. The efficacy of these protocols is based mostly on the antitumor effects of GVM, with toxicity spared due to the lower intensity of the conditioning regimens.

The extent or potency of GVM appears to vary based upon the underlying disease, disease status, and, undoubtedly, unknown essential interactions between the donor and the recipient. Both donor-derived T cells and NK cells appear to have key roles in GVM. In theory, the T-cell response is driven by the presentation of host or tumor antigens to donor T cells, which leads to a clonal expansion of CD8$^+$ cytotoxic T cells specific for the antigen. NK cells also appear to be potent mediators of GVL (12, 13), but differ from T cells in that they can kill tumor cells without the prerequisites of activation and clonal expansion. NK cells express inhibitory receptors known as killer cell immunoglobulin-like receptors (KIRs) which recognize specific inhibitory MHC Class I allele groups (KIR ligands). NK-cell alloreactivity occurs when recipient cells do not express an MHC-I ligand which can engage KIR on the surface of donor NK cells. Overall, it remains unclear if the immunologic mechanisms driving GVM differ from those responsible for GVHD, and current methods are unable to reliably separate the two (14). Ongoing research is focusing on methods to better cultivate GVM without inducing significant GVHD, using approaches such as preemptive post-HSCT treatment with immunomodulatory agents and vaccination protocols against specific tumor antigens. A summary of these approaches is shown in Figure 37-2.

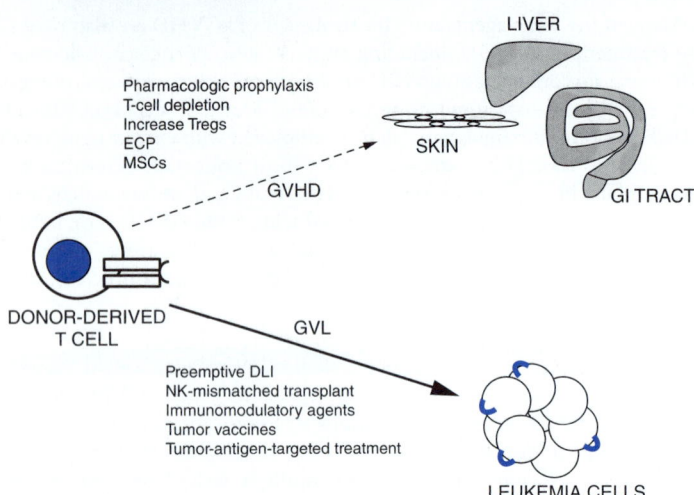

FIGURE 37-2 The promise of HSCT lies in augmenting GVL (thick arrow) while mini-mizing GVHD (dotted arrow). Strategies for minimizing GVHD include pharmacologic agents, T-cell depletion, increasing number of Treg cells, extracorporeal pheresis (ECP), and mesenchymal stem cell (MSC) infusion. Strategies for augmenting GVL include donor-lymphocyte infusion (DLI), increasing number of Treg cells, conducting NK-cell (KIR) mismatched transplants, tumor vaccines, and therapies targeted and tumor-specific antigens.

GVHD PROPHYLAXIS

■ PHARMACOLOGIC APPROACHES

As mentioned previously, the accepted standard pharmacologic approach to prevent GVHD includes a calcineurin inhibitor in combination with several doses of post-HSCT methotrexate. Other agents have been added to this backbone with the hope of preserving GVM, while preventing GVHD more effectively. Several of these agents are highlighted below.

Antithymocyte globulin (ATG) is very commonly given during con-ditioning to help prevent GVHD by depleting donor T cells in vivo. Several different ATG preparations exist, and they differ in their specific-ity and activity. Many US centers routinely employ thymoglobulin (ATG, Genzyme) when using unrelated or mismatched donors (15), although no prospective clinical trials have shown a proven clinical benefit (16). Recently, a large European study using ATG-F (Fresenius) in addition to cyclosporine and methotrexate showed a decreased incidence of both aGVHD and cGVHD without increasing the rate of relapse (17), and a large confirmatory American trial is now underway.

Alemtuzumab is a humanized monoclonal antibody against CD52, a glycophosphatidylinositol (GPI)-anchored glycoprotein expressed on the surface of B and T lymphocytes, NK cells, macrophages, and dendritic cells. *In vitro* pre-treatment of donor cells with alemtuzumab prior to transplant as a form to T-cell depletion has been performed (18). More commonly, alemtuzumab is included in conditioning regimens to provide a form of in vivo T-cell depletion with all matched (19), mismatched (20), and haploidentical (21) donors. Results of these series all show impressively low rates of GVHD, yet there is a clearly higher incidence of infections and possibly relapse of disease.

Sirolimus (rapamycin) has recently emerged as a promising immunosuppressive agent which works through several mechanisms: (1) binding of FK-binding protein 12 (FKBP-12) leading to inhibition of the mTOR pathway, thus blocking activation of B cells and T cells; (2) blocking antigen presentation and dendritic cell maturation; and (3) promoting the development of regulatory T cells. A number of phase II studies suggest that sirolimus may be beneficial in the treatment of both aGVHD and cGVHD, as well as in GVHD prophylaxis (22), and a large national collaborative phase III trial in GVHD prophylaxis has recently finished accrual with results eagerly awaited.

Cyclophosphamide, an alkylating agent used commonly in the treatment of many malignancies, selectively induces apoptosis in proliferating T cells. High-doses (50 mg/kg/day on days +3 and +4 after HSCT) given in the first week after HSCT has been pioneered as a novel method to prevent GVHD and promote tolerance. This was first developed in murine models and has been successfully translated into human patients using both matched related (23) and haploidentical donors (24).

Newer, more experimental, approaches seek to manipulate the cytokine environment. Both antitumor immunity and aGVHD appear to be dominated by a Th1-polarized T-cell response (with key cytokines being IL-1, IL-2, IL-6, IFN-γ, TNF-α), while cGVHD is driven by a Th2-polarized response (with key cytokines being IL-4, IL-5, IL-10). Several attempts have been made, all in preclinical animal models, to alter the cytokine milieu in such a way as to minimize GVHD while preserving GVM. While these approaches are promising, it remains unclear to what extent exogeneous cytokine administration can be safely translated to the human clinical setting.

Anergy refers to the process whereby immune tolerance is induced. Several attempts have been made to induce anergy in donor T cells ("alloanergy") and thereby reduce the incidence of GVHD. Most approaches to doing this focus on blocking the costimulatory signal between host APC and donor T cells by using monoclonal antibodies or fusion proteins (25). In vitro results employing this approach are promising, suggesting that alloreactive T cells are reduced in number without major effect on GVM. Clinical trials of this alloanergization approach are currently in progress.

■ CELL-BASED APPROACHES

Cellular approaches to preventing GVHD have largely centered on strategies attempting to selectively deplete the donor T cell pool of alloreactive T cells. Early strategies employed ex vivo pan-T cell depletion using antisera directed against all T cells. While this approach reduced the incidence of GVHD, relapse rates and infectious complications were increased, leading to comparable rates of overall survival relative to traditional pharmacologic methods. In appropriate clinical settings, ex vivo T-cell depletion remains a very effective method of GVHD prophylaxis (26, 27). However, rigorous T-cell depletion methodology requires significant laboratory expertise and facilities.

Preemptive donor lymphocyte infusion (DLI) has been used in an attempt to augment the GVM effect while minimizing GVHD. When DLI is used for this purpose, it is typically given to patients who have received in vivo or ex vivo T-cell depleted transplants, especially if those patients exhibit evidence of mixed donor-host chimerism posttransplant (28). DLI clearly has the capacity to convert mixed host-donor chimerism to full donor chimerism without causing graft rejection (28, 29). Because the acute inflammation that activates host antigen presentation subsides after the immediate posttransplant period, this technique theoretically reduces allogeneic T-cell reactivity while preserving GVM. In practice, however, the timing of DLI is often coincident with immunosuppression taper, which may also contribute to promoting GVHD.

DLI is also commonly employed as salvage immunotherapy following disease relapse after HSCT. Historically, when given to several patients with relapsed chronic phase CML after HSCT, DLI alone was able to induce remission—one of the earliest examples of a clear GVM effect. Nonetheless, more recent data have shown that DLI is generally ineffective if a significant burden of disease is present for the majority of diseases. Furthermore, there is a significant risk of developing GVHD after DLI (30, 31). Clinical trials are investigating techniques to increase the effectiveness of DLI while suppressing the risk of GVHD. These strategies include the insertion of "suicide" transgenes into donor lymphocytes prior to infusion to allow a simple and controlled means for killing alloreactive T cells after transplantation if significant GVHD develops (32, 33). Other approaches include giving selective populations of DLI and coadministration of specific cytokines to increase GVM activity.

There has been great interest in the regulatory T-cell subset as a means to separate GVL from GVHD. Tregs comprise about 5% of the CD4+ T-cell pool and express high levels of CD25 and FoxP3. In multiple mouse models, Treg cells can potently suppress aGVHD without impairing GVM. Therefore, augmenting the activity or size of the donor Treg cell pool is an attractive way to enhance GVM and minimize GVHD. However, reliable and generalizable methods of ex vivo expansion of Tregs are not currently available, limiting the ability to translate promising preclinical results to the clinical setting although clinical protocols are ongoing (34).

Mesenchymal stem cells (MSCs) are bone marrow derived stromal cells with the capacity to differentiate into fibroblasts, adipocytes, osteoblasts, and chondrocytes. In various preclinical models, MSCs have been shown to stimulate the production of regulatory T cells and suppress development of GVHD. This is likely mediated through the secretion of particular cytokines or growth factors that stimulate Treg cell growth and development. Early clinical data indicated that MSCs were safe for use in humans and may improve outcomes in steroid-resistant acute GVHD (34, 35), and although this has not yet been confirmed in larger prospective studies, use of MSCs remain an active area of investigation.

Extracorporeal photopheresis (ECP) is an immunomodulatory procedure used for the treatment of cGVHD and, more recently, aGVHD. With ECP, the patient undergoes leukapheresis and collected leukocytes are treated with a DNA-intercalating dye. The leukocytes are then exposed to UVA radiation, which causes cells to undergo apoptosis. Following dye treatment and UVA exposure, treated leukocytes are returned to the patient. Data from murine models indicate that ECP acts through several mechanisms: promoting alloreactive lymphocyte apoptosis, increasing numbers of regulatory T cells, and indirectly decreasing the number of donor effector lymphocytes that have never even been exposed to dye or UVA radiation (36). ECP is especially attractive in that it appears to induce less global immunosuppression relative to other therapies.

Umbilical cord blood (UCB) stem cells are the newest source of hematopoietic stem cells used in HSCT. UCB transplantation is attractive as less stringent HLA-matching requirements are required given the intrinsic immunologic immaturity of UCB cells. With the growth of UCB transplantation, several retrospective series have suggested that rates of acute and chronic GVHD are lower compared to adult peripheral blood stem cells or bone marrow, yet relapse rates are lower as well. However, overall rates of survival remain comparable given higher rates of mortality from infections and other complications with UCB transplantation. Nevertheless, it is compelling that rates of relapse are not increased in this setting where GVHD is clearly decreased.

CONCLUSIONS

Hematopoietic stem cell transplantation serves as a powerful technique for both cellular replacement and for cancer immunotherapy. Unfortunately, the immunologic anti-malignancy effects of HSCT are often offset by debilitating effects of GVHD. Work has begun to elucidate the myriad cell types and complex molecular pathways involved in both GVL and GVHD. It is only after understanding the specific immunologic players involved in each of these processes that we will be able to develop therapeutic approaches which can potentially separate them. Although recent approaches have suggested the ability to partially decrease GVHD without increasing infection or disease relapse, future work is clearly needed to further refine HSCT into an adoptive immunotherapy platform with more tolerable morbidity and mortality.

REFERENCES

1. Ball LM, Egeler RM. Acute GVHD: pathogenesis and classification. *Bone Marrow Transplant.* 2008; 41 (Suppl 2): S58–S64.

2. Washington K, Jagasia M. Pathology of graft-versus-host disease in the gastrointestinal tract. *Hum Pathol.* 2009; 40: 909–917.

3. Martin PJ, Schoch G, Fisher L, et al. A retrospective analysis of therapy for acute graft-versus-host disease: initial treatment. *Blood.* 1990; 76: 1464–1472.

4. Westin JR, Saliba RM, De Lima M, et al. Steroid-refractory acute GVHD: predictors and outcomes. *Adv Hematol.* 2011; 2011: 601–953.

5. Martin PJ. Biology of chronic graft-versus-host disease: implications for a future therapeutic approach. *Keio J Med.* 2008; 57: 177–183.

6. Miklos DB, Kim HT, Miller KH, et al. Antibody responses to H-Y minor histocompatibility antigens correlate with chronic graft-versus-host disease and disease remission. *Blood.* 2005; 105: 2973–2978.

7. Sarantopoulos S, Stevenson KE, Kim HT, et al. High levels of B-cell activating factor in patients with active chronic graft-versus-host disease. *Clin Cancer Res.* 2007; 13: 6107–6114.

8. Cutler C, Miklos D, Kim HT, et al. Rituximab for steroid-refractory chronic graft-versus-host disease. *Blood.* 2006; 108: 756–762.

9. Khera N, Storer B, Flowers ME, et al. Nonmalignant late effects and compromised functional status in survivors of hematopoietic cell transplantation. *J Clin Oncol.* 2012; 30: 71–77.

10. Horowitz MM, Gale RP, Sondel PM, et al. Graft-versus-leukemia reactions after bone marrow transplantation. *Blood.* 1990; 75: 555–562.

11. Porter DL, Connors JM, Van Deerlin VM, et al. Graft-versus-tumor induction with donor leukocyte infusions as primary therapy for patients with malignancies. *J Clin Oncol.* 1999; 17: 1234.

12. Ruggeri L, Capanni M, Urbani E, et al. Effectiveness of donor natural killer cell alloreactivity in mismatched hematopoietic transplants. *Science.* 2002; 295: 2097–2100.

13. Ruggeri L, Mancusi A, Capanni M, et al. Donor natural killer cell allorecognition of missing self in haploidentical hematopoietic transplantation for acute myeloid leukemia: challenging its predictive value. *Blood.* 2007; 110: 433–440.

14. Hess AD. Separation of GVHD and GVL. *Blood.* 2010; 115: 1666–1667.

15. Pidala J, Tomblyn M, Nishihori T, et al. ATG prevents severe acute graft-versus-host disease in mismatched unrelated donor hematopoietic cell transplantation. *Biol Blood Marrow Transplant.* 2011; 17: 1237–1244.

16. Soiffer RJ, Lerademacher J, Ho V, et al. Impact of immune modulation with anti-T-cell antibodies on the outcome of reduced-intensity allogeneic hematopoietic stem cell transplantation for hematologic malignancies. *Blood.* 2011; 117: 6963–6970.

17. Finke J, Bethge WA, Schmoor C, et al. Standard graft-versus-host disease prophylaxis with or without anti-T-cell globulin in haematopoietic cell transplantation from matched unrelated donors: a randomised, open-label, multicentre phase 3 trial. *Lancet Oncol.* 2009; 10: 855–864.

18. Barge RM, Starrenburg CW, Falkenburg JH, et al. Long-term follow-up of myeloablative allogeneic stem cell transplantation using Campath "in the bag" as T-cell depletion: the Leiden experience. *Bone Marrow Transplant.* 2006; 37: 1129–1134.

19. Kottaridis PD, Milligan DW, Chopra R, et al. In vivo CAMPATH-1H prevents graft-versus-host disease following nonmyeloablative stem cell transplantation. *Blood.* 2000; 96: 2419–2425.

20. Mead AJ, Thomson KJ, Morris EC, et al. HLA-mismatched unrelated donors are a viable alternate graft source for allogeneic transplantation following alemtuzumab-based reduced-intensity conditioning. *Blood;* 115: 5147–5153.

21. Rizzieri DA, Koh LP, Long GD, et al. Partially matched, nonmyeloablative allogeneic transplantation: clinical outcomes and immune reconstitution. *J Clin Oncol.* 2007; 25: 690–697.

22. Cutler C, Antin JH. Sirolimus immunosuppression for graft-versus-host disease prophylaxis and therapy: an update. *Curr Opin Hematol.* 2010; 17: 500–504.

23. Luznik L, Bolanos-Meade J, Zahurak M, et al. High-dose cyclophosphamide as single-agent, short-course prophylaxis of graft-versus-host disease. *Blood.* 2010; 115: 3224–3230.

24. Brunstein CG, Fuchs EJ, Carter SL, et al. Alternative donor transplantation after reduced intensity conditioning: results of parallel phase 2 trials using partially HLA-mismatched related bone marrow or unrelated double umbilical cord blood grafts. *Blood.* 2011; 118: 282–288.

25. Davies JK, Gribben JG, Brennan LL, et al. Outcome of alloanergized haploidentical bone marrow transplantation after ex vivo costimulatory blockade: results of 2 phase 1 studies. *Blood.* 2008; 112: 2232–2241.

26. Devine SM, Carter S, Soiffer RJ, et al. Low risk of chronic graft-versus-host disease and relapse associated with T cell-depleted peripheral blood stem cell transplantation for acute myelogenous leukemia in first remission: results of the blood and marrow transplant clinical trials network protocol 0303. *Biol Blood Marrow Transplant.* 2011; 17: 1343–1351.

27. Aversa F, Terenzi A, Tabilio A, et al. Full haplotype-mismatched hematopoietic stem-cell transplantation: a phase II study in patients with acute leukemia at high risk of relapse. *J Clin Oncol.* 2005; 23: 3447–3454.

28. Mohamedbhai SG, Edwards N, Morris EC, et al. Predominant or complete recipient T-cell chimerism following alemtuzumab based allogeneic transplantation is reversed by donor lymphocytes and not associated with graft failure. *Br J Haematol.* 2012; 156: 516–522.

29. Dey BR, McAfee S, Colby C, et al. Impact of prophylactic donor leukocyte infusions on mixed chimerism, graft-versus-host disease, and anti-tumor response in patients with advanced hematologic malignancies treated with nonmyeloablative conditioning and allogeneic bone marrow transplantation. *Biol Blood Marrow Transplant.* 2003; 9: 320–329.

30. Roddie C, Peggs KS. Donor lymphocyte infusion following allogeneic hematopoietic stem cell transplantation. *Expert Opin Biol Ther.* 2011; 11: 473–487.

31. Chalandon Y, Passweg JR, Schmid C, et al. Outcome of patients developing GVHD after DLI given to treat CML relapse: a study by the Chronic Leukemia Working Party of the EBMT. *Bone Marrow Transplant.* 2010; 45: 558–564.

32. Di Stasi A, Tey SK, Dotti G, et al. Inducible apoptosis as a safety switch for adoptive cell therapy. *N Engl J Med.* 2011; 365: 1673–1683.

33. Tiberghien P. Use of suicide gene-expressing donor T-cells to control alloreactivity after haematopoietic stem cell transplantation. *J Intern Med.* 2001; 249: 369–377.

34. Li, J-M, Giver CR, Lu Y, et al. Separating graft-versus-leukemia from graft-versus-host disease in allogeneic hematopoietic stem cell transplantation. *Immunotherapy*. 2009; 1: 599–62.

35. Le Blanc K, Frassoni F, Ball L, et al. Mesenchymal stem cells for treatment of steroid-resistant, severe, acute graft-versus-host disease: a phase II study. *Lancet*. 2008; 371: 1579–1586.

36. Paczesny S, Choi SW, Ferrara JLM. Acute graft-versus-host disease: new treatment strategies. *Curr Opin Hematol*. 2009; 16: 427–436.

CHAPTER **38**

Overview of Clinical Bone Marrow Transplantation

Sarah Nikiforow, Thomas R. Spitzer

INTRODUCTION

Bone marrow or hematopoietic cell transplantation (BMT or HCT) is a potentially curative therapy for a wide variety of life-threatening congenital and acquired hematopoietic stem cell disorders and neoplastic diseases. With the development of human leukocyte antigen (HLA) typing to identify suitably matched donors, advances in tolerability and efficacy of conditioning regimens, improvements in supportive care, and advances in the prophylaxis and treatment of graft-versus-host disease (GVHD), clinical HCT became a reality. Many of the initial clinical HCT efforts were directed toward severe aplastic anemia and acute leukemia (which remains the paradigm for allogeneic HCT in adults). However, the demonstration of lasting donor lymphohematopoietic reconstitution, the powerful cytoreductive effect of intensive pretransplantation conditioning therapy, and the exploitation of a potent immunologically-mediated graft-versus-tumor (GVT) effect led to the successful application of HCT as up-front and salvage therapy for the many hematologic malignancies and other disorders shown in Table 38-1. Some applications of HCT are potentially curative, e.g., allogeneic transplantation for acute myeloid leukemia (AML). In other settings, HCT is primarily utilized to lengthen disease-free intervals without expectation of cure, e.g., autologous transplantation for multiple myeloma. In parallel with the above advances, the use of hematopoietic cell transplantation has expanded yearly. In 2009, more than 26,000 transplants were performed worldwide, over 15,000 of these being allogeneic HCTs (1).

The principal functions of HCT are to provide:

1. *Rescue* (i.e., by the infusion of pluripotent hematopoietic progenitor cells in the setting of cytoreductive chemotherapy that eradicates malignant cells but also ablates stem cells and other hematopoietic bone marrow elements)

TABLE 38-1 HEMATOPOIETIC STEM CELL TRANSPLANTATION: SELECTED INDICATIONS

Allogeneic: acquired	Allogeneic: congenital
• Hematologic malignancies 　AML/ALL 　CML/CLL 　Multiple myeloma 　Non-Hodgkin lymphoma 　Hodgkin lymphoma 　MDS 　IMF • Nonmalignant stem cell disorders 　Aplastic anemia 　PNH	• Primary immunodeficiency diseases • Hemoglobinopathies 　Sickle cell anemia 　Thalassemia major • Metabolic diseases 　Gaucher's disease 　Mucopolysaccharidosis 　X-linked adrenoleukodystrophy • Bone marrow failure states 　Fanconi's anemia 　Diamond–Blackfan anemia
Autologous: acquired	• Disorders of phagocytosis 　Osteopetrosis 　Familial hemophagocytic lymphohistiocytosis
• Hematologic malignancies 　AML in CR 　ALL in CR 　Multiple myeloma 　Non-Hodgkin lymphoma 　Hodgkin lymphoma • Selected solid tumors 　Neuroblastoma 　Germ cell tumors • Autoimmune conditions 　SLE 　Scleroderma 　Multiple sclerosis	

ALL, acute lymphoblastic leukemia; AML, acute myeloid leukemia; CLL, chronic lymphocytic leukemia; CML, chronic myeloid leukemia; CR, complete remission; IMF, idiopathic myelofibrosis; MDS, myelodysplastic syndrome; PNH, paroxysmal nocturnal hemoglobinuria; SLE, systemic lupus erythematosis.

2. *Replacement* (i.e., of a diseased hematopoietic stem cell population by healthy stem cells capable of regeneration of multiple hematopoietic lineages)

3. *An immunologic platform* (As mixed lymphohematopoietic chimerism often occurs after less intensive conditioning, HCT may be envisioned as creating an immunologic platform for adoptive cellular therapy. Subsequent manipulation may occur through donor lymphocyte infusions (DLI), expansion, or depletion of T-cell subsets (e.g., regulatory T cells), or

selection of NK and dendritic cell subsets in order to augment GVT effects while minimizing GVHD) (2).

DONOR ORIGIN OF HEMATOPOIETIC STEM CELLS

- *Autologous HCT* or "high-dose chemotherapy with autologous stem cell rescue" refers to the collection from and subsequent reinfusion of hematopoietic progenitor cells into a patient with a solid or hematopoietic malignancy. Preparative intensive-conditioning therapy is given in an effort to reduce the number of malignant cells or to achieve immunoablation in a refractory autoimmune disease. Infusion of the patient's own hematopoietic cells follows in order to *rescue* the patient from the negative effects of myeloablation, namely unacceptable levels of subsequent infectious and hematologic complications.
- *Allogeneic HCT* refers to the *rescue* and *replacement* of hematopoietic stem cells from an HLA-matched or partially matched donor source different from the patient. Allogeneic HCT may occur after myeloablative, reduced-intensity, or nonmyeloablative conditioning therapy. In addition to the cytoreductive effects of the preparative therapy, allogeneic HCT confers a potentially potent *immunologically mediated* response of donor immune cells against host tumor cells (i.e., a GVT effect induced by the interaction of donor T cells with host minor or major histocompatibility antigens or tumor antigens).

STEM CELL SOURCES FOR ALLOGENEIC HCT

Preference has historically been given to "matched" related donors (MRD) who are HLA-identical to the recipient, as determined by molecular class I and II HLA typing. As each sibling inherits two haplotypes, one from each parent, there is a 25% chance that any two full siblings will be genotypically identical. Only 30% of patients will have a matched sibling donor. Therefore, alternative, non-HLA-identical related and unrelated donor sources have been increasingly utilized, now enabling the majority of those without sibling donors to undergo HCT. Because of the increasingly varied sources of progenitor cells transplanted, hematopoietic cell transplantation (HCT) is a more representative term than BMT to describe the current field. Stem cell sources include:

- HLA molecularly "matched" unrelated donors (MUD)
- Unrelated donors molecularly "mismatched" at one or more HLA molecules (MMUD)
- Haploidentical-related donors (i.e., children or siblings, sharing only one inherited HLA haplotype)
- Partially HLA-matched umbilical cord blood (UCB)

Hematopoietic progenitor cells capable of restoring hematopoiesis and immune function following transplantation can be procured from:

- *Bone marrow* (BM; following a bone marrow harvest procedure in the operating room).
- *Peripheral blood* (PB; following "mobilization" with chemotherapy and/or recombinant hematopoietic growth factor(s) and/or CXCR4 antagonists followed by "collection" by pheresis).

- *Umbilical cord* (UCB; following full-term delivery) Given longer times to engraftment and higher rates of infectious complications with use of a single cord, the use of two umbilical cord blood units partially matched to each other is now common in adult HCTs.

CD34, a surface glycoprotein expressed on a small percentage of bone marrow cells is typically employed as a surrogate immunophenotypic marker for the pluripotent hematopoietic stem cell. Suitable numbers of CD34-expressing cells are needed in progenitor cell products to ensure acceptable kinetics of engraftment and sustained hematologic recovery following transplantation. Doses of more than or equal to 2×10^6/kg CD34-expressing progenitor cells are typically required in autologous or adult allogeneic donor products. Requirements are approximately one log lower for umbilical cord products.

PRETRANSPLANT CONSIDERATIONS

Designing an HCT approach for a particular patient requires consideration of the underlying disease and the recipient's medical comorbidities, in addition to details of the transplant itself (3).

- *Disease state:* The achievement of disease control is a significant if not *the* dominant determinant of overall survival in most studies and is usually pursued maximally prior to transplantation. For example, according to outcomes analyses from the Center for International Bone Marrow Transplant Registry (CIBMTR), a patient with AML in first complete remission who undergoes an allogeneic transplant from a matched related donor has a 3-year survival probability of 53% compared with a patient with AML *not* in remission, whose 3-year survival probability is 24% (1).
- *Recipient:* Morbidity and mortality can also arise from transplant-related complications including organ failure secondary to the conditioning regimen, bacterial or viral infections, and both acute and chronic GVHD (in the allogeneic setting) or their treatments. These can lead to peritransplant mortality rates in the range of 1%–5% after autologous HCT and 10%–40% after allogeneic HCT. In recent years, the number and age of eligible recipients have increased significantly through the use of nonmyeloablative and reduced-intensity conditioning regimens with associated lower rates of nonrelapse mortality. In analyses of reduced-intensity conditioning regimens, age *per se* has not been shown to correlate with worse outcomes, and in 2009 more than 30% of allogeneic stem cell transplantations (SCTs) were performed in recipients over the age of 50, even in patients into their seventies (1). In contrast, performance status and comorbidities, specifically pulmonary, cardiac, and hepatic function, have been shown to have an important impact on nonrelapse mortality based on several validated scoring systems in both myeloablative and nonmyeloablative settings (4). Nevertheless, even after successful transplantation, life expectancy, immune function, and quality of life of recipients remain lower than that of age-matched peers.

PREPARATIVE THERAPY AND DONOR SELECTION

Choices of intensity of the conditioning regimen, donor, and type of stem cell source are driven not just by age and availability but more importantly by:

(1) the status and nature of the underlying malignancy, (2) the combination of host comorbidities and treatment toxicities, (3) the reliance on GVT effect needed to prevent relapse in each case, and (4) the desire to avoid complications of GVHD.

- *Intensity of the conditioning regimen*: The options for intensity of conditioning regimens have diversified significantly in the last few years, expanding the eligible recipient pool but also increasing potential confusion over classification. One consensus scheme identifies myeloablative (MA) regimens as those that cause irreversible cytopenias requiring hematopoietic cell support, reduced-intensity (RIC) regimens as those that cause cytopenias of variable duration that may or may not be irreversible, and nonmyeloablative (NMA) regimens as those that lead to minimal cytopenias that will recover without hematopoietic cell support (5). Representative regimens for each intensity level are shown in Table 38-2.

  RIC or NMA conditioning may be more appropriate for an older patient with a malignancy sensitive to a GVT effect, such as an indolent non-Hodgkin lymphoma. However, with less-potent conditioning, the benefit of decreased nonrelapse mortality may be negated by an increased risk of relapse. Reduced-intensity conditioning may be an inferior approach for younger patients with more aggressive hematologic malignancies such as AML. The presence of a GVT effect, upon which NMA and RIC conditioning regimens rely, has been indirectly demonstrated in specific disease settings in the form of higher rates of relapse observed when progenitor cells are received from an HLA-identical twin sibling, lower rates of relapse seen in the presence of GVHD, induction of remission by abrupt withdrawal of immunosuppression and directly observed when remission is reestablished after infusion of donor leukocytes in the setting of relapse (6). A schematic representing the relative role of GVT against various malignancies and the relative potencies of various conditioning regimens is provided in Figure 38-1. No recommendation for pairing of any disease entity with a specific conditioning regimen is implied, but RIC and NMA regimens are now increasingly employed in older patients whose diseases are more sensitive to GVT. While in some disease settings conditioning regimens of differing intensities have yielded similar overall survival, prospective trials are ongoing to define the disease and age subgroups that will benefit most from a particular conditioning regimen.

- *Peripheral blood versus bone marrow-derived stem cells:* A multicenter prospective study concluded that for patients undergoing myeloablative matched *unrelated* donor HCT, the use of PB-derived donor stem cells was associated with an increased incidence of chronic GVHD and no improvement in overall survival when compared to the use of BM-derived stem cells. In a separate study, PB-derived stem cells conferred a survival advantage for HCT with matched *related* donors. How this information will impact the clinical choice of a stem cell source for an individual patient is as yet unclear but the majority of allogeneic stem cells used in transplantation are currently harvested from peripheral blood (7).

- *Alternative stem cell sources:* The use of HLA-mismatched unrelated donors, umbilical cord blood units, and haploidentical sibling donors has

TABLE 38-2 CONDITIONING REGIMENS

MYELOABLATIVE

Cy-TBI[a]	Cyclophosphamide 120 mg/kg (or 3600 mg/m^2) total
	TBI $\geq$1200 cGy
Bu-Cy[b]	Busulfan 0.8 mg/kg IV q6h Days-7, -6, -5, -4
	Cyclophosphamide 120–200 mg/kg total
CBV(Auto)	Cyclophosphamide 750 mg/m^2 q12h Days -6, -5, -4, -3
	BCNU 112.5 mg/m^2 IV daily Days -6, -5, -4, -3
	Etoposide 200 mg/m^2 IV q12h Days -6, -5, -4, -3
BEAM (Auto)	BCNU 300 mg/m^2 IV Day -8
	Etoposide 200 mg/m^2 IV daily Days -7, -6, -5, -4
	Cytarabine 200 mg/m^2 IV q12h on Days -7, -6, -5, -4
	Melphalan 140 mg/m^2 IV on Day -3
High-dose melphalan (auto)	200 mg/m^2 IV total over 1–2 days
Flu-Bu	Fludarabine 40 mg/m^2 IV daily Days -7, -6, -5, -4
	Busulfan 0.8 mg/kg IV q6h or 130 mg/m^2 IV daily Days -7, -6, -5, -4

REDUCED-INTENSITY
(alkylators or TBI reduced by at least 30%)

Flu-Mel	Fludarabine 25 mg/m^2 IV daily Days -6, -5,- 4, -3, -2
	Melphalan 140 mg/m^2 IV Day -1
Flu-Bu	Fludarabine 30 mg/m^2 IV daily Days -5, -4, -3, -2
	Busulfan 0.8 mg/kg IV Daily-BID Days -5, -4, -3, -2
Cy-ATG-Thymic XRT	Cyclophosphamide 150–200 mg/kg total
	700 cGy total

NONMYELOABLATIVE

Flu-Cy	Fludarabine 30 mg/m^2 IV daily × 3–5 days
	Cyclophosphamide 30–60 mg/kg (or 900–2000 mg/m^2) total
TBI +/– Flu	100–200 cGy total
	Fludarabine 90–150 mg/m^2 total
TLI-ATG	800 cGy total

ATG, antithymocyte globulin; cGy, centiGray; TBI, total body irradiation; TLI, total lymphoid irradiation; XRT, x-ray radiation therapy.
[a]Regimens are employed in allogeneic transplants unless indicated by (auto) designation.
[b]Many regimens have been administered with or without ATG.

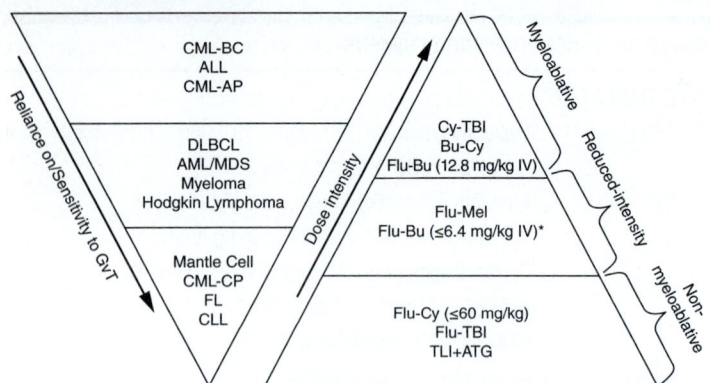

ALL: acute lymphoblastic leukemia: AML: acute myeloid leukemia; CLL: chronic lymphocytic leukemia; CML: chronic myeloid leukemia (AP – acute phase, BC – blast crisis, CP – chronic phase); DLBCL: diffuse large B-cell lymphoma; FL: follicular lymphoma; MDS: myelodysplastic syndrome. ATG: anti-thymocyte globulin; Bu: busulfan; Cy: cytoxan; Flu: bludarabine; Mel: melphalan; TBI: total body irradiation; TLI: total lymphocyte irradiation.
*Original consensus criteria for busulfan-containing regiments: MA 16 mg/kg p.o and RIC ≤8 mg/kg p.o.

FIGURE 38-1 Intensities of graft-versus-tumor effect and conditioning regimens.

greatly expanded the application of HCT and enabled recipients from ethnic populations not well-represented in international bone marrow donor registries to undergo HCT. Since the first successful umbilical cord transplantation in 1988, single and double umbilical cord transplants have been performed with acceptable rates of GVHD and favorable survival profiles compared to other unrelated donor sources. However, this comes at a cost, both literally in terms of $20,000–$30,000 per cord unit and in terms of slower engraftment, higher rates of infectious complications, and lack of availability of donor cells for future immune manipulation.

Transplants from haploidentical-related donors are also becoming more prevalent and offer the option of subsequent donor lymphocyte infusions if indicated. Haploidentical HCT has historically been complicated by higher rates of GVHD and transplant-related mortality requiring aggressive T-cell depletion and immunosuppressive strategies, which potentially compromise any increased GVT effect created by the recipient-donor HLA disparity. However, innovative approaches employing intensified immunosuppression (e.g., posttransplant high-dose cyclophosphamide) have resulted in survival outcomes comparable to those of other alternative donor sources (8). At this point, how to choose among these alternative sources for patients without fully-matched donors is not clear, but retrospective analyses as well as prospective studies are ongoing to better define optimal donor sources for HCT (9).

AUTOLOGOUS HCT

■ INDICATIONS

The principal indications for autologous HCT are chemotherapy-sensitive hematologic malignancies for which other therapies have proven unsuccessful. Prospective randomized trials have demonstrated disease- (or event-)

free survival and/or overall survival advantages for several hematologic malignancies including: (1) recurrent chemotherapy-sensitive aggressive non-Hodgkin lymphoma, (2) recurrent chemotherapy-sensitive indolent non-Hodgkin lymphoma, (3) recurrent Hodgkin lymphoma, and (4) multiple myeloma (Table 38-1). Emerging indications for patients in first remission include mantle cell lymphoma, peripheral T-cell lymphoma, and primary CNS lymphoma; the timing of autologous HCT for multiple myeloma in the era of modern therapies is an active area of investigation. Autologous HCT has also been performed in patients with treatment-refractory autoimmune diseases. Durable remissions have been achieved in patients with systemic lupus erythematosis, scleroderma, multiple sclerosis, and idiopathic thrombocytopenic purpura.

■ TOXICITIES

The risks of high-dose chemotherapy followed by autologous HCT include early toxicities of chemotherapy (e.g., gastrointestinal toxicities, oropharyngeal mucositis, severe pancytopenia with risk of infection and/or hemorrhage, and organ injury such as interstitial pneumonitis and hepatic veno-occlusive disease [VOD]) and late toxicities (particularly secondary malignancies, such as myelodysplastic syndrome or AML, after prior use of alkylating agents). Early (before day 100 post-HCT) mortality after autologous SCT is now <5%. Depending on the underlying disease and the conditioning regimen, late secondary hematologic malignancy risk may be as high as 5%–10%. The specific patterns of toxicity and the pharmacokinetics vary with each high-dose chemotherapy regimen.

■ OUTCOMES

The outcomes of autologous HCT are variable and depend upon the nature and the remission status of the underlying disease. For example, a 3-year disease-free survival probability of approximately 40% has been achieved following autologous HCT for recurrent chemotherapy-sensitive diffuse large B-cell lymphoma (DLBCL) versus 80% for grade III follicular lymphoma. The primary reason for treatment failure is recurrent lymphoma, which occurs in ≥50% of patients with aggressive NHL after HCT. An active area of investigation within NHL is which subgroups of lymphoma might benefit from HCT in first remission versus the relapsed setting. In multiple myeloma, autologous HCT is pursued not for cure but rather to prolong time without symptoms and progression-free and, possibly, overall survival; in this setting, 3-year survival rates are greater than 70% (10).

ALLOGENEIC HCT

■ INDICATIONS

Indications for allogeneic HCT include a variety of congenital disorders (e.g., sickle cell anemia), acquired life-threatening hematopoietic stem cell diseases (e.g., severe aplastic anemia), and a wide variety of malignant diseases (Table 38-1). The majority of allogeneic transplants in adults are performed for AML, MDS, and ALL. Advances in our understanding of the diverse molecular underpinnings of each of these diseases have led to improved risk stratification and decision making as to which patients will benefit from transplantation. At present, allogeneic HCT is recommended or considered for all patients with AML except for those who exhibit core binding factor mutations (i.e., inv(16) or t(8;21)), those with normal cytogenetics carrying a mutated NPM1 and wild-type FLT 3, and possibly those with CEBPa mutations (11). Allogeneic HCT is considered even for older patients given the availability of RIC regimens.

■ TOXICITIES

The early toxicities of myeloablative allogeneic HCT are similar to those of autologous HCT but there is a considerably higher mortality risk, even in the reduced-intensity setting. Selected conditioning regimens are shown in Table 38-2, with use of fludarabine and busulfan-containing regimens in the allogeneic setting increasing in recent years. Some notable complications of any HCT, but particularly of allogeneic HCT, include liver, pulmonary, and renal toxicity. Hepatic VOD is a syndrome characterized by the constellation of weight gain, ascites, right upper quadrant pain, and liver dysfunction often leading to subsequent renal or multiorgan system failure. Data have suggested that defibrotide administration can improve the survival rate in severe VOD from less than 20% to over 40% if started soon after diagnosis (12). Pulmonary complications include diffuse alveolar haemorrhage which usually occurs within 30 days of transplant and idiopathic pneumonia syndrome which typically presents later. Both are treated with high-dose glucocorticoids and potentially anti-TNF agents (e.g., etanercept), but both carry high mortality rates despite aggressive therapy (13). A feared complication that may manifest early or late is thrombotic microangiopathy and nephropathy, which reflects endothelial injury provoked by multiple agents including chemotherapies, infection, GVHD, radiation, and calcineurin inhibitors (14). Care is usually supportive and involves minimizing exacerbating medications and further insults.

■ OUTCOMES

The outcomes of allogeneic HCT vary widely by disease status, conditioning regimen, age, comorbidities, and severity of subsequent GVHD. Probabilities of 3-year overall survival can range from 76% after an MRD transplantation for CML in chronic phase to 19% in Philadelphia chromosome-positive ALL not in remission at the time of an MRD transplant (1).

GRAFT-VERSUS-HOST DISEASE

One of the most challenging and actively investigated sequelae of allogeneic HCT is graft-versus-host disease (GVHD). Patients with acute and especially chronic GVHD have a lower probability of relapse of their underlying malignancy. In some hematologic malignancies, this reduction in relapse probability has translated into an overall survival advantage (e.g., most advanced acute leukemias), especially when GVHD is present to a moderate degree. In other settings, the mortality risk of the GVHD has negated any beneficial antitumor effect and has not conferred a survival advantage after allogeneic transplantation (e.g., "good risk" AML in first remission). (For full discussion of the pathophysiology of and therapies for GVHD, see Chapter 37.)

■ ACUTE GVHD

The risk of an allogeneic HCT recipient developing some degree of acute GVHD ranges from 20% to 80%, depending on histocompatability of the donor and recipient and the GVHD prophylaxis strategy used (15). Acute GVHD is a multiorgan system disease initiated by immunocompetent T cells in the donor graft. The primary targets involved by acute GVHD are the skin (rash), gastrointestinal tract (nausea, vomiting, diarrhea), and liver (jaundice, enzyme elevation).

■ CHRONIC GVHD

Chronic GVHD, which typically presents several months after HCT, occurs in 40%–80% of patients and is manifested by a wider spectrum of organ involvement. Chronic GVHD mimics many classic autoimmune disorders with, for example, sclerodermatous skin changes, a Sjögren's disease-like sicca complex, esophageal dysmotility, and cholestatic hepatopathy. An acute/chronic GVHD overlap syndrome has also been described and is associated with a worse prognosis as compared to chronic GVHD (15). The prognosis of GVHD is related to its stage, which is dependent upon the severity of individual organ involvement, and response to treatment.

■ TREATMENT

GVHD may be effectively prevented by in vivo or ex vivo depletion of T cells from the donor graft. T-cell depletion of a graft, however, is complicated by a higher rate of engraftment failure and a higher risk of relapse (owing to the loss of a GVT effect). An arsenal of immunosuppressive drugs is available to manage GVHD, with calcineurin inhibitor-based combinations being the basis of pharmacoprophylaxis and glucocorticoids being the first-line therapy for both acute and chronic GVHD (Table 38-3). While management of grades I–II acute GVHD is usually successful, more advanced (grades III–IV) GVHD is more difficult to manage, with mortality rates of greater than 50%. Reasons for treatment failure and mortality secondary to GVHD are myriad but opportunistic infections are prominent.

INFECTIOUS COMPLICATIONS AND MONITORING

Many of the advances in HCT over the past three decades have been the result of better prevention of infectious complications and prevention and treatment of GVHD. Anti-infective prophylaxis is now routinely employed given the severely immune compromised state of the peritransplant period and the continued impairment of cellular and humoral immunity which lasts for months to years after transplantation. Guidelines established by the CDC/ASBMT/IDSA recommend (16):

- Quinolone prophylaxis for neutropenia expected to last 7 days or more.
- Antifungal prophylaxis with fluconazole or micafungin preengraftment; prophylaxis with voriconazole or posaconazole after engraftment, particularly in the setting of GVHD.
- Antiviral (CMV, HSV, VZV) prophylaxis with acyclovir or equivalent antiviral therapy.
- Anti-*Pneumocystis* prophylaxis with trimethoprim-sulfamethoxazole.

TABLE 38-3 GVHD-RELATED THERAPIES

Prophylaxis	Treatment
Calcineurin inhibitor: (cyclosporine or tacrolimus) +	Glucocorticoids ±
• Methotrexate or	• Calcineurin inhibitor and/or
• MMF or	• anti-TNF therapy and/or
• Sirolimus versus	• MMF and/or
in or ex vivo T-cell depletion	• Sirolimus and/or
	• Polyclonal (e.g., antithymocyte globulin) or monoclonal T-cell antibodies (e.g., anti-IL2R, anti-IL2, anti-CD3, anti-CD25, anti-CD52)
	• Extracorporeal phototherapy

GVHD, graft-versus-host disease; IL2R, IL-2 receptor; MMF, mycophenolate mofetil; TNF, tumor necrosis factor.

Newer generation broad-spectrum antibiotics, new antiviral agents, and antifungal agents with reduced toxicity and a broader spectrum of coverage are available for patients with suspected or established opportunistic infections.

Cytomegalovirus (CMV), one of the chief infectious causes of mortality in the early allogeneic HCT experience, may be prevented by donor selection (CMV-seronegative donors for CMV-seronegative recipients whenever possible), the routine monitoring for CMV reactivation posttransplant (by PCR-based or antigenemia assays), and the preemptive use of ganciclovir for patients with demonstrated viremia. With the more widespread use of umbilical cord blood donors, an increased incidence of viral infections has been observed (accounting for 30% of deaths), particularly infections with BK virus, EBV and resulting lymphoproliferative diseases, adenovirus, and HHV-6. Neurologic manifestations of HHV-6 have been reported and routine monitoring for EBV and HHV-6 in addition to CMV is advised in UCB settings (17) (Figure 38-2).

Other important supportive care measures include red blood cell and platelet transfusional support. Blood products are irradiated to prevent transfusion-associated GVHD, and third-generation leukocyte reduction filters are used to prevent allosensitization, febrile nonhemolytic transfusion reactions, and CMV transmission. Total parenteral nutrition is often required because of poor oral nutrition resulting from oropharyngeal mucositis and frequent nausea and vomiting.

FUTURE DIRECTIONS

Hematopoietic HCT has become more widely applicable in large part secondary to the expansion of donor sources (i.e., matched or mismatched unrelated donors, haploidentical donors, and umbilical cord blood) and the expansion of eligibility criteria to include many patients who were previously believed to be too old or too ill to have a transplant (i.e., through RIC

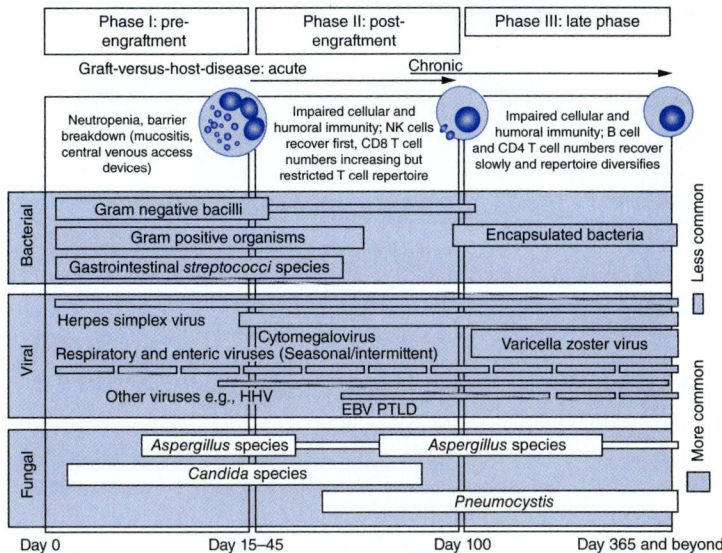

FIGURE 38-2 Immune defenses and susceptibility to infection post HCT. EBV, Epstein-Barr virus; HHV, human herpesvirus 6; NK, natural killer; PTLD, posttransplant lymphoproliferative disease. (From Mackall C, Fry T, Gress R, et al. Background to hematopoietic cell transplantation, including posttransplant immune recovery. *Bone Marrow Transplantation.* 2009; 44: 457–462.)

or NMA conditioning, improved supportive care, etc.). Further improvement in the outcomes of HCT may stem from the approaches listed below:

- *Disease-specific:* More effective eradication of the underlying disease, via targeted or maintenance therapies (e.g., FLT 3-inhibitors, lenalidomide, radiolabeled antibodies, adoptive therapy using chimeric T-cell receptors) and targeting of the malignant, noncycling stem cell.
- *Patient selection:* Improvement in identifying those patients at less risk for relapse in whom transplant-related mortality can be avoided by choosing less-intensive conditioning.
- *Regimen selection:* Clarification of disease and patient populations for whom specific conditioning and stem cell combinations yield the greatest overall survival.
- *Engraftment/immune reconstitution:* Especially for umbilical cord transplants, enhanced immune reconstitution by ex vivo or in vivo expansion or by better selection of units.
- *Separation of GVT from GVHD:* Manipulation of the initial immunologic platform via adoptive immunotherapy to: (1) enhance reactivity to tumor antigens (e.g., via NK- or T-cell or DC subset manipulation) and (2) decrease global alloreactivity (e.g., via depletion of alloreactive T-cell subsets, augmenting regulatory T-cell populations, or insertion of suicide gene cassettes) (18, 19).

Our understanding of the biology of malignant stem cells and characterization of the immune cells involved in GVT and GVHD are continually improving in concert with early-phase clinical trials introducing new classes of agents into the transplant arena (20). Advances in relapse-free and overall survival outcomes following HCT are expected to result from these emerging and promising therapies.

REFERENCES

1. Pasquini MC, Wang Z. Current use and outcome of hematopoietic stem cell transplantation: CIBMTR Summary Slides, 2011. Available at: http://www.cibmtr.org.

2. Parmar S, Fernandez-Vina M, de Lima M. Novel transplant strategies for generating graft-versus-leukemia effect in acute myeloid leukemia. *Curr Opin Hematol.* 2011; 18: 98–104.

3. Deeg HJ, Sandmaier BM. Who is fit for allogeneic transplantation? *Blood.* 2010; 116:4726–4770.

4. Sorror ML. Comorbidities and hematopoietic cell transplantation outcomes. *Hematology Am Soc Hematol Educ Program.* 2010; 237–247.

5. Bacigalupo A, Ballen K, Rizzo D, et al. Defining the intensity of conditioning regimens: working definitions. *Biol Blood Marrow Transplant.* 2009; 15: 1628–1633.

6. Leis J, Porter D. Unrelated donor leukocyte infusions to treat relapse after unrelated donor bone marrow transplantation. *Leuk Lymphoma.* 2002; 43: 9–17.

7. Anasetti C, Logan BR, Lee SJ, et al. Increased incidence of chronic graft-versus-host disease (GVHD) and no survival advantage with Filgrastim-mobilized peripheral blood stem cells (PBSC) compared to bone marrow (BM) transplants from unrelated donors: results of Blood and Marrow Transplant Clinical Trials Network (BMT CTN) Protocol 0201, a phase III, prospective, randomized trial [abstract]. In: ASH Annual Meeting Abstracts. *Blood.* 2011; 118: 3. Abstract #1.

8. Brunstein CG, Fuchs EJ, Carter SL, et al. Alternative donor transplantation after reduced intensity conditioning: results of parallel phase II trials using partially HLA-mismatched related bone marrow or unrelated double umbilical cord blood grafts. *Blood.* 2011; 118: 282–288.

9. Ballen KK, Koreth J, Chen YB, et al. Selection of optimal alternative graft source: mismatched unrelated donor, umbilical cord blood, or haploidentical transplant. *Blood.* 2012; 119:1972–1980.

10. Palumbo A, Attal M, Roussel M. Shifts in the therapeutic paradigm for patients newly diagnosed with multiple myeloma: maintenance therapy and overall survival. *Clin Can Res.* 2011; 17: 1253–1263.

11. Grimwade D, Mrozek K. Diagnostic and prognostic value of cytogenetics in acute myeloid leukemia. *Hematol Oncol Clin N Am.* 2011; 25: 1135–1161.

12. Richardson PG, Soiffer RJ, Antin JH, et al. Defibrotide for the treatment of severe hepatic veno-occlusive disease and multiorgan failure after

stem cell transplantation: a multicenter, randomized, dose-finding trial. *Biol Blood Marrow Transplant.* 2010; 16: 1005–1017.

13. Afessa B, Abdulai RM, Kremers WK, et al. Risk factors and outcome of pulmonary complications after autologous hematopoietic stem cell transplant (HSCT). *Chest.* 2012; 141: 442–450.

14. Laskin BL, Goebel J, Davies SM, Jodele S. Small vessels, big trouble in the kidneys and beyond: hematopoietic stem cell transplantation-associated thrombotic microangiopathy. *Blood.* 2011; 118: 1452–1462.

15. Ferrara JL, Levine JE, Reddy P, Holler E. Graft-versus-host disease. *Lancet.* 2009; 373: 1550–1561.

16. Tomblyn M, Chiller T, Einsele H, et al. Guidelines for preventing infectious complications among hematopoietic cell transplant recipients: a global perspective. *Biol Blood Marrow Transplant.* 2009; 15: 1143–1238.

17. Mackall C, Fry T, Gress R, et al. Background to hematopoietic cell transplantation, including post transplant immune recovery. *Bone Marrow Transplantation.* 2009; 44: 457–462.

18. Alyea EP, DeAngelo DJ, Moldrem J, et al. NCI first international workshop on the biology, prevention, and treatment of relapse after allogeneic hematopoietic stem cell transplantation: report from the committee on prevention of relapse following allogeneic cell transplantation for hematologic malignancies. *Biol Bone Marrow Transplant.* 2010; 16: 1037–1069.

19. Miller JS, Warren EH, van den Brink MRM, et al. NCI first international workshop on the biology, prevention, and treatment of relapse after allogeneic hematopoietic stem cell transplantation: report from the committee on the biology underlying recurrence of malignant disease following allogeneic HSCT: graft-versus-tumor/leukemia reaction. *Biol Bone Marrow Transplant.* 2010; 16: 565–586.

20. Reddy P, de Lima, M, Koreth J. Emerging therapies in hematopoietic stem cell transplantation. *Biol Bone Marrow Transplant.* 2012; 18: S125–S131.

SECTION 8 | GU Oncology

CHAPTER **39**
Renal Cell Carcinoma
M. Dror Michaelson

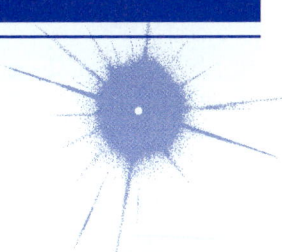

INTRODUCTION

The incidence of renal cell carcinoma (RCC) in the United States has been rising steadily, with an estimated 65,150 cases and 13,680 deaths in 2013 (1). RCC is the 6th most common malignancy in men and the 8th in women with a male-to-female ratio of 1.6:1. The majority of patients are now identified through incidental findings on imaging studies. Fortunately, the prognosis of early stage disease is excellent. However, 25% of patients have advanced disease at initial presentation, and metastatic disease is generally considered incurable. The median survival for patients with metastatic disease historically was 12–15 months, with 5-year survival of 10% (2). However, this appears to have changed over the past decade, as advances in the understanding of RCC biology combined with the development of novel targeted therapies have improved and redefined management of advanced RCC.

ETIOLOGY AND PATHOGENESIS

Numerous environmental, lifestyle, and genetic factors have been linked to the development of RCC, including cigarette smoking and obesity. Different pathologic types of RCC have been identified including clear cell, papillary, chromophobe, collecting duct, medullary, and unclassified RCC (Table 39-1) (2). High-grade variants with spindle cell differentiation are described as having sarcomatoid growth patterns and typically confer a poor prognosis (3). There are important biologic, prognostic, and therapeutic distinctions between these different diseases.

Several hereditary syndromes predispose patients to RCC (4). Insight into Von Hippel Lindau (VHL) disease has formed the foundation of our understanding of clear cell RCC, which accounts for 75% of renal cancer and >90% of metastatic RCC. The VHL tumor suppressor gene is located on chromosome 3, and in the hereditary form of clear cell RCC, one allele is inherited as an abnormal gene. Development of RCC occurs when the second allele is altered by deletion, hypermethylation, or mutational inactivation. Biallelic gene alteration leads to loss of function of the tumor suppressor protein and is observed in nearly 100% of the hereditary cases as well as >75% of sporadic cases of clear cell renal carcinoma. The VHL protein normally functions to inhibit cellular growth and is involved in regulating the expression of several proangiogenic genes. Under normal oxygen conditions, the VHL protein targets the hypoxia-inducible factor (HIF) family of transcription factors for ubiquitination and degradation. Biallelic loss or

501

TABLE 39-1 HISTOLOGIC CHARACTERIZATION

Histologic Cell Type Survival	Frequency (%)	Syndrome	Gene	5 Years
Clear cell	60–75	VHL disease/HP FCRC	VHL/SDHB 3p del	~60%
Papillary	12	HPRC HLRCC	MET FH	~80%
Chromophobe	4	BHD syndrome	BHD	~90%
Oncocytoma	4	BHD syndrome	BHD	Benign
Collecting Duct	<1	–	–	<5%
Medullary	<1	–	Sickle trait	Rare

FCRC, familial clear cell renal cancer; FH, fumarate hydratase; HLRCC, hereditary leiomyomatosis and renal cell cancer; HP, hereditary paraganglioma; HPRC, hereditary papillary renal carcinoma; SDHB, succinate dehydrogenase B.

inactivation of VHL leads to constitutive upregulation of intracellular HIF proteins with subsequent increased expression of downstream gene targets including vascular endothelial growth factor (VEGF), transforming growth factor (TGF), and others.

The pathogenesis of non-clear cell RCC is entirely different. Various other mutations have been linked to development of papillary or chromophobe subtypes of RCC. These include activating mutations of the MET proto-oncogene at 7q31.3, mutations of the Birt-Hogg-Dube gene on chromosome 17, mutations in the fumarate hydratase gene, and others (5).

An additional important intracellular pathway identified in RCC is the mammalian target of rapamycin (mTOR) pathway, and agents that inhibit mTOR have proven efficacy in RCC as well (6). Genetic mutations in this pathway have not been identified in renal cancer.

CLINICAL PRESENTATION

A majority of patients diagnosed with RCC are asymptomatic at the time of presentation. The classic triad of hematuria, abdominal pain, and flank/abdominal mass is observed in fewer than 5% of patients. Patients with RCC may present with a wide range of signs and symptoms including hematuria, anemia, pain, or constitutional symptoms such as weight loss. Paraneoplastic syndromes associated with RCC include polycythemia, nonmetastatic liver enzyme abnormalities (Stauffer syndrome), hypercalcemia, and others.

The cure rate for localized RCC following definitive local therapy is dependent primarily on stage, with >90% long-term disease-free survival for stages 1 and 2, but closer to 50% 5-year disease-free survival for stage 3 (see Tables 39-2 and 39-3). Of those who undergo surgical resection of apparently localized disease, about 33% will eventually develop disease recurrence. RCC can metastasize to nearly any anatomic location but most commonly metastasizes to the lungs, mediastinum, retroperitoneum, adrenals, bone, pancreas, liver, or CNS.

TABLE 39-2 STAGING CLASSIFICATION

Primary tumor (T)

TX	Primary tumor cannot be assessed
T0	No evidence of primary tumor
T1	Tumor 7 cm or less in greatest dimension limited to the kidney
T1a	Tumor 4 cm or less in greatest dimension limited to the kidney
T1b	Tumor more than 4 cm but not more than 7 cm in greatest dimension limited to the kidney
T2	Tumor more than 7 cm in greatest dimension limited to the kidney
T2a	Tumor more than 7 cm but less than or equal to 10 cm in greatest dimension limited to the kidney
T2b	Tumor more than 10 cm limited to the kidney
T3	Tumor extends into major veins or perinephric tissues but not into the ipsilateral adrenal gland and not beyond Gerota's fascia
T3a	Tumor grossly extends into the renal vein or its segmental (muscle containing) branches, or tumor invades perirenal and/or renal sinus fat but not beyond Gerota's fascia
T3b	Tumor grossly extends into the vena cava below the diaphragm
T3c	Tumor grossly extends into the vena cava above the diaphragm or invades the wall of the vena cava
T4	Tumor invades beyond Gerota's fascia (including contiguous extension into the ipsilateral adrenal gland)

Regional lymph nodes (N)

NX	Regional lymph nodes cannot be assessed
N0	No regional lymph node metastasis
N1	Metastasis in regional lymph node(s)

Distant metastasis (M)

M0	No distant metastasis
M1	Distant metastasis

Stage grouping

Stage I	T1	N0	M0
Stage II	T2	N0	M0
Stage III	T1 or T2	N1	M0
	T3	N0 or N1	M0
Stage IV	T4	Any N	M0
	Any T	Any N	M1

(Used with the permission of the American Joint Committee on Cancer [AJCC], Chicago, Illinois. The original source for this material is Edge SB et al [eds]. *AJCC Cancer Staging Manual,* 7th edition. New York, Springer, 2010. www.springeronline.com.)

TABLE 39-3 FIVE-YEAR SURVIVAL CORRELATES CLOSELY WITH TNM STAGING

TNM stage	% 5-Year survival
T1	95
T2	88
T3	59
T4	20
M1	10–20

For diagnostic evaluation of suspected RCC, either CT or MRI of the abdomen is highly sensitive and specific. They have largely replaced intravenous pyelograms. Initial evaluations should also include the following:

- Family history screening for familial syndromes, especially if <50 years of age.
- Chest x-ray or chest CT scan.
- Consider MRI evaluation for involvement of renal vein and inferior vena cava.
- Note that bone scintigraphy and positron emission tomography (PET) scan are insensitive for RCC, and are not routinely recommended.

PROGNOSIS

Prognosis in RCC is closely related to T-N-M staging (Table 39-3). In advanced RCC, prognosis can be stratified according to well-characterized poor risk features. A common classification system in patients undergoing initial therapy for metastatic RCC uses five clinical criteria (Table 39-4) (7):

- Impaired Karnofsky performance status
- Elevated serum lactate dehydrogenase
- Low hemoglobin
- Less than 1-year interval from initial RCC diagnosis to start of systemic therapy
- Elevated serum calcium

It is important to note that prognostic system was developed prior to the availability of targeted therapies. Prognosis for patients beyond initial

TABLE 39-4 PROGNOSTIC FACTORS IN METASTATIC RCC

Risk Group	Number of Risk Factors	Median Survival (Months)	% of Patients
Favorable	0	20	25
Intermediate	1–2	10	53
Poor	3 or more	4	22

Note: Median survival times were estimated prior to the development of targeted therapy.

therapy can also be stratified based on clinical risk factors and has important implications with regard to subsequent therapy (8).

TREATMENT
■ LOCALIZED DISEASE

- *Radical nephrectomy* has long been standard of care for localized RCC, and consists of removal of Gerota's fascia, kidney, ureter, ipsilateral adrenal gland, and adjacent hilar lymph nodes (LNs).
- *Nephron-sparing surgery (partial nephrectomy)* is a preferred alternative in selected patients for whom it is feasible. Multiple case series support long-term outcomes that include cancer control, safety, and feasibility.
- *Percutaneous ablation (radiofrequency ablation [RFA] or cryotherapy)* may be an alternative in selected patients who cannot tolerate definitive surgical resection. Single-center case series have shown excellent outcomes and good tolerability with RFA in tumors <4 cm.

■ ADJUVANT THERAPY

Several studies have evaluated the role of adjuvant therapy for patients with RCC. To date, none has demonstrated benefit. In one study, 283 patients with T3-T4a or N1 disease were randomized to observation or interferon (IFN)-α following nephrectomy and lymphadenectomy (9). After a 10-year median follow-up, there was no difference in overall survival or relapse-free survival. Another randomized study with high-dose interleukin-2 (IL2) compared to observation was terminated early after an interim analysis for futility (10). With the advent of effective targeted therapies, a new generation of adjuvant clinical trials is being carried out in patients at high risk of recurrence. These trials are designed to evaluate efficacy and feasibility of sunitinib, sorafenib, pazopanib, everolimus, and others (11). While results are awaited, the standard of care remains clinical trial participation or active surveillance.

■ METASTATIC DISEASE

RCC is relatively resistant to cytotoxic chemotherapy and to radiation therapy with a median survival that was measured in months until recently. The natural history of advanced RCC is substantially varied, as some cases progress rapidly while others exhibit spontaneous tumor regressions. Immunotherapy with IFN or IL2 has been studied extensively and was the mainstay of systemic therapy prior to the development of targeted agents.

In the wake of new biologic insights, particularly for clear cell RCC, a wave of important therapeutic advances has transformed management of metastatic disease and resulted in improved outcomes for the majority of patients. Between 2005 and 2012, seven new targeted agents were approved by the U.S. FDA for the treatment of advanced RCC (Table 39-5). Nevertheless, curative treatments are still lacking and clinical trial participation should be encouraged whenever possible.

SURGERY

Two prospective phase III randomized trials evaluated the benefit of nephrectomy in patients with metastatic RCC (12, 13). Both studies demonstrated a statistically significant increase in median survival for patients

TABLE 39-5 APPROVED TARGETED AGENTS IN ADVANCED RCC

Agent	Target	Phase III Patient Population	Phase III Median PFS (Months)
Sunitinib	VEGF receptor	Front line good/intermediate	11
Pazopanib	VEGF receptor	Front line good/intermediate	11
Axitinib	VEGF receptor	Second line	6.7
Sorafenib	VEGF receptor	Second line	4.7–5.5*
Bevacizumab	VEGF ligand	Front line good/intermediate	8.4–10.2†
Temsirolimus	mTOR	Front line poor risk	5.5
Everolimus	mTOR	Second line following TKI	4.0

*Based on two phase III trials.
†In combination with interferon, based on two phase III trials.
mTOR, mammalian target of rapamycin; PFS, progression free survival; TKI, tyrosine kinase inhibitor; VEGF, vascular endothelial growth factor.

treated with nephrectomy followed by IFN when compared with IFN alone. The results of these studies support the role of nephrectomy in selected patients with good performance status. The role of nephrectomy in the era of targeted therapy has not been prospectively established but appears to be beneficial (14). Randomized studies are ongoing.

Surgical management of solitary metastases, both synchronous and metachronous, should be strongly considered in selected patients.

CHEMOTHERAPY

Metastatic RCC is refractory to cytotoxic chemotherapeutic agents in multiple phase II trials (15). Attempts to combine cytokine therapy with cytotoxic agents have not led to clearly improved outcomes and should not be used outside of clinical trials. More recently, combinations of cytotoxic chemotherapy with targeted therapy are being investigated but should generally not be considered outside of clinical trial participation. An exception may be rare histologic subtypes of RCC such as sarcomatoid or collecting duct cancers, in which use of chemotherapy may be beneficial.

IMMUNOTHERAPY

Until 2005, high-dose IL2 was the only approved treatment for metastatic RCC in the United States. While the overall response rate to IL2 is only 10%–15%, the major appeal of high-dose IL2 is the small but measurable rate of durable complete responses (16). The major limitation to treatment with high-dose IL2, other than low response rate, is the morbidity and mortality of treatment side effects including severe hypotension and capillary leak syndrome. High-dose IL2 should only be administered in experienced centers with the necessary monitoring and supportive measures available.

TARGETED THERAPY

Improved understanding of tumorigenesis in clear cell RCC has led to novel therapeutic approaches aimed at inhibiting the VEGF and mTOR pathways (Table 39-5). Bevacizumab, a monoclonal antibody against VEGF ligand, was evaluated in a randomized phase II study (17). There was a significant difference in time to progression: 2.5 months in the placebo arm compared with 4.8 months in the high-dose arm. This proof of concept study of single-agent VEGF inhibition opened up an entirely new approach to RCC. Since then, five antiangiogenic agents have gained approval on the strength of proven efficacy in phase III trials, including sunitinib, pazopanib, axitinib, sorafenib, and bevaizumab (18–23). Additional experimental agents targeting this pathway are under late stages of investigation, including tivozanib, dovitinib, aflibercept, and others.

Sunitinib is a multitargeted tyrosine kinase inhibitor (TKI) of the VEGF receptor and other receptors, and was tested in a randomized phase III trial versus IFN in the first-line treatment of metastatic clear cell RCC (19). Sunitinib demonstrated an improvement in progression-free survival (PFS) of 11 versus 5 months, and in overall response rate of 47% versus 12% in comparison to IFN (24). On the basis of this study, sunitinib is considered the reference standard for initial therapy of good and intermediate-risk advanced RCC. Sunitinib is typically administered at 50 mg daily on a 4-week on/2-week off schedule, which is likely superior to continuous dosing at a lower dosage (25). Pazopanib is another tyrosine kinase inhibitor of the VEGF receptor, among others, and had a similar 11-month PFS in front-line treatment of advanced RCC (21). Bevacizumab combined with IFN was superior to IFN alone in two similar phase III trials (22, 23), although the single-agent activity of bevacizumab in front-line therapy has not yet been fully defined.

Sorafenib, an inhibitor of the VEGF receptor in addition to b-raf and other targets, demonstrated a significant improvement in PFS compared with placebo in second-line treatment of RCC following cytokines (18). A second-generation TKI, axitinib, which has greater specificity for the VEGF receptor, was tested in a head-to-head study with sorafenib. Axitinib was superior to sorafenib with a median PFS of 6.7 versus 4.7 months in second-line treatment (20).

Adverse effects are commonly observed with VEGF-targeted agents and often limit dosing (Table 39-6). Attempts at combination therapy with targeted agents to date have appeared to increase toxicity without a clear benefit in efficacy (26, 27). The most frequently observed side effects with antiangiogenic drugs include hypertension, fatigue, diarrhea, hand-foot syndrome, hypothyroidism, and others.

The mTOR pathway has also emerged as an important target in advanced RCC. Temsirolimus is an mTOR inhibitor that is administered intravenously once weekly. In a phase III trial of patients with poor-risk RCC, temsirolimus significantly improved overall survival compared with IFN (10.9 vs. 7.3 months) (28). Rash, peripheral edema, hyperglycemia, and hyperlipidemia were the most common side effects. Everolimus is an oral mTOR inhibitor, and demonstrated improved PFS versus placebo in patients previously treated with antiangiogenic therapy (4.0 vs. 1.9 months) (29).

TABLE 39-6 COMMON ADVERSE EFFECTS OF TARGETED AGENTS IN ADVANCED RCC

Adverse Event	Bevacizumab	Sunitinib	Sorafenib	Pazopanib	Axitinib	Temsirolimus	Everolimus
Fatigue	+	++	+	+	+	+	+
Rash	–	–	+	–	–	+	+
Hand-foot syndrome	–	+	++	+	–	–	–
Hypertension	++	+	++	+	++	–	–
Diarrhea	–	+	+	+	+	+	+
Stomatitis	–	+	–	–	–	+	+
LFT elevation	–	+	–	++	–	+	+
Metabolic syndrome	–	–	–	–	–	+	+
Proteinuria	++	–	–	–	–	–	–
Pneumonitis	–	–	–	–	–	+	+

Adverse effects were similar to those with temsirolimus, including a low-but-measurable incidence of pneumonitis (8% any grade, 3% grade ≥3 with everolimus). On the basis of this study, everolimus has been considered a standard option for second-line therapy following failure of antiangiogenic therapy in advanced RCC.

FUTURE DIRECTIONS

Localized RCC is generally effectively treated with either open or laparoscopic surgery. Increasingly used nephron-sparing approaches include partial nephrectomy and percutaneous ablation. Adjuvant medical therapy is an area of active research, but currently surveillance remains standard of care following definitive local therapy. While the treatment of advanced RCC has been transformed by the advent of targeted therapy, novel therapies aimed at achieving durable complete responses are urgently needed. Mechanisms of resistance to VEGF therapy, including alternative antiangiogenic pathways such as angiopoietin or fibroblast growth factor signaling or c-met activation, are the subject of current study that may provide insights with therapeutic implications. Novel immunotherapy approaches, such as those targeting CTLA4 and PD-1 inhibition, preliminarily appear to be promising. Additional clinical trials are evaluating sequential and combination therapy with targeted agents and immunotherapy or chemotherapy. Finally, identification of predictive factors of response, along with biomarker development, remains a crucial area of research for guiding selection of optimal therapy in individual patients.

REFERENCES

1. Siegel R, Naishadham D, Jemal A. Cancer statistics, 2013. *CA Cancer J Clin.* 2013; 63: 11–30.

2. Linehan WM, Bates SE, Yang JC. Cancer of the kidney. In Devita V, Lawrence T, Rosenberg S (eds.), *Cancer: Principles and Practice of Oncology* (7th ed). Philadelphia, Lippincott Williams & Wilkins, 2011, 1161–1182.

3. Cheville JC, Lohse CM, Zincke H, et al. Sarcomatoid renal cell carcinoma: an examination of underlying histologic subtype and an analysis of associations with patient outcome. *Am J Surg Pathol.* 2004; 28: 435–441.

4. Iliopoulos O, Eng C. Genetic and clinical aspects of familial renal neoplasms. *Semin Oncol.* 2000; 27: 138–149.

5. Linehan WM. The genetic basis of kidney cancer: implications for management and use of targeted therapeutic approaches. *Eur Urol.* 2012; 61: 896–898.

6. Voss MH, Molina AM, Motzer RJ. mTOR inhibitors in advanced renal cell carcinoma. *Hematol Oncol Clin North Am.* 2011; 25: 835–852.

7. Motzer RJ, Mazumdar M, Bacik J, et al. Survival and prognostic stratification of 670 patients with advanced renal cell carcinoma. *J Clin Oncol.* 1999; 17: 2530–2540.

8. Heng DY, Xie W, Regan MM, et al. Prognostic factors for overall survival in patients with metastatic renal cell carcinoma treated with vascular endothelial growth factor-targeted agents: results from a large, multicenter study. *J Clin Oncol.* 2009; 27: 5794–5799.

9. Messing EM, Manola J, Wilding G, et al. Phase III study of interferon alfa-NL as adjuvant treatment for resectable renal cell carcinoma: an Eastern Cooperative Oncology Group/Intergroup trial. *J Clin Oncol.* 2003; 21: 1214–1222.

10. Clark JI, Atkins MB, Urba WJ, et al. Adjuvant high-dose bolus interleukin-2 for patients with high-risk renal cell carcinoma: a cytokine working group randomized trial. *J Clin Oncol.* 2003; 21: 3133–3140.

11. Smaldone MC, Fung C, Uzzo RG, et al. Adjuvant and neoadjuvant therapies in high-risk renal cell carcinoma. *Hematol Oncol Clin North Am.* 2011; 25: 765–791.

12. Flanigan RC, Salmon SE, Blumenstein BA, et al. Nephrectomy followed by interferon alfa-2b compared with interferon alfa-2b alone for metastatic renal-cell cancer. *N Engl J Med.* 2001; 345: 1655–1659.

13. Mickisch GH, Garin A, van Poppel H, et al. Radical nephrectomy plus interferon-alfa-based immunotherapy compared with interferon alfa alone in metastatic renal-cell carcinoma: a randomised trial. *Lancet.* 2001; 358: 966–970.

14. Choueiri TK, Xie W, Kollmannsberger C, et al. The impact of cytoreductive nephrectomy on survival of patients with metastatic renal cell carcinoma receiving vascular endothelial growth factor targeted therapy. *J Urol.* 2011; 185: 60–66.

15. Yagoda A, Petrylak D, Thompson S. Cytotoxic chemotherapy for advanced renal cell carcinoma. *Urol Clin North Am.* 1993; 20: 303–321.

16. McDermott DF, Regan MM, Clark JI, et al. Randomized phase III trial of high-dose interleukin-2 versus subcutaneous interleukin-2 and interferon in patients with metastatic renal cell carcinoma. *J Clin Oncol.* 2005; 23: 133–141.

17. Yang JC, Haworth L, Sherry RM, et al. A randomized trial of bevacizumab, an anti-vascular endothelial growth factor antibody, for metastatic renal cancer. *N Engl J Med.* 2003; 349: 427–434.

18. Escudier B, Eisen T, Stadler WM, et al. Sorafenib in advanced clear-cell renal-cell carcinoma. *N Engl J Med.* 2007; 356: 125–134.

19. Motzer RJ, Hutson TE, Tomczak P, et al. Sunitinib versus interferon alfa in metastatic renal-cell carcinoma. *N Engl J Med.* 2007; 356: 115–124.

20. Rini BI, Escudier B, Tomczak P, et al. Comparative effectiveness of axitinib versus sorafenib in advanced renal cell carcinoma (AXIS): a randomised phase 3 trial. *Lancet.* 2011; 378: 1931–1939.

21. Sternberg CN, Davis ID, Mardiak J, et al. Pazopanib in locally advanced or metastatic renal cell carcinoma: results of a randomized phase III trial. *J Clin Oncol.* 2010; 28: 1061–1068.

22. Escudier B, Pluzanska A, Koralewski P, et al. Bevacizumab plus interferon alfa-2a for treatment of metastatic renal cell carcinoma: a randomised, double-blind phase III trial. *Lancet.* 2007; 370: 2103–2111.

23. Rini BI, Halabi S, Rosenberg JE, et al. Phase III trial of bevacizumab plus interferon alfa versus interferon alfa monotherapy in patients with metastatic renal cell carcinoma: final results of CALGB 90206. *J Clin Oncol.* 2010; 28: 2137–2143.

24. Motzer RJ, Hutson TE, Tomczak P, et al. Overall survival and updated results for sunitinib compared with interferon alfa in patients with metastatic renal cell carcinoma. *J Clin Oncol.* 2009; 27: 3584–3590.

25. Motzer RJ, Hutson TE, Olsen MR, et al. Randomized phase II trial of sunitinib on an intermittent versus continuous dosing schedule as first-line therapy for advanced renal cell carcinoma. *J Clin Oncol.* 2012; 30: 1371–1377.

26. Feldman DR, Baum MS, Ginsberg MS, et al. Phase I trial of bevacizumab plus escalated doses of sunitinib in patients with metastatic renal cell carcinoma. *J Clin Oncol.* 2009; 27: 1432–1439.

27. Negrier S, Gravis G, Perol D, et al. Temsirolimus and bevacizumab, or sunitinib, or interferon alfa and bevacizumab for patients with advanced renal cell carcinoma (TORAVA): a randomised phase 2 trial. *Lancet Oncol.* 2011; 12: 673–680.

28. Hudes G, Carducci M, Tomczak P, et al. Temsirolimus, interferon alfa, or both for advanced renal-cell carcinoma. *N Engl J Med.* 2007; 356: 2271–2281.

29. Motzer RJ, Escudier B, Oudard S, et al. Efficacy of everolimus in advanced renal cell carcinoma: a double-blind, randomised, placebo-controlled phase III trial. *Lancet.* 2008; 372: 449–456.

CHAPTER **40**

Localized Prostate Cancers

Jason A. Efstathiou, Phillip J. Gray, Douglas M. Dahl

EPIDEMIOLOGY

In the United States, an estimated 238,590 men will be diagnosed with prostate cancer in 2013 with 29,720 deaths attributable to prostate cancer (1). These statistics highlight a paradox of prostate cancer. Although it is the second leading cause of cancer death for men in the United States, only a relatively small percentage of men diagnosed with prostate cancer will die of their disease. This chapter will present guidelines for the management of localized prostate cancer. It will describe the controversies associated with prostate-specific antigen (PSA) screening, describe the work up and staging of prostate cancer, and finally discuss treatment options for localized disease.

PROSTATE-SPECIFIC ANTIGEN (PSA)

PSA is an abundant exocrine protein of the prostate, which has function in seminal clot lysis. Serum PSA measurement is a useful, although highly controversial, biomarker commonly used as a screening tool for prostate cancer. In addition to prostate cancer, PSA elevations may be the result of a

TABLE 40-1 AGE-SPECIFIC PSA RANGES

PSA Values (ng/ml)	Age
0.0–0 2.5	40–49
0.0–3.5	50–59
0.0–4.5	60–69
0.0–6.5	70–79

variety of nonmalignant conditions including benign prostatic hypertrophy, inflammation, or urinary tract infection. Traditionally, 4.0 ng/ml has been considered the upper limit of normal for serum PSA; however, recent data demonstrate that many men with a serum PSA in the normal range have prostate cancer if biopsied (2). Conversely, many men with elevated PSA levels do not. As PSA normally rises with age, an age-specific algorithm may be a more effective screening approach. Age-specific PSA normal ranges have been shown to aid in finding important early cancer in younger men and avoiding unnecessary procedures and over-diagnosis in older men (Table 40-1).

CURRENT RECOMMENDATIONS FOR SCREENING

Prostate cancer screening is a controversial topic with several large recent studies informing the debate over the benefits of screening (3–5). Although PSA screening has led to the detection of earlier stage prostate cancer, it is not clear if this has led to better outcomes for screened men. Many screen-detected cancers may be incidental cancers that would have never resulted in clinical sequelae within the man's lifetime. Given this lack of clear evidence, the United States Preventative Service Task Force has recently recommended against routine PSA screening, concluding that "many men are harmed as a result of prostate cancer screening and few, if any, benefit" (6). This recommendation has met significant resistance from the urologic and oncologic communities (7, 8). These groups point out the difficulty of interpreting PSA screening studies, given high levels of contamination, and that this broad recommendation may not apply to young healthy men. As such, The American Cancer Society and the National Comprehensive Cancer Network (NCCN) currently recommend a careful discussion between the patient and his physician before proceeding with screening. The American Urological Association (AUA) has released a similar guidelines calling for shared decision making about PSA screening between providers and patients age 55–69 (available: http://www.auanet.org/education/guidelines/prostate-cancer-detection.cfm). For men who elect screening, PSA and digital rectal examination (DRE) should be offered every 1–2 years. Continued screening is most appropriate in men with a life expectancy of at least 10 years. Factors that increase the risk of prostate cancer include sub-Saharan African descent or history of prostate cancer in a first-degree relative before the age of 65 years. In men with these risk factors, screening should begin at age 40 years.

■ DIGITAL RECTAL EXAMINATION (DRE)

Although the majority of prostate cancer is detected by PSA screening, others are diagnosed based on an abnormal DRE even in the setting of a normal PSA. Both PSA and DRE should be incorporated into the screening process. A palpable nodule or a discrete indurated area constitutes a suspicious DRE that should prompt further evaluation.

DIAGNOSIS

Prostate cancer is diagnosed exclusively by the use of a transrectal ultrasound guided needle biopsy (**Figure 40-1**). This is an outpatient office-based procedure performed under local anesthetic. It has a very low-complication rate estimated at 1 serious complication per 1000 procedures. There is no radiographic modality adequate for diagnosis without the use of biopsy. Ultrasound may show a hypoechoic area that corresponds to localized carcinoma, but this is an unreliable finding. The proper technique for prostate biopsy has been well studied. The standard approach is a systematic sampling of all areas of the prostate in a grid pattern (**Figure 40-2**). Most urologists employ a technique of sampling 6–12 regions of the prostate. The cancer detection rate is substantially higher with a 10–12 core biopsy technique.

■ GLEASON SCORE

The histologic grading of prostate cancer is described using the Gleason scoring system (**Table 40-2**) (9, 10). This system assigns two numeric scores to the carcinoma. As there is often heterogeneity within the cancer, the first score describes the dominant pattern and the second the secondary pattern. For example, Gleason 3 + 4 indicates the primary pattern is 3. Gleason 4 + 3 indicates that the higher grade predominates. This is clinically important

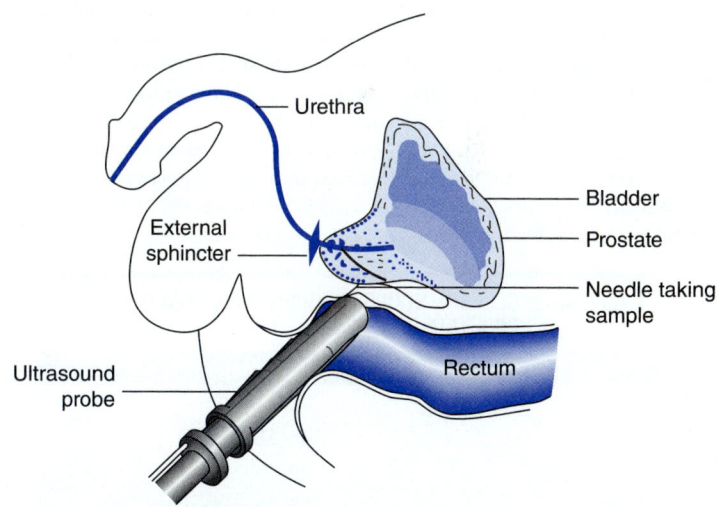

FIGURE 40-1 Transrectal ultrasound guided biopsy.

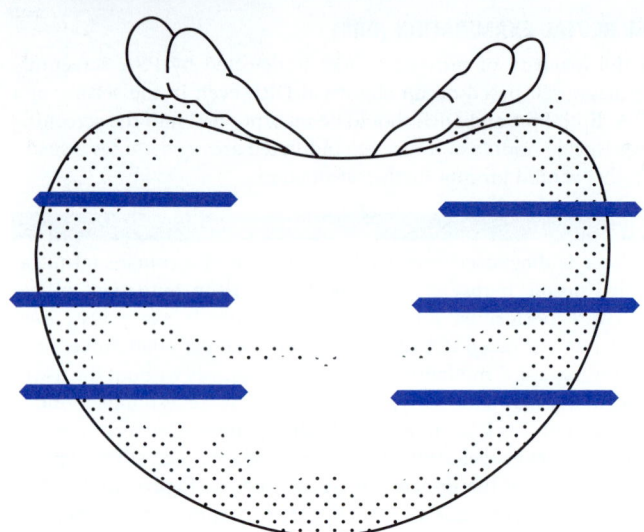

FIGURE 40-2 Sextant biopsy pattern.

because prognosis is substantially related to the primary Gleason score. In discussing prostate cancer staging, the Gleason sum, that is, the sum of the individual scores, is commonly referenced. Although the Gleason sum is one of the most important prognostic features, the primary and secondary scores should also be reported as they may refine a patient's prognosis. For instance, Gleason sum of 3 + 4 and 4 + 3 are both 7, although the latter cancer has a worse prognosis.

In the absence of prostate cancer, there are other common histologic findings that warrant consideration. Atypical small acinar proliferation (ASAP) frequently represents an inadequately sampled carcinoma escaping definitive diagnosis. A repeat biopsy is indicated. High-grade prostatic intraepithelial neoplasia (HGPIN) is commonly found on prostate biopsies. The significance of this finding is controversial. Standard practice calls for continued close monitoring and rebiopsy of these patients. Perineural invasion (PNI) is a finding often reported in men who have prostate cancer. Some investigators believe this is associated with a higher risk of extraprostatic tumor spread, but this has been an inconsistent finding.

TABLE 40-2 GLEASON SCORE FREQUENCY FOR PSA DETECTED PROSTATE CANCERS

Gleason Score	Percentage
2–4	<5
5–6	45–50
7	30–35
8–10	15–20

STAGING

The most important independent variables used in staging prostate cancer are the patient's PSA, the DRE findings, and the Gleason score. Using these clinical features, significant prognostic judgment can be made. The Partin tables assess the likelihood of pathologic stage based on these clinical variables. They are very useful in counseling patients about appropriate treatment options (available at: http://urology.jhu.edu/prostate/partintables.php). Metastatic workup includes a CT scan of the abdomen and pelvis to assess for pelvic and retroperitoneal lymphadenopathy. A bone scan may pick up bone metastases. Because of the extremely small likelihood of positive findings, these studies are rarely useful in early stage disease. In general, these studies are indicated only in patients with either Gleason 4 + 3 or higher cancer, PSA greater than 10, or clinical high local stage tumor (T2b or higher).

Endorectal MRI has been extensively studied for its role in local staging of prostate cancer. While its sensitivity for detecting subtle extra-capsular extension is higher than that of ultrasound, the clinical implications of such findings remain unclear.

■ MANAGEMENT OPTIONS

Definitive local treatment is primarily a curative strategy in patients with localized disease, but it is occasionally employed to prevent symptoms from locally advanced disease even in men with evidence of distant metastasis.

■ WATCHFUL WAITING/ACTIVE SURVEILLANCE

Prostate cancer frequently behaves in an indolent fashion. Watchful waiting or active surveillance is an attractive strategy for men with less than a 10-year life expectancy or with low-volume Gleason 3 + 3 disease. Population-based studies suggest only a tiny minority of men with Gleason 3 + 3 carcinoma will develop metastatic or life-threatening disease within 10 years if left untreated (11). Despite this, a randomized trial performed in Europe demonstrated that radical prostatectomy reduced the risk of death, metastatic dissemination, and local progression as opposed to watchful waiting in men with early prostate cancer (12). As the majority of these men did not have screen-detected cancers, this study may not fully represent the population with prostate cancer in the United States. A more recent study of patients with PSA screening-detected cancers showed no benefit to prostatectomy except for men with high Gleason grade or PSA greater than 10 ng/ ml (13). Active surveillance, a different concept than watchful waiting, relies on serial PSA follow-up and repeat biopsies allowing significant cancers to declare themselves early in follow-up. Patients with significant cancers are offered treatment in a timely fashion, while patients with indolent prostate cancer are spared radical treatment and the associated sequelae. Prostate cancer specific survival of 97% at 10 years have been reported and up to 70% of men are able to avoid treatment (14). Multidisciplinary care has been shown to increase rates of active surveillance usage in low-risk patients (15).

■ RADICAL PROSTATECTOMY

Radical prostatectomy is the standard surgical procedure comprising complete removal of the prostate and seminal vesicles. This procedure is done using several different approaches. Radical retropubic prostatectomy involves a midline incision from the umbilicus to symphysis pubis. Radical perineal prostatectomy is performed through a midline incision between the scrotum and the anus. Minimally invasive surgical approaches are now in wide use. A laparoscopic approach through the lower abdomen can be accomplished by standard laparoscopic technique or with the aid of a surgical robot. In skilled hands, the mortality and major morbidity rates with any of these procedures are extremely low. Major potential complications of surgical removal of the prostate are urinary incontinence, erectile dysfunction, significant hemorrhage, and bladder neck contracture. In properly selected patients, severe incontinence occurs in less than 1% of cases. Mild stress urinary incontinence in which the patient may require pads in his underwear to catch some occasional urinary leakage is found in less than 10% of patients who are treated at high-volume centers. Erectile dysfunction rates vary widely with patients' preoperative sexual function, the choice of surgical approach (nerve sparing or non-nerve sparing), and the patient's age. In early stage disease, bilateral nerve sparing surgery may result in preservation of erectile function in up to 80% of younger men with normal preoperative sexual function. More aggressive surgical resection that includes one of the paired neurovascular bundles, which run posterolaterally to the prostate, results in less than 50% of patients recovering spontaneous erectile function. If both nerve bundles are sacrificed, spontaneous erectile function is unlikely to recover. Bladder neck contracture results when dense scar tissue obstructs the point of anastomosis of the urethra and bladder. This may result in acute urinary retention in the early postoperative period. Repeated urologic procedures may be necessary to restore adequate urinary function. Significant hemorrhage may be encountered during radical prostatectomy. It has been common practice for surgeons to bank autologous blood prior to radical prostatectomy. Blood loss on average is much reduced with perineal and robotic approaches to radical prostatectomy. Regional pelvic lymph nodes are routinely sampled during radical retropubic and laparoscopic radical prostatectomy. It is not possible to sample pelvic lymph nodes through the perineal approach.

■ RADIATION THERAPY OPTIONS

External Beam Radiation Therapy

External beam radiation therapy has a well-established track record in the management of localized and locally advanced prostate cancer (16–18). It is a noninvasive form of treatment delivered in daily fractions over the course of several weeks. Modern trials have demonstrated that higher doses, on the order of 79 Gy, are more efficacious for cancer control when external radiation is used as monotherapy and can be delivered without a decrement in patient-reported quality of life (19–21). Conformal radiation therapy utilizing CT or MRI planning is necessary for the safe delivery of sufficient radiation dose in this setting. Daily prostate imaging (i.e., image-guided therapy) using transabdominal ultrasound, radiographic visualization of implanted fiducial markers, electromagnetic transponders or cone-beam CT allows more accurate targeting of the prostate. This facilitates the delivery of high radiation doses to the prostate while minimizing dose to nontarget tissue, such as the bladder and rectum, that is the primary cause of late morbidity.

A variety of external beam radiation techniques are acceptable forms of treatment including multifield 3D conformal radiation, intensity modulated radiation therapy (IMRT), and proton beam radiation therapy. Currently such treatment is typically delivered over the course of 8–9 weeks; however, several trials studying the efficacy of shorter (i.e., hypofractionated) courses are ongoing. Potential toxicity of external beam radiation therapy include acute changes to bowel habits (e.g., looser stools) and increased urinary frequency/urgency as well as potential radiation proctitis, cystitis, and urethritis, though the rates of significant late complications are less than 10%. Similar to surgery, erectile dysfunction is a common side effect of treatment, although it typically manifests later. Rates of erectile dysfunction vary with patient age and the presence of medical comorbidities, particularly cardiovascular disease, obesity, diabetes, and smoking.

Prostate Brachytherapy

Prostate brachytherapy is another common treatment modality for early prostate cancer. As monotherapy, prostate brachytherapy may be less effective in patients with Gleason grade 7 or higher, palpable cancer, or PSA greater than 10 (22). For well-selected patients, brachytherapy may be more attractive than a protracted course of external beam radiation. Modern prostate brachytherapy is typically delivered under transrectal ultrasound guidance using a transperineal approach (**Figure 40-3**). As modern series have matured, results have been comparable to surgical and external beam radiation for early stage disease. Commonly, this procedure is performed in an operating room under either general or spinal anesthesia. An ultrasound probe is placed in the rectum, and needles containing radioactive seeds are guided into the prostate using a transperineal template or grid. These seeds typically contain either iodine-125 or palladium-103, whose half-lives are 60 and 17 days, respectively. They remain in the prostate permanently and deliver the full dose of radiation over several months. This procedure is termed transperineal permanent low-dose rate (LDR) prostate brachytherapy. It differs from high-dose rate (HDR) brachytherapy where temporary catheters are placed in the prostate using a similar placement technique. The catheters serve as avenues for an HDR radioactive wire, which contains a high-activity source, typically iridium-192. High-dose rate brachytherapy requires the delivery of several fractions, necessitating repeated catheter placement. This treatment is most frequently combined with external radiation but is also used as monotherapy.

The most troublesome acute side effects of brachytherapy are obstructive urinary symptoms including urgency and frequency. Poorly selected patients with larger prostates or preexisting obstructive symptoms are at risk of urinary retention. Late sequelae include radiation urethritis, cystitis, and proctitis, which may result in prolonged symptoms or bleeding. Erectile dysfunction is another common side effect with rates comparable to external beam radiation.

Role of Androgen Deprivation Therapy

The benefit of the addition of androgen deprivation therapy (ADT) to external radiation for patients with intermediate-risk or more advanced prostate cancer has been demonstrated in several large randomized studies.

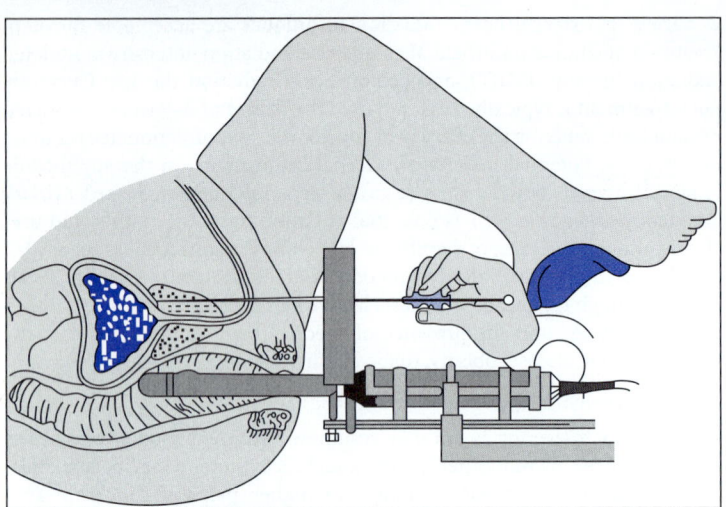

FIGURE 40-3 Ultrasound guided transperineal permanent prostate implant technique.

Most have demonstrated an overall survival benefit, while all have demonstrated a benefit in terms of biochemical and local control, decreased distant metastasis, and prostate cancer-specific survival. For patients with the highest risk of recurrence (Gleason score ≥8 or extraprostatic extension), these trials suggest a benefit to a prolonged course of ADT prior to, during, and after radiation (2–3 years in total) (23, 24). A short course of ADT preceding and continuing to the end of radiation (4–6 months in total) is considered appropriate in those with intermediate-risk disease (25–27). Patients treated in all of these studies were treated with lower radiation doses than commonly used in current practice. Comparative studies of dose escalation with or without ADT are ongoing. There is no evidence that ADT is of any benefit for low-risk patients. Side effects of androgen deprivation therapy include erectile dysfunction, loss of libido, hot flashes, fatigue, weight gain (gain of fat mass, loss of muscle mass), elevated triglycerides, decreased insulin sensitivity, and accelerated loss of bone mineral density.

■ OTHER OPTIONS

Cryotherapy

Liquid nitrogen delivered through probes in the perineum guided by transrectal ultrasonography has been employed to treat localized prostate cancer (28). This procedure is FDA approved and being used in the United States. Its efficacy and safety are far less certain than with the above-mentioned surgical or radiation therapy techniques, given lack of sufficient long-term follow-up data. Significantly more research efforts will be required to establish this technique as an acceptable alternative.

High Intensity Focused Ultrasound (HIFU)

High intensity focused ultrasound is an investigational technology that employs a transrectal probe to deliver very intense focused pulses of ultrasound energy through the rectal wall into the prostate. Several centers have explored its use; however, it remains an investigational technique. Serious complications of urinary retention or rectal-urethral fistula have been reported in early series. Its efficacy as an oncologic procedure remains unproven.

REFERENCES

1. Siegel R, Naishadham D, Jemal A. Cancer statistics, 2013. *CA Cancer J Clin*. 2013; 63: 11–30.

2. Thompson IM, Pauler DK, Goodman PJ, et al. Prevalence of prostate cancer among men with a prostate-specific antigen level < or =4.0 ng per milliliter. *N Engl J Med*. 2004; 350: 2239–2246.

3. Schroder FH, Hugosson J, Roobol MJ, et al. Prostate-cancer mortality at 11 years of follow-up. *N Engl J Med*. 2012; 366: 981–990.

4. Crawford ED, Grubb R 3rd, Black A, et al. Comorbidity and mortality results from a randomized prostate cancer screening trial. *J Clin Oncol*. 2011; 29: 355–361.

5. Hugosson J, Carlsson S, Aus G, et al. Mortality results from the Goteborg randomised population-based prostate-cancer screening trial. *Lancet Oncol*. 2010; 11: 725–732.

6. USPSTF. Screening for Prostate Cancer: U.S. Preventive Services Task Force; http://www.uspreventiveservicestaskforce.org/prostatecancerscreening.htm. 2012; http://www.uspreventiveservicestaskforce.org/prostatecancerscreening.htm. Accessed September 6, 2012.

7. Basch E, Oliver TK, Vickers A, et al. Screening for prostate cancer with prostate-specific antigen testing: American society of clinical oncology provisional clinical opinion. *J Clin Oncol*. 2012; 30: 3020–3025.

8. Messing EM, Albertsen P, Andriole GL Jr., et al. The Society of Urologic Oncology's reply to the US Preventative Services Task Force's recommendation on PSA testing. *Urol Oncol*. 2012; 30: 117–119.

9. Albertsen PC, Hanley JA, Barrows GH, et al. Prostate cancer and the Will Rogers phenomenon. *J Natl Cancer Inst*. 2005; 97: 1248–1253.

10. Albertsen PC, Hanley JA, Gleason DF, et al. Competing risk analysis of men aged 55 to 74 years at diagnosis managed conservatively for clinically localized prostate cancer. *JAMA*. 1998; 280: 975–980.

11. Albertsen PC, Hanley JA, Fine J. 20-year outcomes following conservative management of clinically localized prostate cancer. *JAMA*. 2005; 293: 2095–2101.

12. Bill-Axelson A, Holmberg L, Ruutu M, et al. Radical prostatectomy versus watchful waiting in early prostate cancer. *N Engl J Med*. 2011; 364: 1708–1717.

13. Wilt TJ, Brawer MK, Jones KM, et al. Radical prostatectomy versus observation for localized prostate cancer. *N Engl J Med*. 2012; 367: 203–213.

14. Klotz L, Zhang L, Lam A, et al. Clinical results of long-term follow-up of a large, active surveillance cohort with localized prostate cancer. *J Clin Oncol*. 2010; 28: 126–131.

15. Aizer AA, Paly JJ, Zietman AL, et al. Multidisciplinary care and pursuit of active surveillance in low-risk prostate cancer. *J Clin Oncol.* 2012; 30: 3071–3076.

16. Warde P, Mason M, Ding K, et al. Combined androgen deprivation therapy and radiation therapy for locally advanced prostate cancer: a randomised, phase 3 trial. *Lancet.* 2011; 378: 2104–2111.

17. Widmark A, Klepp O, Solberg A, et al. Endocrine treatment, with or without radiotherapy, in locally advanced prostate cancer (SPCG-7/SFUO-3): an open randomised phase III trial. *Lancet.* 2009; 373: 301–308.

18. Kuban DA, Thames HD, Levy LB, et al. Long-term multi-institutional analysis of stage T1-T2 prostate cancer treated with radiotherapy in the PSA era. *Int J Radiat Oncol Biol Phys.* 2003; 57: 915–928.

19. Zietman AL, Bae K, Slater JD, et al. Randomized trial comparing conventional-dose with high-dose conformal radiation therapy in early-stage adenocarcinoma of the prostate: long-term results from proton radiation oncology group/American College of Radiology 95-09. *J Clin Oncol.* 2010; 28: 1106–1111.

20. Kuban DA, Tucker SL, Dong L, et al. Long-term results of the M.D. Anderson randomized dose-escalation trial for prostate cancer. *Int J Radiat Oncol Biol Phys.* 2008; 70: 67–74.

21. Talcott JA, Rossi C, Shipley WU, et al. Patient-reported long-term outcomes after conventional and high-dose combined proton and photon radiation for early prostate cancer. *JAMA.* 2010; 303: 1046–1053.

22. D'Amico AV, Whittington R, Malkowicz SB, et al. Biochemical outcome after radical prostatectomy, external beam radiation therapy, or interstitial radiation therapy for clinically localized prostate cancer. *JAMA.* 1998; 280: 969–974.

23. Bolla M, de Reijke TM, Van Tienhoven G, et al. Duration of androgen suppression in the treatment of prostate cancer. *N Engl J Med.* 2009; 360: 2516–2527.

24. Horwitz EM, Bae K, Hanks GE, et al. Ten-year follow-up of radiation therapy oncology group protocol 92-02: a phase III trial of the duration of elective androgen deprivation in locally advanced prostate cancer. *J Clin Oncol.* 2008; 26: 2497–2504.

25. Jones CU, Hunt D, McGowan DG, et al. Radiotherapy and short-term androgen deprivation for localized prostate cancer. *N Engl J Med.* 2011; 365: 107–118.

26. Denham JW, Steigler A, Lamb DS, et al. Short-term neoadjuvant androgen deprivation and radiotherapy for locally advanced prostate cancer: 10-year data from the TROG 96.01 randomised trial. *Lancet Oncol.* 2011; 12: 451–459.

27. D'Amico AV, Chen MH, Renshaw AA, et al. Androgen suppression and radiation vs radiation alone for prostate cancer: a randomized trial. *JAMA.* 2008; 299: 289–295.

28. Donnelly BJ, Saliken JC, Brasher PM, et al. A randomized trial of external beam radiotherapy versus cryoablation in patients with localized prostate cancer. *Cancer.* 2010; 116: 323–330.

CHAPTER **41**
Metastatic Prostate Cancer
Matthew R. Smith

INCIDENCE

Prostate cancer is the most commonly diagnosed cancer in men and a leading cause of cancer death. In the United States, there were approximately 238,590 new prostate cancer cases and 29,790 deaths in 2013 (1). Incidence and mortality rates for prostate cancer are highly variable worldwide.

Prostate cancer incidence in the United States increased steadily throughout the second half of the 20th century. This increase appears related to the increase in life expectancy and associated rise in number of older men at risk for prostate cancer. Other factors including widespread use of prostate-specific antigen (PSA) screening also appear to have contributed to the increase in annual prostate cancer incidence. PSA screening identified a large number of prevalent cases of asymptomatic prostate cancer. The annual incidence of prostate cancer peaked at approximately 350,000 cases in 1993. After declining in the late 1990s, the annual incidence of prostate cancer has slowly increased. In contrast to the striking variations in annual rates of prostate cancer diagnosis, prostate cancer mortality rates have declined since 1990.

SPECTRUM OF ADVANCED DISEASE

Prostate cancer preferentially spreads to regional lymph nodes and bone. Clinically significant metastases to liver, lung, or other visceral organs are less common. Bone scans using technetium-99m methylene diphosphonate (^{99m}Tc MDP) are routinely used to assess skeletal involvement. Computed tomography scans or magnetic resonance imaging scans are used to assess regional lymph nodes.

The spectrum of advanced disease has markedly changed in recent decades. Prostate cancer screening with serum PSA has been accompanied by a dramatic stage migration, and now less than 10% of men in the United States have radiographic evidence of metastases at initial diagnosis. Additionally, PSA testing is routinely used for surveillance after surgery or radiation therapy for early stage disease. As a result, advanced prostate cancer now includes men with rising serum PSA levels as the only indication of disease progression after prior treatment for early stage disease.

ANDROGEN DEPRIVATION THERAPY
■ HYPOTHALAMIC-PITUITARY-GONADAL AXIS

Prostate cancers ubiquitously express the androgen receptor and require androgens for growth and survival. Testosterone synthesized by the Leydig cells of the testis is the primary source of androgens in men. Leydig cell synthesis of testosterone is regulated by luteinizing hormone (LH) of pituitary origin.

The release of LH is regulated by gonadotropin-releasing hormone (GnRH) from the hypothalamus. Levels of circulating testosterone are maintained within normal limits by negative feedback at the level of the hypothalamus and pituitary.

Approximately 98% of plasma testosterone is present in a biologically inactive protein bound form. Free testosterone enters cells by diffusion across the cell membrane. In some tissues, including the brain, pituitary, and kidney, unmodified testosterone is bound by the androgen receptor. In other tissues, including the prostate, seminal vesicles, epididymis, adrenals, liver, and skin, testosterone is efficiently converted to dihydrotestosterone (DHT) by membrane-bound 5α-reductase type II. DHT binds the androgen receptor with approximately threefold greater affinity than testosterone. In adipose tissue, testosterone is converted to estradiol by cytochrome p450-dependent aromatization.

Under the influence of pituitary adrenocorticotropin (ACTH), the adrenal glands produce androstenedione, dehydroepiandosterone (DHEA), and dehydroepiandosterone sulfate (DHEA-S). These compounds, collectively known as the adrenal androgens, have relatively weak androgenic activity. Androstenedione can be converted to testosterone in peripheral tissues and in the prostate. In normal men, the adrenal cortex is a minor source of androgen production. Residual adrenal androgens, however, may be important in promoting disease progression in men with advanced prostate cancer following medical or surgical castration.

◼ GnRH AGONISTS AND ANTAGONISTS

The mainstay of treatment for metastatic prostate cancer is androgen deprivation therapy (Table 41-1). Permanent androgen deprivation can be accomplished by bilateral orchiectomies. Reversible methods of androgen deprivation therapy include diethylstilboestrol (DES), GnRH agonists, and GnRH antagonists. DES suppresses pituitary LH production resulting in castrate testosterone levels. Administration of GnRH agonists causes an initial stimulation of pituitary LH production and rise in serum testosterone levels. Chronic administration of GnRH agonists causes downregulation of pituitary GnRH receptors and prompt suppression of testicular androgen production. GnRH antagonists directly inhibit pituitary GnRH receptors, producing castrate testosterone levels without an initial rise.

The various forms of androgen deprivation therapy have similar efficacy. A meta-analysis of 10 randomized controlled trials, for example, concluded

TABLE 41-1 FORMS OF ANDROGEN DEPRIVATION THERAPY

Class	Agents	Mechanism of Action
GnRH agonist	Leuprolide acetate goserelin	Downregulation of GnRH receptors
GnRH antagonist	Degarelix	Inhibition of GnRH receptors
Estrogen	Diethylstilbestrol	Suppression of pituitary luteinizing hormone production

that bilateral orchiectomies and GnRH agonists produce equivalent progression-free and overall survival (2). GnRH agonists have become the most prevalent form of androgen deprivation therapy because they are convenient, are potentially reversible, and lack the psychological implications of bilateral orchiectomies. DES is not routinely used because it causes increased risk of thromboembolic events.

Androgen deprivation therapy achieves prompt marked decline in PSA in nearly all cases and symptomatic improvement in most men with disease-related symptoms. For men with bone metastases, the median time to disease progression is 12–18 months and median survival is 24–30 months. In men without radiographic evidence of metastases, response duration and survival are substantially longer. The median survival for men with receiving adjuvant therapy for regional lymph node metastases, for example, is greater than 10 years.

For men without clinical or radiographic evidence of metastases, the optimal timing of androgen deprivation therapy is controversial (3). Three randomized controlled trials have compared immediate versus delayed androgen deprivation therapy for men with locally advanced disease or regional lymph node metastases. Early primary androgen deprivation therapy improved survival for men with locally advanced nonmetastatic prostate cancer. Adjuvant androgen deprivation therapy improves survival for men with locally advanced prostate cancer treated with radiation therapy and men with lymph node-positive prostate cancer treated with radical prostatectomy and pelvic lymphadenectomy. The effects of early androgen deprivation therapy on clinical outcomes for men with "PSA-only"disease are unknown.

Most adverse effects of androgen deprivation therapy are due to severe gonadal steroid deficiency. These adverse effects include loss of lidido, hot flashes, fatigue, and osteoporosis. Androgen deprivation therapy also increases fat mass and decreases insulin sensitivity. Consistent with these adverse effects, androgen deprivation therapy is associated with greater risk for diabetes. Some but not all studies have linked androgen deprivation therapy to greater risk for myocardial infarction.

■ COMBINED ANDROGEN BLOCKADE

Nonsteroidal antiandrogens including bicalutamide, flutamide, and nilutamide competitively inhibit the binding of testosterone and DHT to the androgen receptor. These nonsteroidal antiandrogens bind to the androgen receptor with <2% of the affinity of DHT. Monotherapy with nonsteroidal antiandrogens is inferior to castration for metastatic prostate cancer, likely due to their relatively low binding affinity.

The combination of androgen deprivation therapy with an antiandrogen, termed combined androgen blockade, has the potential advantage of inhibiting testicular androgen production and blocking the action of residual adrenal androgens. Three meta-analyses concluded that combined androgen blockade is associated with a small survival benefit compared to androgen deprivation therapy alone (4), although combined androgen blockade is also associated with greater side effects than androgen deprivation alone.

TABLE 41-2 FDA APPROVED THERAPIES FOR CASTRATION-RESISTANT PROSTATE CANCER

Agent	Class	Clinical Benefit
Docetaxel	Chemotherapy	Improved progression-free and overall survival
Cabazitaxel	Chemotherapy	Improved progression-free and overall survival
Mitoxantrone	Chemotherapy	Pain relief
Sipuleucel-T	Immunotherapy	Improved overall survival
Abiraterone acetate	Androgen biosynthesis inhibitor	Improved progression-free and overall survival
Enzalutamide	Androgen-receptor-signaling inhibitor	Improved progression-free and overall survival
Strontium-89	Radiopharmaceutical	Pain relief
Samarium-153	Radiopharmaceutical	Pain relief
Zoledronic acid	Osteoclast-targeted therapy	Decreased skeletal-related events
Denosumab	Osteoclast-targeted therapy	Decreased skeletal-related events

MANAGEMENT OF CASTRATION-RESISTANT DISEASE

Most men with metastatic prostate cancer experience disease progression within a few years of initiating androgen deprivation therapy—a disease state termed castration-resistant prostate cancer. Rising serum levels of PSA are usually the first indication of disease progression.

The landscape of clinical management for castration-resistant prostate cancer has changed dramatically in recent years. Currently, there are five therapies (docetaxel, cabazitaxel, sipuleucel-T, abiraterone acetate, and enzalutamide) approved by the United States Food and Drug Administration for metastatic castration-resistant based on improved overall survival. A randomized controlled trial of radium-223 reported survival benefit in men with metastatic castration-resistant disease. Additional therapies are approved based on prevention or relief of symptoms (Table 41-2).

CHEMOTHERAPY

Docetaxel is the standard first-line chemotherapy for prostate cancer. In two randomized controlled trials of men with metastatic castration-resistant prostate cancer, docetaxel was associated with improved progression-free and overall survival compared to mitoxantrone plus prednisone (5, 6). Cabazitaxel, a semisynthetic taxane analog designed to overcome taxane resistance, is standard second-line chemotherapy for prostate cancer. In a randomized controlled trial of men with metastatic castration-resistant prostate cancer and disease progression despite prior docetaxel, cabazitaxel plus prednisone was associated with improved progression-free and overall survival compared to mitoxantrone plus prednisone (7).

IMMUNOTHERAPY

Sipuleucel-T is the first therapeutic anticancer vaccine approved by the Food and Drug Administration. Sipuleucel-T is an autologous cellular product in which antigen-presenting cells, obtained by leukapheresis, are enriched and pulsed with a granulocyte macrophage colony-stimulating factor/prostatic acid phosphatase fusion protein. In a randomized controlled trial of men with asymptomatic or minimally symptomatic metastatic castration-resistant prostate cancer, sipuleucel-T was associated with improved overall survival but not time to progression compared to placebo vaccine (8).

INHIBITION OF ANDROGEN BIOSYNTHESIS

Abiraterone acetate is a specific and irreversible inhibitor of CYP17, a key enzyme in gonadal and extragonadal androgen biosynthesis. In a randomized controlled trial of men with metastatic castration-resistant prostate cancer and disease progression despite prior docetaxel, abiraterone acetate plus prednisone improved progression-free and overall survival compared to placebo plus prednisone (9). In a subsequent randomized controlled trial of men with metastatic castration-resistant prostate cancer and no prior chemotherapy, abiraterone acetate plus prednisone was also associated with improved progression-free and overall survival compared to placebo plus prednisone. Other androgen biosynthesis inhibitors, including oreteronel, are in clinical development.

◼ NOVEL ANTIANDROGENS

Enzalutamide is a novel androgen receptor antagonist that blocks androgen binding and prevents nuclear translocation and recruitment of coactivators. In a randomized controlled trial of men with metastatic castration-resistant prostate cancer and disease progression despite prior docetaxel, enzalutamide improved progression-free and overall survival compared to placebo. A randomized controlled trial of enzalutamide in men with metastatic castration-resistant prostate cancer and no prior chemotherapy is ongoing. Other highly active androgen receptor antagonists are in clinical development.

◼ BONE-SEEKING RADIOPHARMACEUTICALS

Strontium-89 chloride and samarium-153 are beta-emitting radiopharmaceuticals indicated for relief of pain in patients with osteoblastic bone metastases. The effects of strontium-89 and samarium-153 on disease progression and survival are not well studied.

Radium-223 is an investigational alpha-emitting radiopharmaceutical in development for the treatment of metastatic prostate cancer. In contrast to beta-emitters, radium-223 has a shorter range and higher linear energy transfer. In a randomized controlled trial of men with castration-resistant prostate cancer and bone metastases, radium-223 was associated with improved progression-free and overall survival compared to placebo.

OSTEOCLAST-TARGETED THERAPY

Bone metastases are a major cause of morbidity for men with prostate cancer. Complications of bone metastases include pain, fractures, and spinal cord compression. Although they appear osteoblastic by radiographic imaging, most bone metastases are characterized by excess osteoclast number and activity.

Two osteoclast-targeted therapies (zoledronic acid, denosumab) are approved to reduce the risk of skeletal related events (pathologic fractures, spinal cord compression, or surgery or radiation to bone) in men with castration-resistant prostate cancer and bone metastases. In a randomized controlled trial of men with metastatic castration-resistant prostate cancer, zoledronic acid was associated with lower rates of skeletal related events compared to placebo (10). In a randomized controlled trial in metastatic castration-resistant prostate cancer, denosumab was superior to zoledronic acid for prevention of skeletal related events (11).

REFERENCES

1. Siegel R, Naishadham D, Jemal A. Cancer statistics, 2013. *CA Cancer J Clin*. 2013; 63: 11–30.

2. Seidenfeld J, Samson DJ, Hasselblad V, et al. Single-therapy androgen suppression in men with advanced prostate cancer: a systematic review and meta-analysis. *Ann Intern Med*. 2000; 132: 566–577.

3. Loblaw DA, Virgo KS, Nam R, et al. Initial hormonal management of androgen-sensitive metastatic, recurrent, or progressive prostate cancer: 2007 Update of an American Society of Clinical Oncology Practice Guideline. *J Clin Oncol*. 2007; 25: 1596–1605.

4. Sharifi N, Gulley JL, Dahut WL. Androgen deprivation therapy for prostate cancer. *JAMA*. 2005; 294: 238–244.

5. Petrylak DP, Tangen CM, Hussain MH, et al. Docetaxel and estramustine compared with mitoxantrone and prednisone for advanced refractory prostate cancer. *N Engl J Med*. 2004; 351: 1513–1520.

6. Tannock IF, de Wit R, Berry WR, et al. Docetaxel plus prednisone or mitoxantrone plus prednisone for advanced prostate cancer. *N Engl J Med*. 2004; 351: 1502–1512.

7. de Bono JS, Oudard S, Ozguroglu M, et al. Prednisone plus cabazitaxel or mitoxantrone for metastatic castration-resistant prostate cancer progressing after docetaxel treatment: a randomised open-label trial. *Lancet*. 2010; 376: 1147–1154.

8. Kantoff PW, Higano CS, Shore ND, et al. Sipuleucel-T immunotherapy for castration-resistant prostate cancer. *N Engl J Med*. 2010; 363: 411–422.

9. de Bono JS, Logothetis CJ, Molina A, et al. Abiraterone and increased survival in metastatic prostate cancer. *N Engl J Med*. 2011; 364: 1995–2005.

10. Saad F, Gleason DM, Murray R, et al. A randomized, placebo-controlled trial of zoledronic acid in patients with hormone-refractory metastatic prostate carcinoma. *J Natl Cancer Inst.* 2002; 94: 1458–1468.

11. Fizazi K, Carducci M, Smith M, et al. Denosumab versus zoledronic acid for treatment of bone metastases in men with castration-resistant prostate cancer: a randomised, double-blind study. *Lancet.* 2011; 377: 813–822.

CHAPTER **42**

Bladder Cancer

Richard J. Lee

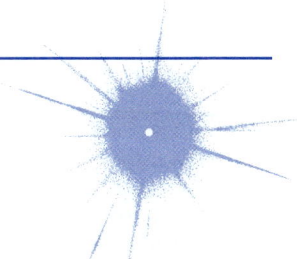

EPIDEMIOLOGY AND RISK FACTORS

More than 350,000 new cases of bladder cancer are diagnosed per year worldwide. In the United States, bladder cancer is the 4th most common cancer, with 72,570 new cases in 2013 (1). Bladder cancer is three times more common in men (54,610 cases) than women (17,960 cases). There will be an estimated 15,210 deaths from bladder cancer in 2013. The median age at diagnosis is 65 years.

The best established risk factor for bladder cancer development is tobacco use, which is linked to 50% of bladder cancer cases (2). Carcinogens from tobacco are filtered from the blood into urine, and have sustained contact with urothelial cells lining the bladder, ureter, and renal pelvis. Tobacco-related cancer risk is dose dependent and diminishes with tobacco cessation. Pelvic irradiation and exposure to the chemotherapeutic cyclophosphamide also increase the risk of developing bladder cancer. In some areas of the world, chronic bladder inflammation caused by schistosomiasis is linked to a squamous cell subtype of bladder cancer.

CLINICAL PRESENTATION AND DIAGNOSIS

Hematuria is the most common presenting symptom for bladder cancer. Hematuria may be gross or microscopic and is often painless, unless associated with clots and obstruction. Evaluation of asymptomatic patients for microscopic hematuria has not been an effective screening test for detection of bladder cancer.

When bladder cancer is suspected, workup should include urine cytology, cystoscopy, and an upper tract imaging study. Urine cytology has a sensitivity of 40%–60% with a specificity of greater than 90%. Spiral computed tomography (CT) can evaluate the upper urothelial tracts (renal pelvis and ureter), renal parenchyma, and lymph nodes. The definitive diagnosis can only be established by biopsy via transurethral resection of the bladder tumor (TURBT). Fluorescence in situ hybridization (FISH) of specific genes cannot be used to diagnose bladder cancer in the absence of a tissue biopsy, and the role of FISH in management of bladder cancer patients is not well established.

Transitional cell (urothelial) carcinoma is the most common subtype of bladder cancer (>90%), and can arise in other organs lined by transitional epithelium, including renal pelvis, ureter, and the proximal two-thirds of the urethra. Other histologic subtypes include squamous cell carcinoma (3% of bladder tumors in the United States), adenocarcinoma (2%; includes tumors at the bladder dome originating from the urachal remnant), and small cell tumors (1%). Further classification of transitional cell carcinoma subtypes includes the particularly aggressive micropapillary and sarcomatoid histologies. The remainder of this chapter will discuss management of transitional cell carcinoma.

STAGING

Urinary bladder cancer can be grouped into three general categories by stage at presentation: non-muscle-invasive (formerly described as superficial), muscle-invasive, and metastatic. Each differs in clinical behavior, primary management, and outcome.

The primary bladder tumor is staged according to the depth of invasion into the bladder wall or beyond (see **Figure 42-1**). During TURBT, the visible tumor is resected along with sampling of involved or adjacent muscularis propria, to assess for the presence of muscle invasion. Non-muscle-invasive tumors include papillary mucosal tumors (Ta), flat mucosal tumors (carcinoma in situ [CIS], or Tis), and tumors involving the lamina propria (T1). Tumors that invade the muscularis propria layer comprise T2 disease. Tumors that penetrate beyond the muscle layer to the serosa are classified as T3. Tumors that involve contiguous pelvic structures such as the prostate, vagina, uterus, or pelvic/abdominal walls are classified as stage T4.

Patients with muscle-invasive bladder cancer require further staging workup beyond the initial abdominopelvic CT scan, including chest CT,

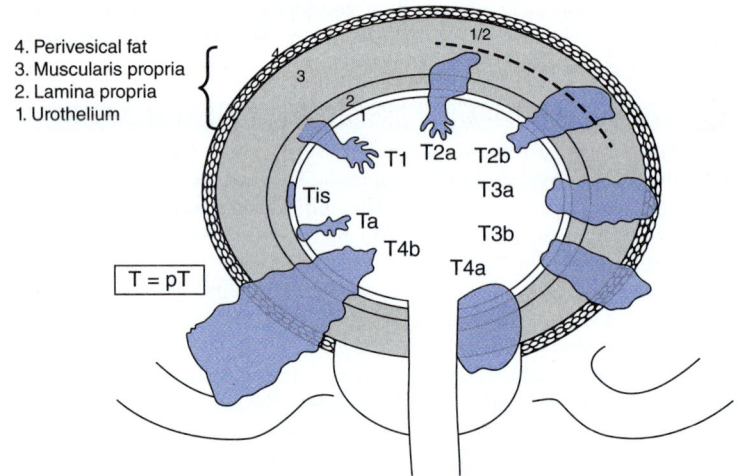

FIGURE 42-1 Primary bladder tumor staging. (Adapted from Reference 3.)

TABLE 42-1 FIVE-YEAR SURVIVAL RATE BY STAGE

Stage	5-Year Survival Rate
0	98%
I	88%
II	63%
III	46%
IV	15%

Source: National Cancer Institute Surveillance Epidemiology and End Results (SEER) Database.

complete blood count, blood chemistries, and consideration of a bone scan. Although the presence of urinary bladder cancer is associated with upper tract disease in <5% of cases, careful evaluation of the upper tracts is warranted due to the "field defect" from carcinogen exposure throughout the urothelium.

In the absence of lymph node or distant metastasis, T stage determines anatomic stage. Stage 0 disease constitutes Ta and Tis tumors. Stage I and II cancers have T1 and T2 tumors, respectively. Stage III cancers include T3 tumors and T4a tumors (involvement of prostate, uterus, or vagina). Stage IV cancers include T4b tumors (invading pelvic or abdominal wall), and tumors of any T stage that include lymph node or distant metastasis. Survival by stage is described in Table 42-1.

MANAGEMENT

■ NON-MUSCLE-INVASIVE BLADDER CANCER (TA, TIS, T1)

Non-muscle-invasive tumors constitute 70% of new diagnoses. Approximately 15%–20% of these patients will eventually progress to stage T2 or worse disease. Up to 70% of patients diagnosed with non-muscle-invasive cancer will have a local recurrence following initial therapy. Low-grade tumors and low-stage (Ta) disease tend to have a lower recurrence rate at about 50%, with a 5% rate of progression to higher stage disease. However, high-risk disease (high-grade disease, multifocal disease, or T1 disease) has a 70% recurrence rate and a 30% progression rate to stage T2+ disease. Due to high recurrence and progression rates, these patients require close urologic follow-up indefinitely, initially consisting of cystoscopy and urine cytology every 3 months. Fewer than 5% of patients with non-muscle-invasive bladder cancer will develop metastatic disease without exhibiting evidence of muscle invasion during the course of surveillance, underscoring the importance of close follow-up.

Patients at high risk for development of progressive or recurrent disease are generally considered candidates for adjuvant intravesical therapy. In general, this group includes patients with T1 tumors, multifocal CIS, high-grade tumors, or rapidly recurrent disease following initial resection. Standard options for intravesical therapy include immunologic agents such as Bacillus Calmette-Guérin (BCG) with or without interferon, or chemotherapy agents such as mitomycin C or doxorubicin. The goal of therapy is to decrease the rate of recurrence and progression.

Radical cystectomy of non-muscle-invasive bladder cancer is occasionally considered for patients with frequent recurrences, multiple tumors despite intravesical therapy, or intolerance of intravesical therapy.

■ MUSCLE-INVASIVE BLADDER CANCER (T2-4)

Surgical Approaches

The standard of care for muscle-invasive bladder cancer is radical cystectomy with bilateral pelvic lymph node dissection. In female patients, an anterior exenteration is performed, which includes removal of the bladder and urethra (the urethra may be spared if uninvolved and an orthotopic bladder reconstruction is to be performed), the ventral vaginal wall, and the uterus. In male patients, when the prostate stroma is involved with cancer or when there is concomitant CIS of the urethra, a cystoprostatourethrectomy is the treatment of choice.

Urinary diversion techniques include formation of an ileal conduit or construction of an orthotopic neobladder, an internal urinary reservoir that can drain via the urethra or abdominal wall. The morbidity of cystectomy is significant, with one case series at a high-volume center describing 64% of cases with one or more complications, 26% requiring readmission to the hospital, and 2.7% 90-day mortality (4).

The probability of survival from bladder cancer following cystectomy is determined by the pathologic stage of the disease. Five-year overall survival (OS) is markedly influenced by the presence of lymph node involvement. In contemporary series, survival for pathologic T2 disease ranges from 59% to 72%, whereas T3/T4 disease survival ranges from 26% to 58%. Node positive disease survival rates range from 26% to 35% (5–7).

Selective Bladder-Preserving Approaches

An alternative to radical cystectomy with lymph node dissection is organ preservation with trimodality therapy in selected patients. This approach requires the use of early cystectomy at the first sign of failure of local control. Successful approaches have evolved over the past three decades following the initial reports of the effectiveness of cisplatin against transitional cell carcinoma. Trials in the United States and Europe have evaluated various schedules of concurrent chemoradiotherapy with or without neoadjuvant or adjuvant chemotherapy, with iterative improvements in the treatment regimens concurrent with improved radiation techniques. Radiosensitizing drugs studied in these series, either singly or in various combinations, include cisplatin, carboplatin, paclitaxel, 5-fluorouracil, mitomycin C, and gemcitabine.

A phase III trial of 360 patients evaluated radiation therapy with or without 5FU and mitomycin C chemotherapy (8). Subjects largely had clinical T2-T4a disease. Subjects were also randomized to either whole-bladder or modified-volume radiation therapy. The primary endpoint of locoregional disease-free survival favored chemoradiotherapy at 2 years (67% vs. 54%;

$p = 0.03$). Five-year OS also favored chemoradiotherapy, but the difference was not statistically significant (48% vs. 35%; $p = 0.16$).

The long-term outcomes of the approach at Massachusetts General Hospital via the Radiation Therapy Oncology Group (RTOG) was updated (9). Successive protocols involving 348 patients with clinical T2-T4a disease were combined. In summary, 72% of patients had complete response (CR) to induction chemoradiotherapy. Five-year OS was 52%. For clinical stage T2 disease (54% of subjects), the 5-year OS rate was 61%, as opposed to 41% for patients with T3-T4 disease. Greater than 70% of subjects retained their native bladder. Predictors of outcome include clinical T stage and CR to induction therapy.

The University of Erlangen has published the largest bladder-sparing study to date, involving 415 subjects that included 89 subjects with "high-risk T1" disease (10). This group included 126 patients who received radiation without any chemotherapy. The CR rate of all 415 patients was 72%. The 10-year disease-specific survival was 42%, and more than 80% of these survivors preserved their bladders.

The currently open North American protocol for bladder-sparing treatment (RTOG 0712) is a randomized phase II study comparing induction chemoradiotherapy with cisplatin plus 5FU with twice-daily radiation treatment, versus gemcitabine with once-daily radiation treatment. Consolidation chemoradiotherapy and adjuvant chemotherapy are given to subjects whose post-induction evaluation reveals <T1 disease; if ≥T1 disease is found, subjects proceed to prompt radical cystectomy followed by adjuvant chemotherapy.

Bladder preserving trimodality therapy should be one of the approaches considered in the treatment of selected patients with muscle-invasive bladder cancer. For example, eligible patients should have transitional cell carcinoma histology, absence of hydronephrosis, and tumors that can be maximally resected at TURBT. Published reports indicate comparable survival rates with contemporary cystectomy series (Table 42-2). This approach requires closely coordinated care among urologic surgeons, radiation oncologists, and medical oncologists. Patient-reported quality of life is favorable (11).

TABLE 42-2 FIVE-YEAR OVERALL SURVIVAL RATES ACROSS CONTEMPORARY STUDIES EVALUATING RADICAL CYSTECTOMY AND BLADDER PRESERVATION STRATEGIES

	Cystectomy			Trimodality Therapy		
	MSKCC (5)	USC (6)	SWOG (12)	Erlangen (10)	United Kingdom (8)	MGH/ RTOG (9)
Stage	pT2-4a	pT2-4a	pT2-4a	cT2-4	cT2-4a*	cT2-4a
N	181	633	307	326	360	348
5y OS	41%	48%	50%	45%	48%	52%

*1 subject had T1 disease.

■ EVOLVING ROLE FOR PERIOPERATIVE CHEMOTHERAPY

Neoadjuvant Chemotherapy

Radical cystectomy for muscle-invasive bladder cancer fails to cure a significant proportion of patients, suggesting that micrometastatic disease exists in many cases at the time of initial diagnosis. The goals of neoadjuvant chemotherapy are to eradicate micrometastatic disease and improve cure rates.

Two prospective studies have influenced the use of neoadjuvant chemotherapy. Southwest Oncology Group (SWOG) 8710 was a randomized controlled trial of 317 subjects comparing neoadjuvant methotrexate, vinblastine, doxorubicin, cisplatin (MVAC) chemotherapy preceding radical cystectomy, versus cystectomy alone (12). Neoadjuvant chemotherapy prolonged median survival (77 vs. 46 months, $p = 0.06$) and improved 5-year OS (57% vs. 43%, $p = 0.06$), but these effects were not statistically significant. There were higher rates of pathologic CR with chemotherapy (38% vs. 15%, $p < 0.001$). The International Collaboration of Trialists study was a randomized controlled trial of 976 subjects comparing neoadjuvant cisplatin, methotrexate, vinblastine (CMV) chemotherapy or no chemotherapy, preceding local therapy (13). Local therapy in this trial could include radical cystectomy, radiation therapy, or low-dose radiation with radical cystectomy. The initial report did not demonstrate a statistically significant difference in outcome. With longer follow-up, 10-year OS was significantly improved by neoadjuvant chemotherapy (36% vs. 30%, $p = 0.037$) (13).

A meta-analysis of 11 randomized trials reported by the Advanced Bladder Cancer Meta-Analysis Collaboration found an absolute 5-year OS benefit of 5% favoring neoadjuvant platinum-based chemotherapy (HR: 0.86; CI: 0.77–0.95; $p = 0.003$) (14). Careful discussion of the potential benefits and risks of neoadjuvant chemotherapy is warranted during planning for radical cystectomy, and may be of particular importance to those patients at highest risk for disseminated disease. Ongoing studies are evaluating dose-dense MVAC, gemcitabine-cisplatin doublet, and targeted therapies, among others, as neoadjuvant regimens.

Adjuvant Chemotherapy

The advantage of adjuvant, as opposed to neoadjuvant, chemotherapy is the selection of patients at highest risk for disease recurrence using pathologic staging. Node-positive disease or pathologic T3-4 stages are clear risk factors for disease progression. Unfortunately, there are no data to support adjuvant chemotherapy in resected bladder cancer. Trials that have attempted to evaluate adjuvant chemotherapy were underpowered or closed early due to poor accrual. Disadvantages to adjuvant chemotherapy include the delay to systemic therapy during surgery and recovery, high rates of postoperative complications that increase the delay to chemotherapy (4), and lack of clinical endpoints that allow assessment of response to treatment. Despite the lack of evidence demonstrating improved cure rates, investigators generally agree that in the face of high-risk pathologic features, adjuvant chemotherapy is worthy of consideration.

■ METASTATIC DISEASE

Bladder cancer typically spreads first to pelvic lymph nodes. Lymphatic and hematogenous spread can also produce metastases to distant organs, including lungs, bones, liver, and brain. The prognosis of metastatic bladder cancer is poor, with a median survival of 12–14 months.

Compared with other solid tumors, transitional cell carcinoma is particularly sensitive to chemotherapy. Numerous agents are active as single agents in bladder cancer, including cisplatin, carboplatin, docetaxel, doxorubicin, 5FU, gemcitabine, ifosfamide, paclitaxel, pemetrexed, methotrexate, vinblastine, and vinflunine. In contemporary trials, overall response rates to first-line chemotherapy are as high as 50%–80%. Moreover, a small but measurable minority of responding patients manifest a CR. Among these patients, some durable responses are observed. For most patients, however, the duration of response to chemotherapy is brief (median, 4–6 months), and thus the impact of chemotherapy on OS has been disappointing.

The standard chemotherapy regimen for advanced bladder cancer has been MVAC, developed at Memorial Sloan-Kettering Cancer Center in the 1980s. The response rate to MVAC is 40%–65%, and there is improved progression-free and OS compared with either single-agent cisplatin or cisplatin, cyclophosphamide, doxorubicin (CISCA). CR is seen in 15%–25% of patients.

The combination of gemcitabine and cisplatin (GC) showed promise in early phase clinical trials in terms of response rate with modest side effects (15). A phase III randomized controlled trial of GC compared to standard MVAC evaluated 405 subjects with metastatic bladder cancer. Median survival was statistically comparable (GC: 13.8 months; MVAC: 14.8 months; $p = 0.75$) (16). The response rates were 49% for the GC arm and 46% for the MVAC arm. The toxic death rate was 1% for subjects receiving GC, compared with 3% for subjects receiving MVAC. On this basis, GC is broadly considered a standard first-line choice for metastatic bladder cancer, and has been used for both neoadjuvant and adjuvant purposes.

Other chemotherapy regimens have been tested, largely as second-line treatments after first-line cisplatin-containing chemotherapy. Addition of paclitaxel to GC did not significantly increase OS in untreated patients (17). Vinflunine conferred a survival advantage (6.9 vs. 4.3 months, $p = 0.040$) compared with best supportive care in a phase III randomized controlled trial in subjects who progressed after first-line platinum-containing chemotherapy (18). The combination of paclitaxel and gemcitabine has been examined in numerous small studies as second-line therapy, with response rates up to 40% (19). Vinorelbine with gemcitabine is another active regimen with a 39% overall response rate in a small study ($n = 31$) (20).

The use of targeted therapies has revolutionized treatment in many solid tumors. Potential molecular targets in bladder cancer have been identified including HER2, FGFR3, and VEGF, among others. The role of bevacizumab, an antiangiogenesis antibody, is currently being evaluated in combination with GC chemotherapy in a randomized phase III trial sponsored by CALGB.

FUTURE DIRECTIONS

Numerous unanswered questions in bladder cancer management remain. For non-muscle-invasive disease, can patients at highest risk for disease progression be identified and treated prior to development of metastatic disease? For localized, muscle-invasive disease, which patients are optimally treated with neo-adjuvant chemotherapy? Which patients can have bladder preservation using trimodality approaches? For advanced or metastatic disease, can survival be improved using targeted therapies either as single agents or in combination with chemotherapy? In this era of rapid advances in molecular understanding of cancers, will the power of molecular biology improve survival and cure rates for this common malignancy?

REFERENCES

1. Siegel R, Naishadham D, Jemal A. Cancer statistics, 2013. *CA Cancer J Clin.* 2013; 63: 11–30.

2. Freedman ND, Silverman DT, Hollenbeck AR, et al. Association between smoking and risk of bladder cancer among men and women. *JAMA.* 2011; 306: 737–745.

3. *AJCC Cancer Staging Handbook,* 6th ed. New York: Springer; 2002. p. 370.

4. Donat SM, Shabsigh A, Savage C, et al. Potential impact of postoperative early complications on the timing of adjuvant chemotherapy in patients undergoing radical cystectomy: a high-volume tertiary cancer center experience. *Eur Urol.* 2009; 55: 177–186.

5. Dalbagni G, Genega E, Hashibe MIA, et al. Cystectomy for bladder cancer: a contemporary series. *J Urol.* 2001; 165: 1111–1116.

6. Stein JP, Lieskovsky G, Cote R, et al. Radical cystectomy in the treatment of invasive bladder cancer: long-term results in 1,054 patients. *J Clin Oncol.* 2001; 19: 666–675.

7. Madersbacher S, Hochreiter W, Burkhard F, et al. Radical cystectomy for bladder cancer today: a homogeneous series without neoadjuvant therapy. *J Clin Oncol.* 2003; 21: 690–696.

8. James ND, Hussain SA, Hall E, et al. Radiotherapy with or without chemotherapy in muscle-invasive bladder cancer. *N Engl J Med.* 2012; 366: 1477–1488.

9. Efstathiou JA, Spiegel DY, Shipley WU, et al. Long-term outcomes of selective bladder preservation by combined-modality therapy for invasive bladder cancer: the MGH experience. *Eur Urol.* 2012; 61: 705–711.

10. Rodel C, Grabenbauer GG, Kuhn R, et al. Combined-modality treatment and selective organ preservation in invasive bladder cancer: long-term results. *J Clin Oncol.* 2002; 20: 3061–3071.

11. Zietman AL, Sacco D, Skowronski URI, et al. Organ conservation in invasive bladder cancer by transurethral resection, chemotherapy and radiation: results of a urodynamic and quality of life study on long-term survivors. *J Urol.* 2003; 170: 1772–1776.

12. Grossman HB, Natale RB, Tangen CM, et al. Neoadjuvant chemotherapy plus cystectomy compared with cystectomy alone for locally advanced bladder cancer. *N Engl J Med.* 2003; 349: 859–866.

13. International Collaboration of Trialists on behalf of the Medical Research Council Advanced Bladder Cancer Working Party. International phase III trial assessing neoadjuvant cisplatin, methotrexate, and vinblastine chemotherapy for muscle-invasive bladder cancer: long-term results of the BA06 30894 trial. *J Clin Oncol.* 2011; 29: 2171–2177.

14. Vale CL. Neoadjuvant chemotherapy in invasive bladder cancer: update of a systematic review and meta-analysis of individual patient data: advanced bladder cancer (ABC) meta-analysis collaboration. *Eur Urol.* 2005; 48: 202–206.

15. Kaufman D, Raghavan D, Carducci M, et al. Phase II trial of gemcitabine plus cisplatin in patients with metastatic urothelial cancer. *J Clin Oncol.* 2000; 18: 1921–1927.

16. von der Maase H, Hansen SW, Roberts JT, et al. Gemcitabine and cisplatin versus methotrexate, vinblastine, doxorubicin, and cisplatin in advanced or metastatic bladder cancer: results of a large, randomized, multinational, multicenter, phase III study. *J Clin Oncol.* 2000; 18: 3068–3077.

17. Bellmunt J, von der Maase H, Mead GM, et al. Randomized phase III study comparing paclitaxel/cisplatin/gemcitabine and gemcitabine/cisplatin in patients with locally advanced or metastatic urothelial cancer without prior systemic therapy: EORTC Intergroup Study 30987. *J Clin Oncol.* 2012; 30: 1107–1113.

18. Bellmunt J, Theodore C, Demkov T, et al. Phase III trial of vinflunine plus best supportive care compared with best supportive care alone after a platinum-containing regimen in patients with advanced transitional cell carcinoma of the urothelial tract. *J Clin Oncol.* 2009; 27: 4454–4461.

19. Albers P, Park SI, Niegisch G, et al, for the AUOBCG. Randomized phase III trial of 2nd line gemcitabine and paclitaxel chemotherapy in patients with advanced bladder cancer: short-term versus prolonged treatment (German Association of Urological Oncology [AUO] trial AB 20/99). *Ann Oncol.* 2011; 22: 288–294.

20. Turkolmez K, Beduk Y, Baltaci S, et al. Gemcitabine plus vinorelbine chemotherapy in patients with advanced bladder carcinoma who are medically unsuitable for or who have failed cisplatin-based chemotherapy. *Eur Urol.* 2003; 44: 682–686.

CHAPTER **43**
Testicular Cancer

Timothy Gilligan

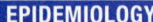

EPIDEMIOLOGY

Although testis cancer is rare when viewed across the lifespan, it is the most common malignancy in men aged 20–35 years. Thanks to the high cure rate of the disease, however, it represents fewer than 5% of cancer deaths during those ages. In 2013, there were about 7,920 new cases and 370 deaths from testicular cancer. Incidence is relatively stable while mortality has been in decline. The declining mortality rate is attributed to the development of curative chemotherapy for advanced disease, improved treatment algorithms, earlier stage at presentation, and a growing proportion of seminomas relative to nonseminomas. The U.S. male lifetime risk of being diagnosed with testis cancer is between 3 and 4 in 1000. Testis cancer is exceedingly rare in African American men, whose incidence of the disease is one-fifth that of white Americans.

Major risk factors for testis cancer include cryptorchidism, and a family history or personal history of testicular cancer. Having a brother with testis cancer raises a man's risk about 8- to 10–fold, whereas testis cancer in the father raises the son's risk fourfold. The risk for testis cancer in men with cryptorchidism is estimated to be 10–15 times higher than in the general population, resulting in a roughly 2%–3% lifetime risk of testis cancer. Prepubertal orchiopexy is strongly recommended in men with cryptorchidism to reduce the risk of testis cancer. Men who have had testis cancer have about a 2%–3% risk of developing a second cancer in the contralateral testis.

PATHOLOGY

The vast majority of testicular neoplasms are germ cell tumors (GCTs), which include the following subcategories:

- Seminoma
- Embryonal carcinoma
- Teratoma
- Yolk sac tumor (also known as endodermal sinus tumor)
- Choriocarcinoma

Choriocarcinomas and teratomas in men are different diseases from gestational choriocarcinomas and gestational teratomas in women. In contrast, ovarian GCTs in women and pediatric GCTs are similar but not identical to testicular GCTs in post-pubescent males. For management purposes, GCTs in men are divided into pure seminomas and nonseminomas. Pure seminomas may contain no other GCT elements. Nonseminomas, in contrast, usually consist of a mixture of two or more GCT subtypes and one of these subtypes may be seminoma.

Serum tumor markers (STMs) are elevated in over half of all testis cancer patients. STMs are more likely to be elevated in advanced stage than localized disease. The following STMs all play a critical role in the diagnosis, staging, and management of testicular cancer:

- Alpha-fetoprotein (AFP) (half-life = 5–7 days)
- Human chorionic gonadotropin (HCG) (half-life = 24–36 h)
- Lactate dehydrogenase (LDH)

One critical fact is that seminomas do not produce AFP. Elevated serum AFP therefore precludes a diagnosis of seminoma regardless of the histopathology unless an alternative source for the AFP is clearly identified. Likewise, a post-orchiectomy HCG greater than 1000 IU/L would be considered inconsistent with pure seminoma by many GCT experts.

The degree of elevation of STMs following orchiectomy but prior to other treatment affects stage and prognosis. Similarly, a slower than expected rate of decline of AFP and HCG during chemotherapy is associated with a worse prognosis. Persistently elevated STMs following orchiectomy indicate the presence of metastatic disease (unless a compelling alternative explanation is identified), while rising STMs are often the earliest indication of relapse.

GCTs are not the only cause of elevated AFP, HCG, and LDH. Elevations of AFP are seen in hepatocellular carcinoma, hepatitis, and cancers of the stomach, colon, rectum, and other gastrointestinal sites. AFP can be elevated due to hepatotoxicity from chemotherapy, so elevations of AFP at the conclusion of treatment cannot always be interpreted as indicative of residual disease or relapse. Elevations of HCG are seen in biliary, pancreatic, and many other cancers, but in non-GCT neoplasms, the elevation is typically mild. Hypogonadism resulting in elevated serum gonadotropins can result in elevations of serum HCG assays due to assay cross reactivity with luteinizing hormone and due to pituitary production of HCG. In such a scenario, the elevation of HCG should resolve with supplemental testosterone. Elevations of LDH are seen in a host of cancers and other diseases, including lymphoma, liver disease, myocardial infarction, and other conditions associated with cell death.

DIAGNOSIS AND STAGING

Testis cancer typically presents with a painless or painful testicular mass. Less common presenting symptoms include gynecomastia, gynecodynia, testicular atrophy, infertility, and, in advanced stage disease, back pain, supraclavicular adenopathy, thromboembolic events, or respiratory symptoms. If a testicular tumor is suspected from the history and/or physical examination, a scrotal ultrasound should be ordered to evaluate both testicles. If the ultrasound indicates that a tumor is present, the following steps should be performed:

- Measure serum AFP, HCG, LDH
- Radical/inguinal orchiectomy
- CT scan of the abdomen and pelvis
- Chest x-ray if the CT of the abdomen/pelvis and serum tumor markers are normal

TABLE 43-1 STAGE I IS FURTHER SUBDIVIDED BASED ON TUMOR STAGE

IA	T1	Limited to testis with or without invasion of tunica albuginea, epididymis and rete testis
IB	T2	Lymphovascular invasion or invasion of the tunica vaginalis
	T3	Invasion of the spermatic cord
	T4	Invasion of the scrotum
IS	any	T stage plus elevated markers

- Chest CT if the CT of the abdomen/pelvis shows nodal or visceral metastases or if post-orchiectomy STMs are elevated
- If any STM was elevated before orchiectomy, recheck STMs after orchiectomy
- Brain MRI or CT in patients with post-orchiectomy AFP or HCG >5000 or signs or symptoms intracranial metastases

■ STAGING

Testicular cancer divides into three stages:

I. Limited to the testis, spermatic cord, and scrotum (Table 43-1)

II. Metastatic disease to retroperitoneal and/or pelvic lymph nodes and STMs normal or mildly elevated (Table 43-2)

III. Regional nodal metastases plus moderately to highly elevated STMs and/or visceral or distant nodal metastases

Although patients with persistently elevated STMs following orchiectomy are technically labeled stage I if there is no radiographic evidence of metastatic disease (stage IS), they are treated as stage III patients for presumed micrometastatic disease.

Stage III is subdivided based on the level of STMs and the location of metastases. Treatment decisions about advanced stage disease are based on the International Germ Cell Consensus Classification system that divides patients into risk categories (Table 43-3) (1).

TABLE 43-2 STAGE II IS SUBDIVIDED BASED ON THE NUMBER AND SIZE OF ENLARGED LYMPH NODES

IIA	Fewer than 6 enlarged nodes, none measuring more than 2 cm in greatest diameter
IIB	Any node between 2 and 5 cm or more than 5 enlarged nodes with none greater than 5 cm
IIC	A nodal mass greater than 5 cm

TABLE 43-3 INTERNATIONAL GERM CELL CONSENSUS CLASSIFICATION SYSTEM RISK CATEGORIES

GOOD PROGNOSIS	
Nonseminoma	Seminoma
Testis/retroperitoneal primary	Any primary site
and	and
No nonpulmonary visceral metastases	No nonpulmonary visceral metastases
and	and
All of the following:	Normal AFP, any HCG, any LDH
AFP <1000 ng/ml	
HCG <5000 mIU/ml	
LDH <1.5 × upper limit of normal (ULN)	
5-Year progression-free survival = 89%	5-Year progression-free survival = 82%
5-Year overall survival = 92%	5-Year overall survival = 86%
INTERMEDIATE PROGNOSIS	
Nonseminoma	Seminoma
Testis/retroperitoneal primary	Any primary site
and	and
No nonpulmonary visceral metastases	Nonpulmonary visceral metastases
and	and
Any of the following:	Normal AFP, any HCG, any LDH
AFP ≥1000 and ≤ 10,000 ng/ml	
HCG ≥5000 and ≤50,000 mIU/ml	
LDH ≥1.5 × ULN and ≤10 × ULN	
5-Year progression-free survival = 75%	5-Year progression-free survival = 67%
5-Year overall survival = 80%	5-Year overall survival = 72%
POOR PROGNOSIS	
Nonseminoma	Seminoma
Mediastinal primary	
and/or	
Nonpulmonary visceral metastases	No seminoma patients classified as poor prognosis
and/or	
Any of the following:	
AFP >10,000 ng/ml	
HCG >50,000 mIU/ml	
LDH >10 × ULN	
5-Year progression-free survival = 41%	
5-Year overall survival = 48%	

TREATMENT

Treatment for testis cancer that includes chemotherapy, para-aortic or pelvic radiation therapy, or retroperitoneal lymph node dissection can render men infertile. Men who wish to preserve their fertility should be advised to bank semen prior to treatment. Men receiving bleomycin chemotherapy as part of their treatment must be advised to alert health-care providers to this fact in the future if they undergo surgery so that perioperative precautions can be taken. These include minimizing exposure to supplemental oxygen and IV fluids during surgery and the perioperative period.

◼ STAGE I AND II SEMINOMAS

Stage I Seminoma

Stage I seminomas carry an outstanding prognosis with fewer than 1% of patients expected to die as a result of the disease. There are three management options for these patients and they result in indistinguishable long-term survival rates (2):

- Surveillance
- Single agent carboplatin chemotherapy
- External beam radiation therapy

Each option has distinct risks and benefits.

Numerous studies have reported that surveillance produces survival rates indistinguishable from those associated with radiation therapy and carboplatin chemotherapy, although no randomized controlled trials of surveillance have been published. The relapse rate for stage I patients managed with surveillance following orchiectomy is about 18% compared to 4% after radiation therapy. The vast majority of relapsing surveillance patients can be cured with radiation therapy at the time of relapse while almost all of the others can be cured with chemotherapy. Risk factors for relapse during surveillance include a large tumor (e.g., >4 cm) and invasion of the rete testis (3). Risk of relapse is about 10%, 16%, and 32% for men with zero, one, or both risk factors, respectively. A common surveillance schedule is to perform a physical examination, chest x-ray, serum tumor marker measurement, and an abdominopelvic CT scan at the following intervals:

- Years 1–3:   every 4 months
- Years 4–5:   every 6 months
- Years 6–10:   annually

An alternative to surveillance is carboplatin chemotherapy given as either one or two cycles at a dose of an AUC of 7. A randomized trial comparing a single dose of carboplatin to external beam radiation reported no difference in relapse rate (4). Studies of two cycles of carboplatin have reported lower relapse rates of about 2% (5, 6). Very limited long-term follow-up for patients treated with carboplatin is available, but disease-specific survival in reported series is 100%. Little is known about the hypothetical risk of late relapse and late toxicity (Table 43-4).

Once widely used, radiation therapy became less popular after long-term follow-up studies reported an excess risk of developing secondary malignancies and an increased risk of cardiovascular disease and death.

TABLE 43-4 OUTCOMES FOR STAGE I SEMINOMA IN PUBLISHED SERIES

	N	Relapses	Relapse Rate (%)	5-Year DSS (%)
Surveillance	1756	276	16	99.5
Carboplatin (two cycles)	795	13	1.6	100
Radiation	4630	175	3.8	99.7

DSS, disease-specific survival.

Stage II Seminoma

Treatment of stage II seminoma has never been investigated in well-designed, adequately powered randomized trials. Currently, stage IIA patients typically receive radiation therapy, stage IIC patients are treated with cisplatin-based chemotherapy for disseminated disease, and stage IIB patients can be treated with either approach. The cure rate for IIA/IIB disease is 90%–95% and for IIC is 85%–90% (7). There has been a trend toward treating all stage II seminoma patients with chemotherapy (3 cycles of BEP or 4 cycles of EP), but there are no randomized controlled trials comparing these approaches.

■ STAGE I AND II NONSEMINOMATOUS GERM CELL TUMORS

Stage I NSGCT

Persistently elevated STMs usually indicate distant metastases. Men with stage I NSGCTs who have persistently elevated STMs should be treated as stage III patients using cisplatin-based chemotherapy. Stage I NSGCTs in men with normal post-orchiectomy STMs can be managed successfully with any of the following three strategies (6, 8):

Surveillance

Retroperitoneal lymph node dissection

One or two cycles of BEP chemotherapy (BEP = bleomycin, etoposide, cisplatin)

Each results in a disease-specific survival of about 99%. Men on surveillance face a 30% risk of relapse on average, but the risk is higher for men with lymphovascular invasion and/or a predominance of embryonal carcinoma. Surveillance requires frequent doctor visits and medical tests (Table 43-5).

Retroperitoneal lymph node dissection reduces the risk of relapse and permits more accurate staging. The operation should be performed by a highly experienced surgeon in order to avoid incomplete resections and/or unnecessary side effects such as infertility. If no cancer is found at surgery, the risk of relapse is 5%–10%. If cancer is found, adjuvant chemotherapy is often recommended, particularly if the pathological stage is IIB or IIC. Adjuvant chemotherapy with two cycles of BEP or EP following retroperitoneal lymph node dissection reduces the relapse risk to about 1%.

Given as primary treatment following orchiectomy, one or two cycles of BEP chemotherapy for stage Ia or Ib disease results in a relapse risk of less than 3%. Primary chemotherapy is thus the most effective treatment at preventing relapses. However, there is some concern that these patients

TABLE 43-5 SURVEILLANCE SCHEDULE FOR CLINICAL STAGE I NONSEMINOMA

Year 1:	Monthly visits for PE, STMs, CXR.	Abdominopelvic CT at months 3 and 9
Year 2:	Bimonthly PE, STMs, CXR	Abdominopelvic CT at month 18
Year 3:	PE, STMs, CXR every 3 mo	Abdominopelvic CT at month 30
Year 4:	PE, STMs, CXR every 4 mo	Abdominopelvic CT at month 42
Year 5:	PE, STMs, CXR every 6 mo	Abdominopelvic CT at month 60
Years 6+:	PE, STMs, CXR, annually	Consider abdominopelvic CT every 2 y until 10 y out

PE, physical examination.

may be at increased risk of late relapse due to incompletely treated cancers or unresected teratomatous elements. There is also concern about late toxicity from BEP such as secondary malignancies, cardiovascular disease, and neurotoxicity. As a result, the question of optimal management of stage I NSGCT remains contentious.

Stage II NSGCT

Treatment of stage II NSGCTs depends on the extent of the disease. A significant number of men with radiographic evidence of low volume (IIA) disease, and normal STMs will turn out to have benign pathological findings at surgery and will thus be pathological stage I. One main goal of RPLND in clinical stage IIA patients is to obtain accurate staging and avoid administering unnecessary chemotherapy. An alternative to RPLND for low volume stage IIA disease is close observation with subsequent chemotherapy in the event of progression. Stage II patients undergoing RPLND should be warned that they will probably be advised to undergo postoperative chemotherapy with two cycles of BEP or EP chemotherapy.

Men with bulkier nodal disease on CT scans (IIB or IIC) and/or mildly elevated STMs (S1) are generally treated with three cycles of BEP or four cycles of EP chemotherapy. RPLND in the setting of elevated STMs is associated with a very high risk of relapse. Men undergoing chemotherapy for stage II NSGCT should be warned that they will probably be advised to undergo a post-chemotherapy RPLND to resect any residual GCT.

ADVANCED STAGE TESTIS CANCER

■ FIRST-LINE CHEMOTHERAPY

First-line chemotherapy for testicular cancer is usually curative and optimal regimens have been well defined in randomized controlled trials. Deviations from standard care are to be avoided. The following guidelines should be followed:

- Avoid treatment delays and dose reductions
- Monitor for pulmonary toxicity if administering bleomycin
- Recommend sperm banking prior to chemotherapy

First-line chemotherapy for good-risk patients:
- Three cycles of BEP chemotherapy (9, 10) OR
- Four cycles of EP chemotherapy

First-line chemotherapy for intermediate-risk and poor-risk patients:
- Four cycles of BEP chemotherapy OR
- Four cycles of VIP (etoposide, ifosfamide, cisplatin) chemotherapy (10–12)

■ SALVAGE CHEMOTHERAPY

Salvage chemotherapy produces a substantially lower cure rate (25%–50%) than first-line chemotherapy. In this setting, patients with pure seminomas patients have substantially better outcomes than those with NSGCTs. The proper role, if any, for high-dose chemotherapy in this setting remains unclear.

Salvage chemotherapy regimens (10):
- Four cycles of VeIP (vinblastine, ifosfamide, cisplatin)
- Four cycles of TIP (paclitaxel, ifosfamide, cisplatin)
- Two cycles of high-dose carboplatin and etoposide chemotherapy with autologous peripheral stem cell rescue

Third-line chemotherapy:
- Cisplatin, gemcitabine, paclitaxel
- Gemcitabine, paclitaxel
- Gemcitabine, oxaliplatin

MANAGEMENT OF RESIDUAL MASSES

■ NONSEMINOMAS

Residual masses following chemotherapy in patients with NSGCTs may consist of fibrosis (45%–50%), teratoma (40%–45%), or viable cancer (10%). Radiographic imaging, including PET, cannot reliably distinguish these entities. If left unresected, teratomatous elements of NSGCTs can transform into carcinomas, sarcomas, and other cancers. When surgically feasible, all residual post-chemotherapy masses in patients with NSGCTs should be resected (10, 13). This can include excision of pulmonary, hepatic, and retroperitoneal masses. Persistent elevation of serum tumor markers following chemotherapy is not a contraindication to resection, but salvage chemotherapy is preferred as initial treatment if markers are rising. Thorough post-chemotherapy resections can be technically difficult and risky; referral to a highly experienced surgeon is appropriate (13).

■ SEMINOMAS

Residual masses following chemotherapy in men with seminomas are usually benign. Masses smaller than 3 cm on CT scan can be observed. Masses larger than 3 cm should be evaluated with an FDG PET scan. Observation is appropriate for FDG-negative masses, but FDG-avid masses should be biopsied or resected; if residual disease is histopathologically confirmed, it should be treated with salvage chemotherapy.

REFERENCES

1. International Germ Cell Cancer Collaborative Group. International germ cell consensus classification: a prognostic factor-based staging system for metastatic germ cell cancers. *J Clin Oncol.* 1997; 15: 594–603.

2. Krege S, et al. European consensus conference on diagnosis and treatment of germ cell cancer: a report of the second meeting of the European Germ Cell Cancer Consensus Group (EGCCCG): part I. *Eur Urol.* 2008; 53: 478–496.

3. Warde P, et al. Prognostic factors for relapse in stage I seminoma managed by surveillance: a pooled analysis. *J Clin Oncol.* 2002; 20: 4448–4452.

4. Oliver RT, et al. Randomized trial of carboplatin versus radiotherapy for stage I seminoma: mature results on relapse and contralateral testis cancer rates in MRC TE19/EORTC 30982 study (ISRCTN27163214). *J Clin Oncol.* 2011; 29: 957–962.

5. Oliver RT, et al. Radiotherapy versus single-dose carboplatin in adjuvant treatment of stage I seminoma: a randomised trial. *Lancet.* 2005; 366: 293–300.

6. Tan, A. and T. Gilligan. Controversies in the management of early-stage germ cell tumors. *Curr Oncol Rep.* 2009; 11: 235–243.

7. Chung PW, Bedard P. Stage II seminomas and nonseminomas. *Hematol Oncol Clin North Am.* 2011; 25: 529–541, viii.

8. Powles T. Stage I nonseminomatous germ cell tumor of the testis: more questions than answers? *Hematol Oncol Clin North Am.* 2011; 25: 517–527, viii.

9. Saxman SB, et al. Long-term follow-up of a phase III study of three versus four cycles of bleomycin, etoposide, and cisplatin in favorable-prognosis germ-cell tumors: the Indian University experience. *J Clin Oncol.* 1998; 16: 702–706.

10. Krege S, et al. European consensus conference on diagnosis and treatment of germ cell cancer: a report of the second meeting of the European Germ Cell Cancer Consensus Group (EGCCCG): part II. *Eur Urol.* 2008; 53: 497–513.

11. de Wit R, et al. Four cycles of BEP vs four cycles of VIP in patients with intermediate-prognosis metastatic testicular non-seminoma: a randomized study of the EORTC Genitourinary Tract Cancer Cooperative Group. European Organization for Research and Treatment of Cancer. *Br J Cancer.* 1998; 78: 828–832.

12. Nichols CR, et al. Randomized comparison of cisplatin and etoposide and either bleomycin or ifosfamide in treatment of advanced disseminated germ cell tumors: an Eastern Cooperative Oncology Group, Southwest Oncology Group, and Cancer and Leukemia Group B Study. *J Clin Oncol.* 1998; 16: 1287–1293.

13. Nguyen CT, Stephenson AJ. Role of postchemotherapy retroperitoneal lymph node dissection in advanced germ cell tumors. *Hematol Oncol Clin North Am.* 2011; 25: 593–604, ix.

CHAPTER **44**
Esophageal and Gastric Cancer
Lawrence S. Blaszkowsky

The incidence of esophageal cancer has steadily increased while the incidence of gastric cancer has decreased in the United States for over a half century. Over the past several decades, the incidence of tumors in the distal esophagus/gastroesophageal junction and cardia is rising. The highest rates of esophageal cancer are found in East Asia, Eastern Africa, and Southern Africa. Over half of all gastric cancers occur in developing countries with the highest incidence in East Asia, South America (Andes Region), and Eastern Europe. Following migration to areas of lower risk, subsequent generations experience a risk approaching that of the surrounding population, implicating an important role for environmental factors on the development of gastric cancer. In the United States, there were estimated to be 17,990 new cases of esophageal cancer and 15,210 deaths in 2013. The estimated new cases and deaths of gastric cancer were 21,600 and 10,990, respectively (1). Advances in prevention, early detection, aggressive surgery, the use of adjuvant therapy, and more effective antineoplastic agents will hopefully reduce the incidence and improve survival.

PATHOLOGY

- Esophageal
  - Squamous cell carcinoma: decreasing incidence and may arise throughout the esophagus
  - Adenocarcinoma: increasing incidence and arises in the distal esophagus and gastroesophageal junction
- Gastric
  - Intestinal type (expanding): characterized by the formation of distinct glands, and typically involves the cardia, corpus, or antrum. It is often associated with multifocal (atrophic) gastritis and intestinal metaplasia of the antrum, as well as pernicious anemia, older age, male sex, and various environmental factors, including *Helicobacter pylori*. There has been a dramatic decrease in the incidence of this form of gastric cancer in developing countries.
  - Diffuse type (infiltrative): often presents as linitis plastica. It is characterized by poorly organized clusters or signet-ring cells (mucin containing). They often arise in the corpus and affect a generally young population. There is a propensity for these tumors to develop in patients with superficial gastritis related to *H. pylori* without atrophy or metaplasia, as well as those who have the type A blood group. Familial clusters are common. These tumors generally tend to be more aggressive than the intestinal type.

RISK FACTORS

- Esophageal
  - Squamous cell: cigarette smoking, alcohol, achalasia, tylosis, caustic stricture (i.e., lye), prior radiation.
  - Adenocarcinoma: Barrett's esophagus due to GERD, smoking, obesity, higher socioeconomic class, Caucasian, male.
- Gastric
  - Diets rich in salty or smoked foods, nitroso compounds, low in vegetable and antioxidants.
  - *H. pylori* infection, which is dependent on genotype and host factors (polymorphisms).
  - Smoking increases the risk by about 1.5-fold.
  - Atrophic gastritis increases the risk by nearly sixfold.
  - Prior gastric surgery with the highest risk at 15–20 years. The risk is greater following Billroth II than Billroth I anastomosis.
  - Ionizing radiation was associated with a relative risk of 3.7 in survivors of the Japanese atomic bomb.
  - Blood group A is associated with a 20% higher incidence.
  - Low-socioeconomic group results in an increase in distal cancers, whereas high-socioeconomic group increases the risk of proximal cancers.
  - Epstein-Barr virus associated gastric cancer is related to DNA methylation of promoter genes of various cancer-associated genes. They may have a more favorable prognosis.
  - Several familial syndromes have been associated with a predisposition to gastric cancer: Lynch syndrome, E-cadherin (CDH1) mutation (diffuse type), familial adenomatous polyposis, and Peutz-Jeghers syndrome.

SIGNS AND SYMPTOMS

Progressive dysphagia leading to weight loss is the most common symptom of esophageal cancer. Abdominal pain and weight loss are common presenting complaints in gastric cancer. Nausea and vomiting are more commonly seen with distal gastric cancers, whereas early satiety is more common with linitis plastica tumors. Gastric cancers may bleed, leading to hematemesis, melena, and anemia. Malignant ascites, resulting in increased abdominal girth, are more commonly seen in patients with linitis plastica.

DIAGNOSIS AND STAGING EVALUATION

- Physical examination may be remarkable for cachexia, abdominal distension, hepatomegaly in the case of liver metastases, and lymphadenopathy.
- Upper GI series may demonstrate a stricture in the esophagus, a filling defect along the gastric wall, or decreased distensibility of the stomach due to a linitis plastica tumor.
- Esophagogastroduodenoscopy is the mainstay of diagnosis. Deep biopsies are often necessary if linitis plastica of the stomach is suspected as the tumor tends to infiltrate the submucosa. A single biopsy of a malignant ulcer has a 70% sensitivity rate of diagnosis and seven biopsies increase the sensitivity in gastric cancer to 98%.

- Endoscopic ultrasound aids in determining the depth of invasion, which may be important for determination of the need for neoadjuvant therapy or clinical trial considerations.
- CT scan of the chest, abdomen, and pelvis is important for the identification of metastatic disease.
- Bone scan is typically reserved for patients with symptoms suggesting osseous metastases.
- PET scan is commonly used to detect metastatic disease for esophageal cancer. The role in gastric cancer has not entirely been defined.
- Laparoscopy may detect occult peritoneal or hepatic metastases too small to be appreciated by CT scan and is often considered if imaging studies raise concern for peritoneal disease or in the case of bulky adenopathy.
- Tumor markers including CEA and CA 19-9 are sometimes helpful in monitoring patients with adenocarcinoma but are frequently not elevated.

STAGING (AJCC)

The American Joint Committee on Cancer is the system used for esophageal and gastric cancer staging in most countries (2). The seventh edition utilizes a separate staging system for squamous cell and adenocarcinoma of the esophagus and also incorporates grade. T stage is based on depth of invasion and N stage is based on total number of involved lymph nodes rather than location (unless distant lymph node). See Tables 44-1 and 44-2. The Siewert-Stein classification is based on the location of a tumor about the GE junction (3). A type I tumor has its center within 1–5 cm above the anatomic GE junction. A type 2 tumor is centered between 1 cm above and 2 cm below the GE junction. A type 3 tumor is centered 2–5 cm below the GE junction, in the cardia. Tumors arising in the cardia, within 5 cm, and invading the esophagus are staged according to esophageal cancer, whereas tumors located in the cardia of the stomach and not invading the GE junction are staged as gastric cancer.

TREATMENT OF LOCALIZED DISEASE

■ SURGICAL AND INVASIVE APPROACHES

Esophageal Cancer

Less than half of all patients presenting with a new diagnosis of esophageal cancer have disease that is potentially resectable. The type of intervention offered to these patients may depend upon the depth of invasion of the tumor, location, comorbidities, and the preference of the surgeon. In patients with high-grade dysplasia or superficial cancers (i.e., T1a), particularly in those who are felt to be at high risk for esophagectomy, radiofrequency ablation, argon plasma coagulation, or photodynamic therapy (PDT) may be considered.

- Transhiatal esophagectomy: involves an upper midline laparotomy and left neck incision. A cervical anastomosis is created by a gastric pull-up. There is a limited ability to do thoracic lymphadenectomy.
- Ivor-Lewis transthoracic esophagectomy: involves a right thoracotomy and a laparotomy with an intrathoracic anastomosis. This procedure may be modified with a left thoracotomy for GE junction tumors.

TABLE 44-1　TNM AND AJCC STAGING FOR ESOPHAGEAL CANCER

Primary Tumor (T)

Tx	Primary tumor cannot be assessed
T0	No evidence of primary tumor
Tis	High-grade dysplasia
T1	Tumor invades lamina propria, muscularis mucosae, or submucosa
T1a	Tumor invades lamina propria or muscularis mucosae
T1b	Tumor invades submucosa
T2	Tumor invades muscularis propria
T3	Tumor invades adventia
T4	Tumor invades adjacent structures
T4a	Resectable tumor invading pleura, pericardium, or diaphragm
T4b	Unresectable tumor invading other adjacent structures, such as aorta, vertebral body, trachea, etc

Regional Nodes

N0	No regional lymph node metastases
N1	Metastases in 1–2 regional lymph nodes
N2	Metastases in 3–6 regional lymph nodes
N3	Metastases in 7 or more regional lymph nodes

Distant Metastases

M0	No distant metastases
M1	Distant metastases

Anatomic Stage/Prognostic Group (Squamous cell carcinoma)

Stage	T	N	M	Grade	Location
0	Tis	N0	M0	1, X	Any
IA	T1	N0	M0	1, X	Any
IB	T1	N0	M0	2-3	Any
	T2-3	N0	M0	1, X	Lower, X
IIA	T2-3	N0	M0	1, X	Upper, middle
	T2-3	N0	M0	2-3	Lower, X
IIB	T2-3	N0	M0	2-3	Upper, middle
	T1-2	N1	M0	Any	Any
IIIA	T1-2	N2	M0	Any	Any
	T3	N1	M0	Any	Any
	T4a	N0	M0	Any	Any
IIIB	T3	N2	M0	Any	Any
IIIC	T4a	N1-2	M0	Any	Any
	T4b	Any	M0	Any	Any
	Any	N3	M0	Any	Any

(*continued*)

TABLE 44-1 TNM AND AJCC STAGING FOR ESOPHAGEAL CANCER (CONTINUED)

IV	Any	Any	M1	Any	Any

Anatomic Stage/Prognostic Group (Squamous cell carcinoma)

Stage	T	N	M	Grade
0	Tis	N0	M0	1, X
IA	T1	N0	M0	1-2, X
IB	T1	N0	M0	3
	T2	N0	M0	1-2, X
IIA	T2	N0	M0	3
IIB	T3	N0	M0	Any
	T1-2	N1	M0	Any
IIIA	T1-2	N2	M0	Any
	T3	N1	M0	Any
	T4a	N0	M0	Any
IIIB	T3	N2	M0	Any
IIIC	T4a	N1-2	M0	Any
	T4b	Any	M0	Any
	Any	N3	M0	Any
IV	Any	Any	M1	Any

TABLE 44-2 TNM AND AJCC STAGING FOR GASTRIC CANCER

Primary Tumor (T)

Tx	Primary tumor cannot be assessed
T0	No evidence of primary tumor
Tis	Carcinoma in situ, intraepithelial tumor without lamina propria invasion
T1	Tumor invades lamina propria, muscularis mucosae or submucosa
T1a	Tumor invades lamina propria or muscularis mucosae
T1b	Tumor invades submucosa
T2	Tumor invades muscularis propria
T3	Tumor invades subserosal connective tissue without invasion of visceral peritoneum or adjacent structures
T4	Tumor invades serosa (visceral peritoneum) or adjacent structures
T4a	Tumor invades serosa
T4b	Tumor invades adjacent structures

(continued)

TABLE 44-2 TNM AND AJCC STAGING FOR GASTRIC CANCER (CONTINUED)

Regional Nodes

N0	No regional lymph node metastases
N1	Metastases in 1–2 regional lymph nodes
N2	Metastases in 3–6 regional lymph nodes
N3	Metastases in 7 or more regional lymph nodes
N3a	Metastases in 715 regional lymph nodes
N3b	Metastases in greater than 15 regional lymph nodes

Distant Metastases

M0	No distant metastases
M1	Distant metastases

Anatomic Stage/Prognostic Group

Stage	T	N	M
0	Tis	N0	M0
IA	T1	N0	M0
IB	T2	N0	M0
	T1	N1	M0
IIA	T3	N0	M0
	T2	N1	M0
	T1	N2	M0
IIB	T4a	N0	M0
	T3	N1	M0
	T2	N2	M0
	T1	N3	M0
IIIA	T4a	N1	M0
	T3	N2	M0
	T2	N3	M0
IIIB	T4b	N0-N1	M0
	T4a	N2	M0
	T3	N3	M0
IIIC	T4b	N2-N3	M0
	T4a	N3	M0
IV	Any	Any	M1

Gastric Cancer

Approximately 50% of gastric cancers present with locoregional disease. The 5-year survival of patients with gastric cancer is only 15%–20%, but in those with disease only involving the stomach, the 5-year survival is 50%. Survival falls to about 20% once the regional nodes are involved by tumor. Curative surgery typically consists of a subtotal or total gastrectomy. Although the incidence of gastric cancer has been decreasing, the incidence of proximal gastric cancer and cancer of the gastroesophageal (GE) junction have dramatically increased. These more proximal tumors are associated with a poorer prognosis than their distal counterparts.

- Distal tumors: tumors arising in the distal two-thirds of the stomach are typically amenable to subtotal gastrectomy.
- Proximal tumors are usually managed with a total gastrectomy.
- Linitis plastica tumors are diffusely infiltrative, more commonly seen in the young, and typically metastatic at the time of diagnosis. If surgery is indicated, a total gastrectomy is the preferred operation.

LYMPH NODE DISSECTION

The magnitude of lymph node dissection required has remained a contentious area of debate in the surgical management of gastric cancer. For many years, the Japanese have advocated for an extended lymph node dissection in which the lymph nodes of the perigastric (D1 dissection), in addition to the lymph nodes of the hepatic, left gastric, celiac, splenic arteries, and splenic hilum (D2 dissection), as well as the nodes in the porta hepatis and periaortic areas (D3 dissection), are removed. Proponents of the extended lymph node dissection argue that patients will be more accurately staged, leading to a better stage-related survival. Such aggressive dissections may require a distal pancreatectomy and splenectomy, leading to considerable additional morbidity. Randomized trials have failed to demonstrate an improvement in survival for the more aggressive D3 dissections. In a 15-year follow-up of the Dutch D1D2 trial, D2 lymphadenectomy was associated with a lower locoregional recurrence and gastric cancer-related death rate than D1 surgery (4). The D2 dissection is associated with higher morbidity and mortality. As a result, there has been a move away from performing distal pancreatectomy and splenectomy. At least 15 lymph nodes should be removed.

ROLE OF DEFINITIVE CHEMORADIATION

Tumors arising in the cervical esophagus are generally not amenable to surgical resection and are primarily treated with definitive chemoradiation (Table 44-3). The Radiation Therapy Oncology Group (RTOG)-8501 study demonstrated an improvement in median survival for those who received chemoradiation with 5-fluorouracil (5-FU), cisplatin, and 50 Gy compared to 64 Gy of radiation alone (5). The 5-year survival of the chemoradiation group was 27% compared to 0% in the radiation alone group. The PRODIGE 5/ACCORD17 Trial showed that FOLFOX (5-FU, leucovorin, and oxaliplatin) with radiation was equally efficacious and less toxic than 5-FU, cisplatin, and radiation (6). Surgical series utilizing neoadjuvant chemoradiation have demonstrated pathologic response rates of

TABLE 44-3 DEFINITIVE CHEMORADIATION FOR ESOPHAGEAL CANCER

Author	Treatment	Survival
RTOG 8501	FU, CDDP + XRT	Median 14.1 mo, 5 y 27% (<0.0001)
	Radiation	Median 9.3 mo, 5 y 0%
PRODIGE5	FOLFOX + XRT	Median 20.2 mo
	FU, CDDP + XRT	Median 17.5 mo

CDDP, cisplatin; FOLFOX- 5-luorouracil, leucovorin and oxaliplatin; FU, 5-fluorouracil; XRT-radiation therapy.

nearly 22%–40%, making chemoradiation a legitimate alternative to surgical resection (7–9).

ROLE OF NEOADJUVANT AND ADJUVANT THERAPY

Despite advances in staging and operative techniques, the long-term survival for patients undergoing resection for esophageal and gastric cancer remains well under 50%. Investigators have evaluated the role of chemotherapy and radiation in both the preoperative (neoadjuvant) and postoperative (adjuvant) setting.

■ ESOPHAGEAL CANCER

Most cases of esophageal cancer diagnosed in the United States are locally advanced. Neoadjuvant chemoradiation with 5-FU and cisplatin in combination with radiotherapy has been considered the standard of care based on a 113-patient trial by Walsh et al. (7), Table 44-4. In this study, there was an improvement in median survival from 11 to 16 months with the administration of neoadjuvant therapy. The pathologic complete response rate (pCR) was 22%. In Cancer and Leukemia Group B (CALGB) 9781, a

TABLE 44-4 NEOADJUVANT CHEMORADIATION FOR ESOPHAGEAL AND GASTROESOPHAGEAL JUNCTION CANCER

Author	Treatment	Survival
Walsh	FU/CDDP + XRT, Surgery	Median 16 mo ($P = 0.01$), 2 y 37%, 3 y 32% ($P = 0.01$)
	Surgery	Median 11 mo, 2 y 26%, 3 y 6%
CALGB 9781	FU/CDDP + XRT, Surgery	Median 4.5 y ($P = 0.002$), 5 y 39% ($P < 0.008$)
	Surgery	Median 1.8 y, 5 y 16%
CROSS	Paclitaxel, carboplatin +XRT, Surgery	Median 49.4 mo ($P = 0.003$), 5 y 47%
	Surgery	Median 24 mo, 5 y 34%

CDDP, cisplatin; FU, 5-fluorouracil; XRT- radiation.

similar regimen of 5-FU and cisplatin in combination with 50.4 Gy of radio-therapy resulted in a median survival of 4.5 years compared to 1.8 years for those who did not receive neoadjuvant therapy (8). The pCR rate was 40%. Chemoradiation with 5-FU and cisplatin is a very toxic regimen. The operative mortality in the treatment arms of the Walsh and CALGB trials was 12% and 4%, respectively. The Chemoradiotherapy for Oesophageal Cancer Followed by Surgery Study (CROSS) compared weekly paclitaxel, carboplatin, and radiotherapy followed by surgical resection to resection alone (9). The median survival was 49 months compared to 24 months in the surgery-alone arm, with a pCR of 29%. There was no difference in operative mortality between the two treatment arms. The role of postoperative therapy for this patient population has not been established. Due to the toxicity of the neoadjuvant therapy and morbidity of the surgery, it may be challenging for patients to tolerate additional chemotherapy postoperatively. In Intergroup (INT)-0113, the administration of pre- and postoperative 5-FU and cisplatin did not result in an improvement in survival, but did result in a lower R0 resection rate (10). In contrast, the Medical Research Council (MRC) trial of preoperative 5-FU and cisplatin resulted in an improvement in R0 resection rate (60% vs. 54%) and survival (16.8 vs. 13.3 months) compared to surgery alone (11).

■ GASTRIC CANCER

Many randomized trials prior to 2000 comparing surgery versus radiation or chemotherapy failed to demonstrate an improvement in survival; however, meta-analyses have suggested a benefit. The Gastrointestinal Intergroup Study 0116 randomized 556 patients with GE junction and gastric cancers postoperatively to receive bolus 5-FU and leucovorin by the Mayo Clinic schedule for one cycle, followed by an abbreviated course of 5-FU and leucovorin for two cycles with 45 Gy of radiation, and then completing with two more cycles of 5-FU and leucovorin, versus no further therapy (12). The median overall, 3-year survival and disease-free survival favored the adjuvant therapy group: 36 months, 50%, and 30 months versus 27 months, 41%, and 19 months, respectively. Although a D2 resection was recommended, only 10% had such an extensive surgery and 54% had a D0 resection, which would be considered an inadequate surgery. Since this study was conceived, more effective chemotherapy regimens have been developed. This study established a new standard of care for the management of patients with resected gastric cancer. The CALGB 80101 compared epirubicin, cisplatin, and 5-FU (ECF) to the treatment arm of INT-0116 in CALGB (13). Both arms received radiation therapy, but instead of administering it with bolus 5-FU and leucovorin, 5-FU is administered as a continuous infusion. There was no difference in survival. Gastrectomy is major surgery, and many patients are unable to complete the prescribed chemoradiation due to postoperative complications or impaired performance status. A major criticism of the INT-0116 study is the inadequate lymph node sampling, and it is suggested that radiation may be more beneficial in such a population. In the Medical Research Council Adjuvant Gastric Infusional Chemotherapy (MAGIC) trial, 237 patients with lower esophageal and gastric cancers were randomized to receive three cycles of ECF prior to and following surgery, versus surgery alone (14). Patients underwent endoscopic ultrasound as part of their preoperative staging. The median, 5-year and progression-free survivals favored the treatment arm: 24 months, 36%, and 19 months, versus 20 months, 23%, and 13 months, respectively. A significant reduction in tumor size was also appreciated: 5 cm versus 3 cm. The capecitabine and oxaliplatin adjuvant study in stomach cancer (CLASSIC) study randomized 1035 Korean patients who underwent a D2 dissection to receive adjuvant chemotherapy or observation alone and showed an improvement in 3-year disease-free survival (74% vs. 59%, $P < 0.0001$) (15). In the same population, the ARTIST trial evaluated the addition of capecitabine chemoradiation to capecitabine and cisplatin adjuvant therapy. Although there was no improvement in disease-free survival for the entire group, the subgroup of patients who received chemoradiation and had lymph node metastases at the time of surgery had a superior disease-free survival (16). Adjuvant therapy is considered the standard of care, but the exact role of radiation therapy and the superiority of neoadjuvant versus postoperative adjuvant therapy are yet to be determined.

■ GASTROESOPHAGEAL JUNCTION CANCER

GE junction cancers are typically included in clinical trials of esophageal cancer and gastric cancer. INT-0116, MAGIC, CALGB 9781, and CROSS trials all included these patients and resulted in an improvement in survival for the treatment arm. This group of patients is often managed differently based on the bias of the institution and whether they are cared for by thoracic or gastrointestinal multidisciplinary teams. One could argue that the more proximal GE junction tumors be treated with chemoradiation. In a patient with bulky adenopathy, a neoadjuvant chemotherapy approach may be favored. The general trend is to treat GE junction cancers with neoadjuvant chemoradiation. As with esophageal cancer, the benefit of additional postoperative chemotherapy has not been determined.

MANAGEMENT OF ADVANCED AND METASTATIC DISEASE

The median survival for patients with metastatic esophageal and gastric cancer is approximately 4 months if no treatment is offered. Esophageal cancer most commonly metastasizes to the liver, lung, lymph nodes, and bone. GE junction and gastric cancer most commonly metastasize to the liver, abdominal cavity, and lymph nodes (perigastric, retroperitoneal, left supraclavicular, and left axillary), but also metastasize to the ovaries (Krukenberg tumor), lung, and bone. Gastric cancer in particular may result in a microangiopathic hemolytic anemia and may infiltrate the bone marrow. Patients may experience complications related to the primary tumor that require intervention. These include pain, dysphagia, early satiety, nausea, and vomiting due to obstruction, and bleeding. These may be managed conservatively with pain medications, promotility agents, stent placement, and external beam radiation. Esophageal cancers found proximal to the carina may result in a tracheoesophageal fistula causing aspiration pneumonia. Palliative resection may improve symptom control and perhaps survival, but there is no proven benefit in performing total gastrectomy for gastric cancer in the setting of metastatic disease. Management of malignant ascites may be challenging in these patients, requiring frequent paracenteses if not permanent peritoneal catheter placement. Malignant ascites is more commonly seen in young patients, particularly women, and in those with poorly differentiated or signet-ring cell carcinoma of the stomach. Hepatic metastases are more commonly seen in patients with well to moderately differentiated tumors, and more frequently in males. Systemic chemotherapy is the cornerstone of therapy for these patients. Several randomized trials have now demonstrated an improvement in survival for those receiving chemotherapy.

■ SYSTEMIC THERAPY

Chemotherapy

Multiple chemotherapy agents have documented activity in this disease. These include 5-FU (and capecitabine), S1, cisplatin, oxaliplatin, irinotecan, epirubicin, paclitaxel, and docetaxel. Single-agent response rates are generally up to 20%. Many combinations have been tested, and most of them contain 5-FU as the backbone (Table 44-5). Based on these studies, ECF and DCF have been considered standard regimens. The TAX 325 trial reported a very highly adverse event rate, including 82% grade 3–4 neutropenia and a 30-day mortality (post-last infusion) of about 12% and a toxic death rate of 6.3% (17). Modifications have been made to this regimen to reduce the toxicity. An unfavorable feature of the ECF regimen is the need to wear the infusional 5-FU continuously, without break. The REAL-2 trial demonstrated noninferiority for the substitution of capecitabine for 5-FU and oxaliplatin for cisplatin (18). The substitution of oxaliplatin for cisplatin resulted in reduced toxicity. The actual benefit of epirubicin remains a question. In CALGB 80403/ECOG1206, the activity of FOLFOX was similar to ECF and appeared superior to the combination of irinotecan and cisplatin (19). All arms of this study also included cetuximab. Consequently, FOLFOX or CAPOX is generally the favored first-line therapy. It also makes itself more amenable to combination with other agents in clinical trials. There is no defined second-line therapy for esophagogastric cancer, but the Japanese Oncology Group randomized patients who received 5-FU and cisplatin in the first line to weekly paclitaxel or irinotecan every 2 weeks (20). There was a nonsignificant improvement in response rate and survival for patients receiving paclitaxel.

TABLE 44-5 SYSTEMIC CHEMOTHERAPY

Author	Regimen	RR (%)	PFS/TTP (Months)	Survival (Months)
REAL-2	ECF	40.7	6.2	9.9
	ECX	46.4	6.7	9.9
	EOF	42.4	6.5	9.3
	EOX	47.9	6.7	11.2
V325	CF	25	3.7	8.6
	DCF	37	5.6	9.2

C, cisplatin; D, docetaxel; E, epirubicin; F, 5-fluorouracil; X, capecitabine.

Targeted Therapy

Several targeted agents have been tested in esophagogastric cancer. Approximately 20% of esophagogastric cancers are HER2 positive as defined by IHC 3+ or IHC 2+ with confirmatory FISH positivity. HER2 positivity is more common in intestinal compared to diffuse gastric cancers. Trastuzumab has been FDA approved for use in combination with cisplatin and a fluoro-pyrimidine (5-FU or capecitabine) for patients with GE junction and gastric cancer expressing HER2. The ToGA trial demonstrated an improvement in response rate (47% vs. 35%) and survival (13.8 vs. 11.1 months) to the addition of trastuzumab (21). In the AVAGAST trial, the vascular endothelial growth factor (VEGF) inhibitor bevacizumab was added to cisplatin and capecitabine (22). Although there was an improvement in response rate and progression-free survival, the improvement in survival was not significant. On subgroup analysis, patients in the Americas appeared to benefit most, with those in Asia benefitting least. Ramucirumab is a fully human IgG1 monoclonal antibody receptor antagonist designed to bind the extracellular domain of vascular endothelial growth factor (VEGF) receptor-2, thereby blocking the interaction of VEGF ligands (VEGF-A, VEGF-C, and VEGF-D) and inhibiting receptor activation. The REGARD trial reported at GI ASCO in January 2013 randomized 355 patients with metastatic adenocarcinoma of the stomach or GE junction who had progressed on first-line fluoropyrimidine and a platinum to ramucirumab or placebo. Patients assigned to ramucirumab experienced significantly longer median OS (5.2 months vs. 3.8 months; HR = 0.776; 95% CI, 0.603–0.998) and PFS (2.1 months vs. 1.3 months; HR = 0.483; 95% CI, 0.376–0.620) than patients assigned to placebo (23). The role of VEGF inhibition in esophagogastric cancer is evolving. In the REAL-3 trial, the addition of panitumumab to epirubicin, oxaliplatin, and capecitabine had a detrimental impact in overall survival (24). MET has recently become a target of interest in gastric cancer. MET is expressed in up to 74% and amplified in up to 23% of gastric cancers. In a randomized phase II trial of the MET inhibitor rilotumumab in combination with epirubicin, cisplatin, and capecitabine (ECX), there was an improvement in overall survival in patients with high expression of MET compared to those receiving only ECX (25). The importance of MET in esophagogastric cancer will be determined in subsequent randomized trials.

REFERENCES

1. Siegel R, Naishadham, D, Jemal A. Cancer statistics 2013. *CA Cancer J Clin.* 2013; 63: 11–30.

2. American Joint Committee on Cancer. In Edge, SB, Byrd, DR, Compton, CC, et al (eds). *AJCC Cancer Staging Handbook,* 7th edition. Springer, New York, 2010.

3. Siewert JR, Stein HJ. Classification of adenocarcinoma of the oesophagogastric junction. *Br J Surg.* 1998; 85: 457.

4. Songun I, Puttere H, Kranenbarg EM, et al. Surgical treatment of gastric cancer: 15-year follow-up results of the randomised nationwide Dutch D1D2 trial. *Lancet Oncol.* 2010; 11: 439–449.

5. Al-Saraaf M, Martz K, Herskovic A, et al. Progress report of combined chemoradiotherapy versus radiotherapy alone in patients with esophageal cancer: an intergroup study. *J Clin Oncol.* 1997; 15: 277–284.

6. Conroy T, Galais M-P, Raoul JL, et al. Phase III randomized trial of definitive chemoradiotherapy with FOLFOX or cisplatin and fluorouracil in esophageal cancer: final results of the PRODIGE 5/ACCORD 17 trial. *ProcASCO.* 2012; 30, LBA4003.

7. Walsh TN, Noonan N, Hollywood D, et al. A comparison of multimodal therapy and surgery for esophageal adenocarcinoma. *N Engl J Med.* 1996; 335: 462–467.

8. Tepper J, Krasna MJ, Niedzwiecki D, et al. Phase III trial of trimodality therapy with cisplatin, 5-fluorouracil, radiotherapy, and surgery compared with surgery alone for esophageal cancer: CALGB 9781. *J Clin Oncol.* 2008; 26: 1086–1092.

9. van Hagen P, Hulshof MCCM, van Lanschot JJB, et al. Preoperative chemoradiation for esophageal or junction cancer. *N Engl J Med.* 2012; 366: 2074–2084.

10. Kelsen DP, Ginsberg R, Pajak T, et al. Chemotherapy followed by surgery compared with surgery alone for localized esophageal cancer. *N Engl J Med.* 1998; 339: 1979–1984.

11. Medical Research Council Oesophageal Cancer Working Party. Surgical resection with or without preoperative chemotherapy in oesophageal cancer: a randomized controlled trial. *Lancet.* 2002; 359: 1727–1733.

12. MacDonald JS, Smalley SR, Benedetti J, et al. Chemoradiotherapy after surgery compared with surgery alone for adenocarcinoma of the stomach or gastroesophageal junction. *N Engl J Med.* 2001; 345: 725–730.

13. Fuchs CS, Tepper JE, Niedzwiecki D, et al. Postoperative adjuvant chemoradiation for gastric or gastroesophageal junction (GEJ) adenocarcinoma using epirubicin, cisplatin, and infusional (CI) 5-FU (ECF) before and after CI 5-FU and radiotherapy (CRT) compared with bolus 5-FU/LV before and after CRT: intergroup trial CALGB 80101. *ProcASCO.* 2011; 29: 256s, abstract 4003.

14. Cunningham D, Allum WH, Stenning SP, et al. Perioperative chemotherapy versus surgery alone for resectable gastroesophageal cancer. *N Engl J Med.* 2006; 355: 11–20.

15. Bang Y-J, Kim Y-W, Yang H-K, et al. Adjuvant capecitabine and oxaliplatin for gastric cancer after D2 gastrectomy (CLASSIC): a phase 3 open-label, randomised controlled trial. *Lancet.* 2012; 379: 315–321.

16. Lee J, Lim DH, Ki S, et al. Phase III trial comparing capecitabine plus cisplatin versus capecitabine plus cisplatin with concurrent capecitabine radiotherapy in completely resected gastric cancer with D2 lymph node dissection: the ARTIST trial. *J Clin Oncol.* 2011; 30: 268–273.

17. van Cutsem E, Moiseyenko VM, Tjulandin S, et al. Phase III study of docetaxel and cisplatin plus fluorouracil compared with cisplatin and fluorouracil as first-line therapy for advanced gastric cancer: a report of the V325 study group. *J Clin Oncol.* 2006; 24: 4991–4997.

18. Cunningham D, Starling N, Rao S, et al. Capecitabine and oxaliplatin for advanced esophagogastric cancer. *J Clin Oncol.* 2008; 358: 36–46.

19. Enzinger PC, Burtness B, Hollis D, et al. CALGB80403/ECOG1206: a randomized phase II study of three standard chemotherapy regimens (ECF, IC, FOLFOX) plus cetuximab in metastatic esophageal and GE junction cancer. *ProcASCO.* 2010; 28: 15s, abstract 4006.

20. Ueda S, Hironaka S, Yasui H, et al. Randomized phase III study of irinotecan (CPT-11) versus weekly paclitaxel for advanced gastric cancer refractory to combination chemotherapy of fluoropyrimidine plus platinum: WJOG4007 trial. *ProcASCO.* 2012; 30, abstract 4002.

21. Bang Y-J, van Cutsem E, Feyereislova A, et al. Trastuzumab in combination with chemotherapy versus chemotherapy alone for treatment of Her-2 positive advanced gastric or gastro-oesophageal junction cancer (ToGA): a phase III, open label, randomised controlled trial. *Lancet.* 201; 376: 687–697.

22. Ohtsu A, Shah MA, van Cutsem E, et al. Bevacizumab in combination with chemotherapy as first-line therapy in advanced gastric cancer: a randomized double-blind placebo-controlled phase III study. *J Clin Oncol.* 2011; 29: 3968–3976.

23. Fuchs CS, Tomasek J, Cho JY, et al. REGARD: a phase III, randomized, double-blind trial of ramucirumab and best supportive care (BSC) versus placebo and BSC in the treatment of metastatic gastric or gastroesophageal junction (GEJ) adenocarcinoma following disease progression on first-line platinum- and/or fluoropyrimidine-containing combination therapy. *J Clin Oncol.* 2012; 30 (suppl 34), abstr LBA5.

24. Waddell TS, Chau I, Barbachano Y, et al. A randomized multicenter trial of epirubicin, oxaliplatin, and capecitabine plus panitumumab in advanced esophagogastric cancer (REAL3). *ProcASCO.* 2012; 30, abstract LBA4000.

25. Oliner KS, Tang R, Anderson A, et al. Evaluation of MET pathway biomarkers in a phase II study of rilotumumab (AMG 102) or placebo in combination with epirubicin, cisplatin, and capecitabine (ECX) in patients with locally advanced or metastatic gastric or esophagogastric junction cancer. *ProcASCO.* 2012; 30, abstract LBA4005.

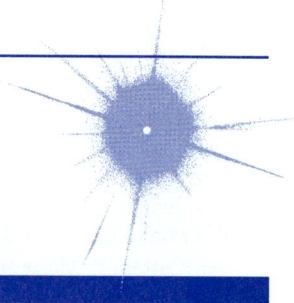

CHAPTER **45**
Pancreatic Cancer

Jeffrey W. Clark

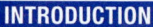

INTRODUCTION

For most patients, pancreatic adenocarcinoma remains highly lethal and is the fourth leading cause of deaths from cancer in the USA. Less than 5% survive 5 years after diagnosis. Surgical resection is the only curative treatment.

However, the cure rate with surgery is only 18%–25% and most patients are not surgical candidates. Patients with unresectable disease can have symptoms palliated by chemotherapy and/or radiation therapy. However, these have not significantly impacted 5-year survival. Improved understanding of pancreatic cancer biology continues to provide new therapeutic ideas. Trials are evaluating whether new approaches to earlier diagnosis or improvements in radiation therapy, chemotherapy (including targeted therapy), and/or immunotherapy (e.g., vaccines, therapy aimed at inhibiting negative immunoregulatory proteins) can impact survival.

INCIDENCE AND EPIDEMIOLOGY

- Approximately 45,000 individuals develop pancreatic cancer yearly in the United States with over 38,000 dying from the disease.
- Increases with age, slight male predominance, increased incidence in African Americans, variation in prevalence by world region (higher in western Europe, Scandinavia, the United States, and New Zealand) (1).
- Risk factors for pancreatic adenocarcinoma include (1–3):
  Environmental
  - Cigarette smoking, history of diabetes mellitus, previous radiation therapy to the pancreas as treatment for other malignancies (such as Hodgkin's disease, or testicular cancer) and chronic pancreatitis (especially that due to genetic risk factors); increased body mass index and heavy alcohol consumption (but not light consumption) may be risk factors.
  Genetic
  - Mutations in p16; mismatched repair genes (hMSH2 and hMLH1); BRCA1 (rare pancreatic cancers); BRCA2; PALB2 (a BRCA associated protein), STK11/LKB1 (Peutz-Jeghers syndrome); ataxia telangectasia (AT); p53 (Li-Fraumeni syndrome); APC (familial adenomatous polyposis); von Hippel-Lindau (VHL); cationic trypsinogen (PRSS1 gene); and cystic fibrosis transmembrane regulator (CFTR) genes (2–4).
- Families with increased risk of pancreatic cancer without as yet defined genetic abnormalities.
- Overall, approximately 5%–10% of patients with pancreatic cancer will have a first-degree relative who develops pancreatic cancer (2–4).

PATHOLOGY

Normal pancreatic cell types include ductal, acinar, endocrine/neuro-endocrine, connective tissue support, endothelial, and lymphocytes. Malignancies can arise from each cell type. In adults, approximately 90% are adenocarcinomas derived from duct cells with approximately two-thirds arising in the head, and one-third being in the body/tail or multicentric (5–7). Other histologic subtypes of ductal origin include pleomorphic carcinomas, giant cell carcinomas, microglandular adenocarcinomas, and cystic neoplasms. Cystic neoplasms comprise a small but increasingly identified subgroup of pancreatic tumors (7). They can be divided into serous cyst adenomas (usually benign) and mucinous cystadenocarcinomas. A higher percentage of these tumors occur in middle-aged women as compared to ductal adenocarcinomas. They appear to be divided into a group that has benign or borderline malignant cells with good prognosis and a group with carcinoma that metastasizes widely and has a prognosis similar to that of other ductal adenocarcinomas. Pancreatic papillary cystic tumors tend to occur in women of reproductive years with relatively better prognosis after surgical excision. There are also noncystic mucin-producing tumors of the pancreas that tend to have a better prognosis after surgical excision. Acinar cell carcinomas make up 1%–2% of pancreatic cancers. Acinar cell tumors occur most commonly in the elderly, but they also occur in younger patients and comprise a higher percentage of tumors seen in children, who have a better prognosis (8). Overall, adult patients with acinar cell carcinomas tend to have a slightly better clinical course than those with ductal adenocarcinomas. Uncommon pancreatic tumors include pancreatic inflammatory tumors and small cell undifferentiated carcinomas. Tumors with mixed histologies including adenosquamous carcinomas and carcinosarcomas can occur and tend to have a poor prognosis. Pancreatoblastomas are rare neoplasms arising from multipotential cells that can differentiate into mesenchymal, endocrine, or acinar cells, which occur primarily in children, although rare cases can occur in adults. They frequently have elevated alpha feto protein levels and are potentially curable when localized. Metastatic pancreaticoblastomas are often responsive to chemotherapy. Other pancreatic tumors found in children include solid pseudopapillary tumors, pancreatic endocrine/neuroendocrine neoplasms, and acinar cell tumors (8).

Pancreatic neuroendocrine cell cancers (PNET) comprise approximately 5%–10% of pancreatic tumors (9). Although associated with longer survival than pancreatic adenocarcinomas, they frequently metastasize. Lymphomas, sarcomas, and other mesenchymal tumors (e.g., teratomas, schwannomas, and neurofibromas) make up only a small proportion of pancreatic cancers (less than 2%). Their biology is similar to that of malignancies of similar histology arising in other areas of the body.

A wide variety of neoplasms can metastasize to the pancreas, including breast, lung, melanoma, renal, gastrointestinal, and other sites.

BIOLOGY OF PANCREATIC ADENOCARCINOMA

Pancreatic adenocarcinomas have frequently invaded locally and/or metastasized by the time initially detected. Local spread is directly to soft tissues and adjacent organs (5, 6). They tend to metastasize widely including lymph nodes, liver, peritoneum, lungs, adrenal glands, and, less commonly, bone and brain.

The biology of pancreatic ductal adenocarcinoma has provided targets for earlier diagnosis, potential therapy, and possible avenues for prevention in the future (3, 4, 10, 11). As is true of most tumors, there is a complex pattern of genetic changes with variation between different tumors. Frequent mutations have been found in proteins involved in cell signaling pathways (especially K-ras [70%–90%]) as well as a number of tumor suppressor genes (especially p53, p16, and DPC4/Smad4). A number of growth factor receptor families, including insulin-like growth factor receptors, the epidermal growth factor receptors (EGFRs), and fibroblast growth factor receptors, are highly expressed in a proportion of pancreatic adenocarcinomas.

The life span of cells normally is limited by shortening of telomeric DNA at chromosomal ends. Telomerase (the enzyme important in maintaining telomeric DNA at chromosomal ends) activity is elevated in a high percentage of pancreatic carcinomas.

The potential role of some of the mutations found in familial pancreatic cancer (e.g., BRCA2, PALB2, or mismatched repair genes) in the development of nonhereditary pancreatic cancers is unclear (3, 4, 10, 11). The frequency of these mutations in sporadic cases is low. Tumors that have mutations in mismatched repair genes but not Ras genes are characterized by the appearance of "pushing borders" on histopathology and a better prognosis.

In addition to genetic changes, epigenetic factors, alterations in metabolic processes, suppression of host immune response, hypoxia-induced changes in tumor cells and the microenvironment, and the complexity of the tumor microenvironment all play important roles in development, survival, proliferation, and metastatic spread of pancreatic cancer (10, 11). These all offer potential targets to improve treatment.

PRESENTING SYMPTOMS AND SIGNS

The initial symptoms produced by pancreatic cancer are insidious. Most patients have nonspecific symptoms for several months prior to diagnosis. Tumors in the head of the pancreas sometimes produce obstruction of the bile duct and therefore jaundice at a relatively earlier stage, although most of these tumors are still unresectable. Fatigue, weight loss, anorexia, abdominal pain, back pain, jaundice/light stools/dark urine/pruritus (for head lesions), nausea, vomiting, early satiety, dyspnea, and glucose intolerance are the most common presenting symptoms. Depression is seen in a significant percentage of patients. There is a relatively high incidence of blood clot formation and some patients present with thrombophlebitis. Patients who develop portal or splenic vein obstruction can present with hematemesis (due to varices) or ascites. Ascites may also be due to metastatic disease to the peritoneum.

DIAGNOSTIC WORKUP

The diagnosis should be considered in individuals who present with the above symptoms, especially with several symptoms. A careful history should be obtained including review for the above symptoms, history of cigarette smoking or other risk factors, and a family history. Physical exam should include evaluation for evidence of weight loss, lymph node enlargement (especially in the supraclavicular or periumbilical areas), jaundice, hepatosplenomegaly, ascites, peripheral edema, and evidence of coagulopathy. For most patients, findings on physical exam are nonspecific.

Laboratory tests should include a complete blood count (CBC) and liver function tests, although, in general, laboratory studies are nonspecific and not particularly helpful in making a diagnosis. CA19-9 is the most useful tumor marker and is elevated in 70%–90% of patients with advanced disease. Although not useful as a screening tool due to relative nonspecificity, it is helpful in following a patient's therapeutic response. Although less frequent, CEA is occasionally elevated in patients who do not have CA19-9 elevations and can be used to follow response to therapy.

Radiological evaluation plays a key role in the diagnosis (12). Computerized tomographic (CT) scans currently are the most commonly used modality for assessing for a pancreatic mass, potential vascular invasion, and determining whether the tumor has metastasized. Alternatively, MRI can be utilized. Pulmonary metastases in the absence of abdominal metastases are relatively uncommon but can occur, and CT imaging of the chest is also important.

Pathology is ultimately required to make a diagnosis. Biopsies of either the pancreas or nodal lesions can be obtained at the time of endoscopic ultrasound (EUS). These theoretically carry less potential risk of peritoneal seeding than percutaneous biopsies. Although ideally a diagnosis can be made preoperatively, for patients with a potentially resectable pancreatic mass, surgery is often necessary in any case even if the initial fine needle biopsy was not diagnostic. For patients with unresectable disease, percutaneous biopsy under radiological guidance of either the pancreas itself or a metastatic lesion is usually obtained.

STAGING AND TREATMENT DECISIONS

The American Joint Commission on Cancer (AJCC) staging system with the TNM format is utilized to group patients into stages I–IV (5). Although different stages by the TNM classification have prognostic significance (i.e., survival decreases with increasing stage), for purposes of treatment decisions, there are three groups of patients that need to be defined: potentially resectable, localized but unresectable, and metastatic. Once pancreatic cancer is diagnosed, the most important question is whether it is potentially resectable. Unless findings on physical exam or radiological studies indicate that the disease is already metastatic, findings from CT/MRI scans, including a careful evaluation of the question of vascular involvement by the tumor, are usually the critical factors in helping determine potential resectability. Tumors are generally considered unresectable if there is: (1) metastatic disease, (2) encasement or occlusion by the tumor of the superior mesenteric vein (SMV) or SMV–portal vein confluence, or (3) direct involvement by the tumor of the aorta, celiac plexus, inferior vena cava (IVC), or the superior mesenteric artery (SMA). FDG positron emission tomography (PET) scanning has been shown to have good sensitivity in detecting potentially metastatic disease and may be helpful when findings from CT scans are equivocal, but a definitive role has not yet been established. As newer approaches combining CT or MRI with PET imaging are developed and enhanced, they may allow the best features of each technique to be combined for staging patients.

EUS is increasingly being utilized as part of staging. This can be combined with endoscopic retrograde cholangiography (ERCP) for stent placement allowing both diagnostic information and a palliative approach for maintaining bile duct patency in patients who do not have potentially resectable disease.

If preliminary staging findings indicate a potentially resectable tumor, then the next step is either consideration of neoadjuvant treatment (discussed later) or proceeding with laparoscopic staging or exploratory laparotomy with resection, if possible. There remains debate about the exact value of laparoscopic staging before planned surgery as improvements in imaging techniques (especially MRI, CT, and PET) enhance the ability to detect small metastatic lesions in the peritoneal cavity. At the present time, it continues to be utilized by many surgeons.

SURGERY

There are four main surgical approaches for resecting pancreatic cancer depending on the exact nature of the disease (6–8). These are: (1) the pancreaticoduodenectomy (Whipple's procedure with various modifications that are utilized by different surgeons), (2) total pancreatectomy, (3) regional or extended pancreatectomy, and (4) distal pancreatectomy and splenectomy. Pancreaticoduodenectomies are the most commonly performed procedure for lesions in the head of the pancreas or peri-ampullary lesions. Distal pancreatectomy with splenectomy is usually used for body and tail lesions. Laparoscopic approaches are being used with increased frequency, and their exact role is being defined in ongoing studies. Morbidity and mortality after surgery for pancreatic cancer have significantly declined with most major centers reporting mortality rates less than 2%–5%. Median survival is approximately 18 months with approximately 20% of patients alive at 5 years. Features associated with a lower cure rate include increased tumor size, positive margins, or positive lymph nodes.

Palliative surgical approaches to delay or prevent biliary and duodenal obstruction are utilized for patients who undergo exploration but are not resectable. The major alternatives to surgical palliation of biliary and gastrointestinal obstruction are endoscopically placed stents. Stenting of the gastrointestinal tract itself remains of somewhat limited efficacy, although improvements in stents have allowed this to be used more commonly.

CHEMOTHERAPY ± RADIATION IN THE ADJUVANT OR NEOADJUVANT SETTING

Clinical trials have not yet established a definitive role for preoperative, intraoperative, or postoperative radiation therapy utilized alone for improving survival of patients who have resected pancreatic cancer (13, 14). Intraoperative radiotherapy (IORT) may increase local control rate but has not yet been shown to affect overall survival in randomized trials. Improvements in delivery of IORT make this an area of continued study. Even when local control can be achieved with radiation therapy, the primary issue remains that the majority of patients die from metastatic disease. Adjuvant or neoadjuvant trials have utilized combined modality therapy integrating surgery and chemotherapy ± radiation (14–16). A randomized GI Tumor Study Group (GITSG) trial of combined postoperative treatment (external beam radiation therapy [EBRT] with chemotherapy [5-FU]) and subsequent nonrandomized trials at a number of centers suggest that adjuvant or neoadjuvant chemotherapy and radiation therapy may lead to a longer survival than surgery alone. In contrast, recent randomized trials from Europe have not shown a statistically significant improvement in survival for combined chemotherapy and radiation therapy, although they have shown a survival benefit for chemotherapy alone.

Thus, despite trials suggesting benefit, overall evidence remains inconclusive as to whether adjuvant combined chemotherapy plus radiation therapy produces a long-term survival advantage for resected pancreatic cancer patients over that seen with chemotherapy alone. In an attempt to better define the roles of radiation and chemotherapy in this setting, additional studies are currently ongoing. Since a number of studies have shown same survival benefit for chemotherapy, there is general consensus that adjuvant chemotherapy is of value. In the United States, combined chemoradiation therapy is also usually given, often after completion of adjuvant chemotherapy if restaging shows no evidence of metastatic disease.

A number of studies have evaluated the potential for neoadjuvant chemotherapy (primarily 5-FU or gemcitabine based) alone or combined with EBRT to enhance the ability to adequately deliver adjuvant therapy to a higher percentage of patients than can be done in the postoperative setting and potentially to convert what appear to be unresectable lesions to resectable ones. Most of these studies indicate an overall ability to resect approximately 10%–15% of lesions that were deemed unresectable prior to therapy. Since it is not possible to be certain what percentage of these patients would have been resectable without neoadjuvant therapy, the magnitude of the benefit cannot be absolutely defined. However, the potential benefit of neoadjuvant therapy utilizing current chemotherapy approaches appears to be relatively limited for this purpose. At present, the emphasis of those pursuing neoadjuvant therapy is focused on trying to define better therapeutic approaches, especially incorporating newer agents or combinations. Early trials utilizing the FOLFIRINOX (combined 5-FU, leucovorin, irinotecan, and oxaliplatin) chemotherapy regimen suggest that it may increase the number of patients with borderline resectable diseases who may become resectable (17). However, randomized studies are needed to establish whether neoadjuvant therapy can increase the percentage of borderline resectable patients who can subsequently have their tumors resected or would lead to enhanced overall survival as compared with postoperative adjuvant therapy.

PATIENTS WITH LOCALIZED BUT UNRESECTABLE DISEASE

■ CHEMOTHERAPY ± RADIATION THERAPY FOR UNRESECTABLE PATIENTS

Definitive radiation therapy is not curative for the vast majority of patients whose tumors cannot be resected. However, it can palliate symptoms (especially pain) and possibly lead to a small survival prolongation. Addition of 5-FU-based chemotherapy may increase survival over that seen with radiation therapy alone but this benefit is modest. A recent phase III trial has shown that gemcitabine plus radiation followed by gemcitabine alone produced a survival advantage compared to gemcitabine alone (18). In contrast, an earlier randomized, phase III trial utilizing different agents in combination with the radiation (5-FU plus cisplatin) had shown a survival advantage for patients receiving gemcitabine alone as compared to those who received initial chemoradiation followed by maintenance gemcitabine, possibly because of the difficulty of delivering adequate doses of gemcitabine to patients with prior chemoradiation (19). Given results from different phase III trials, at the present time, acceptable approaches include: (1) chemotherapy alone, or (2) chemotherapy given alone for a specified period in addition to combined chemoradiation therapy. A potentially attractive approach is to give chemotherapy alone for the initial 4–6 months followed by a consideration of combined chemotherapy and radiation for those patients who do not have metastatic disease upon restaging. To try to improve on the results seen with either 5-FU or gemcitabine in this setting, FOLFIRINOX is being explored for its role in locally advanced disease both alone and followed by combined chemoradiation.

CHEMOTHERAPY FOR METASTATIC DISEASE

Overall, median survival of patients with metastatic pancreatic cancer is short with ranges of 5–11 months in most large series (20–23). The most active single agents produce response rates in the 5%–20% range, and there is minimal impact of treatment on 5-year survival. Clinical benefit may be seen in a slightly higher percentage of patients with approximately 25% achieving short-term clinical benefit with gemcitabine, which is the standard single agent based on a randomized trial that showed a slight survival advantage as compared with 5-fluorouracil (5-FU) (19–22).

Other agents with some activity against pancreatic cancer include 5-FU (including oral capecitabine), taxanes, oxaliplatin, cisplatin, camptothecins (e.g., irinotecan), and erlotinib (small molecule epidermal growth factor receptor [EGFR] inhibitor). A number of combinations of agents with gemcitabine have been evaluated in phase III studies compared to gemcitabine alone, but only two have shown an overall survival advantage: (1) gemcitabine and erlotinib, although the evidence for additional benefit is modest (increase of approximately 2 weeks in median survival with erlotinib) (21–23), and (2) gemcitabine and nab-paclitaxel (abraxane) (24). The combination of gemcitabine and nab-paclitaxel increased the median survival as compared to gemcitabine alone (8.5 vs. 6.7 months). The single biggest step forward in standard treatment of unresectable pancreatic cancer has been the demonstration that FOLFIRINOX provides a significant survival advantage as compared to gemcitabine alone (11.1 vs. 6.8 months, respectively) (20). FOLFIRINOX or gemcitabine plus nab-paclitaxel can have significant toxicity, including febrile neutropenia, and should only be utilized in patients who are likely to tolerate them (e.g., good performance status and few comorbidities). Gemcitabine alone (or combined with erlotinib) could be considered for patients who would not be candidates for more aggressive therapy because of decreased performance status or comorbid factors. Better understanding of the basic biology of pancreatic cancer, preclinical studies, and clinical trials should help guide the next steps in improving therapy.

HORMONAL AND IMMUNOTHERAPY

There is no evidence for significant antitumor benefit for either hormonal or immunotherapy. The utilization of vaccines and other immunotherapeutic approaches for patients with resected pancreatic cancer as well as for patients with metastatic disease are currently being extensively studied, although there is not yet clear evidence for benefit (21).

FUTURE THERAPEUTIC DIRECTIONS

Given the limited effectiveness of current approaches against pancreatic cancer, continued studies to better understand disease biology and clinical trials are vital in making progress (10, 11). Perhaps most promising for the future are therapies based on increased understanding of the biological processes important for proliferation, survival, or metastasis of neoplastic pancreatic cells and the role of the tumor microenvironment in this process. Compounds developed using biochemical and molecular biological approaches to target these are already providing new agents and combinations for testing in the treatment of this disease.

MANAGEMENT OF SYMPTOMS

Supportive care and management of symptoms are vitally important in maintaining the quality of life of pancreatic cancer patients. The majority of patients will develop significant pain at some point. Management includes some combination of opioids, nonsteroidals, acetaminophen, gabapentin, or other analgesic agents. Celiac plexus blocks can be utilized if abdominal or back pain cannot be controlled by medication, and evidence suggests that the pain is due to tumor involvement of the celiac plexus. Malnutrition is a significant problem. Pancreatic enzymes can sometimes help ameliorate malabsorption. Antacids may be useful in both enhancing the benefit of pancreatic enzymes and decreasing reflux symptoms. Megestrol acetate, dronabinol, or glucocorticoids can help stimulate appetite in some patients. There is a relatively high incidence of depression. This is often in the setting of increased anxiety, fatigue, and loss of any ambition making it more difficult to treat. A multidisciplinary approach to palliate symptoms can be very helpful, including pain and/or palliative care teams.

NEUROENDOCRINE PANCREATIC TUMORS

Tumors arising in islet cells make up less than 10% of pancreatic cancers (8). Different functional tumors (with symptoms related to the specific hormone(s) that are produced) can occur or they may be nonfunctional. Poorly differentiated tumors tend to metastasize early and have a poor prognosis. These are usually treated similarly to small cell lung cancer with etoposide plus cisplatin with a reasonable initial response rate but with eventual relapse in the majority of patients. Types of well or moderately well differentiated tumors include insulinomas, glucagonomas, somatostatinomas, gastrinomas, VIPomas (vasointestinal polypeptide), PPomas (pancreatic polypeptide), GRFomas (growth hormone releasing factor), ACTHomas (adrenocorticotropin), carcinoids, tumors that produce hypercalcemia, and nonfunctioning tumors. Tumors can produce more than one peptide hormone, and the hormone that predominates can change over time. Except for insulinomas (which have a lower risk of metastasizing), they have similar clinical features and are malignant in the majority of cases. They tend to metastasize to lymph nodes and liver. Certain of these tumors can occur as part of multiple endocrine neoplasia syndrome I (MEN-I). MEN-I is an autosomal dominant trait that is associated with tumors or hyperplasia of multiple endocrine organs, often including pancreatic endocrine tumors (most frequently gastrinomas or insulinomas).

General treatment principles are similar for most of these well or moderately well-differentiated tumors, although there are specific aspects of each that need to be addressed as well. Treatment includes surgical resection when that can be done especially for cure. Even when curative surgery may not be feasible, palliative cytoreduction (by surgery and/or radiofrequency ablation [RFA]) may be of value in controlling symptoms. Symptoms can sometimes be ameliorated utilizing agents that block the effects of produced hormones. Many of these tumors can have symptoms somewhat palliated by somatostatin analogs. Although somatostatin analogs do not significantly increase long-term survival, they can markedly improve quality of life and can improve progression-free survival. A number of chemotherapeutic agents have some activity against these tumors. However, they are not curative, and overall activity of any one agent or combination is limited. Two agents (everolimus, an inhibitor of mTOR, which is a kinase in the PI3-kinase pathway; and sunitinib, an inhibitor of multiple kinases including growth factor receptors important for tumor associated angiogenesis) have shown a progression-free survival advantage in phase III trials and are approved in the United States for treatment of patients with metastatic neuroendocrine cancers (9). Dacarbazine (or its oral equivalent temozolamide) has moderate activity, and this continues to be explored both alone and in combination with other agents. Hepatic arterial embolization or chemoembolization can palliate symptoms in patients with functional tumors and a significant tumor burden in the liver. Radiolabeled octreotide is being pursued as a potential means of relatively specifically targeting those tumors that are positive on octreotide scan. There is evidence of antitumor activity, although the exact clinical value of this approach has not yet been established.

LYMPHOMAS AND SARCOMAS

Lymphomas and sarcomas arising within the pancreas are both uncommon neoplasms. The most important issue is establishing the diagnosis histologically, so that appropriate staging and therapeutic decisions can be made. These malignancies behave with a similar clinical course to tumors of the same histology arising in other organs.

METASTATIC LESIONS

Since metastases to the pancreas can occur from a number of primary sites, it is important to determine the histology of pancreatic lesions by biopsy if feasible. Metastatic tumors should be treated based on the primary tumor site.

SUMMARY

Pancreatic adenocarcinoma remains a disease with poor long-term survival. Curative surgery is only achievable in a relatively small percentage of patients. Clearly, improvements in earlier diagnosis (including more sensitive approaches for detecting the disease at an early stage) and continued development and evaluation of novel treatment approaches are needed. Clinical trials are evaluating the efficacy of approaches combining new antitumor agents, radiation therapy, and surgery. Chemotherapeutic agents are being studied alone or in combinations with each other or newer agents (e.g., targeted agents, vaccines) for treatment of patients with metastatic disease.

Despite limited clinical progress, significant advances in information about cellular and molecular biology of pancreatic cancers have been made. The nature of biological mechanisms (such as angiogenesis) important for growth and metastasis of cancers within the host are being elucidated. Increased knowledge about the molecular origins and progression of pancreatic cancer has led to evaluation of novel approaches specifically targeting proteins important for cancer cell proliferation or survival. These include vaccines, gene therapy, monoclonal antibodies, and small-targeted molecules, including agents targeting pathways downstream of mutant KRAS, given the high frequency of KRAS mutations in pancreatic adeno-carcinomas. Improved understanding of how the immune system functions and, therefore, how it might be utilized to control malignant cells has led to renewed efforts to try to develop effective immunotherapy, including vaccines or approaches to overcome tumor-induced inhibition of immune function. Continued development of these exciting new approaches is needed to improve treatment of this usually fatal disease. Enhanced under-standing of the biology of pancreatic cancer should also provide avenues to pursue for prevention and earlier detection with prospects for decreasing deaths from pancreatic cancer.

REFERENCES

1. Chang KJ, Parasher G, Christie C, et al. Risk of pancreatic adenocar-cinoma: disparity between African Americans and other race/ethnic groups. *Cancer.* 2005; 103: 349–357.

2. Maisonneuve P, Lowenfels AB. Epidemiology of pancreatic cancer: an update. *Dig Dis.* 2010; 28: 645–656.

3. Klein AP. Genetic susceptibility to pancreatic cancer. *Mol Carcinog.* 2012; 51: 14–24.

4. Hruban RH, Klein AP, Eshleman JR, et al. Familial pancreatic cancer: from genes to improved patient care. *Expert Rev Gastroenterol Hepatol.* 2007; 1: 81–88

5. Adsay NV, Bagci P, Tajiri T, et al. Pathologic staging of pancreatic, ampullary, biliary, and gallbladder cancers: pitfalls and practical limita-tions of the current AJCC/UICC TNM staging system and opportuni-ties for improvement. *Semin Diagn Pathol.* 2012; 29: 127–141.

6. Warshaw AL, Lillemoe KD, Fernandez-del Castillo C. Pancreatic sur-gery for adenocarcinoma. *Curr Opin Gastroenterol.* 2012; 28: 488–493.

7. Valsangkar NP, Morales-Oyarvide V, Thayer SP, et al. 851 resected cys-tic tumors of the pancreas: a 33-year experience at the Massachusetts General Hospital. *Surgery.* 2012; 152(3 Suppl 1): S4–S12.

8. Marchegiani G, Crippa S, Malleo G, et al. Surgical treatment of pancre-atic tumors in childhood and adolescence: uncommon neoplasms with favorable outcome. *Pancreatology.* 2011; 11: 383–389.

9. Ellison TA, Edil BH. The current management of pancreatic neuroendocrine tumors. *Adv Surg.* 2012; 46: 283–296.

10. Hidalgo M. New insights into pancreatic cancer biology. *Ann Oncol.* 2012; 23 Suppl 10: x135–x138.

11. Yachida S. Novel therapeutic approaches in pancreatic cancer based on genomic alterations. *Curr Pharm Des.* 2012; 18: 2452–2463.

12. Tamm EP, Balachandran A, Bhosale PR, et al. Imaging of pancreatic adenocarcinoma: update on staging/resectability. *Radiol Clin North Am.* 2012; 50: 407–428.

13. Zygogianni GA, Kyrgias G, Kouvaris J, et al. Intraoperative radiation therapy on pancreatic cancer patients: a review of the literature. *Minerva Chir.* 2011; 66: 361–369.

14. Kimple RJ, Russo S, Monjazeb A, et al. The role of chemoradiation for patients with resectable or potentially resectable pancreatic cancer. *Expert Rev Anticancer Ther.* 2012; 12: 469–480.

15. Chaulagain CP, Ng J, Wazer D, et al. Adjuvant therapy of pancreatic cancer. *JOP.* 2012; 13: 349–353.

16. Herreros-Villanueva M, Hijona E, Cosme A, et al. Adjuvant and neoadjuvant treatment in pancreatic cancer. *World J Gastroenterol.* 2012; 18: 1565–1572.

17. Hosein PJ, Macintyre J, Kawamura C, et al. A retrospective study of neoadjuvant FOLFIRINOX in unresectable or borderline-resectable locally advanced pancreatic adenocarcinoma. *BMC Cancer.* 2012; 12: 199.

18. Loehrer PJ Sr, Feng Y, Cardenes H, et al. Gemcitabine alone versus gemcitabine plus radiotherapy in patients with locally advanced pancreatic cancer: an Eastern Cooperative Oncology Group trial. *J Clin Oncol.* 2011; 29: 4105–4112.

19. Chauffert B, Mornex F, Bonnetain F, et al. Phase III trial comparing intensive induction chemoradiotherapy (60 Gy, infusional 5-FU and intermittent cisplatin) followed by maintenance gemcitabine with gemcitabine alone for locally advanced unresectable pancreatic cancer. Definitive results of the 2000-01 FFCD/SFRO study. *Ann Oncol.* 2008; 19: 1592–1599.

20. Conroy T, Desseigne F, Ychou M, et al. FOLFIRINOX versus gemcitabine for metastatic pancreatic cancer. *N Engl J Med.* 2011; 364: 1817–1825.

21. Lowery MA, O'Reilly EM. New approaches to the treatment of pancreatic cancer: from tumor-directed therapy to immunotherapy. *BioDrugs.* 2011; 25: 207–216.

22. Giuliani F, Di Maio M, Colucci G, et al. Conventional chemotherapy of advanced pancreatic cancer. *Curr Drug Targets.* 2012; 13: 795–801.

23. Tokh M, Bathini V, Saif MW. First-line treatment of metastatic pancreatic cancer. *JOP.* 2012; 13: 159–162.

24. Von Hoff DD, et al. Abstract: LBA #148: Final results of a randomized phase III study of weekly nab-paclitaxel plus gemcitabine versus gemcitabine alone in patients with metastatic adenocarcinoma of the pancreas. ASCO GI 2013.

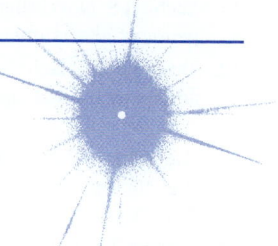

CHAPTER **46**

Cholangiocarcinoma and Gallbladder Cancers

Janet E. Murphy, Andrew X. Zhu

INTRODUCTION

Biliary tract cancers (BTCs) are invasive carcinomas that arise from the epithelial lining of the gallbladder and bile ducts. Cholangiocarcinomas are cancers arising in the intrahepatic, perihilar, or distal biliary tree, exclusive of cancers of the gallbladder and ampulla of Vater (**Figure 46-1**). Tumors involving the proper hepatic duct bifurcation are collectively referred to as Klatskin tumors, and are subdivided further using the Bismuth-Corlette Classification based on involvement of the left and right hepatic ducts, and focality versus multifocality of the tumor (1).

The vast majority of cholangiocarcinomas and gallbladder cancers (GBCs) are adenocarcinoma. While anatomically these malignancies are related, each has a distinct clinical presentation, molecular features, metastatic pattern, and prognosis. This group of tumors is characterized by local invasion, extensive regional lymph node metastasis, vascular encasement, and, especially with GBC, distant metastasis. Complete surgical resection offers the only chance for cure; rates of surgical resectability vary by primary location. Extrahepatic cholangiocarcinomas have the highest resectability rates compared to Klatskin and intrahepatic tumors (2). Among GBCs, only 10% of patients present with T1 tumors (those confined to the gallbladder muscle wall) unless they are found incidentally at cholecystectomy (3). Among those patients who do undergo "curative" resection, recurrence rates are high. BTCs have a poor prognosis; their 5-year survival rates are 5%–10% or less. The median survival of patients with unresectable or metastatic BTC at diagnosis is less than a year.

EPIDEMIOLOGY AND RISK FACTORS

Assessing incidence and prevalence of cholangiocarcinoma is difficult because intrahepatic cholangiocarcinoma is grouped with hepatocellular carcinoma. Collectively, there are an estimated 28,700 liver and intrahepatic bile duct cancers annually in the United States. Approximately 10%–15% of these tumors are estimated to be intrahepatic cholangiocarcinoma (4, 5). Extrahepatic bile duct and gallbladder cancers are grouped together. They

Classification of Cancers of the Human Biliary Tract

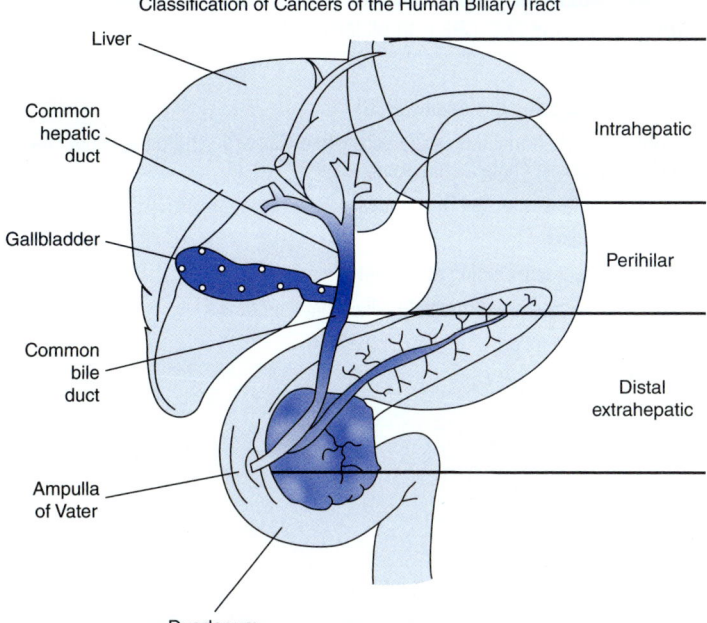

FIGURE 46-1 Classification of biliary tract cancers. (From de Groen PC, Gores GJ, LaRusso NF, et al. *N Engl J Med.* 1999; 341. Copyright © 1999 Massachusetts Medical Society. All rights reserved.)

total about 13,000 new cases annually in the United States, of which 9810 cases are extrahepatic cholangiocarcinoma, the remainder primary GBC (4). For unclear reasons, the incidence of intrahepatic cholangiocarcinoma has been rising over the past two decades in Europe and North America, Asia, Japan, and Australia. The risk factors for cholangiocarcinoma and GBC are shown in Table 46-1. For cholangiocarcinoma, these factors include primary sclerosing cholangitis (PSC), congenital abnormalities of the biliary tree (Caroli's syndrome, congenital hepatic fibrosis, choledochal cysts), parasitic infection of the liver flukes of the genera *Clonorchis* and *Opisthorchis*, hepatolithiasis, toxic exposures including radiologic contrast agent thorotrast (a radiologic contrast agent banned in the 1960s for its carcinogenic properties), Lynch syndrome II and multiple biliary papillomatosis, and possibly hepatitis C infection (6).

PSC is strongly associated with ulcerative colitis (UC). The incidence of colitis is around 90% in patients with PSC. Nearly 30% of cholangiocarcinomas are diagnosed in patients with UC and PSC. The annual incidence of cholangiocarcinoma in patients with PSC has been estimated to be between 0.6% and 1.5% per year, and lifetime risk is 10%–15% (7). Cholangiocarcinoma develops at a significantly younger age (between the ages of 30 and 50 years) in patients with PSC than in patients without PSC.

TABLE 46-1 RISK FACTORS FOR BILIARY TRACT CANCERS

Cholangiocarcinoma

  Primary sclerosing cholangitis (PSC)

  Congenital abnormalities of the biliary tree (Caroli's syndrome, congenital hepatic fibrosis, choledochal cysts)

  Parasitic infection of the liver flukes

  Hepatolithiasis

  Toxic exposures including thorotrast

  Lynch syndrome II and multiple biliary papillomatosis

  Hepatitis C infection

Gallbladder cancer

  Gallstones

  Porcelain gallbladder

  Gallbladder polyps

  Chronic salmonella infection

  Congenital biliary cysts

  Abnormal pancreaticobiliary duct junction

In the United States, GBC is the fifth most common GI cancer, and the most common involving the biliary tract (8). Among both Southwestern Native Americans and in Mexican-Americans, GBC is the most common GI malignancy (9). Worldwide, there is a prominent geographic variability in GBC incidence that correlates with the prevalence of cholelithiasis. High rates of GBC are seen in Chile, Bolivia, Japan, and Southeast Asia (10). Incidence steadily increases with age. Women are affected two to six times more often than men, and GBC is more common in Caucasians than in blacks (11).

For GBC, several conditions associated with chronic inflammation are considered risk factors, which include gallstone disease, porcelain gallbladder, gallbladder polyps, chronic salmonella infection, congenital biliary cysts, and abnormal pancreaticobiliary duct junction.

Gallstones are present in 70%–90% of patients with GBC, and there appears to be a relationship between gallstones and the development of GBC (12). Those with symptomatic gallbladder disease, larger gallstones, and longer duration of cholelithiasis have higher risks for the development of GBC. It should be noted that despite the increased risk of GBC in patients with gallstones, the overall incidence of GBC in patients with cholelithiasis is only 0.5%–3%.

An increased risk of GBC has been described in workers in industries involved in manufacture or processing of oil, paper, chemicals, shoes, textiles, and cellulose acetate fiber, and in miners exposed to radon. An association between medications and GBC has yet to be established.

PATHOLOGY

The majority of bile duct and gallbladder cancers are adenocarcinoma, although other histologic types are occasionally found, including small cell cancer, squamous cell carcinoma, lymphoma, and sarcoma. The molecular pathology is not well understood in these diseases. A subset of intrahepatic cholangiocarcinomas harbor mutations in the metabolic enzyme isocitrate dehydrogenase 1 (IDH1), which may prove to be a druggable target in the future (13).

CLINICAL FEATURES

The clinical presentations may vary depending on the location of the disease. Extrahepatic cholangiocarcinomas usually become symptomatic when the tumor obstructs the biliary drainage system, causing painless jaundice. Common symptoms include pruritus, abdominal pain (a constant dull ache in the right upper quadrant), weight loss, and fever. Patients with underlying PSC and cholangiocarcinoma tend to present with declining performance status and cholestasis. Other symptoms related to biliary obstruction include clay-colored stools and dark urine. Patients with intrahepatic cholangiocarcinomas usually present with a history of dull right upper quadrant pain and weight loss, an elevated serum alkaline phosphatase, and normal or only slightly elevated serum bilirubin levels.

Patients with early invasive GBC are most often asymptomatic, or have nonspecific symptoms that mimic or are due to cholelithiasis or cholecystitis. The diagnosis of GBC should be considered if compression of the common hepatic duct by an impacted stone in the gallbladder neck is identified (the Mirizzi syndrome). Patients with more advanced GBC may present with abdominal pain, anorexia, nausea, or vomiting, malaise, and weight loss.

DIAGNOSIS

■ IMAGING

Ultrasound (US) is often used as the initial imaging test due to its easy availability. Intrahepatic cholangiocarcinomas would appear as a mass lesion on US. Perihilar and extrahepatic cancers may not be readily detected, especially if small but indirect signs (biliary ductal dilatation throughout the obstructed liver segments) may point toward the diagnosis.

Computed tomography (CT) is useful for detecting intrahepatic tumors, assessing the level of biliary obstruction, and confirming the presence of liver atrophy and distant metastases. Ductal dilatation in both hepatic lobes with a contracted gallbladder suggests a Klatskin tumor, which sits at the bifurcation of the common, left, and right hepatic ducts, while a distended gallbladder without dilated intrahepatic or extrahepatic ducts suggests cystic duct obstruction by a stone or tumor. A distended gallbladder with dilated intrahepatic and extrahepatic ducts is more typical of tumors involving the common bile duct because the obstructive segment is more distal. Dilatation of the ducts within an atrophied hepatic lobe, in conjunction with a hypertrophic contralateral lobe (the atrophy–hypertrophy complex), suggests invasion of the portal vein (14).

Magnetic resonance cholangiopancreatography (MRCP) is a noninvasive technique for evaluating the intrahepatic and extrahepatic bile ducts (**Figure 46-2**). Unlike conventional endoscopic retrograde pancreatography (ERCP), MRCP does not require contrast material to be administered into the ductal system, thus avoiding the morbidity associated with endoscopic procedures and contrast administration. MRCP has advantages over CT because it not only images the liver parenchyma and intrahepatic lesions but also creates a three-dimensional image of the biliary tree (allowing assessment of the bile ducts both above and below a stricture) and vascular structures. MRCP provides information about disease extent and potential resectability that is comparable to the combined information obtained from CT, cholangiography, and angiography.

Direct cholangiography involves an injection of radiographic contrast material to opacify the bile ducts; it can be performed by ERCP or via a percutaneous approach (percutaneous transhepatic cholangiogram [PTC]) (**Figure 46-3**). However, MRCP and dynamic CT have largely replaced invasive cholangiography in patients thought to have a hilar cholangiocarcinoma. Cholangiography may still be indicated if the suspected level of obstruction is distal, or if preoperative drainage of the biliary tree is needed.

Endoscopic ultrasound (EUS) can be helpful in the diagnosis of distal bile duct cancer. It can visualize the extent of the primary tumor and the status of regional lymph nodes, and guide the fine needle aspiration and biopsy of primary tumors and enlarged nodes. EUS is more accurate for imaging the gallbladder than is extracorporeal US. The role of positron emission tomography (PET) scan in bile duct cancers is being investigated.

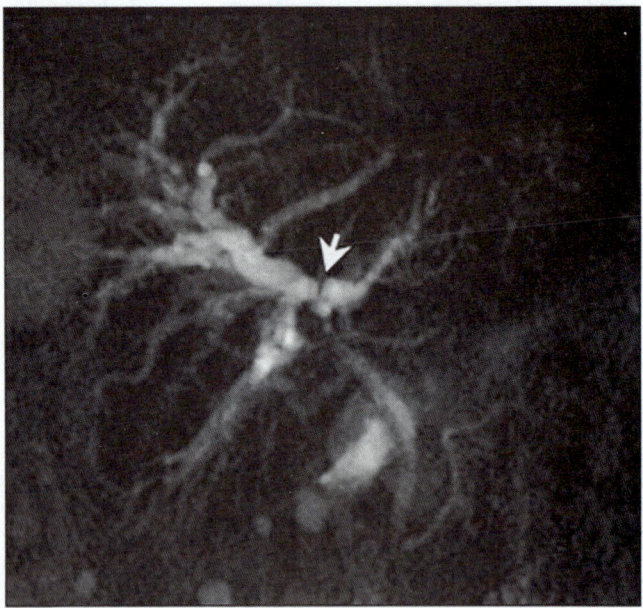

FIGURE 46-2 Klatskin tumor shown on MRCP.

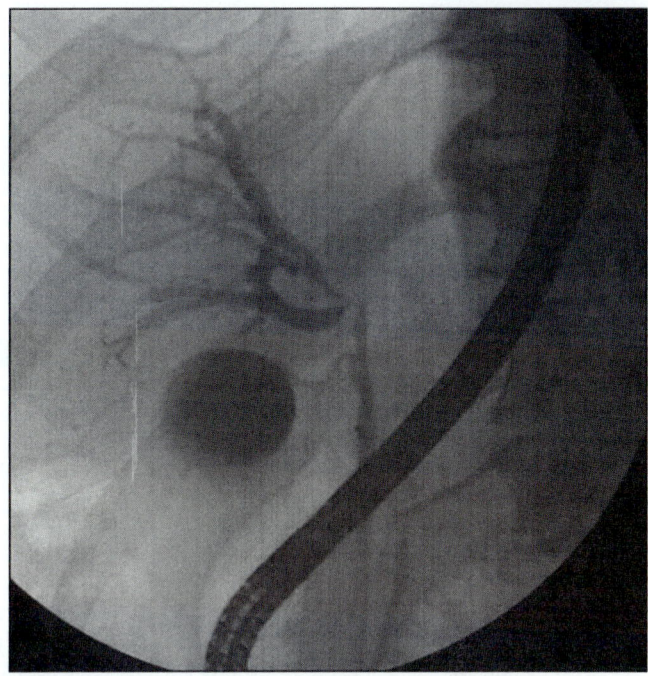

FIGURE 46-3 Klatskin tumor shown by ERCP cholangiography.

■ BIOPSY

Establishing a tissue diagnosis in bile duct cancers can be challenging. Sampling of bile by PTC or ERCP alone will only have a 30% positive rate in detecting malignant cells by cytology for cholangiocarcinoma (15). EUS-guided sampling of bile for cytologic analysis will have a sensitivity of 73% for the diagnosis of GBC (16). The diagnostic yield can be increased if the suspected lesion is biopsied or brushings taken from the duct for cytologic examination. The necessity of establishing a tissue diagnosis prior to surgery depends upon the clinical situation. For patients with characteristic findings of malignant biliary obstruction or mass lesion, a preoperative biopsy may not be necessary. Cholecystectomy should be strongly considered for patients with gallbladder polyps >1 cm as they are likely to contain an invasive cancer. A tissue diagnosis should be obtained for patients who would undergo chemotherapy or radiation therapy, or participate in a therapeutic clinical trial. It should be considered for patients with biliary strictures of clinically indeterminate origin, for example, in patients with a history of biliary tract surgery, bile duct stones, or PSC.

■ SERUM MARKERS

Although not specific for cholangiocarcinoma, the presence of certain tumor markers in the serum or bile of patients with cholangiocarcinoma may be of diagnostic value. Serum levels of carcinoembryonic antigen

(CEA) are neither sufficiently sensitive nor specific to diagnose cholangiocarcinoma. Serum levels of cancer antigen (CA) 19-9 are widely used, particularly for detecting cholangiocarcinoma in patients with PSC. However, the accuracy of serum CA 19-9 as a tumor marker for cholangiocarcinoma is variable in different studies depending on the cut-off values used with a sensitivity of 53%–79% and specificity of 98%–100%. The presence of cholangitis and cholestasis may influence the optimal cut-off CA 19-9 value that best discriminates between benign or malignant biliary tract diseases, as benign blockages of the biliary tree can cause significant CA 19-9 elevation. CEA or CA 19-9 levels are not diagnostically useful for GBC because of lack of specificity and sensitivity.

STAGING AND PROGNOSTIC SCORING SYSTEMS

The tumor staging systems for intrahepatic and extrahepatic cholangiocarcinoma are slightly different, and they are both based upon the TNM system devised by the American Joint Committee on Cancer (AJCC).

The current TNM classification schemes for both hilar and distal cholangiocarcinoma have undergone multiple revisions through the AJCC staging criteria (the preferred classification in the United States). The 2010 staging revisions (Table 46-2) separated intrahepatic, hilar (Klatskin), and extrahepatic cholangiocarcinoma (17).

GBC staging underwent revision in 2010 as well, with T stage reflecting the degree of invasion out of the gallbladder. T1 tumors invade the lamina propria (T1a) or muscular layer (T1b), T2 invades perimuscular tissue, T3 invades serosa or adjacent organs, and T4 invades the main portal vein or hepatic artery, or more than two adjacent organs. T4 reflects unresectable disease and overall was redefined as stage IVA disease. Nodal status is staged similarly to Klatskin tumors, with N1 nodes defined as proximal and N2 nodes defined as more distant locoregional spread.

TREATMENT

Surgery represents the only potentially curative treatment modality in BTCs. Fewer than 30% of patients with cholangiocarcinoma have surgically resectable disease. The resectability rates are higher for distal cholangiocarcinomas and lower for proximal (particularly perihilar) tumors. Absolute contraindications to surgery include liver or peritoneal metastases, ascites, encasement or occlusion of major vessels including portal vein and hepatic arteries, and extensive involvement of the regional lymph nodes. The surgical procedure required for definitive resection varies depending on the sites and extent of disease. For distal cholangiocarcinoma, a pancreaticoduodenectomy (Whipple procedure) is required. For perihilar cholangiocarcinomas, bile duct resection alone leads to high local recurrence rates due to early involvement of the confluence of the hepatic ducts and the caudate lobe branches. For intrahepatic cholangiocarcinoma, hepatic resection is indicated with intent to achieve negative margins.

For patients known to have GBC preoperatively, a simple cholecystectomy is usually not recommended. Rather, many surgical oncologists recommend a radical or extended cholecystectomy that includes removal of the gallbladder plus at least 2 cm of the gallbladder bed. In addition,

TABLE 46-2 HIGHLIGHTS OF 2010 AJCC STAGING FOR CHOLANGIOCARCINOMA

Tumor Type	Intrahepatic Cholangiocarcinoma	Perihilar (Klatskin)	Extrahepatic Cholangiocarcinoma
T stage	T1 tumors are solitary and lack vascular invasion	T1 tumors are those confined to the bile duct	T1 tumors are confined to the extrahepatic bile duct
	T2a tumors are solitary but have vascular invasion. T2b signifies multiple tumors, with or without vascular invasion	T2a tumors invade to surrounding adipose tissue (i.e., are clear of the liver parenchyma itself) while T2b tumors invade hepatic parenchyma	T2 tumors invade past the bile duct wall
	T3 tumors perforate into visceral peritoneum or involve the liver structures directly	T3 tumors invade unilateral branches of the portal vein or hepatic artery	T3 tumors invade neighboring viscera (gallbladder, pancreas, duodenum)
	T4 tumors invade the duct with longitudinal growth detected on gross and microscopic examination	T4 tumors invade the main portal vein, common hepatic artery, or other extensive vascular involvement	T4 tumors invade vasculature (celiac axis, SMA)
N stage	Nodal status for intrahepatic cholangiocarcinoma is either N0 (no nodes) vs. N1 (regional nodal involvement)	N1 nodes in hilar tumors are those along the cystic duct, common bile duct, hepatic artery, and portal vein. N2 nodes are metastatic to periaortic, pericaval, superior mesenteric artery, and/or celiac artery regions	Like intrahepatic tumors, extrahepatic nodal status is defined simply as N0 vs. N1 (regional nodes positive)

dissection of the regional lymph nodes from the hepatoduodenal ligament behind the second portion of the duodenum, head of the pancreas, and the celiac axis is recommended if a GBC is known or suspected. If a GBC is known to invade the liver, resection of the involved liver (segment or lobe) is often performed.

For patients who are diagnosed incidentally at the time of cholecystectomy, reexploration and radical resection is warranted if disease extent is T2 or greater. This benefit is based on the fact that more than 50% of patients with ≥T2 or greater disease will have positive nodes upon reexploration. The benefit of reexploration for patients with incidentally diagnosed T1 disease is more controversial as the incidence of liver invasion and nodal metastases is less. While simple cholecystectomy may be sufficient for many patients with T1 lesions, reexploration should be considered for patients with T1b disease (tumor invading the muscularis layer).

PROGNOSIS AND THE ROLE OF ADJUVANT THERAPY

The outcome for patients undergoing resection of a primary bile duct or gallbladder cancer depends upon the stage of disease. The 5-year survival rate for patients with completely resected bile duct and gallbladder cancers is in the range of 20%–50%. Due to the rarity of bile duct and gallbladder cancer, the role of adjuvant radiation therapy has not been definitively evaluated in randomized trials. Most studies consist of small, heterogeneous groups of patients seen in single institutions. Several retrospective series and small phase II studies suggest superior outcomes for patients who receive postoperative chemoradiotherapy (CRT). In the absence of definitive prospective data, for resected GBC, National Comprehensive Cancer Network (NCCN) guidelines recommend adjuvant 5FU-based CRT or 5FU or gemcitabine chemotherapy except for very early disease (T1bN0). For intrahepatic cholangiocarcinoma, for R0 resection (complete resection to negative margins), recommendations are for observation or clinical trial, but since recurrence rates are high, some centers offer adjuvant chemotherapy even in the absence of data, particularly with high-risk features such as vascular invasion or positive nodes. For R1 or R2 resections (resection with residual microscopic positive margins or gross residual disease, respectively), NCCN recommends re-resection, CRT, or chemotherapy. For resected extrahepatic cholangiocarcinoma, guidelines are similar to ampullary or pancreas cancer; chemotherapy and/or CRT are recommended, particularly in the setting of residual disease and/or positive nodes.

Prioritizing systemic disease control versus local control depends on patterns of failure. While both GBC and cholangiocarcinoma have high rates of local recurrence, GBC has a more prevalent pattern of metastatic spread. In one series of 97 patients with resectable GBC, distant recurrence (+/– local recurrence) was found in 85% of patients (18). For this reason, systemic chemotherapy is often prioritized in resected GBC.

■ LOCALLY ADVANCED, UNRESECTABLE DISEASE

For patients with locally advanced unresectable biliary tract and gallbladder cancer, radiation, usually given in combination with concurrent 5FU-based chemotherapy, can offer palliation and may improve local control. However, the overall impact of chemoradiation on survival is unknown. Locally advanced disease sits on the spectrum of true metastatic disease and doublet gemcitabine-cisplatin chemotherapy as demonstrated in the ABC-02 study (19), which has defined the standard of care for advanced disease, is considered the standard in these patients as well.

■ THERAPY FOR ADVANCED DISEASE

Systemic chemotherapy for BTC occasionally improves symptoms and may improve survival when compared to a historical series of supportive care alone. In one earlier study, patients with advanced biliary and pancreatic cancer were randomized to best supportive care alone or best supportive care plus chemotherapy with 5FU, etoposide, and leucovorin (FELV) (20). The median survival for the chemotherapy arm was significantly higher compared to best supportive care alone for all patients (6.5 vs. 2.5 months, $P < 0.01$). Since response rates to chemotherapy for biliary tract and gallbladder adenocarcinoma are similar, most recent studies have combined patients from both sites of origin. Several single agents have been tested with response rate of less than 20%, and these include 5FU, gemcitabine, capecitabine, irinotecan, and docetaxel. In 2010, the landmark ABC-02 trial defined the standard of care for locally advanced and metastatic BTC (19). This multicenter phase III trial randomized 410 patients with GBC, cholangiocarcinoma, and ampullary cancer (25% who had locally advanced disease) to gemcitabine (day 1, 8, 15 every 28 days) versus gemcitabine + cisplatin (day 1, 8 every 21 days). Combination therapy demonstrated superior progression free survival (8 vs. 5 months) and overall survival (11.7 vs. 8.1 months) with comparable toxicity. Gemcitabine plus a platinum (cisplatin or oxaliplatin) has become the standard of care in the first-line treatment of good performance status patients with advanced BTC. Nonetheless, these tumors remain a highly lethal group of malignancies and clinical trials incorporating biologic and targeted therapies are ongoing.

REFERENCES

1. Bismuth H, Nakacue R, Diamond T. Management strategies in resection for hilar cholangiocarcinoma. *Ann Surg.* 1992; 215: 31–38.

2. Nakeeb A, Pitt HA, Sohn TA, et al. Cholangiocarcinoma. a spectrum of intrahepatic, perihilar, and distal tumors. *Ann Surg.* 1996; 224: 463–473.

3. Fong Y, Wagman L, Gonen M, et al. Evidence-based gallbladder cancer staging: changing cancer staging by analysis of data from the National Cancer Database. *Ann Surg.* 2006; 243: 767–771.

4. Siegel R, Naishadham D, Jemal A. Cancer statistics, 2012. *CA Cancer J Clin.* 2012; 62: 10–29.

5. Patel T. Increasing incidence and mortality of primary intrahepatic cholangiocarcinoma in the United States. *Hepatology.* 2001; 33: 1353–1357.

6. Shaib YH, El-Serag HB, Davila JA, et al, Risk factors of intrahepatic cholangiocarcinoma in the United States: a case-control study. *Gastroenterology.* 2005; 128: 620–626.

7. Lee YM, Kaplan MM. Primary sclerosing cholangitis. *N Engl J Med.* 1995; 332: 924–933.

8. Carriaga MT, Henson DE. Liver, gallbladder, extrahepatic bile ducts, and pancreas. *Cancer.* 1995; 75: 171–190.

9. Diehl AK. Epidemiology of gallbladder cancer: a synthesis of recent data. *J Natl Cancer Inst.* 1980; 65: 1209–1214.

10. Randi G, Franceschi S, La Vecchia C. Gallbladder cancer worldwide: geographical distripbution and risk factors. *Int J Cancer.* 2006; 118: 1591–1602.

11. Scott TE, Carroll M, Cogliano FD, et al. A case-control assessment of risk factors for gallbladder carcinoma. *Dig Dis Sci.* 1999; 44: 1619–1625.

12. Paraskevopoulous JA, Dennison AR, Ross B, et al. Primary carcinoma of the gallbladder: a 10-year experience. *Ann R Coll Surg Engl.* 1992; 74: 222–224.

13. Borger DR, Tanabe KK, Fan KC, et al. Frequent mutation of isocitrate dehydrogenase (IDH)1 and IDH2 in cholangiocarcinoma identified through broad-based tumor genotyping. *Oncologist.* 2012; 17: 72–79.

14. Hann LE, Getrajdman GI, Brown KT, et al. Hepatic lobar atrophy: association with ipsilateral portal vein obstruction. *AJR Am J Roentgenol.* 1996; 167: 1017–1021.

15. Desa LA, Akosa AB, Lazzara S, et al. Cytodiagnosis in the management of extrahepatic biliary stricture. *Gut.* 1991; 32: 1188–1191.

16. Mohandas KM, Swaroop VS, Gullar SU, et al. Diagnosis of malignant obstructive jaundice by bile cytology: results improved by dilating bile duct strictures. *Gastrointest Endosc.* 1994; 40: 150–154.

17. Edge SB, Byrd DR, Compton CC, et al (eds). *American Joint Committee on Cancer Staging Manual*, 7th edition. Springer, New York, 2010.

18. Jarnigan WR, Ruo L, Little SA, et al. Patterns of initial disease recurrence after resection of gallbladder carcinoma and hilar cholangiocarcinoma: implications for adjuvant therapeutic strategies. *Cancer.* 2003; 98: 1689–1700.

19. Valle J, Wasan H, Palmer DH, et al. Cisplatin plus gemcitabine versus gemcitabine for biliary tract cancer. *N Engl J Med.* 2010; 362: 1273–1281.

20. Glimelius B, Hoffman K, Sjoden PO, et al. Chemotherapy improves survival and quality of life in advanced pancreatic and biliary cancer. *Ann Oncol.* 1996; 7: 593–600.

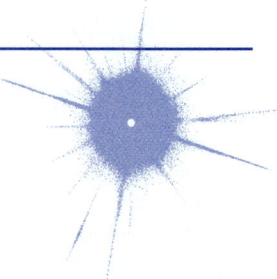

CHAPTER **47**

Colon Cancer

David P. Ryan

EPIDEMIOLOGY

■ STATISTICS

In the United States, 102,480 new cases of colon cancer were expected in 2013 (men 50,090; women 52,390) (1), and 40,340 new cases of rectal cancer were expected in 2013 (men 23,590; women 16,750). Colorectal cancer is the second leading cause of cancer-related death in the United States with 50,830 deaths annually. Age is a major risk factor in developing colon cancer. The lifetime risk of developing colorectal cancer is approximately 5% with the vast majority of cancers occurring after age 50 years. The overall incidence has been falling perhaps due to screening.

■ EPIDEMIOLOGIC ASSOCIATIONS

The vast majority of colorectal cancers are sporadic and not familial. Epidemiologic studies demonstrate an increased risk of colorectal cancer with the following conditions/characteristics:

- Family history of colorectal cancer is associated with an increased risk of developing colorectal cancer. If one first-degree family member had colorectal cancer, the risk increases 1.7-fold
- Western/urbanized societies
- Diet high in red or processed meat
- Increased bowel anaerobic flora
- Diabetes mellitus/insulin resistance: the risk of colon cancer may be 30% higher in diabetics compared with nondiabetics
- Inflammatory bowel disease. Increased incidence is seen with both Crohn's disease and ulcerative colitis and is associated with the severity, extent, and duration of disease affecting the colon. The risk of colon cancer in ulcerative colitis is approximately 10% at 10-year duration, 20% at 20-year duration, and >35% at 30-year duration. Total colectomy eliminates the risk of colon cancer
- Cigarette smoking
- Alcohol consumption
- Ureterosigmoidostomy
- *Streptococcus bovis* bacteremia
- Prior pelvic radiation

■ INHERITED SYNDROMES

Fewer than 10% of colon cancers are known to be associated with an inherited predisposition to colon cancer. The most common inherited syndromes are FAP and HNPCC. The MYH gene mutations are associated with an inherited predisposition to colon cancer as well (2).

Familial Adenomatous Polyposis (FAP)

Most cases of FAP are due to mutations in the APC gene on chromosome 5q21. These mutations are inherited in an autosomal dominant fashion.

APC is a tumor suppressor gene whose product interacts with critical cell proliferation genes in part by its interaction with transcription factor, beta catenin.

FAP is associated with hundreds to thousands of polyps throughout the colon. Fewer polyps and a later onset of colorectal cancer characterize an attenuated form of FAP. The use of COX-2 inhibitors can result in regression of some polyps.

By age 10 years, 15% of carriers will have adenomas; by age 20 years, 75% will have adenomas; and by age 30 years more than 90% will have adenomas. Screening of first-degree relatives should be done by age 10 years. Treatment is a total proctocolectomy.

FAP accounts for <1% of colon cancers and is associated with congenital hypertrophy of the retinal pigment, desmoid tumors (Gardner's syndrome), and brain tumors (Turcot's syndrome).

Hereditary Nonpolyposis Colon Cancer (HNPCC)

HNPCC is due to mutation in mismatch repair genes (e.g., MLH1, MSH2), which leads to microsatellite instability and errors in DNA replication. Inherited in an autosomal dominant fashion, HNPCC may account for up to 6% of all colon cancers. The median age for development of colon cancer is less than 50 years. Right-sided tumors are much more common than left-sided tumors. HNPCC is associated with endometrial cancer, ovarian cancer, upper gastrointestinal cancers, and transitional cell cancers of the renal pelvis/ureter.

An individual is likely to belong to a family with HNPCC and require genetic testing if: (1) three or more relatives have had colon cancer (or another cancer associated with HNPCC such as uterine, small bowel, ure-thral, or renal pelvic cancer) and at least one of the relatives is a first-degree relative, (2) two or more generations of the family have colon cancer, or (3) one or more relatives were diagnosed with colon cancer before age 50 years. Screening should begin by age 21 years in affected patients and be done at least every 5 years thereafter.

These criteria for identifying HNPCC are referred to as the Amsterdam II Criteria. The Bethesda criteria modify the Amsterdam II Criteria to include in the evaluation those patients who have had family members with adenomatous colonic polyps in addition to colon cancers.

MYH

MYH is a base excision repair gene located on the short arm of chromosome 1. Homozygous mutations in MYH have been associated with a syndrome manifesting itself as multiple colonic polyps and colorectal cancer. It is inherited in an autosomal recessive fashion. MYH mutations are thought to account for less than 1% of colorectal cancers.

PRIMARY PREVENTION AND SCREENING

■ PREVENTION STRATEGIES

Nonsteroidal anti-inflammatory drugs (NSAIDs), calcium, folate, and estrogens prevent the development of polyps, but there is no clear prevention of cancer. Their role is unknown in the patient who is getting adequately screened (3).

Antioxidants do not prevent colon cancer and conflicting data exist for the preventive ability of calcium, vitamin D, and statins. Diets high in fiber do not prevent colon cancer and diets high in red/processed meat and low in fish have been associated with an increased risk of colon cancer. However, physical activity may have a protective effect.

■ SCREENING

Most colorectal cancers arise from adenomatous polyps. The progression of adenomatous polyps from small polyps, to larger polyps, to dyspastic

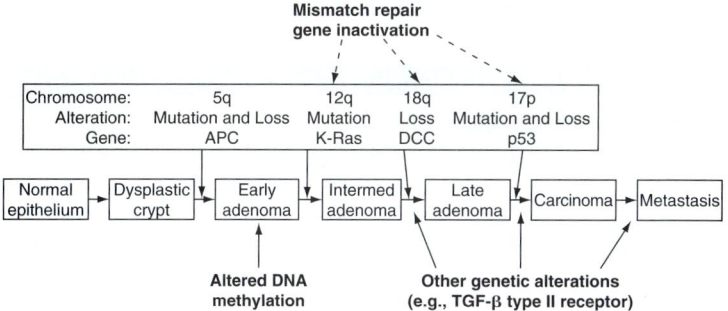

FIGURE 47-1 Vogelgram model of colon carcinogenesis.

polyps, and finally to cancer occurs over at least a 10-year period. Villous adenomas have a higher rate of progression to colon cancer than tubular or hyperplastic polyps. This progression is due to a series of acquired mutations as outlined by the work of Bert Vogelstein. It is generally felt that only 1% of polyps will progress through this sequence to form a cancer. This progression is due to a series of acquired mutations and is often referred to as the Vogelgram model after Bert Vogelstein, who initially described these events (**Figure 47-1**). The purpose of screening is to detect polyps before they turn into cancer. Guidelines for screening take into account the effectiveness, sensitivity, specificity, cost, and morbidity of the test (4).

Approximately 3%–6% of Americans undergoing colonoscopic screening in their 50s will have a colon cancer, dysplastic polyp, or villous adenoma. Over the last 20 years, there has been a movement away from barium enema as the screening tool of choice toward endoscopic screening. The preferred method (i.e., flexible sigmoidoscopy vs. colonoscopy) is controversial, but it is clear that colonoscopy is a more effective means of detecting any polyps in the colon. Any diagnosis of a polyp on sigmoidoscopy should prompt a full colonoscopy examination.

For patients without a family history of colon cancer, the United States Multisociety Task Force recommends screening patients beginning at age 50 years with annual fecal occult blood test as well as sigmoidoscopy every 5 years.

Alternatively, the task force recommended screening colonoscopy beginning at age 50 years and repeated every 10 years in those patients without any colonic pathology.

For patients with two or more affected first-degree relatives or any first-degree relative with colon cancer under the age of 60 years, screening should begin by age 40 years or at least 10 years younger than the age at which the affected family member was diagnosed.

Some experts recommend colonoscopy rather than FOBT and sigmoidoscopy on the basis of the following facts: (1) the combination of FOBT and sigmoidoscopy has a sensitivity of 75%; that is, it will miss 25% of lesions, (2) approximately 2% of asymptomatic adults at age 50 years will have a precancerous or cancerous proximal colonic lesion and have a totally normal sigmoidoscopy (5, 6). However, recent studies suggest that colonoscopy may not be as protective against death from right-sided colon cancer as it is for left-sided colon cancer (7).

PRESENTATION AND STAGING

■ SIGNS AND SYMPTOMS

Approximately 50% of colon cancers are found in the right side of the colon that is different than 50 years ago when the majority of tumors were found on the left side of the colon. The reason for this change is not known. The presenting symptoms depend on the location of the tumor. Obstruction, perforation, change in stool character, and hematochezia are more common with left-sided tumors. Fe-deficiency anemia is more common with right-sided tumors.

■ STAGING OF COLON CANCER

The process of staging a colon cancer is based on the American Joint Committee on Cancer (AJCC) TNM system and replaces the previous Duke's and Astler-Collier's systems (Table 47-1).

TREATMENT

■ SURGICAL MANAGEMENT

At presentation, the initial evaluation should consist of routine chemistries and a complete blood count. An elevated carcinoembryonic antigen (CEA) preoperatively is associated with a poor prognosis. The routine use of imaging is controversial. It is reasonable to obtain CT scans of the chest, abdomen, and pelvis to evaluate for the presence of metastatic disease.

For patients with stage I, II, or III colon cancer, surgical resection of the colon cancer is the mainstay of therapy. Open colectomy or laparoscopic colectomy is equally effective. For patients with stage IV colon cancer who are not considered candidates for cure, resection of the primary lesion can be based upon the symptoms of the patient. In the asymptomatic patient, surgical resection of the primary tumor is not necessary and can be deferred until the patient experiences local symptoms. Some patients will die of metastatic disease without ever experiencing symptoms from the primary tumor.

■ STAGE 1

Surgical resection cures >90% of patients with stage 1 colon cancer. Adjuvant therapy is not recommended. Patients should undergo surveillance colonoscopy 1 year after the diagnosis and then again in 3–5 years. Patients with more than two first-degree relatives with colon cancer, a first-degree relative with colon cancer under the age of 50 years, or who are under 50 years themselves, should undergo evaluation in a genetic/high-risk clinic.

■ STAGE 2

Surgical resection cures approximately 80% of patients with stage 2 colon cancer. The use of adjuvant chemotherapy is controversial and is currently not recommended by the American Society of Clinical Oncology. Randomized studies have not shown a statistically significant benefit for

TABLE 47-1 COLORECTAL CARCINOMA STAGING SYSTEM OF THE
AMERICAN JOINT COMMITTEE ON CANCER, 7TH EDITION

Primary tumor (T)

TX	Primary tumor cannot be assessed
T0	No evidence of primary tumor
Tis	Carcinoma in situ: intraepithelial or invasion of lamina propria*
T1	Tumor invades submucosa
T2	Tumor invades muscularis propria
T3	Tumor invades through the muscularis propria into pericolorectal tissues
T4a	Tumor penetrates to the surface of the visceral peritoneum•
T4b	Tumor directly invades or is adherent to other organs or structures△

Regional lymph node (N)◊

NX	Regional lymph nodes cannot be assessed
N0	No regional lymph node metastasis
N1	Metastasis in 1–3 regional lymph nodes
N1a	Metastasis in one regional lymph node
N1b	Metastasis in 2–3 regional lymph nodes
N1c	Tumor deposit(s) in the subserosa, mesentery, or nonperitonealized pericolic or perirectal tissues without regional nodal metastasis
N2	Metastasis in 4 or more regional lymph nodes
N2a	Metastasis in 4–6 regional lymph nodes
N2b	Metastasis in 7 or more regional lymph nodes

Distant metastasis (M)

M0	No distant metastasis
M1	Distant metastasis
M1a	Metastasis confined to one organ or site (eg, liver, lung, ovary, nonregional node)
M1b	Metastases in more than one organ/site or the peritoneum

Anatomic stage/prognostic groups§

Stage	T	N	M	Dukes¥	MAC¥
0	Tis	N0	M0	-	-
I	T1	N0	M0	A	A
	T2	N0	M0	A	B1
IIA	T3	N0	M0	B	B2
IIB	T4a	N0	M0	B	B2
IIC	T4b	N0	M0	B	B3

(*continued*)

TABLE 47-1 COLORECTAL CARCINOMA STAGING SYSTEM OF THE AMERICAN JOINT COMMITTEE ON CANCER, 7TH EDITION (CONTINUED)

IIIA	T1-2	N1/N1c	M0	C	C1
	T1	N2a	M0	C	C1
IIIB	T3-T4a	N1/N1c	M0	C	C2
	T2-T3	N2a	M0	C	C1/C2
	T1-T2	N2b	M0	C	C1
IIIC	T4a	N2a	M0	C	C2
	T3-T4a	N2b	M0	C	C2
	T4b	N1-N2	M0	C	C3
IVA	Any T	Any N	M1a	-	-
IVB	Any T	Any N	M1b	-	-

*This includes cancer cells confined within the glandular basement membrane (intraepithelial) or mucosal lamina propria (intramucosal) with no extension through the muscularis mucosae into the submucosa.

*Direct invasion in T4 includes invasion of other organs or other segments of the colorectum as a result of direct extension through the serosa, as confirmed on microscopic examination (e.g., invasion of the sigmoid colon by a carcinoma of the cecum) or, for cancers in a retroperitoneal or subperitoneal location, direct invasion of other organs or structures by virtue of extension beyond the muscularis propria (i.e., respectively, a tumor on the posterior wall of the descending colon invading the left kidney or lateral abdominal wall; or a mid or distal rectal cancer with invasion of prostate, seminal vesicles, cervix, or vagina).

△Tumor that is adherent to other organs or structures, grossly, is classified cT4b. However, if no tumor is present in the adhesion, microscopically, the classification should be pT1-4a depending on the anatomical depth of wall invasion. The V and L classifications should be used to identify the presence or absence of vascular or lymphatic invasion, whereas the PN site-specific factor should be used for perineural invasion.

◊A satellite peritumoral nodule in the pericolorectal adipose tissue of a primary carcinoma without histologic evidence of residual lymph node in the nodule may represent discontinuous spread, venous invasion with extravascular spread (V1/2), or a totally replaced lymph node (N1/2). Replaced nodes should be counted separately as positive nodes in the N category, whereas discontinuous spread or venous invasion should be classified and counted in the site-specific factor category tumor deposits (TD).

§cTNM is the clinical classification, and pTNM is the pathologic classification. The y prefix is used for those cancers that are classified after neoadjuvant pretreatment (e.g., ypTNM). Patients who have a complete pathologic response are ypT0N0cM0 that may be similar to Stage Group 0 or I. The r prefix is to be used for those cancers that have recurred after a disease-free interval (rTNM).

ᵞDukes stands for the Dukes staging classification and MAC stands for the modified Astler-Coller staging system.

Used with the permission of the American Joint Committee on Cancer (AJCC), Chicago, Illinois. The original source for this material is Edge SB et al (eds). *AJCC Cancer Staging Manual,* 7th edition. New York, Springer, 2010.

the use of adjuvant chemotherapy in patients with stage 2 colon cancer. However, many experts advocate for the use of adjuvant chemotherapy in high-risk patients, because these patients carry a greater than 20% risk of dying from recurrent disease. Patients with stage 2 colon cancer who are considered high risk carry the following features:

- T4 disease
- Presentation with perforation or obstruction
- Inadequate nodal evaluation; the American College of Pathology recommends that at least 12 regional lymph nodes be examined for the presence of nodal metastases
- Poorly differentiated tumors

Patients with microsatellite unstable (or MSI-high) tumors have a favorable prognosis that may supersede any poor risk feature. Many experts argue against treating patients with MSI-high tumors with adjuvant chemotherapy

For type of adjuvant chemotherapy see stage 3 section.

■ STAGE 3

Surgical resection cures approximately half of patients with stage 3 colon cancer. Patients with N1 disease can expect a cure rate with surgery alone of approximately 60%–70%. Patients with N2 disease can expect a cure rate of 30% with surgery alone. Adjuvant chemotherapy is recommended for all patients with stage 3 colon cancer at improved overall survival.

Standard treatment can consist of 6 months of 5-fluorouracil (5-FU) and leucovorin. Six months of capecitabine, an oral fluoropyrimidine, has equivalent efficacy to intravenous 5-FU and leucovorin. Recently, the addition of oxaliplatin to intravenous 5-FU and leucovorin has been associated with an improved disease-free survival compared with 5-FU and leucovorin for patients with stage 2 and 3 colon cancer. Subset analysis of patients with stage 2 disease did not reveal a statistically significant advantage in disease-free survival or overall survival for patients receiving FOLFOX compared with 5-FU and leucovorin. Subset analyses in patients with stage 3 disease demonstrated a significant improvement in disease-free and overall survival.

■ STAGE 4

All patients with isolated liver or lung metastases should be evaluated by a surgical specialist for consideration of resection of the metastases. Approximately 30% of patients undergoing complete resection of isolated liver or lung metastases will be cured (8).

For patients in whom a curative resection cannot be done, the median survival is approximately 6–8 months without chemotherapy and 2 years with chemotherapy. Approximately 10%–20% of patients who undergo aggressive chemotherapy will live for 5 years.

Until 1997, 5-FU was the only active chemotherapy. Studies demonstrated that the addition of folinic acid (leucovorin) to 5-FU improved the response rates and time to tumor progression. Since 1997, irinotecan, oxaliplatin, bevacizumab, and cetuximab have been approved for use in patients with metastatic colon cancer. The major randomized studies are presented in Table 47-2.

First-line chemotherapy for patients with metastatic disease of consists of either FOLFOX (5-FU, leucovorin, oxaliplatin) or FOLFIRI (5-FU,

TABLE 47-2 MAJOR PHASE 3 STUDIES IN STAGE 4 COLON CANCER

Common Title	Regimen	No. of Patients	Median Survival (Months)
Saltz study (9)	IFL	221	14.8
	5-FU/LV	236	12.6
			$p = 0.04$
N9741 (10)	FOLFOX	264	19.5
	IFL	267	15.0
			$p = 0.0001$
Tournigand study (11)	FOLFOX	111	21.5
	FOLFIRI	109	20.4
			$p = 0.9$
Bevacizumab study (12)	IFL	411	20.3
	IFL/Bevacizumab	402	15.6
			$p = 0.00004$

FOLFIRI, infusional + bolus 5-FU, leucovorin, irinotecan; FOLFOX, infusional + bolus 5-FU, leucovorin, oxaliplatin; IFL, irinotecan, 5-FU, leucovorin.

leucovorin, irinotecan) with bevacizumab. Second-line chemotherapy typically consists of either an irinotecan-based regimen if FOLFOX was used as the first-line regimen or an oxaliplatin-based regimen if FOLFIRI was used as the first-line regimen. The addition of bevacizumab in second-line chemotherapy regimens when bevacizumab was a component in first-line regimens is associated with an improvement in overall survival. The addition of aflibercept to FOLFIRI in second-line treatment of patients with metastatic colorectal cancer is associated with an improved overall survival benefit compared with FOLFIRI alone. Cetuximab and panitumumab are approved for use either alone or in combination with chemotherapy for patients with metastatic colorectal cancer. Cetuximab and panitumumab are not effective in kras mutant colorectal cancers and their use is restricted to patients who have kras wild-type colorectal cancers. The combination of cetuximab or panitumumab with bevacizumab containing chemotherapy regimens is associated with worse survival outcomes. Capecitabine is often substituted for 5-FU and leucovorin in the FOLFOX regimens. The use of regorafenib in the chemotherapy-refractory setting improves overall survival by 1.4 months compared with the use of a placebo.

REFERENCES

1. Jemal A, Siegel R, Ward E, et al. Cancer statistics, 2013. *CA Cancer J Clin.* 2013; 63: 11–30.
2. Lynch HT, de la Chapelle A. Hereditary colorectal cancer. *N Engl J Med.* 2003; 348: 919–932.

3. Janne PA, Mayer RJ. Chemoprevention of colorectal cancer. *N Engl J Med.* 2000; 342: 1960–1968.

4. Winawer S, Fletcher R, Rex D, et al. Colorectal cancer screening and surveillance: clinical guidelines and rationale-update based on new evidence. *Gastroenterology.* 2003; 124: 544–560.

5. Imperiale TF, Wagner DR, Lin CY, et al. Risk of advanced proximal neoplasms in asymptomatic adults according to the distal colorectal findings. *N Engl J Med.* 2000; 343: 169–174.

6. Lieberman DA, Weiss DG, Bond JH, et al. Use of colonoscopy to screen asymptomatic adults for colorectal cancer. Veterans Affairs Cooperative Study Group 380. *N Engl J Med.* 2000; 343: 162–168.

7. Baxter NN, Warren JL, Barrett MJ, et al. Association between colonoscopy and colorectal cancer mortality in a US cohort according to site of cancer and colonoscopist specialty. *J Clin Oncol.* 2012; 30: 2664–2669.

8. Fong Y, Fortner J, Sun RL, Brennan MF, Blumgart LH. Clinical score for predicting recurrence after hepatic resection for metastatic colorectal cancer: analysis of 1001 consecutive cases. *Ann Surg.* 1999; 230: 309–318; discussion 18–21.

9. Saltz LB, Cox JV, Blanke C, et al. Irinotecan plus fluorouracil and leucovorin for metastatic colorectal cancer. Irinotecan Study Group. *N Engl J Med.* 2000; 343: 905–914.

10. Goldberg RM, Sargent DJ, Morton RF, et al. A randomized controlled trial of fluorouracil plus leucovorin, irinotecan, and oxaliplatin combinations in patients with previously untreated metastatic colorectal cancer. *J Clin Oncol.* 2004; 22: 23–30.

11. Tournigand C, Andre T, Achille E, et al. FOLFIRI followed by FOLFOX6 or the reverse sequence in advanced colorectal cancer: a randomized GERCOR study. *J Clin Oncol.* 2004; 22: 229–237.

12. Hurwitz H, Fehrenbacher L, Novotny W, et al. Bevacizumab plus irinotecan, fluorouracil, and leucovorin for metastatic colorectal cancer. *N Engl J Med.* 2004; 350: 2335–2342.

CHAPTER **48**
Rectal Cancer

Theodore S. Hong

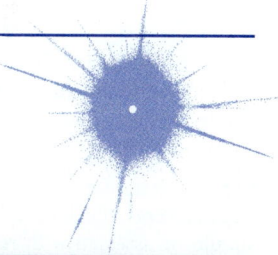

EPIDEMIOLOGY

In 2013 there were approximately 143,000 Americans diagnosed with colon and rectal cancer. Approximately 2/3 will involve the colon and 1/3 the rectum. Epidemiological factors and pathogenesis are similar for rectal cancer as for colon cancer.

ANATOMY

The rectum is generally divided into three portions: lower rectum, mid-rectum, and upper rectum. The distances from the anal verge are approximations and may vary with flexible endoscopic techniques.

- Lower rectum: 4–8 cm from anal verge
- Mid-rectum: 8–12 cm from anal verge
- Upper-rectum: 12–16 cm from anal verge
- Anal canal: 4 cm in length

■ IMPORTANT LANDMARKS

Dentate Line

The dentate line is the transition point between the squamous mucosa of the anus/perineum and the columnar mucosa of the rectum. Below the dentate line, the lymph drainage flows through the inguinal nodes and has implications for treatment.

Rectum/Sigmoid Boundary

In contrast to the sigmoid colon, peritoneum does not cover the circumference of the rectum. Rectal cancer has higher rates of local failure following surgery than colon cancer and requires aggressive local treatment.

Generally, rectal tumors should be no less than 6–7 cm from anal verge if a sphincter sparing operation is to be attempted in order to preserve muscle function while obtaining adequate margins.

DIAGNOSIS AND STAGING

■ DIAGNOSIS

Presenting Symptoms

The majority of patients diagnosed with rectal cancer present with symptoms, although many are nonspecific and this may lead to a delay in diagnosis. Common symptoms include bleeding (gross or occult), constitutional symptoms, abdominal pain, changes in stool caliber, and changes in bowel habits.

WORKUP

When cancer is in the differential diagnosis, the workup entails history and physical including digital rectal examination (DRE), complete blood count, liver and renal function tests, carcinoembryonic antigen (CEA), and endoscopy.

DRE   DRE should be used to assess the location of the tumor in relation to the anal verge, the dentate line, and the anal sphincter. If possible, the tumor should be assessed with respect to anal sphincter involvement, circumferential extent, and possible fixation to normal structures. Baseline sphincter tone should be assessed.

Rigid proctosigmoidoscopy   This is used both to assess the location of the tumor (especially when nonpalpable), and to take biopsies for tissue diagnosis.

■ STAGING

Staging system

Rectal cancer is staged using clinicopathological parameters and classified using the AJCC TNM system (see Table 47-1). Preoperative staging is used for prognostic purposes and to estimate the risk of recurrence after surgery to guide adjuvant therapy.

T and N Stage

Endorectal ultrasound and MRI are commonly used to assess the extent of the primary tumor. Nodal status can be determined using MRI, CT, and EUS, but may be difficult to assess radiographically.

Endorectal Ultrasound (Eus)

EUS is able to distinguish the five layers of the rectal wall with good spatial resolution. The accuracy for T stage ranges from 67% to 97% with a propensity to overstage tumors as indicated by a reported specificity of 24% for peri-rectal penetration. EUS is operator dependent and associated with a fast learning curve (1, 2).

Magnetic Resonance Imaging (Figure 48-1)

When MRI is used for primary determination of T stage, a surface phased array coil is employed enabling differentiation of rectal wall layers. Accuracy is operator dependant with interrater accuracies in one study of 67% and 83%. MRI can also be used for preoperative assessment of the likely circumferential margin (CFM) following surgery. The accuracy of N stage evaluation is similar to that of CT in that both are based on size criteria (3).

Assessment of Metastatic Disease

Computed tomography (CT) CT is used primarily for preoperative assessment of metastatic disease in the lungs, liver, or abdomen. It is less useful for the assessment of T stage with accuracy rates of only 33%–77% resulting from the inability to distinguish layers of rectal wall. The sensitivity for detection of nodal disease ranges from 45% to 73% (1).

Residual or Recurrent Disease

Positron emission tomography may be used for the assessment of residual or recurrent disease and may be helpful in areas of scarring or radiation changes (1).

TREATMENT

A general treatment algorithm is included in **Figure 48-2**.

■ SURGICAL MANAGEMENT

Local Excision

A number of criteria must be met in order to proceed with local excision. These include T1 without evidence of nodal disease, tumor within 4–6 cm of the anal verge, and involvement of less than 40% of circumference of

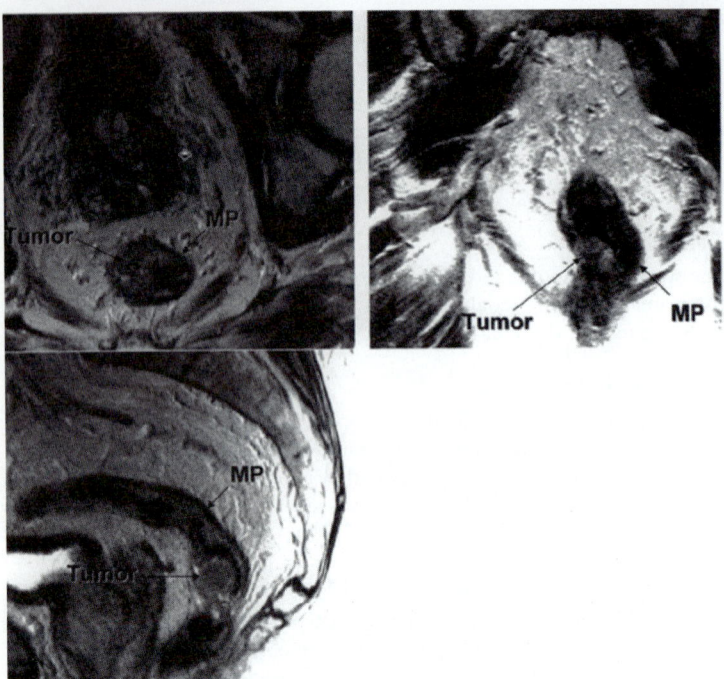

FIGURE 48-1 (Clockwise from lower left) sagittal, axial, and coronal T2 weighted MRI of the pelvis showing a rectal tumor invading through the muscularis propria (MP) making this a T3 lesion.

bowel wall. Histopathological limitations include well to moderately differentiated histology and no evidence of lymphovascular invasion. Local excision techniques must be full-thickness excisions. These include transanal excision, posterior proctoctomy, and transsphincteric excision. The role of local excision for T2 tumors is highly controversial.

ABDOMINAL PERINEAL RESECTION (APR)

An APR is a nonsphincter sparing operation requiring both an abdominal and perineal incision and a permanent colostomy. It is the standard procedure for tumor removal when the lower extent of the tumor does not allow for sphincter preservation with adequate tumor margins (traditional margin is 5 cm, although 2-cm margins have been used). The entire rectum along with the sphincter apparatus is removed through the perineum.

LOW ANTERIOR RESECTION (LAR)

LAR involves the mobilization of the entire rectum and complete resection of the involved segment of the rectum encompassing the tumor with a margin. The remaining ends are reanastomosed, so that no permanent colostomy is required.

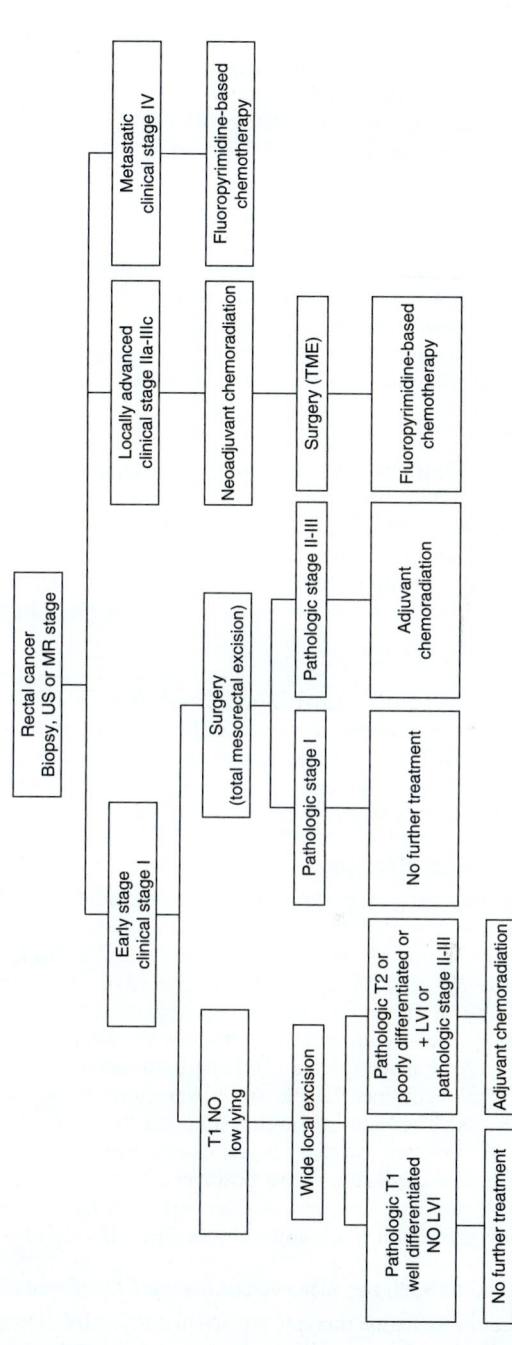

FIGURE 48-2 Treatment algorithm. The type of surgery (LAR, APR) depends on the location of the tumor and the ability to spare the anal sphincter while maintaining adequate surgical margins. Chemoradiation consists of 5FU given concurrently with radiation to a pelvic field.

593

Total Mesorectal Excision (Tme)

Prior to TME, traditional surgical techniques invaded tissue planes during blunt dissection. The CFM status following surgery correlates with the risk of local recurrence. TME requires sharp dissection under direct visualization to remove the entire rectal mesentery along with the peri-rectal fat as one discrete unit. This procedure has improved outcomes (4).

Combined Modality Therapy

Combined modality therapy is considered either when the risk of local recurrence is significant (stage II–III disease) or in an attempt to covert an APR to a sphincter sparing operation. When chemotherapy and radiation are used in addition to surgery for local disease control, fluoropyrimidine-based chemotherapy must be used for systemic therapy following surgery. Major adjuvant and neoadjuvant trials are listed in Table 48-1.

Neoadjuvant Therapy

Although survival was identical between the two arms, the Dutch Colorectal Cancer Group trial showed that in patients undergoing surgery with TME, preoperative radiation was associated with decreased rates of local recurrence (5). Trials with preoperative chemoradiation improved on the results of preoperative radiation. Chemoradiation has also been used preoperatively to convert tumors requiring APR into sphincter sparing procedures.

Adjuvant Therapy

In the mid-1980s, the Gastrointestinal Tumor Study Group (GITSG) showed that adjuvant chemoradiation was associated with a survival benefit when compared with no further treatment following surgery (6). This and other trials led the NIH to recommend adjuvant chemoradiotherapy for patients with stage II or III disease in 1990.

Neoadjuvant versus Adjuvant Therapy

The question of whether pre- or postoperative chemoradiation provided the most benefit was asked by the German Rectal Cancer Study Group. At 5 years of follow-up, preoperative chemoradiation was associated with a lower rate of local recurrence (6% vs. 13%), a lower rate of grade 3 or 4 acute toxic effects (27% vs. 40%), and lower rate of long-term toxic effects (14% vs. 24%). There was no difference in overall survival. Preoperative chemoradiation also allowed for greater sphincter sparing (7). Long-term follow-up of this study confirms the local recurrence benefit with preoperative therapy at 10 years (7.1% vs. 10.1%) (8). The National Surgical Adjuvant Breast and Bowel Project (NSABP) R-03 also demonstrated a 5-year disease-free survival benefit with preoperative chemoradiation versus postoperative chemoradiation (64.7% vs. 53.4%) (9). Standard preoperative chemoradiation includes 50.4 Gy in 1.8 Gy fractions given with continuous infusion 5FU (225 mg/m^2).

Preoperative Short Course Radiation Alone versus Standard Chemoradiation

Preoperative short course radiation therapy, as given in the Dutch Colorectal Cancer Group trial, has been compared to preoperative chemoradiation, as

TABLE 48-1 MAJOR ADJUVANT AND NEOADJUVANT TRIALS

Study	Arms	Local Control (%)	Overall Survival (%)
Pre-TME era			
GITSG (6, 8)	No adjuvant	55 (recurrence rate, med fu 80 mos)	27 (9 y)
	Adjuvant RT	48	
	Adjuvant chemo	46	
	Adjuvant chemo/RT	33	54 ($p = 0.01$)
Swedish Rectal Cancer Trial (12)	Surgery alone	73 (5 y)	48 (5 y)
	Neoadjuvant RT	89 ($p < 0.001$)	58 ($p = 0.004$)
TME era			
Dutch Colorectal Cancer Study (3)	Surgery alone	91.8 (2 y)	82 (2 y)
	Neoadjuvant RT	97.6 ($p < 0.001$)	82 ($p = 0.84$)
German Rectal Cancer Study (7)	Neoadjuvant chemoradiation	94 (5 y)	76 (5 y)
	Adjuvant chemoradiation	87 ($p = 0.006$)	74 ($p = 0.8$)
NSABP R-03 (9)	Neoadjuvant chemoradiation	89 (5 y)	75 (5 y)
	Adjuvant chemoradiation	89 ($p = 0.693$)	66 ($p = 0.065$)
Polish Rectal Study (10)	Neoadjuvant short course radiation	91 (4 y)	67.2 (4 y)
	Neoadjuvant chemoradiation	86 ($p = 0.170$)	66.2 ($p = 0.960$)
TROG 01.04 (11)	Neoadjuvant short course radiation	93 (3 y)	74 (5 y)
	Neoadjuvant chemoradiation	96 ($p = 0.24$)	70 ($p = 0.62$)

given in the German Rectal Study and NSABP R-03. Short course radiation uses five fractions of radiation alone (5 Gy × 5), with surgery the following week. Two randomized trials show no difference in survival, local control, or late toxicity (10, 11).

Unresectable Disease

Neoadjuvant chemoradiation can be used to convert unresectable disease into resectable disease. If there is residual disease or if there is a strong possibility of positive margins, intraoperative radiation therapy (IORT) may be considered.

Recurrent Disease

There are no clear data on the management of recurrent disease. If surgical resection is possible with negative margins, long-term survival is possible. Reirradiation can be associated with high rates of complications as a function of the radiation dose and time interval from prior treatment.

Metastatic Disease

The foundation of the treatment of metastatic disease is fluoropyrimidine-based chemotherapy and is similar to the treatment of metastatic colon cancer (see chapter on colon cancer for details).

SURVEILLANCE AND FOLLOW-UP

- *History and physical.* Every 3–6 months for the first 3 years, every 6 months for years 4 and 5, and at the discretion of the physician thereafter.
- *Proctosigmoidoscopy.* Every 6 months for 5 years in patients not treated with radiation.
- *CEA.* Every 3 months for 3 years; fluorouracil-based chemotherapy may cause false elevation.
- *Chest/Abdomen/Pelvic CT* should be considered once a year for 3 years.

REFERENCES

1. Goh V, Halligan S, Bartram CI. Local radiological staging of rectal cancer. *Clin Radiol.* 2004; 59: 215–226.
2. Carmody BJ, Otchy DP. Learning curve of transrectal ultrasound. *Dis Colon Rectum.* 2000; 43: 193–197.
3. Beets-Tan RG, Beets GL, Vliegen RF, et al. Accuracy of magnetic resonance imaging in prediction of tumour-free resection margin in rectal cancer surgery. *Lancet.* 2001; 357: 497–504.
4. Bolognese A, Cardi M, Muttillo IA, et al. Total mesorectal excision for surgical treatment of rectal cancer. *J Surg Oncol.* 2000; 74: 21–23.
5. Kapiteijn E, Marijnen CA, Nagtegaal ID, et al. Preoperative radiotherapy combined with total mesorectal excision for resectable rectal cancer. *N Engl J Med.* 2001; 345: 638–646.
6. Thomas PR, Lindblad AS. Adjuvant postoperative radiotherapy and chemotherapy in rectal carcinoma: a review of the Gastrointestinal Tumor Study Group experience. *Radiother Oncol.* 1988; 13: 245–252.
7. Sauer R, Becker H, Hohenberger W, et al. Preoperative versus postoperative chemoradiotherapy for rectal cancer. *N Engl J Med.* 2004; 351: 1731–1740.
8. Sauer R, Liersch T, Merkel S, et al. Preoperative versus postoperative chemoradiotherapy for locally advanced rectal cancer: results of the

German CAO/ARO/AIO-04 randomized phase III trial after a median follow-up of 11 years. *J Clin Oncol.* 2012; 30: 3827–3833.

9. Roh MS, Colangelo LH, O'Connell MJ, et al. Preoperative multimodality therapy improves disease-free survival in patients with carcinoma of the rectum: NSABP R-03. *J Clin Oncol.* 2009; 27: 5124–5130.

10. Ngan SY, Burmeister B, Fisher RJ, et al. Randomized trial of short-course radiotherapy versus long-course chemoradiation comparing rates of local recurrence in patients with T3 rectal cancer: Trans-Tasman Radiation Oncology Group Trial 01.04. *J Clin Oncol.* 2012; 30: 3827–3833.

11. Bujko K, Nowacki MP, Nasierowska-Guttmejer A, et al. Long-term results of a randomized trial comparing preoperative short-course radiotherapy with preoperative conventionally fractionated chemoradiation for rectal cancer. *Br J Surg.* 2006; 93: 1215–1223.

12. Swedish Rectal Cancer Trial. Improved survival with preoperative radiotherapy in resectable rectal cancer. *N Engl J Med.* 1997; 336: 980–987.

CHAPTER 49
Anal Cancer

Jennifer Wo

Anal cancer is responsible for approximately 2.1% of digestive system malignancies with 6230 new cases estimated in the United States in 2012 (1). Anal cancer was once believed to be caused by chronic inflammation of the anal canal and treated with abdominoperineal resection (APR). Research has now shown that the development of anal cancer is associated with human papillomavirus (HPV) infection and has a pathophysiology similar to that of cervical cancer. Concurrent chemotherapy and external beam radiation therapy (EBRT) regimens have essentially replaced APR as primary treatment and have allowed for a great majority of patients to be cured with preservation of the anal sphincter.

ANATOMY AND HISTOLOGY

The anal canal extends from the junction of the puborectalis portion of the levator ani muscle and the external anal sphincter to the anal verge. The length of the canal averages 4 cm. The anal canal is divided by the transitional zone, or dentate line, which represents the transition from squamous mucosa to glandular mucosa. There is no easily identifiable landmark between the rectum and anus, so clinicians should rely on the pathologic classification of tumors in this area rather than surgical or endoscopic classification. Anal cancers are primarily keratinizing or non-keratinizing squamous cell carcinomas. Adenocarcinomas of the anal canal comprise about 20% of anal tumors, and share the natural history of rectal adenocarcinomas and should be treated as such.

There are two sites of lymphatic drainage from the anal canal. Tumors above the dentate line drain to the perirectal and perivertebral nodes, while tumors below the dentate line drain to the inguinal and femoral lymph nodes. For this reason, patients who present with anal masses should undergo examination of the inguinal lymph nodes, and patients who present with squamous cell cancers in the inguinal lymph nodes should be evaluated for primary anal tumors.

EPIDEMIOLOGY

The incidence of anal cancer has been rising in the United States. In a review of the SEER database from 1973 to 2000, the incidence of anal cancer in men and women has risen from 1.06 and 1.39 per 100,000 persons to 2.04 and 2.06 per 100,000 persons (2). In 2013, an estimated 7,060 cases were diagnosed in the United States. Although the incidence of anal cancer has risen in both sexes, the rate of rise for men is higher, particularly in patients diagnosed with HIV (3, 4). This increase in incidence may be due to better screening techniques and an increased rate of risk factors for anal cancer within the U.S. population that has occurred over time. Survival for patients with anal cancer is consistently worse for men compared to women and for black patients compared to white patients. Several risk factors have been associated with anal cancer:

- HPV infection
- History of genital warts
- Lifetime number of sexual partners
- Receptive anal intercourse
- History of cervical dysplasia or cancer
- History of previous sexually transmitted disease
- Human immunodeficiency virus (HIV) infection
- Cigarette smoking
- Chronic immunosuppression

Anal cancer risk factors mirror risk factors of sexually transmitted diseases, and are due to the link between HPV and anal cancer. Similar to cervical dysplasia and cancer, HPV can cause premalignant anal squamous intraepithelial lesions (ASIL), which can be low grade (LSIL) or high grade (HSIL). Progression of ASIL to invasive anal cancer is influenced by HIV seropositivity, low CD4 count, infection with multiple HPV serotypes, serotype of HPV infection, and high levels of DNA of high-risk serotypes. As with cervical cancer, HPV type 16 is the most frequently isolated serotype in HSIL and invasive anal cancer, present in 30%–75% of cases, and HPV types 6, 11, and 18 are present in 10% of cases.

Although not completely clear, there does seem to be a relationship between HIV infection and anal cancer. Multiple studies have suggested that anal cancer is increasingly prevalent in people with HIV infection (3, 4). Studies have noted an increase in the incidence of HPV infection, ASIL, HSIL, and anal cancer in HIV positive patients compared to HIV negative patients. However, it is difficult to control for separate risk factors including receptive anal intercourse and prior HPV infection in these studies. Unlike traditional AIDS-related malignancies, risk of anal cancer in HIV positive patients does not seem to correlate with worsening immunosuppression. In addition, the incidence of anal cancer has continued to increase in the age of widespread use of highly active antiretroviral therapy (HAART) (4), while the incidence of AIDS-related malignancies such as Kaposi's sarcoma and non-Hodgkin lymphoma has decreased. A possible explanation is that HAART allows for longer survival with HIV, but does not control HPV infection, allowing more time for HPV infection to create progressive dysplasia.

Individuals with non-HIV causes of chronic immunosuppression, such as renal transplant patients and patients on chronic glucocorticoid therapy, appear to be at an increased risk for ASIL and anal cancer, typically associated with persistent HPV infection. Several case-controlled studies have also noted an increased risk of anal cancer in smokers, particularly current smokers. Cigarette smoking is thought to act as a co-carcinogen.

SCREENING

Given the known high-risk groups for anal cancer, several studies have addressed screening in these populations. Similar to the cervical Papanicolaou smear, anal swabs for cytology are a possible screening method for ASIL and anal cancer. Sensitivity of anal cytology is in the range of 50%–80%, with sensitivity being higher in the HIV positive population. Studies of the potential cost-effectiveness of screening have found that screening HIV positive and HIV negative homosexual and bisexual men every 2–3 years would be cost effective and have life expectancy benefits (5, 6). Other groups where possible benefit of screening has been suggested include all HIV positive individuals, women with a history of cervical dysplasia or cancer, and transplant recipients.

With the development of HPV vaccines, there has been burgeoning interest in the use of the quadrivalent HPV vaccine in the prevention of anal cancer, particularly among high-risk patients. In one study of 602 healthy men who have sex with men (MSM) in the 16–26 year age group, men randomized to receive the quadrivalent HPV vaccine had a lower rate of anal intraepithelial neoplasia (13 per 100 person-years) compared with the placebo group (17.5 per 100 person-years). The rate of grade 2 or 3 AIN associated with oncogenic HPV infection was reduced by 54% in the vaccinated group (7). The vaccine was 94% efficacious against persistent anal HPV-16, and 100% against persistent anal HPV-18 infection. The vaccine was also found to decrease the 2-year recurrence rate of precancerous high-grade anal intraepithelial neoplasia (8). Longer follow-up will be necessary to determine whether this will translate into decreased incidence of anal cancer.

DIAGNOSIS

Diagnosis of anal cancer is based on clinical symptoms, physical exam, and biopsy. Patients can present with symptoms of pain, itching, bleeding, discharge, or anal irritation. Patients may also have tenesmus or, with larger tumors, obstructive-type symptoms. Physical exam should include a rectal exam to fully assess the size and location of the tumor and inguinal lymph node exam. Biopsy confirmation to assess histology of the anal mass as well as fine needle aspiration of enlarged inguinal lymph nodes should also be performed. Transanal ultrasonography may be used to evaluate depth of tumor invasion. CT scanning of the abdomen and pelvis can also be used to assess tumor size, invasion, lymph node involvement, and metastatic disease. PET scans or integrated PET/CT scans have also been shown to improve the sensitivity of detecting inguinal lymph node and distant metastases, which may impact treatment recommendations and radiation treatment fields (9, 10).

STAGING

The American Joint Committee on Cancer (AJCC) and the International Union Against Cancer have established a tumor-node-metastasis (TNM) staging system for anal cancer (Table 49-1). Since the primary treatment modality for anal cancer is nonsurgical, staging is based on physical exam, fine needle aspiration of suspicious lymph nodes, and radiologic data. For this reason, the AJCC staging system is based on tumor size rather than depth of invasion. Patients with T1 or T2 lesions have an 80%–90% 5-year survival rate, whereas patients with T4 lesions have less than a 50% 5-year survival rate. For patients with lymph node metastases, the 5-year survival rate is significantly worse at 25%–40%. At presentation, 50%–60% of patients have a T1 or T2 lesion, and 12%–20% are node-positive. The probability of nodal spread is directly related to tumor size and location.

TREATMENT

Before 1980, APR, a surgery removing the anorectum and creation of a permanent colostomy, was the treatment of choice for tumors of the anal canal. Surgical series prior to 1980 found the overall 5-year survival rate after an APR to range between 40% and 70%. Patients with large tumors and nodal metastases had poorer outcomes. In an attempt to improve surgical outcome, Nigro and colleagues at Wayne State evaluated preoperative chemotherapy with 5-fluorouracil (5-FU) 1000 mg/m² continuous infusion days 1–4 and 29–32 and mitomycin 10–15 mg/m² day 1 combined with EBRT to 30 Gy (11). Unexpectedly, the investigators found that the first three patients who received treatment achieved complete responses. Multiple confirmatory studies have found that combined chemoradiation therapy results in a 70%–86% 5-year colostomy-free survival rate and a 72%–89% 5-year overall survival rate. (See Table 49-2 for suggested diagnosis and treatment options.)

■ CHEMORADIATION VERSUS RADIATION THERAPY ALONE

Two phase III studies have evaluated the relative benefit of chemoradiation compared to radiation therapy alone.

- *UKCCCR*: The Anal Cancer Trial Working Party of the United Kingdom Coordination Committee on Cancer Research (UKCCCR) randomized 585 patients with anal cancer to EBRT (45 Gy of EBRT with either a 15 Gy external beam boost or a 25 Gy brachytherapy boost) or the same radiation therapy in combination with concurrent 5-FU (1000 mg/m² continuous infusion for 4 days or 750 mg/m² continuous infusion for 5 days during the first and last weeks of radiation therapy) and mitomycin (12 mg/m² day 1) (12). Chemoradiation improved local control (39%

TABLE 49-1 ANAL CARCINOMA STAGING SYSTEM OF THE AMERICAN JOINT COMMITTEE ON CANCER 7TH EDITION (2009)

Primary tumor (T)

TX	Primary tumor cannot be assessed
Tis	Carcinoma in situ
T0	No evidence of primary tumor
T1	Tumor 2 cm or less in greatest dimension
T2	Tumor more than 2 cm but not more than 5 cm in greatest dimension
T3	Tumor more than 5 cm in greatest dimension
T4	Tumor of any size invades adjacent organ(s), e.g., vagina, urethra, bladder; direct invasion of the rectal wall, perirectal skin, subcutaneous tissue, or the sphincter muscle(s) is not classified as T4

Lymph node (N)

NX	Regional lymph nodes cannot be assessed
N0	No regional lymph node metastases
N1	Metastasis in perirectal lymph node(s)
N2	Metastasis in unilateral internal iliac and/or inguinal lymph node(s)
N3	Metastasis in perirectal and inguinal lymph nodes and/or bilateral internal iliac and/or inguinal lymph nodes

Distant metastasis (M)

M0	No distant metastasis
M1	Distant metastasis

Stage grouping

Stage 0	Tis	N0	M0
Stage I	T1	N0	M0
Stage II	T2	N0	M0
	T3	N0	M0
Stage IIIA	T1	N1	M0
	T2	N1	M0
	T3	N1	M0
	T4	N0	M0
Stage IIIB	T4	N1	M0
	Any T	N2	M0
	Any T	N3	M0
Stage IV	Any T	Any N	M1

Source: Used with the permission of the American Joint Committee on Cancer (AJCC), Chicago, IL, USA. The original source for this material is Edge SB et al (eds). *AJCC Cancer Staging Manual,* 7th edition. New York, Springer, 2010.

TABLE 49-2 SUGGESTED DIAGNOSIS AND TREATMENT ALGORITHM FOR ANAL CANCER

Physical exam

Assessment of primary tumor size

Assessment of inguinal lymph nodes

Biopsy

Anal tumor

– If squamous cell cancer, proceed with algorithm

– If adenocarcinoma, treat as rectal adenocarcinoma

Inguinal lymph node(s)

– If enlarged on physical exam or seen radiographically

Radiology

Transanal ultrasound

– Can evaluate tumor depth and local lymph nodes

CT scan

– Can evaluate tumor size, local and distant lymph nodes, metastases

PET scan

– Can evaluate local and distant lymph nodes, metastases

Treatment

Chemoradiation

5-FU 1000 mg/m^2 continuous infusion days 1–4, 29–32

Mitomycin 10 mg/m^2 days 1, 29

External beam radiation therapy to primary tumor, perirectal lymph nodes, and inguinal lymph nodes (total dose depending on T and N stag, primary tumor to receive 50.4 Gy or higher)

Posttreatment assessment

Physical exam beginning 6–8 wk after completion of chemoradiation

Biopsy any progressive disease

Any persistent abnormalities 6 mo after completion of treatment should be biopsied

Persistent/recurrent disease

Salvage APR

Salvage chemoradiation

Salvage APR may be used for persistent/recurrent disease after salvage chemoradiation

Metastatic disease

Systemic chemotherapy

5-FU/cisplatin

Possible utility of carboplatin, doxorubicin, irinotecan, and cetuximab

(continued)

TABLE 49-2 SUGGESTED DIAGNOSIS AND TREATMENT ALGORITHM FOR ANAL CANCER (CONTINUED)

Posttreatment follow-up

For complete remission, surveillance every 3–6 mo for 5 y:

Digital rectal examination

Anoscopy

Inguinal node palpation

For T3/T4 or node positive disease, consider restaging CT of chest/abdomen/pelvis for 3 y

vs. 61%) and disease-specific survival (28% vs. 39%), but 3-year overall survival was not statistically significantly different between the two arms (58% vs. 65%).

• *EORTC*: The European Organization for Research and Treatment of Cancer (EORTC) randomized 110 patients with anal cancer to radiation therapy (45 Gy of EBRT with either a 15 Gy or a 30 Gy external beam boost) or the same radiation therapy in combination with concurrent 5-FU (750 mg/m^2 continuous infusion on days 1–5 and 29–33) and mitomycin (15 mg/m^2 day 1) (13). Similar to the UKCCCR study, the chemoradiation therapy improved local control (39% vs. 58%), with a 32% higher colostomy-free rate in the chemoradiation arm. However, 3-year overall survival was not statistically significantly different between the two groups (65% vs. 72%). In this study, skin ulceration and nodal involvement were poor prognostic indicators, and women had better local control and survival than men.

These European trials showed that, compared to radiation therapy alone, chemoradiation offers patients a better chance of achieving local control, disease-free survival, and colostomy-free survival, but does not improve overall survival, possibly because of the impact of APR as salvage therapy. At present, combined modality therapy with chemoradiation is standard of care.

ROLE OF MITOMYCIN

The Radiation Therapy Oncology Group (RTOG) and Eastern Cooperative Oncology Group (ECOG) have evaluated the role of mitomycin in the combined modality regimen. Mitomycin is not a known radiation sensitizer, and its renal, pulmonary, and bone marrow toxicity have raised concerns about its safety. In this trial, 310 patients were randomized to EBRT (45–50.4 Gy) with either 5-FU (continuous infusion 1000 mg/m^2 days 1–4 and 29–32) alone or the same 5-FU schedule with mitomycin 10 mg/m^2 for 2 doses (14). Patients who received mitomycin had significant improvements in colostomy-free survival (59% vs. 71%) and disease-free survival (51% vs. 73%), but not overall survival or disease specific survival. On subset analysis, the addition of mitomycin to patients with T3 or T4 tumors did not have a significant impact on outcome. Toxicity was higher in the mitomycin arm, with significantly increased grade 4 and 5 toxicities (7% vs. 23%), with four patients in the mitomycin arm having fatal neutropenic sepsis versus 1 in the 5-FU only arm. From these results, the investigators concluded that despite the added toxicities, mitomycin plays a significant role in combined modality therapy for anal cancer. 5-FU, mitomycin, and EBRT remain the standard of care chemoradiation treatment for anal cancer.

■ ROLE OF CISPLATIN

Platinum compounds were not available when combination chemoradiation regimens were originally tested, but since have become an active component of chemotherapy regimens for squamous cell cancers. For this reason, they are being evaluated for treatment of anal cancers. Multiple preliminary studies combined 5-FU, cisplatin, and EBRT in the treatment of anal cancers with promising results. Based on these results, Intergroup trial RTOG 98-11 randomized 682 patients to either 5-FU 1000 mg/m^2 days 1–4 and 29–32, mitomycin 10 mg/m^2 days 1 and 29, and EBRT or an induction course of chemotherapy with 5-FU 1000 mg/m^2 on days 1–4 and 29–32 with cisplatin 75 mg/m^2 on days 1 and 29, with EBRT starting day 57 and 5-FU 1000 mg/m^2 on days 57–60 and 85–88 and cisplatin 75 mg/m^2 on days 57 and 85 (10). In the initial publication of 5-year results, with a median follow-up of 2.51 years, there was no significant difference in 5-year rates of disease-free survival or overall survival between treatment arms. However, there was a significantly lower colostomy rate for mitomycin-based therapy compared to cisplatin-based treatment (10% vs. 19%, $p = 0.02$). Additionally, mitomycin-C was significantly associated with higher grade 3 or 4 hematologic toxicity (61% vs. 42%, $p < 0.001$) (15). Long-term update of RTOG 98-11 presented in 2011 now demonstrates that treatment in the mitomycin-C arm yields a significant improvement in 5-year disease-free survival (68% vs. 58%, $p < 0.005$) and 5-year overall survival (78% vs. 70%, $p < 0.02$) compared to cisplatin (16). 5-FU and mitomycin were also associated with a nonsignificant trend toward less locoregional failure (20% vs. 27%, $p = 0.092$) and lower colostomy rates (cumulative rates of 12% vs. 17%, $p = 0.075$) (16). The results of this study, however, are confounded by the administration of two cycles of induction 5-FU and cisplatin in the cisplatin arm. A recent secondary analysis of RTOG 87-04 and 98-11 found that longer total treatment time predicted for higher rates of colostomy failure, locoregional failure, and worse disease-free survival (17). Therefore, it can be argued that induction chemotherapy, which extended overall treatment time, and not the substitution of cisplatin for mitomycin, was responsible for yielding worse disease outcomes. The ongoing ACT II trial is a 2×2 randomized study that aims to more directly address the question of: (1) cisplatin versus mitomycin-C in definitive chemoradiation, and (2) the role of two cycles of maintenance cisplatin/5-FU after chemoradiation. Preliminary analysis demonstrated no difference in complete response rate (94% vs. 95%, $p = 0.53$, mitomycin and cisplatin, respectively). As expected, patients treated with mitomycin-C experienced more acute grade 3/4 hematologic toxicities (25% vs. 13%, $p < 0.001$), but not neutropenic sepsis (3.1% vs. 3.2%, $p = 0.93$) (18). Currently, the combination of 5-FU, mitomycin, and radiation therapy remains standard of care (15).

ROLE OF INTENSITY MODULATED RADIATION THERAPY

Due to the ability to "shape" radiation beams around clinical target volumes, intensity modulated radiation therapy (IMRT) has been shown to reduce treatment-related toxicity to surrounding normal tissue. To prospectively investigate the benefit of IMRT, RTOG 05-29 launched a multi-institutional phase II evaluation of dose-painted IMRT in combination with 5-FU and mitomycin-C. The study included T2-4, N0-3 anal canal cancer patients treated to a range of 42–54 Gy depending on T stage, N stage, and degree of nodal involvement. With a total of 52 patients accrued, dose-painted IMRT reduced grade 3+ genitourinary and gastrointestinal toxicity (22% vs. 36%, $p = 0.014$), and grade 3+ dermatologic toxicity 20% vs. 47%, $p < 0.001$) when compared to RTOG 98-11. Additionally, IMRT yielded a shorter median duration of RT treatment (43 days vs. 49 days, $p < 0.001$) and shorter median duration of treatment break due to toxicity (0 vs. 3 days, $p < 0.001$). With a median follow-up of 23 months, the 2-year locoregional failure and colostomy rates were 20% (95% CI: [9%, 31%]) and 8% (95% CI: [0.4%, 15%]), respectively. The 2-year OS and DFS were 88% (95% CI: [75%, 94%]) and 77% (95% CI: [62%, 86%]), respectively (19). Based on these preliminary results, the authors have proposed that dose-painted IMRT should be the platform for all future studies, potentially allowing for investigation of dose escalation. The current guidelines under RTOG 05-29 prescribe the primary tumor to 54 Gy, gross lymph node disease to 50.4 Gy, and uninvolved inguinal and iliac lymph nodes to 45 Gy.

LOCALLY ADVANCED TUMORS

Patients with larger tumors, T3/4, or with more extensive nodal metastases (N2/3) comprise a group of patients at higher risk for treatment failure. Only about 50% of these patients will be cured with standard therapy. The Cancer and Leukemia Group B (CALGB) evaluated the regimen of induction chemotherapy with 5-FU (1000 mg/m² continuous infusion days 1–4 and 29–32) and cisplatin (75 mg/m² on days 1 and 29) followed by chemoradiation with 5-FU and mitomycin. Induction chemotherapy resulted in 8 complete and 21 partial responses. After induction, combined-modality, and boost therapy, 37 (82%) of 45 assessable high-risk patients achieved a complete response. After 4 years of follow-up, 68% of patients are alive, 61% are disease free, and 50% are colostomy and disease free (20).

Despite these promising results, the role of induction chemotherapy has fallen out of favor in light of the results of RTOG 98-11 (discussed above), which demonstrated worse disease-free survival and overall survival among patients randomized to receive two cycles of induction 5-FU/cisplatin followed by cisplatin-based chemoradiation (16). The UNICANCER ACCORD 03 trial also failed to find a benefit with the addition of induction chemotherapy. In this study, 307 patients with tumors ≥40 mm or <40 mm and N1-3M0 were randomized to receive: (1) two cycles of induction 5-FU 800 mg/m² on days 1–4 and 29–32; and cisplatin 80 mg/m² IV on days 1 and 29, chemoradiation (45 Gy in 25 fractions) followed by standard dose boost (15 Gy), (2) two cycles of induction chemotherapy, chemoradiation and high dose boost (20–25 Gy), (3) chemoradiation and standard dose boost, or (4) chemoradiation and high dose boost. With a median follow-up of

50 months, the addition of induction chemotherapy did not impact 5-year colostomy-free survival (77% vs. 75%, $p = 0.37$) (21).

■ TREATMENT COMPLICATIONS

Complications of chemoradiation therapy for anal cancer include acute and chronic toxicities. Acute toxicities include diarrhea, desquamation and erythema, mucositis, pain, and myelosuppression. Late toxicities include anal ulcers, stricture/stenosis, fistulae, incontinence, and necrosis. Colostomy may be required for these late effects in 6%–12% of patients (22). The risk of these complications increases with radiation dose.

■ TREATMENT OF PATIENTS WITH HIV

The combination of chemotherapy and radiation therapy is generally well tolerated and effective in HIV positive patients. However, treatment-related toxicity appears to be more common in these patients. It is controversial whether CD4 counts correlate with increased toxicity. Occasionally, diverting colostomy or APR is used to manage local treatment toxicity in these patients. Blood counts should also be followed closely in these patients, with dose reductions or treatment breaks used as necessary. Although patients with HIV may be at higher risk for treatment-related toxicity, overall survival appears to be the same between HIV-positive and HIV-negative patients (23). Current clinical practice recommendations are to treat HIV-positive patients at full chemotherapy and radiation dose, with added surveillance of possible treatment-related toxicities including dermatitis and hematologic toxicities.

■ PERSISTENT OR RECURRENT DISEASE

Response to treatment is assessed approximately 6–8 weeks after completion of chemoradiation therapy. Whether the response to treatment should be assessed by physical exam alone or in combination with a biopsy is controversial. Squamous cell carcinomas tend to regress slowly over 3–12 weeks after the completion of therapy. In an Intergroup study evaluating the role of mitomycin in combination with 5-FU, patients had follow-up biopsies 6 weeks after completion of therapy (14). Residual disease was found in 11% of patients. In this trial, patients with residual disease were treated with a salvage regimen of 5-FU plus cisplatin with 9 Gy of EBRT. Fifty-five percent of those patients achieved a complete response. It was unclear whether this high-salvage rate was due to the additional therapy or that the anal tumors in these patients were simply slower to regress after the completion of the original therapy. There is no consensus on the use and timing of biopsy in patients who have had a complete clinical response to therapy. Recently, results of the ACTII study were presented at the American Society of Clinical Oncology (24). Patients without progressive disease were observed up to 26 weeks post completion of chemoradiation. There was continued regression of disease after week 11 and up to week 26. Week 26 complete response rate was a better predictor of progression-free survival than complete response at week 11. It is reasonable to wait until week 26 to define a patient as having persistent disease as long as there is no evidence of progressive disease.

- *Persistent disease.* The treatment for persistent anal cancer is APR. In the UKCCCR trial, 29 patients who had achieved less than 50% response to primary therapy underwent salvage APR (12). Forty percent of the patients who underwent salvage APR eventually had local relapse.

  Salvage chemoradiation therapy has also been evaluated (14). Twenty-two patients on the Intergroup study evaluating the role of mitomycin C were labeled as having persistent disease. These patients received salvage 5-FU, cisplatin, and 9 Gy EBRT. Ten patients continued to have persistent disease and 9 of the 10 underwent salvage APR. Six of the nine patients who underwent salvage APR eventually had disease recurrence. Of the 12 patients who were disease free after salvage chemoradiation, 4 required subsequent APR and remain disease free. In retrospect it is possible that these patients would have had continued regression of disease as was seen in the ACTII trial. Therefore, salvage chemoradiation for persistent disease is generally not recommended.

- *Recurrent disease.* The majority of patients who have recurrent disease recur locally. As with persistent disease, these patients are candidates for salvage APR or chemoradiation. Approximately 50% of patients with recurrent disease who undergo salvage APR will be rendered disease free. There have been no formal trials of salvage chemoradiation in the setting of recurrent disease, but the salvage chemoradiation regimen used to treat patients with persistent disease has been extrapolated to this setting by some practitioners.

■ METASTATIC DISEASE

Distant recurrence occurs in 10%–17% of patients who receive chemoradiation therapy. The most common site of distant metastasis is the liver. No known cure exists for metastatic anal cancer, and there are limited data on active regimens for these patients. Cisplatin plus 5-FU is the most active regimen, although single agent therapy with carboplatin, doxorubicin, and irinotecan may have some clinical activity. There is little information about the response of metastatic anal cancer to more recent chemotherapy agents, such as taxanes, gemcitabine, or irinotecan.

CONCLUSIONS

Remarkable progress has been made in understanding the pathophysiology and treatment of anal cancer in the past 30 years. HPV has been clearly implicated in the development of the majority of anal cancers. Screening programs may allow for the diagnosis of anal dysplasia prior to progression to invasive cancer. The use of sphincter-sparing chemoradiation therapy has remarkably improved the quality of life and survival for patients with anal cancer. We await the results of ACT II trial; however, currently, definitive chemoradiation with 5-fluorouracil and mitomycin-C remains the standard of care.

REFERENCES

1. Siegel R, Naishadham D, Jemal A. Cancer statistics, 2013. *CA Cancer J Clin.* 2013; 63: 11–30.

2. Johnson LG, et al. Anal cancer incidence and survival: the surveillance, epidemiology, and end results experience, 1973-2000. *Cancer.* 2004; 101: 281–288.

3. Chaturvedi AK, et al. Risk of human papillomavirus-associated cancers among persons with AIDS. *J Natl Cancer Inst.* 2009; 101: 1120–1130.

4. Chiao EY, et al. A population-based analysis of temporal trends in the incidence of squamous anal canal cancer in relation to the HIV epidemic. *J Acquir Immune Defic Syndr.* 2005; 40: 451–455.

5. Goldie SJ, et al. The clinical effectiveness and cost-effectiveness of screening for anal squamous intraepithelial lesions in homosexual and bisexual HIV-positive men. *JAMA.* 1999; 281:1822–1829.

6. Goldie SJ, et al. Cost-effectiveness of screening for anal squamous intraepithelial lesions and anal cancer in human immunodeficiency virus-negative homosexual and bisexual men. *Am J Med.* 2000; 108: 634–641.

7. Palefsky JM, et al. HPV vaccine against anal HPV infection and anal intraepithelial neoplasia. *N Engl J Med.* 2011; 365: 1576–1585.

8. Swedish KA, Factor SH, Goldstone SE. Prevention of recurrent high-grade anal neoplasia with quadrivalent human papillomavirus vaccination of men who have sex with men: a nonconcurrent cohort study. *Clin Infect Dis.* 2012. 54: 891–898.

9. Cotter SE, et al. FDG-PET/CT in the evaluation of anal carcinoma. *Int J Radiat Oncol Biol Phys.* 2006; 65: 720–725.

10. Sveistrup J, et al. Positron emission tomography/computed tomography in the staging and treatment of anal cancer. *Int J Radiat Oncol Biol Phys.* 2012; 83: 134–141.

11. Nigro ND, Vaitkevicius VK, Considine B Jr. Combined therapy for cancer of the anal canal: a preliminary report. *Dis Colon Rectum.* 1974; 17: 354–356.

12. UK Co-ordinating Committee on Cancer Research. Epidermoid anal cancer: results from the UKCCCR randomised trial of radiotherapy alone versus radiotherapy, 5-fluorouracil, and mitomycin. UKCCCR Anal Cancer Trial Working Party. *Lancet.* 1996; 348: 1049–1054.

13. Bartelink H, et al. Concomitant radiotherapy and chemotherapy is superior to radiotherapy alone in the treatment of locally advanced anal cancer: results of a phase III randomized trial of the European Organization for Research and Treatment of Cancer Radiotherapy and Gastrointestinal Cooperative Groups. *J Clin Oncol.* 1997; 15: 2040–2049.

14. Flam M, et al. Role of mitomycin in combination with fluorouracil and radiotherapy, and of salvage chemoradiation in the definitive non-surgical treatment of epidermoid carcinoma of the anal canal: results of a phase III randomized intergroup study. *J Clin Oncol.* 1996; 14: 2527–2539.

15. Ajani JA, et al. Fluorouracil, mitomycin, and radiotherapy vs fluorouracil, cisplatin, and radiotherapy for carcinoma of the anal canal: a randomized controlled trial. *JAMA.* 2008; 299: 1914–1921.

16. Gunderson LL. Long-term Update of U.S. GI Intergroup RTOG 98-11 phase III trial for anal carcinoma: comparison of concurrent chemoradiation with 5FU-mitomycin versus 5FU-cisplatin for disease-free and overall survival. In Gastrointestinal Cancer Symposium, American Society of Clinical Oncology. 2011; San Francisco, CA.

17. Ben-Josef E, et al. Impact of overall treatment time on survival and local control in patients with anal cancer: a pooled data analysis of Radiation Therapy Oncology Group trials 87-04 and 98-11. *J Clin Oncol.* 2010; 28: 5061–5066.

18. James R, Wan S, Glynne-Jones R, et al. A randomized trial of chemoradiation using mitomycin-C or cisplatin, with or without maintenance cisplatin/5FU in squamous cell carcinoma of the anus (ACT II). In ASCO Annual Meeting. 2009. JCO.

19. Kachnic LA, Winter K, Myerson R, et al. Early efficacy results of RTOG 0529: a phase II evaluation of dose-painted IMRT in combination with 5-fluorouracil and mitomycin-C for the reduction of acute morbidity in carcinoma of the anal canal. *IJROBP.* 2010; 78: 855.

20. Meropol NJ, et al. Induction therapy for poor-prognosis anal canal carcinoma: a phase II study of the cancer and Leukemia Group B (CALGB 9281). *J Clin Oncol.* 2008; 26: 3229–3234.

21. Peiffert D, et al. Induction chemotherapy and dose intensification of the radiation boost in locally advanced anal canal carcinoma: final analysis of the randomized UNICANCER ACCORD 03 trial. *J Clin Oncol.* 2012; 30: 1941–1948.

22. Sunesen KG, et al. Cause-specific colostomy rates after radiotherapy for anal cancer: a Danish multicentre cohort study. *J Clin Oncol.* 2011; 29: 3535–3540.

23. Chiao EY, et al. Human immunodeficiency virus-associated squamous cell cancer of the anus: epidemiology and outcomes in the highly active antiretroviral therapy era. *J Clin Oncol.* 2008; 26: 474–479.

24. Glynne-Jones R, James R, Meadows H, et al. Optimum time to assess complete clinical response following chemoradiation using mitomycin C or cisplatin, with or without maintenance CisP/5FU in squamous cell carcinoma of the anus: results of ACT II. *J Clin Oncol.* 2012; 30 (suppl): 4004.

CHAPTER **50**
Malignant Mesothelioma

Lee M. Krug, Pasi A. Jänne

BACKGROUND

Malignant mesothelioma is a rare malignancy arising from the mesothelial cells of the pleural or peritoneal surfaces. Mesothelioma can arise from the pleura (pleural mesothelioma), peritoneum (peritoneal mesothelioma), pericardium (pericardial mesothelioma), or *tunica vaginalis* (testicular mesothelioma). In the United States, there are approximately 3000 new cases of mesothelioma reported annually. Eighty percent of these occur as pleural mesothelioma, and this will be the focus of this chapter.

The development of mesothelioma is most clearly associated with prior asbestos exposure (1). Asbestos was (and continues to be in some parts of the world) an important and affordable industrial resource due to its resistance to heat and combustion. Asbestos was used in shipbuilding, in car brakes, in the production of cement, and as insulation. There are two main forms of asbestos known as amphiboles and chrysotile. Amphiboles are long thin asbestos fibers and are felt to be the most carcinogenic of the asbestos fibers. Chrysotile asbestos has also been associated with mesothelioma, although the frequency may be less than with amphibole asbestos (1). The latency period between the time of asbestos exposure to development of mesothelioma can be 20–40 years. These unique features reflect the population of patients who develop mesothelioma including asbestos miners, plumbers, pipefitters, or those who worked in shipbuilding industries. In the United States, mesothelioma is a disease of Caucasian men reflecting the population of asbestos workers in the 1960s and early 1970s. The median age of patients diagnosed with mesothelioma is in the mid-60s, although, in the Surveillance Epidemiology and End Results (SEER) database from the United States, the median age is over 70 years. Approximately 80% of patients who develop mesothelioma are men. Women who develop mesothelioma also may have worked in industries that used asbestos, although there are reports of secondary exposure for example from clothing of spouses who worked directly with asbestos (2). The estimated incidence of mesothelioma worldwide also reflects the use of asbestos in different regions of the world. It is estimated that the cumulative worldwide incidence of mesothelioma will not peak for another 10–20 years. However, in the United States some estimates suggest that this may have already occurred, while in Europe, Australia, and Japan, where common asbestos use occurred until much later than in the United States, the incidence may not peak for another 15–20 years (3). In addition, asbestos is still extensively

611

used in many developing countries suggesting that the worldwide incidence of mesothelioma will continue to rise.

Other etiologic factors besides asbestos can also increase the risk of developing mesothelioma. For example, numerous cases have been reported in patients who have previously received ionizing radiation such as that used to treat Hodgkin lymphoma or other malignancies (4). Genetic factors may also play a role. Germline mutations in the BRCA-associated protein-1 (BAP1) gene were reported in two families with multiple affected generations (5). Mutations in this gene also increase the risk of developing other malignancies such as uveal melanoma and renal cell carcinoma, suggesting this is part of a newly described cancer predisposition syndrome (6–8). The prevalence of BAP1 germline mutations as an underlying cause for mesothelioma remains unknown, however.

CLINICAL PRESENTATION

The most common clinical presentation of malignant pleural mesothelioma includes dyspnea on exertion and shortness of breath. These clinical symptoms often lead physicians to obtain a chest x-ray where a unilateral pleural effusion is noted (**Figure 50-1**). Mesothelioma is rarely an incidental

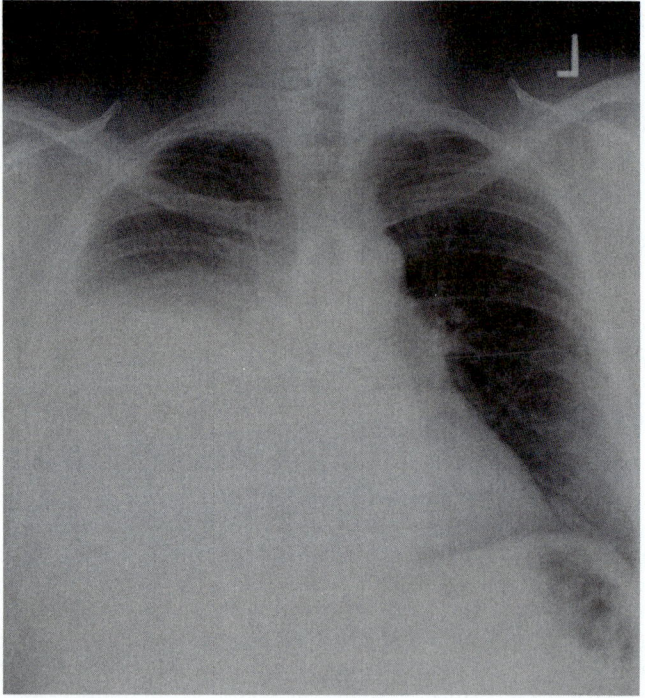

FIGURE 50-1 Anterior-posterior chest radiograph of a patient with newly diagnosed malignant mesothelioma. A large right-sided pleural effusion can be appreciated in this chest x-ray.

TABLE 50-1 SIGNS AND SYMPTOMS OF MALIGNANT MESOTHELIOMA

Mesothelioma Related	Constitutional*
Dyspnea	Weight loss
Chest pain	Anorexia
Discordant chest wall expansion	Night sweats
Palpable chest wall mass	

*The constitutional symptoms are often associated with mesothelioma, but are not specific to the disease.

finding on a routine chest x-ray. Patients can also present with non-pleuritic chest pain. This symptom is important to elicit from patients as those who present with chest pains often have disease extending into the chest wall and thus they are clearly not surgical candidates. Other presenting signs and symptoms include discordant chest wall expansion, weight loss, night sweats, and the presence of a palpable subcutaneous mass (Table 50-1 and Figure 50-2).

DIAGNOSTIC EVALUATION

The presentation of a patient with a new pleural effusion often leads to a thoracentesis to evaluate the nature of the effusion. The pleural effusions in mesothelioma are usually cytologically negative, and patients frequently

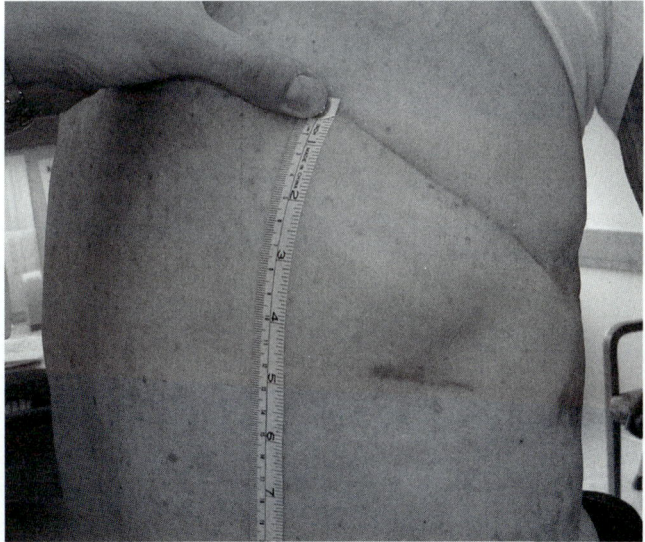

FIGURE 50-2 Subcutaneous chest wall mass in a patient with mesothelioma. This painful subcutaneous mass appeared a few months following surgical exploration.

undergo repeated thoracenteses in order to establish the diagnosis of mesothelioma. Due to the frequent nature of cytologically negative effusions, cytology is not a reliable method to diagnose mesothelioma. In addition, cytologic specimens are often insufficient to determine the histologic subtype of mesothelioma, which itself provides prognostic information.

The diagnostic procedure of choice for mesothelioma is a thoracoscopic biopsy. There are several advantages to this approach. First, it provides the surgeon the ability to assess the extent of tumor on the visceral and parietal pleura. Second, a biopsy of the involved area can be obtained under direct visualization. This is critical to make an accurate histologic diagnosis. Finally, thoracoscopy provides the ability to also perform a pleurodesis, which can help control recurrent pleural effusions. It is important to note that mesothelioma can grow along and through previous biopsy sites (e.g., see Figure 50-2). Thus if a patient is being considered for future a pneumonectomy, it will be important to mark and excise en bloc the prior biopsy site.

The pathologic evaluation of malignant mesothelioma can be challenging and the disease can sometimes be confused pathologically with adenocarcinoma of the lung. However, several immunohistochemical markers can help distinguish adenocarcinoma from malignant mesothelioma (Table 50-2) (9). Unlike adenocarcinomas, mesotheliomas do not express thyroid transcription factor 1 (TTF-1) or carcinoembryonic antigen (CEA). In contrast, mesotheliomas do express the Wilms tumor-1 (WT-1) protein and calretinin, which are not expressed by lung adenocarcinomas. In addition to the pathologic diagnosis of mesothelioma, it is important to distinguish the histologic subtype of mesothelioma. The most common histologic subtype is epithelial mesothelioma and accounts for approximately 60% of all mesotheliomas. Other subtypes of mesothelioma include sarcomatoid mesothelioma and mixed (containing components of both epithelial and sarcomatoid) type mesothelioma. The main reason to determine the histologic subtype of mesothelioma is that patients with sarcomatoid mesothelioma have a much worse prognosis than those with epithelial mesothelioma and may not be ideal candidates for aggressive surgical resection.

Three main imaging modalities, computed tomography (CT), positron emission tomography (PET), and magnetic resonance imaging (MRI),

TABLE 50-2 IMMUNOHISTOCHEMICAL MARKERS USED TO DISTINGUISH MALIGNANT MESOTHELIOMA FROM LUNG ADENOCARCINOMA

	Mesothelioma	Adenocarcinoma
Cytokeratin	Positive	Positive
CEA	Negative	Positive
TTF-1	Negative	Positive
Calretinin	Positive	Negative
WT-1	Positive	Negative

CEA, carcinoembryonic antigen; TTF-1, thyroid transcription factor 1; WT-1, Wilms tumor antigen.

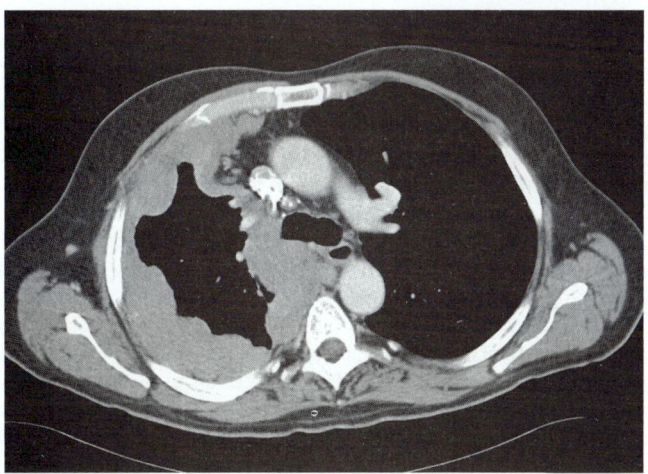

FIGURE 50-3 Computed tomography (CT) appearance of mesothelioma. A thickened circumferential pleural rind is seen on chest CT in this patient with epithelial mesothelioma.

are used to evaluate patients with newly diagnosed mesothelioma. Contrast enhanced CT scanning often reveals a thickened lobulated circumferential pleural rind (**Figure 50-3**) with or without the presence of a concurrent pleural effusion. CT scanning can also help identify the presence of pleural plaques, a sign of previous asbestos exposure, and whether the disease extends into the intralobular fissures. However, CT scanning is not very accurate in determining chest wall invasion or transdiaphragmatic extension of mesothelioma. These features are important to determine, especially if the patient is being considered for surgery. MRI can occasionally be used in this situation to identify chest wall invasion (**Figure 50-4**) as well as transdiaphragmatic invasion

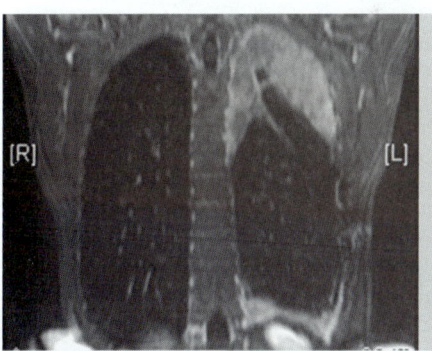
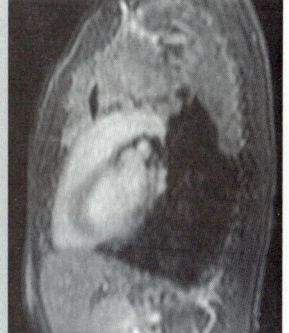

FIGURE 50-4 Coronal (*left*) and sagittal (*right*) MRI images of the left hemithorax of a patient with newly diagnosed malignant mesothelioma. The MRI images help to define mesothelioma invading into the chest wall on the lateral side in the left hemithorax.

(10), although some studies have not found it superior to CT imaging (11). FDG-PET scanning has also recently been evaluated for its clinical utility as most mesotheliomas are PET avid. Analogous to lung cancer, FDG-PET scanning can identify occult metastatic disease in patients who are otherwise potential surgical candidates (12) and may have prognostic significance (13). However, its utility in defining locoregional disease and the role of FDG-PET scanning in advanced mesothelioma remain to be determined.

Soluble mesothelin-related protein (SMRP) is a serum marker for mesothelioma. Mesothelin is a cell surface protein present on mesothelial cells. It can remain membrane bound or be shed into the serum and be detected using an ELISA assay (14). In a study using this assay, 37/44 (84%) of patients with mesothelioma had elevated levels of SMRP compared to 3/160 (2%) of patients with other lung or pleural diseases. In addition, 7 of 40 patients exposed to asbestos had elevated levels of SMRP. Interestingly within 1–5 years, 3 of the 7 patients developed mesothelioma, which suggested that SMRP could also serve as a screening test for asbestos-exposed individuals. However, in a larger cohort of exposed patients who developed mesothelioma, SMRP levels from banked serum samples obtained prior to the diagnosis were elevated in only 17 of 106 people (15). SMRP levels do seem to correlate with disease status, declining after surgery or with response to chemotherapy, suggesting a possible utility for monitoring in conjunction with imaging (16).

STAGING

The goal of staging is to stratify prognosis and to identify patients who are potential candidates for surgery. The most widely accepted staging system is the International Mesothelioma Interest Group (IMIG) system, which is a tumor-node-metastases (TNM) staging system (17). Mesothelioma is a difficult disease to accurately stage based on radiographic imaging and, since it is typically limited to the ipsilateral pleura at diagnosis, staging is often only possible at the time of surgery. Since diffuse chest wall invasion (T4 disease) implies that the tumor is unresectable, this confers a poor prognosis and is qualified as stage IV, even in the absence of distant metastatic disease.

PROGNOSTIC FACTORS

There is no known curative treatment modality for mesothelioma. The median survival of newly diagnosed patients ranges from 6 to 18 months. The disease course (even untreated) can be highly variable and thus several prognostic systems have been developed in order to identify patient subsets with different prognoses. The two main prognostic systems are the Cancer and Leukemia Group B (CALGB) prognostic groups and the European Organization for Research and Treatment of Cancer (EORTC) prognostic factors and prognostic scores (18, 19). Patients with sarcomatoid mesothelioma, those with a poor performance status, and those who present with chest pain (indicative of disease invasion into the chest wall) are ones with a poor prognosis. In addition, patients with evidence of a systemic inflammatory response to their mesothelioma manifested by either an increased white blood cell (WBC) or platelet count also tend to have a poorer prognosis.

TREATMENT

There is no standard therapeutic approach for malignant mesothelioma. One of the limitations in this disease is the lack of randomized clinical trials comparing different treatment modalities. Treatment approaches to mesothelioma vary significantly and range from palliative care to chemotherapy to aggressive surgical approaches based on the patient's age, comorbid medical conditions, and performance status.

IMPACT OF TREATMENT

The true impact of any therapeutic modality in malignant mesothelioma is presently undefined. Some of the reasons behind this include the rarity of the disease, the paucity of randomized studies, heterogeneity within the pathologic subclasses of mesothelioma, imbalance of prognostic factors, and difficulties in assessing response to therapy using computed tomography and other radiographic imaging modalities. The natural history of mesothelioma can be variable and thus benefits seen in clinical trials may be biased by patient selection.

SURGERY

Surgery is a therapeutic option for some patients with malignant mesothelioma. One of the rationales for performing surgery is that mesothelioma is a disease that tends to spread locally into adjacent structures such as the chest wall and the mediastinum before spreading to systemic sites. Thus local treatments such as surgery may offer therapeutic and palliative benefits to patients. Two main surgical approaches, an extrapleural pneumonectomy (EPP) and a pleurectomy/decortication (P/D), have been used to treat mesothelioma (20). An EPP is an en bloc resection of the parietal pleura, lung, pericardium, and diaphragm (21). The diaphragm and pericardium are then reconstructed with the use of a Gortex patch. In contrast, a P/D (or an extended P/D) is a resection of the parietal and mediastinal pleura and involved visceral and diaphragmatic pleura and pericardium (20). The lung however remains in place. It is unclear if either operation adheres to the principles of oncology surgery as no margin of uninvolved tissue is typically resected.

Several controversies exist regarding surgery for mesothelioma. The first is whether surgery improves survival or quality of life in patients with malignant mesothelioma. No randomized trial has ever addressed this question, although the Mesothelioma and Radical Surgery (MARS) trial conducted in the United Kingdom attempted to do so (21). The trial was designed to test the feasibility of randomizing patients to get surgery with an EPP or not. All patients were planned to receive chemotherapy first. Out of 112 patients enrolled on the trial, 50 were eligible and agreeable to randomization. Surgical mortality was higher than expected, with 4 patients dying postoperatively. The median survival in the EPP arm (14.4 months) was lower than in the no surgery arm (19.5 months), although the sample size was not powered for this comparison.

A second surgical dilemma is how to best identify patients benefiting from surgery and to choose the most appropriate operation for those patients. The patients most likely to benefit from surgery are those with epithelial histology in whom there is no N2 lymph node involvement (22). In general, patients who are eligible for an EPP operation are younger with healthy cardiopulmonary reserve. Patients who undergo a P/D are often older with other comorbid medical illnesses. In addition, patients with minimal pleural disease and those whose tumors do not extend into the interlobular pleural surfaces may be more appropriate candidates for a P/D operation. Although there have been no prospective studies comparing the two different surgical approaches, a retrospective analysis that included 663 patients suggested that patients who underwent P/D had an improved survival compared with patients who had an EPP (23). These data, along with the results of the MARS trial, have caused thoracic surgeons to shy away from EPPs in recent years. Nonetheless, most surgeons agree that, regardless of the type of operation, the goal should be maximal tumor cytoreduction (24).

Despite surgery, mesothelioma recurs in nearly all individuals. The pattern of recurrence depends to some degree on the type of operation. For patients who have undergone an EPP, local recurrences (within the operated thoracic cavity) do occur, although systemic recurrences begin to predominate. In contrast, in patients who have undergone a P/D, local recurrences are more common (25).

CHEMOTHERAPY

Historically, mesothelioma was considered a disease refractory to systemic chemotherapy. In fact, most, if not all, chemotherapy agents have been tested in clinical trials for patients with mesothelioma (26). The agents with the most consistent single agent anti-tumor activity include antifolates, platinum agents (cisplatin and carboplatin), vinorelbine, and gemcitabine. Arguably the most important phase III clinical trial in mesothelioma compared the combination of cisplatin and pemetrexed to cisplatin alone as initial treatment for patients with malignant mesothelioma. This study demonstrated a response rate of 41% and a median survival of 12.1 months for the combination arm, which were significantly better than in the cisplatin alone arm (16.7% and 9.3 months, respectively) (27). This trial was the basis for the FDA approval of cisplatin/pemetrexed in malignant mesothelioma and helped establish this combination as the standard first-line chemotherapy regimen. Other platinum-based chemotherapy combinations such as cisplatin/raltitrexed, cisplatin/gemcitabine, and carboplatin/pemetrexed have also been studied and are active combination treatment regimens for this disease (28–31). There are virtually no data on second-line treatment of mesothelioma and this remains an active area of investigation.

RADIATION

Radiation has a limited therapeutic role for most patients with mesothelioma. Radiation is often used in the palliative setting to treat a painful site of chest wall invasion. It has been also used to prophylactically treat a surgical or biopsy site due to the risk of tumor seeding along the tract. In addition for patients who undergo an EPP, radiation is used in the postoperative treatment of the hemithorax (32, 33). Since the surgical margins following EPP are often involved with mesothelioma (or in very close proximity), radiation provides an opportunity to decrease local recurrence. Patients treated with early-stage mesothelioma and hemithoracic radiation have a lower chance of recurrence within the operated thoracic cavity, although they still remain at high risk for systemic recurrence. Adjuvant radiation therapy is much more challenging following a P/D since the intact lung increases the risk of radiation pneumonitis, although newer techniques using intensity modulated radiation therapy have allowed pleural radiation to be administered safely (34).

COMBINED MODALITY THERAPY

Surgery alone is ineffective therapy for pleural mesothelioma due to the inability to eradicate all microscopic disease, resulting in a high risk of both local and systemic recurrence. As such, various approaches have been developed to incorporate chemotherapy and/or radiation into a multimodality treatment plan for fit patients with resectable disease. The most widely studied approach involves induction chemotherapy followed by EPP, and then hemithoracic radiation. In the largest study conducted in the United States (35), 54 of the 77 patients initially enrolled were able to undergo surgical resection, and 44 completed all planned therapy. The median survival for all patients enrolled was 16.8 months, although the median survival for patients who completed all planned therapy was 29.1 months with a 2-year survival rate of 62%. Several other groups have reported comparable results (36, 37). However, as described above, enthusiasm for performing EPP has waned after the retrospective report suggesting better survival with P/D over EPP, and the report of the poor outcomes in the initial MARS study. Various groups are exploring ways to improve local control after P/D, with approaches such as pleural radiation, intraoperative heated chemotherapy, and photodynamic therapy (34, 38, 39).

NOVEL THERAPEUTICS

Clearly, the therapeutic options for mesothelioma are limited, and new treatments are desperately needed. A number of clinical trials with targeted agents have failed to demonstrate benefit. For example, both epidermal growth factor receptor (EGFR) inhibitors (gefitinib and erlotinib) and platelet-derived growth factor receptor (PDGFR) inhibitors (imatinib) are inactive in this disease (40-42). Mesotheliomas are vascular tumors, and a number of small molecule angiogenesis inhibitors including vatalanib, sorafenib, and sunitinib have demonstrated a limited degree of single agent activity in this disease (43-45). A randomized phase II clinical trial evaluating bevacizumab (anti-VEGF antibody) in combination with gemcitabine and cisplatin failed to show benefit (46), although a larger phase III trial combining bevacizumab with pemetrexed and cisplatin is ongoing. Preliminary activity of the histone deacetylase inhibitor, vorinostat, in a phase I trial led to a very large phase III study comparing this agent to placebo in patients previously treated with chemotherapy, but the trial drug failed to improve survival (47). Nonetheless, several other biologically relevant therapies are being tested (48). The high, selective expression of mesothelin in mesothelioma tumors has encouraged the development of monoclonal antibodies targeting mesothelin, and various studies have shown hints of therapeutic efficacy. Other classes of drugs being studied include PI3K and mTOR inhibitors, oncolytic viruses, and immunotherapies targeting WT1.

REFERENCES

1. Hodgson JT, Darnton A. The quantitative risks of mesothelioma and lung cancer in relation to asbestos exposure. *Ann Occup Hyg.* 2000; 44: 565–601.

2. Miller A. Mesothelioma in household members of asbestos-exposed workers: 32 United States cases since 1990. *Am J Ind Med.* 2005; 47: 458–462.

3. Robinson BW, Lake RA. Advances in malignant mesothelioma. *N Engl J Med.* 2005; 353: 1591–1603.

4. De Bruin ML, Burgers JA, Baas P, et al. Malignant mesothelioma after radiation treatment for Hodgkin lymphoma. *Blood.* 2009; 113: 3679–3681.

5. Testa JR, Cheung M, Pei J, Below JE, et al. Germline BAP1 mutations predispose to malignant mesothelioma. *Nat Genet.* 2011; 43: 1022–1025.

6. Harbour JW, Onken MD, Roberson ED, et al. Frequent mutation of BAP1 in metastasizing uveal melanomas. *Science.* 2010; 330: 1410–1413.

7. Abdel-Rahman MH, Pilarski R, Cebulla CM, et al. Germline BAP1 mutation predisposes to uveal melanoma, lung adenocarcinoma, meningioma, and other cancers. *J Med Genetics.* 2011; 48: 856–859.

8. Murali R, Wiesner T, Scolyer RA. Tumours associated with BAP1 mutations. *Pathology.* 2013; 45: 116–126.

9. Husain AN, Colby T, Ordonez N, et al. Guidelines for pathologic diagnosis of malignant mesothelioma: 2012 update of the consensus statement from the International Mesothelioma Interest Group. *Arch Pathol Lab Med.* 2012.

10. Stewart D, Waller D, Edwards J, Jeyapalan K, Entwisle J. Is there a role for pre-operative contrast-enhanced magnetic resonance imaging for radical surgery in malignant pleural mesothelioma? *Eur J Cardiothorac Surg.* 2003; 24: 1019–1024.

11. Heelan RT, Rusch VW, Begg CB, et al. Staging of malignant pleural mesothelioma: comparison of CT and MR imaging. *AJR Am J Roentgenol.* 1999; 172: 1039–1047.

12. Flores RM, Akhurst T, Gonen M, Larson SM, Rusch VW. Positron emission tomography defines metastatic disease but not locoregional disease in patients with malignant pleural mesothelioma. *J Thorac Cardiovasc Surg.* 2003; 126: 11–16.

13. Flores RM, Akhurst T, Gonen M, et al. Positron emission tomography predicts survival in malignant pleural mesothelioma. *J Thorac Cardiovasc Surg.* 2006; 132: 763–768.

14. Robinson BW, Creaney J, Lake R, et al. Mesothelin-family proteins and diagnosis of mesothelioma. *Lancet.* 2003; 362: 1612–1616.

15. Creaney J, Olsen NJ, Brims F, et al. Serum mesothelin for early detection of asbestos-induced cancer malignant mesothelioma. *Cancer Epidemiol Biomarkers Prev.* 2010; 19: 2238–2246.

16. Wheatley-Price P, Yang B, Patsios D, et al. Soluble mesothelin-related Peptide and osteopontin as markers of response in malignant mesothelioma. *J Clin Oncol.* 2010; 28: 3316–3322.

17. Rusch VW. A proposed new international TNM staging system for malignant pleural mesothelioma. From the International Mesothelioma Interest Group. *Chest.* 1995; 108: 1122–1128.

18. Herndon JE, Green MR, Chahinian AP, et al. Factors predictive of survival among 337 patients with mesothelioma treated between 1984 and 1994 by the Cancer and Leukemia Group B. *Chest.* 1998; 113: 723–731.

19. Curran D, Sahmoud T, Therasse P, et al. Prognostic factors in patients with pleural mesothelioma: the European Organization for Research and Treatment of Cancer experience. *J Clin Oncol.* 1998; 16: 145–152.

20. Rice D, Rusch V, Pass H, et al. Recommendations for uniform definitions of surgical techniques for malignant pleural mesothelioma: a consensus report of the international association for the study of lung cancer international staging committee and the international mesothelioma interest group. *J Thorac Oncol.* 2011; 6: 1304–1312.

21. Treasure T, Lang-Lazdunski L, Waller D, et al. Extra-pleural pneumonectomy versus no extra-pleural pneumonectomy for patients with malignant pleural mesothelioma: clinical outcomes of the Mesothelioma and Radical Surgery (MARS) randomised feasibility study. *Lancet Oncol.* 2011; 12: 763–772.

22. Sugarbaker DJ, Flores RM, Jaklitsch MT, et al. Resection margins, extrapleural nodal status, and cell type determine postoperative long-term survival in trimodality therapy of malignant pleural mesothelioma: results in 183 patients. *J Thorac Cardiovasc Surg.* 1999; 117: 54–63; discussion 5.

23. Flores RM, Pass HI, Seshan VE, et al. Extrapleural pneumonectomy versus pleurectomy/decortication in the surgical management of malignant pleural mesothelioma: results in 663 patients. *J Thorac Cardiovasc Surg.* 2008; 135: 620–626, 6 e1-3.

24. Rusch V, Baldini EH, Bueno R, et al. The role of surgical cytoreduction in the treatment of malignant pleural mesothelioma: Meeting Summary of the International Mesothelioma Interest Group Congress, September 11-14, 2012, Boston, Mass. *J Thorac Cardiovasc Surg.* 2013.

25. Janne PA, Baldini EH. Patterns of failure following surgical resection for malignant pleural mesothelioma. *Thorac Surg Clin.* 2004; 14: 567–573.

26. Krug LM. An overview of chemotherapy for mesothelioma. *Hematol Oncol Clin North Am.* 2005; 19: 1117–1136.

27. Vogelzang NJ, Rusthoven JJ, Symanowski J, et al. Phase III study of pemetrexed in combination with cisplatin versus cisplatin alone in patients with malignant pleural mesothelioma. *J Clin Oncol.* 2003; 21: 2636–2644.

28. van Meerbeeck JP, Gaafar R, Manegold C, et al. Randomized phase III study of cisplatin with or without raltitrexed in patients with malignant pleural mesothelioma: an intergroup study of the European

Organisation for Research and Treatment of Cancer Lung Cancer Group and the National Cancer Institute of Canada. *J Clin Oncol.* 2005; 23: 6881–6889.

29. Byrne MJ, Davidson JA, Musk AW, et al. Cisplatin and gemcitabine treatment for malignant mesothelioma: a phase II study. *J Clin Oncol.* 1999; 17: 25–30.

30. Ceresoli GL, Castagneto B, Zucali PA, et al. Pemetrexed plus carboplatin in elderly patients with malignant pleural mesothelioma: combined analysis of two phase II trials. *British J Cancer.* 2008; 99: 51–56.

31. Santoro A, O'Brien ME, Stahel RA, et al. Pemetrexed plus cisplatin or pemetrexed plus carboplatin for chemonaive patients with malignant pleural mesothelioma: results of the International Expanded Access Program. *J Thorac Oncol.* 2008; 3: 756–763.

32. Rusch VW, Rosenzweig K, Venkatraman E, et al. A phase II trial of surgical resection and adjuvant high-dose hemithoracic radiation for malignant pleural mesothelioma. *J Thorac Cardiovasc Surg.* 2001; 122: 788–795.

33. Yajnik S, Rosenzweig KE, Mychalczak B, et al. Hemithoracic radiation after extrapleural pneumonectomy for malignant pleural mesothelioma. *Int J Radiat Oncol Biol Phys.* 2003; 56: 1319–1326.

34. Rosenzweig KE, Zauderer MG, Laser B, et al. Pleural intensity-modulated radiotherapy for malignant pleural mesothelioma. *Int J Radiat Oncol Biol Phys.* 2012; 83: 1278–1283.

35. Krug LM, Pass H, Rusch V, et al. A multicenter U.S. trial of neoadjuvant pemetrexed plus cisplatin followed by extrapleural pneumonectomy and hemithoracic radiation for stage I-III malignant pleural mesothelioma. *J Clin Oncol.* 2007; 25: abstr 7561.

36. Weder W, Stahel RA, Bernhard J, et al. Multicenter trial of neo-adjuvant chemotherapy followed by extrapleural pneumonectomy in malignant pleural mesothelioma. *Ann Oncol.* 2007; 18: 1196–1202.

37. Van Schil PE, Baas P, Gaafar R, et al. Trimodality therapy for malignant pleural mesothelioma: results from an EORTC phase II multicentre trial. *Eur Respir J.* 2010; 36: 1362–1369.

38. Richards WG, Zellos L, Bueno R, et al. Phase I to II study of pleurectomy/decortication and intraoperative intracavitary hyperthermic cisplatin lavage for mesothelioma. *J Clin Oncol.* 2006; 24: 1561–1567.

39. Friedberg JS, Culligan MJ, Mick R, et al. Radical pleurectomy and intraoperative photodynamic therapy for malignant pleural mesothelioma. *Annals of Thoracic Surgery.* 2012;93:1658-1665; discussion 65-67.

40. Govindan R, Kratzke RA, Herndon JE, et al. Gefinib in patients with malignant mesothelioma: a phase II study by the Cancer and Leukemia Group B (CALGB 30101). *Proc Am Soc Clin Onc (ASCO).* 2003; 22: 630 (abstr 2535).

41. Garland LL, Rankin C, Gandara DR, et al. Phase II study of erlotinib in patients with malignant pleural mesothelioma: a Southwest Oncology Group Study. *J Clin Oncol.* 2007; 25: 2406–2413.

42. Mathy A, Baas P, Dalesio O, van Zandwijk N. Limited efficacy of ima-tinib mesylate in malignant mesothelioma: a phase II trial. *Lung Cancer.* 2005; 50: 83–86.

43. Dubey S, Janne PA, Krug L, et al. A phase II study of sorafenib in malig-nant mesothelioma: results of Cancer and Leukemia Group B 30307. *J Thorac Oncol.* 2010; 5: 1655–1661.

44. Jahan T, Gu L, Wang X, et al. Vatalanib in patients with previously untreated advanced malignant mesothelioma: preliminary analysis of a phase II study by the Cancer and Leukemia Group B (CALGB 30107). *Lung Cancer.* 2005; 49: S222 (abstr P-403).

45. Nowak AK, Millward MJ, Creaney J, et al. A phase II study of intermit-tent sunitinib malate as second-line therapy in progressive malignant pleural mesothelioma. *J Thorac Oncol.* 2012; 7: 1449–1456.

46. Kindler HL, Karrison TG, Gandara DR, et al. Multicenter, double-blind, placebo-controlled, randomized phase II trial of gemcitabine/cisplatin plus bevacizumab or placebo in patients with malignant meso-thelioma. *J Clin Oncol.* 2012; 30: 2509–2515.

47. Krug LM, Curley T, Schwartz L, et al. Potential role of histone deacety-lase inhibitors in mesothelioma: clinical experience with suberoylani-lide hydroxamic acid. *Clin Lung Cancer.* 2006; 7: 257–261.

48. Zauderer MG, Krug LM. Novel therapies in phase II and III trials for malignant pleural mesothelioma. *J Natl Compr Canc Netw.* 2012; 10: 42–47.

CHAPTER **51**
Non-Small Cell Lung Cancer

Justin F. Gainor, Jeffrey A. Engelman

INTRODUCTION

EPIDEMIOLOGY

Lung cancer is the leading cause of cancer-related mortality in the United States, with an estimated 160,000 deaths annually. Although lung cancer deaths have been declining among men since the early 1990s, lung cancer mortality has only recently begun to decline in women, likely reflecting gender differences in cigarette smoking and tobacco cessation patterns over the last 50 years. Cigarette smoking is the strongest modifiable risk factor for the development of lung cancer, accounting for 85%–90% of cases (1). Furthermore, smokers have a 20-fold increased risk of death from lung cancer compared to non-smokers. Still, other risk factors exist, including asbestos exposure, ionizing radiation, and exposure to carcinogenic chemi-cals and minerals. Research is ongoing regarding dietary and genetic risk factors.

TABLE 51-1 DISTRIBUTION OF LUNG CANCER BY HISTOLOGY

Histology	Estimated Prevalence
Non-small cell lung cancer (NSCLC)	85%
Adenocarcinoma	40%
Squamous cell carcinoma	20%
Large cell	3%
Other NSCLC[a]	22%
Small cell lung cancer	15%

[a]Includes NSCLC not otherwise specified (NOS).
Adapted from Howlader N, Noone AM, Krapcho M, et al. (eds.). *SEER Cancer Statistics Review, 1975-2009,* National Cancer Institute. Bethesda, MD. Available at http://seer.cancer.gov/csr/1975_2009_pops09/.

Lung cancer is traditionally divided into two major classes: small cell lung cancer and non-small cell lung cancer (NSCLC). NSCLC accounts for approximately 85% of lung cancer cases. NSCLC can be further classified based upon histopathologic designations that include adenocarcinoma, squamous cell carcinoma (SqCC), and large cell carcinoma. Historically, SqCC was the most frequent type of NSCLC; however, adenocarcinoma has become twice as common as SqCC in the last 40 years, perhaps reflecting changes in cigarette composition over this time period (Table 51-1). Recently, the classification of lung adenocarcinoma was revised to provide more uniform terminology and diagnostic criteria across multidisciplinary providers (2). Notably, this revised classification scheme eliminated the category of bronchioloalveolar cell carcinoma (BAC).

■ PRESENTATION

The majority of patients with NSCLC are symptomatic at diagnosis. The most common symptoms arising from the primary tumor are cough, dyspnea, blood-tinged sputum, and chest pain. Local extension of the tumor within the chest can cause pleural or pericardial effusions, chest pain, hoarseness, brachial plexopathy, Horner's syndrome, and superior vena cava syndrome. Metastatic disease may present with weight loss, neurologic symptoms, or bony pain. Paraneoplastic syndromes such as syndrome of inappropriate antidiuretic hormone secretion (SIADH), Cushing's syndrome (ectopic corticotropin secretion), and Lambert-Eaton myasthenic syndrome are more commonly associated with small cell lung cancer, but NSCLC may be associated with hypercalcemia of malignancy or hypertrophic pulmonary osteoarthropathy.

■ SCREENING

Given the global burden of lung cancer deaths, a number of different screening strategies have been explored in order to improve lung cancer detection and survival. In the last three decades, multiple randomized trials using screening chest radiographs with or without sputum cytology failed to show reductions in lung cancer mortality (3–5). More recently, several small trials have suggested that low-dose helical computed tomography (CT) detected more nodules and early-stage lung cancers compared to chest radiography. These results prompted several large randomized screening trials using low-dose CTs, including the National Lung Cancer Screening Trial (NLST) and the ongoing Dutch-Belgian randomized lung cancer screening trial (NELSON). In 2011, results from the NLST were published, demonstrating a 20% relative risk reduction in lung cancer mortality among high-risk patients undergoing annual screening with low-dose CT compared to chest radiographs (6). High-risk patients in the NLST were between 55 and 74 years of age, were current or former smokers (quit ≤15 years), had at least a 30 pack-year smoking history, and had no prior history of lung cancer. Although several organizations have since recommended lung cancer screening using low-dose helical CTs based upon these data, the U.S. Preventative Services Task Force has not endorsed screening to date.

◼ STAGING AND PROGNOSIS

The primary determinant of prognosis in NSCLC is stage at diagnosis. Stage is defined by the size of the primary tumor and involvement of regional lymph nodes and metastatic sites via the American Joint Committee on Cancer TNM system (Table 51-2). Significant revisions to this system were implemented in 2009.

All NSCLC patients should undergo a contrast-enhanced chest CT scan extending through the liver and adrenal glands, as well as a whole body PET scan to identify occult metastases. MRI of the brain is also encouraged. In the absence of metastatic disease, the nodal (N) status is the most important determinant of overall stage and therefore of prognosis. Thus, management decisions often depend on N staging. Nodal involvement may be assessed by clinical means such as CT and PET scan, or more accurately by pathologic evaluation via biopsy. CT scans have a sensitivity of 61% and a specificity of 79% for detection of involved mediastinal nodes in NSCLC, while PET scan is slightly better with a sensitivity of 85% and a specificity of 90% (7). Nevertheless, in the absence of obvious metastatic disease, pathologic assessment of mediastinal lymph nodes via mediastinoscopy is a vital component of NSCLC staging. Recently, alternative approaches to mediastinal lymph node sampling have been advanced, such as endobronchial ultrasound and esophageal ultrasound (8).

EARLY STAGE NSCLC
◼ SURGERY

Surgical resection of the tumor and draining lymph nodes is the cornerstone of therapy for stages I–II NSCLC and provides the greatest likelihood of cure. The type of surgery performed depends on tumor size, location, overall health of the patient, and local practice standards. Pulmonary resections are classified as anatomic if they encompass the draining lymphovascular structures, as in pneumonectomy, lobectomy, and segmentectomy, or non-anatomic, as in wedge resection. Resections can be performed through a standard thoracotomy incision, or in some cases through a smaller incision with video thoracoscopic assistance. Complete resection with a clean

TABLE 51-2 TNM STAGING FOR NSCLC

Primary Tumor (T)

TX	Primary tumor cannot be assessed, or tumor proven by the presence of malignant cells in sputum or bronchial washings but not visualized by imaging or bronchoscopy
T0	No evidence of primary tumor
Tis	Carcinoma in situ
T1	Tumor <3 cm in greatest dimension, surrounded by lung or visceral pleura, without bronchoscopic evidence of invasion more proximal than the lobar bronchus[a]
T1a	Tumor <2 cm in greatest dimension
T1b	Tumor >2 cm but <3 cm in greatest dimension
T2	Tumor >3 cm but <7 cm
	Involves main bronchus >2 cm distal to the carina
	Invades visceral pleura
	Associated with atelectasis or obstructive pneumonitis that extends to the hilar region but does not involve the entire lung
T2a	Tumor >3 cm but <5 cm in greatest dimension
T2b	Tumor >5 cm but <7 cm in greatest dimension
T3	Tumor >7 cm or one that directly invades any of the following: parietal pleura, chest wall (including superior sulcus tumors), diaphragm, phrenic nerve, mediastinal pleura, parietal pericardium; or tumor in the main bronchus <2 cm distal to the carina but without involvement of the carina; or associated atelectasis or obstructive pneumonitis of the entire lung or separate tumor nodule(s) in the same lobe
T4	Tumor of any size that invades any of the following: mediastinum, heart, great vessels, trachea, recurrent laryngeal nerve, esophagus, vertebral body, carina, separate tumor nodule(s) in a different ipsilateral lobe

Regional Lymph Nodes (N)

NX	Regional lymph nodes cannot be assessed
N0	No regional lymph node metastases
N1	Metastasis in ipsilateral peribronchial and/or ipsilateral hilar lymph nodes and intrapulmonary nodes, including involvement by direct extension
N2	Metastasis in ipsilateral mediastinal and/or subcarinal lymph node(s)
N3	Metastasis in contralateral mediastinal, contralateral hilar, ipsilateral or contralateral scalene, or supraclavicular lymph node(s)

Distant Metastasis (M)

M0	No distant metastasis
M1	Distant metastasis
M1a	Separate tumor nodule(s) in a contralateral lobe, tumor with pleural nodules or malignant pleural (or pericardial) effusion[b]
M1b	Distant metastasis (in extrathoracic organs)

(continued)

TABLE 51-2 TNM STAGING FOR NSCLC (CONTINUED)

Anatomic Stage/Prognostic Groups

Stage	T	N	M
Occult Carcinoma	TX	N0	M0
Stage 0	Tis	N0	M0
Stage IA	T1a	N0	M0
	T1b	N0	M0
Stage IB	T2a	N0	M0
Stage IIA	T2b	N0	M0
	T1a	N1	M0
	T1b	N1	M0
	T2a	N1	M0
Stage IIB	T2b	N1	M0
	T3	N0	M0
Stage IIIA	T1a	N2	M0
	T1b	N2	M0
	T2a	N2	M0
	T2b	N2	M0
	T3	N1	M0
	T3	N2	M0
	T4	N0	M0
	T4	N1	M0
Stage IIIB	T1a	N3	M0
	T1b	N3	M0
	T2a	N3	M0
	T2b	N3	M0
	T3	N3	M0
	T4	N2	M0
	T4	N3	M0
Stage IV	Any T	Any N	M1a
	Any T	Any N	M1b

[a]The uncommon superficial spreading tumor of any size with its invasive component limited to the bronchial wall, which may extend proximally to the main bronchus, is also classified as T1a.
[b]Most pleural (and pericardial) effusions with lung cancer are due to tumor. In a few patients, however, multiple cytopathologic examinations of pleural (pericardial) fluid are negative for tumor, and the fluid is nonbloody and is not an exudate. Where these elements and clinical judgment dictate that the effusion is not related to the tumor, the effusion should be excluded as a staging element and the patient should be classified as M0.

Used with the permission of the American Joint Committee on Cancer (AJCC), Chicago, Illinois. The original source for this material is Edge SB et al (eds). *AJCC Cancer Staging Manual*, 7th edition. New York, Springer, 2010.

margin is the strongest predictor of cure after NSCLC surgery; hence, the location and size of the tumor partially dictate the required operation.

An additional consideration is the amount of lung parenchyma to be resected and the resultant morbidity and mortality. A randomized study of peripheral stage IA NSCLC tumors treated with lobectomy versus a limited surgery (segmentectomy or wedge) found that limited surgery was associated with an increased risk of local recurrence and a trend toward inferior survival. The methodology of this study has been criticized due to its statistical design (e.g., lack of intention to treat in primary analysis), lack of modern staging techniques (e.g., CT, PET), and limited long-term, postoperative pulmonary function reporting (9). Nonetheless, lobectomy is the preferred operation for NSCLC unless tumor characteristics or patient comorbidities dictate otherwise. Hospital surgical volume also correlates inversely with perioperative mortality.

■ MEDICALLY INOPERABLE PATIENTS

Patients with early-stage NSCLC and excessive surgical risk due to medical comorbidities are termed "medically inoperable." Characteristics such as current smoking, poor exercise capacity, weight loss, and severe COPD are associated with high-surgical risk. Advanced age alone should not preclude an otherwise fit patient from surgery as retrospective analyses suggest survival among elderly patients is similar to younger patients after resection of early stage NSCLC (10, 11).

Options for medically inoperable patients include standard radiation therapy (RT), stereotactic body radiotherapy (SBRT), radiofrequency ablation (RFA), or observation. Standard RT yields about one-third to one-half the cure rate achieved surgically, with a 5-year OS of 20%–30% for stage I NSCLC (12). More recently, the introduction of SBRT, also known as stereotactic ablative radiotherapy (SABR), has changed the approach to medically inoperable patients with early-stage NSCLC. SBRT involves the delivery of precise, high-dose radiation over a single or limited number of dose fractions. In observational studies of SBRT, medically inoperable patients with early-stage NSCLC experienced local tumor control rates of greater than 90% and a 3-year OS of nearly 60% following treatment with SBRT (13). No randomized trials have been performed comparing SBRT and standard RT. However, based upon historical comparisons of local tumor control rates, SBRT is generally considered standard of care for patients with early-stage NSCLC who are deemed medically inoperable or who decline surgical resection. Studies comparing SBRT versus sublobar surgical resection in high-risk patients (i.e., able to tolerate sublobar resection but not lobectomy) are ongoing.

■ ADJUVANT TREATMENT

Despite surgery, 50%–60% of patients with early-stage NSCLC will relapse and die from their lung cancer. Postoperative, or adjuvant, chemotherapy and RT aim to decrease the risk of local and distant recurrence. Adjuvant RT can decrease local recurrence rates but does not impact overall survival. A large meta-analysis even suggested adjuvant RT could increase the risk of death for stage I and II patients (14). In general, adjuvant RT is not standard of care treatment, but it may be considered for specific patients with positive or close surgical margins or with incidentally discovered stage III disease at the time of resection.

Distant metastases are the most common source of treatment failure following potentially curative surgery in early-stage NSCLC, providing a rationale for adjuvant chemotherapy. In 1995, a large meta-analysis suggested that adjuvant cisplatin-based chemotherapy conferred a survival benefit in patients undergoing resection for NSCLC, although this difference was not statistically significant (15). Subsequently, multiple randomized trials have demonstrated a 3%–15% improvement in survival with cisplatin-based adjuvant chemotherapy. In 2008, data from five of these trials were combined in the Lung Adjuvant Cisplatin Evaluation (LACE) meta-analysis (16). In this pooled analysis of 4584 patients with over 5 years of follow-up, adjuvant cisplatin-based chemotherapy was associated with an absolute survival benefit of 5.4% at 5 years. This benefit was most pronounced in patients with stage II and III disease and those with favorable performance status. In these patient populations, cisplatin-based adjuvant chemotherapy is therefore considered standard of care. Based upon subgroup analyses from available randomized trials, some patients with stage IB NSCLC (e.g., tumor size >4 cm) may also benefit from adjuvant chemotherapy.

■ STAGE III NSCLC

Stage III NSCLC, or locally advanced disease, encompasses a heterogeneous group of tumors. The vast majority of patients with stage IIIA disease are so designated because of N2 lymphadenopathy, meaning involvement of the ipsilateral mediastinal or subcarinal nodes (Figure 51-1). In general, treatment of stage IIIA NSCLC requires multiple therapeutic modalities. Based upon patient and tumor characteristics, treatment may consist of induction chemotherapy followed by surgery, concurrent chemoradiotherapy followed by surgery, or definitive chemoradiation without surgery. Unfortunately, clinical trials comparing such approaches have been limited by patient heterogeneity, poor accrual, and imprecise staging. Thus, the optimal management approach is still controversial, particularly with respect to induction strategies. Indeed, in a 2010 survey of practice patterns for stage IIIA NSCLC among the National Comprehensive Cancer Network (NCCN) member institutions, 50% of institutions reported use of induction chemotherapy as the predominant treatment approach while 50% reported using neoadjuvant chemoradiotherapy in a majority of cases (17).

Another area of controversy in the management of stage IIIA disease is the role of surgical resection following induction therapy. As noted above, treatment approaches for stage IIIA tumors include definitive concurrent chemoradiation or induction therapy (e.g., neoadjuvant chemotherapy or neoadjuvant chemoradiation) followed by surgical resection. The U.S. Intergroup 0139 trial was designed to assess the role of surgical resection as part of these strategies (18). This trial randomized 429 patients with stage IIIA NSCLC and positive N2 nodes to definitive cisplatin-based chemoradiotherapy or neoadjuvant chemoradiotherapy followed by surgery. An interim analysis showed no difference in survival between the two arms. However, the definitive chemoradiotherapy arm had a higher rate of local

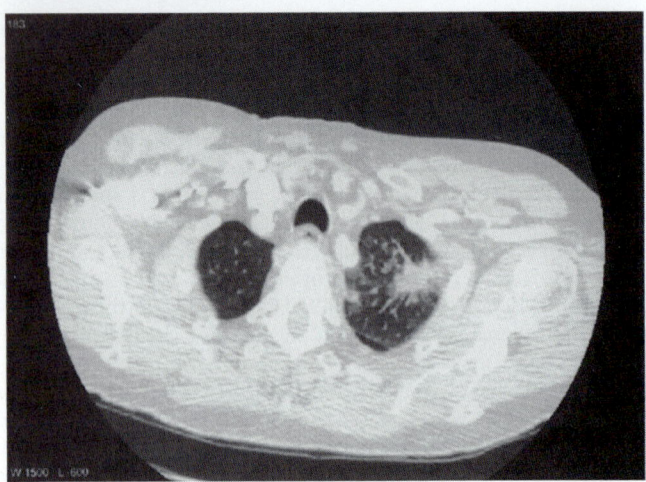

A

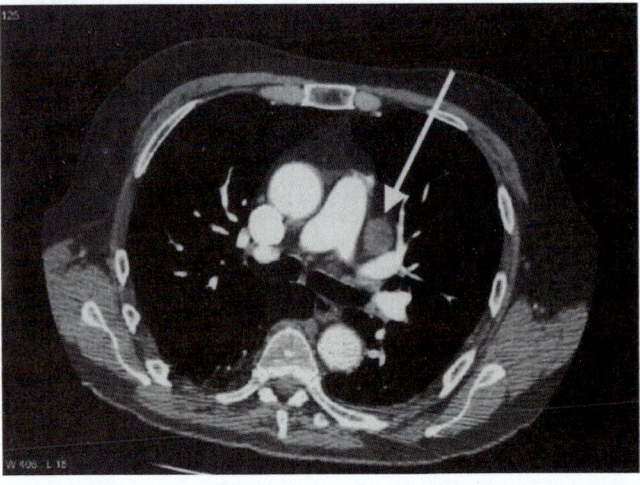

B

FIGURE 51-1 Clinical stage IIIA NSCLC. Panel A shows a spiculated left upper lobe primary tumor. Panel B shows bulky ipsilateral mediastinal lymphadenopathy (*arrow*).

recurrence, while the surgical arm had more early deaths due to perioperative complications, especially among patients requiring pneumonectomy. In fact, a subgroup analysis of the patients undergoing lobectomy and matched nonsurgical controls showed an increased median survival in the lobectomy group (34 months) compared to the definitive chemoradiotherapy group (22 months, $p = 0.002$). The interpretation of these data has been that tumors amenable to lobectomy likely benefit from neoadjuvant therapy, but tumors requiring pneumonectomy should be treated by definitive chemoradiotherapy without surgery. If there is progressive disease or clinical decline during neoadjuvant treatment, the prognosis is poor and resection should no longer be considered.

Locally advanced NSCLC also encompasses stage IIIB disease. Stage IIIB tumors are by definition unresectable, either due to involvement of vital structures or due to spread to the contralateral lymphatic system. In general, the standard of care for patients with stage IIIB disease and a good performance status is definitive, concurrent chemoradiation. This is based upon randomized trial data demonstrating that cisplatin-based chemotherapy given prior to RT results in improved survival compared to RT alone (5-year OS 17% vs. 6%, respectively) (19, 20). Furthermore, cisplatin-based chemotherapy given concurrently with RT is superior to sequential chemotherapy and RT (5-year OS 15.8% vs. 8.9%, respectively) (19, 21). In the United States, the most commonly used chemotherapy regimens in this setting are: (1) cisplatin and etoposide, and (2) weekly carboplatin and paclitaxel. Currently, the combination of cisplatin and pemetrexed with concurrent radiation is also being evaluated in ongoing clinical trials for patients with stage IIIB nonsquamous NSCLCs.

■ PANCOAST TUMORS

Approximately 5% of lung cancers are located in the superior sulcus and are termed pancoast tumors. This designation encompasses tumors of various stages, but they share distinct presenting signs and symptoms, such as arm pain, numbness, and weakness from involvement of the brachial plexus. Limited space in the superior sulcus makes immediate surgical resection technically difficult. As a result, pancoast tumors were historically treated with neoadjuvant RT followed by surgery, although this approach yielded 5-year OS rates of only 30%. The success of neoadjuvant chemoradiotherapy in stage III NSCLC led to a single-arm, phase II trial of this approach in patients with pancoast tumors with T3-4 and N0-1 status (22). A total of 110 patients received neoadjuvant chemoradiotherapy followed by surgery. Five-year OS was 44%, an improvement compared to historical findings with RT and surgery. Interestingly, pathologic complete and near-complete responses exceeded radiographic complete response rates, suggesting that there are often residual abnormalities on CT scan that do not contain viable tumor tissue.

ADVANCED NSCLC

Approximately 40% of patients with NSCLC present with advanced or stage IV disease. Advanced NSCLC is an incurable condition, and the goals of treatment are both to extend life and to palliate. In general, treatment decisions for advanced NSCLC are based upon a number of factors, including tumor histology, patient performance status (PS), and the patient's overall medical condition. Additionally, in the last decade, management approaches for NSCLC have undergone a significant paradigm shift, with an emphasis on stratifying patients based upon the molecular characteristics of their tumors. Such strategies have been informed by the recent success of targeted therapies in patients with genetic alterations in the EGFR and anaplastic lymphoma kinase (ALK). We will begin this section with a discussion of standard first-line chemotherapy in advanced NSCLC, after which we will address these emerging molecular targets (see "Targeted Therapy for NSCLC").

■ FIRST-LINE CHEMOTHERAPY FOR ADVANCED NSCLC

Chemotherapy is a mainstay of treatment for patients with advanced NSCLC. Early evidence of the benefits of chemotherapy in advanced disease came in the form of a 1995 meta-analysis of 11 trials, which demonstrated an approximate 2-month improvement in overall survival with platinum-based chemotherapy compared to best supportive care (15). Several additional studies have since confirmed this survival advantage and shown that chemotherapy improves quality of life for patients with advanced NSCLC and a good performance status (ECOG PS 0 or 1).

In general, standard management for advanced NSCLC consists of two-drug platinum-based combination regimens (doublets). Cisplatin-based regimens appear to offer a slight OS benefit compared to carboplatin-based regimens (23); however, this difference is clinically significant only in the treatment of early-stage disease, when cure is possible. Thus, in the United States, most clinicians prefer to use carboplatin for advanced disease because it has a more favorable side-effect profile.

A number of clinical trials have attempted to identify the optimal doublet for advanced NSCLC. In 2002, results from a phase III randomized trial comparing four different platinum-based doublets were published (24). In this study of 1155 patients with advanced NSCLC, no differences in overall survival were observed among those receiving cisplatin/paclitaxel, cisplatin/gemcitabine, cisplatin/docetaxel, or carboplatin/paclitaxel. Each doublet produced response rates of nearly 20% and a median survival of approximately 8 months.

Until recently, clinicians choose between platinum-based doublets based upon local practice patterns and patient preferences regarding side-effect profiles and schedules of administration. However, several randomized phase III trials have since highlighted the importance of tumor histology as an important determinant in treatment decisions. In a recent phase III non-inferiority trial comparing cisplatin/gemcitabine versus cisplatin/pemetrexed in 1725 previously untreated patients, there was no difference in median OS between the two arms (25). In preplanned subgroup analysis, however, patients with adenocarcinoma histology treated with cisplatin/pemetrexed had a significant improvement in median OS compared to those treated with cisplatin/gemcitabine (12.6 vs. 10.9 months). Conversely, in patients with SqCC histology, cisplatin/gemcitabine produced superior survival compared to cisplatin/pemetrexed (median OS 10.8 vs. 9.4 months). Thus, pemetrexed is now approved as part of first-line treatment in advanced, nonsquamous NSCLC.

In recent years, multiple randomized trials have tried to improve upon the results of platinum-based doublet chemotherapy. Initial attempts to add a third chemotherapeutic agent resulted in increased toxicity without a benefit in survival. More recently, efforts have included adding monoclonal antibodies. Bevacizumab is a monoclonal antibody that targets vascular endothelial growth factor (VEGF). In 2006, results from the landmark ECOG 4599 trial were published, demonstrating an OS benefit with the addition of bevacizumab to carboplatin/paclitaxel chemotherapy (26). Median survival was 10.3 months in the chemotherapy arm and 12.3 months in the chemotherapy plus bevacizumab arm. The population eligible for ECOG 4599 was relatively selective, excluding patients with brain metastases, those with SqCC histology, and those with significant risks of bleeding or thrombosis. Nevertheless, ECOG 4599 represents a major advance in the primary treatment of NSCLC as it is the first randomized trial to show a median survival of greater than 1 year. The triplet regimen with bevacizumab is now considered standard of care treatment for patients who match the study eligibility criteria.

■ MAINTENANCE THERAPY

First-line chemotherapy should be discontinued at the time of disease progression. For patients who respond or have disease stabilization with chemotherapy, continuation of a platinum-based doublet beyond 4–6 cycles does not appear to improve OS. However, there has recently been renewed interest in the notion of maintenance therapy, which aims to prolong the duration of disease control (either response or stable disease) following completion of a predefined number of induction chemotherapy cycles. Two different maintenance strategies have emerged. *Continuation maintenance* describes treatment with at least one of the initial agents from the induction regimen, typically the non-platinum compound. *Switch maintenance* refers to the introduction of a new drug that was not used as part of the induction regimen.

Various agents have been evaluated in the maintenance setting, including multiple non-platinum cytotoxic agents as well as molecularly targeted therapies, such as VEGF and EGFR inhibitors. In recent randomized phase III trials, both gemcitabine and pemetrexed have demonstrated improvements in progression-free survival (PFS) when administered as continuation maintenance, although only pemetrexed has conferred an OS benefit (27). Bevacizumab is often commonly administered as continuation maintenance therapy as well. This is based upon the study design of ECOG 4599 (see "First-Line Chemotherapy for Advanced NSCLC"); however, no prospective comparisons of maintenance bevacizumab versus placebo have been performed. Phase III trials evaluating the combination of maintenance pemetrexed with or without bevacizumab are ongoing.

In randomized trials evaluating switch maintenance, several agents have produced improvements in PFS; however, only pemetrexed and the EGFR inhibitor erlotinib have produced significant improvements in OS (28, 29). Comparisons among these trials are limited by differences in induction chemotherapy regimens, patient eligibility, tumor histology, trial endpoints, and recommendations regarding treatment regimens at the time of progression. Ultimately, selection of appropriate maintenance therapy depends on a number of factors, including patient performance status, quality of life, the molecular characteristics of the tumor, response to induction chemotherapy, and tolerability of therapy.

■ TARGETED THERAPY FOR NSCLC

In recent years, significant advances have been made in understanding NSCLC at a molecular level. It is now recognized that "driver" oncogenes, the function of which are central role to the growth and viability of cancer cells, can be readily identified in approximately half of lung adenocarcinomas (30). Cancers harboring such mutations are often dependent or "addicted" to the corresponding oncogenic pathways for survival, providing the rationale for using therapies designed to inhibit these signaling pathways. In NSCLC, two archetypal examples of molecular targets are EGFR and ALK. As will be discussed more fully below, the success of targeted therapies in patients with genetic alterations in *EGFR* and *ALK* has resulted in a significant paradigm shift in the management of NSCLC, placing emphasis on tumor genotyping in routine clinical practice.

Gefitinib and erlotinib are oral small molecule tyrosine kinase inhibitors (TKIs) that target EGFR. In trials of these agents in the second- and third-line setting, both were associated with response rates of approximately 10% in genetically unselected patient populations. In 2004, however, somatic mutations in *EGFR* were discovered to predict responsiveness to EGFR TKIs (31, 32). Subsequent screening efforts identified *EGFR* mutations in approximately 10%–30% of NSCLC patients, with lower frequencies in Caucasian patients and higher frequencies in patients of East Asian descent. These mutations are associated with an improved prognosis as well as a number of clinical and pathologic features, including lack of smoking history, East Asian ethnicity, female gender, and adenocarcinoma histology.

In the first-line setting, treatment with gefitinib or erlotinib is associated with response rates of approximately 75% in patients with *EGFR* mutations. Furthermore, randomized trials have demonstrated improvements in PFS, tolerability, and quality of life in EGFR-positive patients treated with EGFR TKIs compared to conventional first-line chemotherapy. One such study was the Iressa Pan-Asia Study (IPASS), which randomized 1217 patients with advanced NSCLC to first-line treatment with either gefitinib or carboplatin/paclitaxel (33). The study population was composed of East Asian patients with pulmonary adenocarcinoma who were never or former smokers, characteristics typically associated with sensitivity to EGFR TKIs. In the overall study population, treatment with gefitinib significantly prolonged PFS compared to chemotherapy. Similarly, in the subset of patients with *EGFR* mutations, gefitinib resulted in an improved PFS compared to chemotherapy (9.5 vs. 6.3 months). However, among EGFR wild-type patients, gefitinib produced a significantly shorter PFS compared to chemotherapy (1.5 vs. 6.5 months), underscoring the importance of *EGFR* mutations, not clinical characteristics, in predicting benefit to gefitinib. Thus, tumor genotyping for *EGFR* mutations is now considered standard of care in advanced NSCLC.

Like *EGFR* mutations, chromosomal rearrangements involving the *ALK* gene define a distinct molecular subset of NSCLC first identified in 2007 (34). *ALK* rearrangements are found in approximately 4%–6% of patients with NSCLC. These alterations are essentially mutually exclusive with mutations in other oncogenic drivers, such as *EGFR* and *KRAS*. *ALK* translocations are also associated with unique clinical and pathologic features, including younger age, adenocarcinoma histology, and lack of smoking history. Importantly, *ALK* rearrangements confer marked sensitivity to the ALK TKI crizotinib. In early clinical trials in patients with *ALK* rearrangements, crizotinib was associated with response rates of 60% and a median PFS

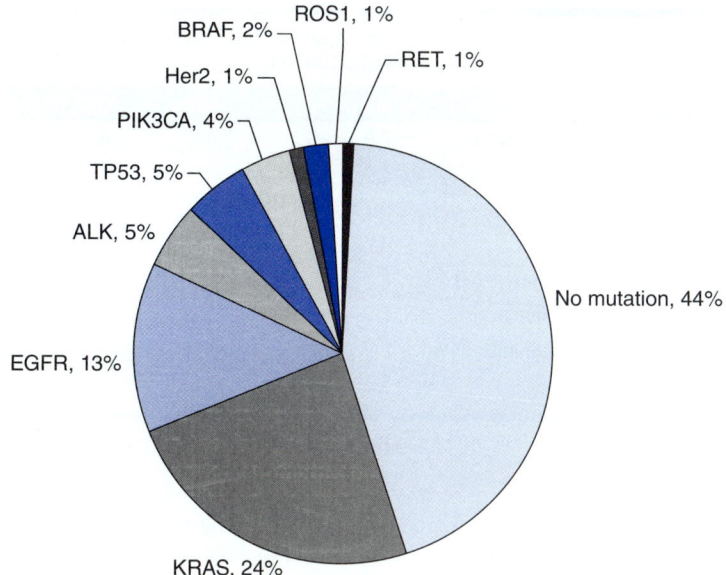

FIGURE 51-2 Distribution of driver mutations identified in lung adenocarcinomas to date.

of 8–10 months (35). Based upon these high rates of response, crizotinib received accelerated approval by the U.S. Food and Drug Administration (FDA) in August 2011. Randomized clinical trials comparing crizotinib and conventional chemotherapy in the first- and second-line settings are ongoing, but crizotinib has already emerged as the standard of care for patients with advanced NSCLC harboring *ALK* rearrangements. Recently, crizotinib has also shown activity in a separate molecular cohort of patients harboring rearrangements in *ROS1*, which is present in approximately 1% of NSCLC (36).

The recent success of EGFR and ALK TKIs in NSCLC has validated the paradigm of stratifying and treating patients based upon molecular characteristics. Efforts are underway to find additional oncogenic driver mutations as well as identify novel therapies for existing targets (**Figure 51-2**).

▊ SECOND- AND THIRD-LINE TREATMENT FOR NSCLC

In patients with a reasonable performance status following disease progression, second-line treatment can be considered. The expected response rate to second-line therapy is only 10%, approximately half that of first-line therapy. There are currently three single-agent treatments approved for second-line NSCLC therapy: docetaxel, pemetrexed, and erlotinib (**Table 51-3**). Both docetaxel and erlotinib treatments confer an OS benefit compared to supportive care in this setting, and outcomes with pemetrexed are equivalent to docetaxel with a better toxicity profile (37–39). All published studies have found that patients that responded to first-line therapy are more likely to benefit from second-line therapy compared to primary refractory patients.

TABLE 51-3 RANDOMIZED TRIALS OF SECOND-LINE SINGLE-AGENT TREATMENTS IN ADVANCED NSCLC

Author	Treatment	MS (Months)	p-Value	ORR (%)
Shepherd	Docetaxel	7.0	0.047	6
	BSC	4.6		0
Shepherd	Erlotinib	6.7	<0.001	9
	BSC	4.7		0
Hanna	Pemetrexed	8.3	NS	9
	Docetaxel	7.9		9
Thatcher	Gefitinib	5.6	NS	–
	BSC	5.1		–

BSC, best supportive care; MS, median survival; NS, not significant; ORR, objective response rate; –, not reported.

The current practice after progression on first-line therapy is to treat with sequential single agents if the patient is an appropriate candidate for active treatment. When available, patients should be considered for participation in clinical trials.

SPECIAL CONSIDERATIONS IN NSCLC MANAGEMENT

OLIGOMETASTATIC DISEASE

One percent of NSCLC cases present with "oligometastatic NSCLC," meaning a primary lung tumor that meets criteria for resection in conjunction with a solitary and resectable metastatic site, most commonly in the brain or adrenal gland. Highly selected patients may achieve long-term disease control by an aggressive approach including surgical resection of both the primary and metastatic disease. Patients selected for such an approach should have a good PS and are often treated initially with chemotherapy to demonstrate disease response or stability before proceeding with surgery.

ELDERLY PATIENTS

Those over the age of 70 years make up half the NSCLC patient population. Lack of participation of older patients in clinical trials and biases in physician treatment patterns against aggressive treatment for the elderly have led to overall poorer outcomes for this population. Recently, an increased interest in studying elderly cancer patients has generated an extensive literature suggesting that "fit" elderly NSCLC patients derive equivalent benefit from cancer treatment compared to younger patients. The challenge is to determine which elderly patients are "fit." No standard measure of fitness exists, but a patient with a good PS, a limited number of comorbidities, who is living independently and has the ability to perform the activities of daily living should generally be managed as per the standard of care for younger patients. Elder-specific clinical trials have also confirmed the benefit of single-agent chemotherapy in this population, with improvement in survival and quality of life compared to supportive care alone (40).

TABLE 51-4 SUMMARY OF STANDARD TREATMENT FOR NSCLC, BY STAGE

Stage	Treatment
IA	Surgery
IB	Surgery ± adjuvant platinum-based chemotherapy[a]
IIA, IIB	Surgery and adjuvant platinum-based chemotherapy
IIIA	If lobectomy possible, neoadjuvant chemoradiotherapy and surgery
	If lobectomy not possible, definitive chemoradiotherapy
IIIB	Definitive chemoradiotherapy
IV	Systemic therapy[b]

[a]Adjuvant chemotherapy should be considered for certain patients with stage IB disease (e.g., tumors >4 cm)
[b]Choice of initial systemic therapy should be made based upon performance status, medical comorbidities, tumor histology, and the molecular characteristics of the tumor.

■ PS2 PATIENTS

ECOG PS ≥2 is one of the strongest predictors of poor prognosis in NSCLC and also predicts for increased toxicity with chemotherapy treatment. The optimal therapy for such patients is unclear, as they have been excluded from participation in most clinical trials. For patients with advanced NSCLC, single-agent chemotherapy treatment and supportive care alone are reasonable options.

SUMMARY

NSCLC is a common and aggressive cancer. Treatment has advanced over the last decade and promising novel therapies are in development. A summary of standard treatment recommendations by stage can be found in Table 51-4.

REFERENCES

1. The health consequences of smoking: a report of the Surgeon General. Atlanta, (GA): U.S. Department of Health and Human Services, Centers for Disease Control and Prevention, National Center for Chronic Disease Prevention and Health Promotion, Office on Smoking and Health; Washington, D.C., 2004.

2. Travis WD, Brambilla E, Noguchi M, et al. International association for the study of lung cancer/american thoracic society/european respiratory society international multidisciplinary classification of lung adenocarcinoma. *J Thorac Oncol.* 2011; 6: 244–285.

3. Melamed MR, Flehinger BJ, Zaman MB, et al. Screening for early lung cancer. Results of the Memorial Sloan-Kettering study in New York. *Chest.* 1984; 86: 44–53.

4. Marcus PM, Bergstralh EJ, Fagerstrom RM, et al. Lung cancer mortality in the Mayo Lung Project: impact of extended follow-up. *J Natl Cancer Inst.* 2000; 92: 1308–1316.

5. Oken MM, Hocking WG, Kvale PA, et al. Screening by chest radiograph and lung cancer mortality: the Prostate, Lung, Colorectal, and Ovarian (PLCO) randomized trial. *JAMA*. 2011; 306: 1865–1873.

6. Aberle DR, Adams AM, Berg CD, et al. Reduced lung-cancer mortality with low-dose computed tomographic screening. *N Engl J Med*. 2011; 365: 395–409.

7. Gould MK, Kuschner WG, Rydzak CE, et al. Test performance of positron emission tomography and computed tomography for mediastinal staging in patients with non-small-cell lung cancer: a meta-analysis. *Ann Intern Med*. 2003; 139: 879–892.

8. Annema JT, van Meerbeeck JP, Rintoul RC, et al. Mediastinoscopy vs endosonography for mediastinal nodal staging of lung cancer: a randomized trial. *JAMA*. 2010; 304: 2245–2252.

9. Ginsberg RJ, Rubinstein LV. Randomized trial of lobectomy versus limited resection for T1 N0 non-small cell lung cancer. Lung Cancer Study Group. *Ann Thorac Surg*. 1995; 60: 615–622; discussion 22–23.

10. Sawada S, Komori E, Nogami N, et al. Advanced age is not correlated with either short-term or long-term postoperative results in lung cancer patients in good clinical condition. *Chest*. 2005; 128: 1557–1563.

11. Cerfolio RJ, Bryant AS. Survival and outcomes of pulmonary resection for non-small cell lung cancer in the elderly: a nested case-control study. *Ann Thorac Surg*. 2006; 82: 424–429; discussion 9–30.

12. Rowell NP, Williams CJ. Radical radiotherapy for stage I/II non-small cell lung cancer in patients not sufficiently fit for or declining surgery (medically inoperable): a systematic review. *Thorax*. 2001; 56: 628–638.

13. Timmerman R, Paulus R, Galvin J, et al. Stereotactic body radiation therapy for inoperable early stage lung cancer. *JAMA*. 2010; 303: 1070–1076.

14. Postoperative radiotherapy in non-small-cell lung cancer: systematic review and meta-analysis of individual patient data from nine randomised controlled trials. PORT Meta-analysis Trialists Group. *Lancet*. 1998; 352: 257–263.

15. Chemotherapy in non-small cell lung cancer: a meta-analysis using updated data on individual patients from 52 randomised clinical trials. Non-small Cell Lung Cancer Collaborative Group. *BMJ*. 1995; 311: 899–909.

16. Pignon JP, Tribodet H, Scagliotti GV, et al. Lung adjuvant cisplatin evaluation: a pooled analysis by the LACE Collaborative Group. *J Clin Oncol*. 2008; 26: 3552–3559.

17. Martins RG, D'Amico TA, Loo BW, et al. The management of patients with stage IIIA non-small cell lung cancer with N2 mediastinal node involvement. *J Natl Compr Canc Netw*. 2012; 10: 599–613.

18. Albain KS, Swann RS, Rusch VW, et al. Radiotherapy plus chemotherapy with or without surgical resection for stage III non-small-cell lung cancer: a phase III randomised controlled trial. *Lancet*. 2009; 374: 379–386.

19. Dillman RO, Seagren SL, Propert KJ, et al. A randomized trial of induction chemotherapy plus high-dose radiation versus radiation alone in stage III non-small-cell lung cancer. *N Engl J Med*. 1990; 323: 940–945.

20. Dillman RO, Herndon J, Seagren SL, et al. Improved survival in stage III non-small-cell lung cancer: seven-year follow-up of cancer and leukemia group B (CALGB) 8433 trial. *J Natl Cancer Inst*. 1996; 88: 1210–1215.

21. Furuse K, Fukuoka M, Kawahara M, et al. Phase III study of concurrent versus sequential thoracic radiotherapy in combination with mitomycin, vindesine, and cisplatin in unresectable stage III non-small-cell lung cancer. *J Clin Oncol*. 1999; 17: 2692–2699.

22. Rusch VW, Giroux DJ, Kraut MJ, et al. Induction chemoradiation and surgical resection for superior sulcus non-small-cell lung carcinomas: long-term results of Southwest Oncology Group Trial 9416 (Intergroup Trial 0160). *J Clin Oncol*. 2007; 25: 313–318.

23. Ardizzoni A, Boni L, Tiseo M, et al. Cisplatin- versus carboplatin-based chemotherapy in first-line treatment of advanced non-small-cell lung cancer: an individual patient data meta-analysis. *J Natl Cancer Inst*. 2007; 99: 847–857.

24. Schiller JH, Harrington D, Belani CP, et al. Comparison of four chemotherapy regimens for advanced non-small-cell lung cancer. *N Engl J Med*. 2002; 346: 92–98.

25. Scagliotti GV, Parikh P, von Pawel J, et al. Phase III study comparing cisplatin plus gemcitabine with cisplatin plus pemetrexed in chemotherapy-naive patients with advanced-stage non-small-cell lung cancer. *J Clin Oncol*. 2008; 26: 3543–3551.

26. Sandler A, Gray R, Perry MC, et al. Paclitaxel-carboplatin alone or with bevacizumab for non-small-cell lung cancer. *N Engl J Med*. 2006; 355: 2542–2550.

27. Paz-Ares L, de Marinis F, Dediu M, et al. Maintenance therapy with pemetrexed plus best supportive care versus placebo plus best supportive care after induction therapy with pemetrexed plus cisplatin for advanced non-squamous non-small-cell lung cancer (PARAMOUNT): a double-blind, phase 3, randomised controlled trial. *Lancet Oncol*. 2012; 13: 247–255.

28. Ciuleanu T, Brodowicz T, Zielinski C, et al. Maintenance pemetrexed plus best supportive care versus placebo plus best supportive care for non-small-cell lung cancer: a randomised, double-blind, phase 3 study. *Lancet*. 2009; 374: 1432–1440.

29. Cappuzzo F, Ciuleanu T, Stelmakh L, et al. Erlotinib as maintenance treatment in advanced non-small-cell lung cancer: a multicentre, randomised, placebo-controlled phase 3 study. *Lancet Oncol*. 2010; 11: 521–529.

30. Heist RS, Engelman JA. Snapshot: non-small cell lung cancer. *Cancer Cell*. 2012; 21: 448.e2.

31. Lynch TJ, Bell DW, Sordella R, et al. Activating mutations in the epidermal growth factor receptor underlying responsiveness of non-small-cell lung cancer to gefitinib. *N Engl J Med*. 2004; 350: 2129–2139.

32. Paez JG, Jänne PA, Lee JC, et al. EGFR mutations in lung cancer: correlation with clinical response to gefitinib therapy. *Science.* 2004; 304: 1497–1500.

33. Mok TS, Wu YL, Thongprasert S, et al. Gefitinib or carboplatin-paclitaxel in pulmonary adenocarcinoma. *N Engl J Med.* 2009; 361: 947–957.

34. Soda M, Choi YL, Enomoto M, et al. Identification of the transforming EML4-ALK fusion gene in non-small-cell lung cancer. *Nature.* 2007; 448: 561–566.

35. Kwak EL, Bang YJ, Camidge DR, et al. Anaplastic lymphoma kinase inhibition in non-small-cell lung cancer. *N Engl J Med.* 2010; 363: 1693–1703.

36. Bergethon K, Shaw AT, Ou SH, et al. ROS1 rearrangements define a unique molecular class of lung cancers. *J Clin Oncol.* 2012; 30: 863–870.

37. Shepherd FA, Dancey J, Ramlau R, et al. Prospective randomized trial of docetaxel versus best supportive care in patients with non-small-cell lung cancer previously treated with platinum-based chemotherapy. *J Clin Oncol.* 2000; 18: 2095–2103.

38. Hanna N, Shepherd FA, Fossella FV, et al. Randomized phase III trial of pemetrexed versus docetaxel in patients with non-small-cell lung cancer previously treated with chemotherapy. *J Clin Oncol.* 2004; 22: 1589–1597.

39. Shepherd FA, Rodrigues Pereira J, Ciuleanu T, et al. Erlotinib in previously treated non-small-cell lung cancer. *N Engl J Med.* 2005; 353: 123–132.

40. Gridelli C. The ELVIS trial: a phase III study of single-agent vinorelbine as first-line treatment in elderly patients with advanced non-small cell lung cancer. Elderly Lung Cancer Vinorelbine Italian Study. *The Oncologist.* 2001; 6 (Suppl 1): 4–7.

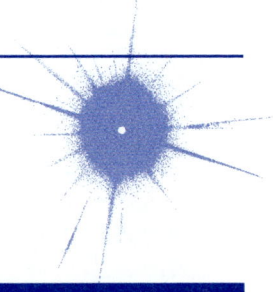

CHAPTER **52**

Small Cell Lung Cancer

Anna F. Farago, Rebecca Suk Heist

EPIDEMIOLOGY

Lung cancer is the leading cause of cancer-related mortality in the United States with over 172,000 new cases and over 163,000 deaths in 2005 with over 225,000 new cases and 160,000 deaths in 2013. Approximately 14% of lung cancers diagnosed between 2005 and 2009 were small cell lung cancer (SCLC), with the remainder being various subtypes of non-small cell lung cancer (NSCLC) such as adenocarcinoma, squamous cell, and large cell, among others. The proportion of new lung cancers diagnosed that are SCLC has been declining over the past few decades. The reasons for this are unclear but may relate at least in part to the changing composition of cigarettes and inhalation patterns.

SCLC is associated with cigarette smoking in the vast majority of cases. Both duration of smoking and number of cigarettes per day are directly correlated with lung cancer risk. Patients who quit smoking decrease their lung cancer risk, although not to never-smoking levels (1).

PATHOLOGY

SCLC is a type of high-grade neuroendocrine lung cancer. The neuroendocrine lung tumors encompass a diverse spectrum that ranges widely in prognosis, from low-grade typical carcinoids and intermediate-grade atypical carcinoids to the higher-grade cancers including large cell neuroendocrine cancer and SCLC. SCLC and large cell neuroendocrine cancer behave similarly and have similar prognoses.

Pathologically, SCLC is defined as "a proliferation of small cells (<4 lymphocytes in diameter) with unique and strict morphologic features, scant cytoplasm, ill-defined borders, finely granular salt and pepper chromatin, absent or inconspicuous nucleoli, frequent nuclear molding, and a high mitotic count" (2). Immunohistochemical staining is generally positive for epithelial cell markers such as keratin and epithelial membrane antigen. In addition, neuroendocrine markers such as chromogranin A and synaptophysin are positive in the majority of SCLCs.

CLINICAL PRESENTATION

Most patients present with symptoms that are related to the intrathoracic bulk of disease or widespread dissemination. Cough, dyspnea, weight loss, and weakness are the most common presenting symptoms (3).

In addition, a variety of paraneoplastic syndromes are observed with SCLC. The ectopic production of hormones is a common culprit for the endocrine paraneoplastic disorders, which include hyponatremia (due to ectopic production of antidiuretic hormone), Cushing's syndrome (ectopic corticotropin production), and acromegaly (ectopic growth hormone releasing hormone). Neurologic paraneoplastic syndromes such as Lambert-Eaton myasthenic syndrome are caused by autoantibody-mediated damage to the nervous system. Treatment of the underlying tumor can help control these paraneoplastic syndromes; in addition, medical management of symptoms may be indicated (see Table 52-1).

DIAGNOSIS AND STAGING

Radiographically, SCLCs tend to present as central hilar masses with bulky mediastinal lymphadenopathy. Given the central location of most SCLCs, the diagnosis is usually made by pathologic analysis of a bronchoscopic or endoscopic biopsy sample. Alternatively, percutaneous CT-guided biopsies provide another means of obtaining tissue for diagnosis.

Once the diagnosis of SCLC is made, accurate staging is important for treatment planning. SCLC is traditionally categorized into either limited stage or extensive stage disease, as described by the Veteran's Administration Lung Group. Limited stage is typically defined as disease that involves one

TABLE 52-1   CLINICAL PRESENTATION

Symptoms and Signs	%
Local	
Cough	50
Dyspnea	40
Chest pain	35
Hemoptysis	20
Hoarseness	10
Distant	
Weight loss	50
Weakness	40
Anorexia	30
Paraneoplastic syndromes	15
Fever	10
Paraneoplastic syndromes	
Hyponatremia	15
Ectopic corticotropin	2–5
Acromegaly	<1
Lambert-Eaton	3
Encephalitis/subacute sensory neuropathy	<1
Cancer-associated retinopathy	<1

Adapted from Reference 3.

hemithorax or disease that is encompassable within one radiotherapy port; using the TNM staging system, this corresponds to T any, N any, M0, excluding T3-4 due to multiple nodules that do not fit within a tolerable radiation field. Extensive stage is any disease that extends beyond these parameters. The majority of patients present with extensive stage disease.

The staging workup is designed to establish whether a patient has metastatic disease, since this will substantially alter both the prognosis and treatment plan. The workup should include a CT of the chest with extension into the abdomen to evaluate the liver and adrenals, which are common sites of metastasis. Brain imaging should be performed since the CNS is a frequent site of spread. Both head CT and brain MRI are commonly used, but MRI is preferred for its greater sensitivity for detecting metastatic disease. Bone scan should be performed to assess for bony metastases. PET scans are increasingly being used for staging purposes, but its exact role is not yet clearly defined.

TREATMENT FOR LIMITED STAGE SCLC

Limited stage SCLC is treated with a combination of chemotherapy and radiation, which typically yields a response rate of greater than 80% (complete response 40%–60%) and median survival of 14–20 months. Surgery is not typically attempted due to the high early dissemination rate and poor overall survival at 5 years. Occasionally, patients present with a T1-2N0M0 cancer that is surgically resected on the presumption of NSCLC. These patients still need adjuvant chemotherapy after resection with appropriate SCLC regimens.

Combination chemotherapy and radiation remain the standard of care for limited stage SCLC. In terms of chemotherapy, cisplatin and etoposide is the standard regimen used. A randomized phase III trial demonstrated better survival among limited stage SCLC patients treated with cisplatin and etoposide in combination with radiation compared with the regimen of cyclophosphamide, epirubicin, and vincristine with radiation (4). As the cisplatin/etoposide regimen is easily combined with radiation, with little mucosal toxicity and less hematologic toxicity than other regimens, it remains the standard of care.

The addition of radiation to chemotherapy improves survival, and approximately 5% more patients are alive at 2 and 3 years when treated with combination chemoradiation versus chemotherapy alone (5). The early incorporation of radiation appears to yield better results than waiting until later in the treatment course. Several trials have addressed the timing of thoracic radiation. The National Cancer Institute of Canada randomized 308 patients receiving chemotherapy to early thoracic radiation (starting with the second cycle of chemotherapy) versus late thoracic radiation (starting with the sixth cycle). There was no difference in the total cumulative chemotherapy dose delivered between the two arms, but both progression-free survival and overall survival were improved in the early radiation arm (6). Multiple meta-analyses have also examined the benefits of early versus late thoracic radiation, and most favor early radiation (7–12). There is a suggestion that completing radiation within 30 days of starting any therapy, without compromising chemotherapy dosing, may be most beneficial.

Hyperfractionated radiation also appears to improve outcomes. Turrisi et al. randomized 417 patients with limited SCLC to cisplatin/etoposide given with either daily (qd) radiation (45 Gy total, 1.8 Gy fractions) or twice-daily (bid) radiation (45 Gy total, 1.5 Gy fractions). Patients on the bid dose schedule had better median survival (23 months for bid, vs. 19 months for qd) and 5-year survival (26% vs. 16%). Significantly worse toxicities were noted with the bid regimen, including grade III esophagitis, which occurred in 27% of this population versus 11% of the qd dosed population (13).

Not all centers have adopted the hyperfractionated dosing, however, and the question of whether hyperfractionation or total dose of radiation is more important remains debated. Choi et al. tested escalating radiation doses in both the qd and bid schedules. The bid total dose was limited to 55 Gy while the qd dose went up to 70 Gy. In long-term follow-up, both median survival (24 months vs. 29.8 months) and 5-year survival (20% vs. 36%) favored qd dosing (14).

Current NCCN guidelines recommend that radiation be delivered concurrently with chemotherapy in limited stage SCLC, starting within the first two cycles of chemotherapy. Either twice-daily dosing of radiation (to a total dose of 45 Gy in 1.5 Gy fractions) or once-daily dosing (to a total dose of 60-70 Gy) is acceptable (15).

PROPHYLACTIC CRANIAL IRRADIATION

Prophylactic cranial irradiation (PCI) should be considered in both limited and extensive stage disease where there has been response.

PCI has been shown to improve overall survival at 3 years by approximately 5% (from 15.3% to 20.7%). In addition, PCI decreases the incidence of future brain metastases by approximately 25% (from 58.6% without PCI to 33.3% with PCI) (16). Slotman et al. have examined PCI in patients with extensive stage disease who had a response to chemotherapy. PCI reduced the risk of brain metastases at 1 year from 40.4% to 14.6%, and improved median overall survival from 5.4 to 6.7 months (17). Typical doses range from 24 to 30 Gy. High-dose (36-Gy) PCI resulted in no significant reduction in brain metastases and a significant increase in mortality compared to standard dose (25 Gy) in patients with limited stage disease (18).

TREATMENT FOR EXTENSIVE STAGE SCLC

Chemotherapy is the mainstay of treatment for extensive stage SCLC. As in limited stage SCLC, the combination of cisplatin and etoposide is one of the most widely used regimens in the United States. Response rates range from 60% to 70%, but the overall survival remains poor, with less than 5% of extensive SCLC patients alive at 2 years. Median survival is between 9 and 11 months.

A phase III trial in Japan raised a great deal of interest in a new combination of cisplatin and irinotecan for treatment of extensive SCLC, showing a significant improvement in median survival among patients treated with cisplatin/CPT11 versus cisplatin/etoposide (12.8 months vs. 9.4 months) (19). However, a follow-up U.S. study failed to show a significant difference in response or survival between the two regimens (20).

Numerous studies have attempted to alternate chemotherapy regimens or add a third agent, but none of these strategies have proven more effective than the doublet of cisplatin/etoposide. In addition, attempts to administer high-dose therapy with autologous bone-marrow transplantation have not shown a significant benefit in the phase III setting.

Therefore, cisplatin/etoposide remains the standard regimen in extensive SCLC. A total of four to six cycles are usually delivered, as prolonged maintenance chemotherapy has not shown any significant survival benefit and increases the toxicity risk. Since chemotherapy in the extensive stage setting is palliative in nature, carboplatin is often substituted for cisplatin to minimize toxicity. A meta-analysis of four trials comparing cisplatin- and carboplatin-based chemotherapy in first-line treatment found no differences in overall survival, progression-free survival, or response rate, although there were differences in the toxicity profiles (21).

TREATMENT FOR REFRACTORY OR RELAPSED SCLC

Patients whose disease recurs within 3 months of completing initial chemotherapy or who have progressive disease during treatment are considered to have "refractory" disease. Patients whose disease recurs beyond 3 months of initial therapy are considered to have "relapsed" disease. Although refractory and relapsed patients are generally treated with similar second-line regimens, their prognoses are significantly different: patients with refractory disease have much poorer response to additional therapies.

Median survival after SCLC recurrence ranges from 2 to 6 months. Therefore, the goals of salvage chemotherapy and a focus on palliation must be carefully discussed with patients and families.

For patients who have failed carboplatin/etoposide or cisplatin/etoposide, topotecan is commonly used as second-line therapy. In a phase II trial administering single-agent topotecan to patients who progressed after first-line chemotherapy, overall response rate was 22%. Patients who had relapsed disease had higher complete and partial response rates (13% CR, 24% PR) compared with patients who had refractory disease (2% CR, 4% PR) (22). In a phase III trial administering single-agent oral topotecan or best supportive care to patients with recurrent disease after first-line chemotherapy, survival was prolonged in the topotecan group (25.9 weeks vs. 13.9 weeks) and quality of life deterioration was slowed (23). Furthermore, oral and IV topotecan offer similar response rates, survival, and tolerability among patients with relapsed disease (24). Other agents with activity include irinotecan, taxanes, and gemcitabine. Single-agent therapy is generally preferred over combination therapies, as minimizing toxicities in this palliative setting is important. Enrollment on clinical trials is encouraged, as none of the above regimens are extremely successful.

MOLECULAR FEATURES OF SCLC

Recently, the molecular alterations underlying SCLC are becoming better understood. Loss of the tumor suppressor genes TP53 and RB1 is nearly universal among SCLC tumors and cell lines (25–29). Amplification of at least one MYC family member (most commonly MYCL1 and N-MYC) also occurs in the majority of tumors (30–32). Altered expression of bcl-2 and c-kit has also been reported in SCLC (33–35), with c-kit mutations reported in a small minority (36). Multiple bcl-2 inhibitors and the c-kit inhibitor imatinib have been tested in SCLC, but have not shown significant activity to date; it is possible that the clinical trials have not pinpointed the optimal subset of patients to treat or the optimal combination of agents (37–39). Heterozygous loss of PTEN is also commonly seen (40), but homozygous deletions and point mutations are less common (28, 41). Although not yet tested clinically, it is possible that PI3K inhibitors may be useful in targeting this subset of patients. While beta-specific inhibitors may be of particular interest for PTEN-deficient tumors (42), there are also reports of p110-alpha inhibition being important to impairing growth of SCLC (43), and clinical testing in genetically defined subsets of patients may be informative.

More recent whole genome and whole exome sequencing efforts have confirmed what has been known historically and identified a variety of other gene mutations that occur in SCLC tumors and/or cell lines, including alterations predicted to influence signaling pathways and histone modifications (28–29). The clinical significance of such alterations is not yet clear, but is an area of active investigation (44–45).

REFERENCES

1. Alberg AJ, Samet JM. Epidemiology of lung cancer. *Chest*. 2003; 123: 21S–49S.

2. Brambilla E, Travis WD, Colby TV, Corrin B, Shimosato Y. The new World Health Organization classification of lung tumours. *Eur Respir J*. 2001; 18: 1059–1068.

3. Jackman DM, Johnson BE. Small-cell lung cancer. *Lancet*. 2005; 366: 1385–1396.

4. Sundstrom S, Bremnes RM, Kaasa S, et al. Cisplatin and etoposide regimen is superior to cyclophosphamide, epirubicin, and vincristine regimen in small-cell lung cancer: results from a randomized phase III trial with 5 years' follow-up. *J Clin Oncol*. 2002; 20: 4665–4672.

5. Pignon JP, Arriagada R, Ihde DC, et al. A meta-analysis of thoracic radiotherapy for small-cell lung cancer. *N Engl J Med*. 1992; 327: 1618–1624.

6. Murray N, Coy P, Pater JL, et al. Importance of timing for thoracic irradiation in the combined modality treatment of limited stage small cell lung cancer. The National Cancer Institute of Canada Clinical Trials Group. *J Clin Oncol*. 1993; 11: 336–344.

7. Fried DB, Morris DE, Poole C, et al. Systemic review evaluating the timing of thoracic radiation therapy in combined modality therapy for limited stage small cell lung cancer. *J Clin Oncol*. 2004; 22: 4837–4845.

8. Huncharek M, McGarry R. A meta-analysis of the timing of chest irradiation in the combined modality treatment of limited-stage small cell lung cancer. *The Oncologist*. 2004; 9: 665–672.

9. De Ruysscher D, Pijls-Johannesma M, Vansteenkiste J, et al. Systematic review and meta-analysis of randomised, controlled trials of the timing of chest radiotherapy in patients with limited-stage, small-cell lung cancer. *Ann Oncol*. 2006; 17: 543–552.

10. Spiro SG, James LE, Rudd RM, et al. Early compared with late radiotherapy in combined modality treatment for limited disease small-cell lung cancer: a London Lung Cancer Group multicentre randomized clinical trial and meta-analysis. *J Clin Oncol*. 2006; 24: 3823–3830.

11. Pijls-Johannesma M, De Ruysscher D, Lambin P, et al. Early versus late chest radiotherapy in patients with limited-stage small cell lung cancer (review). *The Cochrane Library*. 2010; 12: 1–40.

12. De Ruysscher D, Pijls-Johannesma M, Bentzen, SM, et al. Time between the first day of chemotherapy and the last day of chest radiation is the most important predictor of survival in limited-disease small-cell lung cancer. *J Clin Oncol*. 2006; 24: 1057–1063.

13. Turrisi AT, Kim K, Blum R, et al. Twice-daily compared with once-daily thoracic radiotherapy in limited small-cell lung cancer treated concurrently with cisplatin and etoposide. *N Engl J Med*. 1999; 340: 265–271.

14. Choi NC, Herndon JE, Rosenman J, et al. Phase I study to determine the maximum-tolerated dose of radiation in standard daily and hyperfractionated-accelerated twice-daily radiation schedules with concurrent chemotherapy for limited-stage small-cell lung cancer. *J Clin Oncol*. 1998; 16: 3528–3536.

15. National Comprehensive Cancer Network. *Clinical Practice Guidelines in Oncology version 2.2013*. 2012.

16. Auperin A, Arriagada R, Pignon JP, et al. Prophylactic cranial irradiation for patients with small cell lung cancer in complete remission. *N Engl J Med*. 1999; 341: 476–484.

17. Slotman B, Faivre-Finn C, Kramer G, et al. Prophylactic cranial irradiation in extensive small-cell lung cancer. *N Engl J Med*. 2007; 357: 664–672.

18. Le Péchoux C, Dunant A, Senan S, et al. Standard-dose versus higher-dose prophylactic cranial irradiation (PCI) in patients with limited-stage small-cell lung cancer in complete remission after chemotherapy and thoracic radiotherapy (PCI 99-01, EROTC 22003-08004, RTOG 0212, and IFCT 99-01): a randomised clinical trial. *Lancet Oncol*. 2009; 10: 467–474.

19. Noda K, Nishiwaki Y, Kawahara M, et al. Irinotecan plus cisplatin compared with etoposide plus cisplatin for extensive stage small cell lung cancer. *N Engl J Med*. 2002; 346: 85–91.

20. Hanna N, Bunn PA, Langer C et al. Randomized phase III trial comparing irinotecan/cisplatin with etoposide/cisplatin in patients with previously untreated extensive-stage disease small-cell lung cancer. *J Clin Oncol*. 2006; 24: 2038–2043.

21. Rossi A, Di Maio M, Chiodini P, et al. Carboplatin- or cisplatin-based chemotherapy in first-line treatment of small-cell lung cancer: the COCIS meta-analysis of individual patient data. *J Clin Oncol*. 2012; 30: 1692–1698.

22. Ardizzoni A, Hansen H, Dombernowsky P, et al. Topotecan, a new active drug in the second-line treatment of small cell lung cancer: a phase II study in patients with refractory and sensitive disease. *J Clin Oncol*. 1997; 15: 2090–2096.

23. O'Brien MER, Ciuleanu T-E, Tsekov H, et al. Phase III trial comparing supportive care alone with supportive care with oral topotecan in patients with relapsed small-cell lung cancer. *J Clin Oncol*. 2006; 24: 5441–5447.

24. Eckardt JR, von Pawel J, Pujol J-L, et al. Phase III study of oral compared with intravenous topotecan as second-line therapy in small-cell lung cancer. *J Clin Oncol*. 2007; 25: 2086–2092.

25. Wistuba II, Gazdar AF, Minna JD. Molecular genetics of small cell lung carcinoma. *Semin Oncol*. 2001; 28: 3–13.

26. Harbour JW, Lai SL, Whang-Peng J, et al. Abnormalities in structure and expression of the human retinoblastoma gene in SCLC. *Science*. 1988; 241: 353–357.

27. Yokota J, Akiyama T, Fung YK, et al. Altered expression of the retinoblastoma gene in small cell carcinoma of the lung. *Oncogene*. 1988; 3: 471–475.

28. Peifer M, Fernandez-Cuesta L, Sos ML, et al. Integrative genome analyses identify key somatic driver mutations of small-cell lung cancer. *Nat Gen*. 2012; 44: 1104–1110.

29. Rudin CM, Durinck S, Stawiski EW, et al. Comprehensive genomic analysis identifies SOX2 as a frequently amplified gene in small-cell lung cancer. *Nat Genet*. 2012; 44: 1111–1116.

30. Wong AJ, Ruppert JM, Eggleston J, et al. Gene amplification of c-myc and n-myc in small cell carcinoma of the lung. *Science*. 1986; 233: 461–464.

31. Johnson BE, Makuch RW, Simmons AD, et al. myc family DNA amplification in small cell lung cancer patients' tumors and corresponding cell lines. *Cancer Res*. 1988; 48: 5163–5166.

32. Brennan J, O'Connor T, Makuch RW, et al. myc family DNA amplification in 107 tumors and tumor cell lines from patients with small cell lung cancer treated with different combination chemotherapy regimens. *Cancer Res*. 1991; 51: 1708–1712.

33. Kaiser U, Schilli M, Haag U, et al. Expression of bcl-2- protein in small cell lung cancer. *Lung Cancer*. 1996; 15: 31–40.

34. Sekido Y, Obata Y, Ueda R, et al. Preferential expression of c-kit protooncogene transcripts in small cell lung cancer. *Cancer Res*. 1991; 51: 2416–2419.

35. Rygaard K, Nakamura T, Spang-Thomsen M. Expression of the proto-oncogenes c-met and c-kit and their ligands, hepatocyte growth factor/scatter factor and stem cell factor, in SCLC cell lines and xenografts. *Br J Cancer*. 1993; 67: 37–46.

36. Boldrini L, Ursino S, Gisfredi S, et al. Expression and mutational status of c-kit in small-cell lung cancer: prognostic relevance. *Clin Cancer Res*. 2004; 10: 4101–4108.

37. Rudin CM, Hann CL, Garon EB, et al. Phase II study of single-agent navitoclax (ABT-263) and biomarker correlates in patients with relapsed small cell lung cancer. *Clin Cancer Res*. 2012; 18: 3163–3169.

38. Paik PK, Rudin CM, Pietanza MC, et al. A phase II study of obatoclax mesylate, a Bcl-2 antagonist, plus topotecan in relapsed small cell lung cancer. *Lung Cancer*. 2011; 74: 481–485.

39. Johnson BE, Fischer T, Fischer B, et al. Phase II study of imatinib in patients with small cell lung cancer. *Clin Cancer Res*. 2003; 9: 5880–5887.

40. Virmani AK, Fong KM, Kodagoda D, et al. Allelotyping demonstrates common and distinct patterns of chromosomal loss in human lung cancer types. *Genes Chromosomes Cancer*. 1998; 21: 308–319.

41. Forgacs E, Biesterveld EJ, Sekido Y, et al. Mutation analysis of the PTEN/MMAC1 gene in lung cancer. *Oncogene*. 1998; 17: 1557–1565.

42. Wee S, Widerschain D, Maira SM, et al. PTEN deficient cancers depend on PI3KCB. *Proc Natl Acad Sci USA*. 2008; 105: 13057–13062.

43. Wojtalla A, Fisher B, Kotelevets N, et al. Targeting the phosphoinositide 3-kinase p110-a isoform impairs cell proliferation, survival, and tumor growth in small cell lung cancer. *Clin Cancer Res*. 2012; 19: 96–105.

44. Byers LA, Wang J, Nilsson MB, et al. Proteomic profiling identifies dysregulated pathways in small cell lung cancer and novel therapeutic targets including PARP1. *Cancer Discov*. 2012; 2: 798–811.

45. Sos ML, Dietlein F, Peifer M, et al. A framework for identification of actionable cancer genome dependencies in small cell lung cancer. *Proc Natl Acad Sci*. 2012; 109: 17034–17039.

CHAPTER **53**
Thymoma
Panos Fidias

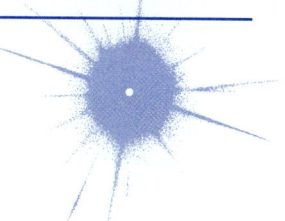

INTRODUCTION

Thymoma is a rare disease, with an incidence of only 0.13 per 100,000 person-years (1). However, it is the most common tumor of the anterior mediastinum, representing approximately 30% of anterior mediastinal lesions and 20% of all mediastinal tumors in adults. Based on Surveillance, Epidemiology and End Results (SEER) data from 1973 to 2006 the incidence is similar between males and females. Interestingly, the incidence in the United States is higher in African Americans and especially Asian/Pacific Islanders compared to whites or Hispanics. The median age at presentation is around 50 years and it peaks in the seventh decade. Approximately one-third of patients are asymptomatic at presentation, one-third have symptoms from local extent of their tumor, and one-third present with paraneoplastic syndromes, typically myasthenia gravis (MG).

HISTOLOGIC CLASSIFICATION

Thymomas are tumors derived from the thymic epithelium. In 1989 Muller-Hermelink and Kirchner proposed a classification based on the similarity of the morphologic appearance of the tumor to normal thymic compartments. This classification subdivided tumors into medullary, mixed, predominantly cortical, cortical, and well-differentiated thymic carcinoma.

In an attempt to standardize the histologic diagnosis of thymoma, the World Health Organization (WHO) published its own classification in 1999, which subdivided tumors into six types: A, AB, B1, B2, B3, and C. Type A tumors have neoplastic cells with spindle or oval appearance, whereas type B tumors have cells with an epithelioid or dendritic appearance. Types B1, B2, and B3 correspond to the predominantly cortical, cortical, and well-differentiated thymic carcinoma, respectively. Tumors combining type A and type B1 or rarely B2 features are classified as type AB. In the 2004 WHO classification update, thymic carcinomas (type C tumors in the 1999 WHO classification) include tumors with histology foreign to thymic tissues and are termed according to their differentiation (such as squamous cell carcinomas, mucoepidermoid, basaloid carcinoma, etc.), including carcinomas with neuroendocrine histology (2).

Thymic carcinomas have distinct morphology and immunophenotype; they present at more advanced stages and have a significantly inferior prognosis compared to other thymoma types. For that reason, some authors propose that well-differentiated thymic carcinomas should be designated as "atypical thymomas," not to be confused with (type C) thymic carcinomas, which will not be considered in this chapter.

GENETIC ALTERATIONS

In an era of personalized medicine and targeted treatment, thymomas remain for the most part outside of the spotlight. Although genetic alterations do occur, there has been no specific molecular target identified, which would be appropriate for therapeutic interventions. Random case reports have described responses to various tyrosine kinase small molecule inhibitors, but these were mostly confined to thymic carcinomas, and for those patients with thymoma who responded, no corresponding genetic alteration was identified in the tumor (3, 4). Allelic imbalances are very low for types A and AB (7%–8%), but increase to 20% for more advanced histologic types (B2 and B3) (5). Interestingly, type A component within an AB tumor is genetically distinct from type A tumors. The most frequent abnormality affects chromosome 6p21.3, which is an MHC locus, and 6q25.2–25.3, suggesting the presence of a yet unidentified tumor suppressor gene in these locations.

STAGING

The most widely used staging system was introduced by Masaoka in 1981, and was modified in 1994, allowing microscopic invasion into, but not through, the capsule to be classified as stage I (Table 53-1). Another staging system used by French groups, the Groupe d'Etudes des Tumeurs Thymiques (GETT) classification is based on the extent of disease but also on the extent of surgical resection (complete, partial, or biopsy). Both staging systems have been shown to be prognostic of overall survival in multiple studies. In a study of 149 patients with non-metastatic thymomas staged both with the Masaoka and GETT systems, there was an 88% concordance between the two systems. A tentative WHO classification based on tumor, node, metastasis (TNM) has also been proposed but is not widely used.

MYASTHENIA GRAVIS

Myasthenia gravis (MG) is the most common paraneoplastic disease associated with thymoma. Evoli reported on 207 patients with MG from Italy. Of the 188 patients with tumor that could be classified, 87% had type B thymomas

TABLE 53-1 MASAOKA CLINICAL STAGING OF THYMOMA

Stage	Description
I	Macroscopically and microscopically completely encapsulated (tumor invading into but not through the capsule is also included)
II	A. Microscopic transcapsular invasion
	B. Macroscopic invasion into surrounding fatty tissue or grossly adherent to but not through mediastinal pleura or pericardium
III	Macroscopic invasion into neighboring organs (i.e., pericardium, great vessels, or lung)
IV	A. Pleural or pericardial dissemination
	B. Lymphogenous or hematogenous metastasis

(B1 in 22.3%, B2 in 55.3%, B3 in 3.1%, and combined B2/B3 in 6.3%), which is similar to findings from other authors showing that thymoma is primarily associated with cortical histology. Interestingly, 13 patients developed MG 0.5–10 years following thymectomy. Out of 189 patients with adequate follow-up only 17 patients had achieved drug-free remission. As a result, some patients with thymoma succumb to complications of MG, rather than their malignant disease. In the study by Evoli et al. eight deaths were attributed to MG and seven deaths to progression of thymoma (6). Similarly, in a series from Mayo Clinic 13% of patients died of thymoma and 16% of myasthenia. Despite its contribution to the morbidity and mortality of thymoma patients, MG is not an independent predictor either of recurrence or of survival.

OTHER PARANEOPLASTIC SYNDROMES

Up to 50% of patients with pure red cell aplasia (PRCA) have thymoma, whereas less than 10% of patients with thymoma have PRCA. In 17 cases reported by Masaoka et al, who were treated with resection of their tumor, 6 patients benefited from surgery. More recently, the combination of octreotide and prednisone has also been found to be effective in the treatment of PRCA. Hypogammaglobulinemia is an uncommon complication of thymoma, but up to 10% of patients with acquired hypogammaglobulinemia will have an associated thymoma (Good syndrome). Unfortunately, surgery does not reliably return immunoglobulin levels to normal levels.

TREATMENT

■ RESECTABLE DISEASE

Surgery remains the only known curative therapy for thymoma. The definition of resectable thymomas includes not only early stage disease (stages I and II) but also more advanced cases where the bulk of the tumor can be removed. Obviously, criteria for unresectability vary among different centers, but extensive mediastinal infiltration or significant bilateral pleural-based tumor would be considered inoperable by most surgeons.

Rates of complete resection based on Masaoka stage and WHO classification are shown in Tables 53-2 and 53-3. Long-term outcome for resected thymomas is dependent both on Masaoka stage and WHO classification. Multivariate analyses in various studies have inconsistently shown that

TABLE 53-2 RATES OF COMPLETE RESECTION ACCORDING TO MASAOKA STAGE

Author	*N*	Stage I (%)	Stage II (%)	Stage III (%)	Stage IV (%)
Blumberg	118	100.0	73.0	56.0	78.0
Nakahara	141	100.0	100.0	73.0	0.0
Kondo	1049	100.0	100.0	84.6	41.6
Okumura	194	100.0	100.0	89.2	0.0

TABLE 53-3 RATES OF COMPLETE RESECTION ACCORDING TO WHO CLASSIFICATION TYPE

Author	N	WHO A (%)	WHO AB (%)	WHO B1 (%)	WHO B2 (%)	WHO B3 (%)
Kondo	100	100.0	100.0	100.0	100.0	92.0
Kim	108	100.0	88.0	100.0	90.6	55.0
Okumura	273	100.0	98.7	94.5	90.7	92.3
Park	150	100.0	92.3	100.0	90.0	65.2

additional factors can have independent prognostic value, such as tumor size, incomplete resection, and invasion of great vessels for stage III patients.

In evaluating the effectiveness of therapy, long-term follow-up is paramount, given the risk of late recurrences. Additionally, disease-specific survival, rather than overall survival, should be the primary end point, since death from thymoma can account for as low as 21% of all causes of death in large studies.

Stage I tumors have an exceptionally favorable outcome following surgery, with 5-, 10-, and 20-year survivals in the 90%–100% range. Survival decreases for more advanced tumors, with the most significant difference usually manifested between stages II and III.

Similarly, survival is excellent for WHO types A and AB, while survival rates drop significantly for types B2 and B3. WHO type B1 seems to have an intermediate prognosis (Tables 53-4 and 53-5).

TABLE 53-4 TEN-YEAR SURVIVAL OF PATIENTS WITH THYMOMA ACCORDING TO MASAOKA STAGE

Author	N	I (%)	II (%)	III (%)	IV (%)
Kim	108	95.0	81.3	46.2	N/A
Park*	150	100.0	88.2	63.0	22.5
Rea	132	84.0	82.0	51.0	0.0
Kondo*	1320	100.0	98.4	88.7	70.6
Nagawaka	130	100.0	100.0	76.0	47.0
Okumura†	243	89.0	91.0	49.0	0.0
Blumberg*	118	95.0	70.0	50.0	100.0
Maggi	241	86.9	64.3	59.9	39.6
Nakahara	141	100.0	84.4	77.2	46.6
Rena	178	94.0	88.0	66.0	N/A

*Five-year survival data.
†Twenty-year survival data.
N/A, not available.

TABLE 53-5 TEN-YEAR SURVIVAL OF PATIENTS WITH THYMOMA ACCORDING TO WHO CLASSIFICATION

Author	N	A (%)	AB (%)	B1 (%)	B2 (%)	B3 (%)
Fang	204	68.5	68.5	68.5	36.7	36.7
Kondo	100	100.0	100.0	83.1	83.1	35.7
Park*	150	100.0	93.2	88.9	82.4	71.3
Rea	132	100.0	90.0	78.0	33.0	35.0
Nagawaka	130	100.0	100.0	86.0	85.0	38.0
Okumura†	243	100.0	87.0	91.0	59.0	36.0
Rena	178	95.0	90.0	85.0	71.0	40.0

*Five-year survival data.
†Twenty-year survival data.

ADJUVANT THERAPY

It is widely accepted that the cure rate of patients with encapsulated thymomas is excellent with surgery alone. However, in more advanced disease, the results reported in surgical series have included a variable percentage of patients undergoing adjuvant therapy, primarily radiation. Several institutions have consistently prescribed radiation therapy for all invasive tumors (stages II and above), while others have selected patients for additional therapy based on the judgment of the thoracic surgeon or the radiation oncologist. Retrospective comparisons of patients who did and did not receive adjuvant therapy are therefore subject to selection bias and cannot be considered conclusive.

Curran et al. showed that following complete resection, 6/18 patients with stage II and 2/3 patients with stage III thymomas recurred in the absence of radiation, whereas none of 5 patients with radiation experienced a recurrence. However, only one patient in the radiation group had stage II disease. In a review of the literature up to that date, the authors demonstrated a 28% recurrence in the absence of radiation and a 5% recurrence rate when radiation was administered (7). In another study of 241 patients with thymoma from the University of Torino, Italy, Maggi et al. reported that 11 of 55 patients with invasive thymoma and no adjuvant therapy recurred, compared to 3 of 21 with adjuvant therapy (mostly radiation therapy) (8). However, subsequent studies have shown little benefit for postoperative radiation therapy.

In the largest retrospective study reported to date, 1320 patients from 115 Japanese centers were reviewed. Complete resection was performed in 247 stage II and in 170 stage III patients, and adjuvant radiation therapy was given to 43.3% and 74.5% of stage II and III patients, respectively. Recurrence rates for patients with and without radiation therapy were 4.7% versus 4.1% in stage II and 23% versus 26% for stage III patients (9). In a series of patients with stage III thymomas from Massachusetts General Hospital (MGH), 54% of recurrences occurred in the pleura (10). Similarly, in a study by Nakagawa et al. 6 out of 12 recurrences occurred in the pleura. Given the high propensity for such pleural dissemination, Haniuda et al. reviewed the efficacy of adjuvant radiation therapy in

70 patients undergoing complete resection of thymoma based on the degree of "pleural factor" defined as follows: p0, no adhesion to mediastinal pleura; p1, fibrous adhesion to the mediastinal pleura without tumor invasion; and p2, microscopic invasion of the mediastinal pleura. In p0 stage II patients no recurrence was observed regardless of radiation therapy. However, in p2 stage II tumors 3 out of 4 patients recurred, even in the presence of adjuvant radiation. Radiation appeared to be helpful in stage II p1 tumors, where none of 6 patients undergoing adjuvant therapy relapsed, compared to 4 out of 11 patients treated with surgery alone (11). Ogawa et al. examined the results of 103 patients with completely resected thymoma treated with adjuvant radiation therapy. The pleura was the most common site of recurrence, which was seen in 12 of 17 patients with relapsed disease. While no pleural recurrences were seen among the 70 patients without pleural invasion in their surgical specimen, 12 out of 38 patients with pleural invasion experienced such a recurrence (12). Therefore, it appears that radiation therapy cannot adequately treat tumors at high risk for the most common site of recurrence.

Newer studies have also evaluated the role of WHO classification in determining risk of relapse following adjuvant therapy. Ströbel et al. reported on 228 thymoma patients treated with primary surgery with or without adjuvant therapy (13). The study also included a small proportion of thymic carcinomas with squamous cell histology (4.8%). Postoperative therapy was quite uncommon in WHO type A thymomas (3 out of 20) but was very frequent in type B3 (15 out of 22). The main finding of the study was that recurrences following complete resection were rare among tumors of type A, AB, or B1, even in stages II and III (2 out of 33), while they were more frequent in stage III tumors of types B2 and B3 (5 out of 18). These results are also supported by data from MGH, which showed no recurrences among 73 patients with types A and AB thymoma (14). How to approach early stage unfavorable histology thymomas is a more difficult issue. Chen identified WHO types B2, B3, and C as independent poor prognostic categories within stages I and II tumors. He observed 4 deaths among 24 patients, compared to only 2 deaths in 78 patients with types A, AB, and B1. However, it is known that thymic carcinomas have distinct natural history and a worse prognosis compared to "pure" thymomas (15). Results in patients with B2 and B3 histology alone are more encouraging: there was only one recurrence out of 37 stage I/II patients in a recent study from Germany.

Exploring the role of adjuvant therapy in tumors of cortical histology (B2 and B3), Ströbel showed that in stage II tumors there were no tumor relapses among those patients who received adjuvant radiation versus one relapse in 16 patients without further treatment. The relapse rate for stage III patients was 0% for the 5 patients who underwent adjuvant therapy, compared to 33% for the patients without adjuvant treatment (13). Chen also reported that adjuvant therapy did not improve survival for types A, AB, and B1, whereas it had a statistically significant benefit for types B2, B3, and C (5-year survival 85.5% vs. 48.3%). Given the independent prognostic value of stage and WHO classification, several authors have proposed treatment algorithms and risk stratification schemes following primary surgery, which take both parameters into consideration.

■ UNRESECTABLE DISEASE

When complete, or near complete, resection cannot be performed, surgical procedures have ranged from biopsy alone to a variable degree of debulking approaches. Some studies have shown that debulking is superior to biopsy, but other studies have found no difference in survival. It is clear, however, that patients can still experience long-term survival when treated with radiation therapy with or without the addition of chemotherapy.

Ninety patients from 10 French centers were treated with partial resection (31 patients), biopsy (55 patients), or complete resection (4 patients with stage IVa disease and pleural implants). Radiation dose ranged from 30 to 70 Gy with a median dose of 50 Gy. Sequential platinum-based chemotherapy was added to 59 patients, while 3 patients received preoperative radiation and chemotherapy. The 5- and 10-year disease-free survival was 60% and 36% for partial resection, compared to 38% and 31% for biopsy alone (16).

An American Intergroup study evaluated the combination of cyclophosphamide, doxorubicin, cisplatin (CAP) followed by radiation therapy at a dose of 54 Gy in 23 patients with limited-stage unresectable thymoma, including 2 patients with thymic carcinoma. All, but one, of the patients had gross residual disease postoperatively. The overall response rate to induction chemotherapy was 69.6% (CR: 5 patients, PR: 11 patients) and the 5-year overall survival was 52.5% (17).

Based on the encouraging results of radiation and radio-chemotherapy, many centers have approached unresectable or borderline resectable thymic tumors with a multimodality treatment plan. Kim et al. from the M.D. Anderson Cancer Center treated 22 patients deemed to be unresectable with neoadjuvant chemotherapy, followed by surgery, postoperative radiation, and consolidation chemotherapy. Eleven patients had stage III, 10 patients had stage IVa, and one patient had stage IVb thymoma. The induction program consisted of cyclophosphamide, doxorubicin via continuous infusion, cisplatin, and prednisone, and it resulted in an overall response rate of 77% (CR: 3 patients, PR: 14 patients). Radiation dose for 16 patients was 60 Gy, and for the remaining patients it was 50 Gy. Twenty-one patients underwent surgery and 16 (76%) had a complete resection. Six of these patients had a more than 80% necrosis in the surgical specimen. The progression-free survival (PFS) at 7 years was 77%. Only one patient died of progressive thymoma with a median follow-up of 50.3 months (18).

Bretti et al. reported their results with neoadjuvant therapy in 33 patients who could not undergo upfront surgery for stage III-IV thymoma. Eight patients received radiation at a dose of 30 Gy in 15 fractions (24 Gy if more than 30% of the lung volume had to be included). The remaining patients received 4 cycles of chemotherapy, either ADOC (doxorubicin 40 mg/m², cisplatin 50 mg/m² on day 1, vincristine 0.6 mg/m² on day 2, and cyclophosphamide 700 mg/m² on day 4) or cisplatin and VP-16 (100 mg/m² on day 1 and 100 mg/m² on days 1–3, respectively). Surgery could be attempted on 17 patients, and a total of 12 patients were able to have a complete resection following induction treatment (1 patient post radiation, 11 patients post chemotherapy). These patients had shorter PFS (56.9 months vs. not reached yet) but similar overall survival compared to a cohort of 20 patients with stage III-IV thymoma, which could be completely resected at the time of diagnosis. The patients who could not be resected were given 50–60 Gy postoperatively, but had a 5-year PFS of only about 10% (19). Venuta et al. treated patients with stage III disease on a multimodality program: 30 patients with resectable disease underwent adjuvant chemotherapy and radiation (40 Gy for complete resection and 50–60 Gy for incomplete resection), while 15 patients judged to be unresectable were given neoadjuvant cisplatin-based chemotherapy. Eleven patients out of the 45 had thymic carcinoma. Overall, 10 patients had a response to the induction regimen (CR: 2 patients, PR: 8 patients, overall RR 67%). Complete resection was possible in 87% of patients; however, only 1 patient had a complete pathologic response (7%). Interestingly, the 10-year overall survival of patients receiving induction treatment was 90%, compared with 71% for patients considered initially resectable (20).

From the above studies it is reasonable to recommend an initial chemotherapy or chemoradiation approach, followed by an attempt to resect the disease for patients who present initially with unresectable thymomas (Table 53-6). In our practice, we often utilize either CAP or ADOC as preoperative chemotherapy. If we select a combined modality approach, we utilize cisplatin and etoposide concurrently with radiation.

TABLE 53-6 RESULTS FOR PATIENTS PRESENTING WITH UNRESECTABLE THYMOMA TREATED EITHER WITH DEFINITIVE RADIATION (OR CHEMORADIATION) OR WITH INDUCTION CHEMOTHERAPY

Author	N	Compl Res (%)	5-Year OS (%)	10-Year OS (%)	5-Year DFS (%)	10-Year DFS (%)
Definitive therapy						
Mornex	90	4.4	51	39	–	–
Ciernik	31	0.0	45	28	–	–
Loehrer	23	0.0	52.5	–	54.3	–
Urgesi	44	0.0	–	–	–	–
Krueger	12	8.3	57.0	–	–	–
Induction therapy						
Macchiarini	7	57	80 (2-year)	–	–	–
Bretti	33	36	–	–	–	–
Venuta	15	87	–	90 (9-year)	–	–
Rea	16	68.7	70 (3-year)	–	–	–
Kim	22	72.7	95	79 (7-year)	77	77 (7-year)

Compl res, complete resection; DFS, disease specific survival; OS, overall survival.

RECURRENT OR METASTATIC DISEASE

Recurrent disease amenable to reoperation should be approached surgically. Although there are no large comparative studies, there is evidence of long-term disease-free survival following aggressive therapy of recurrent tumors. Systemic therapy is the only option for patients with extrathoracic disease or with tumors that have progressed despite all available local measures (Table 53-7). Multiple case reports and small series have demonstrated that thymoma is a responsive malignancy to single agent chemotherapy.

Interestingly, significant responses have also been observed with the use of glucocorticoids, even in cases unresponsive to other modalities. Although it is widely accepted that glucocorticoids act mainly on the lymphoid population of the tumor, responses have been seen in primarily epithelial thymomas as well. Glucocorticoids may be even more efficacious in combination with octreotide. In a study by Palmieri et al. 16 patients with chemotherapy refractory thymoma were given prednisone (0.6 mg/kg/day for 3 months, 0.2 mg/kg/day during follow-up) and octreotide (1.5 mg/day or 30 mg every 14 days for the long-acting analog lanreotide). Six patients had thymic carcinoma, and half of them had progressive small cell neuroendocrine carcinoma. The response rate was 37%, including one patient with complete response. The median time to progression was 14 months, and the median survival time for the group was 15 months. The estimated 2-year survival is approximately 30% (21). Response to therapy did not appear to correlate with histology.

The Eastern Cooperative Oncology Group (ECOG) designed a study with the same combination therapy, but evaluated single agent octreotide initially (at a dose of 1.5 mg/kg daily), and only added prednisone (at a dose of 0.6 mg/kg daily) for patients with stable disease after 2 months of octreotide therapy. The study accrued 38 assessable patients with thymoma (32 patients), thymic carcinoma (5 patients), or thymic carcinoid (1 patient). At the end of the 2 months there were four partial responses, but the addition of prednisone resulted in six additional partial responses and two complete responses for an overall response rate of 30.3% for the combination. Only patients with typical histology responded to therapy. The 2-year overall survival was 75.7% (22). It appears, therefore, that glucocorticoids add to the activity of octreotide. In a case report, a patient with type B3 thymoma progressive after 6 months of octreotide treatment was given prednisone 50 mg/day in addition to long-acting octreotide. After 7 months of combination therapy the patient achieved a complete remission.

EGFR immunoreactivity is observed in thymomas, and overexpression of EGFR is associated with more aggressive thymic tumors (B2 and B3). Based on this observation, 26 patients with previously treated thymoma or thymic carcinoma were treated with gefitinib at a dose of 250 mg daily. Only one response was seen, which lasted for 5 months. None of the five patients who underwent DNA sequencing, including the patient who responded, harbored an EGFR mutation (23).

Among 18 patients treated with imatinib in two different studies, only 2 had typical thymoma and none responded. C-KIT mutations are rare, even in thymic carcinomas, and are essentially never seen in thymomas, even if they overexpress c-KIT by immunohistochemistry (24).

TABLE 53-7 RESULTS OF CHEMOTHERAPY IN PATIENTS WITH ADVANCED THYMOMA

Author	Therapy	N	Carcinoma (%)	Chemo Naive (%)	RR (%)	MST (Months)	2-Year OS (%)	5-Year OS
Palmieri	Octreotide prednisone	16	37.5	0.0	37.0	15.0	~30	N/a
Loehrer	Octreotide prednisone	38	16.0	0.0	30.3	N/A	75.7	N/A
Fornasiero	ADOC	37	0.0	97.2	91.8	15.0	N/a	N/A
Loehrer	CAP	30	3.3	100.0	50.0	37.7	64.5	32.0%
Loehrer	VIP	28	29.0	100.0	32.0	31.6	70.0	N/A
Chahinian	Various	9	0.0	N/A	44.4	N/A	N/A	N/A
Göldel	Various	22	N/A	100.0	50.0	N/A	N/A	N/A
Giaccone	EP	16	0.0	100.0	56.0	51.6	N/A	50.0%
Kurup	Iressa	26	27.0	0.0	3.8	N/A	N/A	N/a

ADOC, doxorubicin, cisplatin, vincristine, cyclophosphamide; CAP, cyclophosphamide, doxorubicin, cisplatin; EP, etoposide, cisplatin; MST, median survival time; N/A, not available; OS, overall survival; RR, response rate; VIP, etoposide, ifosfamide, cisplatin.

Combination chemotherapy has been studied extensively in the treatment of advanced thymoma. More commonly, patients received cisplatin-based regimens; however, responses have been reported with other regimens, such as cyclophosphamide, doxorubicin, vincristine (CAV), or CAV with the addition of prednisone ± bleomycin (CAVP ± Bleo). In a retrospective review of 123 patients treated on five ECOG trials, combination chemotherapy was associated with a higher response rate ($p < 0.0001$) and survival ($p = 0.035$) compared to single agent cisplatin. Fornasiero et al. reported on 37 patients treated with ADOC (cisplatin 50 mg/m^2 and doxorubicin 40 mg/m^2 on day 1, vincristine 0.6 mg/m^2 on day 3, and cyclophosphamide 700 mg/m^2 on day 4) over a period of 13 years. The overall response rate was impressive at 92%, with 43% complete remission rate. Seven patients were confirmed to have complete response pathologically following thoracotomy. The median duration of response was 12 months, and the median survival was 15 months (25). A similar regimen, CAP (cisplatin 50 mg/m^2, doxorubicin 50 mg/m^2, and cyclophosphamide 500 mg/m^2), was given to 30 patients with advanced thymoma. Although the response rate was lower than ADOC at 50%, the median survival time was much more impressive (37.7 months), questioning the value of vincristine in this setting (26). Successful retreatment with the same regimen in two patients relapsing 14 and 60 months after completion of initial therapy has been reported. Based on the promising activity demonstrated by single agent ifosfamide, 28 evaluable patients were treated with VIP (etoposide 75 mg/m^2, ifosfamide 1.2 g/m^2, and cisplatin 20 mg/m^2 days 1–4). Unfortunately, response rate and survival statistics did not appear superior to previous regimens (RR 32%, response duration 11.9 months, median survival time 31.6 months, and 2-year overall survival of 70%) (27). The European Organization for the Research and Treatment of Cancer (EORTC) evaluated the combination of cisplatin (60 mg/m^2 day 1) and etoposide (120 mg/m^2 days 1–3) on 16 chemotherapy-naive patients. The observed response rate was 56%, the duration of response was 40 months, the median survival time was 51.6 months, and the 5-year overall survival was 50% (28).

More recently, ECOG evaluated another non-anthracycline regimen consisting of carboplatin at an AUC of 6 and paclitaxel at a dose of 225 mg/m^2 every 3 weeks for a maximum of 6 cycles (29). They enrolled 46 patients, 13 of whom had type C thymic carcinoma. Unfortunately, the investigators grouped the 10 patients with B3 thymoma together with the type C patients. Results from treatment such as response rates (42.9% vs. 21.7%), PFS (16.7 vs. 5.0 months), and median overall survival (not reached vs. 20 months) were, as expected, all superior within the thymoma group.

CONCLUSIONS

Thymoma is a rare disease, but is highly curable with surgery when complete resection can be achieved. Even for unresectable patients, long-term survival is feasible with the combination of chemotherapy and radiation. There is considerable excitement about the use of neoadjuvant approaches in marginally resectable patients, but more studies are required in this group of patients. Metastatic disease should be treated with cisplatin-based regimens, but no "standard" therapy exists, and new agents need to be evaluated. More importantly, better insight into the biology of the disease is needed. The standardization of pathology has provided valuable prognostic information, but more refined prognostic and predictive markers, including molecular markers, are desperately needed.

REFERENCES

1. Engels EA. Epidemiology of thymoma and associated malignancies. *J Thorac Oncol.* 2010; 5: S260–S265.

2. World Health Organization Classification of Tumors. Pathology and genetics of tumours of the lung, pleura, thymus and heart. In Travis WD, Brambilla E, Muller-Hermelink HK, et al. (eds.). IARC Press, 2004, 341.

3. Chuah C, Lim TH, Lim AS, et al. Dasatinib induces a response in malignant thymoma. *J Clin Oncol.* 2006; 24: e56–e58.

4. Strobel P, Hartmann M, Jakob A, et al. Thymic carcinoma with over-expression of mutated KIT and the response to imatinib. *N Engl J Med.* 2004; 350: 2625–2626.

5. Strobel P, Hohenberger P, Marx A. Thymoma and thymic carcinoma: molecular pathology and targeted therapy. *J Thorac Oncol.* 2010; 5: S286–S290.

6. Evoli A, Minisci C, Di Schino C, et al. Thymoma in patients with MG: characteristics and long-term outcome. *Neurology.* 2002; 59: 1844–1850.

7. Curran WJ Jr, Kornstein MJ, Brooks JJ, et al. Invasive thymoma: the role of mediastinal irradiation following complete or incomplete surgical resection. *J Clin Oncol.* 1988; 6: 1722–1727.

8. Maggi G, Casadio C, Cavallo A, et al. Thymoma: results of 241 operated cases. *Ann Thorac Surg.* 1991; 51: 152–156.

9. Kondo K, Monden Y. Therapy for thymic epithelial tumors: a clinical study of 1,320 patients from Japan. *Ann Thorac Surg.* 2003; 76: 878–884; discussion 884–885.

10. Myojin M, Choi NC, Wright CD, et al. Stage III thymoma: pattern of failure after surgery and postoperative radiotherapy and its implication for future study. *Int J Radiat Oncol Biol Phys.* 2000; 46: 927–933.

11. Haniuda M, Morimoto M, Nishimura H, et al. Adjuvant radiotherapy after complete resection of thymoma. *Ann Thorac Surg.* 1992; 54: 311–315.

12. Ogawa K, Uno T, Toita T, et al. Postoperative radiotherapy for patients with completely resected thymoma: a multi-institutional, retrospective review of 103 patients. *Cancer.* 2002; 94: 1405–1413.

13. Strobel P, Bauer A, Puppe B, et al. Tumor recurrence and survival in patients treated for thymomas and thymic squamous cell carcinomas: a retrospective analysis. *J Clin Oncol.* 2004; 22: 1501–1509.

14. Wright CD, Kessler KA. Surgical treatment of thymic tumors. *Semin Thorac Cardiovasc Surg.* 2005; 17: 20–26.

15. Chen G, Marx A, Wen-Hu C, et al. New WHO histologic classification predicts prognosis of thymic epithelial tumors: a clinicopathologic study of 200 thymoma cases from China. *Cancer.* 2002; 95: 420–429.

16. Mornex F, Resbeut M, Richaud P, et al. Radiotherapy and chemotherapy for invasive thymomas: a multicentric retrospective review of 90 cases. The FNCLCC trialists. Federation Nationale des Centres de Lutte Contre le Cancer [erratum appears in *Int J Radiat Oncol Biol Phys*. 1995; 33: 545]. *Int J Radiat Oncol Biol Phys*. 1995; 32: 651–659.

17. Loehrer PJ Sr, Chen M, Kim K, et al. Cisplatin, doxorubicin, and cyclophosphamide plus thoracic radiation therapy for limited-stage unresectable thymoma: an intergroup trial. *J Clin Oncol*. 1997; 15: 3093–3099.

18. Kim ES, Putnam JB, Komaki R, et al. Phase II study of a multidisciplinary approach with induction chemotherapy, followed by surgical resection, radiation therapy, and consolidation chemotherapy for unresectable malignant thymomas: final report. *Lung Cancer*. 44: 369–379, 2004.

19. Bretti S, Berruti A, Loddo C, et al. Multimodal management of stages III-IVa malignant thymoma. *Lung Cancer*. 2004; 44: 69–77.

20. Venuta F, Rendina EA, Longo F, et al. Long-term outcome after multimodality treatment for stage III thymic tumors. *Ann Thorac Surg*. 2003; 76: 1866–1872; discussion 1872.

21. Palmieri G, Montella L, Martignetti A, et al. Somatostatin analogs and prednisone in advanced refractory thymic tumors. *Cancer*. 2002; 94: 1414–1420.

22. Loehrer PJ, Sr., Wang W, Johnson DH, et al. Octreotide alone or with prednisone in patients with advanced thymoma and thymic carcinoma: an Eastern Cooperative Oncology Group Phase II Trial [erratum appears in *J Clin Oncol*. 2004; 22: 2261]. *J Clin Oncol*. 2004; 22: 293–299.

23. Kurup A, Burns M, Dropcho S, et al. Phase II study of gefitinib treatment in advanced thymic malignancies. *J Clin Oncol*. 2005; 23: 381S. (abstract 7068).

24. Kelly RJ, Petrini I, Rajan A, et al. Thymic malignancies: form clinical management to targeted therapies. *J Clin Oncol*. 2011: 29: 4820–4827.

25. Fornasiero A, Daniele O, Ghiotto C, et al. Chemotherapy for invasive thymoma. A 13-year experience. *Cancer*. 1991; 68: 30–33.

26. Loehrer PJ Sr, Kim K, Aisner SC, et al. Cisplatin plus doxorubicin plus cyclophosphamide in metastatic or recurrent thymoma: final results of an intergroup trial. The Eastern Cooperative Oncology Group, Southwest Oncology Group, and Southeastern Cancer Study Group. *J Clin Oncol*. 1994; 12: 1164–1168.

27. Loehrer PJ Sr, Jiroutek M, Aisner S, et al. Combined etoposide, ifosfamide, and cisplatin in the treatment of patients with advanced thymoma and thymic carcinoma: an intergroup trial. *Cancer*. 2001; 91: 2010–2015.

28. Giaccone G, Ardizzoni A, Kirkpatrick A, et al. Cisplatin and etoposide combination chemotherapy for locally advanced or metastatic thymoma. A phase II study of the European Organization for Research and Treatment of Cancer Lung Cancer Cooperative Group. *J Clin Oncol*. 1996; 14: 814–820.

29. Lemma GL, Lee JW, Aisner SC, et al. Phase II study of carboplatin and paclitaxel in advanced thymoma and thymic carcinoma. *J Clin Oncol*. 2011; 29: 2060–2065.

CHAPTER **54**
Ovarian Cancer
Richard T. Penson

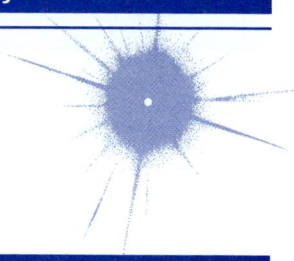

INTRODUCTION

Ovarian cancer remains the most lethal of gynecologic malignancies in developed countries. Initial management is aimed at maximal cytoreduction by surgery either before or after chemotherapy. Sequential palliative chemotherapy has enabled women to live with recurrent disease for years before suffering and dying with bowel obstruction. Despite advances, effective screening and cure remains elusive for most women.

INCIDENCE

Epithelial cancer of the ovary is the fifth most common tumor of women in the United States after cancer of the breast, colon, lung, and endometrium. It is the most lethal gynecologic malignancy, with approximately 22,240 cases and 14,030 deaths each year (1, 2). One in 70 of American women will develop ovarian cancer sometime during their lifetime. In premenopausal women ovarian cancer is uncommon and found in less than 5% of adnexal masses; indeed, only 30% of adnexal masses are malignant in postmenopausal women.

EPIDEMIOLOGY OF EPITHELIAL OVARIAN CANCER

The majority of ovarian cancer presents in postmenopausal women with only 10%–15% of cancers occurring in premenopausal patients. Median age at diagnosis is reported between 60 and 65 years. Possible risk factors identified in case controlled studies include white race, nulliparity, infertility, high fat diet, lactose, paracetamol, and asbestos contaminated talc. Oral contraceptives, pregnancy, tubal ligation, and lactation reduce the risk. The association with early menarche, late menopause, and nulliparity suggests that uninterrupted "incessant" ovulation may predispose to malignancy. The oral contraceptive pill may offer some protective benefit in preventing ovarian cancer in high-risk populations. However, hormone replacement therapy appears to double the risk of death from ovarian cancer. Initial reports of increased risks from fertility drugs have not been confirmed.

FAMILIAL OVARIAN CANCER

The vast majority of ovarian cancer is sporadic. However, a family history of ovarian cancer increases the risk of developing ovarian cancer two- to three-fold, and it is estimated that 5%–15% of all epithelial ovarian cancer cases result from inherited predisposition. Approximately 75% of these families

TABLE 54-1 GENETIC PREDISPOSITION SYNDROMES

Incidence	Lifetime Risk	Germline	Mutation
Sporadic	90% of ovarian cancer	1.4% lifetime	None
HBOC	10% of ovarian cancer	BRCA1 40%–60%	BRCA1 chromosome 17q
		BRCA2 15%–40%	BRCA2 chromosome 13q
HNPCC	Rare	3.5 × increase	MSH2, MLH1, PMS2

HBOC, hereditary breast ovarian cancer syndrome; HNPCC, hereditary non-polyposis colon cancer syndrome.

are linked to the breast ovarian cancer syndrome with loss of function of the tumor suppressor genes BRCA1 and BRCA2, involved in DNA repair, and inherited in an autosomally dominant fashion. Hereditary breast-ovarian cancer syndrome (HBOC) accounts for 65%–75% of all hereditary ovarian cancer cases, and is defined variably but typically with at least three cases of early onset (<60 years) breast or ovarian cancer. Mutations in BRCA1 (located on chromosome 17q) and BRCA2 (13q) are associated with a 40%–60% lifetime risk of ovarian cancer. The founder mutations 185delAG, and 5382insC in BRCA1, and 6174delT in BRCA2 are present in 2.5% of Ashkenazi women.

Hereditary non-polyposis colon cancer syndrome (HNPCC, Lynch syndrome [type II]) results from mismatch repair (MSH2, MLH1, and PMS2) gene defects, low penetrance allele, and modifier gene defects. The American founder mutation is deletion of exons 1–6 of MSH2. HNPCC accounts for approximately 10%–15% of all hereditary ovarian cancer cases. A diagnosis of HNPCC can be made using the Amsterdam Criteria (colon cancer diagnosis in ≥3 relatives, one of whom is a first-degree relative of the other two, and one diagnosis before age 50 years). The risk of developing ovarian cancer associated with HNPCC appears to be associated with an approximately 3.7-fold increase in lifetime risk of developing ovarian cancer. The inherited predisposition syndromes are summarized in Table 54-1.

Women from high-risk families should have genetic counseling and gene testing. At the present time a similar number of women elect biannual pelvic examinations, transvaginal ultrasound, and CA125 with no proven effect on mortality, as we have a prophylactic risk reducing salpingo-oophorectomy (RRSO), which reduces the lifetime risk of ovarian cancer by 95% (3).

BIOLOGY

Although commonly termed "epithelial," the embryologic origin of ovarian cancer is mesodermal, from the peritoneal surface of the ovary. Previously, subepithelial inclusion cysts that form after ovulation were thought to be the initial focus of dyplastic change, but compelling evidence points to the fimbria of the fallopian tube as the origin of perhaps 50% of tumors. Primary peritoneal and fallopian tube carcinomas (5%) are rare, and behave and are treated in an identical fashion.

Tumor cells predominantly spread transcelomically to the pelvic structures, exfoliating and following the circulation of the peritoneal fluid throughout the abdomen. Cells also metastasize by lymphatic and hematogenous routes. Extraperitoneal metastases are rare, but with increasing number of patients living for a protracted time, up to two-fifths of patients will develop metastases in the liver, lung, or the central nervous system during the later stages of their disease.

The majority of epithelial cancers are serous or papillary with a similar appearance to the lining of the fallopian tube (4, 5). Endometrioid carcinoma is associated with synchronous endometrial carcinoma and endometriosis, and therefore more commonly present early, and have a better prognosis. Clear cell tumors have a particularly poor prognosis, are commonly associated with thromboses, and have distinct genetics that link the disease with other clear cell tumors. Mucinous tumors are more commonly bilateral and can be associated with pseudomyxoma peritonei and mucocele of the appendix. Brenner's tumor has a histologic pattern similar to transitional cell carcinoma. Molecular evidence has confirmed that carcinosarcomas, previously called malignant mixed Müllerian tumors have a clonal proliferation of the epithelial element rather than being collision tumors and are treated as epithelial cancers. In women under the age of 40 years, but rarely in older patients, 60%–70% of non-benign ovarian neoplasms are borderline tumors, a neoplasm that has distinctly malignant cytological features without invasion. Ovarian tumor pathology is summarized in Table 54-2.

TABLE 54-2 OVARIAN CANCER PATHOLOGY

Histologic Subgroup	Histologic Subtype
Benign	Serous, mucinous
Epithelial ovarian cancer	Serous papillary (70%)
	Endometrioid (20%)
	Clear cell (10%)
	Mucinous (rare)
	Brenner (transitional cell)
	Carcinosarcoma or malignant mixed Müllerian tumor (MMMT)
Borderline	Tumor or low malignant potential (serous or mucinous)
sex cord-stromal	Granulosa
	Sertoli-Leydig
	Thecoma-fibroma
Germ cell	Dysgerminoma (female equivalent of seminoma)
	Benign or malignant teratoma
	Yolk sac, embryonal, and choriocarcinoma
Metastatic	Krukenberg's (breast, colorectal and gastric)

NON-EPITHELIAL OVARIAN MALIGNANCIES

Non-epithelial ovarian cancer accounts for <10% of ovarian tumors. The commonest of these, germ cell tumors represent almost 70% of ovarian tumors in the first two decades of life, with one-third of these being malignant. These rare tumors disseminate early and the doubling time of the tumor can be very short. The tumor markers βHCG and αFP are important in the treatment and surveillance of germ cell tumors. Dysgerminoma, essentially the female equivalent of testicular seminoma, is exquisitely sensitive to platinum, and this is now favored over the traditional treatment of radiotherapy. Teratoma is probably most effectively treated with combination platinum-based chemotherapy such as BEP (bleomycin, etoposide, and cisplatin) and surgical removal of residual masses. Yolk sac, embryonal, and choriocarcinoma subtypes are rarer, curable, and require specialized care.

Sex-cord-stromal tumors account for even fewer ovarian malignancies. Granulosa cell tumors are typically relatively low grade, secrete estrogen and in juveniles, tumors may be associated with pseudo-precocity. The tumors secrete estradiol, Müllerian inhibiting substance, and dimeric inhibin, which serve as tumor markers. Sertoli-Leydig tumors are associated with the production of androgens. Thecomas and fibromas are rare and non-functional tumors.

EPITHELIAL OVARIAN MALIGNANCIES

■ DIAGNOSIS

The presentation of ovarian cancer is typically subtle, persistent (>2 weeks) abdominal or pelvic pain; bloating, nausea, change in bowel habit, as well as urinary and constitutional symptoms are typical of peritoneal involvement by advanced disease while early stage ovarian cancer is generally asymptomatic (Table 54-3). Unfortunately, most symptomatic women do not have a prompt diagnosis, and indeed it is not uncommon for these women to be misdiagnosed with irritable bowel syndrome, hiatal hernia, diverticulosis, or endometriosis. Pelvic examination remains an essential part of the examination of women complaining of abdominal symptoms.

TABLE 54-3 CLASSICAL PRESENTATIONS

Late
Adnexal mass (solid, complex, elevated CA125)
Ascites
Pleural effusion, adnexal mass and adenocarcinoma of unknown primary
Screening
Sister Mary Joseph's nodule (umbilical metastasis)
Paraneoplastic syndrome: Trousseau's syndrome (thrombosis), cerebellar degeneration, dermatomyositis, Leser-Trélat (Seborrheic keratoses), palmer fasciitis
Krukenberg's tumor (breast, gastric, or colorectal primary)

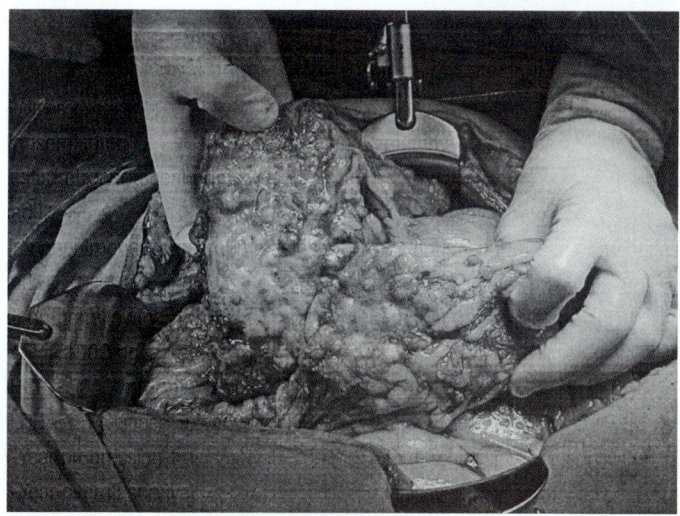

FIGURE 54-1 Advanced ovarian cancer. (Courtesy of Dr. Arlan Fuller.)

The diagnosis and initial management of ovarian cancer is surgical (Figure 54-1). Premenopausal women with a smooth, unilateral, mobile, cystic adnexal masses up to 8 cm can be managed conservatively with the use of oral contraceptives and serial ultrasound, typically performed at 6 weeks and at a different time of the menstrual cycle, as luteal cysts are common. In postmenopausal women, cystic masses larger than 5 cm in diameter warrant a tissue diagnosis. In postmenopausal women with a CA125 greater than 35 U/ml, adnexal masses are malignant in 80% of cases, although this should not be confused with the finding of a raised CA125 in an asymptomatic postmenopausal woman, as perhaps only 1 in 7 will have ovarian cancer. Occasionally there is uncertainty about the site of the primary and colonoscopy and mammography are appropriate. As early disease is typically asymptomatic, over 75% of tumors present as advanced stage disease (International Federation of Gynecology and Obstetrics [FIGO]) stage III/IV) (Table 54-4).

The surface glycoprotein CA125 (gene MUC-16) is found at elevated levels in the blood of >80% of patients with epithelial ovarian cancer (abnormal >35 u/ml) (6). CA125 is not useful in screening for occult carcinoma but can be used as a tumor marker. Human epididymis protein 4 (HE4) is another marker elevated in ovarian cancer and when both markers are elevated, adnexal masses are more often malignant. High levels of both markers are associated with disease bulk. Changes in levels correlate with response to therapy or disease progression. The OVA1™ diagnostic is the first FDA-approved blood test to evaluate the likelihood that an ovarian mass is malignant using 5 tumor markers including CA125.

The differential diagnosis of adnexal masses includes simple hemorrhagic physiologic cysts (follicular or corpus luteal); endometrioma; theca luteal

TABLE 54-4 OVARIAN CANCER STAGING (FIGO 1987)

Stage I: Limited to Ovaries (10%)	
IA	One ovary, no ascites, intact capsule, no tumor on external surface
IB	Both ovaries, no ascites, intact capsule, no tumor on external surface
IC	One or both ovaries with capsular involvement, ruptured capsule, ascites, or positive peritoneal washings
Stage II: Pelvic Extension (5%)	
IIA	To uterus or fallopian tubes
IIB	To other pelvic organs (e.g., bladder, rectum, or vagina)
IIC	Pelvic extension with factors as in IC
Stage III: Upper Abdominal Involvement and/or Positive Lymph Nodes (70%)	
IIIA	Microscopic seeding outside of abdominal peritoneum with negative lymph nodes
IIIB	Gross deposits less than 2 cm with negative lymph nodes
IIIC	Gross deposits greater than 2 cm and/or positive lymph nodes
Stage IV: Distant Metastases (pleural effusion, liver parenchyma, etc.) (15%)	

cysts; benign, malignant, or metastatic tumors; and extraovarian masses such as paraovarian or peritoneal cysts and pedunculated fibroids, extopic pregnancy, hydrosalpinx, tuboovarian, diverticular, or appendiceal abscesses.

SCREENING

Screening for ovarian cancer is an attractive proposition because of the significant morbidity and mortality associated with advanced disease, the availability of apparently sensitive and specific diagnostic tests (ultrasound and CA125), and the better outcome for patients with early-stage disease. However, there is no evidence at the present time that screening improves survival. The serum marker CA125 has been shown to be elevated in only 50% of patients with stage I disease, but in 90% of stage II–IV ovarian cancers. CA125 has a sensitivity of 20%–58% and a specificity of 97%–99%. With a 1/70 lifetime risk, ovarian cancer is present in 1/2000 postmenopausal women and therefore the false-positive rate (1%–3%) for CA125 is unacceptably high, given the morbidity of laparotomy. In the largest study reported to date in 21,935 UK postmenopausal healthy women, the death rate was apparently halved by screening (18 of 10,977 vs. 9 of 10,958). However, this was not statistically significant ($p = 0.083$), and the massive U.S. study, Prostate, Lung, Colorectal, and Ovary Cancer Screening Trial (PLCO), in 150,000 subjects failed to confirm a survival advantage, with a 15% serious complication rate from laparotomy (7). There continues to be speculation about whether the sensitivity of screening can be improved by the use of a panel of markers such as HE-4, ROCA (Risk of Ovarian Cancer Algorithm), which evaluates change in CA125 over time, or proteinomics. At the present time, screening is only recommended in high-risk populations (+ve family history or BRCA carriers), where prophylactic surgery has a far greater impact on the risk.

MANAGEMENT OF EARLY STAGE OVARIAN CANCER

Approximately 2000–3000 patients a year in the United States will have disease confined to pelvis. While this group accounts for only 15% of ovarian cancer cases, more than half of all cured patients come from this group. Adequate staging requires that a surgeon with subspeciality expertise perform an exploratory laparotomy, total abdominal hysterectomy and bilateral salpingo-oophorectomy, omentectomy, careful examination of the peritoneal surfaces of the liver, diaphragm, pericolic gutters, and pelvic sidewalls with multiple biopsies and sampling of ascitic fluid and peritoneal washings with para-aortic and pelvic lymph node sampling. Patients diagnosed with apparently early-stage ovarian cancer without adequate staging should undergo reexploration for definitive staging.

The overall 5-year survival of patients with apparent stage I epithelial cancer was about 60% in earlier reports. With accurate staging, and migration of patients with clinically occult nodal or omental metastases to stage III, survival of stage I patients is now commonly reported as ≥90%. Approximately 30%–46% of cancers that appear to be confined to the pelvis (stages I and II) have occult metastatic disease in the upper abdomen or lymph nodes (stage III). In patients with stage IA and IB disease of low grade (well differentiated), no adjuvant treatment is warranted. For all other patients with high-risk histology or grade, adjuvant treatment is recommended with platinum-based chemotherapy based on Gynecologic Oncology Group (GOG-95), International Collaboration in Ovarian Neoplasia (ICON I), and the European Organization for the Research and Treatment of Cancer (EORTCs) ACTION study (8).

GOG-157 compared 3 with 6 cycles of carboplatin and paclitaxel in early-stage disease. While more cycles were associated with more toxicity, there was a survival advantage in serous tumors and so most patients still receive 6 cycles of chemotherapy if tolerated.

MANAGEMENT OF ADVANCED STAGE OVARIAN CANCER

The principle of therapy for patients with advanced ovarian cancer is to cytoreduce (debulk) with surgery and chemotherapy to a state of minimal residual disease. For some patients this will translate into cure, but for the majority of patients, it delays symptomatic relapse. Current standard of care has been defined as cytoreductive surgery and 6 cycles of a taxane with either cisplatin or carboplatin chemotherapy. Five-year survival rates for patients treated with platinum-based regimens are approximately 20%–40%. Figure 54-2 illustrates a treatment algorithm for advanced ovarian cancer.

■ CYTOREDUCTIVE SURGERY

Meigs and Griffith are credited with the concept that successful surgical debulking to a residual tumor size of ≤1.5 cm maximum diameter results

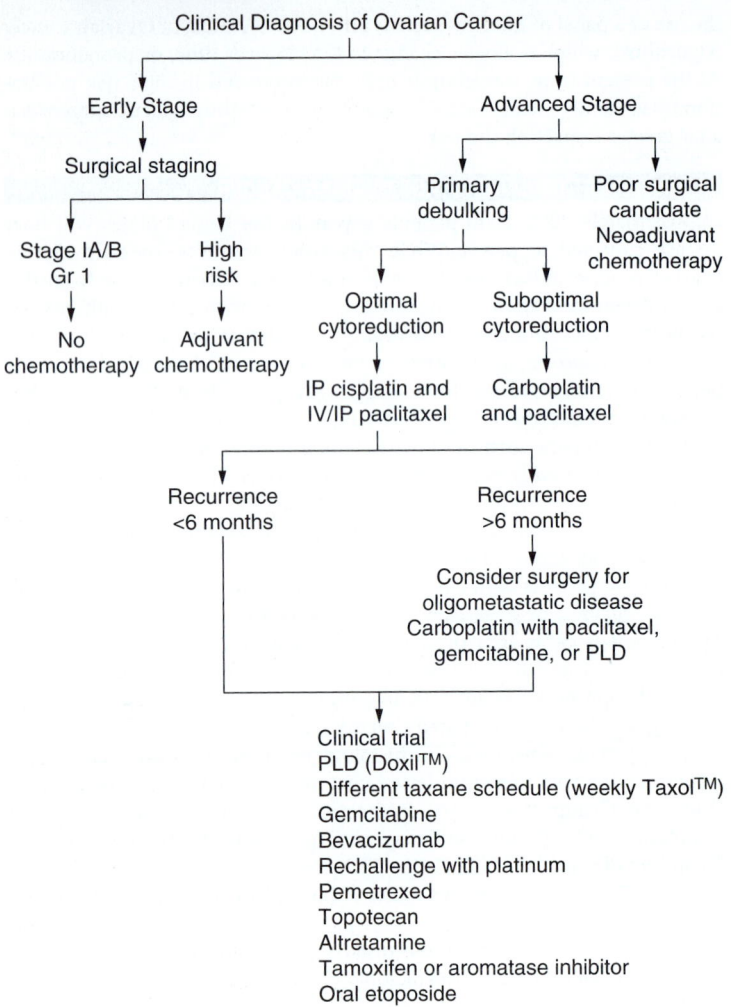

FIGURE 54-2 Treatment algorithm for ovarian cancer.

in superior survival, and that the volume left after surgery is more predictive of survival than the volume that enters the OR. More contemporary studies now strive for even smaller tumor volumes (<1 cm) called "optimal cytoreduction." Surgical cytoreduction has two main advantages. First, it improves physiology with the immediate correction of the functional disorders and pain associated with bowel and ureteral obstruction, also improving the profound protein loss associated with exudative ascites. Second, optimal debulking can remove 90% to many logs of tumor cells, thereby reducing the volume of residual disease to be treated by systemic or intraperitoneal chemotherapy.

In theory cytoreduction may remove de novo chemotherapy-resistant clones and facilitate drug delivery, having removed tumor with a compromised blood supply. Multiple retrospective studies have demonstrated that patients with tumors that can be cytoreduced to minimal residual disease survive longer. However, this may simply reflect the biology of the tumor.

Van der Burg reported a 33% reduction in the risk of death ($p = 0.008$) in a phase III study of interval cytoreduction (after #3 cycles of chemotherapy) in patients with initially suboptimally cytoreduced disease (>1 cm). However, this advantage cannot be replicated if the initial attempt at debulking was performed by a gynecologic oncologist who has already made a maximal attempt at cytoreduction (9). Standard of care is an attempt at debulking by a gynecologic oncologist in every patient with advanced disease.

◼ NEOADJUVANT CHEMOTHERAPY AND INTERVAL CYTOREDUCTIVE SURGERY

There is now level I evidence that supports equivalent survival and less morbidity when surgery is delayed until after #3 of primary or "neoadjuvant" chemotherapy. Vergote randomized 632 patients with bulky (>5 cm in 75% and >10 cm in 62%) stage IIIC or IV epithelial ovarian carcinoma, fallopian-tube carcinoma, or primary peritoneal carcinoma to primary debulking surgery followed by platinum-based chemotherapy or to neoadjuvant platinum-based chemotherapy followed by interval debulking surgery (10). Optimal debulking (to ≤1 cm) was achieved in 42% with primary debulking and in 82% at interval debulking. Postoperative rates of adverse effects and mortality were higher after primary debulking, but survival was the same in both groups ($p = 0.01$ for noninferiority). Complete resection of all macroscopic disease (at primary or interval surgery) was the strongest independent variable in predicting overall survival.

◼ FIRST-LINE CHEMOTHERAPY

Chemotherapy plays an essential role in advanced stage ovarian cancer. Over the last 40 years, tumor response rates (shrinkage of the tumor by more than 50%) have increased from the 20% range with single agent melphalan used in the 1970s to 75% in recent studies using platinum with a taxane. Although overall survival has improved very little, median survival time has significantly increased over the last few decades, and the overall median survival of patients with suboptimally debulked advanced stage disease has nearly tripled over the past quarter century, coincident with an almost fourfold improvement in chemotherapy response rates. While some of this benefit is certainly due to improvements in supportive care and improved surgical staging, the primary reason for this improvement is modern chemotherapy, which is both less toxic and more effective. Following the model of Hodgkin's disease, combination therapy logically followed single agent therapy with cyclophosphamide-based combinations, which produced response rates of approximately 35%. In the 1980s, cisplatin and subsequently carboplatin, non-classical alkylators, were demonstrated to have very significant activity in ovarian carcinoma with response rates of approximately 60%, thus redefining the combinations of chemotherapy used for advanced disease, with a significant survival advantage proven in 1986. Meta-analysis of randomized trials prior to 1991 concluded that cisplatin regimes were superior to non-cisplatin regimes, cisplatin combinations were superior to cisplatin alone, and cisplatin and carboplatin were equally effective.

Paclitaxel (Taxol™), initially derived from the Western Pacific yew tree (*Taxus brevofolia*), inhibits microtubule depolymerization and demonstrated significant activity in patients with ovarian cancer refractory to platinum chemotherapy. Following the introduction of pre-medication that prevented a hypersensitivity reaction, McGuire reported a response rate of 24% using paclitaxel in heavily pretreated patients whose tumors were resistant to platinum, and reported a substantial survival advantage replacing cyclophosphamide with paclitaxel, in 410 randomly assigned women with suboptimally debulked advanced ovarian cancer (GOG-111). Cisplatin 75 mg/m^2 and paclitaxel 135 mg/m^2 over 24 h was associated with more alopecia, neutropenia, fever, and allergic reactions, but improved median overall survival from 24 to 38 months ($p < 0.001$) (11). This result was confirmed by OV10, which also demonstrated that combining a 3-h infusion of 175 mg/m^2 paclitaxel with cisplatin produced unacceptable neurotoxicity. Two subsequent studies GOG-132 and ICON II suggested that platinum alone or sequential platinum and paclitaxel may be equally effective. The most common standard of care was defined in GOG-158, which compared cisplatin and paclitaxel with carboplatin and paclitaxel. Six cycles of carboplatin AUC 7.5 and paclitaxel 175 mg/m^2 over 3 h was a convenient outpatient regimen, which produced less gastrointestinal, renal, and metabolic toxicity, leukopenia, and a similar degree of peripheral neuropathy with a median overall survival of 57 months. As this regimen is associated with greater thrombocytopenia, the Area under the Concentration (AUC) Time Curve dosing, based on renal function, is now typically targeted at 5 or 6, and based on the Calvert formula (Total dose [mg] = target AUC [mg/ml/min] × [CrCl + 25] [ml/min]). Many studies have explored dose intensity as a strategy to improve outcomes, but moderate increases in platinum dose, even those that can be achieved by "high dose" chemotherapy, or more cycles of chemotherapy (10 vs. 5, or 12 vs. 6) do not improve survival.

The SCOTROC study demonstrated that docetaxel (Taxotere™) was significantly less neurotoxicity than paclitaxel and equally effective in combination with carboplatin, and is a valid but less used popular alternative to paclitaxel. Dose-dense paclitaxel (weekly therapy at 80 mg/m^2) with carboplatin is associated with more anemia but has been reported to improve overall survival, and confirmatory studies are ongoing. Adding agents or replacing paclitaxel with pegylated liposomally encapsulated doxorubicin (Doxil™), gemcitabine, or topotecan as first-line therapy has been widely investigated but have not improved cure rates.

■ CONSOLIDATION

In patients with suboptimally debulked disease, who are destined to have relapse, maintenance therapy is a rational strategy. GOG-178 compared monthly paclitaxel for 3 months to the same treatment for 12 months. Time to recurrence was delayed by 7 months with longer duration maintenance but the regimen had excess neurotoxicity. Consolidation with other agents such as topotecan have been shown not to improve survival.

GOG-218 and ICON-7 investigated the integration of bevacizumab (Avastin™) in the upfront treatment of advanced ovarian cancer administered with carboplatin and paclitaxel and as consolidation. Bevacizumab is a particularly promising agent as the response rate is highest in recurrent ovarian cancer compared with any other solid tumor. GOG-218 demonstrated a 3.8-month improvement in PFS, while the European study ICON-7, which had a similar design, reported a PFS of only 1.7 months, suggesting an overall survival in "high-risk" patients, although this remains a very controversial strategy (12, 13).

■ INTRAPERITONEAL CHEMOTHERAPY

One way to achieve high concentrations of cytotoxics is regional administration. Intraperitoneal (IP) infusion lends itself to this approach with a very high ratio of IP drug concentration that bathes the tumor compared with systemic concentrations (platinum 10×, paclitaxel 1000×).

Alberts initially reported a randomized trial of cyclophosphamide intravenously with either intraperitoneal or intravenous cisplatin (GOG-104), with an 8-month median survival advantage. Markman reported a second phase III study (GOG-114), which included intravenous paclitaxel with intraperitoneal cisplatin, but also included two initial cycles of moderate dose carboplatin as "medical" cytoreduction. The survival was extended 11 months but at a cost of greater toxicity. The third study (GOG-172) led to an NCI alert about the potential advantage of intraperitoneal therapy in patients with optimally debulked ovarian cancer because of an unprecedented 16-month, the longest ever reported, survival advantage (14). Armstrong's regimen of paclitaxel 135 mg/m^2 over a 24-h period (to reduce neurotoxicity) followed by intraperitoneal cisplatin 100 mg/m^2 on day 2 with intraperitoneal paclitaxel 60 mg/m^2 on day 8 given every 3 weeks for 6 cycles was associated with more fatigue, hematologic, gastrointestinal, metabolic, and neurologic toxicity, with significantly worse quality of life, but an improvement in median duration of overall survival from 50 to 66 months ($p = 0.03$). The biggest concerns are about catheter complications (infection, pain, and blockage), which are serious in a quarter of patients and prevented 58% of patients completing intraperitoneal therapy in GOG-172. Uptake of IP therapy has been dependent on local expertise.

RECURRENT DISEASE

The majority of patients who achieve a complete remission with first-line platinum-based chemotherapy will ultimately develop recurrent disease. Recurrent ovarian cancer is often considered a chronic disease, since active chemotherapy agents allow patients to live for years with their disease, and quality of life is one of the most important considerations. The definition of relapse is important as a rising CA125 typically has a lead-time of 2–6 months before symptoms develop. Patients with an asymptomatic rising marker can be managed expectantly, as palliative chemotherapy has toxicities. Rustin randomized clinicians and 529 patients to follow up with access to, or blinded to, CA125, and an elevation in marker led to treatment 5 months earlier that did not impact overall survival but did compromise quality of life (15). Treating an asymptomatic patient with a rising CA125 is too early, and waiting until they have bulk disease (>5 cm), which is associated with a poorer response to chemotherapy, may be too late.

The most important factor associated with poor prognosis at time of relapse is a short disease- and platinum-free interval. Platinum-resistant disease is arbitrarily defined as disease that relapses within 6 months of platinum, and platinum-sensitive disease after more than 6 months. Two-thirds of recurrences in the United States fall into this group; localized (oligometastatic on PET/CT scan) disease may be appropriate for surgery, which is being evaluated in GOG-213 and DESKTOP-III, and the role of surgery for recurrence remains controversial.

Rechallenge with a platinum-based combination is appropriate with a platinum-free interval of at least 6 months or a year. ICON 4 (carboplatin and paclitaxel) demonstrated an 18% reduction in risk of death (an absolute difference in 2-year survival of 7% [57 vs. 50%], $p = 0.02$) (16). Meanwhile, the CALYPSO study (carboplatin and pegylated liposomally encapsulated doxorubicin [PLD or Doxil™]) and the AGO studies (carboplatin and gemcitabine) reported only PFS survivals. Concurrent bevacizumab with carboplatin and gemcitabine, followed by consolidation bevacizumab, in the OCEANS study was associated with a particularly long PFS advantage, but it is not clear that this will translate into a survival advantage.

The role of bevacizumab is controversial with no clearly proven survival advantage. However, bevacizumab is very effective against ascites. Toxicities in patients with recurrent disease have included hypertension, proteinuria, as well as arterial thromboses, and one study was halted with 5 of 44 patients developing bowel perforations. Bevacizumab is commonly given as monotherapy or in combination with weekly paclitaxel or metronomic low-dose oral cyclophosphamide.

Subsequent recurrences are typically treated with sequential single agent palliative chemotherapy. There are many options such as pegylated liposomally encapsulated doxorubicin hydrochloride (PLD or Doxil™), topotecan, a different taxane schedule (weekly Taxol™), rechallenge with platinum, gemcitabine, altretamine, or oral etoposide. Hormonal therapy, often tamoxifen, can be effective in ER +ve tumors. Many patients are appropriate for clinical trials, and an exciting number of agents are being investigated.

Obstructive symptoms typically herald the last chapter of patients' lives. The constellation of difficult-to-treat symptoms requires multiprofessional care. Surgery should be limited to patients with chemotherapy-responsive disease, and for others a gastric venting tube (G-tube) alleviates vomiting. Total parenteral nutrition does not substantially alter the clinical course. Steroids and Otreotide™ may provide symptom relief. Attending to end of life issues is a vital part of holistic care.

TABLE 54-5 NOVEL THERAPIES IN CLINICAL TRIALS FOR EPITHELIAL OVARIAN CANCER

Class	Targets	Examples
PARP inhibitor	BER	Olaparib
		Veliparib (ABT-888)
Antiangiogenic	VEGF	Bevacizumab (Avastin™)
	VEGFR-2	Pazopanib (Votrient™)
		Trebananib
	Angiopoietins	AMG-386
Minor groove binder	DNA	Trabectedin (Yondelis™)
Monoclonal antibodies	EpCAM and CD-3	Catumaxomab (Removab™)
	Folate Receptor	Farletuzumab (MORAb-003)
	HER2/neu	Pertuzumab (Omnitarg™)
	EGFR	Cetuximab (Erbitux™)
Small molecule	PIK3CA	BYL-719
	AKT	MK-2206
	Aurora Kinase	MLN-8237
	BRAF	AZD-6244 (Selumetinib™)
	MEK	GDC-0973
	mTOR	Everolimus (Afinitor™)
Vaccines		Polyvalent, NY-ESO-1, ICT-140
CAM		Acupuncture, Flaxseed

◼ NOVEL APPROACHES

Genetic abnormalities underlie the development and progression of cancer. Tumors are increasingly recategorized by gene mutation or pathway activation, such as *BRAF* in low-grade serous tumors, which when treated with targeted therapy may be associated with better outcomes than chemotherapy. Patients with inherited BRCA mutations have "synthetic lethality" in that further inhibition of DNA repair with a PARP inhibitor triggers apoptosis and a response in approximately a third of these tumors. *PIK3CA* looks to be an important target in clear cell and endometrioid tumors. Table 54-5 lists some exciting new agents in late stages of development, with the hope that the impact of novel biologics will more than match the improvement in outcomes with radical surgery and the introduction of platinum.

PROGNOSIS

With modern surgical cytoreduction followed by as little as 18 weeks of chemotherapy, overall survival rates at 5 years exceed 40%. Stage, grade, histologic subtype, age, and whether the patient can be optimally surgically cytoreduced predict prognosis. Although the ultimate long-term prognosis

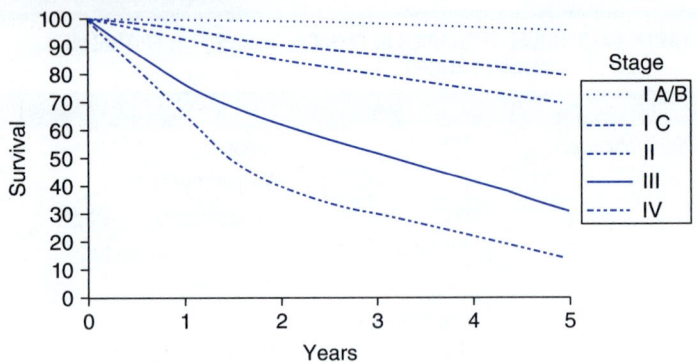

FIGURE 54-3 Overall survival for patients with ovarian cancer.

TABLE 54-6 KEY POINTS

1. The presentation of ovarian cancer is often subtle.

2. A strong family history of breast or ovarian cancer should prompt consideration of gene testing and risk reducing salpingo-oophorectomy.

3. Surgical staging and cytoreduction is essential in the successful management of ovarian cancer and should be undertaken by a trained Gynecologic Oncologist.

4. Combination taxane and platinum chemotherapy is standard and should be delivered intraperitoneally in patients with optimally cytoreduced disease.

5. Chemotherapy provides effective palliation with an increasing number of therapeutic options.

---

of patients with advanced disease remains poor, current therapy often provides excellent palliation for these women for many years (Table 54-6). Figure 54-3 illustrates the overall survival of patients with ovarian cancer.

REFERENCES

1. Cannistra S, McGuire W. Progress in the management of gynecologic cancer. *J Clin Oncol.* 2007: 2865–2866.

2. Siegel R, Naishadham D, Jemal A. Cancer statistics, 2013. *CA Cancer J Clin.* 2013; 63: 11–30.

3. Kauff ND, Satagopan JM, Robson ME, et al. Risk-reducing salpingo-oophorectomy in women with a BRCA1 or BRCA2 mutation. *N Engl J Med.* 2002; 346: 1609–1615.

4. Levanon K, Crum C, Drapkin R. New insights into the pathogenesis of serous ovarian cancer and its clinical impact. *J Clin Oncol.* 2008; 26: 5284–5293.

5. Young RH, Scully RE. Differential diagnosis of ovarian tumors based primarily on their patterns and cell types. *Semin Diagn Pathol.* 2001; 18: 161–235.

6. Bast RC Jr, Klug TL, St John E, et al. A radioimmunoassay using a monoclonal antibody to monitor the course of epithelial ovarian cancer. *N Engl J Med.* 1983; 309: 883–887.

7. Buys SS, Partridge E, Black A, et al. Effect of screening on ovarian cancer mortality: the Prostate, Lung, Colorectal and Ovarian (PLCO) Cancer Screening Randomized Controlled Trial. *JAMA.* 2011; 305: 2295–2303.

8. Colombo N, Guthrie D, Chiari S, et al. International Collaborative Ovarian Neoplasm trial 1: a randomized trial of adjuvant chemotherapy in women with early-stage ovarian cancer. *J Natl Cancer Inst.* 2003; 95: 125–132.

9. van der Burg ME, van Lent M, Buyse M, et al. The effect of debulking surgery after induction chemotherapy on the prognosis in advanced epithelial ovarian cancer. Gynecological Cancer Cooperative Group of the European Organization for Research and Treatment of Cancer. *N Engl J Med.* 1995; 332: 629–634.

10. Vergote I, Trope CG, Amant F, et al. Neoadjuvant chemotherapy or primary surgery in stage IIIC or IV ovarian cancer. *N Engl J Med.* 2010; 363: 943–953.

11. McGuire WP, Hoskins WJ, Brady MF, et al. Cyclophosphamide and cisplatin compared with paclitaxel and cisplatin in patients with stage III and stage IV ovarian cancer. *N Engl J Med.* 1996; 334: 1–6.

12. Burger RA, Brady MF, Bookman MA, et al. Incorporation of bevacizumab in the primary treatment of ovarian cancer. *N Engl J Med.* 2011; 365: 2473–2483.

13. Perren TJ, Swart AM, Pfisterer J, et al. A phase 3 trial of bevacizumab in ovarian cancer. *N Engl J Med.* 2011; 365: 2484–2496.

14. Armstrong DK, Bundy B, Wenzel L, et al. Intraperitoneal cisplatin and paclitaxel in ovarian cancer. *N Engl J Med.* 2006; 354: 34–43.

15. Rustin GJ, van der Burg ME, Griffin CL, et al. Early versus delayed treatment of relapsed ovarian cancer (MRC OV05/EORTC 55955): a randomised trial. *Lancet.* 2010; 376: 1155–1163.

16. Parmar MK, Ledermann JA, Colombo N, et al. Paclitaxel plus platinum-based chemotherapy versus conventional platinum-based chemotherapy in women with relapsed ovarian cancer: the ICON4/AGO-OVAR-2.2 trial. *Lancet.* 2003; 361: 2099–2106.

CHAPTER **55**

Primary Squamous Carcinoma of the Uterine Cervix: Diagnosis and Management

Olivia Foley, Marcela G. del Carmen

INTRODUCTION

Squamous cell carcinoma of the uterine cervix comprises an estimated 80% of all cervical cancers. The other histologies include adenocarcinoma (15%) and adenosquamous carcinomas (3%–5%), with only a small fraction of all cervical cancers having neuroendocrine or small cell histology. This chapter will focus on the diagnosis and management of primary squamous cell carcinoma of the uterine cervix. Amongst all malignancies, cervical cancer is the second most common cancer affecting women, with an estimated 52% case-fatality rate (1). Worldwide, cervical cancer is the most common gynecologic malignancy, accounting for 529,800 new cases (9%) and 273,200 deaths (8%) (1, 2). In developed countries, cervical cancer ranked tenth most common type of cancer in women (9.0/100,000 women) and below the top 10 causes of cancer mortality (3.2/100,000 deaths) (3). An estimated 86% of new cervical cancer cases are seen in the developing world, ranking as the second most common type of cancer (17.8/100,000 women) and cause of cancer deaths (99.8/100,000 deaths) (3). The highest incidence rates worldwide are observed in sub-Saharan Africa, Latin America and the Caribbean, South-Central Asia, and Southeast Asia (1). One-third of the cervical cancer burden in the world is experienced in South-Central Asia. Lastly, although cervical cytology is an excellent screening instrument for pre-invasive disease, the false negative rate for detecting invasive carcinoma is relatively high, reportedly 50%.

■ INCIDENCE

The incidence of invasive cervical cancer is related to age, with a mean age at the time of diagnosis of 48 years in the United States (3). The reported age-adjusted incidence of cervical cancer in the United States in girls under 20 years of age is 0.1 per 100,000, 1.5 per 100,000 in women aged 20–24 years, and 11.0 per 100,000 for women aged 30 to over 85 years (3).

■ EPIDEMIOLOGY

Patients with squamous cell carcinoma of the cervix share the same risk factors as patients with cervical intraepithelial neoplasia or dysplasia (4). These factors include:

- Early onset of sexual activity
- Multiple sexual partners
- High-risk sexual partners

- History of sexually transmitted diseases
- Tobacco use
- Multiparity
- Low socioeconomic status
- Immunosuppression
- Previous history of vulvar or vaginal dysplasia

Perhaps the most significant risk factor for developing squamous cell cervical cancer is lack of cervical cytological screening. It is critical to underscore that infection with certain subtypes of the human papillomavirus (HPV) has been identified as the central causative factor in the development of cervical neoplasia (4). High-risk oncogenic types can be detected in almost all cervical cancers (4). Although most HPV infections are transient, chronic persistent HPV infection with the oncogenic subtypes is the central causative factor in the development of cervical neoplasia. The virus alone, however, is not sufficient to cause cervical neoplasia or cancer (4).

CLINICAL MANIFESTATIONS

■ SYMPTOMS

Because early cervical cancer is usually asymptomatic, screening is critical. Common symptoms, when they occur, include abnormal vaginal bleeding, bleeding after intercourse, and a vaginal discharge (watery, mucoid, malodorous, or even purulent). In the setting of advanced disease, patients may complain of back pain radiating to the lower extremities or pelvic pain. Other symptoms seen in the setting of advanced disease include bowel and urinary symptoms, such as hematuria, hemotochezia, or stool/urine passage *per* vagina.

■ PHYSICAL EXAMINATION

Findings at the time of physical examination may range from a normal appearing cervix to a grossly abnormal cervix with an exophytic, plaque-like, indurated, ulcerated, or endophytic lesion. Findings encountered in patients with regionally advanced stage disease include parametrial, paracervical, or vaginal involvement, lower extremity edema, and inguinal adenopathy. Distant disease may be manifest in ascites, pleural effusions, and supraclavicular adenopathy.

PATTERNS OF SPREAD

Squamous cell carcinoma of the cervix may spread via direct extension as well as lymphatic and hematogenous dissemination. It can spread directly to the parametria, uterine corpus, vagina, bladder, rectum, and peritoneal cavity. Although prior dictum described a predictable pattern of lymphatic spread, sentinel node mapping has demonstrated that the first site of metastasis may involve any one of the pelvic lymph node chains.

DIAGNOSIS

Squamous cell carcinoma of the uterine cervix is staged clinically based on the criteria delineated by the International Federation of Gynecology and Obstetrics (FIGO). Table 55-1 reflects the staging FIGO changes made in 2009.

TABLE 55-1 STAGING OF CERVICAL CANCER BASED ON CRITERIA FROM THE INTERNATIONAL FEDERATION OF GYNECOLOGY AND OBSTETRICS (FIGO)

IA_1 Confined to the cervix, diagnosed only by microscopy with invasion of <3 mm in depth and lateral spread <7 mm
IA_2 Confined to the cervix, diagnosed with microscopy with invasion of >3 mm and < 5 mm with lateral spread <7 mm
IB_1 Clinically visible lesion or greater than A_2, <4 cm in greatest dimension
IB_2 Clinically visible lesion, >4 cm in greatest dimension
IIA_1 Involvement of the upper two-thirds of the vagina, without parametrial invasion, <4 cm in greatest dimension
IIA_2 >4 cm in greatest dimension
IIB With parametrial involvement
IIIA Extension to the distal 1/3 of the vagina
IIIB Sidewall extension, hydronephrosis, or non-functioning kidney
IVA Extension to bladder/rectal mucosa[a]
IVB Distant metastasis

[a]Bullous edema alone is not sufficient.

■ CLINICAL STAGING PROCEDURES

After histological confirmation of an invasive cancer, a thorough physical examination is mandated. This survey should include careful inspection of the cervix, assessment of its size, and careful examination of the entire vagina. Cervical tumor size and parametrial involvement are best evaluated through a rectovaginal examination. The inguinal and supracervical regions should be inspected for the presence of adenopathy. It is reasonable to arrange for an examination under anesthesia in order to better appreciate the extent of local disease and to facilitate patient comfort. The following studies and procedures are allowed by FIGO as part of the staging of cervical cancer:

- Chest x-ray
- Intravenous pyelogram
- Barium enema
- Skeletal x-rays
- Colposcopy/biopsies
- Cervical conization
- Cystoscopy
- Proctoscopy

Other optional studies and procedures that can be obtained, but cannot alter FIGO staging, include the following:

- Computed tomography
- Magnetic resonance imaging
- Positron emission tomography (PET)

TABLE 55-2 FIVE-YEAR SURVIVAL FOR SQUAMOUS CELL CARCINOMA OF THE UTERINE CERVIX BASED ON FIGO STAGING

FIGO Stage	5-Year Survival
IA	98%
IB_1	90%
IB_2	80%
IIA	73%
IIB	67%
IIIA	45%
IIIB	36%
IVA	4%

Adapted from information contained in Reference 5.

- Ultrasonography
- Radionucleotide scanning
- Laparoscopy
- Laparotomy

■ PROGNOSIS

Prognosis for squamous cell carcinoma of the uterine cervix is influenced by numerous tumor-related factors, including stage, tumor volume, depth of invasion, lymph node involvement, lymph-vascular space involvement, histologic subtype, and tumor grade. FIGO tumor stage correlates well with 5-year survival (Table 55-2) (5). Lymph nodal status is also an important prognostic factor. Five-year survival in the presence of pelvic lymph node involvement is 45%–60% (6). Five-year survival in the setting of para-aortic lymph node involvement is estimated to be 15%–30% (7). The number of involved lymph nodes also plays a critical role. In the presence of one involved pelvic lymph node, the recurrence risk in 35% (7). When 2 or 3 pelvic lymph nodes are involved, the risk of recurrence is 59% and 69%, respectively (7).

TREATMENT

Treatment options for squamous cell carcinoma of the uterine cervix include surgery, chemoradiation therapy, and chemotherapy. Both surgical intervention and definitive radiation therapy with concomitant chemotherapy are appropriate alternatives for the treatment of early stage cervical cancer, including FIGO stage IIA (8).

■ SURGERY

For women with stage IA_1 lesions, surgical treatment may be in the form of a loop electrosurgical excision procedure (LEEP) or cervical conization (if they desire to preserve fertility) or an extrafascial hysterectomy (8). For certain selected patients who want to preserve fertility and with stage IA_2/IB_1 lesions, a radical trachelectomy with lymphadenectomy may be an alternative to a radical hysterectomy. A radical trachelectomy involves removal of the entire cervix and the parametria, with placement of a cerclage in order to allow preservation of the uterine corpus with a competent vaginal-uterine junction (8). The radical trachelectomy can be performed abdominally or vaginally, and combined with a laparoscopic or open therapeutic lymphadenectomy. The radical trachelectomy appears to be a reasonable alternative for women with stage IA_2/IB_1 lesions desiring fertility preservation with tumors less than 2 cm in size, absence of lymph vascular space involvement, and absence of lymph nodal disease. The experience with this procedure indicates that it results in a similar oncologic outcome as a radical hysterectomy but allows for the possibility of future pregnancies.

For patients with stage IA_2 lesions, surgical treatment may be in the form of a type II or modified hysterectomy (8). During this type of hysterectomy, the uterine artery is ligated where it crosses over the ureter, the uterosacral and the cardinal ligaments are divided midway toward their attachment to the sacrum and the pelvic side wall, respectively, and the upper one-third of the vagina is resected. For stage IB_1, IB_2, and IIA lesions, the recommended surgical treatment is a type III or radical hysterectomy. During this procedure, the uterine artery is ligated at its origin from the internal iliac artery. The uterosacral and the cardinal ligaments are divided at their insertion into the sacrum and the pelvic sidewall, respectively, and the upper one-half of the vagina is divided.

In premenopausal women, surgery, as compared to radiation therapy as the alternative treatment modality, offers the advantage of ovarian preservation and may avoid vaginal stenosis. It also allows for "debulking" of enlarged lymph nodes and may allow for the individualization and tailoring of the radiation treatment fields.

Part of the surgical treatment of cervical cancer for stage IA_2-IIA includes a lymphadenectomy. For women with stage IA_2 and small IB_1 tumors, a pelvic lymphadenectomy should be performed at the time of hysterectomy (8). For those with enlarged lymph nodes, macroscopic stage IB_1, IB_2, or IIA tumors, or those with histologic confirmation of metastatic nodal disease at the time of frozen section, the surgical intervention should include both a pelvic and para-aortic lymphadenectomy.

■ PRIMARY RADIATION THERAPY

Since the oncologic results are similar, radical surgery and definitive radiation therapy are acceptable treatment modalities for stage IA, IB, and non-bulky IIA lesions (8). For women undergoing definitive treatment with radiation therapy, the use of concomitant cisplatin-based chemotherapy is also recommended. The progression-free survival and overall survival advantage of concomitant chemoradiotherapy over radiation alone in patients with early and locally advanced cervical cancer has been demonstrated in at least five randomized, controlled clinical trials and a meta-analysis.

Radiation therapy can be delivered in the form of external beam radiation or brachytherapy. Brachytherapy allows for treatment of centrally located disease, primarily the cervix, the vagina, and the parametria. It can be delivered via an intracavitary or interstitial needle system. The intracavitary systems include uterine tandems, vaginal colpostats, and vaginal cylinders. External beam radiation therapy involves radiation of the entire pelvis, with doses ranging from 4500 to 5000 cGy, given in daily fractions over several weeks (usually 180 cGy/fraction). As noted earlier, radiation therapy is administered with concomitant chemotherapy using cisplatin (40 mg/m^2/ week) (8). In a recent study of patients with bulky stage IIB to IVA, a novel regimen of concurrent cisplatin plus gemcitabine with radiation therapy followed by brachytherapy and adjuvant gemcitabine plus cisplatin significantly improved outcomes, with notable increased but acceptable toxicity, when compared to standard cisplatin-based chemoradiation therapy (9).

■ ADJUVANT CHEMORADIOTHERAPY

Patients with localized cervical cancer treated primarily with surgery and who have tumors with either intermediate- or high-risk factors for disease recurrence should receive adjuvant chemoradiotherapy (10). High-risk factors include positive or close resection margins, positive lymph nodes, and microscopic parametrial involvement (10). Intermediate-risk factors for disease recurrence include tumor size, deep stromal invasion, or the presence of lymph vascular space involvement (10). The recommended regimen includes radiation therapy with the use of concomitant cisplatin (40 mg/m^2/ week) (8, 10, 11).

POST-TREATMENT SURVEILLANCE

After completion of their treatment plan, patients should be evaluated every 3 months for the first 2 years, every 6 months for the subsequent 3 years, and annually thereafter. Evaluation should include a thorough review of systems and physical examination and a Pap smear at the time of each surveillance visit. Most vaginal recurrences are asymptomatic and may be only recognized through a Pap smear. For women with stage IIB or greater, an annual chest x-ray is recommended. Any palpable mass needs to be biopsied to rule out the presence of recurrent disease.

CONCLUSIONS

Squamous cell cancer of the cervix is staged clinically and can be treated through primary surgical therapy or radiation therapy with concomitant chemotherapy. The choice of treatment modality depends on numerous factors including the patient's general condition, stage of disease, and desire for fertility preservation. stage IA$_1$ tumors may be treated with a cervical conization or LEEP or with an extrafascial hysterectomy. Stage IA$_2$ lesions may be treated with a modified radical hysterectomy and pelvic lymphadenectomy. The surgical treatment of choice for stage IB$_1$, IB$_2$, and small IIA lesions is a radical hysterectomy with a pelvic lymphadenectomy. Chemoradiation therapy may be offered to these patients instead of primary surgical therapy. Patients with stage IIB-IV disease should be treated with chemoradiation therapy. It is estimated that approximately 50% of recurrences from squamous cell carcinoma of the cervix occur within a year of completing treatment. Treatment options for recurrent disease depend on the modality of therapy utilized in the primary setting. Women treated surgically may be candidates for radiation therapy or systemic chemotherapy.

Women treated initially with chemoradiation may be candidates for surgical resection or systemic chemotherapy at the time of disease recurrence. The choice of surgical treatment in the recurrent setting is generally limited to those women who are candidates for exenterative surgery. These patients are limited to those who have a central recurrence following primary treatment, in the absence of distant metastasis.

REFERENCES

1. Ferlay J, Shin HR, Bray F, et al. GLOBOCAN 2008 v1.2, Cancer Incidence and Mortality Worldwide: IARC CancerBase No. 10 [Internet] Lyon, France: International Agency for Research on Cancer, 2010. Available from: http://globocan.iarc.fr. Accessed February 8, 2012.

2. Jemal A, Bray F, Center MM, et al. Global cancer statistics. *CA Cancer J Clin.* 2011; 61: 69–90.

3. Ries LAG, Melbert D, Krapcho M, et al. *SEER Cancer Statistics Review, 1975-2004.* National Cancer Institute; Bethesda, MD. 2007; 2: 302–316.

4. Castle PE, Wacholder S, Lorincz AT, et al: A prospective study of high-grade cervical neoplasia risk among human papillomavirus-infected women. *J Natl Cancer Inst.* 2002; 94: 1406–1414.

5. Benedet JL, Odicino F, Maisonneuve P, et al . Carcinoma of the cervix uteri. *J Epidemiol Biostat.* 2001; 6: 7–43.

6. Averette HE, Nguyen HN, Donato DM, et al. Radical hysterectomy for invasive cervical cancer: a 25-year prospective experience with the Miami technique. *Cancer.* 1993; 71: 1422–1437.

8. Tanaka Y, Sawada S, Murata T. Relationship between lymph node metastases and prognosis in patients irradiated postoperatively for carcinoma of the uterine cervix. *Acta Radiol Oncol.* 1984; 23: 455–459.

9. Committee on Practice Bulletins-Gynecology. Diagnosis and treatment of cervical carcinomas, number 35, May 2002. *Obstet Gynecol.* 2002; 99: 855–867.

10. Duenas-Gonzalez JJ, Zarba JC, Alcedo P, et al. A Phase III study comparing concurrent gemcitabine (Gem) plus cisplatin (Cis) and radiation followed by adjuvant Gem plus Cis versus concurrent Cis and radiation in patients with stage IIB to IVA carcinoma of the cervix. *J Clin Oncol.* 2009; 27: 18s.

11. Peters WA III, Liu PY, Barrett RJ II, et al . Concurrent chemotherapy and pelvic radiation therapy compared with pelvic radiation therapy alone as adjuvant therapy after radical surgery in high-risk early-stage cancer of the cervix. *J Clin Oncol.* 2000; 18: 1606–1613.

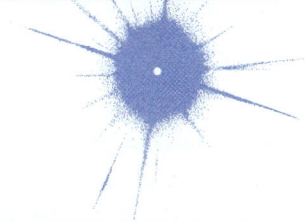

CHAPTER **56**
Uterine Cancer
Don S. Dizon

INCIDENCE

Each year, over 49,000 women are diagnosed with uterine cancer, and approximately 8000 women succumb to the disease (1). The vast majority of uterine tumors are adenocarcinomas. Less than 5% of these are uterine sarcomas.

ENDOMETRIAL ADENOCARCINOMA

■ EPIDEMIOLOGY

Endometrial adenocarcinoma is more commonly diagnosed among older women with the peak incidence occurring in the sixth decade of life. It is also more commonly diagnosed in white women compared to non-white women. These cancers can be broadly categorized into two types based on clinical and pathologic factors (2):

- **Type I** endometrial carcinomas follow an estrogen-dependent pathway. The precursor lesion is atypical hyperplasia. These tumors comprise the majority of endometrial cancers, are limited to the uterus, and have a favorable prognosis.
- **Type II** endometrial carcinomas appear to develop independent of estrogen exposure. They occur more frequently among black women and arise in a background of atrophic endometrium. Compared to type I endometrial cancers, women tend to be diagnosed at an older age and at a later stage. They also confer a poorer overall prognosis.

■ RISK FACTORS

Risk factors for the development of type I endometrial cancer include states related to excess estrogen stimulation. This includes nulliparity, unopposed estrogen administration, tamoxifen exposure, polycystic ovarian syndrome, and obesity. Higher parity, smoking, and use of estrogen-progestin hormonal contraception are known to decrease risk. In contrast, specific risk factors for type II endometrial cancer have not been identified.

Genetic factors contribute to only about 10% of endometrial cancers, mostly due to hereditary nonpolyposis colorectal cancer (HNPCC), also known as Lynch syndrome, and, to a lesser degree, Cowden syndrome. Both of these genetic conditions follow autosomal dominant inheritance patterns. While it is not clear if individuals with BRCA 1 and 2 mutations have increased risk, there does seem to be higher risk for patients with breast cancer, perhaps because of shared risk factors.

■ PATHOGENESIS

There is no single molecular event that gives rise to endometrial cancer. However, type I and type II endometrial carcinomas are associated with distinct molecular changes: type I endometrial adenocarcinomas are associated with mutations involving the PTEN pathway or show evidence of microsatellite instability (3). Type II tumors are associated with p53 mutations and mutations involving HER2/neu (3, 4).

■ HISTOPATHOLOGY

The World Health Organization classifies endometrial adenocarcinoma into multiple types including endometrioid, serous, and clear cell, among the more common variants (5). Another variant of endometrial carcinoma is carcinosarcoma, which is considered a high-risk histology.

Endometrioid carcinoma is the most common endometrial cancer, comprising 75%–80% of all cases. These cancers occur with varying degrees of differentiation, characterized histologically by grade. Well (grade 1) to moderately (grade 2) differentiated endometrioid carcinomas are considered type I endometrial carcinomas. Under the microscope they may have varying degrees of complexity, such as back-to-back, cribiform, or confluent growth (5). In contrast, poorly differentiated (grade 3) endometrioid adenocarcinomas are more aggressive tumors and some experts classify them as a type II tumor. Grade 3 endometrioid adenocarcinomas are characterized by at least 50% of a solid growth pattern or prominent nuclear atypia (5).

Serous carcinomas (previously referred to as papillary serous) account for 5%–10% of endometrial cancer. These cancers are typically irregular in histologic appearance with branching papillae and single cells characterized by large prominent nucleoli (5). These tumors are characteristic of type II endometrial carcinoma. They are uniformly aggressive, regardless of stage.

Clear cell carcinomas are characterized by clear cytoplasm and are associated with a high degree of cytological atypia. Typical architectural patterns include solid, papillary, and tubolocystic variants. As with serous carcinomas, clear cell carcinomas are also considered a type II tumor. They are aggressive variants, which may not respond well to chemotherapy (6).

Undifferentiated carcinomas of the endometrium are characterized by specific findings, including: a predominantly noncohesive proliferative pattern, heterogeneously sized monotonous cells without marked nuclear pleomorphism, and lacking glandular differentiation (5). These tumors are also marked by brisk mitotic activity and extensive evidence of necrosis.

Carcinosarcomas are metaplastic carcinomas composed of epithelial (carcinomatous) and mesenchymal (sarcomatous) elements. The sarcomatous element is histologically defined as being either homologous (i.e., sarcoma arising from tissue native to the uterus) or heterologous (i.e., sarcoma element that is not native to the uterus). Metastatic lesions due to carcinosarcoma most commonly comprise of the epithelial element.

■ CLINICAL PRESENTATION

The classic presenting sign of endometrial cancer is abnormal uterine bleeding. However, other symptoms can be seen, including bloating, pelvic pain, or dyspareunia. However, type II endometrial cancers may not present with symptoms until advanced disease is present, at which time, systemic symptoms (nausea, vomiting, change in bowel habits, anorexia) may be present.

■ DIAGNOSIS

The diagnosis of endometrial cancer is usually made based on endometrial biopsy or dilation and curettage. If the sampling is negative but clinical suspicion of a malignancy is high, however, further evaluation is warranted. This can be performed by repeat endometrial sampling (preferably, biopsy), by diagnostic hysteroscopy, or with pelvic imaging (typically, ultrasound or MRI).

■ STAGING

Endometrial carcinoma, which includes carcinosarcoma, is surgically staged using the Federation of Gynecology and Obstetrics (FIGO) staging system. The staging technique requires total hysterectomy and bilateral salpingo-oophorectomy. Whether or not lymphadenectomy is required for all cases of endometrial adenocarcinoma remains controversial (7).

■ PROGNOSTIC FACTORS

The prognosis of newly diagnosed endometrial cancer are illustrated by the delineation of tumors into risk groups, used for both prognostication and for informing treatment decisions:

Low-risk—These include tumors with low-risk features including low to intermediate grade, minimal to no myometrial invasion, and absence of lymphovascular space invasion (LVSI). These patients have an excellent prognosis following surgery and expected survival is over 90%.

Intermediate-risk—These include cancers confined to the uterus with myometrial invasion (stage IA or IB) or occult cervical stromal invasion (stage II). These patients have approximately an 80% chance of overall survival. Additional factors further divide this group into high- and low-intermediate risk disease, including deep myometrial invasion, grade 2 or 3 differentiation, or the presence of lymphovascular invasion (LVSI). *High-intermediate risk* criteria used by the Gynecologic Oncology Group for trial purposes include patients of any age with all three pathologic factors (grade 2 or 3, outer 1/3 invasion, LVSI), patients 50–69 years old with two factors, or patients who are 70 years or older with only one factor (8). In the absence of these additional risk factors, patients are considered to have *low-intermediate risk*.

High-risk—Women with clear cell or serous carcinomas and women with carcinosarcoma constitute the high-risk group, regardless of stage at diagnosis. This also includes women with stage III endometrial cancer that has been optimally resected. These patients are at an increased risk for both recurrence and death.

■ ADJUVANT TREATMENT

Low and low intermediate risk—Women with low- or low intermediate-risk endometrial cancer have an excellent prognosis following surgery alone. As such, the risks of adjuvant radiation therapy likely outweigh any benefit of treatment. In addition, adjuvant endocrine therapy is not indicated. A meta-analysis of adjuvant progestin therapy showed no benefit in the risk of mortality at 5 years compared with postoperative surveillance (9).

High intermediate-risk—Women with high intermediate-risk warrant adjuvant therapy due to an elevated risk of a local recurrence. For most patients, vaginal brachytherapy is sufficient. This was demonstrated in the Post Operative Radiation Therapy for Endometrial Cancer (PORTEC 2) trial, which compared pelvic to vaginal brachytherapy and showed that these treatments were equivalent and resulted in similar rates of locoregional or distant recurrence (10, 11).

There is no indication for adjuvant chemotherapy in this select group of women. However, a randomized trial being conducted by the Gynecologic Oncology Group (GOG 249) aims to characterize the benefit of combined modality treatment (vaginal brachytherapy plus carboplatin/paclitaxel chemotherapy) compared to whole pelvic radiation (12).

High-risk—Women with high-risk disease should be treated with adjuvant systemic chemotherapy, which has replaced the use of radiation therapy. This was based on the results of GOG 122, a randomized phase III trial that compared whole abdominal radiotherapy to 8 cycles of cisplatin and doxorubicin chemotherapy (AP) in stage III/IV disease with minimal residual tumor burden following surgery (13). Chemotherapy significantly increased progression-free (hazard ratio 0.71, 95% CI 0.55–0.91) and overall survival (HR 0.68, 95% CI 0.52–0.89). This translated to 5-year progression-free survival rates of 42% versus 38%, and overall survival rates of 53% and 42% for chemotherapy versus radiation, respectively.

Whether or not combining chemotherapy with adjuvant radiation therapy can improve outcomes is not known. This is being evaluated in GOG 258, which is open for women with high-risk endometrial cancer and compares concomitant cisplatin and tumor-directed irradiation followed by carboplatin and paclitaxel versus carboplatin and paclitaxel alone (14).

Approach to early stage serous or clear cell carcinoma—Regardless of stage, patients with serous or clear cell carcinoma are at an increased risk of relapse and death compared to those with similarly staged type I endometrioid cancers. Therefore, adjuvant therapy is generally warranted for stage I or II disease, although women with serous carcinoma limited to the endometrium may be appropriate candidates for surveillance (15). Clear cell carcinoma may be less sensitive to chemotherapy (6). Thus, it would be reasonable to treat clear cell cancers with local radiation therapy alone in an effort to reduce the risk of recurrence.

Carcinosarcoma—Adjuvant treatment is usually administered for carcinosarcoma. One exception may be for stage IA disease, in which the prognosis is good following surgical cytoreduction. However, for stage IB and higher disease, adjuvant chemotherapy is routinely administered. Based on GOG 232B, carboplatin and paclitaxel has largely replaced ifosfamide-based treatment in the adjuvant setting (16).

The benefit of chemotherapy rather than RT was demonstrated in GOG 150, in which 206 women with stage I–IV disease were randomized to whole abdominal irradiation (WAI) or to 3 cycles of ifosfamide plus cisplatin (17). Compared to WAI, chemotherapy resulted in a lower risk of death (HR 0.79, 95% CI 0.5–1.2) and a significantly lower risk of recurrence (HR 0.79, 95% CI 0.5–0.8).

METASTATIC DISEASE

There is no single paradigm for the approach to women with metastatic disease. The options depend on the extent of metastatic disease:

- Recurrence in the vaginal apex—Patients with endometrial cancer have a less than 10% risk for a local recurrence in the vaginal apex. However, these women are candidates for local therapy with radiation therapy (if not previously administered) or surgical excision. However, resection may require pelvic exenteration to ensure complete resection of disease.
- Recurrence in the pelvis—Patients with locally advanced recurrent disease may be candidates for cytoreduction or pelvic exenteration. However, a complete re-staging is important to ensure the extent of disease is identified and that complete resection is feasible.
- Extraabdominal metastatic disease—Patients with disease outside of the pelvis are best managed with chemotherapy. The approach to these patients depends on whether adjuvant chemotherapy was administered. There is no evidence of a platinum-free interval for patients with endometrial cancer.

MEDICAL TREATMENT OPTIONS

■ COMBINATION CHEMOTHERAPY

The standard combination regimen for the first-line treatment of metastatic disease was doxorubicin, cisplatin, and paclitaxel (TAP). This was shown on GOG 177, which compared TAP to AP among women with recurrent or metastatic endometrial carcinoma (18). Compared to AP, TAP resulted in a significant improvement in the overall response rate (57% vs. 34%), progression-free survival (8 vs. 5 months), and overall survival (15 vs. 12 months). However, it came at the expense of a higher rate of grade 3 neuropathy (12% vs. 1%).

More recently, the results of GOG 209, which compared carboplatin and paclitaxel to the TAP in patients with previously untreated, recurrent, advanced, or metastatic endometrial carcinoma (excluding carcinosarcoma), were reported (19). As presented at the 2012 Society for Gynecologic Oncology's Annual Meeting, there was no significant difference in overall response rate (51% in both arms), progression-free survival (13 months in both arms), and overall survival (median, 37 vs. 40 months, respectively). We await longer follow-up of this trial.

■ SINGLE AGENT CHEMOTHERAPY

Multiple agents are active in previously treated endometrial carcinoma, although response durations are relatively short and median overall survival on clinical trials is typically less than 12 months. These include ixabepilone (20), ifosfamide (21), topotecan (22), and oxaliplatin (23). All patients with progressive endometrial cancer should consider enrollment in an appropriately designed randomized trial.

■ ENDOCRINE THERAPY

For patients with limited symptoms related to metastatic disease, endocrine therapy is a reasonable alternative to chemotherapy. While most studies suggest hormonal manipulation is effective in low-grade tumors, there is some evidence that higher grade cancers respond to treatment. For example, medroxyprogesterone (800 mg/day) results in a 40%, 15%, and 2% response rate in patients with grade 1, 2, or 3 cancer, respectively (24). However, the regimen of medroxyprogesterone (160 mg/day) alternating monthly with tamoxifen (40 mg/day) resulted in a 38%, 24%, and 22% response rate, respectively (25).

UTERINE SARCOMA

■ INCIDENCE AND EPIDEMIOLOGY

Uterine sarcoma comprises a heterogeneous group of tumors, including leiomyosarcoma, endometrial stromal sarcoma, and adenosarcoma among the more common variants. These tumors are rare with an incidence of 3%–7% per 100,000 in the United States (26).

As with carcinosarcoma, black women have an increased risk of leiomyosarcoma compared to white women. In addition, tamoxifen treatment appears to increase the risk of sarcoma, although the absolute risk is very small (17 per 100,000 women taking tamoxifen) (27).

■ CLINICAL PRESENTATION

Uterine sarcomas typically present due to pelvic pressure or vaginal bleeding. Women may also present due to a vaginal discharge or dyspareunia. Most cases do not present as a rapidly expanding uterine mass, despite common teachings. **Endometrial stromal sarcomas** typically affect women in their late 40s. Up to 30% have evidence of metastatic disease at presentation. Lung is the most common site of metastatic disease.

Adenosarcomas present in the same population as endometrial stromal sarcomas and are also hormone receptor positive in the vast majority. The recurrence risk is lower than that for endometrial stromal sarcoma.

Leiomyosarcomas typically are diagnosed in women in their 50s. Regardless of stage, the recurrence risk is uniformly high, ranging from 40% to 70% within 3 years of diagnosis.

■ DIAGNOSIS

The diagnosis of uterine sarcoma requires histological confirmation. It is not uncommon for the diagnosis to be made following a simple hysterectomy for a benign procedure.

■ HISTOLOGY

Endometrial stromal sarcoma—Histologically endometrial stromal sarcomas have a low mitotic rate and lack evidence of atypia or necrosis. Hormone receptors are positive in the vast majority (70%–95%) and approximately 70%–80% of endometrial stromal sarcomas are associated with a genetic mutation consisting of the JAZF1/JJAZ1 gene fusion encoding a product associated with cell survival and proliferation (28).
Adenosarcoma—Unlike endometrial stromal sarcoma, these sarcomas are associated with a benign epithelial component. Approximately 90% express hormone receptors. However, the presence of sarcomatous overgrowth typically signifies a more aggressive variant.

Leiomyosarcoma—The histologic appearance of leiomyosarcoma shows variably uniform bundles of smooth muscle cells exhibiting a high mitotic rate.

■ SURGICAL STAGING

For patients with histologically confirmed uterine sarcoma diagnosed by endometrial sampling, hysterectomy should be performed. The role of BSO is controversial and it is not clear if an oophorectomy improves survival, particularly in women with uterine confined endometrial stromal sarcoma or leiomyosarcoma (29–32). Lymphadenectomy should only be performed in patients with evidence of extrauterine involvement.

TREATMENT OF UTERINE SARCOMA

Adjuvant radiation therapy has no impact on survival outcomes. This was shown in a phase III study conducted by the European Organization for the Research and Treatment of Cancer (EORTC) in which 224 patients (103 with leiomyosarcoma, 91 with carcinosarcoma, and 28 with endometrial stromal sarcoma) were randomly assigned to RT vs. observation (33). Disease-free survival was similar (50% vs. 45% with RT vs. observation) as was overall survival (58% vs. 56%).

While chemotherapy has been shown to reduce the rate of recurrence, there is no evidence of a survival benefit with adjuvant administration (34). A large international phase II study (SARC 005) is evaluating a sequential treatment approach in uterine leiomyosarcoma (35). All patients get 4 cycles of docetaxel and gemcitabine followed by reimaging. Those patients without evidence of disease progression then proceed with doxorubicin for 4 cycles. As reported, the rate of progression-free survival at 3 years is 57%. Median progression-free survival and overall survival have not been reached.

■ RECURRENT UTERINE SARCOMA

For patients who present with a oligometastatic disease, surgical resection should be considered. Otherwise, systemic therapy is the only option for patients who desire further treatment. Active agents, which are used alone or as part of a combination regimen, include gemcitabine (with or without docetaxel) (36, 37), ifosfamide (38, 39), temazolamide (40), paclitaxel (41), and doxorubicin (42). There is some evidence that aromatase inhibitors may be active in leiomyosarcomas, although the evidence is fairly limited (43).

REFERENCES

1. Siegel R, Naishadham D, and Jemal A. Cancer Statistics, 2013. *CA Cancer J Clin.* 2013; 63: 11–30.

2. Bokham JV. Two pathologic types of endometrial carcinoma. *Gynecol Oncol.* 1983; 10: 237–246.

3. Cao QJ, Belbin T, Socci N, et al. Distinctive gene expression profiles by cDNA microarrays in endometrioid and serous carcinomas of the endometrium. *Int J Gynecol Pathol.* 2004; 23: 321–329.

4. Kovalev S, Marchenko ND, Gugliotta BG, et al. Loss of p53 function in uterine papillary serous carcinoma. *Hum Pathol.* 1998; 29: 613–619.

5. Bartosch C, Maneul Lopes J, Oliva E. Endometrial carcinomas: a review emphasizing overlapping and distinctive morphological and immuno-histochemical features. *Adv Anat Pathol.* 2011; 18: 415–437.

6. Varughese J, Hui P, Lu Y, et al. Clear cell cancer of the uterine corpus: the association of clinicopathologic parameters and treatment on disease progression. *J Clin Oncol.* 2011; 200: 628084.

7. Dowdy SC, Borah BJ, Bakkum-Gamez JN, et al. Prospective assessment of cost, morbidity, and survival associated with lymphadenectomy in low risk endometrial cancer. *J Clin Oncol.* 2012; 30: abstr 5004.

8. Keys HM, Roberts JA, Brunetto VL, et al. A phase III trial of surgery with or without adjunctive external pelvic radiation therapy in inter-mediate risk endometrial adenocarcinoma: A Gynecologic Oncology Group Study. *Gynecol Oncol.* 2004; 92: 744–751.

9. Martin-Hirsch PP, Bryant A, Keep SL, et al. Adjuvant progestagens for endometrial cancer. *Cochrane Database Syst Rev.* 2011; 6:CD001040.

10. Nout RA, Smit VT, Putter H, et al. Vaginal brachytherapy versus pelvic external beam radiotherapy for patients with endometrial cancer of high-intermediate risk (PORTEC-2): an open-label, non-inferiority, randomised trial. *Lancet.* 2010; 375: 816–823.

11. The ASTEC/EN.5 writing committee. Adjuvant external beam radio-therapy in the treatment of endometrial cancer (MRC ASTEC and NCIC CTG EN.5 randomised trials): pooled trial results, systematic review, and meta-analysis. *Lancet.* 2009; 373: 137–146.

12. Pelvic Radiation Therapy or Vaginal Implant Radiation Therapy, Paclitaxel, and Carboplatin in Treating Patients With High-Risk Stage I or Stage II Endometrial Cancer. http://clinicaltrials.gov/show/NCT00807768. Accessed September 25, 2012.

13. Randall ME, Filiaci VL, Muss H, et al. Randomized phase III trial of whole-abdominal irradiation versus doxorubicin and cisplatin chemo-therapy in advanced endometrial carcinoma: a Gynecologic Oncology Group Study. *J Clin Oncol.* 2006; 24: 36–44.

14. Carboplatin and Paclitaxel With or Without Cisplatin and Radiation Therapy in Treating Patients With Stage I, Stage II, Stage III, or Stage IVA Endometrial Cancer. http://clinicaltrials.gov/show/NCT00942357. Accessed September 25, 2012.

15. Kelly MG, O'Malley DM, Hui P, et al. Improved survival in surgical stage I patients with uterine papillary serous carcinoma (UPSC) treated with adjuvant platinum-based chemotherapy. *Gynecol Oncol.* 2005; 98: 353–359.

16. Powell MA, Fillaci VL, Rose PG, et al. Phase II evaluation of paclitaxel and carboplatin in the treatment of carcinosarcoma of the uterus: a Gynecologic Oncology Group Study. *J Clin Oncol.* 2010; 28: 2727–2731.

17. Wolfson AH, Brady MF, Rocereto T, et al. A gynecologic oncology group randomized phase III trial of whole abdominal irradiation (WAI) vs. cisplatin-ifosfamide and mesna (CIM) as post-surgical therapy in stage I-IV carcinosarcoma (CS) of the uterus. *Gynecol Oncol.* 2007; 107: 177–185.

18. Fleming, G, Brunetto, V, Cella D, et al. Phase III trial of doxorubicin plus cisplatin with or without paclitaxel plus filgrastim in advanced endometrial carcinoma: a gynecologic oncology group study. *J Clin Oncol.* 2004; 22: 2159–2166.

19. Miller D, Filiaci V, Fleming G, et al. Randomized phase III noninferiority trial of first line chemotherapy for metastatic or recurrent endometrial carcinoma: a Gynecologic Oncology Group Study. *Gynecol Oncol.* 2012; 125: 771.

20. Dizon DS, Blessing JA, McMeekin DS, et al. Phase II trial of ixabepilone as second-line treatment in advanced endometrial cancer: gynecologic oncology group trial 129-P. *J Clin Oncol.* 2009; 27: 3104–3108.

21. Sutton GP, Blessing JA, DeMars LR, et al. A phase II Gynecologic Oncology Group trial of ifosfamide and mesna in advanced or recurrent adenocarcinoma of the endometrium. *Gynecol Oncol.* 1996; 63: 25–27.

22. Wadler S, Levy DE, Lincoln ST, et al. Topotecan is an active agent in the first-line treatment of metastatic or recurrent endometrial carcinoma: Eastern Cooperative Oncology Group Study E393. *J Clin Oncol.* 2003; 21: 2110–2114.

23. Fracasso PM, Blessing JA, Molpus KL, et al. Phase II study of oxaliplatin as second-line chemotherapy in endometrial carcinoma: a Gynecologic Oncology Group Study. *Gynecol Oncol.* 2006; 103: 523–526.

24. Podratz KC. Hormonal therapy in endometrial carcinoma. *Recent Results Cancer Res.* 1990; 118: 242–251.

25. Fiorica JV, Brunetto VL, Hanjani P, et al. Phase II trial of alternating courses of megestrol acetate and tamoxifen in advanced endometrial carcinoma: a Gynecologic Oncology Group Study. *Gynecol Oncol.* 2004; 92: 10–14.

26. Brooks SE, Zhan M, Cote T, et al. Surveillance, epidemiology, and end results analysis of 2677 cases of uterine sarcoma 1989-1999. *Gynecol Oncol.* 2004; 93: 204–208.

27. Wickerham DL, Fisher B, Wolmark N, et al. Association of tamoxifen and uterine sarcoma. *J Clin Oncol.* 2002; 20: 2758–2760.

28. Chiang S, Oliva E. Cytogenetic and molecular aberrations in endometrial stromal tumors. *Hum Pathol.* 2011; 42: 609–617.

29. Shah JP, Bryant CS, Kumar S, et al. Lymphadenectomy and ovarian preservation in low-grade endometrial stromal sarcoma. *Obstet Gynecol.* 2008; 112: 1102–1108.

30. Kapp DS, Shin JY, Chan JK. Prognostic factors and survival in 1396 patients with uterine leiomyosarcomas: emphasis on impact of lymphadenectomy and oophorectomy. *Cancer.* 2008; 112: 820–830.

31. Dos Santos LA, Garg K, Diaz JP, et al. Incidence of lymph node and adnexal metastasis in endometrial stromal sarcoma. *Gynecol Oncol.* 2011; 121: 319–322.

32. Riopel J, Plante M, Renaud MC, et al. Lymph node metastases in low-grade endometrial stromal sarcoma. *Gynecol Oncol.* 2004; 96: 402–406.

33. Reed NS, Mangioni C, Malmström H, et al. Phase III randomised study to evaluate the role of adjuvant pelvic radiotherapy in the treatment of uterine sarcomas stages I and II: an European Organisation for Research and Treatment of Cancer Gynaecological Cancer Group Study (protocol 55874). *Eur J Cancer.* 2008; 44: 808–818.

34. Omura GA, Blessing JA, Major F, et al. A randomized clinical trial of adjuvant adriamycin in uterine sarcomas: a Gynecologic Oncology Group Study. *J Clin Oncol.* 1985; 3: 1240–1245.

35. Hensley ML, Wathen K, Maki RG, et al. 3-year follow-up of SARC005: Adjuvant treatment of high risk primary uterine leiomyosarcoma with gemcitabine/docetaxel (GT), followed by Doxorubicin (D). Presented at the 2011 Connective Tissue Oncology Society Meeting, Chicago, IL. (Poster #78).

36. Hensley ML, Blessing JA, Mannel R, et al. Fixed-dose rate gemcitabine plus docetaxel as first-line therapy for metastatic uterine leiomyosarcoma: a Gynecologic Oncology Group phase II trial. *Gynecol Oncol.* 2008; 109: 329–334.

37. Look KY, Sandler A, Blessing JA, et al. Phase II trial of gemcitabine as second-line chemotherapy of uterine leiomyosarcoma: a Gynecologic Oncology Group (GOG) Study. *Gynecol Oncol.* 2004; 92: 644–647.

38. Homesley HD, Filiaci V, Markman M, et al. Phase III trial of ifosfamide with or without paclitaxel in advanced uterine carcinosarcoma: a Gynecologic Oncology Group Study. *J Clin Oncol.* 2007; 25: 526–531.

39. Sutton G, Kauderer J, Carson LF, et al. Adjuvant ifosfamide and cisplatin in patients with completely resected stage I or II carcinosarcomas (mixed mesodermal tumors) of the uterus: a Gynecologic Oncology Group study. *Gynecol Oncol.* 2005; 96: 630–634.

40. Talbot SM, Keohan ML, Hesdorffer M, et al. A phase II trial of temozolomide in patients with unresectable or metastatic soft tissue sarcoma. *Cancer.* 2003; 98: 1942–1946.

41. Gallup DG, Blessing JA, Andersen W, et al. Evaluation of paclitaxel in previously treated leiomyosarcoma of the uterus: a gynecologic oncology group study. *Gynecol Oncol.* 2003; 89: 48–51.

42. Judson I, Radford JA, Harris M, Blay JY, et al. Randomised phase II trial of pegylated liposomal doxorubicin (DOXIL/CAELYX) versus doxorubicin in the treatment of advanced or metastatic soft tissue sarcoma: a study by the EORTC Soft Tissue and Bone Sarcoma Group. *Eur J Cancer.* 2001; 37: 870–877.

43. O'Cearbhaill R, Zhou Q, Iasonos A, et al. Treatment of advanced uterine leiomyosarcoma with aromatase inhibitors. *Gynecol Oncol.* 2010; 116: 424–429.

CHAPTER **57**

Breast Oncology: Clinical Presentation and Genetics

Amy Comander, Tessa Cigler, Paula D. Ryan

EPIDEMIOLOGY

In the United States, breast cancer is the most commonly diagnosed cancer among women and is second only to lung cancer as the leading cause of cancer-related deaths in women (1). In 2013, approximately 234,000 women will be diagnosed with breast cancer in the United States and 40,000 women will die of the disease. An estimated 2200 men will be diagnosed with breast cancer this year. In the United States, the lifetime probability of developing breast cancer is one in eight (2). Since 1975, breast cancer mortality rates have declined. This decline in mortality is largely attributable to increased use of screening mammography, as well as advances in adjuvant therapy.

RISK FACTORS

Approximately half of women diagnosed with breast cancer have identifiable risk factors besides age and gender. There are specific hormonal and reproductive factors that may increase risk for breast cancer. In addition, a number of lifestyle, diet, and environmental factors confer an increased risk of breast cancer. A personal or family history of breast cancer, as well as a history of benign breast disease, also increases a woman's risk of developing breast cancer.

■ ENDOGENOUS ESTROGEN EXPOSURE/REPRODUCTIVE FACTORS

It is known that hormonal and reproductive factors influence breast cancer risk. Prolonged exposure to estrogen is associated with an increased risk of breast cancer (3). Estrogen exposure is increased by early menarche, late menopause, and nulliparity, or greater than 30 years of age at birth of the first child. Breastfeeding confers a protective effect on breast cancer risk.

In postmenopausal women, the main source of estrogen is dehydroepiandrosterone (DHEA), which is produced in the adrenal gland and subsequently metabolized to estradiol and estrone. In postmenopausal women, higher serum levels of estrogen correlate with increased breast cancer risk. Higher bone mineral density and increased mammographic breast density, perhaps surrogates for increased long-term exposure to endogenous estrogen, have also been associated with increased breast cancer risk.

■ EXOGENOUS ESTROGEN EXPOSURE

The role of exogenous estrogen on breast cancer risk is complicated and has been extensively studied. It is generally accepted that past oral contraceptive

(OC) use does not result in any significant increase in breast cancer risk in women over 40 years of age. The data on OC use in women with a family history of breast cancer are conflicting. One study suggested that there was an increased risk of breast cancer among women who took OC prior to 1975 (higher dose formulations) and who also had a first degree relative with breast cancer.

Another study, the Women's Health Initiative (WHI) evaluation of estrogen replacement therapy (ERT) in postmenopausal women, supports a modestly increased associated risk of breast cancer in women taking combined estrogen and progestin therapy (4). Risk appears to rise with increasing duration of use. Short-term use of ERT (less than 4–5 years), however, has not been definitively associated with increased breast cancer risk. In contrast, recent data from the WHI study has shown that use of estrogen alone by postmenopausal women with prior hysterectomy actually decreased the risk of breast cancer (5). At present, the different effects of estrogen plus progestin versus estrogen alone on breast cancer risk are not completely understood.

■ LIFESTYLE

Weight and body mass index (BMI) are considered risk factors for breast cancer, although they have opposite influences on pre- and postmenopausal breast cancer. In postmenopausal women, in whom the primary source of estrogen is metabolism of adrenal androgens to estrogens in fatty tissues, obesity is associated with higher serum concentrations of bioavailable estrogen and an increased risk of breast cancer.

In premenopausal women, studies suggest an inverse association between obesity and breast cancer. Obesity is often associated with longer menstrual cycles and increased anovulatory cycles, resulting in less total estrogen exposure and a lower risk of breast cancer.

The relationship between exercise and breast cancer risk remains unsettled. Some data suggest that increased activity levels among postmenopausal women confer a reduced risk of breast cancer. This may be due to the reduction in BMI or the reduced serum estrogen levels associated with exercise.

■ DIET

There is strong epidemiological evidence that breast cancer risk is higher among women who consume moderate to high levels of alcohol (>=3 drinks/day), compared to women who abstain. In the large prospective Nurse's Health Study, even a low level of alcohol consumption (equivalent to 3–6 glasses of wine per week) was modestly but significantly associated with an increased risk of breast cancer, with a relative risk of 1.15 (95% CI, 1.06–1.24; 333 cases/100,000 person-years) (6). Data also suggest that risk of breast cancer increases linearly with cumulative lifetime alcohol intake, which, in turn, is associated with increased endogenous estrogen levels.

Studies examining fat consumption and breast cancer risk have yielded mixed results, with several case control and cohort studies suggesting at most a modest increase in risk with increased dietary fat consumption.

■ ENVIRONMENTAL

The strongest known environmental risk factor for breast cancer is ionizing radiation. Moderate to high doses of ionizing radiation to the chest at a young age such as that given for treatment of Hodgkin's disease pose a significant risk for the development of breast cancer later in life. The highest risk of breast cancer appears in individuals exposed during prepubertal and pubertal years.

■ BENIGN BREAST DISEASE

Benign breast diseases are classified as proliferative or nonproliferative lesions. Non-proliferative lesions are not associated with increased breast cancer risk. Proliferative lesions without atypia such as hyperplasia, sclerosing adenosis, diffuse papillomatosis, radial scar, and complex fibroadenomas result in a small increase in relative risk estimated between 1.5 and 2.0. Proliferative lesions with atypia (atypical ductal hyperplasia, atypical lobular hyperplasia, flat epithelial atypia, and lobular carcinoma in situ) confer an increased risk of invasive breast cancer.

■ RISK FACTORS FOR MALE BREAST CANCER

Male breast cancer risk factors include a family history of breast cancer, BRCA2 mutations, Klinefelter's syndrome, chronic liver disease, and testicular conditions such as orchitis, cryptorchidism, and testicular injury. Increased risk of male breast cancer is felt to be due to an imbalance between estrogenic and androgenic influences.

RISK ASSESSMENT

Two useful models to assess breast cancer risk in women not suspected of having a hereditary predisposition to breast cancer (see Breast Cancer Genetics) are the Gail model and the Claus model (7). The Gail model derives age-specific breast cancer risk estimates for women based on their age at menarche, age at first live birth, number of previous breast biopsies, presence of atypical hyperplasia in prior breast biopsy, and number of first-degree relatives with breast cancer. By including only first-degree relatives, the Gail model tends to underestimate risk in women with strong family histories of breast cancer. A breast cancer risk assessment tool based on the Gail model can be accessed at http://www.cancer.gov/bcrisktool. The Claus model derives age-specific breast cancer risk estimates for women with at least one relative with breast cancer.

BREAST CANCER GENETICS

While 20%–30% of women with breast cancer have at least one relative with a history of breast cancer, only 5%–10% of women with breast cancer have an identifiable hereditary predisposition. Most of the known hereditary breast cancers are due to mutations in the BRCA1 or BRCA2 genes, which also predispose to ovarian cancer. Rare mutations in other genes including PTEN, p53, CDH1, and STK 11 are also associated with increased breast cancer risk (Table 57-1).

■ BRCA1 AND BRCA2

BRCA1 and BRCA2 genes were cloned in 1994 and 1995, respectively. BRCA1 and BRCA2 are autosomal dominant genes that are believed to act as tumor suppressor genes. They play a role in cellular response to DNA damage and are involved with double-stranded DNA repair (8). BRCA1

TABLE 57-1 BREAST CANCER SUSCEPTIBILITY GENES

Gene	Syndrome	Associated Malignancies
BRCA1	Hereditary breast and ovarian cancer	Breast and ovarian cancer
BRCA2	Hereditary breast and ovarian cancer	Breast and ovarian cancer
TP53	Li-Fraumeni syndrome	Soft tissue and osteosarcomas, breast cancer, brain tumors, adrenal cortical carcinoma, leukemia
PTEN	Cowden's	Hamartomas, benign and malignant tumors of the thyroid, breast, and endometrium
STK11	Peutz-Jeghers	Breast, gastrointestinal, ovarian, testicular, uterine, endometrial cancers
CHEK2	–	Breast cancer

maps to chromosome 17q21, whereas BRCA2 maps to chromosome 11. The prevalence of mutations in either BRCA1 or BRCA2 varies among ethnic groups. A noticeably higher frequency of about 1 in 40 (2.5%) has been observed among individuals of Ashkenazi Jewish ancestry, compared to less than 1% in the general population.

Inherited mutations in either BRCA1 or BRCA2 predispose female carriers to breast and ovarian cancer. Male carriers of BRCA2 mutations are at increased risk of developing breast cancer or prostate cancer. Pancreatic cancer, stomach cancer, and melanoma can also be seen in BRCA1 or BRCA2 mutation carriers. In general, it is estimated that the lifetime risk of developing breast cancer varies between 50% and 80% for a woman carrying either a BRCA1 or a BRCA2 mutation, and between 5% and 10% for a male mutation carrier. The lifetime risk of ovarian cancer among female BRCA1 carriers is estimated to be between 30% and 45%, while that of female BRCA2 carriers ranges from 10% to 20%. BRCA1-associated breast cancers are usually high-grade tumors that stain negative for estrogen and progesterone receptors, and do not overexpress HER2/neu. BRCA2-associated breast cancers have a spectrum of pathologic and molecular features similar to that of sporadic breast cancers.

GENETIC TESTING FOR BRCA1 AND BRCA2 MUTATIONS

The decision to pursue genetic testing for a BRCA1 or BRCA2 mutation is complex, since a positive test result has implications for both the individual as well as for family members. The general consensus is that an individual is usually offered testing if her risk of carrying a deleterious mutation is at least 10%. BRCAPRO is a predictive algorithm frequently used in high-risk clinics. It can be downloaded from http://www4.utsouthwestern.edu/breasthealth/cagene/.

While there are no standardized criteria, family histories suggestive of the presence of BRCA1 or BRCA2 mutations include two or more relatives affected with breast cancer, usually with a predominance of early onset cases (less than 50 years of age), ovarian cancer, male breast cancer, and evidence of transmission in two or more generations or through male relatives. A personal history of breast cancer diagnosed at age less than 40 years, invasive ovarian cancer, bilateral breast cancer, or both breast and ovarian cancers are also characteristic of BRCA1 or BRCA2 mutation carriers. In addition, individuals of Ashkenazi Jewish ancestry with breast cancer and relatives of known mutation carriers are at increased risk of carrying a BRCA1 or BRCA2 mutation and should be considered for testing (9, 10).

The National Comprehensive Cancer Network (NCCN) has established criteria for which individuals should be referred for BRCA1/BRCA2 genetic testing. These criteria are listed in Table 57-2. The NCCN recommends consideration of genetic testing for an individual from a family with a known deleterious BRCA1/BRCA2 mutation. Individuals with a diagnosis of breast ≤45 years should be referred for genetic testing. Other criteria include a breast cancer diagnosis ≤50 years with a close relative with breast cancer ≤50 years, a history of ovarian cancer at any age, or two breast primaries when the first was diagnosed prior to age 50 years. The NCCN also recommends that individuals diagnosed with triple negative breast cancer at age <60 years be considered for genetic testing. Individuals with male breast cancer should be referred for testing, as well as women with a personal history of epithelial ovarian/fallopian tube/primary peritoneal cancer.

Before undergoing genetic testing, individuals must receive careful counseling regarding the potential clinical, psychological, and legal ramifications associated with testing. The implications of both a positive and negative test result should be reviewed carefully. At-risk family members based on family pedigree should be identified, and individuals with a positive test result should be encouraged to share this information with their relatives.

MANAGEMENT OF BRCA MUTATION CARRIERS

Several strategies exist for risk reduction among BRCA mutation carriers. Bilateral prophylactic mastectomy, the most effective method to reduce breast cancer risk among carriers, should be offered to all women with BRCA1 or BRCA2 mutations. Residual breast cancer risk following surgery is <10%. Prophylactic bilateral salpingo-oophorectomy (BSO) should also be offered to women with BRCA1 or BRCA2 mutations. In addition to reducing risk of ovarian cancer by 90%, BSO has been shown to reduce the risk of breast cancer by approximately 50% in premenopausal mutation carriers who have not undergone prophylactic surgery.

Women who elect not to undergo prophylactic mastectomies need to be closely screened for breast cancer. In general, guidelines for mutation carriers suggest annual screening mammograms beginning at 25–30 years of age, clinical breast exams twice a year, and monthly breast self-examinations. Breast MRI is more sensitive than mammography in detecting breast cancers in high-risk women at the cost of a higher false-positive rate (11). The American Cancer Society guidelines for breast screening recommend annual MRI screening as an adjunct to mammography in BRCA mutation

TABLE 57-2 NATIONAL COMPREHENSIVE CANCER NETWORK CRITERIA FOR CONSIDERATION OF BRCA1/2 GENETIC TESTING

Individual from a family with a known deleterious BRCA1/BRCA2 mutation
Personal history of breast cancer plus one or more of the following:
• Diagnosed age ≤45 years
• Diagnosed ≤50 years with ≥1 close blood relative with breast cancer ≤50 years and/or ≥1 close blood relative with epithelial ovarian cancer at any age
• Two breast primaries when first breast cancer diagnosis occurred ≤50 years
• Diagnosed ≤60 years with a triple negative breast cancer
• Diagnosed ≤50 years with a limited family history
• Diagnosed at any age, with ≥2 close blood relatives with breast and /or epithelial ovarian cancer at any age
• Close male blood relative with breast cancer
• For an individual of ethnicity associated with a higher mutation frequency (e.g., Ashkenazi Jewish), no additional family history may be required
Personal history of epithelial ovarian cancer
Personal history of male breast cancer
Personal history of pancreatic cancer at any age with ≥2 close blood relatives with breast and/or ovarian cancer and/or pancreatic cancer at any age
Family history only:
• First- or second-degree blood relative meeting any of the above criteria
• Third-degree blood relative with breast cancer and/or ovarian cancer with ≥2 close blood relatives with breast cancer (at least one breast cancer ≤50 years) and/or ovarian cancer

National Comprehensive Cancer Network, v.1.2012 (www.ncc.org).

carriers (12). Clinical guidelines suggest that MRI screening start by age 25 years.

For those women who elect not to undergo prophylactic BSO, ovarian cancer screening with twice yearly transvaginal ultrasounds and measurements of CA-125 tumor marker is recommended. It is cautioned, however, that these measures are of unproven efficacy.

BREAST CANCER SCREENING IN GENERAL POPULATION

Most North American expert groups recommend breast cancer screening with mammography with or without clinical breast examination every year for women over age 50 years and every 1–2 years for women aged 40–49 years. In 2009, the U.S. Preventive Services Task Force (USPSTF) revised its breast cancer screening guidelines and recommended against routine screening mammography in women aged 40–49 years (13). After much controversy, the USPSTF revised its recommendation and recommended that the decision to start regular biennial screening mammography before the age of

50 years should be individualized for each patient. Several expert groups do not explicitly state at what age breast cancer screening should stop. The USPSTF recommends mammographic screening until age 74 years; other groups recommend that women over age 75 years consult with their physician regarding the role of screening.

Although clinical breast examination (CBE) is generally recommended, its independent role is difficult to determine as most studies included both mammography and CBE. There are few randomized trials to date to guide recommendations regarding breast self-examination (BSE). Limited data suggest that BSE may aid in the diagnosis of cancers at early stages when tumors are more amenable to conservative local therapy. Correct technique of BSE appears to be an important factor. While there is some belief that women with first-degree relatives with histories of breast cancer, particularly premenopausal breast cancer, should undergo screening at an earlier age, mortality data to support this recommendation do not yet exist. BRCA1 and BRCA2 carriers are advised to undergo more intensive screening as detailed above.

DIAGNOSIS

Breast cancer is most often diagnosed by biopsy of a palpable breast mass or biopsy of a mammographic abnormality. Definitive diagnostic evaluation should be promptly initiated for any breast abnormality and pursued until resolution. Lesions in men should be evaluated similarly to those in women. In addition, a dominant breast mass in a pregnant or lactating woman should not be automatically attributed to hormonal changes; diagnostic evaluation should be pursued. In the presence of a persistent breast nodule, physical examination alone or a normal mammogram cannot exclude malignancy. It is generally recommended that mammography be included as part of the evaluation of a palpable breast mass in any woman 30 years of age or older in order to evaluate the size and radiologic features of the mass in question as well as to detect other clinically occult lesions in either breast.

■ PALPABLE BREAST MASS

In women 30 years or older, most experts agree that any dominant mass should be evaluated by physical exam, mammography, and ultrasound. Imaging guided core needle biopsy can be performed if the lesion is suspicious and visible on an imaging study. If it is not easily targeted, then it should be referred to a surgeon for definitive diagnostic biopsy. It is important to note that negative mammogram does not exclude breast cancer.

For women younger than 30 years, initial evaluation is done by physical exam and ultrasound followed by ultrasound guided biopsy or surgical referral for definitive diagnosis. Although some believe that benign solid masses can be distinguished from malignant solid masses using ultrasound, many feel that these should be evaluated with needle or excisional biopsy. Palpable lesions can be aspirated under clinical guidance, and if fluid is drained and the mass resolves, this is good evidence of a simple cyst. If ultrasound demonstrates a simple cyst, no further intervention is needed. Symptomatic cysts can be aspirated to provide symptomatic relief, although they often recur. Non-simple cysts (complex) that appear to contain both fluid and solid tissue should undergo excisional biopsy following needle localization in order to evaluate the entire cyst. Alternatively, consideration

TABLE 57-3 TMN STAGING SYSTEM FOR BREAST CANCER

Primary tumor (T)

TX—Primary tumor cannot be assessed

T0—No evidence of primary tumor

Tis—Carcinoma in situ

Tis (DCIS)—Ductal carcinoma in situ

Tis (LCIS)—Lobular carcinoma in situ

Tis (Paget's)—Paget's disease of the nipple not associated with invasive carcinoma and/or carcinoma in situ (DCIS and/or LCIS) in the underlying breast parenchyma. Carcinomas in the breast parenchyma associated with Paget's disease are categorized based on the size and characteristics of the parenchymal disease, although the presence of Paget's disease should still be noted.

T1—Tumor ≤20 mm in greatest dimension

    T1mi—Tumor ≤1 mm in greatest dimension

    T1a—Tumor >1 mm but ≤5 mm in greatest dimension

    T1b—Tumor >5 mm but ≤10 mm in greatest dimension

    T1c—Tumor >10 mm but ≤20 mm in greatest dimension

T2—Tumor >20 mm but ≤50 mm in greatest dimension

T3—Tumor >50 mm in greatest dimension

T4—Tumor of any size with direct extension to the chest wall and/or skin (ulceration or skin nodules). Note: Invasion of the dermis alone does not qualify as T4.

    T4a—Extension to the chest wall, not including only pectoralis muscle adherence/invasion

    T4b—Ulceration and/or ipsilateral satellite nodules and/or edema (including peau d'orange) of the skin, which do not meet the criteria for inflammatory carcinoma

    T4c—Both (T4a and T4b)

    T4d—Inflammatory carcinoma

Regional lymph nodes: clinical classification (N)

NX—Regional lymph nodes cannot be assessed (e.g., previously removed)

N0—No regional lymph node metastases

N1—Metastases to movable ipsilateral level I,II axillary lymph nodes(s)

N2—Metastases to ipsilateral level I, II axillary lymph node(s) fixed or matted, or in clinically detected ipsilateral internal mammary nodes in the absence of clinically evident axillary lymph node metastases

    N2a—Metastases to ipsilateral level I, II axillary lymph node(s) fixed to one another (matted) or to other structures

    N2b—Metastases only in clinically detected ipsilateral internal mammary nodes and in the absence of clinically evident level I, II axillary lymph node metastases

(*continued*)

TABLE 57-3 TMN STAGING SYSTEM FOR BREAST CANCER (CONTINUED)

N3—Metastases to ipsilateral infraclavicular (level III axillary) lymph node(s) with or without level I, II axillary lymph node involvement; or in clinically detected ipsilateral internal mammary lymph node(s) with clinically evident level I, II axillary lymph node metastases; or metastases in ipsilateral supraclavicular lymph nodes with or without axillary or internal mammary lymph node involvement

  N3a—Metastases in ipsilateral infraclavicular lymph node(s)

  N3b—Metastases in ipsilateral internal mammary lymph node(s) and axillary lymph nodes

  N3c—Metastases in ipsilateral supraclavicular lymph nodes

Regional lymph nodes: pathologic classification (pN)

Classification is based on axillary lymph node dissection (ALND) with or without sentinel lymph node dissection (SLND). Classification based solely on SLND without ALND should be designated (sn) [e.g., pN0 (i+) (sn)].

pNX—Regional lymph nodes cannot be assessed (e.g., previously removed, or not removed for pathologic study)

pN0—No regional lymph node metastasis identified histologically

  pN0 (i–)—No histologic nodal metastases histologically, negative immunohistochemistry (IHC)

  pN0 (i+)—Malignant cells in regional lymph node(s) no greater than 0.2 mm (detected by H&E or IHC including ITC)

  pN0 (mol–)—No regional lymph node metastases histologically, negative molecular findings (RT-PCR)

  pN0 (mol+)—Positive molecular findings (RT-PCR), but no regional lymph node metastases detected by histology or IHC

pN1—Micrometastases; or metastasis in 1–3 axillary lymph node(s); and/or in internal mammary nodes with metastases detected by SLND but not clinically apparent

  pN1mi—Micrometastases (greater than 0.2 mm and/or more than 200 cells, but none greater than 2.0 mm)

  pN1a—Metastases in 1–3 axillary lymph nodes, at least one metastasis greater than 2.0 mm

  pN1b—Metastases to internal mammary nodes with micrometastases or macrometastases detected by sentinel lymph node biopsy but not clinically detected

  pN1c—Metastases in 1–3 axillary lymph node(s) and in internal mammary lymph nodes with micrometastases or macrometastases detected by SLND but not clinically detected.

pN2—Metastases in 4–9 axillary lymph nodes or in clinically detected internal mammary lymph nodes in the absence of axillary lymph node metastases

  pN2a—Metastases in 4–9 axillary lymph nodes (at least one tumor deposit >2 mm)

  pN2b—Metastases in clinically detected internal mammary lymph nodes in the absence of axillary lymph node metastases

(*continued*)

TABLE 57-3 TMN STAGING SYSTEM FOR BREAST CANCER (CONTINUED)

pN3—Metastasis in 10 or more axillary lymph nodes, or in infraclavicular (level III axillary) lymph nodes, or in clinically detected ipsilateral internal mammary lymph nodes in the presence of one or more positive level I, II axillary nodes; or in more than 3 axillary lymph nodes and in internal mammary lymph nodes with micrometastases or macrometastases detected by SLND but not clinically detected; or in ipsilateral supraclavicular lymph nodes

pN3a—Metastases in 10 or more axillary lymph nodes (at least one tumor deposit greater than 2.0 mm), or metastases to the infraclavicular (level III axillary) lymph nodes

pN3b—Metastases in clinically detected ipsilateral internal mammary lymph nodes in the presence of one or more positive axillary nodes; or in more than 3 axillary lymph nodes and in internal mammary lymph nodes with micrometastases or macrometastases detected by sentinel lymph node biopsy but not clinically detected

pN3c—Metastases in ipsilateral supraclavicular lymph nodes

Distant metastases (M)

M0—No clinical or radiographic evidence of distant metastases

cM0 (i+)—No clinical or radiographic evidence of distant metastases, but deposits of molecularly or microscopically detected tumor cells in circulating blood, bone marrow, or other nonregional nodal tissue that are no larger than 0.2 mm in a patient without symptoms or signs of metastases

M1—Distant detectable metastases as determined by classic clinical and radiographic means and/or histologically proven larger than 0.2 mm

TMN stage groupings for breast cancer

Stage 0—Tis N0 M0

Stage IA—T1 N0 M0

Stage IB—T0 N1mi M0; T1 N1mi M0

Stage IIA—T0 N1 M0; T1 N1 M0; T2 N0 M0

Stage IIB—T2 N1 M0; T3 N0 M0

Stage IIIA—T0 N2 M0; T1 N2 M0; T2 N2 M0; T3 N1 M0; T3 N2 M0

Stage IIIB—T4 N0 M0; T4 N1 M0; T4 N2 M0

Stage IIIC—Any T N3 M0

Stage IV—Any T Any N M1

Used with the permission of the American Joint Committee on Cancer (AJCC), Chicago, Illinois. The original source for this material is Edge SB et al (eds). *AJCC Cancer Staging Manual,* 7th edition. New York, Springer, 2010.

can be given to ultrasound guided biopsy. However, if this is performed, a clip should be placed so that if additional evaluation is needed there is a marker to guide further intervention since the biopsy may render it difficult to visualize the lesion. In cases where physical exam and breast imaging are consistent with fibrocystic breast tissue, an FNA may be considered. Whether or not FNA is performed, all such patients should be seen in follow-up at 2 months to ensure stability.

■ ABNORMAL MAMMOGRAM

Women who present with an abnormal screening mammogram in the absence of a palpable breast mass also require prompt evaluation. The work up usually depends on the recommendation of the radiologist interpreting the mammogram. The degree of abnormality is categorized using the Breast Imaging and Reporting Data System (BI-RADS).

STAGING SYSTEM

Breast cancer is most commonly staged according to the TMN staging system. The staging system, published by the American Joint Committee on Cancer (AJCC), was modified in 2010 (Table 57-2) (14). Five-year survival rates are highly correlated with tumor stage, ranging from 99% for women with stage 0 disease to 14% for women with stage IV disease.

STAGING EVALUATION

Initial evaluation of any woman with newly diagnosed breast cancer should include a thorough history and physical exam. The physical exam should be focused on palpation of each breast, lymph nodes, and abdomen, and assessment of the skin for potential disease involvement. Additional workup includes bilateral mammography and routine blood tests, including a complete blood count and liver function tests. Abnormal lab values or signs or symptoms of metastatic disease should prompt further evaluation with chest x-ray; CT scan of the chest, abdomen, and pelvis; and bone scan.

For asymptomatic women with early stage breast cancer (stages I and II), radiographic studies such as chest x-ray; CT scan of the chest, abdomen, and pelvis; and bone scan have a low-diagnostic yield and are not generally recommended. In contrast, all women with stage III disease should undergo evaluation with CT scan of the chest, abdomen, and pelvis, and bone scan. While PET scans can identify sites of metastatic breast cancer, routine PET scans are not recommended for staging of localized breast cancer.

REFERENCES

1. Siegel R, Naishadham J, Jemal A, Cancer statistics, 2013. *CA Cancer J Clin*. 2013; 63: 11–30.

2. Howlader N, Noone AM, Krapcho M, et al. SEER Cancer Statistics Review, 1975-2009 (Vintage 2009 Populations), National Cancer Institute. Bethesda, MD, http://seer.cancer.gov/csr/1975_2009 _pops09/, based on November 2011 SEER data submission, posted to the SEER web site, 2012.

3. Clemons M, Goss P. Estrogen and the risk of breast cancer. *N Engl J Med*. 2001; 344: 276–285.

4. Chlebowski RT, Hendrix SL, Langer RD, et al. Influence of estrogen plus progestin on breast cancer and mammography in healthy postmenopausal women: the Women's Health Initiative Randomized Trial. *JAMA*. 2003; 289: 3243–3253.

5. Anderson GL, Chlebowski RT, Aragaki AK, et al. Conjugated equine oestrogen and breast cancer incidence and mortality in postmenopausal women with hysterectomy: extended follow-up of the

Women's Health Initiative randomised placebo-controlled trial. *Lancet Oncol.* 2012; 13: 476–486.

6. Chen WY, Rosner B, Hankinson SE, et al. Moderate alcohol consumption during adult life, drinking patterns, and breast cancer risk. *JAMA.* 2011; 306: 1884–1890.

7. Armstrong K, Eisen A, Weber B. Assessing the risk of breast cancer. *N Engl J Med.* 2000; 342: 564–571.

8. Narod SA, Foulkes WD. BRCA1 and BRCA2: 1994 and beyond. *Nat Rev Cancer.* 2004; 4: 665–676.

9. Narod SA, Offit K. Prevention and management of hereditary breast cancer. *J Clin Oncol.* 2005; 23: 1656–1663.

10. Genetic risk assessment and BRCA mutation testing for breast and ovarian cancer susceptibility: recommendation statement. U.S. Preventive Services Task Force. *Ann Intern Med.* 2005; 143: 355–361.

11. Liberman L. Breast cancer screening with MRI—what are the data for patients at high risk? *N Engl J Med.* 2004; 351: 497–500.

12. Saslow D, Boetes C, Burke W, et al. for American Cancer Society Breast Cancer advisory group. American Cancer Society Guidelines for Breast Screening with MRI as an Adjunct to Mammography. *CA Cancer J Clin.* 2007; 57: 75–89.

13. Calonge N, Petitti DB, DeWitt TG, et al. Screening for breast cancer: U.S. Preventive Services Task Force recommendation statement. *Ann Intern Med.* 2009; 151: 716–726.

14. American Joint Committee on Cancer (AJCC) Cancer Staging Manual, Seventh Edition. In SB Edge, DR Byrd, CC Compton, et al. (eds.). Springer, New York, 2010, pp. 345–376.

CHAPTER **58**

Localized Breast Cancer

Beverly Moy

Breast cancer is considered "localized" if it is technically possible to excise cancerous tissue, if the tumor does not involve the skin or structures deep to the breast, and if the tumor has not metastasized beyond the axillary or internal mammary lymph nodes.

A variety of prognostic and predictive factors influence the choice of treatment of localized breast cancer, including the status of cancer in the axillary lymph nodes, tumor size, hormone receptor status, HER2/neu status, and a woman's age or menopausal status.

PROGNOSTIC AND PREDICTIVE FACTORS

- **Lymph node involvement**—Fluid from the breast tissue normally drains into lymph nodes located in the axilla, and cancerous involvement of these nodes is an indication of the likelihood that breast cancer has spread and could be present in distant organs. Women with node-positive breast cancer are generally offered chemotherapy, hormone therapy, or both after local treatment, even if the tumor was completely removed. The type of systemic treatment that is recommended depends upon whether the breast cancer expresses hormone receptors and/or the protein HER2/neu.

- **Size and extent of the tumor**—In addition to lymph node status, the prognosis of a breast cancer depends upon its size, since larger tumors (<2 cm) recur more often. In some cases, chemotherapy may be given before surgery to shrink a large tumor (>5 cm) or one that has grown into the chest wall.

- **Histology**—There are several histologic types of breast cancer. However, from the standpoint of treatment, the most important distinction is between invasive and noninvasive (in situ) breast cancer. The surgical treatment of in situ cancers is similar to that of invasive cancers, but axillary nodal dissection is generally not recommended.

- **Hormone receptor status**—Estrogen receptor (ER) and progesterone receptor (PR) assays are routinely performed by pathologists on tumor material. Women with hormone receptor-positive tumors benefit from postoperative endocrine treatments such as tamoxifen, or in postmenopausal women, the aromatase inhibitors (anastrozole, letrozole, or exemestane). For premenopausal women, ovarian ablation or suppression can be considered, but evidence regarding its efficacy from randomized clinical trials is currently lacking. Hormone therapy is not beneficial for women with hormone receptor-negative tumors.

- **HER2/neu status**—Assays for HER2/neu status are routinely performed on the tumor material. Women with invasive tumors that overexpress HER2/neu benefit from postoperative trastuzumab, a monoclonal antibody directed at HER2/neu.

- **Age and/or menopausal status**—Women who are under the age of 50 years or premenopausal at the time of breast cancer diagnosis derive more benefit from adjuvant systemic chemotherapy than postmenopausal women. Postmenopausal women have a lesser absolute benefit in reduction of recurrence risk than premenopausal women but still can have some benefit from adjuvant chemotherapy.

SURGERY FOR LOCALIZED BREAST CANCER

Generally, surgical options for women with localized breast cancer include breast conserving therapy (BCT) and irradiation or mastectomy.

- **BCT**—BCT offers women the option of preserving the breast without compromising survival. The tumor is surgically removed to achieve clear tumor-free margins without removing excess amounts of normal breast tissue. BCT is followed by radiation therapy (RT), either to the entire breast or just to the original tumor site (partial breast irradiation) to eradicate residual disease. BCT plus radiation provides a survival outcome equivalent to mastectomy but allows women to preserve the breast (1).
  - **Absolute contraindications to BCT:**
    - Persistently positive resection margins after re-excision attempts
    - Multicentric disease with two or more primary tumors in separate breast quadrants

- Diffuse malignant-appearing microcalcifications on mammography
- History of prior RT to the breast or chest wall that precludes further RT
- Inflammatory breast cancer
- **Relative contraindications to BCT:**
  - History of connective tissue disease (particularly scleroderma) because RT is generally tolerated poorly
  - Large tumor or small breast that would lead to a significantly poor cosmetic outcome
- **Mastectomy**—Mastectomy refers to the surgical removal of the breast. There are several different types of mastectomy.
  - **Radical mastectomy**: is the most extensive surgical procedure and is no longer routinely performed nor is it indicated. The breast is removed along with the pectoralis major and minor muscles and some overlying skin (at least 4 cm on each side of the tumor biopsy site), and there is an en bloc resection of all axillary contents, including lymph nodes beyond the subclavian vein.
  - **Modified radical mastectomy**: removes the entire breast and includes an axillary dissection, in which the level I and II axillary lymph nodes are also removed. Most women who have mastectomies today for invasive breast cancer have modified radical mastectomies.
  - **Simple or total mastectomy**: removes the entire breast and a small amount of skin but does not remove the axillary lymph nodes. A total mastectomy is appropriate for women with ductal carcinoma in situ (DCIS) and for women seeking prophylactic mastectomies—that is, breast removal in order to prevent any possibility of breast cancer occurring. In prophylactic simple mastectomy, overlying skin and nipple may be spared.

MANAGEMENT OF THE REGIONAL LYMPH NODES

Axillary lymph node dissection (ALND) has traditionally been used to manage localized breast cancer both to prevent an axillary recurrence and to provide prognostic information. Axillary metastases are an important indicator of the need for adjuvant systemic therapy and postmastectomy RT.

Complications of ALND include:

- Injury or thrombosis of the axillary vein
- Injury to the motor nerves
- Lymphedema of the upper extremity
- Seroma formation
- Shoulder dysfunction
- Loss of sensation

Sentinel node biopsy (SLNB) is routinely used for women with breast cancer without palpable axillary lymphadenopathy. SLNB is possible because breast tumor cells migrating from a primary tumor drain to one or a few axillary lymph nodes before involving other axillary nodes. Injection of a vital blue dye and/or radioactive colloid in the breast area permits intraoperative identification of the sentinel lymph node(s). The status of the SLN accurately predicts the status of the remaining regional nodes (2).

RADIATION THERAPY (RT) FOR LOCALIZED BREAST CANCER

RT is routinely delivered after BCT and may also be indicated after mastectomy, particularly for large primary tumors. The intent of RT is to eradicate subclinical residual disease and to minimize local recurrence rates. RT should be considered in almost all subgroups of women with breast cancer. Even in patients with the lowest risk disease with the most favorable prognostic features (e.g., low grade tumor, ER+, small size), whole breast RT reduces the rate of local recurrence by 75% regardless of whether adjuvant systemic therapy is used (3).

RT after BCT may be avoided in two circumstances:

- Elderly women taking hormonal therapy for ER+ breast cancer—In women over age 70 years with ER+ tumors no larger than 2 cm, RT decreased the rate of in-breast recurrence by 75%, but the overall rate of local recurrence in these women taking tamoxifen is so low that very few actually benefit from RT (4).
- Well-differentiated DCIS—If the resection margins are adequate, it is possible that RT can be avoided but this is very controversial.

Postmastectomy RT in women with larger (≥ 5 cm) tumors or axillary lymph node-positive disease reduces the risk of locoregional recurrence, increases disease-free survival, and reduces the risk of dying from breast cancer. Women with ≥ 5 cm tumors or ≥ 4 positive axillary lymph nodes are routinely offered postmastectomy RT. The benefit of RT for women with 1–3 positive lymph nodes is uncertain. The treatment field usually includes the chest wall and supraclavicular and infraclavicular regions.

ADJUVANT SYSTEMIC THERAPY

Adjuvant systemic therapy is the administration of hormonal therapy, chemotherapy, and/or trastuzumab (a humanized monoclonal antibody directed against HER2/neu) after definitive local therapy for breast cancer. Adjuvant therapy significantly reduces the risk of both recurrence and death from breast cancer.

Hormonal Therapy—Hormonal therapy is directed toward reducing estrogen and thereby blocking the growth of cancer cells that require estrogen to proliferate. Hormone receptor (ER and/or PR)-positive breast cancer requires estrogen to grow while hormone receptor-negative breast cancers are not dependent on estrogen for growth. Therefore, hormonal therapy is only effective in hormone receptor-positive breast cancers. Hormonal therapies include:

- **Tamoxifen**—an oral selective estrogen receptor modulator (SERM).
- **Aromatase inhibitors** (letrozole, anastrozole, or exemestane)—only for postmenopausal women. In premenopausal women, these drugs are ineffective as inhibition of aromatase results in reduced feedback of estrogen to the hypothalamus and pituitary, leading to increased gonadotropin secretion and increased ovarian production of estrogen.
- **Fulvestrant**—an injectable pure anti-estrogen.
- **Ovarian function suppression or ablation**—via surgical removal of the ovaries, irradiation of the ovaries, or use of luteinizing hormone releasing hormone analogs (e.g., goserelin or leuprolide).

Benefits of hormonal therapy—Data from the Early Breast Cancer Trialists Collaborative Group (EBCTCG) showed that 5 years of tamoxifen reduces the annual risk of breast cancer recurrence by about 40% and decreases the annual risk of death by about 35% in patients with ER-positive localized breast cancer (5). Adjuvant tamoxifen followed by aromatase inhibitor is one of the standard options for *postmenopausal* women with ER-positive localized breast cancer and is the *only* standard option for *premenopausal* women with ER-positive localized breast cancer.

Aromatase inhibitors for postmenopausal women—Several randomized clinical trials of postmenopausal women with localized hormone receptor-positive breast cancer have shown that adjuvant use of aromatase inhibitors, either used upfront or sequenced after tamoxifen, is superior to tamoxifen alone or placebo in terms of disease-free survival and rates of contralateral breast cancer (6–8). An aromatase inhibitor should be considered as a component of adjuvant hormonal therapy in all postmenopausal women with hormone receptor-positive breast cancer (9).

Side effects of hormonal therapy generally include vasomotor complaints and vaginal discharge and/or atrophy. Although rare, tamoxifen is also associated with an increased risk of uterine cancer, thromboembolic events, and cerebral vascular accidents. Aromatase inhibitors are also associated with loss of bone density, increased risk of bone fractures, musculoskeletal aches, and modestly increased cholesterol.

Chemotherapy—Adjuvant chemotherapy is generally recommended for:

- Women with hormone receptor-negative breast cancer, particularly if they have positive lymph nodes, larger tumors, or other adverse features

- Women with node-positive breast cancer, regardless of hormone receptor status.

- Women with HER2/neu overexpressed breast cancer with trastuzumab
  Adjuvant chemotherapy can benefit both premenopausal and postmenopausal women with localized breast cancer irrespective of hormone receptor status, although the absolute magnitude of benefit is greater in younger as compared to older women. The EBCTCG 2000 overview (5) concluded that adjuvant administration of two or more chemotherapy agents:

- For women under age 50 years and with node positive disease, chemotherapy reduces the risk of relapse by 37% and death by 30%. This results into a 10% absolute improvement in 15-year survival.

- For women ages 50–69 years, chemotherapy reduces the risk of relapse by 19% and death by 12%. This results in a 3% absolute improvement in 15-year survival.

- For women over age 70 years, the benefits of chemotherapy are uncertain because few studies include women in this age group.

The benefit of adding chemotherapy to hormonal therapy for women with hormone receptor-positive, node-negative breast cancer is unclear.

There are many choices of adjuvant chemotherapy regimens (Table 58-1). There is a modest but significant additional benefit for anthracycline-containing regimens such as (doxurobicin plus cyclophosphamide, or AC) compared to nonanthracycline-containing regimens

TABLE 58-1 COMMON ADJUVANT CHEMOTHERAPY REGIMENS FOR HER2/NEU NON-OVEREXPRESSING EARLY STAGE BREAST CANCER

Regimen	Cycle Number and Duration (Days)	Cytoxan (mg/m²)	Methotrexate (mg/m²)	5-FU (mg/m²)	Doxorubicin/Epirubicin (mg/m²)	Paclitaxel (P) or Docetaxel (D) (mg/m²)
Oral CMF	6 × 28	100, PO days 1–14	40, IV days 1, 8	600, IV days 1, 8	–	–
IV FAC	6 × 28	400, IV day 1	–	400, IV days 1, 8	40, IV day 1	
CAF	6 × 21	500, IV day 1	–	500, IV day 1	50, IV day 1	
AC	4 × 21	600, IV day 1	–	–	60, IV day 1	
AC-T	4(AC), 4(T) ×21	600, IV day 1	–	–	60, IV day 1	P: 175, IV day 1
Dose dense AC-T	4(AC), 4(T) ×14	600, IV day 1	–	–	60, IV day 1	P: 175, IV day 1
TAC	6 × 21	500, IV day 1	–	–	50, IV day 1	D: 75, IV day 1
Oral CEF	6 × 28	75, PO days 1–14	–	500, IV days 1, 8	Epirubicin 60, IV days 1, 8	–
IV FEC	6 × 21	500, IV day 1	–	–	Epirubicin 100, IV day 1	–
Docetaxel plus cyclophosphamide	4 × 21	600, IV day 1	–	–	–	D: 75, IV day 1

(such as cyclophosphamide, methotrexate, plus fluorouracil [CMF]). A taxane is often considered for premenopausal and postmenopausal women with node-positive breast cancer.

Side effects of chemotherapy—Acute side effects include temporary hair loss, nausea, vomiting, fatigue, mucositis, and diarrhea. Cardiomyopathy caused by anthracyclines is rare and increases in frequency at higher cumulative doses of the drug. Anthracyclines and alkylating agents are also potential carcinogens and can rarely cause secondary leukemias.

Trastuzumab—Approximately 20% of breast cancers overexpress the HER2/neu protein. Trastuzumab is a humanized anti-HER2/neu monoclonal antibody and improves response rate and survival in women with HER2/neu overexpressed metastatic breast cancer. The addition of trastuzumab to adjuvant chemotherapy has also been shown to significantly improve disease-free survival and overall survival in women with localized HER2/neu overexpressed breast cancer (10). However, combined trastuzumab and chemotherapy treatment regimens are associated with a small but significant increase in cardiotoxicity, particularly when used with anthracyclines. Trastuzumab is generally recommended in addition to an anthracycline and taxane-based regimen for women with node-positive breast cancer. The benefit of trastuzumab in women with high-risk, node-negative breast cancer is uncertain but is also generally recommended. Trastuzumab should not be given concurrently with an anthracycline outside of a clinical trial due to excessive cardiotoxicity risks.

REFERENCES

1. Fisher B, Anderson S, Bryant J, et al. Twenty-year follow-up of a randomized trial comparing total mastectomy, lumpectomy, and lumpectomy plus irradiation for the treatment of invasive breast cancer. *N Engl J Med*. 2002; 347: 1233–1241.

2. Lyman GH, Giuliano AE, Somerfield MR, et al. American Society of Clinical Oncology guideline recommendations for sentinel lymph node biopsy in early-stage breast cancer. *J Clin Oncol*. 2005; 23: 7703–7720.

3. Early Breast Cancer Trialists' Collaborative Group. Effects of radiotherapy and surgery in early breast cancer: an overview of the randomized trials. *N Engl J Med*. 1995; 333: 1444–1455.

4. Hughes KS, Schnaper LA, Berry D, et al. Lumpectomy plus tamoxifen with or without irradiation in women 70 years of age or older with early stage breast cancer. *N Engl J Med*. 2004; 351: 971–977.

5. Early Breast Cancer Trialists' Collaborative Group. Effects of chemotherapy and hormonal therapy for early breast cancer on recurrence and 15-year survival: an overview of the randomized trials. *Lancet*. 2005; 365: 1687–1717.

6. Howell A, Cuzick J, Baum M, et al. Results of the ATAC (Arimidex, Tamoxifen, Alone or in Combination) trial after completion of 5 years' adjuvant treatment for breast cancer. *Lancet*. 2005; 365: 60–62.

7. Goss PE, Ingle JN, Martino S, et al. A randomized trial of letrozole in postmenopausal women after five years of tamoxifen therapy for early-stage breast cancer. *N Engl J Med*. 2003; 349: 1793–1802.

8. Coombes RC, Hall E, Gibson LJ, et al. A randomized trial of exemestane after two to three years of tamoxifen therapy in postmenopausal women with primary breast cancer. *N Engl J Med.* 2004; 350: 1081–1082.

9. Winer EP, Hudis C, Burstein HJ, et al . American Society of Clinical Oncology technology assessment on the use of aromatase inhibitors as adjuvant therapy for postmenopausal women with hormone receptor-positive breast cancer: status report 2004. *J Clin Oncol.* 2005; 23: 619–629.

10. Romond E . Doxorubicin and cyclophosphamide followed by paclitaxel with or without trastuzumab as adjuvant therapy for patients with HER-2 positive operable breast cancer. In *Am Soc Clin Oncol.* 2005. Orlando, FL.

CHAPTER **59**
Metastatic Breast Cancer

Steven J. Isakoff

INTRODUCTION

Since 1990, the annual rate of breast cancer death has been decreasing by approximately 2.2% per year (1). Historically, median survival of patients with metastatic breast cancer (MBC) was estimated to be 18–30 months. Many experts agree that median survival has improved in recent years beyond 30 months, although survival varies significantly by breast cancer subtype. A number of newer active agents have recently been added to the armamentarium against breast cancer, including third-generation aromatase inhibitors, novel antimicrotubule chemotherapy agents, and biologic agents such as lapatinib, pertuzumab, and everolimus. Despite these advances, breast cancer remains the second leading cause of cancer death in women in the United States, with 39,620 women estimated to die of breast cancer in 2013 (1).

■ PROGNOSIS

Several factors contribute to predicting an individual patient's course of disease:

*   Prolonged relapse-free survival of more than 5 years is more favorable.
*   Isolated chest wall or ipsilateral nodal recurrence predicts better outcome than visceral disease.
*   Bone and soft-tissue recurrence is more favorable than visceral or central nervous system disease.
*   The prognosis of HER2-positive MBC is not established but median survival may be well beyond 3 years with the advent of newer HER2-directed strategies (2, 3).
*   The prognosis of triple negative breast cancer (ER/PR/HER2 negative) remains poor with median survival of approximately 1 year (4).

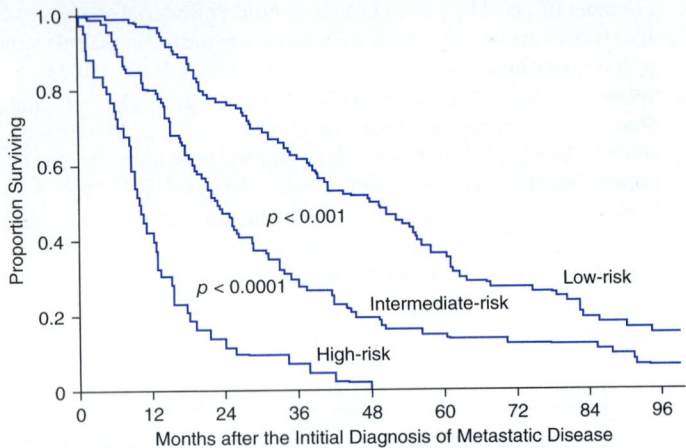

FIGURE 59-1 Prognostic index for patients with metastatic breast cancer. Patients with MBC were stratified into risk groups based on the total sum of individual prognostic factors as follows: (1) adjuvant chemotherapy—add 1 point if received; (2) distant lymph node metastates—add 1 point if present; (3) liver metastases—add 1 point if present; (4) lactate dehydrogenase—add 1 point if >1× normal; (5) disease-free interval—add 2 points if <24 months. Low-risk group ≤1 point, intermediate group = 2–3 points, high risk ≥4 points. (Adapted from Reference 5 with permission.)

- A prognostic index predicts median overall survival of 50, 23, and 11 months for low-, intermediate-, and high-risk groups, respectively (**Figure 59-1**) (5). However, its utility is limited in clinical practice because it does not account for differences in breast cancer subtypes that impact treatment options.
- Up to 2%–3% of patients with favorable characteristics may be long-term survivors with over 20-year survival. Such patients tend to be young, have limited disease, and have a complete response to initial therapy.

■ GOALS OF TREATMENT

Metastatic breast cancer is not considered curable. Therefore, the goals of treatment must carefully balance the risks of treatment-induced toxicity with the expected clinical benefit. Accepted clinical endpoints in the treatment of MBC include prolonged overall survival, improved quality of life (QOL), progression-free survival (PFS), and cancer-related symptom control.

DIAGNOSTIC EVALUATION

Most patients with MBC present with a recurrence following treatment for early-stage breast cancer. Less than 10% of patients present with MBC at the time of initial diagnosis. The most common sites of metastatic recurrence are bone, lungs, liver, and the central nervous system. Up to 50%–75% of patients will have single organ involvement at the time of initial diagnosis with MBC. Local recurrence after mastectomy usually involves the chest wall or overlying skin. In such cases, distant metastatic disease is present in 25%–30% of cases.

Evaluation of patients presenting with recurrent or MBC includes the following (6):

- History and physical exam
- Complete blood count
- Liver function tests
- Chest CT
- Abdomen and pelvis CT (or MRI)
- Positron emission tomography (PET) scan (optional, but of low added value in most cases)
- Bone scan, with subsequent radiographs of areas of concern for fracture
- Biopsy to confirm first metastatic recurrence, with confirmation of hormone receptor and HER2 preferred

Biopsy-proven confirmation of the first metastatic recurrence is preferred. The presence of estrogen receptor (ER), progesterone receptor (PgR), and HER2 overexpression in tumors will influence the selection of therapy. Therefore, biopsy of initial metastatic recurrence is increasingly clinically indicated to confirm ER, PgR, and HER2 status. In addition, patients with a history of breast cancer are at increased risk for secondary non-breast cancers, which may affect treatment selection.

TREATMENT

■ OVERVIEW

A treatment algorithm for MBC is shown in **Figure 59-2**. Although treatment options have improved significantly in recent years, most patients with MBC will eventually succumb to the disease and, therefore, all patients with MBC should be considered for participation in clinical trials.

Selection of initial and subsequent treatment requires consideration of multiple factors:

- Patient goals
- Social support
- ER, PgR, and HER2 status
- Sites of disease
- Comorbid conditions
- Performance status (ECOG or Karnofsky)
- Toxicities of treatments
- Pace of disease progression
- Previous treatment and responses
- Need for concurrent localized therapy (e.g., radiotherapy or surgery for bone or CNS disease)
- Likelihood of response to treatment

■ MONITORING TREATMENT

Treatment may be followed by periodic evaluation of the following:

- History and physical exam—Monthly evaluation for patients with MBC is reasonable to assess for progression and toxicities of treatment, although for patients on endocrine therapy less frequent follow-up may be appropriate.

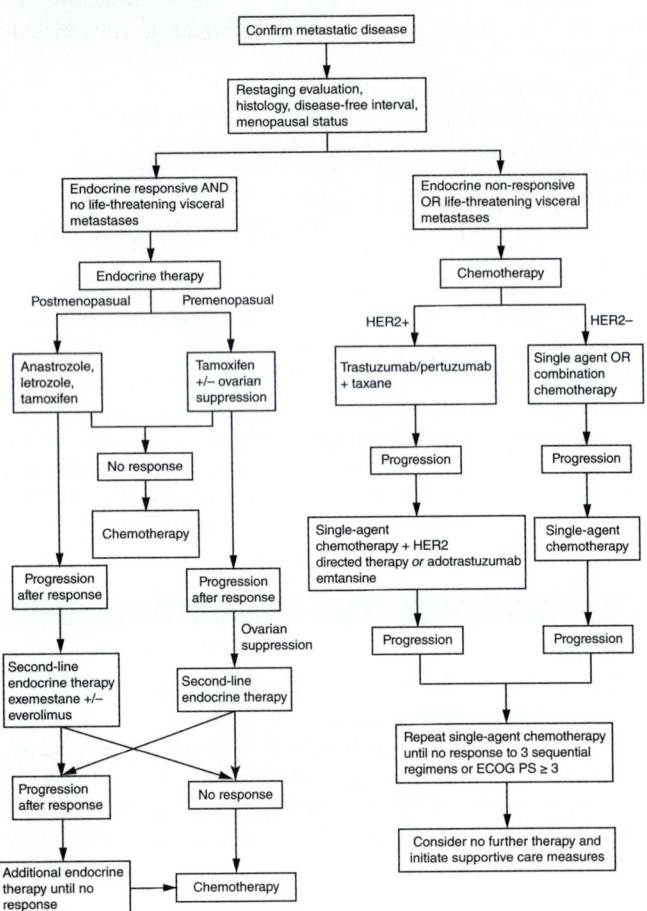

FIGURE 59-2 Treatment algorithm for metastatic breast cancer.

- Serum tumor markers: CA15-3, CA27.29, and CEA—The serum markers CA15-3 and CA 27.29 correlate with the course of disease in 60%–70% of patients, and carcinoembryonic antigen (CEA) levels correlate in 40%. Elevated serum markers prior to treatment initiation allow periodic monitoring of marker levels during the course of treatment. A "flare" reaction often occurs with endocrine therapy causing a rise in serum markers in the first month of treatment. The only recommended use of serum tumor markers is to monitor patients with MBC, according to an expert panel convened by the American Society of Clinical Oncology (7). Although assessment of circulating tumor cells (CTCs) is available for patients with MBC, its utility in routine clinical care remains controversial and most expert panels do not recommend its use.

- Radiographic studies: CT, MRI, PET, bone scans, plain films—Standardized guidelines for radiographic monitoring of patients with MBC are not established and monitoring must be individualized for each patient. Periodic scans in the absence of rising tumor markers or changing symptoms are unlikely to affect survival. Radiographic evaluation is appropriate if symptoms change or tumor markers rise. CT scans are useful to establish a new baseline after maximum response to a given therapy is achieved. PET scans are currently approved for MBC for staging and monitoring response to therapy. However, its value in clinical decision making is not established. Routine use of MRI or CT scans to monitor the central nervous system is not recommended unless a patient has known CNS disease or presents with symptoms suggestive of CNS involvement.

■ ENDOCRINE THERAPY

Endocrine therapy is preferred for most patients with hormone receptor positive MBC. Hormonal agents used in MBC are listed in Table 59-1. The mechanism of action and toxicities are described in more detail in Chapter 11, "Hormonal Agents: Antiestrogens." The following general guidelines apply to selection of hormonal therapy for MBC (Figure 59-2):

- Endocrine therapy should be initial treatment for patients with hormone receptor-positive tumors without symptomatic visceral metastases or rapidly progressive disease.
- The response rates to hormonal therapy for ER+/PgR+, ER+/PgR-, ER-/PgR- are 70%, 40%, and 10%, respectively.
- Patients with primary endocrine resistance generally should proceed directly to chemotherapy.
- Patients who respond to initial endocrine therapy may proceed to additional lines of endocrine therapy until no further response is attained or visceral metastases develop requiring rapid and more effective response. The response rate to second-line endocrine therapy is up to 33% in patients who initially responded to tamoxifen and 15% in patients who had no initial response.
- Tamoxifen is commonly used as first-line hormonal therapy in both pre- and postmenopausal women with MBC. Response rates are as high as 50%–60% and may last on average over 12 months in patients without prior exposure to adjuvant endocrine therapy. A "tamoxifen flare" can result in bone pain and increased metastatic skin lesions in up to 13% of patients. Withdrawal of tamoxifen can induce a secondary withdrawal response. Anastrozole and letrozole are third-generation nonsteroidal aromatase inhibitors (AIs) approved for first-line use in postmenopausal women with MBC and as second-line use after tamoxifen failure. Letrozole is more potent than anastrozole but results in no difference in overall survival.
- Direct comparison of tamoxifen to AIs as first-line therapy in three large randomized studies showed no statistically significant difference in median overall survival (8, 9). However, letrozole produced a longer time to progression (TTP) and a higher overall response rate (8). As a result, AIs are often preferred over tamoxifen as first-line therapy in postmenopausal women with MBC.

TABLE 59-1 HORMONAL AGENTS USED IN MBC

Agent	Regimen
• *Partial antiestrogens*	
– Tamoxifen	20 mg PO daily
– Toremifine	60 mg PO daily
• *Nonsteroidal aromatase inhibitors**	
– Anastrozole	1 mg PO daily
– Letrozole	2.5 mg PO daily
• *Steroidal aromatase inhibitors**	
– Exemestane (± Everolimus)	25 mg PO daily (± 10 mg PO daily)
• *Pure antiestrogens**	
– Fulvestrant	500 mg IM monthly
• *LHRH-agonists*†	
– Goserelin	3.6 mg SC every 28 d
– Leuprolide	3.75 or 7.5 mg IM every 28 d
– Triptorelin^	3.75 mg IM every 28 d
• *Progestin*	
– Megestrol acetate	40 mg PO four times daily
• *Androgens*	
– Fluoxymestrone	10–40 mg PO daily, in divided doses
• *High-dose estrogen*	
– Ethinyl estradiol	2 mg PO three times daily

*Therapy is appropriate for postmenopausal women only or premenopausal women receiving concurrent ovarian suppression.
†Therapy is appropriate for premenopausal women only.
^Not available in the United States.

- Exemestane is a steroidal AI approved for second-line therapy in postmenopausal women with MBC. Exemestane may induce responses in patients with primary resistance to tamoxifen. Although not approved in the United States for first-line therapy in MBC, it is a reasonable choice; exemestane results in prolonged PFS and improved response rates compared to tamoxifen for first-line therapy (10) and has similar efficacy as nonsteroidal AIs.
- Everolimus is an oral rapamycin analogue that inhibits mTOR and is approved in combination with exemestane for ER-positive/HER2-negative MBC following progression on a prior nonsteroidal AI (11). Addition of everolimus resulted in improved PFS (11.0 vs. 4.1 months) and improved response rate (12.6% vs. 1.7%), although no statistically significant improvement in overall survival was observed and toxicity was significantly higher.

- Fulvestrant is approved for postmenopausal MBC and results in similar median survival and TTP as tamoxifen (12, 13). Fulvestrant is similar in efficacy and safety to exemestane following progression on a nonsteroidal AI (14). However, dose of fulvestrant used in prior studies was shown to be inferior to the currently recommended higher dose (15).
- Ovarian suppression (OvS) with the leutinizing hormone-releasing hormone (LHRH) agonists (goserelin, triptorelin, and leuprolide) has equal efficacy to surgical OvS for premenopausal women with MBC. LHRH agonists may cause a flare reaction similar to tamoxifen. Combined tamoxifen and OvS results in higher response rates than OvS alone (39% vs. 30%), without clear survival benefit over sequential therapy.
- Megestrol acetate may have a role in patients who progress on previous therapies but has largely been replaced by the antiestrogens and AIs.
- Estradiol administration at 6 mg orally may be active in ER-positive breast cancer that has previously been treated with antiestrogen therapy and may be an option for appropriate candidates (15, 16).
- In men with hormone receptor-positive MBC, tamoxifen is the preferred initial therapy. Aromatase inhibitors have limited data but do demonstrate activity in men who progress after tamoxifen. The role of GnRH agonists is unclear in men treated with endocrine therapy. Men who are resistant to endocrine therapy or are HER2+ should be treated according to the algorithms below.

■ CHEMOTHERAPY

A treatment algorithm is shown in Figure 59-2 and representative common chemotherapy regimens for MBC are shown in **Tables 59-2** through **59-4** (3, 9–14). The mechanism of action and toxicities of specific chemotherapies are described in more detail section 1, "Classes of Drugs." The following are guidelines for chemotherapy treatment in MBC:

- Patients with visceral metastases, rapidly progressive disease, or hormone-refractory disease may be treated with chemotherapy.
- First-line chemotherapy results in response rates of 30%–60% and improved QOL.
- Combination chemotherapy has higher response rates but more toxicity and no survival benefit over sequential single agents. Second-line chemotherapy should use single agents except in selected patients.
- Factors predicting resistance to chemotherapy include relapse within 12 months of adjuvant chemotherapy, progression on a prior chemotherapy regimen, poor performance status, and multiple sites of visceral disease.
- Concurrent chemotherapy and hormonal therapy for MBC should be avoided.
- Several first-line therapy options are considered reasonable, and the choice of agent should be individualized to balance efficacy, toxicity, and breast cancer subtypes. Such agents include anthracyclines, taxanes, capecitabine, and platinums.
- Liposomal doxorubicin has equal efficacy to standard doxorubicin (17) but allows for increased cumulative dosing.

TABLE 59-2 SINGLE AGENT CHEMOTHERAPY REGIMENS FOR METASTATIC BREAST CANCER

Regimen	Agent	Cycle Length
Doxorubicin	60 mg/m^2 IV day 1	21 d
Doxorubicin—weekly	20 mg/m^2 IV	7 d
Pegylated liposomal doxorubicin	40–50 mg/m^2 IV day 1	28 d
Paclitaxel	175 mg/m^2 IV	21 d
Paclitaxel—weekly	80 mg/m^2 IV	7 d
Nanoparticle albumin-bound paclitaxel	260 mg/m^2 IV day 1	21 d
Docetaxel	75–100 mg/m^2 IV	21 d
Docetaxel—weekly	40 mg/m^2 IV day 1, 8, 15, 22, 29, 36	49 d
Vinorelbine	25–30 mg/m^2 IV	7 d
Capecitabine	1000–1250 mg/m^2 PO twice daily days 1–14	21 d
Gemcitabine	1000–1200 mg/m^2 IV days 1, 8, 15	28 d
Eribulin	1.4 mg/m^2 IV days 1, 8	21 d
Ixabepilone	40 mg/m^2 IV day 1	21 d

- Paclitaxel and docetaxel may be given on weekly or every 3-week schedules. Response rates may be higher with weekly dosing, but overall survival is similar and neurotoxicity is significantly worse. Patients who progress on paclitaxel may respond to docetaxel.
- Nanoparticle albumin-bound (nab)-paclitaxel is approved for treatment of MBC. Benefits include treatment without steroid premedication, shorter infusion times, higher effective administered paclitaxel dose, and lower hematologic toxicity. No difference in overall survival has been shown (18).
- Capecitabine, an oral 5-FU derivative, has response rates up to 28% as monotherapy. The combination of capecitabine and docetaxel showed improved survival (14.5 vs. 11.5 months) compared to single agent docetaxel in patients who progress after anthracycline therapy (19). Intravenous 5-fluorouracil is used in many of the common combination regimens for MBC but rarely as a single agent.
- Single agent vinorelbine has response rates up to 25%–50% and is particularly well tolerated in elderly patients.
- Eribulin is a novel non-taxane antimicrotubule agent recently approved for MBC. In a phase III trial comparing eribulin to physician's treatment choice in MBC patients who received between 2 and 5 prior lines of therapy, overall survival was extended by nearly 3 months (HR 0.81) and a response rate increased from 5% to 12% (20). The short infusion time,

TABLE 59-3 COMBINATION CHEMOTHERAPY REGIMENS FOR METASTATIC BREAST CANCER

Regimen	Agent	Cycle Length
CAF	Cyclophosphamide 100 mg/m^2 PO days 1–14	28 d
	Doxorubicin 30 mg/m^2 IV days 1, 8	
	5-Fluorouracil 500 mg/m^2 IV days 1, 8	
FAC	5-Fluorouracil 500 mg/m^2 IV days 1, 8	21 d
	Doxorubicin 50 mg/m^2 IV day 1	
	Cyclophosphamide 500 mg/m^2 IV day 1	
AC	Doxorubicin 60 mg/m^2 IV day 1	21 d
	Cyclophosphamide 600 mg/m^2 IV day 1	
CMF	Cyclophosphamide 100 mg/m^2 PO days 1–14	28 d
	Methotrexate 40 mg/m^2 IV days 1, 8	
	5-Fluorouracil 600 mg/m^2 IV days 1, 8	
Docetaxel/ Capecitabine	Docetaxel 75 mg/m^2 IV day 1	21 d
	Capecitabine 950 mg/m^2 PO twice daily days	1–14
Docetaxel/ Carboplatin	Docetaxel 75 mg/m^2 IV day 1	21 d
	Carboplatin AUC 6 IV day 1	
GT	Paclitaxel 175 mg/m^2 IV day 1	21 d
	Gemcitabine 1250 mg/m^2 IV day 1, 8	
FEC	5-Fluorouracil 500 mg/m^2 IV days 1, 8	28 d
	Epirubicin 50 mg/m^2 IV days 1, 8	
	Cyclophosphamide 400 mg/m^2 IV day 1, 8	
Ixabepilone/ capecitabine	Ixabepilone 40 mg/m^2 IV day 1	21 d
	Capecitabine 2000mg/m^2 PO day 1–14	
Paclitaxel/ bevacizumab	Paclitaxel 90 mg/m^2 days 1, 8, 15	28 d
	Bevacizumab 10 mg/kg IV days 1, 15	

lack of required premedication, and generally tolerable side-effect profile have been attractive features for its use in MBC.

- Single agent gemcitabine is well tolerated and has response rates up to 40% in chemotherapy-naive patients. Combination with cisplatin, vinorelbine, or paclitaxel results in higher response rates, but also increased toxicity with no improvement in overall survival. Gemcitabine may have a role in third-line therapy and beyond.

- Ixabepilone is a novel epothilone microtubule inhibitor approved as a single agent for MBC after prior anthracycline, taxane, and capecitabine. It is also approved in combination with capecitabine after anthracycline

TABLE 59-4 HER2-DIRECTED REGIMENS

Agent(s)	Regimen	Cycle Length
Trastuzumab (for use in regimens as indicated below)		
Trastuzumab	4 mg/kg IV day 1 followed by 2 mg/kg IV weekly, or 8 mg/kg IV day 1 followed by 6 mg/kg IV every 3 wk	21 d
Single agents with trastuzumab		
Paclitaxel*	175 mg/m^2 IV days 1 or 80 mg/m^2 IV day 1, 8, 15	21 d
Docetaxel*	75-100 mg/m^2 IV day 1 or 35 mg/m^2 IV day 1, 8, 15	21 d
Vinorelbine*	25–30 mg/m^2 IV day 1, 8, 15	21 d
Capecitabine*	Capecitabine 2000 mg/m^2 PO days 1–14	21 d
Pertuzumab/trastuzumab regimens		
Pertuzumab/trastuzumab/ taxane	Pertuzumab 840 mg day 1 followed by 420 mg every 3 wk	21 d
	Trastuzumab 8 mg/kg day 1 followed by 6 mg/kg every 3 wk	
	Docetaxel 75 mg/m^2 day 1 OR Paclitaxel 80 mg/m^2 day 1, 8, 15	
Ado-trastuzumab emtansine		
Ado-trastuzumab emtansine	3.6 mg/kg IV day 1	21 d
Lapatinib regimens		
Capecitabine/lapatinib	Capecitabine 2000 mg/m^2 PO days 1–14	21 d
	Lapatinib 1250 mg PO daily	
Trastuzumab/lapatinib	Trastuzumab 8 mg/kg IV day 1 followed by 6 mg/kg IV every 3 wk	21 d
	Lapatinib 1000 mg PO daily	
Combination chemotherapy regimens		
PCH*	Paclitaxel 175 mg/m^2 IV day 1	21 d
	Carboplatin AUC of 6 IV day 1	
PCH* weekly	Paclitaxel 80 mg/m^2 IV day 1, 8, 15	28 d
	Carboplatin AUC of 2 IV days 1, 8, 15	
TCH*	Docetaxel 75 mg/m^2 IV day 1	21 d
	Carboplatin AUC of 6 IV day 1	

*Each chemotherapy regimen listed may be used with either weekly or every 3-week dosing schedule of trastuzumab as shown for trastuzumab monotherapy.

and taxane treatment (21, 22). Response rates are higher in combination with capecitabine (35%–43%) than as monotherapy (12%). However, despite an improved PFS, no improvement in overall survival is seen with the combination over capecitabine monotherapy.

- Bevacizumab is a monoclonal antibody against vascular endothelial growth factor (VEGF). First-line therapy using paclitaxel plus bevacizumab compared to paclitaxel monotherapy showed a significant improvement in PFS (11.4 vs. 6.1 months) (23). No difference in overall survival was observed. However, subsequent studies reported less robust findings and in 2011 the FDA revoked the breast cancer indication for bevacizumab. The role of bevacizumab in MBC remains undefined and its use with chemotherapy remains controversial. Significant efforts are ongoing to identify biomarkers of response and to identify clinical situations where bevacizumab may be most active.

- Supportive measures should be considered in patients with an ECOG performance status ≥3 or after lack of response to three successive chemotherapy regimens.

■ HER2-DIRECTED THERAPY

Prior to the discovery of HER2-directed therapies, HER2+ MBC had relatively poor survival. However, the development of a number of approved agents, beginning with trastuzumab in the late 1990s, has resulted in significant improvements in overall survival and QOL for patients with HER2+ MBC. Patients with HER2+ breast cancer, defined as overexpression by immunohistochemistry with 3+ staining or amplification by fluorescent in situ hybridization (FISH) ratio ≥2, should receive HER2-directed therapy.

Trastuzumab is a monoclonal antibody that binds to the extracellular domain of HER2 and inhibits tumor growth by a number of possible mechanisms, including inhibition of receptor tyrosine kinase activation and signaling, enhanced receptor internalization and degradation, and antibody-dependent cellular cytotoxicity. Trastuzumab monotherapy has a response rate of at least 35% and 18% as first- and second-line treatment, respectively, in HER2+ patients. Trastuzumab combination therapy with a taxane, platinum, or vinorelbine has higher response rates than monotherapy. Paclitaxel and trastuzumab had higher response rates (41% vs. 17%), TTP (6.9 vs. 3.0 months), and a trend toward overall survival (22.1 vs. 18.4 months) compared to paclitaxel alone (9). Docetaxel combined with trastuzumab has also been shown to be superior to docetaxel alone in HER2+ patients.

Pertuzumab is a new monoclonal antibody that binds to the extracellular domain of HER2 at a distinct location from the binding site of trastuzumab and inhibits HER2-mediated cell signaling primarily by preventing heterodimerization with HER3.

Based on a phase III study demonstrating significant improvements in PFS and overall survival, first-line treatment of HER2+ disease should include combination therapy with trastuzumab and pertuzumab together with a taxane (as shown in Table 59-4) (2, 3). Activity of the trastuzumab/pertuzumab combination beyond first-line therapy was shown in several small studies, but current FDA approval is restricted to first-line use. Nevertheless, use of trastuzumab/pertuzumab combination therapy beyond first line in those patients who have not received prior pertuzumab is reasonable.

With the advent of newer HER2-directed therapies, there are now many options for treatment beyond first-line therapy and the preferred course is not established. However, it is clear that HER2 remains an important therapeutic target beyond first line, and subsequent lines of therapy should include HER2-directed agents as well. The following guidelines may be considered in treatment selection:

- Single agent trastuzumab has not been directly compared to combinations with taxanes leaving combination regimens as the preferred choice. Impressive activity with response rates over 40%–60% has also been shown in combinations of trastuzumab with vinorelbine, paclitaxel plus carboplatin, and gemcitabine, and these are reasonable choices for therapy.

- Continued use of trastuzumab following disease progression beyond first-line therapy has been shown to improve response rates and PFS. Although the benefit of trastuzumab beyond two lines of trastuzumab-based therapy is undefined, it is considered safe and may continue to provide benefit.

- Lapatinib is an oral HER2 and EGF receptor dual kinase inhibitor approved for use in combination with capecitabine after prior anthracycline, taxane, and trastuzumab therapy. In that population, the time to progression improved from 4.4 to 8.4 months in a phase III study comparing capecitabine monotherapy to capecitabine plus lapatinib (24).

- The combination of trastuzumab and lapatinib after prior trastuzumab-based therapy is an active regimen, confirming the importance of continued HER2 blockade beyond first-line therapy and the enhanced activity of dual HER2 blockade. Despite limited improvements in response rates (10.3% vs 6.9%), there was a significant improvement in overall survival of 4.5 months (HR 0.74) with the combination of trastuzumab plus lapatinib compared to lapatinib alone (25).

- In HER2+ patients who are also ER+, the addition of lapatinib to letrozole improved PFS from 3.0 to 8.2 months (26). Similar results were seen with trastuzumab and anastrozole compared to anastrozole alone (PFS 4.8 vs 2.4 months) (27). In selected patients with ER+ and HER2+ MBC, use of an AI with HER2-directed therapy is a reasonable option.

- Ado-trastuzumab emtansine (T-DM1) is a novel antibody-drug conjugate formed by covalent linkage of trastuzumab to DM1, a derivative of the chemotherapy agent maytansine. A phase III trial comparing T-DM1 to capecitabine plus lapatinib in HER2+ patients who received prior trastuzumab and taxane therapy demonstrated a significant improvement in overall survival (31 vs. 25 months) and response rate (44% vs. 31%) with an improved safety and tolerability profile (28).

- Patients with HER2+ MBC may have a higher incidence of brain metastases, with reports of up to 50% of patients developing CNS metastases during the course of their disease. This is likely due to both the lack of CNS penetration of trastuzumab despite effective systemic disease control elsewhere as well as the underlying biology of HER2+ tumors. HER2+ brain metastases may be more sensitive to radiotherapy compared to other subtypes of breast cancer. Capecitabine and lapatinib penetrate the CNS and may have some activity in HER2+ brain metastases that progressed after prior radiotherapy.

- Concurrent administration of trastuzumab and anthracyclines is contraindicated due to cardiotoxicity (29). Trastuzumab following anthracycline treatment also increases the risk of cardiotoxicity, which is often reversible and can be managed medically.

TREATMENT OF THE ELDERLY

The treatment of women over 65 years with MBC is similar to younger women with some exceptions. The elderly are at increased risk for reduced social support structures, reduced tolerance to chemotherapy, and cognitive impairment. Elderly patients without visceral disease or rapid progression may warrant a trial of hormonal therapy, regardless of hormone receptor status, as response rates up to 20% have been reported in elderly patients with hormone receptor-negative tumors. AIs may have higher response rates in the elderly. Cardiac toxicity from doxorubicin is increased in women over 70 years, but is uncommon with liposomal doxorubicin. Methotrexate and capecitabine should be dose-adjusted because of declining renal function. Sequential chemotherapy is preferable because of lower toxicity than combination regimens. Many active agents are particularly well tolerated in the elderly, including capecitabine, vinorelbine, weekly doxorubicin, trastuzumab, pertuzumab, and taxanes.

LOCAL THERAPY IN MBC

In selected patients, specific organ-directed therapy may improve QOL or survival.

Surgery has a limited role in MBC. Patients with a solitary metastasis or oligometastatic disease may be candidates for metastatectomy. Observational studies suggest surgery may improve survival in selected cases, but such studies may be subject to treatment bias. For most patients, metastatectomy should only be considered after a period of demonstrated disease control with systemic therapy.

In patients who present with de novo MBC with a primary breast tumor in situ, the role for mastectomy is controversial. Several retrospective studies suggest improved overall survival with primary breast surgery, but such studies are confounded by selection bias. Symptomatic breast tumors may require palliative breast surgery.

Up to 10%–24% of patients with MBC will develop disease limited to the lung. Surgical resection may improve survival in such patients. More than 50% of solitary pulmonary nodules may represent a primary lung cancer.

Malignant pleural effusions commonly develop in patients with MBC. Talc pleurodesis may help provide temporary symptomatic relief for patients with recurrent effusions. Newer approaches using permanent indwelling draining catheters may be more effective than traditional talc pleurodesis. Alternatively, periodic thoracentesis may be appropriate in patients with slowly accumulating effusions. Therapeutic paracentesis may provide symptomatic relief for patients with malignant ascites. Radiofrequency ablation or surgery is an option in selected patients with limited liver disease.

Up to one-third of the patients who develop brain metastases will have brain-only disease. Resection of solitary brain lesions may improve survival and QOL. The management of epidural spinal cord compression and central nervous system metastases is discussed in Chapter 63, "Metastatic Brain Tumors."

Bone is the most common site of metastatic disease in breast cancer. Patients with identified bone metastases should receive bone-directed agents, including either a bisphosphonate (zoledronic acid 4 mg IV monthly, or pamidronate 90 mg IV monthly) or denosumab (120 mg SC monthly) to reduce the risk of bone events. Radiotherapy is an effective approach to alleviate specific sites of painful bone metastasis. The management of bone metastases is discussed in detail in Chapter 16.

REFERENCES

1. Siegel R, Naishadham D, Jemal A. Cancer statistics, 2013. *CA Cancer J Clin*. 2013; 63: 11–30.

2. Swain SM, Kim SB, Cortés J, et al. Pertuzumab, trastuzumab, and docetaxel for HER2-positive metastatic breast cancer (CLEOPATRA study): overall survival results from a randomised, double-blind, placebo-controlled, phase 3 study. *Lancet Oncol*. 2013; 14(6): 461–471.

3. Baselga J, Cortes J, Kim SB, et al. Pertuzumab plus trastuzumab plus docetaxel for metastatic breast cancer. *N Engl J Med*. 2011; 366: 109–119.

4. Lin NU, Claus E, Sohl J, et al. Sites of distant recurrence and clinical outcomes in patients with metastatic triple-negative breast cancer: high incidence of central nervous system metastases. *Cancer*. 2008; 113: 2638–2645.

5. Yamamoto N, Watanabe T, Katsumata N, et al. Construction and validation of a practical prognostic index for patients with metastatic breast cancer. *J Clin Oncol*. 1998; 16: 2401–2408.

6. Carlson RW. NCCN Breast Cancer Clinical Practice Guidelines. 2012 (updated 2012; cited 2012); Version 3.2012 [available from www.nccn.org].

7. Harris L, Fritsche H, Mennel R, et al. American Society of Clinical Oncology 2007 update of recommendations for the use of tumor markers in breast cancer. *J Clin Oncol*. 2007; 25: 5287–5312.

8. Mouridsen H, Gershanovich M, Sun Y, et al. Phase III study of letrozole versus tamoxifen as first-line therapy of advanced breast cancer in postmenopausal women: analysis of survival and update of efficacy from the International Letrozole Breast Cancer Group. *J Clin Oncol*. 2003; 21: 2101–2109.

9. Bonneterre J, Buzdar A, Nabholtz JM, et al. Anastrozole is superior to tamoxifen as first-line therapy in hormone receptor positive advanced breast carcinoma. *Cancer*. 2001; 92: 2247–2258.

10. Paridaens RJ, Dirix LY, Beex LV, et al. Phase III study comparing exemestane with tamoxifen as first-line hormonal treatment of metastatic breast cancer in postmenopausal women: the European Organisation for Research and Treatment of Cancer Breast Cancer Cooperative Group. *J Clin Oncol*. 2008; 26: 4883–4890.

11. Baselga J, Campone M, Piccart M, et al. Everolimus in postmenopausal hormone-receptor-positive advanced breast cancer. *N Engl J Med.* 2011; 366: 520–529.

12. Howell A, Robertson JF, Abram P, et al. Comparison of fulvestrant versus tamoxifen for the treatment of advanced breast cancer in postmenopausal women previously untreated with endocrine therapy: a multinational, double-blind, randomized trial. *J Clin Oncol.* 2004; 22: 1605–1613.

13. Howell A, Pippen J, Elledge RM, et al. Fulvestrant versus anastrozole for the treatment of advanced breast carcinoma: a prospectively planned combined survival analysis of two multicenter trials. *Cancer.* 2005; 104: 236–239.

14. Chia S, Gradishar W, Mauriac L, et al. Double-blind, randomized placebo controlled trial of fulvestrant compared with exemestane after prior nonsteroidal aromatase inhibitor therapy in postmenopausal women with hormone receptor-positive, advanced breast cancer: results from EFECT. *J Clin Oncol.* 2008; 26: 1664–1670.

15. Di Leo A, Jerusalem G, Petruzelka L, et al. Results of the CONFIRM phase III trial comparing fulvestrant 250 mg with fulvestrant 500 mg in postmenopausal women with estrogen receptor-positive advanced breast cancer. *J Clin Oncol.* 2011; 28: 4594–4600.

16. Ellis MJ, Gao F, Dehdashti F, et al. Lower-dose vs high-dose oral estradiol therapy of hormone receptor-positive, aromatase inhibitor-resistant advanced breast cancer: a phase 2 randomized study. *JAMA.* 2009; 302: 774–780.

17. O'Brien ME, Wigler N, Inbar M, et al. Reduced cardiotoxicity and comparable efficacy in a phase III trial of pegylated liposomal doxorubicin HCl (CAELYX/Doxil) versus conventional doxorubicin for first-line treatment of metastatic breast cancer. *Ann Oncol.* 2004; 15: 440–449.

18. Gradishar WJ, Tjulandin S, Davidson N, et al. Phase III trial of nanoparticle albumin-bound paclitaxel compared with polyethylated castor oil-based paclitaxel in women with breast cancer. *J Clin Oncol.* 2005; 23: 7794–7803.

19. Miles D, Vukelja S, Moiseyenko V, et al. Survival benefit with capecitabine/docetaxel versus docetaxel alone: analysis of therapy in a randomized phase III trial. *Clin Breast Cancer.* 2004; 5: 273–278.

20. Cortes J, O'Shaughnessy J, Loesch D, et al. Eribulin monotherapy versus treatment of physician's choice in patients with metastatic breast cancer (EMBRACE): a phase 3 open-label randomised study. *Lancet.* 2011; 377: 914–923.

21. Sparano JA, Vrdoljak E, Rixe O, et al. Randomized phase III trial of ixabepilone plus capecitabine versus capecitabine in patients with metastatic breast cancer previously treated with an anthracycline and a taxane. *J Clin Oncol.* 28: 3256–3263.

22. Thomas ES, Gomez HL, Li RK, et al. Ixabepilone plus capecitabine for metastatic breast cancer progressing after anthracycline and taxane treatment. *J Clin Oncol.* 2007; 25: 5210–5217.

23. Miller K, Wang M, Gralow J, et al. Paclitaxel plus bevacizumab versus paclitaxel alone for metastatic breast cancer. *N Engl J Med.* 2007; 357: 2666–2676.

24. Geyer CE, Forster J, Lindquist D, et al. Lapatinib plus capecitabine for HER2-positive advanced breast cancer. *N Engl J Med.* 2006; 355: 2733–2743.

25. Blackwell KL, Burstein HJ, Storniolo AM, et al. Overall survival benefit with lapatinib in combination with trastuzumab for patients with human epidermal growth factor receptor 2-positive metastatic breast cancer: final results from the EGF104900 Study. *J Clin Oncol.* 2012; 30: 2585–2592.

26. Johnston S, Pippen J Jr., Pivot X, et al. Lapatinib combined with letrozole versus letrozole and placebo as first-line therapy for postmenopausal hormone receptor-positive metastatic breast cancer. *J Clin Oncol.* 2009; 27: 5538–5546.

27. Kaufman B, Mackey JR, Clemens MR, et al. Trastuzumab plus anastrozole versus anastrozole alone for the treatment of postmenopausal women with human epidermal growth factor receptor 2-positive, hormone receptor-positive metastatic breast cancer: results from the randomized phase III TAnDEM study. *J Clin Oncol.* 2009; 27: 5529–5537.

28. Verma S, Miles D, Gianni L, et al. Trastuzumab emtansine for HER2-positive advanced breast cancer. *N Engl J Med.* 2012; 367: 1783–1791.

29. Slamon DJ, Leyland-Jones B, Shak S, et al. Use of chemotherapy plus a monoclonal antibody against HER2 for metastatic breast cancer that overexpresses HER2. *N Engl J Med.* 2001; 344: 783–792.

CHAPTER **60**

Melanoma

Ryan J. Sullivan, Krista Rubin, Donald Lawrence

EPIDEMIOLOGY, RISK FACTORS, SCREENING, AND PREVENTION

EPIDEMIOLOGY

The incidence of melanoma has dramatically risen over the past several decades and in 2013, an estimated 76,690 new cases and 9,480 deaths were expected in the United States (1). As a result, melanoma is now the fifth and sixth most common malignancy in the United States among men and women, respectively (1).

RISK FACTORS

Risk factors for melanoma include light complexion, poorly tanning skin, and blonde or red hair, which confer a relative risk of 1.3–4.1 (2). Intense, intermittent sun exposure and a history of blistering sunburn appear to confer a greater risk than lower-level, continuous sunlight exposure (3). Both ultraviolet A (UVA) and ultraviolet B (UVB) radiation have been implicated in the pathogenesis of melanoma (4). Exposure to UV radiation via tanning booths and, with psoralen, as a treatment for psoriasis, is associated with an increase in the risk of melanoma (5).

Numerous common nevi are a marker of increased risk, as are atypical nevi (6). Large congenital nevi have a high risk of malignant transformation (lifetime risk 4%–10%) (7–9). Following the diagnosis of melanoma, the probability of developing a second primary melanoma has been estimated to be 5.34% over an interval of 20 years (10).

Melanoma in a first-degree relative confers an increased risk, and about 10% of individuals diagnosed with melanoma have an affected family member (11, 12). However, the magnitude of the risk associated with family history is quite variable. Most families with multiple affected members have no identifiable genetic abnormality. Genes in which germline mutations or polymorphisms have been associated with an increased risk of melanoma include CDKN2A and CDK4, which encode cell cycle regulatory proteins, the melanocortin 1 receptor gene, and the breast cancer susceptibility gene, BRCA2 (relative risk for melanoma, 2.58) (13–16).

The dysplastic nevus syndrome is characterized by numerous atypical nevi and the development of melanoma at an early age (17). The lifetime risk of melanoma approaches 100% in this syndrome. Its genetic basis remains unknown.

■ SCREENING

The majority of melanomas display at least one of the following features:

    A: Asymmetry
    B: Irregularity of borders
    C: Color variegation
    D: Diameter >6 mm
    E: Enlargement or evolution

Ten percent of incident cases of melanoma are classified as having nodular histology and, therefore, lack the characteristic asymmetry, irregularity of border, and color variegation of the more common superficial spreading melanoma. However, nodular melanomas are associated with the poorest survival of all subtypes and account for a disproportionate number of melanoma deaths (18).

Melanoma is highly curable by surgical excision when detected at an early stage (i.e., less than 1 mm in thickness), whereas the risk of mortality rises sharply with thicker lesions (19). The American Academy of Dermatology has sponsored a screening program for over one million individuals. In a subgroup for which pathologic data were available, a presumptive diagnosis of melanoma was made in 0.8% and confirmed in 0.15%. The highest yield was among white males over the age of 50 years, a population that also has the highest risk for mortality from melanoma (20). While no survival data are available from this program, it lends support to the feasibility, and possibly the efficacy, of large-scale screening, as do similar programs in other countries. The overall benefit and cost-effectiveness of screening remain to be determined.

■ PREVENTION

The efficacy of topical sunscreens in the primary prevention of melanoma has not been rigorously demonstrated (21). Effective melanoma prevention strategies will probably involve a combination of education and behavior modification beginning at an early age. Such programs are underway in the United States, Australia, and other endemic areas, but their impact is difficult to gauge at this point.

For decades, although there was a clear link between sun-exposure or recreational exposure to UV radiation (i.e., tanning beds) and melanoma, no definitive, randomized evidence had existed which proved that sunscreen use prevents melanomagenesis (3, 4). It was thought that this may have been be due to the fact that commercially available sunscreens reduce exposure to UVB radiation but not to UVA, that they were inadequately applied, or that they provided a false sense of security leading to more prolonged sun exposure. The first randomized trial rigorously evaluating the use of sunscreen for the prevention of melanoma was reported in 2011 (22). In this study, investigators randomized 1621 participants in Nambour, Australia (ages 25–75 years) to either sunscreen intervention or no sunscreen intervention from 1992 to 1996 and then were followed with questionnaires and/or pathology departments and cancer registries through 2006. A borderline-statistically significant reduction in both total melanomas (HR 0.50, 95% CI 0.271.02; $p = 0.051$) and invasive melanomas

(0.27, 95% CI 0.080.97; $p = 0.045$) in the intervention group. These findings support the long-assumed contention that sunscreen likely prevents the formation of invasive melanoma. In addition, a greater benefit might be expected if such a study such as this were performed in children, given that intense sun exposure and burns in childhood are a strong risk factor for developing melanoma (23). It is unlikely; however, that such a study would be performed given the ethical dilemma of randomizing children to not receive sunscreen intervention in areas of high incidence for melanoma.

PATHOLOGIC FEATURES OF MELANOMA

The likelihood of recurrence and death from melanoma is directly correlated with tumor thickness. Ulceration (the absence of an intact epidermal layer overlying the melanoma) is a powerful adverse prognostic feature. A high mitotic rate is also associated with a poor prognosis, and along with thickness and ulceration are the three factors incorporated into the American Joint Committee on Cancer staging criteria (24, 25).

Melanoma may arise de novo, from a preexisting nevus, or from melanoma in situ, in which the melanocytic proliferation is limited to the epidermis. Radial growth phase melanoma is confined in large part to the epidermis and has a low likelihood of dissemination. The vertical growth phase is characterized by prominent dermal invasion and signals the acquisition of metastatic potential.

Several distinct growth patterns of melanoma are recognized. Superficial spreading melanoma is defined by the presence of both a radial and a vertical growth phase, and accounts for up to 75% of melanomas. Nodular melanomas (15%–25%) are vertical growth phase lesions, located exclusively or predominantly in the dermis. Lentigo maligna melanoma typically arises from a noninvasive precursor lesion (lentigo maligna, or lentigo maligna melanoma in situ) and occurs most frequently on the face, scalp, or neck in older individuals. Acral lentiginous melanoma accounts for only 5% of melanomas but is the most common subtype in non-Caucasians. The sites of highest incidence are the palmar and plantar surfaces. Histologically, these lesions are characterized by the presence of nests of atypical melanocytes at the dermal-epidermal junction, with infiltration of single cells or nests into the dermis.

A minority of melanomas are amelanotic, lacking obvious pigmentation, and mimic a variety of benign entities, often leading to a delay in diagnosis. In other respects their behavior is similar to pigmented melanomas.

The detection of melanocyte-associated antigens by immunohistochemistry may suggest or support the diagnosis of melanoma in difficult cases, such as metastatic cancer of uncertain histogenesis. Immunohistochemistry may also detect small deposits of metastatic melanoma within lymph nodes that are not evident on routine microscopic examination. S-100 is expressed by cells of melanocytic lineage, but also by histiocytes and certain neural tumors. Melan-A is also somewhat nonspecific. Antigens with a higher degree of specificity for melanocytes include tyrosinase, the microphthalmia transcription factor, and a protein in the premelanosome complex targeted by the monoclonal antibody HMB45. None of these antigens, however, can be used to distinguish melanoma from benign melanocytic proliferative processes.

STAGING AND PROGNOSTIC FACTORS

The American Joint Committee on Cancer's 7th edition (2009) staging system for cutaneous melanoma is based on the analysis of prognostic factors in 30,946 patients (19). Stage I and II melanomas is defined as disease without regional lymphatic or systemic spread. The staging of node-negative melanoma is based on the worsening prognosis with increasing thickness of the primary lesion ulceration and, for thin melanomas (≤1 mm), the presence of dermal mitoses (Table 60-1). While the majority of stage I and II melanomas are cured by surgery alone, even melanomas 1 mm or less in thickness, without ulceration or nodal involvement (T1aN0M0) have metastatic potential, and are associated with a 10-year disease-specific mortality rate of approximately 5%–10%. The 10-year survival in patients with thick melanomas (stages IIB and IIC) is 32.3%–53.9%. Ulceration is associated with a relative risk of death of 1.9 in node-negative melanomas.

Stage III melanoma is defined by the presence of satellite and/or in-transit metastases, and/or involvement of regional lymph nodes (Table 60-2) in the absence of systemic metastasis. Lymphatic metastases within 2 cm of the primary lesion are designated satellite metastases; those located more than 2 cm from the primary melanoma, but before the first echelon of draining lymph nodes, are designated in-transit metastases. The burden of tumor in the lymph nodes is predictive of outcome and is represented by the number of nodes involved, and whether the involvement is microscopic (not clinically apparent prior to surgery) or macroscopic (clinically apparent).

While lymphatic involvement is associated with an increased risk of recurrence and death with each T stage subgroup, stage III melanoma is a heterogeneous disease. Specifically, patients with a thin (T1) or intermediate (T2), non-ulcerated melanomas with microscopic nodal involvement have a 10-year survival rate of approximately 70%, while patients with clinically detectable lymphadenopathy, ≥4 involved or matted lymph nodes, in-transit/satellite metastases, and/or ulceration of the primary melanoma and any degree of nodal involvement, have a 10-year survival that ranges from approximately 25% to 45%.

TABLE 60-1 PRIMARY TUMOR STAGE, CUTANEOUS MELANOMA

TX	Primary tumor cannot be assessed
T0	No evidence of primary tumor
Tis	Melanoma in situ
T1	≤1 mm in thickness[*]
T2	1.01–2 mm in thickness[†]
T3	2.01–4 mm in thickness[†]
T4	>4 mm in thickness[†]

[*]a: Non-ulcerated, invasion to anatomic level<IV; b: Ulcerated, or invasion to anatomic level IV or V.
[†]a: Non-ulcerated; b: Ulcerated.
Source: Adapted from Reference 25.

TABLE 60-2 REGIONAL NODAL/LYMPHATIC STAGING OF MELANOMA

NX	Regional lymph nodes cannot be assessed
N0	No regional lymph node/lymphatic metastases
N1a	Metastasis in one regional lymph node, clinically occult
N1a	Metastasis in one regional lymph node, clinically apparent
N2a	Metastases in 2–3 regional lymph nodes, clinically occult
N2b	Metastases in 2–3 regional lymph nodes, clinically apparent
N2c	In-transit/satellite metastases without nodal involvement
N3	Metastases in >4 regional lymph nodes, matted lymph nodes, or in-transit/satellite metastases with nodal involvement

Source: Adapted from Reference 25.

Stage IV melanoma represents distant metastatic spread, and is stratified according to sites of involvement and lactate dehydrogenase level (Table 60-3). Based on these T, N, and M criteria, patients can be grouped according to prognosis (Table 60-4).

Stage-for-stage, advanced age, and male sex are associated with a worse prognosis in melanoma (19). Melanomas of the extremities have a more favorable prognosis than those of the trunk. Head and neck melanomas, particularly those of the scalp and ears, have a worse prognosis than other sites (26).

SURGICAL MANAGEMENT

When a cutaneous lesion is suspected to be melanoma, biopsy techniques should be employed which preserve the pathologist's ability to assess the thickness and depth of invasion of the lesion, that is, conservative excisional biopsy, or punch biopsy. Ablative procedures such as cryotherapy should be avoided.

TABLE 60-3 STAGING OF MELANOMA, DISTANT METASTASES

MX	Distant metastases cannot be assessed
M0	No distant metastases
M1a	Metastases to skin, subcutaneous sites, and/or distant lymph nodes
M1b	Metastases to lung only
M1c	Metastases to all other sites, or to any site with elevated serum lactate dehydrogenase (LDH)

Adapted from Reference 25.

TABLE 60-4 PATHOLOGIC STAGE GROUPING AND PROGNOSIS IN MELANOMA

Stage	TNM	10-Year Survival (%)
Node/lymphatic negative		
IA	T1aN0M0	87.9 ± 1.0
IB	T1bN0M0	83.1 ± 1.5
	T2aN0M0	79.2 ± 1.1
IIA	T2bN0M0	64.4 ± 2.2
	T3aN0M0	63.8 ± 1.7
IIB	T3bN0M0	50.8 ± 1.7
	T4aN0M0	53.9 ± 3.3
IIC	T4bN0M0	32.3 ± 2.1
Node/lymphatic positive		
IIIA	T1-4aN1aM0	63.0 ± 4.4
	T1-4aN2aM0	56.9 ± 6.8
IIIB	T1-4bN1aM0	37.8 ± 4.8
	T1-4bN2aM0	35.9 ± 7.2
	T1-4aN1bM0	47.7 ± 5.8
	T1-4aN2bM0	39.2 ± 5.8
	T1-4(a or b)N2cM0	
IIIC	T1-4bN1bM0	24.4 ± 5.3
	T1-4bN2bM0	15.0 ± 3.9
	T(any)N3M0	18.4 ± 2.5
Metastatic		
IV	T(any)N(any)M1a	15.7 ± 2.9
	T(any)N(any)M1b	2.5 ± 1.5
	T(any)N(any)M1c	6.0 ± 0.9

Adapted from References 24 and 25.

Once the diagnosis of melanoma is established, a wide local excision is the treatment of choice. Five randomized trials have assessed the effect of margins of resection on local recurrence (27–31). For melanomas ≤1 mm in depth, local recurrence was not significantly different with 1 or 3 cm margins; therefore, 1-cm margins are acceptable for thin melanomas. For melanomas greater than 1 mm, the data generally support margins of 2 cm.

Randomized studies have failed to demonstrate a survival benefit for elective lymph node dissection in patients without clinically apparent nodal involvement, and this approach has largely been abandoned. The procedure of sentinel lymph node mapping and selective lymphadenectomy is highly sensitive for the detection of microscopic nodal metastases and has a high negative predictive value. Thus, patients without clinical evidence of nodal involvement (the majority) can be accurately staged without the morbidity of a complete nodal dissection, and patients harboring occult nodal disease can be identified. For patients with a positive sentinel node, a complete dissection of the involved lymph node basin(s) is usually recommended, although the benefit of this procedure has not been formally demonstrated. The detection of occult nodal metastases also identifies patients who may be candidates for adjuvant systemic therapy with interferon-alfa (high-dose or pegylated interferon) or participation in clinical trials.

In the Multicenter Selective Lymphadenectomy Trial, 1327 patients with melanomas 1.2–3.5 mm were randomized to wide excision with sentinel node mapping and biopsy, or wide excision followed by observation (32). Patients found to have positive sentinel nodes underwent completion node dissections. At a median follow-up of 59.8 months, the melanoma specific survival in the two groups was not significantly different (death from melanoma occurred in 13.8% of the observation group and 12.5% of the biopsy group). The benefit of sentinel node biopsy was reflected in risk of regional/nodal recurrence. Patients assigned to sentinel node biopsy had statistically superior disease-free survival compared with those who were observed (78.3% vs. 73.1%). Accounting for either microscopic nodal involvement (in the sentinel node biopsy cohort) or clinically evident nodal involvement (in the observation cohort), the overall rate of lymph node involvement was found to be very similar in both groups. Thus, sentinel node biopsy provided a basis for identifying those patients who warrant further lymph node surgery to prevent a clinically evident and potentially morbid regional recurrence.

ADJUVANT THERAPY FOR HIGH-RISK MELANOMA

The staging criteria described above identify patients at high risk for recurrence and death. Most studies of adjuvant therapies have focused on patients with intermediate thick, ulcerated primary melanomas (T3b), thick primary melanomas (>4 mm), and/or those with nodal involvement (stages IIB, IIC, and III), a group with an expected survival rate of less than 50%. Attempts to identify effective adjuvant therapy have been hampered historically by the absence of systemic therapies that produce meaningful response rates in advanced melanoma.

High-dose interferon alfa-2b (HDI) has been the subject of three phase III trials in high-risk, resected melanoma, yet controversy persists about its efficacy (33–35). A pooled, updated analysis of two of these trials showed a relapse-free survival advantage for HDI versus observation (HR = 1.30, $p < 0.006$) at a median follow-up of 7.2 years but no benefit for HDI in terms of overall survival (36). In a third trial, 880 patients with stage IIB–III melanoma were randomized to HDI or to vaccination with GM2, an immunogenic ganglioside expressed by melanoma cells. At a median follow-up of 2.4 years, there was a statistically significant advantage for HDI in terms of relapse-free and overall survival (35).

The impact of HDI on the risk of relapse seems confined to 20%–30% of patients, and its adverse effects are considerable. Recent investigations suggest a correlation between autoimmunity and a benefit from interferon.

In a cohort of 200 patients receiving HDI, those who developed autoimmune manifestations (vitiligo, thyroid dysfunction, or autoantibodies) had dramatically better outcomes: 7/52 (13.5%) relapsed, and 2/52 (4%) died, as compared with 108/148 (73%) relapses and 80/148 (54%) deaths in patients without autoimmunity ($p < 0.001$) (37). Identifying genetic factors that predispose to autoimmunity may allow selection of patients more likely to benefit from interferon.

Pegylated interferon was evaluated in a large, observation-controlled phase III trial in patients with resected stage III melanoma and demonstrated a statistically significant improvement in relapse-free survival (38). At least 1256 patients were evenly randomized to 5 years of pegylated interferon (6 mcg/kg SC weekly for 8 weeks, followed by 3 mcg/kg weekly for up to 5 years). With 7.6 years of follow-up, a 13% improvement in relapse-free survival was noted in the overall population (HR 0.87, $p = 0.05$). No difference in overall survival was detected (HR 0.96, $p = 0.57$). Subset analysis suggested that more benefit was accrued to those patients with microscopic nodal involvement at study entry compared to those with clinically evident nodal metastases (relapse-free survival HR 0.82, $p = 0.08$). Amongst the subset of patients with microscopic nodal involvement and ulcerated primary tumors (15% of the overall study population), a 28% improvement in relapse-free survival ($p = 0.06$) and 41% improvement in overall survival ($p = 0.006$) were observed. This has prompted a follow-up observation-controlled trial evaluating pegylated interferon in patients with resected, ulcerated stage II melanomas.

METASTATIC MELANOMA

The prognosis for patients with metastatic melanoma is generally poor. The prognosis varies depending on whether the disease is limited to subcutaneous sites and/or lymph nodes (M1a), if the lungs are the only site of visceral metastasis (M1b), or if other sites of visceral metastasis are identified, and/or if the lactate dehydrogenase (LDH) level is elevated (M1c) (19). The 1-year survival rates of M1a, M1b, and M1c are approximately 70%, 60%, and 35%, respectively. Still, melanoma typically disseminates widely, and frequently involves sites that are uncommon in other cancers, such as the GI tract and the skin. Brain metastases are very common and are associated with a median survival of less than 6 months (39).

Treatment options for stage IV melanoma have traditionally been extremely limited, with only dacarbazine (DTIC) and high-dose interleukin 2 (HD IL-2) receiving FDA approval from 1976 to 2011. Recent advances in molecularly targeted therapy and immunotherapy have led to the development of BRAF-targeted agents and a CTLA-4 blocking antibody that have demonstrated survival improvements in phase III trials. A small subset of patients, generally those with a limited extent of metastatic disease (AJCC M1a), may survive for >10 years (24, 25).

■ SURGERY AND LIMB PERFUSION

A small and highly selected group of patients with advanced melanoma may achieve prolonged freedom from relapse after surgical resection of oligo-metastases. The patients who appear most likely to benefit are those with a solitary metastasis involving skin, lungs, distant lymph nodes, or the gastrointestinal tract, those with a long disease-free interval between disease recurrence, and those in whom the metastatic focus can be completely resected. In these patients, 5-year survival rates of 4%–35% have been reported (40–44).

Isolated limb perfusion with melphalan and moderate hyperthermia is an effective treatment for recurrent or unresectable in-transit metastases of an extremity. High concentrations of chemotherapy to the limb can be achieved without excessive systemic exposure by isolation of the circulation, leading to complete responses in greater than 50% of patients (45). As this approach has no effect on subclinical visceral metastases, it is not surprising that no improvement in overall survival has been observed.

◼ CHEMOTHERAPY

Melanoma is refractory to most standard cytotoxic agents. Objective response rates to single-agent chemotherapy are in the range of 51%–55% and are typically of brief duration. Response rates to combination chemotherapy are somewhat higher, but toxicity is increased with the use of multiple agents, and no survival advantage has been demonstrated. DTIC had been considered the "standard" treatment, and temozolomide (Temodar), an oral methylating agent, was also commonly used. In a randomized trial comparing these agents, response rates were similar (13.5% with temozolomide and 12.1% with DTIC). Progression-free survival was slightly longer in the temozolomide arm (1.9 months vs. 1.5 months), but there was no statistical difference in overall survival (7.7 and 6.4 months) (46).

◼ IMMUNOTHERAPY

Patients with metastatic melanoma experience spontaneous remissions, albeit rarely (47). This phenomenon presumably results from an antitumor immune response. As a result, numerous immune-based therapies, including various cytokines and vaccines, have been tested in advanced melanoma with varying results. With nearly every agent/strategy complete regressions have been reported. Still, very few of these therapies demonstrated any meaningful benefit in larger cohorts of patients (48). More recently, inhibitors of immune check points have been developed, which include ipilimumab, a monoclonal antibody that blocks the activity of cytotoxic T-cell antigen 4 (CTLA-4). With the advent of this and other new agents, the promise of immunotherapy in melanoma is now being realized in many patients.

High Dose Interleukin 2

The first approved immunotherapy for advanced melanoma was HD IL-2. IL-2, a type 1 cytokine, is a central regulator of the cellular immune response, inducing activation and proliferation of T cells and NK cells. In vitro, it stimulates the development of lymphokine-activated killer (LAK) cells, which can lyse autologous tumor cells. HD IL-2 (aldesleukin, Proleukin®) treatment has been evaluated extensively in patients with metastatic melanoma. The objective response rate to high-dose IL-2 was 16%, and the complete response rate was 6% in an analysis of 270 patients.

Twelve of the responding patients remained progression free, including 10 patients in continuous complete remission. Five other responding patients remained disease free after surgery or radiation for limited sites of progressive disease (49). Patients with metastases limited to skin and subcutaneous sites appear most likely to benefit (response rate 53.6%) (50). IL-2 treatment is associated with substantial toxicity, including a capillary leak syndrome, hemodynamic instability, and a high risk of infection. As a result, its availability is limited to a small number of highly specialized centers.

Both HD and lower dose IL-2 have been evaluated in various contexts: with adoptive cellular immunotherapy using autologous LAK cells or tumor-infiltrating lymphocytes, with other cytokines, and with chemotherapy agents and vaccines. The great majority of these approaches have demonstrated no clear superiority compared to IL-2 as a single agent (48). One such study, however, did show a significant improvement in response rate and overall survival. Specifically, patients were randomized in a phase III trial to receive either HD IL-2 alone or in combination with a GP100 vaccine (51). While a doubling of response rate and survival was seen in this study, the patients treated with HD IL-2 alone had outcomes that were much worse than previously described and the combination group had outcomes in line with historical and contemporary cohorts of patients treated with HD IL-2. For this reason, despite the purported superiority of this combination, this study has not led to the FDA approval of the GP100 vaccine in combination with HD IL-2 in patients with advanced melanoma.

Ipilimumab

Investigations in immunotherapy have focused on overcoming barriers to generating a sustained and effective antitumor immune response. Cytotoxic T-lymphocyte-associated antigen-4 (CTLA-4) is expressed on activated T cells and serves as an immune checkpoint of T-cell activation (52). When CTLA-4 is engaged by its ligands on antigen presenting cells, the T-cell response is inhibited and anergy may result. Monoclonal antibodies that block the interaction of CTLA-4 with its ligands enhance antitumor immune responses. Complete responses and sustained partial responses have been reported in up to 13% of patients with metastatic melanoma treated with anti-CTLA-4 antibodies, but serious autoimmune toxicity, including enterocolitis and hyphophysitis, has also been observed (53, 54). There appears to be a positive correlation between autoimmune phenomena and response. In comparison to DTIC alone in treatment-naive patients, the combination of ipilimumab (one CTLA-4 antibody) and DTIC improved survival (HR 0.72, $p < 0.001$), with 21% of patients receiving the combination alive at 3 years versus 12% in the chemotherapy arm (55). In comparison to GP100 peptide vaccine alone, ipilimumab monotherapy improved survival in chemotherapy refractory patients by 34% ($p = 0.003$) (56). On the basis of these combined results, ipilimumab monotherapy was approved for use in metastatic melanoma.

PD1/PDL1

A second immune checkpoint that has emerged as a target of monoclonal antibody inhibition is the Programmed Death 1 (PD-1)—Programmed

Death Ligand 1 (PD-L1) pathway. PD1 is a cell surface protein on T cells that interacts with PD-L1 expressed on antigen presenting cells and various tissues to impair T-cell activation (52). Additionally, tumor cells, including approximately 70% of melanomas, may express PD-L1. PD-L1 expression is an important mechanism in the abrogation of antitumor immunity (57). Recently, monoclonal antibodies against both PD-1 and PD-L1 have been introduced into the clinic with highly encouraging results (58, 59). In particular, the anti-PD1 antibody nivolumab (MDX-1106, BMS-936558) has shown excellent activity in patients with melanoma. In the phase I study of this agent, 26 of 94 patients with melanoma treated at five different doses responded to treatment, with half of these responses lasting greater than a year (58). Relatively few serious immune-related adverse events were observed and thus nivolumab, other anti-PD1 antibodies, and anti-PD-L1 antibodies are among the most promising anticancer therapies currently in development.

Tumor Infiltrating Lymphocytes

Harvesting of tumor infiltrating lymphocytes from metastatic tumors, ex vivo expansion, and administration following lymphodepleting therapy (so-called adoptive T-cell therapy) have resulted in long-lasting complete remission in highly selected patients (60). A recent protocol that involves introduction of a new T-cell receptor into harvested lymphocytes, lymphodepleting chemotherapy, and total body irradiation is reported to produce a 72% response rate, with 40% achieving a complete response. This approach remains investigational.

■ TARGETED THERAPY FOR MELANOMA

Recent research has begun to elucidate the genetic abnormalities underlying dysregulated growth, resistance to apoptosis, invasion, and metastasis in melanoma. Substantial molecular heterogeneity has been discovered among melanomas, but a number of mutations occur with high frequency and appear to be critical for survival and proliferation. Activating mutations in the mitogen-activated protein kinase (MAP kinase) signal transduction pathway are found in the large majority of melanomas, most frequently in the serine-threonine kinase BRAF, where a single amino acid substitution (V600E) is present in 40%–50% if metastatic melanoma patients. Activating mutations are found in N-RAS in 15%–30% of cases (61). These mutations are mutually exclusive in the large majority of melanomas. Melanomas lacking mutations in N-RAS or BRAF have been found to harbor abnormalities in cell cycle regulatory genes that may obviate the requirement for an activated MAP kinase pathway, for example, amplification of CCND1 or CDK4, or loss of the tumor suppressor gene CDKN2A (p16) (62). Novel melanoma oncogenes have recently been described, which may serve as therapeutic targets in melanomas that are wild type for BRAF and NRAS (63).

BRAF inhibitor therapy has been established as an effective treatment for melanomas with V600E or V600K BRAF mutations. A survival improvement was documented in comparison to DTIC in treatment-naive patients (HR 0.37, $p < 0.001$), as well as 74% improvement in progression-free survival ($p < 0.001$) (64, 65). BRAF inhibitor therapy is distinguished by a high response rate of 40%–50%, rapid onset of action, and reversible cutaneous and joint toxicity. Single agent MEK inhibition also improves progression-free and overall survival in this population in comparison to chemotherapy (HR for progression-free survival 0.45, $p < 0.001$ and HR for overall survival 0.55, $p = 0.01$) (66). The results of a randomized phase II trial suggest that the addition of a MEK inhibitor to a BRAF inhibitor further improves outcomes, with a 61% improvement in progression-free survival compared to BRAF inhibitor monotherapy ($p < 0.001$) and a response rate of 76% compared to 54% ($p = 0.03$) (67).

The majority of acral lentiginous and mucosal melanomas express wild-type BRAF and N-RAS, but have more diffuse chromosomal gains and losses than other types of melanoma (62). Approximately 20% have mutations or amplification of the gene encoding the receptor tyrosine kinase c-kit (62). Small-molecule signal transduction inhibitors that target the MAP kinase pathway are being evaluated in clinical trials in advanced melanoma. Among a minority of patients with certain activating c-kit mutations, imatinib has produced complete or partial responses (68, 69).

OCULAR AND MUCOSAL MELANOMA

■ OCULAR MELANOMA

The incidence of intraocular melanoma is <1% that of cutaneous melanoma. UV radiation exposure, fair skin, and light eye color have been implicated as risk factors (70). The large majority of uveal melanomas arise in the choroid. Uveal melanomas are often diagnosed on routine funduscopic exam or present with visual symptoms. Small uveal melanomas can be difficult to distinguish from benign nevi and can be followed closely, since some will not progress. Enucleation is reserved for advanced lesions. The majority of uveal melanomas can be treated either by brachytherapy with implantation of radioactive plaques or by charged particle (proton or helium ion) radiotherapy. Local recurrence rates with these modalities are low, and survival rates are similar to those obtained with enucleation (71).

Risk factors for metastatic spread of uveal melanoma include tumor diameter, ciliary body involvement, and scleral or extraocular extension. Uveal melanoma is an aggressive disease, with metastases developing in 34% of patients within 10 years (72). Dissemination tends to be hematogenous, and up to 90% of patients who develop metastases have liver involvement. The mortality rate for metastatic uveal melanoma is 80% 1 year after diagnosis and 95% within 2 years (72).

Somatic genetic alterations in uveal melanoma have recently been defined and are distinct from those found in cutaneous or mucosal melanomas. One of two G-proteins, GNAQ and GNA11, harbors a point mutation that results in constitutive activation in 80%–90% of ocular melanomas (73, 74). A similarly high percentage have inactivating mutations in the BAP1 tumor suppressor gene (75). Therapeutic strategies to counteract the pathogenic effect of these mutations are currently in development.

■ MUCOSAL MELANOMA

Mucosal melanomas are uncommon and aggressive tumors. They typically present at an advanced stage and are associated with a poor prognosis.

The most common sites are the female genitalia, the head and neck (oral and nasal cavities and paranasal sinuses), and the anorectal region. In each of these sites, surgical resection is the mainstay of therapy, but the high risk of distant relapse must be weighed when considering radical surgery.

For anorectal melanomas, sphincter-sparing surgery followed by radiotherapy is a reasonable alternative to abdominoperineal resection. Vulvar melanomas tend to occur in older, Caucasian women. Prognostic factors are similar to those for cutaneous sites, and wide local excision, when feasible, appears to be associated with outcomes similar to radical vulvectomy. Reported 5-year survival rates range from 22% to 54% (76–78). Melanomas of the vaginal mucosa have an extremely poor prognosis, with a reported 5-year survival rate of 14% (79).

For mucosal melanomas of the head and neck, the possibility of cure rests on adequate surgical control of the primary tumor. Even with radical surgery, however, most patients will subsequently relapse and die from their disease. Five-year survival rates of 20%–50% have been reported. Postoperative radiotherapy may decrease the likelihood of local relapse but is unlikely to affect survival, given the high incidence of distant metastases (80).

REFERENCES

1. Siegel R, Naishadham D, Jemal A. Cancer statistics, 2013. *CA Cancer J Clin.* 2013; 63: 11–30.

2. Bliss JM, Ford D, Swerdlow AJ, et al. Risk of cutaneous melanoma associated with pigmentation characteristics and freckling: systematic overview of 10 case-control studies. The International Melanoma Analysis Group (IMAGE). *Int J Cancer.* 1995; 62: 367–376.

3. Lew RA, Sober AJ, Cook N, et al. Sun exposure habits in patients with cutaneous melanoma: a case control study. *J Dermatol Surg Oncol.* 1983; 9: 981–986.

4. Stern RS. The risk of melanoma in association with long-term exposure to PUVA. *J Am Acad Dermatol.* 2001; 44: 755–761.

5. Gallagher RP, Spinelli JJ, Lee TK. Tanning beds, sunlamps, and risk of cutaneous malignant melanoma. *Cancer Epidemiol Biomarkers Prev.* 2005; 14: 562–566.

6. Holly EA, Kelly JW, Shpall SN, et al. Number of melanocytic nevi as a major risk factor for malignant melanoma. *J Am Acad Dermatol.* 1987; 17: 459–468.

7. Quaba AA, Wallace AF. The incidence of malignant melanoma (0 to 15 years of age) arising in "large" congenital nevocellular nevi. *Plast Reconstr Surg.* 1986; 78: 174–181.

8. Egan CL, Oliveria SA, Elenitsas R, et al. Cutaneous melanoma risk and phenotypic changes in large congenital nevi: a follow-up study of 46 patients. *J Am Acad Dermatol.* 1998; 39: 923–932.

9. Marghoob AA, Schoenbach SP, Kopf AW, et al. Large congenital melanocytic nevi and the risk for the development of malignant melanoma. A prospective study. *Arch Dermatol.* 1996; 132: 170–175.

10. Goggins WB, Tsao H. A population-based analysis of risk factors for a second primary cutaneous melanoma among melanoma survivors. *Cancer.* 2003; 97: 639–643.

11. Ostlere LS, Houlston RS, Laing JH, et al. Risk of cancer in relatives of patients with cutaneous melanoma. *Int J Dermatol.* 1993; 32: 719–721.

12. Ford D, Bliss JM, Swerdlow AJ, et al. Risk of cutaneous melanoma associated with a family history of the disease. The International Melanoma Analysis Group (IMAGE). *Int J Cancer.* 1995; 62: 377–381.

13. Bishop DT, Demenais F, Goldstein AM, et al. Geographical variation in the penetrance of CDKN2A mutations for melanoma. *J Natl Cancer Inst.* 2002; 94: 894–903.

14. FitzGerald MG, Harkin DP, Silva-Arrieta S, et al: Prevalence of germline mutations in p16, p19ARF, and CDK4 in familial melanoma: analysis of a clinic-based population. *Proc Natl Acad Sci USA.* 1996; 93: 8541–8545.

15. Landi MT, Bauer J, Pfeiffer RM, et al. MC1R germline variants confer risk for BRAF-mutant melanoma. *Science.* 2006; 313: 521–522.

16. Cancer risks in BRCA2 mutation carriers. The Breast Cancer Linkage Consortium. *J Natl Cancer Inst.* 1999; 91: 1310–1316.

17. Elder DE, Goldman LI, Goldman SC, et al. Dysplastic nevus syndrome: a phenotypic association of sporadic cutaneous melanoma. *Cancer.* 1980; 46: 1787–1794.

18. Pollack LA, Li J, Berkowitz Z, et al. Melanoma survival in the United States, 1992 to 2005. *J Am Acad Dermatol.* 2011; 65: S78–S86.

19. Balch CM, Gershenwald JE, Soong SJ, et al. Final version of 2009 AJCC melanoma staging and classification. *J Clin Oncol.* 2009; 27: 6199–6206.

20. Geller AC, Zhang Z, Sober AJ, et al. The first 15 years of the American Academy of Dermatology skin cancer screening programs: 1985-1999. *J Am Acad Dermatol.* 2003; 48: 34–41.

21. Dennis LK, Beane Freeman LE, VanBeek MJ. Sunscreen use and the risk for melanoma: a quantitative review. *Ann Intern Med.* 2003; 139: 966–978.

22. Green AC, Williams GM, Logan V, et al: Reduced melanoma after regular sunscreen use: randomized trial follow-up. *J Clin Oncol.* 2011; 29: 257–263.

23. Chang YM, Barrett JH, Bishop DT, et al. Sunexposure and melanoma risk at different latitudes: a pooled analysis of 5700 cases and 7216 controls. *Int J Epidemiol.* 2009; 38: 814–830.

24. Balch CM, Soong SJ, Gershenwald JE, et al. Prognostic factors analysis of 17,600 melanoma patients: validation of the American Joint Committee on Cancer melanoma staging system. *J Clin Oncol.* 2001; 19: 3622–3634.

25. Balch CM, Buzaid AC, Soong SJ, et al. Final version of the American Joint Committee on Cancer staging system for cutaneous melanoma. *J Clin Oncol.* 2001; 19: 3635–3648.

26. Lachiewicz AM, Berwick M, Wiggins CL, et al. Survival differences between patients with scalp or neck melanoma and those with melanoma of other sites in the Surveillance, Epidemiology, and End Results (SEER) program. *Arch Dermatol.* 2008; 144: 515–521.

27. Veronesi U, Cascinelli N, Adamus J, et al. Thin stage I primary cutaneous malignant melanoma. Comparison of excision with margins of 1 or 3 cm. *N Engl J Med.* 1988; 318: 1159–1162.

28. Khayat D, Rixe O, Martin G, et al. Surgical margins in cutaneous melanoma (2 cm versus 5 cm for lesions measuring less than 2.1-mm thick). *Cancer.* 2003; 97: 1941–1946.

29. Cohn-Cedermark G, Rutqvist LE, Andersson R, et al. Long term results of a randomized study by the Swedish Melanoma Study Group on 2-cm versus 5-cm resection margins for patients with cutaneous melanoma with a tumor thickness of 0.8–2.0 mm. *Cancer.* 2000; 89: 1495–1501.

30. Balch CM, Soong SJ, Smith T, et al. Long-term results of a prospective surgical trial comparing 2 cm vs. 4 cm excision margins for 740 patients with 1–4 mm melanomas. *Ann Surg Oncol.* 2001; 8: 101–108.

31. Thomas JM, Newton-Bishop J, A'Hern R, et al. Excision margins in high-risk malignant melanoma. *N Engl J Med.* 2004; 350: 757–766.

32. Morton DL, Thompson JF, Cochran AJ, et al. Sentinel-node biopsy or nodal observation in melanoma. *N Engl J Med.* 2006; 355: 1307–1317.

33. Kirkwood JM, Strawderman MH, Ernstoff MS, et al. Interferon alfa-2b adjuvant therapy of high-risk resected cutaneous melanoma: the Eastern Cooperative Oncology Group Trial EST 1684. *J Clin Oncol.* 1996; 14: 7–17.

34. Kirkwood JM, Ibrahim JG, Sondak VK, et al. High- and low-dose interferon alfa-2b in high-risk melanoma: first analysis of intergroup trial E1690/S9111/C9190. *J Clin Oncol.* 2000; 18: 2444–2458.

35. Kirkwood JM, Ibrahim JG, Sosman JA, et al. High-dose interferon alfa-2b significantly prolongs relapse-free and overall survival compared with the GM2-KLH/QS-21 vaccine in patients with resected stage IIB-III melanoma: results of intergroup trial E1694/S9512/C509801. *J Clin Oncol.* 2001; 19: 2370–2380.

36. Kirkwood JM, Manola J, Ibrahim J, et al. A pooled analysis of eastern cooperative oncology group and intergroup trials of adjuvant high-dose interferon for melanoma. *Clin Cancer Res.* 2004; 10: 1670–1677.

37. Gogas H, Ioannovich J, Dafni U, et al. Prognostic significance of auto-immunity during treatment of melanoma with interferon. *N Engl J Med.* 2006; 354: 709–718.

38. Eggermont AM, Suciu S, Testori A, et al. Long-term results of the randomized phase III trial EORTC 18991 of adjuvant therapy with pegylated Interferon alfa-2b versus observation in resected stage III melanoma. *J Clin Oncol.* 2012; 30: 3810–3818.

39. Korn EL, Liu PY, Lee SJ, et al. Meta-analysis of phase II cooperative group trials in metastatic stage IV melanoma to determine progression-free and overall survival benchmarks for future phase II trials. *J Clin Oncol.* 2008; 26: 527–34.

40. Wong JH, Skinner KA, Kim KA, et al. The role of surgery in the treatment of nonregionally recurrent melanoma. *Surgery.* 1993; 113: 389–394.

41. Fletcher WS, Pommier RF, Lum S, et al. Surgical treatment of metastatic melanoma. *Am J Surg.* 1998; 175: 413–417.

42. Karakousis CP, Velez A, Driscoll DL, et al. Metastasectomy in malignant melanoma. *Surgery.* 1994; 115: 295–302.

43. Leo F, Cagini L, Rocmans P, et al. Lung metastases from melanoma: when is surgical treatment warranted? *Br J Cancer.* 2000; 83: 569–572.

44. Agrawal S, Yao TJ, Coit DG. Surgery for melanoma metastatic to the gastrointestinal tract. *Ann Surg Oncol.* 1999; 6: 336–344.

45. Grunhagen DJ, de Wilt JH, van Geel AN, et al. Isolated limb perfusion for melanoma patients—a review of its indications and the role of tumour necrosis factor-alpha. *Eur J Surg Oncol.* 2006; 32: 371–380.

46. Middleton MR, Grob JJ, Aaronson N, et al. Randomized phase III study of temozolomide versus dacarbazine in the treatment of patients with advanced metastatic malignant melanoma. *J Clin Oncol.* 2000; 18: 158–166.

47. Baker HW. Spontaneous regression of malignant melanoma. *Am Surg.* 1964; 30: 825–829.

48. Sullivan RJ, Atkins MB. Cytokine therapy in melanoma. *J Cutan Pathol.* 2010; 371: 60–67.

49. Atkins MB, Lotze MT, Dutcher JP, et al. High-dose recombinant interleukin 2 therapy for patients with metastatic melanoma: analysis of 270 patients treated between 1985 and 1993. *J Clin Oncol.* 1999; 17: 2105–2116.

50. Phan GQ, Attia P, Steinberg SM, et al. Factors associated with response to high-dose interleukin-2 in patients with metastatic melanoma. *J Clin Oncol.* 2001; 19: 3477–3482.

51. Schwartzentruber DJ, Lawson DH, Richards JM, et al. GP100 peptide vaccine and interleukin-2 in patients with advanced melanoma. *N Engl J Med.* 2011; 364: 2119–2127.

52. Pardoll DM. The blockade of immune checkpoints in cancer immunotherapy. *Nat Rev Cancer.* 2012; 12: 252–264.

53. Attia P, Phan GQ, Maker AV, et al. Autoimmunity correlates with tumor regression in patients with metastatic melanoma treated with anti-cytotoxic T-lymphocyte antigen-4. *J Clin Oncol.* 2005; 23: 6043–6053.

54. Ribas A, Camacho LH, Lopez-Berestein G, et al. Antitumor activity in melanoma and anti-self responses in a phase I trial with the anticytotoxic T lymphocyte-associated antigen 4 monoclonal antibody CP-675,206. *J Clin Oncol.* 2005; 23: 8968–8977.

55. Robert C, Thomas L, Bondarenko I, et al. Ipilimumab plus dacarbazine for previously untreated metastatic melanoma. *N Engl J Med.* 2011; 364: 2517–2526.

56. Hodi FS, O'Day SJ, McDermott DF, et al. Improved survival with ipilimumab in patients with metastatic melanoma. *N Engl J Med.* 2010; 363: 1290.

57. Dong H, Strome SE, Salomao DR, et al. Tumor-associated B7-H1 promotes T-cell apoptosis: a potential mechanism of immune evasion. *Nat Med*. 2002; 8: 793–800.

58. Topalian SL, Hodi FS, Brahmer JR, et al. Safety, activity, and immune correlates of anti-PD-1 antibody in cancer. *N Engl J Med*. 2012; 366: 2443–2454.

59. Brahmer JR, Tykodi SS, Chow LQ, et al. Safety and activity of anti-PD-L1 antibody in patients with advanced cancer. *N Engl J Med*. 2012; 366: 2455–2465.

60. Rosenberg SA. Raising the bar: the curative potential of human cancer immunotherapy. *Sci Transl Med*. 2012; 4: 127ps8. doi: 10.1126/scitranslmed.3003634.

61. Davies H, Bignell GR, Cox C, et al. Mutations of the BRAF gene in human cancer. *Nature*. 2002; 417: 949–954.

62. Curtin JA, Fridlyand J, Kageshita T, et al. Distinct sets of genetic alterations in melanoma. *N Engl J Med*. 2005; 353: 2135–2147.

63. Hodis E, Watson IR, Kryukov GV, et al. A landscape of driver mutations in melanoma. *Cell*. 2012; 150: 251–263.

64. Chapman PB, Hauschild A, Robert C, et al. Improved survival with vemurafenib in melanoma with BRAF V600E mutation. *N Engl J Med*. 2011; 364: 2507–2516.

65. Hauschild A, Grob JJ, Demidov LV, et al. Dabrafenib in BRAF-mutated metastatic melanoma: a multicentre, open-label, phase 3 randomised controlled trial. *Lancet*. 2012; 380: 358–365.

66. Flaherty KT, Robert C, Hersey P, et al. Improved survival with MEK inhibition in BRAF-mutated melanoma. *N Engl J Med*. 2012; 367: 107–114.

67. Flaherty KT, Infante JR, Daud A, et al. Combined BRAF and MEK inhibition in melanoma with BRAF V600 mutations. *N Engl J Med*. 2012; 367: 1694–1703.

68. Guo J, Si L, Kong Y, et al. Phase II, open-label, single-arm trial of imatinib mesylate in patients with metastatic melanoma harboring c-Kit mutation or amplification. *J Clin Oncol*. 2011; 29: 2904–2909.

69. Carvajal RD, Antonescu CR, Wolchok JD, et al. KIT as a therapeutic target in metastatic melanoma. *JAMA*. 2011; 305: 2327–2334.

70. Tucker MA, Shields JA, Hartge P, et al. Sunlight exposure as risk factor for intraocular malignant melanoma. *N Engl J Med*. 1985; 313: 789–792.

71. Grin JM, Grant-Kels JM, Grin CM, et al. Ocular melanomas and melanocytic lesions of the eye. *J Am Acad Dermatol*. 1998; 38: 716–730.

72. Diener-West M, Reynolds SM, Agugliaro DJ, et al. Development of metastatic disease after enrollment in the COMS trials for treatment of choroidal melanoma: Collaborative Ocular Melanoma Study Group Report No. 26. *Arch Ophthalmol*. 2005; 123: 1639–1643.

73. Van Raamsdonk CD, Bezrookove V, Green G, et al. Frequent somatic mutations of GNAQ in uveal melanoma and blue naevi. *Nature*. 2009; 457: 599–602.

74. Van Raamsdonk CD, Griewank KG, Crosby MB, et al. Mutations in GNA11 in uveal melanoma. *N Engl J Med.* 2010; 363: 2191–2199.

75. Harbour JW, Onken MD, Roberson ED, et al. Frequent mutation of BAP1 in metastasizing unveal melanomas. *Science.* 2010 Dec 3; 330: 1410–1413.

76. Trimble EL, Lewis JL Jr, Williams LL, et al. Management of vulvar melanoma. *Gynecol Oncol.* 1992; 45: 254–258.

77. Davidson T, Kissin M, Westbury G. Vulvo-vaginal melanoma—should radical surgery be abandoned? *Br J Obstet Gynaecol.* 1987; 94: 473–476.

78. DeMatos P, Tyler D, Seigler HF. Mucosal melanoma of the female genitalia: a clinicopathologic study of forty-three cases at Duke University Medical Center. *Surgery.* 1998; 124: 38–48.

79. Creasman WT, Phillips JL, Menck HR. The National Cancer Data Base report on cancer of the vagina. *Cancer.* 1998; 83: 1033–1040.

80. Mendenhall WM, Amdur RJ, Hinerman RW, et al. Head and neck mucosal melanoma. *Am J Clin Oncol.* 2005; 28: 626–630.

CHAPTER **61**

Soft Tissue and Bone Sarcomas

Edwin Choy, Sam S. Yoon, Francis J. Hornicek,
Thomas F. DeLaney

SOFT TISSUE SARCOMAS

Soft tissue sarcomas (STS) are uncommon malignancies, arising in about 11,410 persons in the United States each year and accounting for 4390 deaths, mostly due to either locoregional recurrence or distant metastasis (1–4). Although malignant tumors of soft tissue are scarce, benign tumors such as lipomas are 100 times more common. STS occur at any age with a median age of around 50-years old, and are equally common in men and women.

STS constitute a highly heterogeneous group of tumors with respect to anatomical distribution, histologic subtype, and clinical behavior (1). STS occur throughout the body, but nearly one-half occur in the extremities, with about one-third occurring in the lower extremity and 15% occurring in the upper extremity. Another one-third of STS occur in the abdomen, and these are equally divided among intra-abdominal visceral sarcomas (primarily gastrointestinal stromal tumors and leiomyosarcomas) and retroperitoneal sarcomas. Other anatomic sites include the head/neck, trunk, and other miscellaneous sites (e.g., heart).

STS are malignant tumors which arise from the mesodermal tissues (e.g., fat, muscle, connective tissue, and vessels) excluding bone and cartilage. In addition, malignant tumors of peripheral nerve sheaths are usually included despite being ectodermal in origin. There are over 50 different histologic subtypes of STS with the most common being liposarcoma, leiomyosarcoma, fibrosarcoma, and synovial sarcoma. Malignant fibrous histiocytoma was historically the most common subtype but the majority of these are now classified as other subtypes including undifferentiated pleomorphic sarcomas. All suspected STS cases should be reviewed by a pathologist experienced in sarcomas given that about 10% of cases originally designated as STS are in fact not STS and about 20% are initially assigned the incorrect histologic subtype (5). While each histologic subtype may have certain specific clinical behaviors, all STS can generally be categorized into low-, intermediate-, and high-grade tumors. Low-grade tumors grow more slowly, can locally recur after resection, but have a low risk of distant metastases (about 5%). High-grade tumors tend to grow more rapidly, can recur locally, and have the added risk of distant metastasis that can approach 50% for large tumors greater than 5–10 cm in largest dimension.

The treatment of STS has advanced significantly over the past few decades. In particular, evidence has accumulated that in addition to surgery, there are important roles for radiation therapy and chemotherapy in the management of some STS patients. Optimal results from more conservative local treatment strategies require a multidisciplinary approach to the overall management of these patients. The team should include not only an experienced and specialized surgeon, but also a radiation oncologist, medical oncologist, pathologist, and diagnostic radiologist expert in the disease. Additional specialists who may be important in the care of these patients include plastic/reconstructive surgeons, physiatrists working with physical and occupational therapists, psychiatrists, psychologists, and social workers. For this relatively uncommon solid tumor that occurs throughout the body and has over 50 histologic subtypes, evaluation and treatment is best done at a tertiary referral center.

ETIOLOGY

The vast majority of STS occur as sporadic tumors in patients with no identified genetic or environmental risk factors. However, certain genetic syndromes are associated with an increased risk of developing sarcomas including neurofibromatosis 1 (NF1, von Recklinghausen's disease), hereditary retinoblastoma, and Li-Fraumeni syndrome. Specific genetic abnormalities, evidenced by nonrandom chromosomal aberrations, are well established in certain STS histologic subtypes, and are often utilized in the definitive diagnosis (Table 61-1).

Radiation is recognized as capable of inducing sarcomas of bone and soft tissue. The frequency increases with radiation dose and with the postradiation observation period. Chemotherapeutic agents are likewise associated with risks of sarcoma induction. STS (primarily lymphangiosarcomas) may be observed following massive and quite protracted edema after axillary lymphadenectomy (Stewart–Treves syndrome). Trauma is rarely a factor in the development of these tumors with the possible exception of desmoid tumors.

STAGING

The Task Force on STS of the American Joint Committee on Cancer (AJCC) Staging and End Result Reporting has established a staging system for STS which is an extension of the TNM system to include G for histological grade (Table 61-2). Grade, size, depth, and presence of nodal or distant metastases are the determinants of stage. Of these, grade is particularly important in staging sarcomas. Some institutions will assign grades 1–3, where grade 1 lesions are considered low grade with minimal metastatic potential and the intermediate grade 2 and high grade 3 lesions are considered high grade and capable of metastatic disease. Other institutions use a 2- or 4-tiered system.

EXTREMITY STS
CLINICAL EVALUATION

The most frequent initial complaint is that of a painless, enlarging mass for a few weeks to several months. Occasionally, pain or tenderness precedes the detection of a mass. With progressive growth of the tumor, symptoms

TABLE 61-1 SOFT TISSUE SARCOMA CHROMOSOMAL TRANSLOCATIONS AND GENES INVOLVED

Histologic Subtype	Translocation	Genes Involved
Alveolar rhabdomyosarcoma	t(2;13) (q35,q14)	PAX3, FKHR
	t(1;13) (p36;q14)	PAX7, FKHR
Alveolar soft part sarcoma	t(X;17) (p11;q25)	TFE2, ASPL
Clear cell sarcoma	t(12;22) (q13;q12)	ATF1, ETF
Dermatofibrosarcoma protuberans	t(17;22) (q22;q13)	COL1A1, PDGFB1
Desmoplastic small round cell tumor	t(11;22) (p13;q12)	WT1, EWS
Ewing's sarcoma/primitive neuroectodermal tumor	t(11;22) (q24;q12)	FLI1, EWS
	t(21;22) (q22;q12)	ERG ,EWS
	t(7;22) (p22;q12)	ETV1, EWS
	t(2;22) (q33;q12)	FEV, EWS
	t(17;22) (q12;q12)	E1AF, EWS
Extraskeletal myxoid chondrosarcoma	t(9;22) (q21–31;q12.2	CHN, EWS
	t(9;17) (q22;q11)	CHN, RBP56
Myxoid/round cell liposarcoma	t(12;16) (q13;p11)	CHOP, TLS
	t(12;22) (q13;q11–q12)	CHOP, EWS
Synovial sarcoma	t(X;18) (p11.2;q11.2)	SSX1 or SSX2, SS18 (SYT)

Adapted from Clark MA, Fisher C, Judson I, Thomas JM. Soft-tissue sarcomas in adults. *N Engl J Med*. 2005; 353: 701–711.

appear which are usually secondary to infiltration of or pressure on adjacent structures. Interestingly, some high-grade sarcomas in the foot or ankle may have been noticed initially several years prior to diagnosis. One should obtain a complete history and physical examination, with particular attention paid to the region of the primary lesion: definition of size, site of origin (superficial or deep, attached to or fixed to deep structures), involvement or discoloration of overlying skin, functional status of vessels and nerves, mass effect on adjacent organs and joints, and presence of distal edema. Laboratory studies need not go beyond a complete blood count and chemistry panel. There are no tumors markers for STS.

For the primary site, the radiographic evaluation should include a CT scan or MRI. The most useful radiologic study to evaluate an extremity or trunk primary site is the MRI, but CT scans can provide supplemental information. A chest CT should be obtained for high-grade tumors to evaluate for lung metastases. A chest x-ray may be adequate for low-grade tumors. The role of PET scans has yet to be defined, but many primary and

TABLE 61-2 AJCC STAGING SYSTEM FOR SOFT TISSUE SARCOMAS

Histological grade of malignancy				
GX	Grade cannot be assessed			
G1	Well differentiated			
G2	Moderately differentiated			
G3	Poorly differentiated			
T Primary tumor				
TX	Primary tumor cannot be assessed			
T0	No evidence of primary tumor			
T1	Tumor 5 cm or less in greatest dimension			
T1a	Superficial tumor			
T1b	Deep tumor			
T2	Tumor greater than 5 cm in greatest dimension			
T2a	Superficial tumor			
T2b	Deep tumor			
N Regional lymph nodes				
NX	Regional lymph nodes cannot be assessed			
N0	No regional lymph nodes metastases			
N1	Regional lymph node metastasis			
M Distant metastasis				
M0	No distant metastasis			
MI	Distant metastasis			
Stage I	A	G1, GX	T1a-1b	N0	M0
	B	G1, GX	T2a-2b	N0	M0
Stage II	A	G2, G3	T1a-1b	N0	M0
	B	G2	T2a-2b	N0	M0
Stage III		G3	T2a-2b	N0	M0
		Any G	Any T	N1	M0
Stage IV		Any G	Any T	Any N	M1

Used with the permission of the American Joint Committee on Cancer (AJCC), Chicago, Illinois. The original source for this material is the AJCC Cancer Staging Manual, Seventh Edition (2010) published by Springer-New York, www.springerlink.com.

metastatic tumors may show increased FDG uptake especially as the grade increases.

An adequate biopsy is required to determine a histologic diagnosis as to tumor type and grade and to determine an optimal treatment strategy. In the majority of cases, the diagnosis can be established by core needle biopsy. Superficial lesions which are readily palpable can be directly biopsied with ultrasound guidance (all lesions should be imaged prior to biopsy), but for tumors which are located at a depth which makes the lesion appear less well defined, a CT-directed approach is advocated. Open biopsies are done less commonly and should be reserved for the uncommon cases where core biopsy is not adequate. The incision for open biopsies should usually be oriented longitudinally such that it can be easily incorporated in the definitive resection. For tumors <3–5 cm in size, and depending on where they are located (i.e., hand or foot are exceptions), an excisional biopsy can sometimes be performed, and incisional biopsies can be performed for larger lesions. Care should be taken to minimize bleeding and contamination of surrounding tissues. Fine needle biopsy can best be employed to confirm metastatic or recurrent tumor when the primary diagnosis is already established.

■ SURGERY AND RADIATION THERAPY

If STS are "shelled out" as is performed for benign tumors such as lipomas, the local recurrence will be up to 90%. Radical resection of tumors with a margin of normal tissue can decrease the local recurrence rate to 10%–30%. However, many extremity STS grow adjacent to major blood vessels and bones, and the standard operation for many STS up until the early 1980s was amputation. Rosenberg et al. at the National Cancer Institute (NCI) published a randomized trial of amputation versus limb-sparing surgery and radiation (both groups received chemotherapy) in 1982 and demonstrated equivalent overall survival with a local recurrence rate of 0% versus 15% (6). Currently limb-sparing surgery can be performed in over 90% of patients with extremity STS, and overall local recurrence rates are often less than 10%.

Several surgical principles should be followed when resecting STS. First, the preoperative imaging studies should be carefully examined to identify the full extent of tumor penetration as well as the relationship of the tumor to adjacent structures. Second, tumors should be resected with an adequate margin of normal tissue if this can be performed without severe morbidity. The distance is variable and probably can be reduced when high-quality margins such as fascia are present as the border. Tissues such as fat or muscle probably require 1–2 cm of normal tissue because of frequent infiltration of the tumor cells within these tissues. One can often accept a few millimeters of fascia margin but should be more concerned about a close margin of fat or muscle. Third, STS usually do not invade the periadventitial tissue of arteries or the periosteum of bone and can often be dissected along these planes. However, some STS actually arise in the vessels or nerves precluding salvage in terms of resection. Surgeons in general must use considerable judgment in resecting STS and careful discussion with bone and soft tissue radiologists prior to the procedure is important. Positive microscopic margins are very strongly associated with an increased risk of local recurrence, and one should strive for negative microscopic margins in all cases unless this would create major or unacceptable morbidity. In such cases one may rely on adjuvant radiation therapy in order to reduce major surgical morbidity, given radiation can usually be delivered in doses to the extremity that can eradicate microscopic residual disease.

Several studies have defined the essential role of radiation therapy in the local control of STS. Another NCI randomized trial published in 1998 comparing limb-spring surgery alone to surgery and external beam radiation (patients with high-grade tumors all received chemotherapy) demonstrated that radiation reduced local recurrence from 20%–33% to 0%–4% (7). The rate of distant recurrence was the same in both groups. Brachytherapy has also been used to deliver radiation. In a randomized trial of surgery alone versus surgery and brachytherapy, local recurrence for high-grade tumors was reduced from 30% to 5% with brachytherapy. At our institution, brachytherapy is often employed for patients who have a local recurrence after prior surgery and radiation, and this allows the delivery of additional radiation while minimizing morbidity. Brachytherapy or intraoperative radiation therapy can also be used at the time of initial surgery and radiation to deliver a focal boost to areas of close or positive surgical margins.

The order of radiation therapy in relation to surgery is a subject of debate between major sarcoma centers. One randomized trial by the Canadian NCI examined preoperative and postoperative radiation therapy and found no difference in local control (8). Complications were twice as high in the preoperative therapy group (35% vs 17%), but tissue fibrosis and other late complications were more frequent in the postoperative radiation group.

There are certain situations such as difficult anatomical location (e.g., pelvis, spine, or base of skull) or major medical comorbidities (e.g., cardiac dysfunction or metastatic lung cancer) in which a conservative surgical procedure may have much apparent risk and radiation alone is delivered. In one study from Memorial Sloan-Kettering, 25 patients were treated by radiotherapy alone, and local control was achieved in 14 of the 25 patients. To achieve a high probability of local control, higher doses than would be used for residual microscopic disease in the range of 70–75 Gy are essential. Among patients receiving ≥63 Gy, Kepka et al. reported local control in 72% of patients with tumors ≥5 cm in size, 42% for lesions >5 cm but ≤10 cm, and only 25% for lesions >10 cm (9). Because high doses are required for control of these unresected lesions, treatment techniques such as proton beam radiation, or even conventional radiation in an intensity-modulated fashion may be required to deliver dose and stay within the constraints of normal tissue tolerance.

Patients with large (>8–10 cm), deep, high-grade sarcomas present more difficult problems in terms of local control and are at significant risk of distant metastasis. Some groups have combined chemotherapy with surgery and radiation therapy strategies. Eilber and Morton have been proponents of a program, which has consisted of intra-arterial doxorubicin followed by rapid fraction hypofractionated radiation therapy (3.5 Gy/fraction, 28 Gy total) and subsequent local excision. Their data have shown local recurrence rates of <10% with survival rates of 74% in stage III tumors. Among these patients, there was a 5% amputation rate. They have since shown that it is not necessary to provide the doxorubicin by an intra-arterial route. Our institution has employed a regimen of preoperative mesna, Adriamycin, ifosfamide, and dacarbazine (MAID) chemotherapy interdigitated with radiation therapy (44 Gy) followed by postoperative MAID chemotherapy for patients with >8 cm, high-grade STS (10). Five-year local control was 92% and 5-year overall survival was 87%. In experimental protocols, hyperthermic isolated limb perfusion (HILP) with chemotherapeutic agents (e.g., tumor necrosis factor alpha, melphalan, and interferon gamma) has used to control large tumors that would otherwise require amputation because of proximity to nerve or blood vessels.

■ ADJUVANT CHEMOTHERAPY

Although surgery and radiotherapy achieve control of the primary tumor in the majority of patients, many patients (especially those with large, high-grade tumors) develop and die of metastatic disease not evident at diagnosis. Doxorubicin and ifosfamide are the most active chemotherapy agents in metastatic STS. For doxorubicin, objective response rates between 20% and 40% have been reported. Several prospective studies using single-agent doxorubicin failed to show an improvement in disease-free or overall survival in patients receiving postoperative chemotherapy compared with surgery alone. The large EORTC study of adjuvant chemotherapy employed CyVADic consisting of cyclophosphamide, vincristine, doxorubicin, and DTIC found improved 7-year recurrence-free survival (56% vs 43%) but no significant difference in overall survival (63% vs 56%) (11). A meta-analysis of 14 randomized trials of doxorubicin-based adjuvant chemotherapy versus no chemotherapy in STS was performed in 1997 (12) and updated in 2008 with three additional studies using ifosfamide with doxorubicin (13). The adjuvant chemotherapy group had a statistically significant improved rate of distant and overall recurrence (OR was 0.67; 95% CI 0.56–0.82; $P = 0.0001$), distant recurrence-free survival (70% vs 60%, $P = 0.003$), but overall survival was only significantly improved in the studies that combined ifosfamide with doxorubicin (OR = 0.56; 95% CI, 0.36–0.85; $P = 0.01$). However, the toxicities associated with these chemotherapeutic agents dictate caution in generalizing adjuvant chemotherapy to all patients (indeed, different sarcoma centers in North America and Europe have varying degrees of enthusiasm for the use of adjuvant chemotherapy), which argues for and favor continuing enrollment of patients in clinical trials where available.

■ RETROPERITONEAL STS

Approximately 10%–15% of soft tissue sarcomas arise in the retroperitoneum. Tumors may be identified on imaging studies for unrelated complaints, or patients may also present with a palpable abdominal mass or with symptoms such as abdominal pain or lower extremity neurologic symptoms. Since the retroperitoneum can accommodate large tumors without symptoms, the average size of tumors in large series is often greater than 10 cm. Upon histologic examination, about two-thirds of tumors are either liposarcomas or leiomyosarcomas, with the remaining tumors distributed among a large variety of other histologic subtypes. Retroperitoneal liposarcomas are further subclassified into well-differentiated/dedifferentiated, myxoid/round cell, and pleomorphic subtypes. Most unifocal tumors in the retroperitoneum that do not arise from adjacent organs will be either benign soft tissue tumors (e.g., schwannomas, paraganglioneuroma, or neurofibroma) or sarcomas. Other malignancies in the differential diagnosis include primary germ cell tumor, metastatic testicular cancer, and lymphoma. Following a careful history and physical examination, radiologic assessment of these tumors is usually performed with an abdominal and pelvic CT scan. Liposarcomas often have a characteristic appearance with large areas of abnormal-appearing fat (well-differentiated liposarcoma) sometimes containing higher-density nodules (dedifferentiated liposarcoma). Patients with high-grade tumors should have a chest CT to evaluate for lung metastases.

The primary treatment for the local control of these tumors is surgical resection (14). The optimal goal of surgical resection is complete gross resection with microscopically negative margins, but this can be difficult to accomplish, and complete gross resection rates in large series are reported to be around 60%. In about three-quarters of cases, complete gross resection requires removal of adjacent viscera. The goal of obtaining negative microscopic margins for large retroperitoneal tumors is frequently not achieved. These tumors are surrounded by a pseudocapsule that often contains microscopic disease, and dissection with a normal tissue margin away from the pseudocapsule is difficult, especially along the posterior aspect of the tumor where it abuts the retroperitoneal fat and musculature. Controversy exists as to the optimal role of radiation therapy for local control of retroperitoneal sarcomas. Those who advocate radiation therapy usually prefer that radiation be delivered preoperatively. With the tumor still in place, normal organs are pushed away from the radiation field, the margin around the tumor at risk of local recurrence is more clearly defined, and the effective radiation dose required to control microscopic disease is likely lower.

In the extremity, the local control of sarcomas treated with total gross resection with positive microscopic margin and adjuvant radiation therapy is about 75%. Typically, positive microscopic margins are treated with a boost of intraoperative, perioperative brachytherapy, or additional postoperative radiation to a total dose of about 60–70 Gy, although some recent data suggest that selected patients such as those with well-differentiated liposarcoma and a focal, planned positive margin following preoperative radiation may not benefit additional postoperative boost radiation (15). It is reasonable to assume that total gross resection of retroperitoneal tumors along with adequate doses of radiation could achieve local control rates similar to that seen for extremity tumors resected with positive microscopic margins. However, unlike the extremity, it is difficult to deliver high doses of radiation to the abdomen. The availability of intensity-modulated radiation therapy, proton beam radiation, and intraoperative radiation therapy may facilitate the efficacy and minimize morbidity of adjuvant radiation therapy for these tumors. In a report from our institution, 29 patients were treated with preoperative radiation to a median dose of 45 Gy and then underwent complete gross resection (16). Intraoperative radiation therapy (IORT) (10–20 Gy) was delivered to 16 of the 29 patients. Local control at

5 years was 83% for patients who received both preoperative and intraoperative radiation therapy and 61% for those who received only preoperative radiation. More recently, we have incorporated the use of preoperative proton beam radiation therapy and/or IMRT along with aggressive anterior surgical resection +/− and intraoperative radiation therapy for retroperitoneal tumors to further minimize to maintain high rates of local tumor control while minimizing morbidity on adjacent structures. In a report of this experience with a median follow-up of 33 months, Yoon et al noted only two local recurrences among 20 patients treated for primary retroperitoneal sarcomas. Among all 28 patients in the series, 28% had surgical complications and 14% had radiation related complications (17).

■ FOLLOW-UP

The intensity of follow-up visits and imaging studies varies between institutions, and can also be varied according to tumor grade. The National Comprehensive Cancer Network (NCCN) published guidelines in 2011 suggesting for low-grade extremity tumors, patients should be evaluated by history and physical examination every 3–6 months for the first 2–3 years, then annually. Chest x-rays should be obtained every 6–12 months. Imaging of the primary tumor site depends on the location and the risk of locoregional recurrence. For superficial tumors, physical examination is often sufficient. For deeper extremity tumors, CT scan or MRI may be performed.

For high-grade lesions, the NCCN guidelines suggest a history a physical examination every 3–6 months for 2–3 years, then every 6 months for the next 2 years, then annually. Chest CT scans or chest x-rays should be obtained at each visit.

METASTATIC DISEASE

While local control of STS can be attained in >90% of patients, up to 50% of patients present with or develop metastatic disease. Median survival after the development of metastatic disease is 8–12 months, although a sizeable minority of patients can live several years if the disease is indolent. The most common site of metastatic disease for extremity and trunk STS is the lung. Intra-abdominal and retroperitoneal sarcomas metastasize with about equal frequency to the lung and liver. STS rarely metastasizes to regional lymph nodes (about 5%) except for certain histologic subtypes including clear cell sarcoma, epithelioid sarcoma, rhabdomyosarcoma, hemangiosarcoma, and synovial sarcoma.

As noted above, doxorubicin and ifosfamide have been demonstrated to be the most active chemotherapy agents in widely disseminated soft tissue sarcoma (18). Response rates range from about 20% to 30%, and there is some evidence that higher doses can result in increased response rates. These two agents carry significant risks of toxicity: doxorubicin dosage is limited by cardiotoxicity and ifosfamide causes hemorrhagic cystitis and nephrotoxicity. Ifosfamide-induced hemorrhagic cystitis can be avoided by adding the protective agent mesna. Another agent with some activity against STS is dacarbazine (DTIC), with reported response rates around 20%. However for metastatic disease, complete responses are uncommon

(<15% even with combination therapy), duration of response averages 8 months, and as yet the higher response rates seen with intense combination therapy have not been proven to provide a survival advantage over that conferred by sequential single agent treatment.

A variety of combination chemotherapy regimens for metastatic disease have been studied in randomized clinical trials. Most of these studies were small and included mixed histologies (see Table 61-3). Most of these trials include doxorubicin (or epirubicin) and an alkylating agent. Overall survival for any combination chemotherapy regimen has not been clearly demonstrated to be superior to doxorubicin alone, but trials have been underpowered due to the rarity of this disease type. A commonly used combination chemotherapy regimen is mesna, adriamycin, ifosfamide, and dacarbazine (MAID). In a large phase II trial, this regimen achieved an overall response rate of 47%. When MAID was compared to the combination of adriamycin and dacarbazine in a randomized trial, the response rate was higher for MAID (32% vs 17%). However, there were more toxic deaths in the MAID group and there was no survival advantage to MAID. Higher doses of chemotherapy can be given with better control of toxicity if granulocyte-colony-stimulating factor (G-CSF) is used.

Other trials evaluating the use of other chemotherapy agents such as docetaxel, gemcitabine, vinorelbine, and topotecan all show modest rates of significant tumor shrinkage. Some histologies may be particularly sensitive to specific agents, such as scalp angiosarcoma to paclitaxel. Another agent that has shown some promise in recent trials against STS is Ecteinascidin 743 (ET-743), which is also known as Yondelis or trabectedin. This drug seems to have particular activity against myxoid liposarcomas and is commercially available in Europe, Asia, and Australia, but it is not yet approved for use in the United States. Patients with metastatic disease should be strongly considered for enrollment in investigational or experimental trials.

Two randomized phase III studies in patients with advanced sarcomas have been performed to demonstrate improvement in progression-free survival. The PALETTE trial randomized 372 patients with metastatic soft tissue sarcoma in 2:1 fashion to receive pazopanib (a multiple tyrosine kinase inhibitor) or placebo (19). The median progression-free survival time was 4.6 months for pazopanib and 1.6 months for placebo. The SUCCEED trial took 711 patients with metastatic sarcoma who experienced stable disease or better to standard chemotherapy to be randomized in 1:1 fashion to either ridaforolimus (an mTor inhibitor) or placebo (20). The median progression-free survival time was 17.7 weeks for ridaforolimus and 14.6 weeks for placebo. This was found to be statistically significant. However, neither trial demonstrated improvement in overall survival. Based on these results, pazopanib was approved for marketing to patients with sarcomas by the FDA. Ridaforolimus was not recommended for FDA approval.

There are currently five other randomized, phase III studies underway at the time this manuscript is being prepared. These include a first-line study of: (1) trabectedin versus doxorubicin, (2) doxorubicin with or without TH-302, (3) doxorubicin with or without palifosfamide, and a third-line

TABLE 61-3 SELECTED RANDOMIZED CHEMOTHERAPY TRIALS FOR METASTATIC SOFT TISSUE SARCOMAS

Investigator/ Group (year)	Regimen	Patients (*n*)	Response Rate (%)	Median Survival (*m*)
Schoenfeld et al. ECOG (1983)	A	54	27	8.5
	CyAV	56	19	7.7
	CyActV	58	11	9.4
Borden et al. ECOG (1987)	A q 3 wks	94	18	8.0
	A q wk	89	16	8.4
	ADtic	92	30	8.0
Borden et al. ECOG (1990)	A	148	17	9.4
	AVd	143	18	9.9
Edmonson et al. ECOG (1993)	A	90	20	<9
	AI	88	34	11
	MAP	84	32	9
Santoro et al. EORTC (1995)	A	263	23	12.0
	AI	258	28	12.7
	CyVADtic	142	28	11.8
Antman et al. CALBG/SWOG (1993)	AD	170	17	12
	AID	170	32	13
Nielsen et al. EORTC (1998)	A	112	14	10.4
	Epi	111	15	10.8
	Epi	111	14	10.4
EORTC meta-analysis (1999)	Any anthracycline-based regimen	2185	26	11.8

A, doxorubicin (Adriamycin); Act, actinomycin; CALGB, Cancer and Leukemia and Group B; Cy, cyclophosphamid; Dtic, dacarbazine; Epi, epirubicin; I, ifosfamide; M, mitomycin C; P, Cisplatin; SWOG, Southwest Oncology Group; V, vincristine; Vd, vindesine.
Adapted from Reference 18.

study of (4) eribulin versus dacarbazine and (5) trabectedin versus dacarbazine. These studies are described in clinicaltrials.gov.

Surgical resection has been performed for isolated STS metastases to the lung or liver. For select patients with STS metastases isolated to the lung, surgical resection (a.k.a. metastasectomy) can be performed, and 5-year survival can approach 20%–30%. Intra-abdominal and retroperitoneal STS metastasize commonly to the liver as well as the lung. Isolated, resectable liver metastases from STS are less common than isolated, resectable lung metastases, but several small series have examined partial hepatectomy for these patients and 5-year survival can reach 30%.

GASTROINTESTINAL STROMAL TUMORS

Gastrointestinal stromal tumors (GIST) are the most common mesenchymal tumor of the gastrointestinal tract and originate from the interstitial cells of Cajal (15). Interstitial cells of Cajal and the vast majority of GIST express c-KIT, which is a 145-kD transmembrane glycoprotein that acts as the receptor for stem cell factor (SCF). Prior to the identification and availability of immunohistochemistry for c-KIT, the majority of GIST were thought to be of smooth muscle origin and termed leiomyomas, leiomyosarcomas, and leiomyoblastomas. It is now known that the majority of stromal tumors of the gastrointestinal tract are GIST. Ninety-five percent of GIST stain positive on immunohistochemistry for c-KIT and the majority of GIST have a mutation in the c-KIT gene. Unlike most other cancers, GISTs seem highly dependent on this single pathway for neoplastic growth.

GIST can occur at nearly all ages, with the median age being around 60. The incidence is roughly equal in men and women. There are roughly 5000 cases per year in the United States. GISTs are located most commonly in the stomach (60%) followed by the small intestine (30%), colon/rectum (5%), and esophagus (5%). These tumors can be found on upper endoscopy, where they appear as submucosal lesions. However, even large GIST of the stomach may not be seen on endoscopy if they are pedunculated or exophytic. Endoscopic biopsy can establish the diagnosis, especially following staining for c-KIT expression. For small bowel tumors, CT-guided biopsy poses the risk of inadequate tissue and spillage of tumor cells and is likely not necessary given most isolated small bowel tumors require resection. Staging workup should include an abdomen and pelvis CT scan to rule out intra-abdominal or liver metastases.

GIST can range from small, pedunculated lesions to large lesions with adherence or invasion of surrounding tissues and organs. Thus the surgical approach can be quite varied but certain principles should be followed. Upon surgical exploration, the liver and peritoneal cavity should be examined for possible metastatic disease. GISTs uncommonly metastasize to lymph nodes so a regional lymphadenectomy is not required. Thus for a pedunculated gastric tumor, wedge resection of the gastric wall along with resection of the tumor is adequate. Some gastric tumors encompass a large portion of the stomach and a formal distal, subtotal, or even total gastrectomy may be required. For small bowel and colon tumors, segmental bowel resection can be performed. Small rectal GIST can be removed through transanal procedures while larger tumors may require low anterior resection or even abdominal-perineal resection, although there are reports of excellent responses using neoadjuvant imatinib and radiation as a means of allowing anal sphincter sparing surgery (21). Some large GISTs with significant necrosis are susceptible to tumor rupture and spillage, which can lead to intraperitoneal spread of disease, and so these tumors should be manipulated carefully. For large GISTs that invade adjacent organs, an en bloc resection of the entire tumor mass should be performed.

Risk of recurrence is most closely related to mitotic rate, size, and location. Table 61-4 shows the estimated risk of recurrence for resected GIST based on these three parameters, mitotic rate, tumor size, and tumor location (22).

TABLE 61-4 PERCENT OF PATIENTS WITH PROGRESSIVE DISEASE BASED ON MITOTIC RATE, SIZE, AND LOCATION

Mitotic Rate (per 50 HPF)	Tumor Size (cm)	Location			
		Stomach	Duodenum	Jejunum/Ileum	Rectum
<5	≤2	0	0	0	0
	2–5	1.9	8.3	4.3	8.5
	5–10	3.6	NA	24	NA
	>10	12	34	52	57
>5	≤2	NA	NA	NA	54
	2–5	16	50	73	52
	5–10	55	NA	85	NA
	>10	86	86	90	71

Adapted from Reference 22.

The most common sites of metastasis are the liver and peritoneal cavity, and less common sites include the lung and bone. Prior to the introduction of imatinib, GISTs were found to be highly resistant to chemotherapeutic agents. Imatinib inhibits both the c-KIT receptor and platelet-derived growth factor receptor (PDGFR) tyrosine kinases. Several large studies have shown imatinib to be highly effective against metastatic GIST, with a partial response rate of about 40% and stable disease rate of about 30% (see Table 61-5). The median time to progression is 19–24 months. Even tumors that are sensitive to imatinib may take months to show a decrease in tumor size on CT scans, and so PET scans have been employed to assess response. GISTs are usually positive on PET scans, and response to imatinib as demonstrated by decrease in PET activity can frequently be seen immediately after initiation of therapy. When resistance to imatinib ultimately develops, the dose can be escalated or other new targeted biologic agents may be considered. The most studied agents include sunitinib, sorafenib, and regorafenib.

The role of surgery for metastatic GIST has yet to be defined. Some investigators surgically resect or debulk imatinib-responsive disease to decrease tumor burden and hypothetically delay the development of imatinib resistance. When resistance to imatinib ultimately develops, the dose can be escalated or other newly targeted biologic agents, which have shown promise for imatinib-resistant GIST, may be considered. The most studied agent is sunitinib, which targets not only c-KIT and PDGFR but also the VEGF receptors, fms-related tyrosine kinase (Flt3), and the Ret oncogene. In a randomized study of 312 patients with imatinib-refractory GIST, sunitinib achieved stable disease for 27.3 weeks while placebo achieved stable disease for 6.4 weeks (23). Sunitinib was FDA approved for second-line therapy of metastatic GIST on January 2006, and Regorafenib was FDA approved for third-line therapy of metastatic GIST on February 2013.

TABLE 61-5 IMATINIB TRIALS FOR METASTATIC GIST

Trial	Phase	Patients (*n*)	Dose (mg/day)	Follow-Up (months)	CR %	PR %	SD %	PD %
Demetri et al.	II	73	400	10	0	36	23	12
US and Finland (2002)		74	600		0	43	18	8
Verweij et al.	III	470	400	25	5	45	32	13
EORTC (2004)		472	800		6	48	32	9
Benjamin et al.	III	361	400	14	NR	43	32	NR
US Intergroup (2003)		360	800		NR	41	32	NR

CR, complete response; PD, progressive disease; PFS, progression-free survival; PR, partial response; SD, stable disease.
Adapted from van der Zwan SM, DeMatteo RP. Gastrointestinal stromal tumor: 5 years later. *Cancer.* 2005; 104: 1781–1788.

DESMOID TUMOR (AGGRESSIVE FIBROMATOSIS)

Desmoid tumors are benign but locally infiltrative neoplasms arising from fibroblastic stromal elements that can grow at variable rates. Although neoplastic and locally aggressive, desmoids do not have the capacity to establish metastatic lesions. Desmoid tumors are uncommon (possibly about 1000 per year in the United States), slightly more common in females than males, and occur predominantly in individuals of 15–60 years of age. There is no significant racial or ethnic distribution. The etiology of desmoid tumors is not known, but these tumors occur commonly in patients with Gardner's syndrome and occur more frequently at sites of trauma or surgery.

Desmoid tumors usually present as a painless or minimally painful mass with a history of slow growth, but can cause symptoms if they impinge on adjacent structures. Desmoid tumors occur at virtually all body sites; most commonly in the torso (shoulder girdle and hip-buttock region) and the proximal aspect of extremities. The location is usually deep in the muscles or along fascial planes. Multiple lesions at distant sites are infrequent; however, additional lesions are not rare on the same extremity following the initial treatment.

The natural history of desmoids can be quite variable. They commonly grow relatively slowly, with periods of comparative stability or even in certain cases temporary regression. Desmoid tumors can be locally progressive with infiltration of adjacent normal tissues and structures. They may become locally malignant and highly destructive of normal tissue leading to the death of the patient. Spontaneous regressions have been observed, and regrowth is not observed in all patients following grossly incomplete surgical resection.

Desmoid tumors may be treated by surgical resection with a wide margin when medically and technically feasible. In recent years, the option to observe initially asymptomatic lesions has also emerged as an appropriate management strategy, with the finding that that approximately 50% of patients with desmoid tumors exhibit spontaneous growth arrest during simple follow-up with either medical therapy only or no therapy at all (24, 25). Since these tumors are benign, treatments with potentially serious late sequelae should be avoided if at all possible. Radiation therapy is an effective option for patients who are not good surgical candidates or decline surgery and, as an adjunctive therapy, for patients with grossly or microscopically positive margins or for those patients with recurrent disease. While some advocate adjuvant radiation for primary disease, our institution generally reserves radiation for patients with recurrent tumors after prior surgery or unresectable tumors that have progressed after observation or simple systemic treatment such as nonsteroidal anti-inflammatory drugs (NSAIDs) because this is a benign disease. Results from a number of centers demonstrate that radiation alone (50 Gy) or radiation combined with surgery in patients with positive margins achieves permanent control of desmoid tumors in approximately 70%–80% of patients (26). We also tend to try to defer the use of radiation as long as possible in pediatric patients, preferring to use any of the multiple systemic agents prior to radiotherapy in the child, in whom radiation may be associated with growth arrest, soft tissue atrophy, and late second malignancies.

There is increasing evidence for a role for systemic therapy in patients whose desmoid tumors cannot be controlled without morbid surgery and/or radiation (27). Increasing experience is accumulating with systemic agents in patients with advanced or recurrent disease, especially at intra-abdominal and abdominal wall sites. There are, for example, a number of anecdotal reports of excellent response to tamoxifen, the antiestrogen toremifine, and progestational agents. There are also documented responses to NSAIDs (most often sulindac) alone or in combination with tamoxifen. Regression is usually partial and may take many months after an initial period of tumor enlargement. Low-dose chemotherapy based upon methotrexate and vinblastine has obtained worthwhile response rates in patients with desmoid tumors, particularly in children. The combination of methotrexate and vinorelbine may produce a similar response to methotrexate and vinblastine with less neurotoxicity. In addition, there are anecdotal reports of doxorubicin-based drug protocols with good responses. For patients with Gardner's syndrome and intra-abdominal desmoid tumor, one should often avoid aggressive surgery given the relatively poor results of surgery and the higher rate of recurrence. Such patients can be treated with tamoxifen, NSAIDs, or low-dose chemotherapy. Surgery is the second option if there is no response.

BONE SARCOMAS

Malignant tumors of the skeletal system are rare. There were an estimated 3010 new bone sarcomas cases in the United States in 2013 with 1440 deaths. The most common primary bone sarcoma is osteosarcoma, followed by chondrosarcoma and Ewing's sarcoma. Osteosarcoma and Ewing's sarcoma occur primarily in childhood and adolescence. Other primary bone sarcomas, including chondrosarcomas, fibrosarcoma, and MFH, occur primarily in adults. Malignant tumors of bone must be differentiated from benign bone and cartilage tumors such as osteochondroma, enchondroma, osteoid osteoma, osteoblastoma, and desmoplastic fibroma, and giant cell tumor of bone and other malignant tumors such as myeloma and metastatic carcinoma. Just as for soft tissue sarcomas, the NCCN has been able to provide guidelines for management.

■ OSTEOSARCOMA

Osteosarcoma is the most common malignant bone tumor (28). Tumors are usually located in the metaphysis of long bone, especially the distal femur, proximal tibia, and proximal humerus. The most common presentation of patients with bone sarcomas is pain or swelling in a bone or near a joint. At the time of presentation, 10%–20% of patients have macroscopic metastatic disease and over 80% of patients likely harbor micrometastatic disease. Osteosarcomas metastasize primarily to the lung (90%) and less commonly to other bone sites (10%). Rarely do they metastasize to lymph nodes except in advanced stages of the disease. On pathologic analysis, the characteristic feature of osteosarcoma is the presence of tumor cell-produced osteoid. Several histologic subtypes of osteosarcomas exist: conventional (including osteoblastic, chondroblastic, and fibroblastic), small cell, radiation induced, sclerosing, extra-osseus, telangiectatic (high-grade aggressive with blood-filled cavities), and juxtacortical (parosteal [low grade] and periosteal [usually intermediate to high grade with cartilage]). The low-grade tumors have a much better prognosis than intermediate- to high-grade tumors, with the former not requiring chemotherapy. Most osteosarcomas are conventional approaching 80% of the total number per year.

Diagnosis and Staging

The radiologic appearance of osteosarcomas and other malignant bone tumors are usually different from that of benign tumors. Benign tumors usually have well-circumscribed borders with no cortical destruction or periosteal reaction. Malignant tumors often have irregular borders, bone destruction, periosteal reaction, and soft tissue extension. Patients should be fully evaluated by history and physical examination, plain radiographs, MRI and CT scan of the primary tumor site, chest CT, and bone scan. The diagnosis can usually be established by CT-guided core biopsy or open incisional biopsy. Often there exists an associated soft tissue component that can be biopsied for presence of most aggressive cells and it avoids producing a hole in the bone. The most commonly used staging system was developed by Enneking et al. and is outlined in Table 61-6 (29).

TABLE 61-6 MUSCULOSKELETAL TUMOR SOCIETY STAGING SYSTEM FOR BONE SARCOMAS

Histological Grade (G)	G1	Low grade
	G2	High grade
Site (T)	T1	Intracompartmental*
	T2	Extracompartmental*
Metastases	M0	No lymphatic or distant metastases
	M1	Lymphatic or distant metastases
Stage I A (G1, T1, M0)		Low-grade tumor, intracompartmental lesion without metastases
Stage IB (G1, T2, M0)		Low-grade tumor, extracompartmental lesion without metastases
Stage IIA (G2, T1, M0)		High grade, intracompartmental lesion without metastases
Stage IIB (G2, T2, M0)		High-grade tumor, extracompartmental lesion without metastases
Stage IIIA (G1/G2, T1, M0)		Any grade tumor, intracompartmental lesion with metastases
Stage IIIB (G1/G2, T2, M0)		Any grade tumor, extracompartmental lesion with metastases

*Compartment is defined as an anatomic structure or space bounded by natural barriers for tumor extension. A compartment can include any individual bone, intra-articular spaces, and any clearly identified facially enclosed space.
Adapted from Reference 29.

Surgery and Radiation

A wide surgical margin is preferred for resection of tumor coordinated with chemotherapy in intermediate- to high-grade osteosarcomas. In the axial locations where tumors tend to be larger when discovered the outcome in general is worse. In the extremities, about 90% of osteosarcomas can be removed using limb-sparing surgery, although amputation is sometimes necessary to achieve a negative surgical margin. Limb-sparing surgery is divided into three components:

1. *Resection of tumor*: Tumors are ideally removed with a rim of normal tissues to obtain a negative gross and microscopic margin. For low-grade lesions in which patients do not get chemotherapy, a marginal margin through the reactive zone may allow for salvage of those neurovascular structure abutting the tumor without jeopardizing local or distant disease.
2. *Skeletal reconstruction*: The skeletal defect is usually reconstructed but not always, especially if the tumor is located in an expendable bone like the proximal fibula. Most defects created by the resection can be reconstructed using a variety of techniques including autologous bone graft, allograft, endoprosthesis, and rotationplasty.
3. *Muscle and soft tissue coverage*: Local muscle, fat, and skin can be mobilized to cover the tumor resection bed and skeletal reconstruction. For larger defects, rotational or free flaps may be required. Areas more prone to infection like the proximal tibia may routinely get a gastrocnemius muscle flap.

Osteosarcomas are relatively resistant to radiation. Radiation therapy is generally not used in the primary treatment of most patients osteosarcomas, but is reserved for patients who refuse definitive surgery, have no good surgical option (i.e., base of skull), have grossly or microscopically positive resection margins, have less than wide resection margins and poor histologic response, have primary lesions in sites with high rates of relapse after surgery including head and neck, spine, or pelvis, present with a pathologic fracture and might be at higher risk of local recurrence, or require palliation. Retrospective reports suggest potential benefit for the addition of radiation therapy in these settings (30). For osteosarcomas in patients with extremity lesions who refused amputation, a combination of chemotherapy and primary radiation therapy (median dose 60 Gy) has been reported to obtain a 5-year local control of 56% in 31 patients; local control was 11/11 in selected patients who had a good response based on imaging and normalization of alkaline phosphatase. However, at our institution, surgical resections of osteosarcomas even in difficult locations requiring internal hemipelvectomy have been performed with acceptable morbidity, and local recurrence risk is substantially decreased. For patients for whom resection has been incomplete (43 patients) or has not been done (12 patients) because no good resection option exists (such as skull base) or in whom resection at such difficult locations as the upper sacrum has been declined, high-dose proton-based radiation or chemoradiation has provided durable local control for 73% of patients in one recent series (31).

Chemotherapy

In the 1970s prior to the use of adjuvant chemotherapy, <20% of osteosarcoma patients treated with surgery alone lived over 5 years. With the introduction of adjuvant chemotherapy (high-dose methotrexate), 5-year survival rates rose to 40%–60%. Prospective randomized trials performed in the 1980s confirmed the utility of adjuvant chemotherapy. Effective agents include high-dose methotrexate, doxorubicin, bleomycin, cyclophosphamide, dactinomycin, vincristine, cisplatin, ifosfamine, and etoposide (Pediatric Oncology Group, POG 8651). Neoadjuvant chemotherapy was originally introduced at Memorial Sloan-Kettering in concert with increased utilization of limb-sparing surgery. Chemotherapy was delivered to patients prior to surgery while awaiting creation of custom prosthetics, and retrospective analysis suggested these patients fared better than those that received postoperative chemotherapy alone. A randomized trial of comparing neoadjuvant and postoperative chemotherapy versus purely postoperative chemotherapy that consisted of alternating courses of high-dose methotrexate with leucovorin rescue, cisplatin and doxorubicin, and bleomycin, cyclophosphamide, and dactomycin given before or after surgical resection showed equivalent 5-year relapse-free survival (61% vs 65%) and limb salvage rates (50% vs 55%).

Currently about 65% of osteosarcoma patients treated with adjuvant chemotherapy attain long-term survival. Most centers deliver chemotherapy in the neoadjuvant setting, and this has several theoretical advantages: (1) early delivery of treatment for micrometastases, (2) increase in limb-salvage rates, and (3) assessment of tumor response. Tumor response to neoadjuvant chemotherapy (>90% tumor necrosis) is the most important prognostic factor for survival, and poor responders can be switched to alternative postoperative chemotherapy regimens. There exists some controversy as to the benefits of switching to alternative chemotherapy regimens in patients with <90% tumor necrosis.

The optimal chemotherapy regimen is still controversial. Many centers offer children, adolescents, and younger adults treatment similar to the POG regimen described above in the neoadjuvant setting. Ifosfamide and etoposide are used in some regimens. Older adults may not tolerate doxorubicin and cisplatin for more than 6 cycles. However, high-dose methotrexate and ifosfamide can also be used for most adults.

Recurrent and Metastatic Disease

Patients with metastatic osteosarcoma have long-term survival ranging from 10% to 40% with chemotherapy and surgery and in some cases radiation therapy. Patients with isolated lung metastases have a more favorable prognosis than those with bone metastases. The most active single agents are high-dose methotrexate, doxorubicin, cisplatin, and ifosfamide, with response rates ranging between 20% and 40%, and a variety of combination regimens have been used. Patients who recur following initial treatment with adjuvant chemotherapy and surgery tend to have chemotherapy-resistant disease. For isolated lung metastases that are few in number and do not invade the pleura, complete resection of all lesions can result in 5-year survival up to 35%. Unresectable metastatic disease can be treated with alternative chemotherapy regimens. Most patients who have already received doxorubicin and cisplatin (with or without high-dose methotrexate) can receive etoposide and ifosfamide with or without carboplatin, and such patients should be considered for enrollment in clinical trials.

■ EWING'S SARCOMA FAMILY OF TUMORS

Ewing's sarcoma was initially described by James Ewing as a tumor that was responsive to radiation treatment, and is rare tumors that arise in bone and less commonly in soft tissue. There is currently a spectrum of neoplastic diseases known as the Ewing's sarcoma family of tumors, which includes Ewing's sarcoma, primitive neuroectodermal tumors (PNET), adult neuroblastoma, malignant small cell tumor of the thoracopulmonary region (Askin's tumor), paravertebral small cell tumor, and atypical Ewing's sarcoma. These tumors are thought to be derived from a common cell of origin, share pathologic characteristics, and often have common chromosomal translocations (Table 61-1). As with osteosarcomas, these tumors primarily occur in adolescents and young adults and present with pain or swelling in a bone or joint. They usually involve flat bones or the metaphyseal and diaphyseal regions of tubular bones. While less than 25% of patients present with overt metastases, the majority of patients likely harbor micrometastatic disease, and the common sites of metastasis are the lung, and bone marrow. Workup and diagnosis are performed in a way similar to that for patients with osteosarcoma, except that bone marrow biopsy may be useful.

The surgical principles used for these tumors are similar to those for osteosarcoma. In contrast to osteosarcoma, the soft tissue mass present with Ewing's sarcoma usually shrinks with preoperative chemotherapy. In osteosarcoma the soft tissue mass will frequently demonstrate changes radiographically but not necessarily in the size of the mass. Deciding whether to use radiation or surgery for local control in the pelvis and axial regions is not always clear. Some groups have even proposed a combination therapy for management of these cases. In general, Ewing's sarcoma/PNET is relatively sensitive to radiation which is often applied to patients with positive surgical margins and for primary radiation local therapy in cases where surgery would be highly morbid. Selection factors make it difficult to determine whether primary radiotherapy results in as good local control as surgery alone or as surgery combined with radiation therapy. The major concern with the use of radiation therapy is the potential for late radiation-induced malignancies, particularly in younger patients. Radiation therapy has also been used in patients with positive surgical margins, although it is generally preferred to avoid surgery if positive margins are anticipated, because the dose generally applied for positive margins (50.4 Gy) is not much lower than that employed for primary radiotherapy alone (55.8 Gy) and the use of radiation therapy alone in this setting is generally expected to result in less morbidity than both surgery and radiotherapy.

For Ewing's sarcoma/PNET, standard chemotherapy includes vincristine, doxorubicin, and cyclophosphamide with or without actinomycin D (VDCA or VDC) alternating with ifosfamide and etoposide (IE). Most current protocols employ 4–6 cycles of chemotherapy over 12 weeks. Usually at least a few of the cycles are given as neoadjuvant chemotherapy preoperatively prior to local treatment with surgery or radiotherapy followed by additional chemotherapy that ultimately approaches close to a year of treatment. With modern multimodality treatment, long-term survival can be achieved in 70%–80% of patients with nonmetastatic disease.

For patients with metastatic disease, high-dose chemotherapy with or without whole body radiation and autologous hematopoietic stem cell support has been used. Patients with metastatic disease have a better prognosis when the lung is involved compared to bone and bone marrow. With chemotherapy, 5-year survival can be 20%–40%. Low-dose bilateral lung radiation can also be used, and isolated lesions in other locations can be controlled with radiation.

■ CHONDROSARCOMAS

Chondrosarcomas are the second most common malignant bone tumor and occur in patients usually in their third to fifth decade of life (32). The most common anatomic locations are the pelvis (31%), femur (21%), and shoulder girdle (13%). They occur in five primary types: 75% are "conventional" chondrosarcomas of either central (arising within a bone) or peripheral (arising from a bone surface) types and 25% are chondrosarcoma variants (mesenchymal, differentiated, and clear cell). The central and peripheral types of chondrosarcoma can be primary tumors or arise secondary to an underlying neoplasm such as a benign cartilage tumors. Most chondrosarcomas are grade I or II and uncommonly metastasize, but grade III lesions have the same metastatic potential as osteosarcomas. In a large single institution series of 344 chondrosarcomas, overall 5-year survival was 77% (33). Local recurrence developed in 20% and distant metastases in 14%. Local recurrence was higher for shoulder and pelvis tumors, high-grade tumors, and tumors with intralesional or marginal resections. High-grade was also an important prognostic factor distant recurrence. These results are similar to those reported by our institution (34).

The primary treatment of chondrosarcomas is surgical resection. These tumors are highly resistant to chemotherapeutic agents, possibly due to their extracellular matrix. Intralesional excision of grade I tumors has been advocated due to their benign behavior, although tumors located in the spine and pelvis can have a more aggressive biology. Grades II and III tumors should be resected with a wide surgical margin. Although it has been stated repeatedly that chondrosarcoma is a radioresistant tumor, several recent reports have demonstrated the effectiveness of conventional radiation therapy for this histology and it has been successfully employed in patients considered to be a high risk for local recurrence such as those with lesions located at complex sites where complete resection would be anticipated to be a problem such as spine, sacral, cranial or skull-base chondrosarcoma, and/or lesions with close or involved surgical margins and/or high-grade lesions (35). High rates of local control of these lesions in the base of skull/cervical spine and lower spine and sacrum with proton radiation therapy have been reported. The indications for radiation therapy for chondrosarcomas include unresectable or subtotally tumors, those resected with positive margins, and recurrent tumors. Because of the need for high radiation doses for control of these tumors and the proximity of radiosensitive critical structures in the skull base, spine, and pelvis, proton beam radiation, which has no exit dose beyond the target, is advantageous for treatment of tumors in these sites (36, 37).

There is no standard chemotherapy for chondrosarcoma, but patients with metastatic disease should be considered for enrollment in clinical trials.

CHORDOMAS

Chordomas are rare tumors that arise from the notochordal remnant in the midline of the neural axis (20). They occur most commonly in the sacrococcygeal region (50%) and base of skull (35%), but can occur in the cervical, thoracic, and lumbar spine regions (15%). Extraxial or parachordomas have been reported in unusual anatomic locations like the tibia and wrist. Sacrococcygeal lesions usually present with local pain. Patient can also have constipation or urinary symptoms. Base of skull lesions usually present with headache, visual changes, or cranial nerve dysfunction. CT scans and MRI are used for radiologic evaluation. CT imaging of the liver and lung should be performed to rule out metastases, and CT-guided biopsy usually establishes the diagnosis.

These tumors do metastasize in about 30% of patients with sacrococcygeal lesions (38) and a lower percentage of patients with skull base lesions, they present formidable local tumor control challenge and the tumors can be lethal due to their location adjacent to vital structures, locally aggressive behavior, and high rate of recurrence. Local control is difficult and local recurrence and complications often lead to death. The best chance at local control for these tumors is with the initial treatment, and such treatment should include aggressive surgical resection if feasible and radiation therapy when extraosseous extension is present. Even in small lesions after radical resection, recurrence rates are as high as 50%–100%, with local control and survival curves following a continuous downward slope in many series. Salvage treatment after local failure rarely is curative. A possible dose-response relationship for conventional radiation treatment has been reported. One of the best results of conventional, postoperative radiation treatment was published by Keisch et al (39). The rate of actuarial disease-free survival at 5 years was significantly better for patients undergoing surgery and radiotherapy (60%) compared to that of patients undergoing surgery only (25%), although patients continued to recur beyond 5 years. Investigators at the Lawrence Berkeley Laboratory (LBL) and our institution have demonstrated promising results for chordomas at the base of skull and cervical spine using charged particle irradiation, although local control is less favorable than with chondrosarcomas. Munzenrider and Liebsch reported that the 10-year local control for skull base tumors was highest for chondrosarcomas, intermediate for chordomas in males, and lowest for chordomas in females (94%, 65%, and 42%, respectively). For cervical spine tumors, 10-year local control rates were not significantly different for chordomas and chondrosarcomas (54% and 48%, respectively), nor was there any significant difference in local control between males and females. Hug et al. reported 5-year rates of local control and survival for lower spine and sacral chordomas of 53% and 50%, respectively, with a mean dose of 74.6 CGE (cobalt gray equivalent). DeLaney et al noted no local recurrences among 23 patients with primary spine chordomas treated with high-dose proton-based radiation (70.2 Gy for microscopic disease and 77.4 Gy for gross disease) with surgery in the majority of patients, although similar treatment resulted in local tumor control in only 3/6 patients with local tumor recurrence after prior surgery A trend for improved local control was noted for primary lesions compared to recurrent tumors, with radiation doses of at least 77 CGE and less residual tumor burden.

There is no standard chemotherapy for chordomas, but for metastatic disease there is some evidence for the use of imatinib, and patients should be considered for enrollment in clinical trials.

REFERENCES

1. Brennan MF, Lewis JL. *Diagnosis and Management of Soft Tissue Sarcoma.* Martin Dunitz, London, 2002.

2. Siegel R, Naishadham D, Jemal A. Cancer statistics, 2013. *CA Cancer J Clin.* 2013; 63: 11–30.

3. http://www.cancer.gov/cancertopics/pdq/treatment/adult-soft-tissue-sarcoma/HealthProfessional. Accessed August 20, 2013.

4. Lewis JJ, Leung D, Woodruff JM, et al. Retroperitoneal soft-tissue sarcoma: analysis of 500 patients treated and followed at a single institution. *Ann Surg.* 1998; 228: 355–365.

5. Lurkin A, Ducimetière F, Vince DR, et al. Epidemiological evaluation of concordance between initial diagnosis and central pathology review in a comprehensive and prospective series of sarcoma patients in the Rhone-Alpes region. *BMC Cancer.* 2010; 10: 150.

6. Rosenberg SA, Tepper J, Glatstein E, et al. The treatment of soft-tissue sarcomas of the extremities: prospective randomized evaluations of (1) limb-sparing surgery plus radiation therapy compared with amputation and (2) the role of adjuvant chemotherapy. *Ann Surg.* 1982; 196: 305–315.

7. Yang JC, Chang AE, Baker AR, et al. Randomized prospective study of the benefit of adjuvant radiation therapy in the treatment of soft tissue sarcomas of the extremity. *J Clin Oncol.* 1998; 16: 197–203.

8. O'Sullivan B, Davis AM, Turcotte R, et al. Preoperative versus postoperative radiotherapy in soft-tissue sarcoma of the limbs: a randomised trial. *Lancet.* 2002; 359: 2235–2241.

9. Kepka L, DeLaney TF, Suit HD, et al. Results of radiation therapy for unresected soft-tissue sarcomas. *Int J Radiat Oncol Biol Phys.* 2005; 63: 852–859.

10. DeLaney TF, Spiro IJ, Suit HD, et al. Neoadjuvant chemotherapy and radiotherapy for large extremity soft-tissue sarcomas. *Int J Radiat Oncol Biol Phys.* 2003; 56: 1117–1127.

11. Bramwell V, Rouesse J, Steward W, et al. Adjuvant CYVADIC chemotherapy for adult soft tissue sarcoma-reduced local recurrence but no improvement in survival: a study of the European Organization for Research and Treatment of Cancer Soft Tissue and Bone Sarcoma Group. *J Clin Oncol.* 1994; 12: 1137–1149.

12. Adjuvant chemotherapy for localised resectable soft-tissue sarcoma of adults: meta-analysis of individual data. Sarcoma Meta-analysis Collaboration. *Lancet.* 1997; 350: 1647–1654.

13. Pervaiz N, Colterjohn N, Farrokhyar F, et al. A systematic meta-analysis of randomized controlled trials of adjuvant chemotherapy for localized resectable soft-tissue sarcoma. *Cancer.* 2008; 113: 573–581.

14. Lewis JJ, Leung D, Woodruff JM, et al. Retroperitoneal soft-tissue sarcoma: analysis of 500 patients treated and followed at a single institution. *Ann Surg.* 1998; 228: 355–365.

15. Al Yami A, Griffin AM, Ferguson PC, et al. Positive surgical margins in soft tissue sarcoma treated with pre-operative radiation: is a postoperative boost necessary? *Int J Rad Oncol Bio Phys.* 2010; 77: 1191–1197.

16. Gieschen HL, Spiro IJ, Suit HD, et al. Long-term results of intraoperative electron beam radiotherapy for primary and recurrent retroperitoneal soft tissue sarcoma. *Int J Radiat Oncol Biol Phys.* 2001; 50: 127–131.

17. Yoon SS, Chen YL, Kirsch DG, et al. Proton-beam, intensity-modulated, and/or intraoperative electron radiation therapy combined with aggressive anterior surgical resection for retroperitoneal sarcomas. *Ann Surg Oncol.* 2010; 17: 1515–1529.

18. Brennan MF, Alektiar KM, Maki RG. Soft tissue sarcoma. In DeVita VT, Hellman S, Rosenberg SA (eds). *Cancer: Principles & Practice of Oncology.* Philadelphia, Lippincott Williams & Wilkins, 2001, pp. 1841–1980.

19. van der Graaf WT, Blay JY, Chawla SP, et al. Pazopanib for metastatic soft-tissue sarcoma (PALETTE): a randomised, double-blind, placebo-controlled phase 3 trial. *Lancet.* 2012; 379: 1879–1886.

20. Chawla SP, Blay J, et al. Results of the phase III, placebo-controlled trial (SUCCEED) evaluating the mTOR inhibitor ridaforolimus (R) as maintenance therapy in advanced sarcoma patients (pts) following clinical benefit from prior standard cytotoxic chemotherapy (CT). Presented at the 2011 Annual Meeting of the American Society of Clinical Oncology.

21. Ciresa M, D'Angelillo RM, Ramella S, et al. Molecularly targeted therapy and radiotherapy in the management of localized gastrointestinal stromal tumor (GIST) of the rectum: a case report. *Tumori.* 2009; 95: 236–239.

22. Joensuu H. Predicting recurrence-free survival after surgery for GIST. *Lancet Oncol.* 2009; 10: 1025.

23. Demetri GD, van Oosterom AT, Garrett CR, et al. Efficacy and safety of sunitinib in patients with advanced gastrointestinal stromal tumour after failure of imatinib: a randomised controlled trial. *Lancet.* 2006; 368: 1329–1338.

24. Bonvalot S, Eldweny H, Haddad V, et al: Extra-abdominal primary fibromatosis: aggressive management could be avoided in a subgroup of patients. *Eur J Surg Oncol.* 2008; 34: 462–468.

25. Fiore M, Rimareix F, Mariani L, et al: Desmoid-type fibromatosis: a front-line conservative approach to select patients for surgical treatment. *Ann Surg Oncol.* 2009; 16: 2587–2593.

26. Nuyttens JJ, Rust PF, Thomas CR Jr, et al. Surgery versus radiation therapy for patients with aggressive fibromatosis or desmoid tumors: a comparative review of 22 articles. *Cancer*. 2000; 88: 1517–1523.

27. Schlemmer M. Desmoid tumors and deep fibromatoses. *Hematol Oncol Clin North Am*. 2005; 19: 565–571.

28. Gebhardt MC, Hornicek FJ. Osteosarcoma and variants. In Bell MJ, et al (eds). *Orthopaedics and Trauma*. Oxford University Press, Oxford, 2002, pp. 224–238.

29. Enneking WF, Spanier SS, Goodman MA. A system for the surgical staging of musculoskeletal sarcoma. *Clin Orthop Relat Res*. 1980; 153: 106–120.

30. DeLaney TF, Park L, Goldberg SI, et al. Radiotherapy for local control of osteosarcoma. *Int J Radiat Oncol Biol Phys*. 2005; 61: 492–498.

31. Ciernik IF, Niemierko A, Harmon DC, et al. Proton-based radiotherapy for unresectable or incompletely resected osteosarcoma. *Cancer*. 2011; 117: 4522–4530.

32. Harsh GR, Janecka IP, Mankin HJ, et al. *Chordomas and Chondrosarcomas of the Skull Base and Spine*. Thieme Medical Publishers, New York, 2003.

33. Bjornsson J, McLeod RA, Unni KK, et al. Primary chondrosarcoma of long bones and limb girdles. *Cancer*. 1998; 83: 2105–2119.

34. Lee FY, Mankin HJ, Fondren G, et al. Chondrosarcoma of bone: an assessment of outcome. *J Bone Joint Surg Am*. 1999; 81: 326–338.

35. Goda JS, Ferguson PC, O'Sullivan B, et al. High-risk extracranial chondrosarcoma: long-term results of surgery and radiation therapy. *Cancer*. 2011; 117: 2513–2519.

36. Rosenberg AE, Nielsen GP, Keel SB, et al. Chondrosarcoma of the base of the skull: a clinicopathologic study of 200 cases with emphasis on its distinction from chordoma. *Am J Surg Pathol*. 1999; 23: 1370.

37. DeLaney TF, Liebsch NJ, Spiro IJ, et al. Proton radiotherapy for spine and paraspinal sarcomas. *Int J Rad Oncol Biol Phys*. 2006; 66: 115.

38. Schwab JH, Healey JH, Rose P, et al. The surgical management of sacral chordomas. *Spine*. 2009; 34: 2700–2704.

39. Keisch ME, Garcia DM, Shibuya RB. Retrospective long-term follow-up analysis in 21 patients with chordomas of various sites treated at a single institution. *J Neurosurg*. 1991; 75: 374–377.

CHAPTER **62**
Primary Brain Tumors

Andrew S. Chi

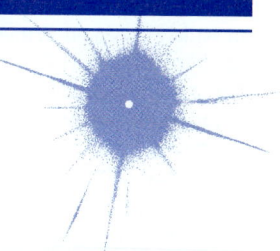

INTRODUCTION

Over 100 types of primary brain tumor are defined by the World Health Organization (WHO), the most commonly accepted classification system (1). Only a few entities account for the bulk of the incidence while the others are rare. The incidence rate of all primary central nervous system (CNS) tumors in the United States (U.S.) is 19.3 cases per 100,000 person-years (2). An estimated 64,530 primary CNS tumors were diagnosed in the United States in 2011. Approximately 24,070 of these tumors were malignant and this subgroup represented 1.46% of all malignant cancers diagnosed in the United States (2, 3).

Although relatively uncommon, primary brain tumors cause a disproportionate amount of morbidity and mortality, with an estimated 14,080 deaths attributed to malignant primary CNS tumors in the United States in 2013 (2). In this chapter we discuss the clinical evaluation of a patient with a suspected primary brain tumor and review the most common adult primary brain tumors encountered by oncologists: gliomas, primary central nervous system lymphomas, and meningiomas.

DIAGNOSIS

■ CLINICAL FEATURES

Patients with primary brain tumors can present suddenly with seizures or subacutely with progressive focal or non-focal neurological symptoms over several weeks to several months. Progressive focal neurological deficits are usually referable to growth of a tumor in a specific brain location. Non-focal symptoms include headache, vomiting, fatigue, cognitive changes, mood disturbances, imbalance, and gait disorder. Less often, patients may present with an acute stroke-like neurological deficit caused by hemorrhage into a previously subclinical tumor.

Headaches result from local irritation of pain-sensitive dura or from increased intracranial pressure (ICP). Headaches from increased ICP due to tumors are usually holocephalic, progressive, often associated with nausea, worse with recumbency, and may awaken a patient from sleep. They may be precipitated by Valsalva maneuvers or coughing. Systemic symptoms such as malaise, anorexia, weight loss, and fever are usually absent, and presence of these symptoms suggests a metastatic rather than primary brain tumor.

■ LABORATORY EVALUATION

Primary brain tumors are not associated with serologic abnormalities, and no widely accepted primary brain tumor-specific systemic marker exists. Lumbar puncture (LP) for cerebrospinal fluid (CSF) analysis is indicated if there is suspicion of CNS metastasis of systemic cancers or leptomeningeal spread of astrocytoma and for staging of certain primary brain tumors that commonly disseminate in the CSF compartment such as primary CNS lymphoma and primitive neuroectodermal tumor. The CSF may demonstrate an elevated protein level and a mild lymphocytic pleocytosis. A lumbar puncture may precipitate brain herniation if there is increased ICP, and therefore should be performed only after reviewing cranial imaging and obtaining neurological consultation.

■ NEUROIMAGING

The diagnosis of a primary brain tumor is suggested by contrast-enhanced cranial imaging with either computerized tomography (CT) or magnetic resonance imaging (MRI). With the exception of skull bone evaluation, MRI is almost always superior to CT and is the imaging modality of choice.

On CT, tumors and associated vasogenic edema usually appear as regions of low attenuation. Areas of increased attenuation may indicate hemorrhage or calcification. On MRI, tumors often have low signal intensity on T1-weighted sequences and high signal intensity on T2-weighted and FLAIR sequences, although signal characteristics vary with specific tumor types (**Figure 62-1**). Abnormal enhancement after the administration of intravenous contrast material on either CT or MRI correlates with areas of blood-brain barrier disruption and abnormal endothelial proliferation, and

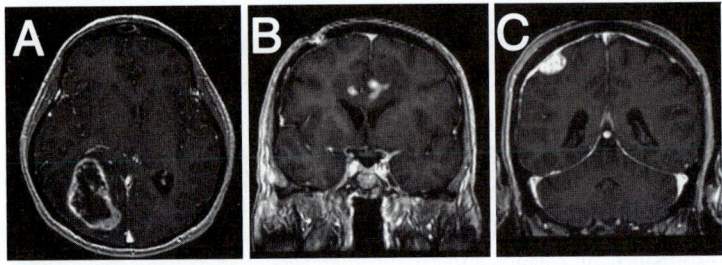

FIGURE 62-1 Magnetic resonance images of primary brain tumors. A. Glioblastoma. Axial T1 contrast-enhanced sequence demonstrating a heterogeneous, peripherally enhancing, centrally necrotic lesion centered in the right temporal-occipital region, causing mass effect on adjacent structures including the corpus callosum and basal ganglia. B. Primary CNS lymphoma. A T1 hypointense mass located in the left cingulate gyrus and subcortical area extending across the corpus callosum and containing several discrete areas of contrast enhancement. C. Meningioma. Coronal T1 contrast-enhanced sequence demonstrates a dural-based, extra-axial mass with intense contrast enhancement and adjacent T1 hypointensity in the brain parenchyma representing vasogenic edema.

is a surrogate for the location of a tumor. In general, contrast enhancement is characteristic of more malignant tumors.

Other technologies such as magnetic resonance spectroscopy and positron emission tomography (PET) are useful in specific situations such as surgical guidance and distinguishing between recurrent tumor and treatment-related necrosis. The gold standard for diagnosis, however, remains tissue biopsy.

GLIOMAS

■ CLASSIFICATION

Gliomas account for 80% of all malignant primary brain tumors and 30% of all brain and CNS tumors in adults (2). They consist of cells that display glial differentiation and resemble glial cells (e.g., astrocytes, oligodendrocytes, and ependymal cells). Gliomas comprise a group of tumor types that includes astrocytoma, oligodendroglioma, mixed oligoastrocytoma, ependymoma and other less common variants. Astrocytomas account for approximately 75% of all gliomas and are most often supratentorial, although they may arise anywhere in the CNS.

The WHO categorizes gliomas into four histological grades (1). Grade I is reserved for rare, relatively benign, and slow-growing histological variants including pilocytic astrocytoma, pleomorphic xanthoastrocytoma, and dysembryoplastic neuroepithelial tumor. These tumors carry an excellent prognosis after surgical resection.

Other gliomas are graded using specific histological criteria: cellularity, nuclear atypia, mitotic activity, vascular proliferation, and necrosis. Gliomas that display only one of these features, usually nuclear atypia, are classified as grade II. Gliomas with two features, usually nuclear atypia and mitotic activity, are classified as grade III. Presence of three features, usually nuclear atypia, mitoses, vascular proliferation and/or necrosis, is classified grade IV and these gliomas are termed glioblastoma. Grade II gliomas are commonly referred to as low-grade gliomas (LGGs) while grade III and IV gliomas are commonly referred to as high-grade gliomas (HGGs) or malignant gliomas (MGs).

■ LOW-GRADE GLIOMA (LGG)

Classification

Most adult low-grade (grade II) gliomas are categorized into three histologically defined subgroups: astrocytoma, oligodendroglioma, and oligoastrocytoma. LGGs are relatively uncommon tumors that typically present between the second and fourth decades. They are highly infiltrative tumors that invade and expand contiguous brain tissue.

Although initially slow growing, LGGs nearly always progress to HGGs despite treatment. Median survival ranges between 5 and 10 years (Table 62-1) (2). Histological subtype is a critical determinant of survival, with oligodendrogliomas having a more indolent course and better responsiveness to therapy than astrocytomas. Mixed oligoastrocytomas have an intermediate outcome. Other factors that negatively impact survival include

TABLE 62-1 SURVIVAL RATES FOR SELECTED PRIMARY BRAIN TUMORS (2)

Histology	10-Year Survival
Astrocytic tumors	
Pilocytic astrocytoma (WHO grade I)	92.1%
Diffuse astrocytoma (WHO grade II)	36.4%
Anaplastic astrocytoma (WHO grade III)	21.9%
Glioblastoma (WHO grade IV)	2.8%
Oligodendroglial tumors	
Oligodendroglioma (WHO grade II)	63.6%
Anaplastic oligodendroglioma (WHO grade III)	34.6%
Mixed glioma	46.4%
Primary CNS lymphoma	21.6%

age >40 years, the presence of preoperative neurologic deficit, tumor size >6 cm in maximal diameter, and tumor crossing the midline (Table 62-2) (4).

Molecular Profiles of LGG

Proliferation indices such as Ki-67 and MIB-1 are often reported; however, their prognostic relevance in LGG is controversial. Somatic genetic markers have become increasingly useful as potential diagnostic and prognostic tools in LGG. Approximately 80%–90% of low-grade oligodendrogliomas have combined loss of heterozygosity (LOH) on chromosomes 1p and 19q, and loss of both markers correlates with longer survival (5).

Recently discovered alterations in *BRAF*, *IDH1*, and *IDH2* appear to be hallmark aberrations in particular grade I and II glioma subtypes. Tandem duplication at 7q34 leading to a fusion between *KIAA1549* and *BRAF* results in constitutively active BRAF activity and is found in approximately 70% of pilocytic astrocytomas (6–8). An activating point mutation in *BRAF* (V600E) is found in an additional 5%–9% of these tumors (9, 10) and in general, RAF alterations occur in ~80% of pilocytic astrocytomas. *BRAF V600E* mutations are frequently observed (~60%) in other relatively benign glioma variants, including pleomorphic xanthoastrocytoma (10) and ganglioglioma (11), while *BRAF* tandem duplications are not found in these tumors.

The vast majority (87%) of grade II gliomas (astrocytomas, oligodendrogliomas, and oligoastrocytomas) harbor point mutations in the R132 position of isocitrate dehydrogenase 1 (*IDH1*) (12) or rarely the analogous codon in *IDH2* (R172) (13). Mutant IDH has altered catalytic activity that results in marked accumulation of 2-hydroxyglutarate in gliomas (14), although the functional consequence of this activity is unclear.

Other than 1p/19q co-deletion, the prognostic significance of these somatic alterations remains unclear. However, several have potential diagnostic utility. Pleomorphic xanthoastrocytomas frequently have *BRAF*

TABLE 62-2 PROGNOSTIC FACTORS FOR SURVIVAL IN SELECTED PRIMARY BRAIN TUMORS

Prognostic Factor	Favorable	Unfavorable
Low-grade (II) glioma		
Age (y)	<40	>40
Largest diameter of the tumor	<6 cm	≥6 cm
Tumor crossing midline	No	Yes
Histology	Oligodendroglioma/mixed glioma	Astrocytoma
Preoperative Neurologic deficit	Absent	Present
High-grade (III or IV) glioma		
Age (y)	<45	>45
Histology	Oligodendroglioma/mixed glioma	Astrocytoma
Functional status (KPS[a])	>70	<70
1p and 19q status (oligodendrogliomas, oligoastrocytomas)	Co-deleted	Not co-deleted
MGMT promoter DNA	Methylated	Unmethylated
IDH1/IDH2	R132 or R172 point mutation	Wild type
Primary CNS Lymphoma (16)		
Age (y)	<60	>60
Functional status (KPS[a])	>70	<70
Lactate dehydrogenase (LDH)	Normal	Elevated
CSF protein concentration	Normal	Elevated
Area of brain involved		Deep[b]

[a]Karnofsky Performance Status Scale.
[b]Periventricular, basal ganglia, brainstem, cerebellum.

V600E mutation, while *BRAF* tandem duplications (typical of pilocytic astrocytomas) and *IDH1/2* mutations (typical of more aggressive grade II gliomas) are rare (10, 13). The vast majority (90%) of *IDH* mutations in gliomas result in an R132H substitution, which can be detected with a highly sensitive and specific monoclonal antibody. A rapid immunohistochemical analysis using the mutant-specific IDH1 antibody can aid diagnostic analysis (15).

Treatment of LGG

Surgery has an important role in obtaining tissue for histological diagnosis and in providing relief from symptoms caused by mass effect on adjacent structures and increased ICP. No prospective, randomized data exist regarding the benefit of extensive resection of LGGs; however, a number of retrospective analyses suggest cytoreductive surgery improves survival (16). Gross total resection is often advocated for, however, the invasiveness of LGGs and their frequent location near eloquent brain regions often precludes complete excision. Therefore, the primary objective is often maximal safe resection.

Adjuvant treatment options include observation, radiation therapy, and chemotherapy. Radiation is a standard component of treatment for LGGs; however, there remains significant controversy regarding the timing of its implementation. A multicenter, randomized phase III trial demonstrated that early radiotherapy after surgery increases the time to tumor progression but not overall survival compared to radiotherapy at the time of tumor progression (17). However, this study did not stratify for known strong prognostic factors such as oligodendroglial histology and 1p/19q status.

Because patients with LGGs may live for many years, the risk of developing radiation-related adverse effects including cognitive impairment (18) and endocrinopathy (pituitary dysfunction) must be carefully considered. Technical advances in imaging and radiation delivery allow more accurate planning of target volumes and may minimize the long-term side effects of radiotherapy. However, prospective studies incorporating cognitive and quality of life assessments are needed to assess the risk of neurotoxicity and the value of longer time-to-progression with modern radiation techniques.

There is limited but emerging evidence that chemotherapy may be effective in treating LGGs, particularly oligodendrogliomas. Procarbazine, lomustine, and vincristine (PCV) combination therapy and temozolomide have been reported in small series to have activity in both newly diagnosed and progressive LGGs. A randomized phase III trial comparing adjuvant radiotherapy versus temozolomide for newly diagnosed LGG is currently accruing (EORTC 22041).

Because subgroups of LGG patients may survive a long time with little or no neurologic deficit and long-term toxicity is a risk with all therapeutic modalities, management of newly diagnosed LGG remains controversial. Treatment is individualized based on a risk score determined from a number of prognostic factors (Table 62-2) (4). Typically, low-risk patients, particularly those with gross-totally resected tumors, are monitored with serial contrast-enhanced MRI scans. Adjuvant radiation is often provided for high-risk patients, particularly in the setting of incomplete resection.

■ MALIGNANT GLIOMAS

Classification and Molecular Profiles of MG

Classification. Malignant gliomas include grade III tumors such as anaplastic astrocytoma, anaplastic oligodendroglioma, and anaplastic oligoastrocytoma, as well as glioblastoma (GBM, grade IV). GBM accounts for 60% of MGs and is the most common adult malignant primary brain tumor (2).

TABLE 62-3 HEREDITARY RISK FACTORS FOR GLIOMAS

Hereditary Syndromes	Gene
Neurofibromatosis 1 (NF1)	*NF1*
Neurofibromatosis 2 (NF2)	*NF2*
Tuberous sclerosis complex (TSC)	*TSC1*; *TSC2*
Nevoid basal cell carcinoma syndrome (NBCCS), Gorlin-Goltz syndrome	*PTC*
Li-Fraumeni syndrome	*TP53*
Brain tumor-polyposis syndrome (BTPS), hereditary nonpolyposis colorectal cancer (HNPCC), Turcot syndrome	DNA mismatch repair (*MLH1, MSH2, PMS1,* and *PMS2*)
Multiple endocrine neoplasia type 1 (MEN1), Wermer syndrome	*MEN1*

The average age at diagnosis of GBM is 64 years, although it can present at any age.

The prognosis of patients with MG remains unsatisfactory (Table 62-1). The median survival of patients with AA is 2–5 years, while the survival is 10–15 months for those with GBM (2). Prognostic factors associated with improved survival include grade III tumors, oligodendroglial histology, younger age, better performance status, and molecular features such as 1p/19q co-deletion, *IDH1/2* mutation (12, 13), and *MGMT* promoter DNA methylation (19, 20) (Table 62-2). Anaplastic oligodendrogliomas, particularly the 50%–70% with 1p/19q co-deletion, have a better prognosis and are perhaps more responsive to treatment than astrocytomas (21).

Molecular profiles of GBM. Most GBMs arise as a result of genetic alterations involving tumor suppressor genes and proto-oncogenes within a progenitor cell, although a rare subgroup of gliomas are associated with certain hereditary syndromes (Table 62-3). At least two distinct clinical and genetic forms of GBM have been described (22). Primary GBMs, which account for the vast majority of cases, arise de novo and typically in older patients. These tumors are associated with increased activity of the epidermal growth factor receptor (EGFR), inactivation of the *PTEN* gene, and normal *TP53* status.

Secondary GBMs arise from malignant transformation of previously known low-grade astrocytomas and typically occur in younger patients. Recently, *IDH1/2* mutation was discovered as a hallmark of secondary GBM, being found in approximately 85% of secondary GBM versus 5% of primary GBM (12, 13). The genetic pathway to secondary GBM is thought to involve early *IDH1/2* mutation (23, 24) followed by mutations of *TP53* and overexpression of platelet-derived growth factor (PDGF) and PDGF receptors (PDGFR) in low-grade astrocytomas. Progression to grade III is associated with inactivation of *RB1* and increased activity of *HDM2*.

Subsequent progression to GBM involves loss of chromosome 10 among other changes (22).

These molecular alterations primarily deregulate two cellular systems: growth factor mediated signaling pathways and the cell cycle. Phenotypic consequences include increased cell proliferation, inhibition of apoptosis, cell invasion, and angiogenesis.

Treatment of Newly Diagnosed MG

Treatment of MGs requires supportive care and multimodality antitumor therapy. Supportive care requirements are often considerable, and include management of cerebral edema, seizures, venous thromboembolism, infections, and cognitive dysfunction.

Definitive antitumor therapy usually begins with maximal safe resection. The decision between biopsy and resection depends on the proximity of the tumor to critical brain regions, the patient's age and functional status, and the degree of mass effect. Resection may also be indicated to relieve symptoms such as local compression or elevated ICP.

Modern intraoperative imaging and physiological monitoring techniques may allow for more extensive resection of tumors located in or near eloquent brain regions. Several retrospective studies suggest extent of resection impacts survival in MG. A prospective, randomized phase III trial investigating the effect of fluorescence guidance on surgical radicality in MG found that patients without residual contrast-enhancing tumor had higher median survival than those with residual enhancing tumor. These studies suggest gross total resection of the contrast-enhancing tumor on MRI improves outcome in MG.

Radiation therapy is the standard adjuvant therapy for newly diagnosed MG (25). Focal conformal radiation (involved-field radiation therapy) is directed at the tumor and a small surrounding margin, typically 2 cm. Limiting radiation fields may reduce the risk of neurotoxicity, and some data suggest most recurrences occur within this margin.

Anaplastic glioma.   Histological and molecular factors such as oligodendroglial histology, 1p/19q status (21, 26, 27), *MGMT* promoter methylation (19), and *IDH1/2* mutation status (13, 28) all have strong prognostic value in anaplastic gliomas (Table 62-2); however, it's unclear whether these factors predict responsiveness to treatment.

Considerable controversy exists regarding the addition of chemotherapy to radiotherapy after surgery for anaplastic glioma. Two randomized, phase III trials in anaplastic oligodendroglial tumors demonstrated no difference in overall survival with the addition of neoadjuvant (26) or adjuvant (27) PCV to radiotherapy compared to radiotherapy alone. However, progression-free survival was longer with chemotherapy, and the majority of the patients in the radiotherapy alone arms received chemotherapy at recurrence. More recently, a phase III trial in anaplastic gliomas demonstrated that adjuvant chemotherapy (PCV or temozolomide) followed by radiation at recurrence was as effective as adjuvant radiation followed by chemotherapy at recurrence (29).

Two randomized, phase III cooperative group trials aim to address questions regarding adjuvant chemotherapy. A four-arm trial for anaplastic gliomas without 1p/19q co-deletion (RTOG 0834) is randomizing between radiation alone, radiation + concurrent temozolomide, radiation + adjuvant temozolomide, and radiation + concurrent and adjuvant temozolomide. A trial for 1p/19q co-deleted anaplastic gliomas is randomizing patients to receive radiation alone, radiation + concurrent and adjuvant temozolomide, or temozolomide alone (NCCTG N0577/RTOG 1071).

Glioblastoma. The current standard of care in the adjuvant setting consists of radiotherapy with concurrent temozolomide (Temodar®), a well-tolerated oral DNA methylating agent, followed by 6 months of post-radiation temozolomide. This regimen was established by a EORTC/NCIC phase III trial that demonstrated an increase in median survival from 12 months with radiotherapy alone to 14.6 months with radiation and concurrent temozolomide followed by 6 cycles of temozolomide (30). A subgroup appeared to derive significant benefit, as the 2-year survival proportion was 26.5% in the temozolomide arm compared to 10% in the radiotherapy-only arm.

The presence of *IDH1/2* mutations (12, 13) and/or *MGMT* promoter methylation (20) is strong positive prognostic factor in GBM. It has been proposed that *MGMT* promoter methylation is predictive of response to temozolomide (20); however, this has not been validated prospectively. Generally temozolomide is given to GBM patients regardless of *MGMT* promoter methylation status.

Intratumoral or intracavitary administration of chemotherapy may increase the exposure of drug to the tumor with reduced systemic toxicity. Implantation of BCNU-impregnated wafers (Gliadel®) at the time of surgical resection is occasionally utilized in patients with newly diagnosed MG. This therapy was associated with a median survival of 13.9 months in a phase III trial while placebo-treated patients survived a median of 11.6 months (31).

Management of elderly patients is challenging due to their poorer prognosis and reduced tolerance of treatment. However, a recent phase III study demonstrated improved survival of MG patients 70 years of age or older with an abbreviated course of radiation compared to best supportive care. Importantly, radiotherapy was not associated with reduced quality of life or cognitive ability in this study (32).

Salvage Therapy

Despite aggressive therapy, nearly all MGs recur. Bevacizumab has gained accelerated FDA approval for use in progressive GBM based on improved objective response proportions (20% and 26%) observed in two historically controlled, single-arm, or non-comparative phase II trials (33, 34). However, the median durations of response were only 4.2 and 3.9 months and most patients ultimately progressed. The addition of bevacizumab to radiation and temozolomide in newly diagnosed GBM is currently being investigated in an ongoing multicenter, randomized trial (RTOG 0825).

No therapy has demonstrated improved survival in a prospective, randomized, controlled trial in the recurrent GBM setting. Because current salvage options have limited efficacy, management of recurrent MG patients is individualized. Tumor location, size, histology, prior therapy, and the general health of the patient are considered.

If surgically accessible, debulking may improve symptoms and allow time for additional therapy. Some evidence suggests that stereotactic radiosurgery (SRS), which delivers a high single dose of radiation to a small (<4 cm) treatment volume, improves survival in recurrent MGs. A number of conventional chemotherapies, including lomustine, BCNU, carboplatin, etoposide, irinotecan, and PCV, are used as salvage agents, although none significantly improves survival. In general, patients with recurrent disease should be considered for clinical trials.

Experimental Therapy

There is a wide array of experimental therapeutic strategies being developed for MGs, including locoregional therapies, radiosensitizers, biological agents, and immunological therapy.

A major focus of clinical development is on molecularly targeted inhibitors of overactive cell signaling pathways, including the receptor tyrosine kinase (e.g., EGFR, PDGFR, and c-MET), RAS/MAPK, and PI3K/AKT pathways. The cell cycle and tumor-associated angiogenesis are also being targeted due to their high frequency of abnormality in MG. Initial targeted therapy clinical trials in MGs have reported modest activity at best, however, with low response rates and no significant increases in survival.

Many factors may have contributed to the limited efficacy seen in these trials; however, the most important may have been the molecular heterogeneity that exists between and within individual MGs. Molecular subsets of responsive tumors have been identified in some targeted inhibitor trials (35, 36), suggesting that increased efficacy with targeted agents may be derived with improved patient stratification. Current efforts are focused on improving molecular profiling of tumors, combinatorial regimens of targeted agents, and combinations of molecularly targeted agents with cytotoxic therapies such as radiation or chemotherapy.

PRIMARY CENTRAL NERVOUS SYSTEM LYMPHOMA

Primary central nervous system lymphoma (PCNSL) is a rare form of non-Hodgkin lymphoma that presents within the CNS without evidence of systemic lymphoma. Most cases are high-grade B-cell lymphoma. PCNSL may affect the brain, spinal cord, leptomeninges, and eyes. They occur commonly in immunocompromised patients, including those with AIDS, autoimmune diseases, and iatrogenic immunosuppression for organ transplants. Tumor cells in immunocompromised patients are invariably associated with Epstein-Barr virus (EBV) infection. Immunocompetent patients with PCNSL usually present after the age of 60 years.

Lesions are most often supratentorial and periventricular, and discrete masses characteristically span the corpus callosum. Immunocompetent patients most often have solitary lesions, whereas AIDS-associated PCNSL is often multicentric. Up to 40% of patients have leptomeningeal involvement, and 20% may have ocular disease. On MRI, lesions are typically hyperintense on T2-weighted or FLAIR images, exhibit diffusion restriction, and markedly enhance after contrast administration (37).

Diagnostic evaluation includes physical examination, slit-lamp examination, serum lactate dehydrogenase levels, human immunodeficiency virus testing, CT scans of the chest/abdomen/pelvis, bone marrow biopsy, contrast-enhanced brain MRI, and LP (Table 62-2). Testicular ultrasonography and contrast-enhanced MRI of the entire spine should be considered if clinically indicated. Diagnosis is established by pathological analysis of CSF, vitreous fluid, or a brain biopsy specimen. CSF studies should include chemistry (glucose and protein), cell counts, cytology, flow cytometry, and PCR for clonal immunoglobulin gene rearrangements or EBV DNA. Brain biopsy remains the gold standard for diagnosis (38).

Due to the relative rarity of PCNSL and the paucity of prospective, randomized trials, the optimal treatment regimen remains controversial. Systemic chemotherapy is effective and has increased the overall survival from 18 months to up to 55 months. High-dose methotrexate (at least 3.5 g/m^2) is the mainstay of therapy and is the most effective drug against PCNSL (39). Methotrexate is given with or without other chemotherapy agents or whole-brain radiation therapy (WBRT). Recently, improved survival was reported in a randomized phase II trial with the addition of high-dose cytarabine to methotrexate (40).

WBRT is often used for consolidation; however, delayed radiation-induced neurotoxicity is an undesirable and irreversible treatment-associated morbidity that is a particularly significant risk for patients over age 60 years. Regimens that may achieve comparable outcomes with less neurotoxicity include reduced dose WBRT (41) and combined chemotherapy consisting of methotrexate, temozolomide, and rituximab with consolidating cytarabine and etoposide without radiation (42).

In younger patients, chemotherapy-only regimens are common, although these approaches may be associated with increased relapse rates. A promising approach is high-dose chemotherapy followed by autologous stem cell transplant without consolidating radiotherapy. One report demonstrated high relapse-free and overall survival rates (43), and a multicenter phase III trial based on this approach is being initiated.

Although most patients eventually recur, salvage therapy may be effective. Chemotherapy options include re-induction with methotrexate, high-dose cytarabine, PCV, topotecan, and temozolomide + rituximab. High-dose chemotherapy followed by autologous stem cell rescue has shown promise in small, non-randomized trials (44).

MENINGIOMAS

Meningiomas arise from the meninges, originating from arachnoidal cap cells of the arachnoidal granulations. These tumors are typically located along the dura of the superior sagittal sinus. Other common locations include the cerebral convexities, base of the brain, sphenoidal ridges, and parasellar areas.

Meningiomas are the most common intracranial non-glial tumor, and constitute up to 34% of all intracranial tumors. An estimated 2%–3% of the population has an incidental asymptomatic meningioma. They occur mostly in middle-aged or elderly patients, with a female preponderance of 2:1 that recedes with age (2). Approximately a third of meningiomas are asymptomatic, diagnosed incidentally or at autopsy. Patients usually present with slowly progressive symptoms due to compression of neighboring brain structures and less commonly with seizures or progressive hydrocephalus.

On contrast-enhanced MRI, meningiomas are characteristically extra-axial, dural-based masses with intense, uniform contrast enhancement. Meningiomas are usually low-grade (grade I) tumors associated with long progression-free survival after gross total resection. Rarely, they have aggressive histopathological features and are classified as atypical (grade II) or anaplastic (grade III) meningiomas. These higher-grade meningiomas have much higher rates of recurrence and may invade the brain or metastasize outside the CNS.

There are several options for management of a newly discovered presumed meningioma on MRI. Small, asymptomatic meningiomas may be observed with serial cranial imaging to monitor for tumor growth. Treatment, usually resection, is recommended if meningiomas are symptomatic and associated with worsening neurological function. Fractionated, conformal radiation therapy or SRS is used for subtotally resected tumors, atypical or malignant meningioma resection cavities (45), or tumors in close proximity to critical brain regions such as the optic apparatus or brainstem.

REFERENCES

1. Louis D, Ohgaki H, Wiestler O, Cavenee W. *WHO Classification of Tumours of the Central Nervous System.* 4th ed. Lyon, France: IARC Press; 2007.

2. CBTRUS. CBTRUS Statistical Report: Primary Brain and Central Nervous System Tumors Diagnosed in the United States in 2004-2007. Central Brain Tumor Registry of the United States (CBTRUS); 2011.

3. United States Cancer Statistics 1999–2007 Cancer Incidence and Mortality Data. Centers for Disease Control and Prevention (CDC) and the National Cancer Institute (NCI); 2007. http://apps.nccd.cdc.gov/uscs/index.aspx. Accessed 2007.

4. Pignatti F, van den Bent M, Curran D, et al. Prognostic factors for survival in adult patients with cerebral low-grade glioma. *J Clin Oncol.* 2002; 20: 2076–2084.

5. Smith JS, Perry A, Borell TJ, et al. Alterations of chromosome arms 1p and 19q as predictors of survival in oligodendrogliomas, astrocytomas, and mixed oligoastrocytomas. *J Clin Oncol.* 2000; 18: 636–645.

6. Sievert A, Jackson E, Gai X, et al. Duplication of 7q34 in pediatric low-grade astrocytomas detected by high-density single-nucleotide polymorphism-based genotype arrays results in a novel BRAF fusion gene. *Brain Pathol.* 2009; 19: 449–458.

7. Pfister S, Janzarik W, Remke M, et al. BRAF gene duplication constitutes a mechanism of MAPK pathway activation in low-grade astrocytomas. *J Clin Invest.* 2008; 118: 1739–1749.

8. Jones D, Kocialkowski S, Liu L, et al. Tandem duplication producing a novel oncogenic BRAF fusion gene defines the majority of pilocytic astrocytomas. *Cancer Res.* 2008; 68: 8673–8677.

9. Schindler G, Capper D, Meyer J, et al. Analysis of BRAF V600E mutation in 1,320 nervous system tumors reveals high mutation frequencies

in pleomorphic xanthoastrocytoma, ganglioglioma and extra-cerebel-lar pilocytic astrocytoma. *Acta Neuropathol.* 2011; 121: 397–405.

10. Dias-Santagata D, Lam Q, Vernovsky K, et al. BRAF V600E mutations are common in pleomorphic xanthoastrocytoma: diagnostic and thera-peutic implications. *PLoS ONE.* 2011; 6: e17948.

11. MacConaill LE, Campbell CD, Kehoe SM, et al. Profiling critical cancer gene mutations in clinical tumor samples. *PLoS ONE.* 2009; 4: e7887.

12. Parsons D, Jones S, Zhang X, et al. An integrated genomic analysis of human glioblastoma multiforme. *Science.* Sep 26 2008; 321: 1807–1812.

13. Yan H, Parsons D, Jin G, et al. IDH1 and IDH2 mutations in gliomas. *N Engl J Med.* 2009; 360: 765–773.

14. Dang L, White DW, Gross S, et al. Cancer-associated IDH1 mutations produce 2-hydroxyglutarate. *Nature.* 2009; 462: 739–744.

15. Camelo-Piragua S, Jansen M, Ganguly A, et al. A sensitive and specific diagnostic panel to distinguish diffuse astrocytoma from astrocytosis: chromosome 7 gain with mutant isocitrate dehydrogenase 1 and p53. *J Neuropathol Exp Neurol.* 2011; 70: 110–115.

16. Smith J, Chang E, Lamborn K, et al. Role of extent of resection in the long-term outcome of low-grade hemispheric gliomas. *J Clin Oncol.* 2008; 26: 1338–1345.

17. van den Bent M, Afra D, de Witte O, et al. Long-term efficacy of early versus delayed radiotherapy for low-grade astrocytoma and oligoden-droglioma in adults: the EORTC 22845 randomised trial. *Lancet.* 2005; 366: 985–990.

18. Douw L, Klein M, Fagel SS, et al. Cognitive and radiological effects of radiotherapy in patients with low-grade glioma: long-term follow-up. *Lancet Neurol.* 2009; 8: 810–818.

19. van den Bent MJ, Dubbink HJ, Sanson M, et al. MGMT Promoter methylation is prognostic but not predictive for outcome to adjuvant PCV chemotherapy in anaplastic oligodendroglial tumors: a report from EORTC Brain Tumor Group Study 26951. *J Clin Oncol.* 2009; 27: 5881–5886.

20. Hegi M, Diserens A, Gorlia T, et al. MGMT gene silencing and ben-efit from temozolomide in glioblastoma. *N Engl J Med.* 2005; 352: 997–1003.

21. Cairncross J, Ueki K, Zlatescu M, et al. Specific genetic predictors of chemotherapeutic response and survival in patients with anaplastic oligodendrogliomas. *J Natl Cancer Inst.* 1998; 90: 1473–1479.

22. Kleihues P, Ohgaki H. Primary and secondary glioblastomas: from concept to clinical diagnosis. *Neuro-oncol.* 1999; 1: 44–51.

23. Lai A, Kharbanda S, Pope WB, et al. Evidence for sequenced molecular evolution of IDH1 mutant glioblastoma from a distinct cell of origin. *J Clin Oncol.* 2011; 29: 4482–4490.

24. Watanabe T, Nobusawa S, Kleihues P, et al. IDH1 mutations are early events in the development of astrocytomas and oligodendrogliomas. *Am J Pathol.* 2009; 174: 1149–1153.

25. Leibel SA, Scott CB, Loeffler JS. Contemporary approaches to the treatment of malignant gliomas with radiation therapy. *Semin Oncol.* 1994; 21: 198–219.

26. Cairncross G, Berkey B, Shaw E, et al. Phase III trial of chemotherapy plus radiotherapy compared with radiotherapy alone for pure and mixed anaplastic oligodendroglioma: Intergroup Radiation Therapy Oncology Group Trial 9402. *J Clin Oncol.* 2006; 24: 2707–2714.

27. van den Bent M, Carpentier A, Brandes A, et al. Adjuvant procarbazine, lomustine, and vincristine improves progression-free survival but not overall survival in newly diagnosed anaplastic oligodendrogliomas and oligoastrocytomas: a randomized European Organisation for Research and Treatment of Cancer phase III trial. *J Clin Oncol.* 2006; 24: 2715–2722.

28. van den Bent MJ, Dubbink HJ, Marie Y, et al. IDH1 and IDH2 mutations are prognostic but not predictive for outcome in anaplastic oligodendroglial tumors: a report of the European Organization for Research and Treatment of Cancer Brain Tumor Group. *Clin Cancer Res.* 2010; 16: 1597–1604.

29. Wick W, Hartmann C, Engel C, et al. NOA-04 randomized phase III trial of sequential radiochemotherapy of anaplastic glioma with procarbazine, lomustine, and vincristine or temozolomide. *J Clin Oncol.* 2009; 27: 5874–5880.

30. Stupp R, Mason W, van den Bent M, et al. Radiotherapy plus concomitant and adjuvant temozolomide for glioblastoma. *N Engl J Med.* 2005; 352: 987–996.

31. Westphal M, Hilt D, Bortey E, et al. A phase 3 trial of local chemotherapy with biodegradable carmustine (BCNU) wafers (Gliadel wafers) in patients with primary malignant glioma. *Neuro-oncol.* 2003; 5: 79–88.

32. Keime-Guibert F, Chinot O, Taillandier L, et al. Radiotherapy for glioblastoma in the elderly. *N Engl J Med.* 2007; 356: 1527–1535.

33. Friedman HS, Prados MD, Wen PY, et al. Bevacizumab alone and in combination with irinotecan in recurrent glioblastoma. *J Clin Oncol.* 2009; 27: 4733–4740.

34. Kreisl T, Kim L, Moore K, et al. Phase II trial of single-agent bevacizumab followed by bevacizumab plus irinotecan at tumor progression in recurrent glioblastoma. *J Clin Oncol.* 2009; 27: 740–745.

35. Mellinghoff I, Wang M, Vivanco I, et al. Molecular determinants of the response of glioblastomas to EGFR kinase inhibitors. *N Engl J Med.* 2005; 353: 2012–2024.

36. Haas-Kogan D, Prados M, Tihan T, et al. Epidermal growth factor receptor, protein kinase B/Akt, and glioma response to erlotinib. *J Natl Cancer Inst.* 2005; 97: 880–887.

37. Eichler A, Batchelor T. Primary central nervous system lymphoma: presentation, diagnosis and staging. *Neurosurg Focus.* 2006; 21: E15.

38. Abrey LE, Batchelor TT, Ferreri AJ, et al. Report of an international workshop to standardize baseline evaluation and response criteria for primary CNS lymphoma. *J Clin Oncol.* 2005; 23: 5034–5043.

39. Batchelor T, Carson K, O'Neill A, et al. Treatment of primary CNS lymphoma with methotrexate and deferred radiotherapy: a report of NABTT 96-07. *J Clin Oncol.* 2003; 21: 1044–1049.

40. Ferreri AJ, Reni M, Foppoli M, et al. High-dose cytarabine plus high-dose methotrexate versus high-dose methotrexate alone in patients with primary CNS lymphoma: a randomised phase 2 trial. *Lancet.* 2009; 374: 1512–1520.

41. Shah G, Yahalom J, Correa D, et al. Combined immunochemotherapy with reduced whole-brain radiotherapy for newly diagnosed primary CNS lymphoma. *J Clin Oncol.* 2007; 25: 4730–4735.

42. Rubenstein J, Johnson J, Jung S, et al. Intensive chemotherapy and immunotherapy, without brain irradiation, in newly diagnosed patients with primary CNS lymphoma: results of CALGB 50202. Paper presented at: 52nd ASH Annual Meeting 2010; Orlando, FL.

43. Illerhaus G, Muller F, Feuerhake F, et al. High-dose chemotherapy and autologous stem-cell transplantation without consolidating radiotherapy as first-line treatment for primary lymphoma of the central nervous system. *Haematologica.* 2008; 93: 147–148.

44. Soussain C, Hoang-Xuan K, Taillandier L, et al. Intensive chemotherapy followed by hematopoietic stem-cell rescue for refractory and recurrent primary CNS and intraocular lymphoma: Societe Francaise de Greffe de Moelle Osseuse-Therapie Cellulaire. *J Clin Oncol.* 2008; 26: 2512–2518.

45. Aghi MK, Carter BS, Cosgrove GR, et al. Long-term recurrence rates of atypical meningiomas after gross total resection with or without postoperative adjuvant radiation. *Neurosurgery.* 2009; 64: 56–60; discussion 60.

CHAPTER **63**

Metastatic Brain Tumors

April F. Eichler

INTRODUCTION

Brain metastasis is a common complication of cancer. Recent population-based data suggest that up to 20% of adults with cancer will develop symptomatic brain metastases during life (1). Autopsy studies indicate that another 25%–30% of patients with disseminated cancer have asymptomatic brain metastases at the time of death. The incidence of brain metastasis varies by primary cancer type, being highest for lung (20%) followed by melanoma (7%), renal (6.5%), breast (5%), and colorectal (1.8%). Prostate, gynecologic, head and neck, and non-melanomatous skin cancers involve the brain parenchyma infrequently. The prevalence of brain metastases has increased in the past three decades. Contributing factors may include more sensitive imaging techniques (gadolinium enhanced MRI), lengthened survival due to more effective systemic therapies, and poor central nervous system (CNS) penetration of many chemotherapeutic and antibody-based agents.

CLINICAL MANIFESTATIONS

Common signs and symptoms of metastatic brain tumors can be classified as either focal or generalized (Table 63-1) (2). Focal symptoms, such as hemiparesis, aphasia, and visual field defects, vary according to location of the tumor. Generalized symptoms, such as headache, confusion, lethargy, nausea, and vomiting, result from increased ICP or hydrocephalus. Metastatic deposits near the ventricular system can cause obstructive hydrocephalus by interruption of normal cerebrospinal fluid (CSF) outflow pathways through the third and fourth ventricles. Obstructive hydrocephalus is of particular concern with posterior fossa tumors. Headaches caused by increased ICP and/or hydrocephalus may have the following characteristics:

- Worse in the morning and with recumbency
- Associated with nausea and vomiting
- Exacerbated by coughing or straining
- Accompanied by confusion or lethargy

The presence of papilledema is very suggestive of increased ICP, although its absence does not exclude it.

EVALUATION

Contrast-enhanced MRI has replaced CT as the study of choice for patients with suspected brain metastasis (Figure 63-1). MRI is more sensitive than

TABLE 63-1 SYMPTOMS AND SIGNS OF BRAIN METASTASIS

Symptoms	%	Signs	%
Headache	49	Mental status change	58
Focal weakness	30	Hemiparesis	59
Mental disturbance	32	Sensory loss	21
Gait ataxia	21	Papilledema	20
Speech difficulty	12	Gait ataxia	19
Visual disturbance	6	Aphasia	18
Sensory disturbance	6	Visual field cut	7
Limb ataxia	6	Limb ataxia	6
		Depressed consciousness	4

Data from Cairncross JG, Kim J-H, Posner JB. Radiation therapy for brain metastases. *Ann Neurol.* 1980; 7: 529–541, and Young DF, Posner JB, Chu F, et al. Rapid-course radiation therapy of cerebral metastases: results and complications. *Cancer.* 1974; 4: 1069–1076.

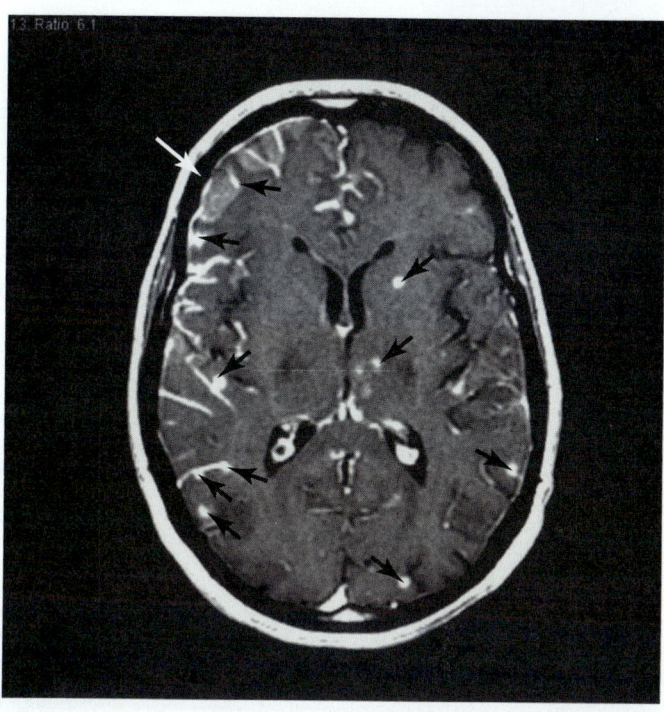

FIGURE 63-1 Gadolinium-enhanced T1-weighted MRI showing multiple small parenchymal metastases (*arrowheads*) and leptomeningeal enhancement (*arrow*) in a patient with non-small cell lung cancer. Spinal fluid was positive for malignant cells.

CT for small lesions, particularly in the brain stem and posterior fossa (**Figure 63-2**). In addition, MRI is better able to distinguish metastatic lesions from alternative diagnoses such as abscess or stroke. All cancer patients with new neurological symptoms should be screened for brain metastases. In patients who cannot undergo MRI because of implanted hardware, morbid obesity, or extreme claustrophobia, a contrast-enhanced CT should be obtained instead. If leptomeningeal enhancement is present, lumbar puncture should be strongly considered to rule out leptomeningeal metastases. Lumbar puncture should not be performed in patients with increased intracranial pressure from obstructive hydrocephalus, lateral shift of midline structures, or any evidence of mass effect in the posterior fossa.

DIFFERENTIAL DIAGNOSIS

The differential diagnosis of a mass lesion in a patient with cancer is broad and includes:

- Primary brain tumor
- Abscess (bacterial, mycobacterial, fungal, parasitic)
- Acute demyelinating plaque

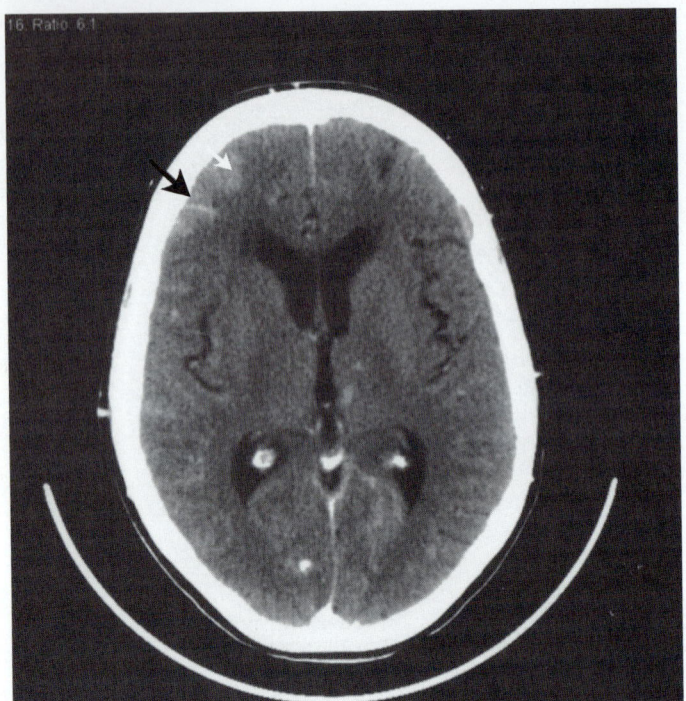

FIGURE 63-2 Contrast-enhanced CT in the same patient showing a single paren-chymal lesion (*arrowhead*) and faint leptomeningeal enhancement (*arrow*). This image demonstrates the decreased sensitivity of CT compared with MRI for detecting small metastases.

- Subacute cerebral infarction
- Primary intracranial hemorrhage

In a study of 54 patients with cancer who underwent biopsy of a single mass lesion, a diagnosis other than metastatic cancer was obtained in 11% (equally divided between primary brain tumor and infection) (3). This study highlights the importance of obtaining pathologic confirmation before proceeding with definitive therapy if the diagnosis is at all uncertain.

MANAGEMENT

SYMPTOMATIC THERAPY

Glucocorticoids

Glucocorticoids should be administered to patients with focal deficits, headache, or other symptoms resulting from peritumoral edema or increased ICP. Glucocorticoids act to restore the integrity of the blood-brain barrier and thereby reduce cerebral edema. Dexamethasone is the most widely used glucocorticoid for this purpose because of its long half-life and minimal mineralocorticoid effects. It is typically given as an intravenous 10 mg loading dose followed by 16 mg/day divided in 2–4 doses (either intravenous or oral). Symptoms should improve within 2–3 days, and higher doses (up to 100 mg/day) may be required in some patients. Adverse effects of glucocorticoids are dose dependent, and therefore the dose should always be tapered to the lowest possible dose required to ameliorate symptoms. Patients taking daily glucocorticoids for longer than 2–4 weeks should receive prophylaxis for *Pneumocystis jiroveci,* typically with trimethoprim/sulfamethoxazole.

Anticonvulsants

Twenty percent to 40% of all brain tumor patients experience a seizure by the time their tumor is diagnosed. In these patients, the need for anticonvulsant therapy is clear. An additional 20%–40% of patients will develop seizures as a complication of their disease. Based on this risk, many physicians choose to start prophylactic anticonvulsants at the time of diagnosis. However, this practice must be weighed against the potential adverse effects of anticonvulsants, which include:

- Allergic reaction, including Stevens-Johnson syndrome
- Hepatic dysfunction
- Cognitive impairment and imbalance
- Myelosuppression
- Alteration of cytochrome P-450 enzyme system

The latter is an important consideration in patients receiving chemotherapeutic and targeted agents that are metabolized by the liver, such as taxanes, vinca alkaloids, and many tyrosine kinase inhibitors. The American Academy of Neurology has published a practice parameter finding no evidence to support the use of prophylactic anticonvulsant medication in patients with brain tumors who have not experienced a seizure (4).

■ DEFINITIVE THERAPY

Treatment of brain metastases is aimed at improving neurologic function, enhancing quality of life, and extending survival. Multiple treatment modalities are now available that may further lengthen survival, including surgery, various forms of radiation therapy, and chemotherapy. Treatment strategies often involve a combination of two or more modalities. The following three factors should be considered when designing a treatment regimen:

- Patient (age, functional status, comorbidities)
- Primary tumor (histology, degree of local control, presence of extracranial metastases)
- Metastatic brain disease (location, size, number)

Surgery

Single lesion. The goal of surgery is to relieve neurologic symptoms, establish a pathologic diagnosis, and achieve local control. Patients with a single metastatic brain deposit and stable extracranial disease show longer survival, improved functional status, and better local control when treated with surgery plus whole brain radiation therapy (WBRT) as compared with

WBRT alone (3, 5). Younger patients (age <60 years) and those with stable extracranial disease show the most benefit from surgery. The majority of patients show symptomatic improvement after resection, often apparent in the immediate postoperative period.

Multiple lesions. When evaluated by contrast enhanced MRI, the majority (70%) of patients with metastatic brain disease have multiple lesions. The role of surgery in these patients is less clear but should be strongly considered in the following circumstances:

- Dominant lesion causing significant symptoms or impending herniation
- Two lesions accessible by a single craniotomy
- Need for pathologic diagnosis
- Young age, good functional status, and stable extracranial disease

Radiotherapy

Radiation therapy has been the cornerstone of treatment for brain metastases since the 1950s. Although surgery is a viable option for selected patients, many patients are not candidates for this intervention or do not wish to undergo an operation. Radiation therapy can be administered safely to most patients with the goal of palliation of neurological symptoms.

Whole brain radiation therapy. Whole brain fractionated external beam radiotherapy is delivered to the entire brain down to the bottom of the C2 vertebral body. A variety of schedules are employed; a widely used dosing regimen consists of 30 Gy delivered in 10 fractions over 2 weeks. WBRT is widely available and results in symptom palliation in many patients when used in combination with glucocorticoids. Short-term side effects of WBRT include fatigue, nausea, anorexia, skin irritation, and hair loss. In long-term survivors, delayed toxicity may result in memory loss, dementia, gait ataxia, incontinence, and/or neuroendocrine dysfunction (e.g., hypothyroidism). The incidence of late neurotoxicity may be reduced by avoiding daily fractions >3 Gy. When administered postoperatively in conjunction with surgical resection of a single lesion, WBRT decreases the likelihood of both local recurrence (10% with postoperative WBRT vs. 46% with surgery alone) and distant recurrence (14% vs. 37%) (6).

Stereotactic radiosurgery. Stereotactic radiosurgery (SRS) is a form of external beam radiation that uses multiple convergent beams to deliver a single high dose of radiation to a discrete target volume. The technique is generally used for lesions up to 3 cm in diameter. Several approaches exist, each of which employs a different source of radiation.

- LINAC, using high-energy x-ray radiation from a linear accelerator (LINAC)
- Gamma knife, using gamma radiation from a fixed array of cobalt-60 sources
- Cyclotron, using protons generated from a large accelerator

For most techniques, precise localization is accomplished using a stereotactic head frame that is anchored to the patient's skull by bone screws (placed under local anesthesia). The treatment itself lasts only minutes, and the frame is removed immediately afterward. Tumors can be safely and effectively treated using a single dose of radiation ranging from 15 to 24 Gy according to lesion size. It is important to note that SRS produces excellent local control for metastases but does not treat "micrometastases" that are not evident on imaging. The addition of SRS to WBRT has been shown to increase survival in patients with single brain metastasis and achieve effective palliation in patients with 1–3 brain metastases (7). Complications of stereotactic radiation include seizures, headache, exacerbation of neurologic deficits, nausea, hemorrhage, and radiation necrosis.

Over the past 5–10 years, SRS alone with deferred WBRT has become a more common therapeutic approach for patients with a limited number of brain metastases. This shift has been driven by the high local control rates achieved by SRS alone as well as concerns about the neurocognitive consequences of WBRT. The evidence base for this practice comes from three recent randomized studies examining various combinations of SRS, surgery, and/or WBRT. In the first, Aoyama et al. randomized 132 patients with 1–4 brain metastases and KPS ≥70 to treatment with SRS alone or SRS plus WBRT (8). Patients receiving SRS plus WBRT had a significant improvement in local and distant control rates in brain as well as need for salvage therapy, compared with patients who received SRS alone. However, overall survival was similar in the two groups. Folstein mini-mental status exam scores before and after treatment indicated no clear detriment in the patients receiving WBRT. Similar findings were reported by the European Organization for Research and Treatment of Cancer (EORTC), in a study in which patients with up to three brain metastases were treated with either surgery or SRS at the discretion of treating physicians, and then randomized to receive either WBRT or observation (9). This study again found no difference in overall survival or duration of functional independence between the two arms but, similar to the Aoyama study, showed an increase in progression free survival and in rates of intracranial control in the combination arm. A third randomized study was stopped early when interim analysis of the primary endpoint of neurocognitive outcome, as assessed by the Hopkins Verbal Learning Test-Revised (HTLV-R) at 4 months, showed that more patients in the combined treatment arm (SRS plus WBRT) experienced a 5-point drop in HTLV-R scores compared with patients receiving SRS alone (52% vs. 24%) (10). The neurocognitive deficits were accompanied by worse survival in the combined treatment arm but improved local and distant control rates in brain.

Taken together, these studies indicate that withholding WBRT at diagnosis and treating with SRS alone in patients with a limited number of brain metastases does not sacrifice overall survival and may be associated with improved neurocognitive outcomes, at least in the first few months after treatment. However, SRS alone is associated with worsened brain control rates and increased need for salvage therapy compared with a combined SRS plus WBRT approach. This emphasizes the need for close serial monitoring and imaging of patients in whom WBRT has been deferred in order to recognize relapse early and thereby minimize neurological decline that is associated with intracranial progression.

Radiosurgery vs. surgery. For single brain metastases, both surgery and radiosurgery are effective options, and thus debate remains regarding which modality should be considered first-line therapy. Randomized trials comparing surgery and radiosurgery have not yet been performed to address this question. For large metastatic tumors with extensive edema and mass effect, surgery is probably superior to radiation for quick and reliable relief of symptoms, provided the lesion can be safely resected. Because even minor swelling in the posterior fossa after radiosurgery can cause hydrocephalus, surgery is often recommended for cerebellar metastases. Radiosurgery has the advantage of being noninvasive and therefore associated with less morbidity and mortality than surgery. Moreover, radiosurgery can be used to treat metastases in surgically inaccessible areas of the brain, such as the brain stem or basal ganglia. Multiple, minimally symptomatic metastases are more simply treated with radiation (WBRT with or without radiosurgery) than surgery.

Chemotherapy

The role of chemotherapy in the treatment of metastatic brain tumors has historically been confined to patients who have failed surgery, WBRT, and radiosurgery. Temozolomide, an oral alkylating agent that is widely used in the treatment of malignant primary brain tumors, has excellent bioavailability and relatively high central nervous system penetration (20% of plasma levels). Multiple studies have examined the effects of concurrent temozolomide and WBRT in patients with newly diagnosed brain metastases, but despite early optimism, large-scale randomized controlled trials have not yet shown a definitive benefit in any cancer subtype. Other agents have shown activity in small trials, but a complete discussion is beyond the scope of this review.

Breast cancer. It is now widely recognized that patients with HER2-positive breast cancer treated with trastuzumab (Herceptin) are at increased risk for isolated CNS progression. This may reflect improved peripheral disease control and patient survival with trastuzumab-based therapy; poor CNS penetration of trastuzumab and relative lack of CNS activity; and/or a predilection for the CNS by HER2-positive cancers. The small molecule HER1/HER2 tyrosine kinase inhibitor, lapatinib, is the most widely studied agent to date for patients with brain metastases from HER2-positive breast cancer. In a multicenter phase II trial of 242 patients with new or progressive intracranial metastatic HER2-positive breast cancer treated with lapatinib monotherapy, objective response rates were seen in 6% of patients and tumor reduction in 21% of patients (11). Combined with capecitabine, lapatinib is associated with higher response rates in this same population, and this combination is an option for patients with HER2-positive disease who have progressive brain metastases after radiation therapy.

Non–small cell lung cancer. Platinum agents such as cisplatin and carboplatin, alone or in combination with other chemotherapeutic agents, have been associated with response rates of 20%–40% in chemotherapy-naive patients, but durability of response is often poor. In patients whose tumors carry activating mutations in the *EGFR* gene, the tyrosine kinase inhibitors erlotinib and gefitinib have shown more promise, perhaps because they have better CNS penetration than traditional chemotherapeutics. The likelihood of response is particularly high in patients with synchronous brain and systemic presentations of *EGFR*-mutated NSCLC, and in patients with small asymptomatic brain metastases, it may be reasonable to start with an EGFR inhibitor and defer brain radiation therapy, so long as close follow-up is provided. Other targeted agents, including angiogenesis inhibitors such as bevacizumab (a monoclonal antibody against vascular endothelial growth factor, VEGF) and receptor tyrosine kinase inhibitors such as sorafenib and sunitinib are currently being evaluated for safety and efficacy in patients with brain metastases.

Melanoma.   Metastatic melanoma is poorly responsive to systemic chemotherapy both intracranially and extracranially. Historically, few trials have evaluated the role of chemotherapy in melanoma patients with brain metastases, with most focusing on fotemustine (in Europe) and TMZ. More recently, antibodies that enhance antitumor immune responses by blocking the interaction of cytotoxic T-lymphocyte-associated antigen (CTLA-4) with its ligands B7.1 and B7.2 have shown clinical benefit in patients with metastatic melanoma. The CTLA-4 monoclonal antibody, ipilumimab, has been associated with objective responses in brain and durable disease control in patients with brain metastases from melanoma. Larger studies are needed to better understand what role ipilumimab should play in relation to radiation therapy for patients with CNS melanoma. Similarly in patients with BRAF-mutant melanoma, ongoing studies will be examining the responsiveness of brain metastases to targeted therapies and the role combined modality therapy.

PROGNOSIS

Historically, patients with untreated brain metastases have a median survival of 1 month. Glucocorticoids improve median survival to 2 months. The addition of WBRT extends median survival to 4–6 months (12). Patients with single brain lesions and limited extracranial disease who are treated with surgery or SRS plus WBRT have a median survival of 10–15 months. Favorable prognostic factors include:

- Absence of systemic disease
- Young age (less than 60 years)
- Good performance status (Karnofsky performance status [KPS] of 70 or greater)
- Long interval from systemic cancer diagnosis to development of brain metastasis
- Surgical resection
- Fewer than three brain lesions
- Certain primary cancer subtypes (HER2-positive breast cancer, EGFR-mutant non-small cell lung cancer)

Patients with brain metastases from breast cancer tend to live longer than patients with other types of cancer that have spread to the brain.

REFERENCES

1. Barnholtz-Sloan JS, Sloan AE, Davis FG, et al. Incidence proportions of brain metastases in patients diagnosed (1973 to 2001) in the metropolitan detroit cancer surveillance system. *J Clin Oncol.* 2004; 22: 2865–2872.

2. Posner JB. *Neurologic Complications of Cancer.* Philadelphia: FA Davis Company; 1995.

3. Patchell RA, Tibbs PA, Walsh JW, et al. A randomized trial of surgery in the treatment of single metastases to the brain. *N Engl J Med.* 1990; 322: 494–500.

4. Glantz MJ, Cole BF, Forsyth PA, et al. Practice parameter: anticonvulsant prophylaxis in patients with newly diagnosed brain tumors. Report of the quality standards subcommittee of the american academy of neurology. *Neurology.* 2000; 54: 1886–1893.

5. Vecht CJ, Haaxma-Reiche H, Noordijk EM, et al. Treatment of single brain metastasis: radiotherapy alone or combined with neurosurgery? *Ann Neurol.* 1993; 33: 583–590.

6. Patchell RA, Tibbs PA, Regine WF, et al. Postoperative radiotherapy in the treatment of single metastases to the brain: a randomized trial. *JAMA.* 1998; 280: 1485–1489.

7. Andrews DW, Scott CB, Sperduto PW, et al. Whole brain radiation therapy with or without stereotactic radiosurgery boost for patients with one to three brain metastases: phase III results of the RTOG 9508 randomised trial. *Lancet.* 2004; 363: 1665–1672.

8. Aoyama H, Shirato H, Tago M, et al. Stereotactic radiosurgery plus whole-brain radiation therapy vs stereotactic radiosurgery alone for treatment of brain metastases: a randomized controlled trial. *JAMA.* 2006; 295: 2483–2491.

9. Kocher M, Soffietti R, Abacioglu U, et al. Adjuvant whole-brain radiotherapy versus observation after radiosurgery or surgical resection of one to three cerebral metastases: results of the EORTC 22952-26001 study. *J Clin Oncol.* 2011; 29: 134–141.

10. Chang EL, Wefel JS, Hess KR, et al. Neurocognition in patients with brain metastases treated with radiosurgery or radiosurgery plus whole-brain irradiation: a randomised controlled trial. *Lancet Oncol.* 2009; 10: 1037–1044.

11. Lin NU, Dieras V, Paul D, et al. Multicenter phase II study of lapatinib in patients with brain metastases from HER2-positive breast cancer. *Clin Cancer Res.* 2009; 15: 1452–1459.

12. Gaspar L, Scott C, Rotman M, et al. Recursive partitioning analysis (RPA) of prognostic factors in three radiation therapy oncology group (RTOG) brain metastases trials. *Int J Radiat Oncol Biol Phys.* 1997; 37: 745–751.

CHAPTER **64**
Paraneoplastic Neurologic Syndromes
Jorg Dietrich

INTRODUCTION

Paraneoplastic neurologic syndromes are heterogenous disorders that can occur in the setting of various types of cancer (1). Paraneoplastic neurologic disorders are commonly caused by immune-mediated mechanisms triggered by an underlying tumor and have to be distinguished from neurological symptoms related to direct tumor invasion, infection, vasculopathy, ischemia, metabolic disturbances, or treatment-related toxicities.

Abnormal antibody or T-cell-mediated responses can target any part of the central, peripheral or autonomic nervous system to cause a diverse range of neurological symptoms. In general, the incidence of paraneoplastic syndromes is less than 1% in the general cancer population, but may be more frequently seen in specific types of cancer, such as small cell lung cancer (SCLC), cancers of the ovary and breast, and thymoma.

The diagnosis of a paraneoplastic neurologic syndrome is primarily clinical. Classical paraneoplastic syndromes (Table 64-1) may develop before the diagnosis of cancer, in a patient with known cancer, or in a patient considered to be in cancer remission. While an extensive search for an underlying tumor is warranted in classical paraneoplastic syndromes, such as paraneoplastic cerebellar degeneration (PCD) or Lambert-Eaton myasthenic syndrome, it may be noteworthy that several neurologic syndromes designated as "paraneoplastic" may also be seen in non-neoplastic autoimmune diseases.

Since paraneoplastic syndromes often herald the diagnosis of cancer, patients may be diagnosed and treated early in the course of the disease. Earlier cancer diagnosis may correlate with a higher likelihood of cure and remission of neurologic symptoms. It remains controversial, however, whether a better prognosis in patients with paraneoplastic syndromes is related to the immune control of the underlying cancer.

PATHOGENESIS

While the detailed pathomechanism of most paraneoplastic syndromes remains elusive, production of antibodies directed against antigens expressed by both tumors and nervous system tissues have been described as a key mechanism in some distinct types of paraneoplastic syndromes (Table 64-2). Antibodies can be directed against cytoplasmic antigens (e.g., Purkinje cells and anterior horn cells) or cell surface proteins (e.g., voltage gated potassium and calcium channels). Immune mechanisms may involve both humoral and T-cell-mediated responses, although the exact contribution of cellular and antibody-mediated mechanisms to the

TABLE 64-1 CLASSICAL PARANEOPLASTIC SYNDROMES OF THE NERVOUS SYSTEM

Syndrome	Symptoms	Common Antibodies
Paraneoplastic cerebellar degeneration	Rapid onset (days to weeks) of truncal and appendicular ataxia, imbalance, dizziness, nausea, diplopia, dysphagia, nystagmus	Anti-Yo, anti-Hu, anti-VGCC, anti-CV2/CRMP5, anti-Ma2, anti-Ri, anti-Tr, anti-GAD, anti-mGluR1
Paraneoplastic encephalomyelitis/limbic encephalitis	Subacute onset of mental status changes, memory deficits, behavioral changes, emotional lability, insomnia, seizures	Anti-Hu, anti-Ma2, anti-CV2/CRMP5, anti-VGKC, anti-Ri, anti-amphiphysin, anti-GABA$_B$R, anti-AMPAR, anti-GAD
Paraneoplastic opsoclonus-myoclonus	Large amplitude ocular saccades (opsoclonus) and other abnormal eye movements alone or in combination with myoclonus; can be associated with hypotonia, irritability, ataxia and encephalopathy	Anti-Hu, anti-Ri, anti-Ma2, anti-amphiphysin
Cancer associated retinopathy	Photosensitivity and visual loss; may start in one eye and frequently progresses to involve both eyes; bilateral blindness may develop over the course of several months	Anti-recoverin
Melanoma associated retinopathy	Rapid onset of visual disturbances with flickering, night blindness and peripheral field visual loss; usually does not progress to full blindness	Anti-bipolar cells of the retina
Stiff person syndrome	Axial stiffness, spine deformities, painful muscle spasms triggered by sudden movements and noise or emotional upset	Anti-amphiphysin, anti-GAD
Dorsal root ganglionitis (subacute sensory neuronopathy)	Abnormal sensations affecting pain, temperature, touch and proprioception	Anti-Hu, anti-CV2/CRMP5, anti-amphiphysin
Sensorimotor polyneuropathy	Motor and sensory deficits, occasionally associated with tremors and gait disorder; may be acute or chronic	Anti-MAG, anti-Hu, anti-CV2/CRMP5, anti-amphiphysin

(*continued*)

TABLE 64-1 CLASSICAL PARANEOPLASTIC SYNDROMES OF THE NERVOUS SYSTEM (CONTINUED)

Syndrome	Symptoms	Common Antibodies
Autonomic neuropathy	Orthostatic hypotension, arrhythmias, impotence, intestinal pseudo-obstruction	Anti-Hu, anti-gAChR
Neuromyotonia	Fasciculations, delayed muscle relaxation, weakness	Anti-VGKC
Lambert Eaton myasthenic syndrome	Proximal muscle weakness, typically improving with repetitive action	Anti-VGCC

disease manifestation remains controversial (2–4). Abnormal antibodies can frequently be detected in serum and cerebrospinal fluid (CSF); however, a direct pathogenic effect of certain antibodies on nervous system tissue or the neuromuscular junction has only been demonstrated in a subset of paraneoplastic disorders. Importantly, some antibodies can also be detected in the absence of a clinical paraneoplastic syndrome (5) (Table 64-3).

TABLE 64-2 WELL-CHARACTERIZED PARANEOPLASTIC ANTIBODIES DIRECTED TO NON-SURFACE ANTIGENS, ASSOCIATION WITH NEUROLOGIC SYNDROMES AND UNDERLYING TUMORS

Antibody	Predominant Syndromes	Commonly Underlying Cancer
Anti-Yo (PCA1 = cdr2)	PCD, POM	Ovarian, breast
Anti-Hu (ANNA-1)	PEM, POM, PCD, autonomic neuropathy, sensory neuronopathy	SCLC, neuroblastoma, seminoma, prostate cancer, others
Anti-Ri (ANNA-2)	PCD, PEM, POM	Breast, Ovarian, SCLC
Anti-amphiphysin	SPS, PEM, sensorimotor neuropathy	Breast, Ovarian, SCLC
Anti-Ma2 (Ta)	PEM, PCD, POM	Testicular, SCLC, others
Anti-Tr	PCD	Hodgkin lymphoma
Anti-CV2/CRMP5	PCD, PEM, chorea, optic neuritis, uveitis, peripheral neuropathy	SCLC, thymoma, others
Anti-recoverin	Cancer associated retinopathy	SCLC

TABLE 64-3 PARTIALLY CHARACTERIZED ANTIBODIES THAT CAN OCCUR WITH AND WITHOUT CANCER ASSOCIATION

Antibody	Predominant Syndromes	Associated Cancer
ANNA-3	Encephalomyelitis, sensory neuropathy	SCLC
Anti-gAChR	Autonomic dysfunction	SCLC
Anti-CASPR2 (anti-VGKC)	Morvan's syndrome, neuromyotonia	Thymoma, others
Anti-AMPAR	Encephalomyelitis	Lung cancer, breast cancer, others
Anti-bipolar cells of the retina	Melanoma-associated retinopathy	Melanoma
Anti-GABA$_B$R	Encephalomyelitis	SCLC
Anti-GAD	Stiff person syndrome, cerebellar syndromes	Thymoma
Anti-mGluR1	Cerebellar degeneration	Hodgkin lymphoma
Anti-LGI1 (anti-VGKC)	Encephalomyelitis	SCLC, thymoma
Anti-NMDAR	Encephalomyelitis, autonomic dysfunction	Teratoma
Anti-VGCC	LEMS, cerebellar degeneration	SCLC, lymphoma
Anti-Zic 4	Cerebellar degeneration	SCLC
GlyR	Encephalomyelitis	Various cancers
PCA-2	Cerebellar degeneration and encephalomyelitis	SCLC

DIAGNOSTIC AND THERAPEUTIC CONSIDERATIONS

The diagnosis of a paraneoplastic neurologic syndrome can be challenging and, in classical syndromes, is usually based on clinical features of the neurologic condition, such as in cerebellar degeneration and Lambert-Easton myasthenic syndrome (1, 6, 7). Neurological symptoms commonly develop in the early stages of cancer and in two-thirds of patients before a cancer diagnosis has been established (1). Therefore, early recognition and treatment of a paraneoplastic neurologic disorder along with treatment of the underlying cancer are critical to reduce neurologic morbidity and to improve overall patient survival. Paraneoplastic neurologic syndromes usually have an acute or subacute onset, but the diagnosis may remain challenging if no typical antibodies are found in serum or CSF (7). As most syndromes and malignancies are associated with more than one specific antibody, screening for a panel of paraneoplastic antibodies may increase the yield to establish a diagnosis (7, 8). In patients with CNS manifestation, antibody screening in CSF is usually recommended, as antibody titers in CSF are generally higher than in serum (9). CSF analysis typically reveals an inflammatory pattern with mild pleocytosis, elevated protein, and evidence of oligoclonal bands. Positron emission tomography (PET) in combination with computed tomography (CT) is helpful in the search for an underlying malignancy (10, 11). Mammography and pelvic ultrasound may be indicated in women with suspected paraneoplastic neurologic syndromes, given the frequent association with breast and gynecologic cancers. Neuroimaging of the brain with magnetic resonance imaging (MRI) may be unremarkable but is abnormal in the majority of patients with encephalomyelitis and limbic encephalitis (1). In cases in which no underlying tumor can be identified but a high clinical suspicion for a classic paraneopolastic syndrome exists, or in patients tested positive for paraneoplastic antibodies in the setting of a less classic form of a paraneoplastic neurologic syndrome, repeat cancer screening studies are recommended every 6 months (7). An underlying malignancy usually can be identified within the first 4 years from onset of neurological symptoms (7).

The most important management goals in patients with paraneoplastic neurologic syndromes are identification and treatment of an underlying cancer. In general, antibody-mediated neurologic disorders affecting the peripheral nervous system will have a higher likelihood of response to treatment and symptom improvement. In these patients, immunomodulatory strategies with intravenous immunoglobulins, plasmapheresis, or immunosuppressants are commonly effective. While most paraneoplastic syndromes affecting the central nervous system generally respond poorly to immunomodulatory therapies, patients with opsoclonus-myoclonus syndrome (12) or limbic encephalitis and presence of anti-NMDAR, anti-AMPAR, or anti-Ma antibodies (13, 14) may show a remarkable benefit from treatment. In patients not actively treated with chemotherapy for an underlying cancer and with progressive neurological decline, more aggressive immunosuppression may be considered, including the use of cyclophosphamide, tacrolimus, azathioprine, and cyclosporine.

SYNDROMES OF THE CENTRAL NERVOUS SYSTEM

■ PARANEOPLASTIC CEREBELLAR DEGENERATION

Paraneoplastic cerebellar degeneration (PCD) is a classical paraneoplastic neurologic syndrome. Symptoms commonly precede tumor diagnosis by months or occasionally years and are characterized by rapidly progressive cerebellar dysfunction. The development of gait dysfunction, appendicular ataxia, and speech dysfunction may develop and progress over the course of days to weeks, unlike in primary degenerative cerebellar disorders, where symptoms develop over months to years. Brain stem and cerebellar dysfunction, including oculomotor symptoms with diplopia, oscillopsia, nystagmus, nausea, and dysphagia are usually irreversible (15, 16). Emotional lability and cognitive deficits may occur, underlining the importance of the cerebellum in mood and cognitive function (17). In addition, patients may develop pyramidal tract signs, posterior column signs, and polyneuropathy, suggesting a more widespread involvement of the nervous system in the pathology of the disease process. The majority of patients develop severe gait difficulties, inability to write and to swallow (18).

PCD is frequently associated with anti-Yo antibodies (Purkinje-cell antibody-1; PCA-1; also termed cerebellar degeneration related-2; cdr2), directed against Purkinje cells of the cerebellum, and usually occurs in patients with breast or ovarian cancer (16, 19). Because presence of anti-Yo antibodies is so frequently associated with underlying breast or ovarian cancer, careful and repeated cancer screening is mandated. Notably, more than two-thirds of patients with anti-Yo-associated cerebellar degeneration do not have a cancer diagnosis at the onset of neurologic symptoms. PCD has also been described in the presence of anti-Hu antibodies and anti-CV2/CRMP5 antibodies and SCLC (20), anti-Tr antibodies and Hodgkin lymphoma (21, 22), or anti-Ri antibodies and breast cancer (23). Interestingly, PCD has also been reported in patients with non-Hodgkin lymphoma and lung cancer without detectable anti-neuronal antibodies (24), and in SCLC patients with evidence of P/Q calcium channel antibodies (25).

As seen in other paraneoplastic neurologic syndromes, CSF analysis may reveal lymphocytic pleocytosis, elevated protein, and oligoclonal bands. At later disease stages neuroimaging with CT or MRI may identify loss of cerebellar architecture and eventually global cerebellar atrophy.

Treatment with plasmapheresis or intravenous immunoglobulins do usually not alter the progressive course of the disease (26), although clinical improvement has been seen in some cases (18, 27), with treatment of the underlying tumor (28, 29), or in some cases of PCD and underlying anti-Tr and anti-Ri antibodies (22, 30).

■ PARANEOPLASTIC ENCEPHALOMYELITIS

Paraneoplastic encephalomyelitis (PEM) may affect multiple sites and levels of the nervous system, including the temporal and frontal lobes, midbrain, pons, cerebellum, spinal cord, dorsal root ganglia, and autonomic nervous system. Patients may therefore present with multiple neurological dysfunctions depending on the site of nervous system involvement. Symptoms usually develop over weeks to months. Involvement of the limbic system is characterized by short-term memory deficits, mood changes, emotional lability, and seizures. Brain stem involvement is classically associated with oculomotor dysfunction, nystagmus, and other cranial nerve palsies, whereas movement disorders are seen with midbrain involvement. Symptoms of autonomic dysfunction, such as cardiac arrhythmias, hypotension, and impaired gastrointestinal motility, can be identified in about 25% of patients. PEM typically occurs in the setting of lung cancer, particularly SCLC with presence of anti-Hu (ANNA-1) antibodies (20). Although less common, other antibodies have been linked to PEM, including anti-Ri antibodies (ANNA-2) in breast and gynecologic cancers (31), anti-CV2/CRMP5 antibodies in SCLC and thymoma (32), anti-amphiphysin antibodies in SCLC (33), anti-Ma2 antibodies in germ cell tumors and other cancers (34–36), and anti-NMDAR antibodies in ovarian teratomas (37, 38).

Diagnosis of PEM is usually clinical and supported by the presence of paraneoplastic antibodies. Neuroimaging studies with MRI frequently reveal T2/Flair signal hyperintensities of affected nervous system sites with and without gadolinium enhancement. In general, PEM is poorly responsive to treatment, although disease stabilization or mild symptom improvement has been reported with combined tumor treatment and immunotherapies, including intravenous immunoglobulins, plasmapheresis, or cyclophosphamide (38, 39).

◾ PARANEOPLASTIC LIMBIC ENCEPHALITIS

Paraneoplastic limbic encephalitis (PLE) is clinically associated with short-term memory deficits, mood disturbances, emotional lability, sleep alterations, behavioral abnormalities, and seizures (40). Symptoms may stabilize or improve over time; however, anterograde amnesia and cognitive deficits frequently persist. PLE typically occurs in the setting of SCLC with presence of anti-Hu antibodies, but can also be seen in presence of other antibodies, such as anti-Ma2, anti-NMDAR, anti-CV2/CRMP5, anti-amphiphysin, and anti-Ri (35, 38, 40–42). Notably, the clinical and radiographic picture of limbic encephalitis can also be seen in non-neoplastic autoimmune disorders characterized by presence of anti-VGKC (43, 44) and anti-AMPAR antibodies (14).

The diagnosis of PLE commonly precedes tumor diagnosis. Although less frequently, tumors other than SCLC have been associated with PLE, such as Hodgkin lymphoma, ovarian cancer, teratomas, testicular cancer, breast cancer, and thymomas.

Pathological findings may reveal perivascular and interstitial lymphocytic infiltrates and microglia activation in limbic structures, including hippocampus, amygdala, cingulate gyrus, and hypothalamus. There may be some overlap with the clinical picture of PEM, and neuropathology may not be restricted to limbic structures.

CSF findings usually demonstrate mild pleocytosis, protein elevation, and oligoclonal bands. Neuroimaging with MRI may infrequently demonstrate unilateral or bilateral T2/Flair signal abnormalities in mesial temporal lobes with or without gadolinium enhancement. Some patients develop progressive temporal lobe atrophy as a delayed consequence of encephalitis. Hypermetabolism in various brain regions may be detectable on PET (45). EEG studies frequently show temporal lobe dysfunction with or without epileptiform activity.

Treatment includes immunotherapy with glucocorticoids, intravenous immunoglobulins, and plasmapheresis. Successful treatment has been described in patients with presence of antibodies directed against surface antigens (41).

◾ PARANEOPLASTIC OPSOCLONUS-MYOCLONUS

Opsoclonus refers to spontaneous, arrhythmic, large-amplitude, and multidirectional eye movements. Myoclonus describes involuntary muscle jerks in extremities and trunk, and usually occurs along with hypotonia, gait difficulties, and irritability. Paraneoplastic opsoclonus-myoclonus syndrome (POM) occurs in 2% of children with neuroblastoma, and nearly 50% of children with POM have underlying neuroblastoma. Since neurologic symptoms frequently precede tumor diagnosis, a search for an underlying malignancy is warranted in all children with POM (46). In adults, POM is associated with SCLC in the majority of cases, but can also be seen with other malignancies. The most commonly identified antibodies include anti-Hu, anti-Ri, anti-Yo, anti-Ma2, and anti-amphiphysin (12, 47).

In women with anti-Ri, opsoclonus also occurs as a separate clinical entity characterized by imbalance, ataxia, and movement disorders, suggesting a more widespread brain stem and midbrain involvement. Symptoms develop within weeks to months. Breast cancer and, to some degree, SCLC are by far the most common tumors in which anti-Ri syndromes develop. Adult patients with opsoclonus without evidence of anti-Ri antibodies usually develop myoclonus, and the underlying cause is commonly SCLC. Gait difficulties, ataxia, encephalopathy, lethargy, and coma may develop.

POM may respond to treatment of the underlying tumor or immunotherapies, including use of steroids, intravenous immunoglobulins, and plasmapheresis. Rituximab has been successfully used in some cases (48).

■ CANCER-ASSOCIATED RETINOPATHY

Cancer-associated retinopathy (CAR) is characterized by acute to subacute onset of photosensitivity and visual loss (49). Symptoms can present monocular, but commonly progress to involve both eyes (50). Exam findings include poor visual acuity, retinal artery narrowing, and scotomata. Blindness eventually develops over the course of months. CAR is associated with antibodies targeting recoverin, a calcium-binding protein on photoreceptors. Most commonly SCLC is the underlying tumor, and visual symptoms usually precede the diagnosis of cancer. Association with other tumors has been reported, including breast, gynecologic, pancreatic, prostate, bladder, colon, non-small cell lung cancer (NSCLC), and lymphoma (18). A distinct entity occurs in patients with metastatic melanoma (melanoma associated retinopathy), in which antibodies reacting with bipolar cells of the retina can be identified. Visual symptoms usually develop in the setting of known metastatic disease, sometimes months to years after initial tumor diagnosis (51).

■ STIFF PERSON SYNDROME

Stiff person syndrome (SPS), also known as stiff man syndrome, is characterized by fluctuating axial stiffness and muscle rigidity that can result in significant spine deformity. Extremities and facial muscles can be involved (52). Loud noise, sudden movement, and emotional upset often exacerbate painful muscle spasms. The remaining neurological exam is usually unremarkable. Notably, symptoms disappear in sleep or under deep anesthesia. Electrophysiologic studies with EMG show continuous motor unit activity in affected muscle groups at rest. Anti-amphiphysin antibodies can be identified in SPS, and both SCLC and breast cancer have been linked to this syndrome. However, SPS more frequently manifests as an autoimmune disorder in the absence of a tumor diagnosis (53). In these patients anti-GAD antibodies are more commonly identified. Treatment strategies include GABA-enhancing agents such as benzodiazepines, gabapentin, and baclofen that are beneficial in limiting painful muscle spasms. Symptoms may improve with treatment of the underlying tumor and with the use of intravenous immunoglobulins (54).

SYNDROMES OF THE PERIPHERAL NERVOUS SYSTEM

■ DORSAL ROOT GANGLIONITIS

Dorsal root ganglionitis, also referred to as subacute sensory neuronopathy, causes impairment of all sensory modalities, including pain, temperature, touch, and proprioception. Most common symptoms are numbness, paresthesias, and pain involving face, trunk, and extremities that develop over the course of days to weeks. Isolated cranial nerves can be affected. Neurological exam demonstrates loss of deep tendon reflexes and vibration sense. Patients may develop gait difficulties due to sensory impairment.

Dorsal root ganglionitis is nearly pathognomonic for paraneoplastic disease and can occur in combination with multifocal PEM (20). SCLC is the most frequent underlying cancer, but this syndrome may also be seen in lymphoma and NSCLC (55). No specific antibodies have been described with this condition; however, the same antibodies that are present in PEM (e.g., anti-Hu and anti-CV2/CRMP5) can be detected in dorsal root ganglionitis. Notably, the differential diagnosis includes symptoms related to Sjogren's syndrome, in which ganglion cell damage also occurs. Unfortunately, most patients with paraneoplastic dorsal root ganglionitis and underlying SCLC do not show meaningful neurologic improvement despite aggressive antitumor and immunotherapy.

■ SENSORY AND SENSORIMOTOR POLYNEUROPATHY

Subacute and chronic peripheral neuropathies may occur for a variety of reasons in cancer patients, such as a treatment complication of chemotherapy, and as a consequence of metabolic disorders. The clinical distinction from paraneoplastic polyneuropathies can be challenging but should be considered in patients without known underlying malignancy (56). A wide variety of neuropathies may result from diverse paraneoplastic antibodies (e.g., anti-MAG, anti-Hu, anti-CV2/CRMP5). The exact pathogenic mechanisms have not been identified in most syndromes, but antibody reaction with peripheral nerve fibers may play a role, resulting in inflammation and possibly secondary demyelination. As a consequence, symptoms are usually complex and may impact both motor and sensory function.

Exam findings may demonstrate gait disorders, plexopathies, and clinical pictures that resemble Guillain-Barre syndrome, chronic inflammatory demyelinating polyneuropathy (CIPD), and anterior horn cell disease. Hodgkin's disease is commonly identified as the underlying cancer. Chronic peripheral neuropathy has also been described in patients with SCLC, melanoma, lymphoma, and plasma cell disorders (55, 57).

The neuropathy seen in POEMS syndrome (P = polyneuropathy, O = organomegaly, E = endocrinopathy, M = elevated IgM protein, and S = skin changes) usually occurs in the setting of myeloma (58). Unlike other paraneoplastic syndromes, the involved antibody is produced by the underlying malignancy and not against it. Amyloidosis associated with hematological malignancies or paraproteinemias may complicate the clinical picture.

Response to therapy is usually unsatisfactory, but may include treatment of the underlying tumor, immunotherapies, radiation to bony lesions in myeloma, and chemotherapy (55). Symptom improvement has been reported in patients with POEMS following peripheral blood stem cell transplantation (59).

■ AUTONOMIC NEUROPATHY

Paraneoplastic syndromes associated with cancer can affect both the sympathetic and parasympathetic autonomic nervous system. Associated clinical symptoms include blood pressure dysregulation and postural hypotension, bowel and bladder dysfunction, arrhythmias, xerostomia, pupillary abnormalities, impotence and erectile dysfunction, diaphoresis, and anhidrosis. Autonomic dysfunction can occur as an isolated syndrome or in combination with encephalomyelitis, sensory neuronopathy, or sensorimotor neuropathy. This syndrome is commonly seen in patients with SCLC and presence of anti-Hu antibodies, but has also been described with other underlying cancers, including Hodgkin lymphoma, thymoma, and carcinoid tumors (18, 60).

Treatment of the underlying cancer may stabilize or improve symptoms. In addition, immunotherapies, plasmapheresis, and rituximab have been successfully used in some patients (61, 62).

SYNDROMES OF THE NEUROMUSCULAR JUNCTION AND MUSCLE

■ LAMBERT-EATON MYASTHENIC SYNDROME

Lambert-Eaton myastenic syndrome (LEMS) is one of the most common paraneoplastic syndromes. SCLC is most frequently identified as underlying cancer (63). LEMS frequently develops before the cancer diagnosis and should raise a high suspicion for an underlying cancer. Development of LEMS after cancer therapy should prompt investigation for tumor recurrence. Antibodies directed against the *P/Q* voltage-gated calcium channels (VGCC) (64) interfere with acetylcholine release at the neuromuscular junction, resulting in predominant proximal muscle weakness, mostly affecting the lower extremities with associated gait difficulties. Other symptoms include xerostomia, generalized fatigue, and autonomic dysfunction (65). The neurologic exam reveals diminished deep tendon reflexes that typically improve with repetitive muscle activity (66). The diagnosis is further supported by EMG studies that show low muscle amplitudes at rest with diminished response at low rate and elevated response at high rates.

Treatment of the underlying cancer in combination with immunotherapies, such as intravenous immunoglobulins and plasmapheresis, may result in symptom improvement. Immunosuppression with azathioprine has been applied in long-term management. In addition, the use of 3,4-diaminopyridine, which facilitates acetylcholine release at the neuromuscular junction, has been associated with clinical benefit (67).

■ NEUROMYOTONIA

Neuromyotonia is the consequence of peripheral nerve hyperexcitability and is characterized by (often painful) muscle cramps, delayed relaxation, fasciculations, and weakness. The autonomic nervous system may also be affected and some patients demonstrate cognitive deficits as well as behavioral and personality changes (Morvan's syndrome). This syndrome occurs in the setting of an underlying cancer or as an autoimmune condition unrelated to malignancy. Antibodies directed against CASPR2 (previously attributed to voltage-gated potassium channels) can be identified in this syndrome (68, 69). Other antibodies such as anti-Hu and anti-amphiphysin have also been identified in this syndrome. Among the cancers commonly underlying this syndrome are thymoma, SCLC, and Hodgkin's disease. The treatment of choice is immunosuppression with plasmapheresis or intravenous immunoglobulins (70). Some patients have demonstrated symptom improvement with anticonvulsants and muscle relaxants.

■ NECROTIZING MYOPATHY, POLYMYOSITIS, AND DERMATOMYOSITIS

Cancer-associated necrotizing myopathy typically starts as painful proximal weakness and rapidly progresses to generalized weakness. Respiratory muscles can be involved. Laboratory studies usually reveal elevated creatinine kinase (CK), and muscle biopsy demonstrates necrotic muscle fibers without significant inflammation. Among the cancers linked to this syndrome are SCLC, breast, prostate, and gastrointestinal malignancies.

In contrast to necrotizing myopathy, biopsy findings in polymyositis and dermatomyositis show significant inflammation. Polymyositis is associated with an elevated cancer risk of up to 20% (18), including non-Hodgkin lymphoma, lung, ovarian, and bladder cancer (71). Dermatomyositis is associated with a higher frequency of malignancies when compared to polymyositis, typically ranging from 20% to 25% (72) and symptom onset should prompt a thorough investigation for an underlying malignancy (7). Patients with inflammatory myopathies typically develop proximal and symmetric muscle weakness over several weeks to months. Patients with dermatomyositis may also demonstrate skin manifestations (73), including an erythematous V-shaped rash over chest and shoulders, a heliotrope upper eyelid rash, and scaling erythema on the extensor surfaces of the extremities ("Grotton's sign"). The most common cancers associated with dermatomyositis are lymphomas, lung, pancreatic, gastrointestinal, and gynecologic malignancies (71, 74). Treatment of inflammatory myopathies consists of treatment of the underlying tumor and immunosuppression with intravenous immunoglobulins, glucocorticoids, azathioprine, cyclosporine, and methotrexate (73, 75, 76).

SUMMARY

Paraneoplastic syndromes are heterogenous disorders with a low incidence in the general cancer population. As many paraneoplastic syndromes occur prior to the diagnosis of cancer, recognition of distinct paraneoplastic syndromes is essential to initiate thorough screening for malignancy. Both humoral and T-cell-mediated immune mechanisms play a role in the pathogenesis of paraneoplastic syndromes. Most important treatment goal is the identification and treatment of the underlying cancer in order to slow or to reverse neurological impairment. While long-term remission of neurological symptoms is infrequently achieved, early recognition of paraneoplastic syndromes is crucial. In general, antibody-mediated disorders affecting the peripheral nervous system have a higher likelihood of response to treatment. Immunomodulatory therapies have been frequently employed, including plasmapheresis, intravenous immunoglobulins, and glucocorticoids. In addition, more aggressive immunosuppressive strategies have proven beneficial in some circumstances, including treatment with rituximab, azathioprine, cyclosporine, and cyclophosphamide.

REFERENCES

1. Darnell RB, Posner JB. *Paraneoplastic Syndromes.* Oxford University Press, New York, NY, 2011.

2. Albert ML, Austin LM, Darnell RB. Detection and treatment of activated T cells in the cerebrospinal fluid of patients with paraneoplastic cerebellar degeneration. *Ann Neurol.* 2000; 47: 9–17.

3. Benyahia B, et al. Cell-mediated autoimmunity in paraneoplastic neurological syndromes with anti-Hu antibodies. *Ann Neurol.* 1999; 45: 162–167.

4. Tanaka M, Tanaka K, Shinozawa K, et al. Cytotoxic T cells react with recombinant Yo protein from a patient with paraneoplastic cerebellar degeneration and anti-Yo antibody. *J Neurol Sci.* 1998; 161: 88–90.

5. Graus F, Saiz A, Dalmau J. Antibodies and neuronal autoimmune disorders of the CNS. *J Neurol.* 2010; 257: 509–517.

6. Graus F, et al. Recommended diagnostic criteria for paraneoplastic neurological syndromes. *J Neurol Neurosurg Psychiatry.* 2004; 75: 1135–1140.

7. Titulaer MJ, et al. Screening for tumours in paraneoplastic syndromes: report of an EFNS task force. *Eur J Neurol.* 2011; 18: 19–e3.

8. Monstad SE, Knudsen A, Salvesen HB, et al. Onconeural antibodies in sera from patients with various types of tumours. *Cancer Immunol Immunother.* 2009; 58: 1795–1800.

9. Rosenfeld MR, Dalmau J. Update on paraneoplastic neurologic disorders. *The Oncologist.* 2010; 15: 603–617.

10. Linke R, Schroeder M, Helmberger T, et al. Antibody-positive paraneoplastic neurologic syndromes: value of CT and PET for tumor diagnosis. *Neurology.* 2004; 63: 282–286.

11. Younes-Mhenni S, et al. FDG-PET improves tumour detection in patients with paraneoplastic neurological syndromes. *Brain.* 2004; 127: 2331–2338.

12. Bataller L, Graus F, Saiz A, et al. Clinical outcome in adult onset idiopathic or paraneoplastic opsoclonus-myoclonus. *Brain.* 2001; 124: 437–443.

13. Dalmau J, et al. Anti-NMDA-receptor encephalitis: case series and analysis of the effects of antibodies. *Lancet Neurol.* 2008; 7: 1091–1098.

14. Lai M, et al. AMPA receptor antibodies in limbic encephalitis alter synaptic receptor location. *Ann Neurol.* 2009; 65: 424–434.

15. Peterson K, Rosenblum MK, Kotanides H, et al. Paraneoplastic cerebellar degeneration. I. A clinical analysis of 55 anti-Yo antibody-positive patients. *Neurology.* 1992; 42: 1931–1937.

16. Shams'ili S, et al. Paraneoplastic cerebellar degeneration associated with antineuronal antibodies: analysis of 50 patients. *Brain.* 2003; 126: 1409–1418.

17. Schmahmann JD, Weilburg JB, Sherman JC. The neuropsychiatry of the cerebellum—insights from the clinic. *Cerebellum.* 2007; 6: 254–267.

18. Darnell RB, Posner JB. Paraneoplastic syndromes affecting the nervous system. *Semin Oncol.* 2006; 33: 270–298.

19. Rojas-Marcos I, et al. Spectrum of paraneoplastic neurologic disorders in women with breast and gynecologic cancer. *Medicine* (Baltimore). 2003; 82: 216–223.

20. Graus F, et al. Anti-Hu-associated paraneoplastic encephalomyelitis: analysis of 200 patients. *Brain*. 2001; 124: 1138–1148.

21. Bernal F, et al. Anti-Tr antibodies as markers of paraneoplastic cerebellar degeneration and Hodgkin's disease. *Neurology*. 2003; 60: 230–234.

22. Graus F, et al. Immunological characterization of a neuronal antibody (anti-Tr) associated with paraneoplastic cerebellar degeneration and Hodgkin's disease. *J Neuroimmunol*. 1997; 74: 55–61.

23. Sutton IJ, Barnett MH, Watson JD, et al. Paraneoplastic brainstem encephalitis and anti-Ri antibodies. *J Neurol*. 2002; 249: 1597–1598.

24. Sabater L, et al. Protein kinase Cgamma autoimmunity in paraneoplastic cerebellar degeneration and non-small-cell lung cancer. *J Neurol Neurosurg Psychiatry*. 2006; 77: 1359–1362.

25. Graus F, et al. P/Q type calcium-channel antibodies in paraneoplastic cerebellar degeneration with lung cancer. *Neurology*. 2002; 59: 764–766.

26. Rojas I, et al. Long-term clinical outcome of paraneoplastic cerebellar degeneration and anti-Yo antibodies. *Neurology*. 2000; 55: 713–715.

27. Phuphanich S, Brock C. Neurologic improvement after high-dose intravenous immunoglobulin therapy in patients with paraneoplastic cerebellar degeneration associated with anti-Purkinje cell antibody. *J Neuro Oncol*. 2007; 81: 67–69.

28. Blaes F, et al. Intravenous immunoglobulins in the therapy of paraneoplastic neurological disorders. *J Neurol*. 1999; 246: 299–303.

29. David YB, et al. Autoimmune paraneoplastic cerebellar degeneration in ovarian carcinoma patients treated with plasmapheresis and immunoglobulin. A case report. *Cancer*. 1996; 78: 2153–2156.

30. Dropcho EJ, Kline LB, Riser J. Antineuronal (anti-Ri) antibodies in a patient with steroid-responsive opsoclonus-myoclonus. *Neurology*. 1993; 43: 207–211.

31. Pittock SJ, Lucchinetti CF, Lennon VA. Anti-neuronal nuclear autoantibody type 2: paraneoplastic accompaniments. *Ann Neurol*. 2003; 53: 580–587.

32. Honnorat J, et al. Onco-neural antibodies and tumour type determine survival and neurological symptoms in paraneoplastic neurological syndromes with Hu or CV2/CRMP5 antibodies. *J Neurol Neurosurg Psychiatry*. 2009; 80: 412–416.

33. Dropcho EJ. Antiamphiphysin antibodies with small-cell lung carcinoma and paraneoplastic encephalomyelitis. *Ann Neurol*. 1996; 39: 659-667.

34. Rosenfeld MR, Eichen JG, Wade DF, et al. Molecular and clinical diversity in paraneoplastic immunity to Ma proteins. *Ann Neurol*. 2001; 50: 339–348.

35. Dalmau J, et al. Clinical analysis of anti-Ma2-associated encephalitis. *Brain*. 2004; 127: 1831–1844.

36. Mathew RM, et al. Orchiectomy for suspected microscopic tumor in patients with anti-Ma2-associated encephalitis. *Neurology*. 2007; 68: 900–905.

37. Vitaliani R, et al. Paraneoplastic encephalitis, psychiatric symptoms, and hypoventilation in ovarian teratoma. *Ann Neurol.* 2005; 58: 594–604.

38. Dalmau J, et al. Paraneoplastic anti-N-methyl-D-aspartate receptor encephalitis associated with ovarian teratoma. *Ann Neurol.* 2007; 61: 25–36.

39. Vernino S, O'Neill BP, Marks RS, et al. Immunomodulatory treatment trial for paraneoplastic neurological disorders. *Neuro Oncol.* 2004; 6: 55–62.

40. Gultekin SH, et al. Paraneoplastic limbic encephalitis: neurological symptoms, immunological findings and tumour association in 50 patients. *Brain.* 2000; 123: 1481–1494.

41. Bataller L, et al. Autoimmune limbic encephalitis in 39 patients: immunophenotypes and outcomes. *J Neurol Neurosurg Psychiatry.* 2007; 78: 381–385.

42. Alamowitch S, et al. Limbic encephalitis and small cell lung cancer. Clinical and immunological features. *Brain.* 1997; 120: 923–928.

43. Pozo-Rosich P, Clover L, Saiz A, et al. Voltage-gated potassium channel antibodies in limbic encephalitis. *Ann Neurol.* 2003; 54: 530–533.

44. Buckley C, et al. Potassium channel antibodies in two patients with reversible limbic encephalitis. *Ann Neurol.* 2001; 50: 73–78.

45. Ances BM, et al. Treatment-responsive limbic encephalitis identified by neuropil antibodies: MRI and PET correlates. *Brain.* 2005; 128: 1764–1777.

46. Pranzatelli MR. The immunopharmacology of the opsoclonus-myoclonus syndrome. *Clin Neuropharmacol.* 1996; 19: 1–47.

47. Luque FA, et al. Anti-Ri: an antibody associated with paraneoplastic opsoclonus and breast cancer. *Ann Neurol.* 1991; 29: 241–251.

48. Pranzatelli MR, Tate ED, Travelstead AL, et al. Immunologic and clinical responses to rituximab in a child with opsoclonus-myoclonus syndrome. *Pediatrics.* 2005; 115: e115–119.

49. Ko MW, Dalmau J, Galetta SL. Neuro-ophthalmologic manifestations of paraneoplastic syndromes. *J Neuro Ophthalmol.* 2008; 28: 58–68.

50. Keltner JL, Thirkill CE. Cancer-associated retinopathy vs recoverin-associated retinopathy. *Am J Ophthalmol.* 1998; 126: 296-302.

51. Lei B, Bush RA, Milam AH, et al. Human melanoma-associated retinopathy (MAR) antibodies alter the retinal ON-response of the monkey ERG in vivo. *Invest Ophthalmol Vis Sci.* 2000; 41: 262–266.

52. Silverman IE. Paraneoplastic stiff limb syndrome. *J Neurol Neurosurg Psychiatry.* 1999; 67: 126–127.

53. Brown P, Marsden CD. The stiff man and stiff man plus syndromes. *J Neurol.* 1999; 246: 648–652.

54. Dalakas MC, et al. High-dose intravenous immune globulin for stiff-person syndrome. *N Engl J Med.* 2001; 345: 1870–1876.

55. Rudnicki SA, Dalmau J. Paraneoplastic syndromes of the spinal cord, nerve, and muscle. *Muscle Nerve.* 2000; 23: 1800–1818.

56. Antoine JC, et al. Carcinoma associated paraneoplastic peripheral neuropathies in patients with and without anti-onconeural antibodies. *J Neurol Neurosurg Psychiatry.* 1999; 67: 7–14.

57. Rudnicki SA, Dalmau J. Paraneoplastic syndromes of the peripheral nerves. *Curr Opin Neurol.* 2005; 18: 598–603.

58. Silberman J, Lonial S. Review of peripheral neuropathy in plasma cell disorders. *Hematol Oncol.* 2008; 26: 55–65.

59. Kuwabara S, et al. Neurologic improvement after peripheral blood stem cell transplantation in POEMS syndrome. *Neurology.* 2008; 71: 1691–1695.

60. Vernino S, Adamski J, Kryzer TJ, et al. Neuronal nicotinic ACh receptor antibody in subacute autonomic neuropathy and cancer-related syndromes. *Neurology.* 1998; 50: 1806–1813.

61. Vernino S, Sandroni P, Singer W, et al. Invited article: autonomic ganglia: target and novel therapeutic tool. *Neurology.* 2008; 70: 1926–1932.

62. Iodice V, et al. Efficacy of immunotherapy in seropositive and seronegative putative autoimmune autonomic ganglionopathy. *Neurology.* 2009; 72: 2002–2008.

63. Titulaer MJ, et al. Screening for small-cell lung cancer: a follow-up study of patients with Lambert-Eaton myasthenic syndrome. *J Clin Oncol.* 2008; 26: 4276–4281.

64. Motomura M, et al. Incidence of serum anti-P/O-type and anti-N-type calcium channel autoantibodies in the Lambert-Eaton myasthenic syndrome. *J Neurol Sci.* 1997; 147: 35–42.

65. O'Suilleabhain P, Low PA, Lennon VA. Autonomic dysfunction in the Lambert-Eaton myasthenic syndrome: serologic and clinical correlates. *Neurology.* 1998; 50: 88–93.

66. Titulaer MJ, et al. The Lambert-Eaton myasthenic syndrome 1988-2008: a clinical picture in 97 patients. *J Neuroimmunol.* 2008; 201–202, 153–158.

67. Wirtz PW. et al. Efficacy of 3,4-diaminopyridine and pyridostigmine in the treatment of Lambert-Eaton myasthenic syndrome: a randomized, double-blind, placebo-controlled, crossover study. *Clin Pharmacol Ther.* 2009; 86: 44–48.

68. Newsom-Davis J, et al. Autoimmune disorders of neuronal potassium channels. *Ann N Y Acad Sci.* 2003; 998: 202–210.

69. Lai M, et al. Investigation of LGI1 as the antigen in limbic encephalitis previously attributed to potassium channels: a case series. *Lancet Neurol.* 2010; 9: 776–785.

70. van den Berg JS, van Engelen BG, Boerman RH, et al. Acquired neuromyotonia: superiority of plasma exchange over high-dose intravenous human immunoglobulin. *J Neurol.* 1999; 246, 623–625.

71. Hill CL, et al. Frequency of specific cancer types in dermatomyositis and polymyositis: a population-based study. *Lancet.* 2001; 357: 96–100.

72. Callen JP, Wortmann RL. Dermatomyositis. *Clin Dermatol.* 2006; 24: 363–373.

73. Mastaglia FL, Garlepp MJ, Phillips BA, et al. Inflammatory myopathies: clinical, diagnostic and therapeutic aspects. *Muscle Nerve*. 2003; 27: 407–425.

74. Callen JP. Relation between dermatomyositis and polymyositis and cancer. *Lancet*. 2001; 357, 85–86.

75. Dalakas MC. The role of high-dose immune globulin intravenous in the treatment of dermatomyositis. *Int Immunopharmacol*. 2006; 6: 550–556.

76. Feist E, Dorner T, Sorensen H, et al. Longlasting remissions after treatment with rituximab for autoimmune myositis. *J Rheumatol*. 2008; 35: 1230–1232.

CHAPTER 65
Thyroid Cancer

Lori J. Wirth, Tito Fojo

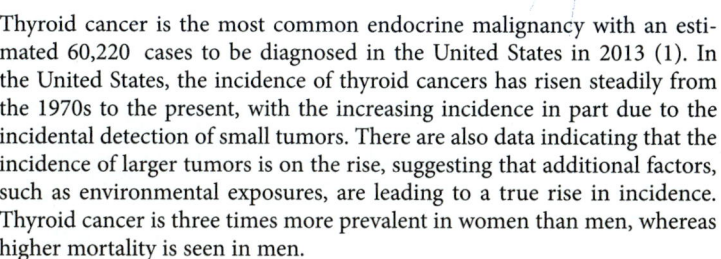

Thyroid cancer is the most common endocrine malignancy with an estimated 60,220 cases to be diagnosed in the United States in 2013 (1). In the United States, the incidence of thyroid cancers has risen steadily from the 1970s to the present, with the increasing incidence in part due to the incidental detection of small tumors. There are also data indicating that the incidence of larger tumors is on the rise, suggesting that additional factors, such as environmental exposures, are leading to a true rise in incidence. Thyroid cancer is three times more prevalent in women than men, whereas higher mortality is seen in men.

There are three major types of thyroid cancer, each with its own unique natural history and approach to treatment: differentiated thyroid cancer (DTC), anaplastic thyroid cancer (ATC), and medullary thyroid cancer (MTC). DTC is the most common, accounting for >90% of all cases, with ATC and MTC accounting for approximately 2% and 5% of cases, respectively.

DIFFERENTIATED THYROID CANCER

There are two predominant subtypes of DTC: papillary thyroid cancer (PTC) and follicular thyroid cancer (FTC), with PTC comprising approximately 85% of cases. Of the multiple staging systems for DTC, the AJCC/UICC TNM system is used most often. Features that impact prognosis most include age >45 years, gross extrathyroidal extension, nodal metastasis, especially with extranodal extension, distant metastasis, FDG avidity, absence of radioiodine uptake, and more aggressive histologic subtypes, such as tall cell, diffuse sclerosing, hobnail, as well as insular or poorly differentiated variants.

There are a variety of genetic alterations seen in DTC, although little overlap is seen in the genetics of PTC and FTC. Alterations in the mitogen-activated protein kinase (MAPK) signaling pathway are common. Mutations in *BRAF* are the most commonly encountered mutations, occurring in 40%–50% of PTCs. *BRAF* mutation is associated with older age, lymph node involvement, distant metastasis, decreased sensitivity to radioiodine, and risk of recurrence. *RET/PTC* rearrangements are the second most common abnormality seen in PTC. In FTC, *RAS* mutations and *PPARG* rearrangements are seen in approximately 50% and 35%, respectively. These molecular changes and others now offer strong rationale for exploring targeted therapies in advanced DTC.

The prognosis of DTC is usually quite good. Most cases can be treated adequately with surgery, frequently followed by radioiodine. Unless there is a contraindication to the procedure, total thyroidectomy is indicated when the primary tumor is >1 cm. Total thyroidectomy addresses the potential for multicentric DTC, facilitates subsequent radioiodine therapy, and allows for subsequent surveillance by serum thyroglobulin levels and radioiodine scanning. Metastasis to cervical nodes is frequent in PTC, while uncommon in FTC. Therefore, prophylactic central compartment neck dissection is usually performed only in PTC. Treatment with radioiodine is indicated for patients with intermediate- and high-risk disease, whereas the role for radioiodine in patients with low-risk disease remains unclear. Beyond surgery and radioiodine, TSH suppression with levothyroxine is employed in most patients to reduce the risk of disease recurrence. The role of external beam radiotherapy (EBRT) in the management of DTC is less clear due to a paucity of prospective data, but in general, patients with unresectable disease in the neck or gross residual disease following surgery may be considered for EBRT.

While long-term overall survival (OS) for DTC is quite good for most patients, approximately 30% will experience disease recurrence. Recurrent disease can involve the thyroid bed or cervical lymph nodes, the trachea, or neck muscles, or can occur distantly. Recurrent disease in the neck is managed with surgery and additional radioiodine, when feasible. In patients with recurrent disease, radioiodine uptake and FDG avidity can be used in risk stratification. Those with FDG-avid disease that does not concentrate radioiodine are at the highest risk for death. Locoregionally recurrent and/or metastatic iodine-refractory DTC not amenable to surgery has traditionally been treated with cytotoxic chemotherapy, although activity is poor and the toxicities are difficult to justify. Studies investigating targeted therapy for iodine-refractory DTC, most notably agents targeting isoforms of the vascular endothelial growth factor receptor (VEGFR), have shown evidence of antitumor activity, while underscoring the difficulties of evaluating anticancer therapies in diseases that are often indolent in nature (Table 65-1). In "differentiated thyroid cancer," 8 VEGFR tyrosine kinase inhibitors (TKIs) have been evaluated in 605 patients: sorafenib, sunitinib, pazopanib, motesanib, selumetinib, axitinib, levanitinib, and vandetanib (2–8). Only one patient has had a complete response, with partial response rates of 2.6%–50% with a median of 18%. Progression-free survival, a difficult endpoint in patients with variably indolent disease, has ranged from 7.4 to 20 months with a median of 13.4 months. One cannot discern major differences amongst all the agents, and randomized trials will be needed to clearly establish the benefit of these therapies. A high incidence of toxicities is evidenced by drug discontinuation and dose adjustments in a median of 20% and 42% of patients, respectively. These high rates of toxicity underscore that these therapies, if shown to be effective, should be reserved only for those with advanced refractory disease, given that in the advanced thyroid cancer patient population, many patients have slow-growing, asymptomatic disease. Thus, the decision when *to* treat and when *not to* treat must be individualized to each patient.

ANAPLASTIC THYROID CARCINOMA

ATC, constituting approximately 2% of all thyroid cancers, remains one of the most lethal of human cancers, with nearly 100% mortality and a median OS of only 5–6 months. ATC can arise de novo or result from the

TABLE 65-1 SELECTED TARGETED THERAPY STUDIES IN ADVANCED THYROID CANCER

Phase of Study/Drug/ Dose	# Patients	RAI-R[a]	ORR[b]	PFS[c]	Duration Rx[d]	Discontinued[e]	Reduced[f]	Reference
Well-differentiated Thyroid Cancers								
P2 Sorafenib 400 mg bid	27	Yes	26%	19.4	6.2	20%	47%	Gupta-Abramson et al., 2008
P2 Sorafenib 400 mg bid	52	Yes	11%	< 16	≈11	26%	55.8%	Kloos et al., 2009
P2 Sorafenib 400 mg bid	31	Yes	25%	13.4	NR	19%	56%	Hoftijzer et al., 2009
P2 Sorafenib 400 mg bid	13	Yes	15%	19	NR	NR	NR	Cabanilas et al., 2010
P2 Sorafenib 400 mg bid	19	Yes	18%	>19	16.5[g]	NR	79%[g]	Ahmed et al., 2011
P2 Sorafenib 400 mg bid	16	Yes	19%	13.5	NR	NR	35%[g]	Capdevila et al., 2012
P1 Sorafenib 400 mg AM/200mg PM[h]	22	Yes	4.5%	20	NR	14%–23%[g]	40%[g]	Hong et al., 2011
P2 Suntinib 50 mg qd 4/6 wk	13	Yes	7.7%	NR	2.9	NR	23.5%	Ravaud et al., 2008
P2 Sunitinib 50 mg qd 4/6 wk	37	Yes	10.8%	NR	NR	NR	NR	Cohen et al., 2008
P2 Sunitinib 37.5 mg daily	29	Yes	24%	12.8[TTP]	8.5[g]	11.4%[g]	60%	Carr et al., 2010
P2 Pazopanib 800 mg qd	39	Yes	46%	11.7	≈11	7.7%	43%	Bible et al., 2010
P2 Motesanib 125 mg qd	93	Yes	14%	9.2	8.1	13%	NR	Sherman et al., 2008

(continued)

TABLE 65-1 SELECTED TARGETED THERAPY STUDIES IN ADVANCED THYROID CANCER (CONTINUED)

Phase of Study/Drug/Dose	# Patients	RAI-R[a]	ORR[b]	PFS[c]	Duration Rx[d]	Discontinued[e]	Reduced[f]	Reference
P2 Selumetinib	39	Yes	2.6%	7.4	3	15.4%	30.8%	Hayes et al., 2012
P2 Axitinib 5 mg bid	45	Yes	31%	18.1[g]	4.8[g]	13%–30%[g]	38%[g]	Cohen et al., 2008
P2 Levantinib 24 mg qd	58	Yes	50%	12.6	NR	23%	35%	Sherman et al., 2011
P2 Vandetanib 300 mg qd	72	Yes	1.4%–8%	11.1	6.3	33%	38%	Leboulleux et al., 2010
Medullary Thyroid Cancer								
P2 Axitinib 5 mg bid	11	NR	18%	18.1[g]	4.8[g]	13%–30%[g]	38%[g]	Cohen et al., 2008
P2 Sorafenib 400 mg bid	21	-	9.5%	17.9	15	23.8%	76%	Lam et al., 2010
P2 Sorafenib 400 mg bid	15	NR	25%	>12	16.5[g]	NR	79%[g]	Ahmed et al., 2011
P2 Sorafenib 400 mg bid	15	-	47%	10.5	NR	NR	35%[g]	Capdevila et al., 2012
P1 Sorafenib 400 mg AM/200 mg PM[h]	13	-	38%	15	NR	14%–23%[g]	40%[g]	Hong et al., 2011
P2 Sunitinib 37.5 mg daily	6	-	50%	12.8[TTP]	8.5[g]	11.4%[g]	60%	Carr et al., 2010
P2 Sunitinib 50 mg qd 4/6 wk	15	-	13.3%	NR	NR	NR	60%	Ravaud et al., 2010

P2 Sunitinib 50 mg qd 4/6 wk	25	Yes	32%	12	NR	NR	NR	DeSouza et al., 2010
P2 Motesanib 125 mg qd	91	-	2%	11.1	8.8	17.6%	NR[i]	Schlumberger et al., 2009
P3 Vandetanib 300 mg qd	231	-	45%	≈30.5	20.8	12.1%	35%	Wells et al., 2010
P1 Cabozantinib, various doses	37	-	27%	NR	NR	NR	NR	Kurzrock et al., 2010
P3 Cabozantinib 140 mg qd	220	-	28%	11.2	NR	27%	79%	Schoffski et al., 2012

P1, phase 1; P2, phase 2; P3, phase 3; NR, not reported; qd, daily; bid, twice a day.

[a]Radio-iodine resistance.

[b]ORR = Overall response rate; only one patient had a complete response; all others had partial responses.

[c]Progression-free survival in months or in some time to progression (TTP) as indicated.

[d]Median duration of treatment.

[e]Percent of patients who had therapy discontinued for toxicity.

[f]Percent of patients who had the starting dose reduced due to poor tolerance.

[g]Values for all patients in study that included several thyroid histologies.

[h]Plus tipifarnib with both drugs administered for 21 d every 28 d.

[i]41% grade 3/4 adverse events.

(continued)

References

1. Gupta-Abramson V, Troxel AB, Nellore A, et al. Phase II trial of sorafenib in advanced thyroid cancer. *J Clin Oncol*. 2008; 26: 4714–4719.
2. Kloos RT, Ringel MD, Knopp MV, et al. Phase II trial of sorafenib in metastatic thyroid cancer. *J Clin Oncol*. 2009; 27: 1675–1684.
3. Hoftijzer H, Heemstra KA, Morreau H, et al. Beneficial effects of sorafenib on tumor progression, but not on radioiodine uptake, in patients with differentiated thyroid carcinoma. *Eur J Endocrinol*. 2009; 161: 923–931.
4. Cabanillas ME, Waguespack SG, Bronstein Y, et al. Treatment with tyrosine kinase inhibitors for patients with differentiated thyroid cancer: the M. D. Anderson experience. *J Clin Endocrinol Metab*. 2010; 95: 2588–2595.
5. Ahmed M, Barbachano Y, Riddell A, et al. Analysis of the efficacy and toxicity of sorafenib in thyroid cancer: a phase II study in a UK based population. *Eur J Endocrinol*. 2011; 165: 315–322.
6. Capdevila J, Iglesias L, Halperin I, et al. Sorafenib in metastatic thyroid cancer. *Endocr Relat Cancer*. 2012; 19: 209–216
7. Hong DS, Cabanillas ME, Wheler J, et al. Inhibition of the Ras/Raf/MEK/ERK and RET kinase pathways with the combination of the multikinase inhibitor sorafenib and the farnesyltransferase inhibitor tipifarnib in medullary and differentiated thyroid malignancies. *J Clin Endocrinol Metab*. 2011; 96: 997–1005.
8. Ravaud A, de la Fouchardiere C, Courbon F, et al. Sunitinib in patients with refractory advanced thyroid cancer: the THYSU phase II trial. Proceedings of the American Society of Clinical Oncology 2008; *J Clin Oncol*. Vol. 26, Abstract 6058.
9. Cohen EE, Needle BM, Cullen KJ, et al. Phase 2 study of sunitinib in refractory thyroid cancer. Proceedings of the American Society of Clinical Oncology 2008; *J Clin Oncol*. Vol. 26, Abstract 6025.
10. Carr LL, Mankoff DA, Goulart BH, et al. Phase II Study of Daily sunitinib in FDG-PET–positive, iodine-refractory differentiated thyroid cancer and metastatic medullary carcinoma of the thyroid with functional imaging correlation. *Clin Cancer Res*. 2010; 16: 5260–5268.
11. Bible KC, Suman VJ, Molina JR, et al. Efficacy of pazopanib in progressive, radioiodine-refractory, metastatic differentiated thyroid cancers: results of a phase 2 consortium study. *Lancet Oncol*. 2010; 11:962–972.
12. Sherman SI, Wirth LJ, Droz JP, et al. Motesanib diphosphate in progressive differentiated thyroid cancer. *N Engl J Med*. 2008; 359: 31–42.
13. Hayes DN, Lucas AS, Tanvetyanon T, et al. Phase II efficacy and pharmacogenomic study of Selumetinib (AZD6244; ARRY-142886) in iodine-131 refractory papillary thyroid carcinoma with or without follicular elements. *Clin Cancer Res*. 2012; 18: 2056–2065.
14. Cohen EE, Rosen LS, Vokes EE, et al. Axitinib is an active treatment for all histologic subtypes of advanced thyroid cancer: results from a phase II study. *J Clin Oncol*. 2008; 26: 4708–4713.
15. Sherman SI, Jarzab B, Cabanillas ME, et al. A phase II trial of the multi-targeted kinase inhibitor, lenvatinib (E7080), in advanced radioiodine (RAI)-refractory differentiated thyroid cancer (DTC). Proceedings of the American Society of Clinical Oncology 2011; *J Clin Oncol*. Vol. 29, Abstract 5503.

16. Leboulleux S, Bastholt L, Krause TM, et al. Vandetanib in locally advanced or metastatic differentiated thyroid cancer (papillary or follicular; DTC): a randomized, double-blind phase II trial. *Ann Oncol* (ESMO Meeting Abstracts). 2010; 21: viii314–viii328.

17. Lam ET, Ringel MD, Kloos RT, et al. Phase II clinical trial of sorafenib in metastatic medullary thyroid cancer. *J Clin Oncol.* 2010; 28: 2323–2330.

18. Ravaud A, de la Fouchardière C, Asselineau J, et al. Efficacy of sunitinib in advanced medullary thyroid carcinoma: intermediate results of phase II THYSU. *The Oncologist.* 2010; 15(2): 212–213.

19. De Souza JA, Busaidy N, Zimrin A, et al. Phase II trial of sunitinib in medullary thyroid cancer (MTC). Proceedings of the American Society of Clinical Oncology 2010; *J Clin Oncol.* Vol. 28, Abstract 5504.

20. Schlumberger MJ, Elisei R, Bastholt L, et al. Phase II study of safety and efficacy of motesanib in patients with progressive or symptomatic, advanced or metastatic medullary thyroid cancer. *J Clin Oncol.* 2009; 27: 3794–3801.

21. Wells SA Jr, Robinson BG, Gagel RF, et al. Vandetanib in patients with locally advanced or metastatic medullary thyroid cancer: a randomized, double-blind phase III trial. *J Clin Oncol.* 2012; 30: 134–141.

22. Kurzrock R, Sherman SI, Ball DW, et al. Activity of XL184 (Cabozantinib), an oral tyrosine kinase inhibitor, in patients with medullary thyroid cancer. *J Clin Oncol.* 2011; 29: 2660–2666.

23. Schoffski P, Elisei R, Müller S, et al. An international double-blind, randomized, placebo-controlled phase III (EXAM) of cabozantinib (XL184) in medullary thyroid cancer patients with documented RECIST progression at baseline. Proceedings of the American Society of Clinical Oncology 2012; *J Clin Oncol.* Vol. 28, Abstract 5508.

dedifferentiation of PTC or FTC. ATC most commonly presents in the seventh decade of life and occurs more in women than in men. Because of the clinical implications of misclassifying ATC, a definitive tissue biopsy, rather than FNA alone, should be performed as part of the diagnosis of ATC, particularly as there is some cytologic overlap with other diagnoses, particularly lymphoma, medullary thyroid carcinoma, and the insular variant of follicular thyroid carcinoma.

ATCs typically harbor multiple genetic abnormalities. In addition to frequent chromosomal gains and losses, gene amplifications and deletions, mutations in *RAS* and *BRAF* are also seen in ATC, suggesting these mutations are early events in carcinogenesis. Late mutations can involve p53, β-catenin, and PIK3CA.

The management of ATC is particularly challenging because most patients present with both extensive locoregional disease and distant metastasis. Long-term survival is essentially limited to patients who have undergone complete resection, often in incidentally discovered disease. Adjuvant chemoradiotherapy, which should be started as soon as the patient has recovered from surgery, is generally administered with the goal to improve locoregional control and prevent death from airway obstruction. Doxorubicin, platinums, and taxanes are the cytotoxic therapies most often given concurrently with radiation.

Taxanes, anthracyclines, and platinums, either as monotherapy and or in combination, are reasonable choices for systemic therapy in ATC patients with locally advanced disease or distant metastasis, although objective response rates are low. Because no clinical trial has shown improvement in OS or quality of life with any systemic regimen, involvement in clinical trials, when available, is encouraged (9).

More effective therapies for ATC are urgently needed. Potential molecular targets under investigation include the ras/RAF/MEK and PI-3K/AKT/mTOR pathways, PPARγ aurora kinases, and "anti-vascular agents" similar to combretastatin. Any targeted therapy shown to be potentially effective will likely require a development strategy that includes cytotoxic chemotherapy due to the rapidly progressive nature of the disease.

MEDULLARY THYROID CARCINOMA

MTC is a rare tumor arising from the thyroid's calcitonin-producing parafollicular C cells. MTC is hereditary in 20%–25% of cases, resulting from germline RET mutation in the familial medullary thyroid carcinoma (FMTC) and multiple endocrine neoplasia (MEN) 2A and B syndromes. The identification of individuals with MTC harboring a germline mutation is critical, since other family members affected by the mutation must be identified and treated. Moreover, patients with MEN2A and B are at risk for pheochromocytoma and primary hyperparathyroidism. Patients with hereditary MTC and MEN2 should be referred for genetic counseling, and all patients with newly diagnosed MTC should undergo genetic testing to establish whether they have sporadic or hereditary disease.

The presentation of MTC is variable and may range from a solitary thyroid nodule to metastatic disease. FNA is the initial test most frequently used to diagnose MTC, with subsequent measurement of serum calcitonin if MTC is suspected. Biochemical screening is generally performed pre-operatively to rule out pheochromocytoma. Surgery plays a central role in the management of MTC. Preoperative neck and chest CT, and liver CT or MRI, is also generally recommended for suspected MTC patients if there is evidence of cervical nodal metastasis or the serum calcitonin is >400 pg/ml. A total thyroidectomy is recommended for all patients with newly diagnosed MTC. Bilateral prophylactic central compartment dissection is generally performed, due to a high rate of occult nodal metastasis, while surgical management of the lateral neck is variable.

The TNM staging system used for MTC does not take into account several prognostic factors, such as postoperative calcitonin and CEA levels or tumor marker doubling times, which are predictive of OS. Surveillance by calcitonin and CEA are recommended to detect persistent or recurrent disease following surgery. Levels are usually not measured until at least 2 months following surgery because of a long half-life and inflammatory effects on calcitonin synthesis.

MTC is not highly responsive to EBRT, although radiotherapy can be considered in the adjuvant setting or for palliation. Historically, cytotoxic chemotherapy was used in metastatic or locally recurrent unresectable MTC, although there is little evidence to support its use. As with well-differentiated thyroid cancers, TKIs targeting the VEGFR isoforms have also been investigated in MTC, including axitinib, sorafenib, sunitinib, and motesanib (Table 65-1) (3,10–12). Generally they have shown much lower response rates than those observed in well-differentiated cancers with similar toxicity profiles. However, there has been greater interest in drugs with putative anti-RET kinase activity (13, 14). Both vandetanib and cabozantinib have received FDA approval for patients with "late-stage (metastatic) medullary thyroid cancer who are ineligible for surgery and who have disease that is growing or causing symptoms." Vandetanib, with demonstrated preclinical activity against RET, as well as VEGFR and EGFR, has been evaluated in an international placebo-controlled phase III study in which 331 patients with sporadic or hereditary locally advanced or metastatic MTC were enrolled (13). PFS was improved from 19 to approximately 31 months. Adverse events including diarrhea, rash, nausea, hypertension, asthenia, and QTc prolongation have been reported and should be managed with dose reductions to 200 and 100 mg, since in many patients these lower doses retain antitumor activity. As with advanced DTC, the side effect profile of TKI treatment that may impact a patient's quality of life needs to be taken into account when treatment decisions are made in these patients who are often minimally symptomatic and have a life measured in years. A second large randomized phase III study investigating another TKI, cabozantinib, in MTC has been successfully completed (14). In the 330 patients enrolled, PFS was significantly improved by cabozantinib, from 4 to 11 months. As with vandetanib and all VEGFR inhibitors, dose adjustments and discontinuations were frequent. Caution should be used when considering cabozantinib since the starting dose of 140 mg used in the MTC trial is no longer being investigated, in large part due to the side effects encountered at this dose. Consequently a lower starting dose might be considered. For both vandetanib and cabozantinib, treatment should be limited to MTC patients with unresectable, locoregionally recurrent, and/or metastatic disease that is progressive or symptomatic, while watchful waiting should continue to be the preferred approach in those patients who are asymptomatic and have indolent, slow-growing disease.

REFERENCES

1. Siegel R, Naishadham D, Jemal A. Cancer Statistics, 2013. *CA Cancer J Clin*. 2013; 63: 11–30.

2. Kloos RT, Ringel MD, Knopp MV, et al. Phase II trial of sorafenib in metastatic thyroid cancer. *J Clin Oncol*. 2009; 27: 1675–1684.

3. Cohen EE, Needle BM, Cullen KJ, et al. Phase 2 study of sunitinib in refractory thyroid cancer. Proceedings of the American Society of Clinical Oncology 2008; *J Clin Oncol*. Vol. 26, Abstract 6025

4. Sherman SI, Wirth LJ, Droz JP, et al. Motesanib Thyroid Cancer Study Group. Motesanib diphosphate in progressive differentiated thyroid cancer. *N Engl J Med*. 2008; 359: 31–42.

5. Hayes DN, Lucas AS, Tanvetyanon T, et al. Phase II efficacy and pharmacogenomic study of Selumetinib (AZD6244; ARRY-142886) in iodine-131 refractory papillary thyroid carcinoma with or without follicular elements. *Clin Cancer Res*. 2012; 18: 2056–2065.

6. Cohen EE, Rosen LS, Vokes EE, et al. Axitinib is an active treatment for all histologic subtypes of advanced thyroid cancer: results from a phase II study. *J Clin Oncol*. 2008; 26: 4708–4713.

7. Sherman SI, Jarzab B, Cabanillas ME, et al. A phase II trial of the multi-targeted kinase inhibitor, lenvatinib (E7080), in advanced radioiodine (RAI)-refractory differentiated thyroid cancer (DTC). Proceedings of the American Society of Clinical Oncology 2011; *J Clin Oncol*. Vol. 29, Abstract 5503.

8. Leboulleux S, Bastholt L, Krause TM, et al. Vandetanib in locally advanced or metastatic differentiated thyroid cancer (papillary or follicular; DTC): a randomized, double-blind phase II trial. *Ann Oncol* (ESMO Meeting Abstracts). 2010; 21: viii314–viii328.

9. Smallridge RC, Ain KB, Asa SL, et al. American Thyroid Association guidelines for management of patients with anaplastic thyroid cancer. *Thyroid*. 2012; 22: 1104–1139.

10. Lam ET, Ringel MD, Kloos RT, et al. Phase II clinical trial of sorafenib in metastatic medullary thyroid cancer. *J Clin Oncol*. 2010; 28: 2323–2330.

11. De Souza JA, Busaidy N, Zimrin A, et al. Phase II trial of sunitinib in medullary thyroid cancer (MTC). Proceedings of the American Society of Clinical Oncology 2010; *J Clin Oncol*. Vol. 28, Abstract 5504.

12. Schlumberger MJ, Elisei R, Bastholt L, et al. Phase II study of safety and efficacy of motesanib in patients with progressive or symptomatic, advanced or metastatic medullary thyroid cancer. *J Clin Oncol*. 2009; 27: 3794–3801.

13. Wells SA Jr, Robinson BG, Gagel RF, et al. Vandetanib in patients with locally advanced or metastatic medullary thyroid cancer: a randomized, double-blind phase III trial. *J Clin Oncol*. 2012; 30: 134–141.

14. Schoffski P, Elisei R, Müller S, et al. An international double-blind, randomized, placebo-controlled phase III (EXAM) of cabozantinib (XL184) in medullary thyroid cancer patients with documented RECIST progression at baseline. Proceedings of the American Society of Clinical Oncology 2012; *J Clin Oncol.* Vol. 28, Abstract 5508.

CHAPTER **66**
Adrenocortical Cancer
Tito Fojo

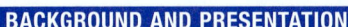

BACKGROUND AND PRESENTATION

Adrenocortical carcinoma (ACC) is a rare malignancy, affecting 1.5–2 persons per million each year (1). ACC is slightly more common in women and has a bimodal age distribution, with a higher incidence in children younger than 5 years and in adults in their 4th and 5th decades of life (1). Despite improved methods of diagnosis, ACC usually presents at an advanced stage and as a result 5-year survival ranges from 20% and 45%.

At the time of disease discovery there may be no symptoms (the tumor may be found incidentally on imaging). In other patients there may be symptoms of hormone excess or complaints referable to an abdominal mass. Hormone excess presents clinically as Cushing's syndrome, virilization, feminization, or, less frequently, hypertension with hypokalemia. Hormone hypersecretion can be found in as many as 73%–79% of ACC patients, although not all patients have symptoms (2). In one study, amongst 45 ACC patients, routine biochemistry documented hormone excess in 33 (73%) with excess glucocorticoid and adrenal androgen in 12, isolated glucocorticoid in 11, isolated adrenal androgen in 7, and 17β-estradiol excess in combination with glucocorticoid and adrenal androgen excess in two and one, respectively. Steroid profiling revealed predominantly immature, early-stage steroid precursors, and their production most likely a consequence of altered expression of steroidogenic enzymes in variably undifferentiated tumors. While the classification of ACCs by hormone profile has limited value, hormone secretion, especially cortisol, may be an independent predictor of poor prognosis (3)—although not all studies agree with this conclusion (4). Older age at diagnosis, stage III (local lymph nodes) and IV (local organ invasion or distant metastases) disease and cortisol hypersecretion are risk factors significantly associated with a shorter survival (3). The poorer prognosis of cortisol-secreting tumors could be attributed to the comorbidity of cortisol hypersecretion, the immunosuppressive effects of excess cortisol possibly favoring development of the tumor and its metastases, or cortisol-mediated metabolic changes that favor the growth of a more aggressive tumor.

GENETICS

Although most ACC lack identifiable risk factors, heredity plays a role in some patients (5). Risk factors include the Li-Fraumeni syndrome (LFS), multiple endocrine neoplasia type 1 (MEN1), familial adenomatous polyposis coli (Gardner syndrome), and the Beckwith-Wiedemann syndrome (BWS) (6). Predisposition is thought to arise from mutations in p53, MEN1, APC, or CDKN1C suppressor genes or dysregulation of the CDKN1C tumor suppressor gene. A unique risk factor has been described in southern and southeastern Brazil. There, a high frequency of an endemic germline p53 R337H mutation is responsible for the highest known incidence of childhood ACC—with a founder germline R337H mutation found in 95% of ACCs reported in young children (7). The frequency of this germline R337H mutation is due to a common ancestor, a conclusion supported by the fact that no case of a de novo R337H mutation has been found (8).

ASSESSMENT/EVALUATION

The initial assessment should determine the extent of disease and whether the tumor is functional. Difficulty in differentiating a benign from a malignant tumor and the risk of seeding tumor argue against a biopsy if the presentation is an isolated adrenal mass without evidence of metastases. Surgical resection can be both diagnostic and therapeutic. Biopsies should be reserved for cases with widespread metastases unlikely to be considered for surgical resection and those in whom there is reason to believe the primary is other than adrenal. Because not all patients present with symptoms of hormonal excess, their hormonal status and the need for steroid replacement should be assessed prior to surgery. Careful assessment may avoid the occurrence of postoperative adrenal insufficiency related to contralateral adrenal involution secondary to tumor hypersecretion of cortisol and suppression of adrenocorticotropic hormone (ACTH) production by the pituitary.

While in the pre-computed tomography (CT) era symptoms of hormone excess most often brought patients to medical attention, increasingly diagnoses are made radiographically, often in asymptomatic patients undergoing evaluation for an unrelated problem. A thin-collimation CT of the chest and abdomen is recommended as the initial imaging technique, with magnetic resonance imaging (MRI) reserved for selected patients. Both CT and MRI can help discriminate benign adenomas from malignant lesions, an important distinction that should be made before any operative intervention. On CT scans, ACCs usually have higher density values (i.e., lower lipid content) and are typically inhomogeneous; on MRI, they are usually isointense with liver on T1 images, with intermediate to high intensity on T2 images (9). MRI is superior in assessing vascular invasion and should be obtained before a surgical resection if there is concern regarding inferior vena cava involvement with right adrenal tumors. The value of [^{18}F] fluorodeoxyglucose (FDG)-positron emission tomography (PET) is not established in routine evaluation or follow-up (10). While imaging might help in discriminating a benign adenoma from a malignant tumor, it is not definitive and cannot differentiate ACC from other tumors that may have similar metabolic activities. Once all information is available, staging

TABLE 66-1 CLASSIFICATION OF ADRENOCORTICAL CARCINOMA, WORLD HEALTH ORGANIZATION (WHO) AND EUROPEAN NETWORK FOR THE STUDY OF ADRENAL TUMORS (ENSAT)

Stage	UICC/WHO	ENSAT
I	T1, N0, M0	T1, N0, M0
II	T2, N0, M0	T2, N0, M0
III	T3, N0, M0	T3–4, N0, M0
	T1–2, N1, M0	T1–4, N1, M0
IV	T3, N1, M0	Any M1
	T4, N0–1, M0	
	Any M1	

UICC, Union Internationale Contre le Cancer; WHO, World Health Organization; ENSAT, European Network for the Study of Adrenal Tumors; T1, tumor ≤5 cm; T2, tumor >5 cm; T3, tumor infiltration in surrounding tissue; T4, tumor invasion in adjacent organs (ENSAT, also venous tumor thrombus in vena cava or renal vein); N0, no positive lymph nodes; M0, no distant metastases; N1, positive lymph nodes; M1, presence of distant metastasis.

is undertaken using the UICC/WHO TNM classification or a revised classification proposed by European Network for the Study of Adrenal Tumors (ENSAT) (11) (Table 66-1). In the latter, stage III includes tumors that infiltrate into surrounding tissue or tumor thrombus in vena cava/renal vein or those that have positive lymph nodes, whereas stage IV is defined by the presence of distant metastasis. The prognostic value of ENSAT staging has been confirmed in an independent cohort from the United States (12).

PATHOLOGY

In the absence of distant metastases or local spread, it may be difficult to distinguish small (less than 6 cm) ACC's from a benign adenoma. Several multi-parametric approaches have been proposed for establishing malignancy. Among these, the Weiss system, first proposed in 1984, is the standard (13). It is based on the presence of nine histopathologic properties associated clinically with metastatic potential or local recurrence. The criteria are related to *tumor structure*: (1) 25% or less clear cells, (2) a "patternless" diffuse architecture, and (3) necrosis; *cytological features*: (4) atypical mitoses, (5) a mitotic rate greater than 5 per 50 high-power fields, and (6) nuclear grade 3 or 4; and *invasive properties*: (7) venous, (8) sinusoidal, and (9) capsular invasion. The individual criterion in the Weiss system are simply given a score of 1 if present and 0 if absent, yielding an overall score from 0 to 9 (Table 66-2). In the initial report 18/19 patients with adrenocortical tumors with a score of 4 or more had a recurrence or metastatic disease, whereas all 24 tumors with scores of 2 or less had a benign clinical course. Subsequently the threshold was lowered from 4 to 3 criteria based on one patient with a recurrent adrenal tumor that exhibited only 3 adverse histologic features. It is unclear whether higher scores above 4 are associated

TABLE 66-2 THE WEISS CRITERIA (THE PRESENCE OF THREE OR MORE CRITERIA HIGHLY CORRELATES WITH MALIGNANCY)

Histological Criteria	1
Nuclear grade[a]	High (grade 3 and 4)
Mitoses[b]	>5 per 50 high-power fields
Atypical mitoses	Yes
Clear cells	Comprise ≤25% of tumor
Diffuse architecture[c]	>33% of tumor
Necrosis	Yes
Venous invasion	Yes
Sinusoidal invasion	Yes
Capsular infiltration	Yes

[a]Grading is based on the Fuhrman nuclear grading system used in renal cell carcinoma (22). High-grade nuclei meet the definition of grades 3 and 4 in the Fuhrman system. This includes enlarged, oval to lobated nuclei with coarsely granular to hyperchromatic chromatin and easily discernible, prominent nucleoli. The grade assigned is based on the most histologically abnormal area present, even if it is only focal.
[b]Evaluate 10 high-power fields in the area of the greatest mitotic activity in each of five slides or a total of 50 high-power fields in fewer slides.
[c]Diffuse = patternless sheets of cells. Nests, cords, or trabeculae are considered nondiffuse.

with an increasingly poor outcome. The latter may not be surprising, since as has been shown, many of the Weiss components including high mitotic rate, tumor necrosis, atypical mitosis, capsular, venous, and adjacent organ invasion, as well as nuclear grade are adverse predictors of tumor-related mortality in a univariate analysis (14).

TREATMENT CONSIDERATIONS: SURGICAL MANAGEMENT

Although surgery is the only potentially curative therapy for ACC, chemotherapy, radiology-guided ablation, and possibly radiotherapy have treatment roles, and management of most patients with ACC requires a multidisciplinary approach, both at presentation and at relapse (15). At presentation, the focus should be on securing a qualified surgical oncologist to perform an open resection that removes all tumors (16). Patients with *incidentalomas* that appear almost certainly benign by imaging can have their adenomas resected laparoscopically. However, tumor seeding at the time of laparoscopy occurs unpredictably and at an unacceptably high rate, even in the hands of experienced surgeons, and in patients with a high suspicion of malignancy, a laparoscopic intervention is not defensible. The role of postoperative irradiation to the surgical field is not resolved, although more recent studies claim high response rates in residual tumor, with little toxicity (17). Thus, pending better data, postoperative radiation should be administered sparingly since it may make a subsequent re-operation technically more difficult. It may be better reserved for a select group of patients after a second or subsequent re-operation.

Even in the hands of a highly skilled surgeon, the most frequent site of recurrence is the adrenal bed. If "sufficient" time has elapsed since the primary resection, a re-operation may be indicated—acknowledging the value of this approach is difficult to estimate since most comparisons are historical and nonrandomized. The "no-surgery cohorts" are likely those with more aggressive disease, not amenable to re-operation. It is also difficult to quantify the benefit of sequential metastasectomies. Admittedly, all published studies are biased in that patients with better prognoses undergo repeated operations. However, the existing literature has convinced most physicians managing patients with metastatic ACC to take an aggressive surgical posture, hoping that it may prolong survival (18).

TREATMENT CONSIDERATIONS: MEDICAL MANAGEMENT

Hypercortisolism should be managed aggressively prior to any surgical intervention or concurrently with systemic chemotherapy. Although control of hormone production may not be possible in most patients, aggressive management may achieve partial or, rarely, complete inhibition of ectopic hormone production. Treatment of hormonal excess should not be delayed even if chemotherapy is planned. Inhibitors of steroid synthesis singly or in combination should be used (6). Mitotane, the cornerstone of any strategy, should be started as soon as possible after the diagnosis is made, with an initial dose of 2 g/day, and gradually increasing to the highest tolerable dose (usually 16 g or less given in 4 divided daily doses). Steady-state levels will not be reached for months. Most patients find mitotane difficult to tolerate, due to anorexia, nausea, lethargy, and dermatitis. Alternative strategies include ketoconazole, an inhibitor of steroid synthesis that can rapidly reduce cortisol production. If ketoconazole is unsuccessful or not tolerated, metyrapone can be used alone or in combination with ketoconazole. In patients unable to take oral medications, an intravenous infusion or bolus of etomidate can be used. With all the above medications, cortisol levels must be monitored, replacing hydrocortisone and mineralocorticoids as needed; patients should wear a bracelet or necklace that will alert emergency personnel to the possibility of adrenal insufficiency.

In addition to its anti-hormonal properties mitotane has measurable antitumor activity in ACC and has been used in patients with locally advanced or metastatic ACC, as well as in the adjuvant setting (6). Even if the extent of tumor reduction is modest, its use should be continued until there is clear evidence of tumor progression. Measurable antitumor activity has been correlated with serum mitotane levels greater than 10–14 mg/l; patients who tolerate lower levels should be continued on therapy (19). It is unclear whether mitotane should be used as an adjuvant after surgical resection. A retrospective non-randomized study reported a better outcome for those receiving adjuvant mitotane, but this benefit was confined to time to recurrence and did not extend to overall survival (20). Most clinicians would agree adjuvant mitotane therapy should be used in patients with large tumors that have many of the features that comprise the Weiss score or if at surgery margins were inadequate or involved with tumor.

For patients in whom surgery is not possible, or in those who experience metastatic disease not amenable to surgical resection or radiology-guided ablation, chemotherapy is indicated. A recently reported randomized trial of 304 patients with advanced ACC compared mitotane plus either a combination of etoposide, doxorubicin, and cisplatin (EDP-mitotane) every 4 weeks or single-agent streptozocin (streptozotocin) every 3 weeks (21). Patients in the EDP-mitotane group had a significantly higher response rate than those in the streptozocin-mitotane group (23.2% vs. 9.2%, $P < 0.001$) and longer median progression-free survival (5.0 months vs. 2.1 months; hazard ratio, 0.55; 95% confidence interval [CI], 0.43–0.69; $P < 0.001$) but not improved overall survival. The results are generally accepted as showing the superiority of EDP-M as first-line therapy. While streptozocin is often used as second-line therapy, new and better therapies are needed.

CONCLUSION

Physicians who treat patients with a diagnosis of ACC will find that reducing the tumor burden and achieving eucortisolism are both very difficult. In a majority of patients with symptoms of hypercortisolism, total control of symptoms cannot be achieved with mitotane or other drugs that suppress cortisol production. At the time of presentation but especially when disease progression occurs, physicians must recognize that uncontrolled hormone production by an ACC has severe consequences. Repeated surgical removal of bulk metastases may palliate symptoms and improve quality of life but is rarely curative. Radiation therapy has unproven benefit as an adjuvant to surgery. Chemotherapy may have useful activity for patients with metastatic disease and progressing on mitotane.

REFERENCES

1. Roman S. Adrenocortical carcinoma. *Curr Opin Oncol.* 2006; 18: 36–42.

2. Arlt W, Biehl M, Taylor AE, et al. Urine steroid metabolomics as a biomarker and tool for detecting malignancy in adrenal tumors. *J Clin Endocrinol Metab.* 2011; 96: 3775–3784.

3. Abiven G, Coste J, Groussin L, et al. Clinical and biological features in the prognosis of adrenocortical cancer: poor outcome of cortisol-secreting tumors in a series of 202 consecutive patients. *J Clin Endocrinol Metab.* 2006; 91: 2650–2655.

4. Terzolo M, Angeli A, Fassnacht M, et al. Adjuvant mitotane treatment for adrenocortical carcinoma. *N Engl J Med.* 2007; 356: 2372–2380.

5. Mazzuco TL, Durand J, Chapman A, et al. Genetic aspects of adrenocortical tumours and hyperplasias. *Clin Endocrinol (Oxf).* 2012; 77: 1–10.

6. Veytsman I, Nieman L, Fojo T. Management of endocrine manifestations and the use of mitotane as a chemotherapeutic agent for adrenocortical carcinoma. *Clin Oncol.* 2009; 27: 4619–4629.

7. Ribeiro RC, Sandrini F, Figueiredo B, et al. An inherited p53 mutation that contributes in a tissue-specific manner to pediatric adrenal cortical carcinoma. *Proc Natl Acad Sci USA.* 2001; 98: 9330–9335.

8. Figueiredo BC, Sandrini R, Zambetti, GP, et al. Penetrance of adrenocortical tumours associated with the germline TP53 R337H mutation. *J Med Genet.* 2006; 43: 91–96.

9. Outwater EK, Siegelman ES, Huang AB, et al. Adrenal masses: correlation between CT attenuation value and chemical shift ratio at MR imaging with in-phase and opposed-phase sequences. *Radiology.* 1996; 200: 749–752.

10. Groussin L, Bonardel G, Silvera S, et al. 18F-fluorodeoxyglucose positron emission tomography for the diagnosis of adrenocortical tumors: a prospective study in 77 operated patients. *J Clin Endocrinol Metab.* 2009; 94: 1713–1722.

11. Fassnacht M, Johanssen S, Quinkler M, et al. Limited prognostic value of the 2004 International Union Against Cancer staging classification for adrenocortical carcinoma: proposal for a revised TNM classification. *Cancer.* 2009; 115: 243–250.

12. Lughezzani G, Sun M, Perrotte P, et al. The European Network for the Study of Adrenal Tumors staging system is prognostically superior to the International Union Against Cancer staging system: a North American validation. *Eur J Cancer.* 2010; 46: 713–719.

13. Lau SK, Weiss LM. The Weiss system for evaluating adrenocortical neoplasms: 25 years later. *Hum Pathol.* 2009; 40: 757–768.

14. Stojadinovic A, Ghossein RA, Hoos A, et al. Adrenocortical carcinoma: clinical, morphologic, and molecular characterization. *J Clin Oncol.* 2002; 20: 941–950.

15. Balasubramaniam S, Fojo T. Practical considerations in the evaluation and management of adrenocortical cancer. *Semin Oncol.* 2010: 37: 619–626.

16. Gaujoux S, Brennan MF. Recommendation for standardized surgical management of primary adrenocortical carcinoma. *Surgery.* 2012; 152: 123–132.

17. Fassnacht M, Hahner S, Polat B, et al. Efficacy of adjuvant radiotherapy of the tumor bed on local recurrence of adrenocortical carcinoma. *J Clin Endocrinol Metab.* 2006; 91: 4501–4504.

18. Datrice NM, Langan RC, Ripley RT, et al. Operative management for recurrent and metastatic adrenocortical carcinoma. *J Surg Oncol.* 2012; 105: 709–713.

19. Baudin E, Pellegriti G, Bonnay M, et al. Impact of monitoring plasma 1,1-dichlorodiphenildichloroethane (o,p'DDD) levels on the treatment of patients with adrenocortical carcinoma. *Cancer.* 2001; 92: 1385–1392.

20. Terzolo M, Angeli A, Fassnacht M, et al. Adjuvant mitotane treatment for adrenocortical carcinoma. *N Engl J Med.* 2007; 356: 2372–2380.

21. Fassnacht M, Terzolo M, Allolio B, et al. FIRM-ACT Study Group. Combination chemotherapy in advanced adrenocortical carcinoma. *N Engl J Med.* 2012; 366: 2189–2197.

22. Fuhrman SA, Lasky LC, Limas C. Prognostic significance of morphologic parameters in renal cell carcinoma. *Am J Surg Pathol.* 1982; 6: 655–663.

CHAPTER **67**
Head and Neck Cancer

Lori J. Wirth, Paul M. Busse, Daniel Deschler

INTRODUCTION

Cancers of the head and neck are composed of a spectrum of malignant neoplasms. Most commonly, however, "head and neck cancer" refers to epithelial carcinomas, squamous cell cancers, and their variant histologic subtypes that arise from the mucosal surfaces of the upper aerodigestive tract and constitute over 85% of the cancers encountered in this region. Those caring for patients with head and neck neoplasms must be conversant with the variable natural histories and approaches to treatment for the many different malignant tumors that arise within this region.

Cancers of the head and neck are traditionally divided into nine distinct anatomic regions from which mucosal cancers originate (Table 67-1). Other neoplastic conditions can arise within these regions and associated areas, such as the base of skull, orbit, and neck itself, including primary tumors of the major or minor salivary glands, the skin, the thyroid or parathyroid glands, and nonepithelial tissues of the neck. Sarcomas and hematologic malignancies are also encountered in the head and neck region. Representative histopathologies encountered in clinical practice are recorded in Table 67-2. This chapter will focus on the most common cancer of the region, namely squamous cell carcinoma of the head and neck (SCCHN).

INCIDENCE AND PREVALENCE

The American Cancer Society estimates that there will be 56,000 new cases of head and neck cancer in the United States in 2013 (excluding thyroid cancers). While head and neck cancer is one of the more curable adult malignancies, the impact of this disease on individuals and society is significant, as it is not measured solely by the low absolute mortality, but also by the acute and chronic functional, cosmetic, and psychological morbidities experienced by patients. Head and neck cancer remains a difficult disease associated with significant rates of both morbidity and mortality.

Surveillance Epidemiology and End Results (SEER) data show that the incidence of head and neck cancer decreased from 1976 to 2009 in a pattern that approximates declines seen for lung cancer. These parallel changes follow the decline in tobacco use. However encouraging these data, several sobering facts must be noted.

For one, significant race-based differences exist in the incidence of head and neck cancer and its treatment outcomes. Not only do head and neck cancers occur with greater frequency in African-Americans compared to Whites, but also there are even greater differences in survival. For example,

TABLE 67-1 HEAD AND NECK PRIMARY SITES

Oral cavity	Mobile tongue to circumvallate papillae, floor of mouth, alveolar ridge, hard palate, and buccal mucosa
Pharynx (3 subsites)	
Nasopharynx	From base of skull to dorsum of soft palate, to choanae of nasal cavities, laterally extending to Eustachian tubes
Oropharynx	From the palatine arches to posterior pharyngeal wall, including soft palate, uvula, and base of tongue, extending inferiorly to larynx
Hypopharynx	Pharyngeal walls posterior and lateral to larynx, including pyriform sinuses
Larynx (3 subsites)	
Supraglottis	Laryngeal structures above true vocal cords, including epiglottis, arytenoids, aryepiglottic folds, false cords, and laryngeal vestibules
Glottis	Restricted to true vocal cords
Subglottis	Larynx below true vocal cords, extending inferiorly 5 mm to cricoid cartilage
Nasal cavity	Nasal vestibule, nasal septum, nasal turbinates, extending to maxillary wall laterally and hard palate inferiorly
Paranasal sinuses	Frontal, sphenoid, ethmoid, and maxillary sinuses

TABLE 67-2 HEAD AND NECK NEOPLASMS

Commonly encountered
- Epithelial lesions:
  - Squamous cell carcinoma arising in the oral cavity, oropharynx, larynx, hypopharynx, nasopharynx, and sinonasal region.
    - Oropharyngeal squamous cell carcinomas are frequently associated with HPV.
    - Nasopharyngeal carcinomas are frequently associated with EBV. WHO type I are well-differentiated, and less often EBV-associated. WHO type II are moderately differentiated. WHO type III are undifferentiated.
  - Premalignant lesions, characterized by dysplasia that may be mild, moderate, or severe, or carcinoma in situ.
  - Squamous papillomas and other verrucous lesions

(*continued*)

TABLE 67-2 HEAD AND NECK NEOPLASMS (CONTINUED)

- Thyroid and parathyroid cancers
  - Differentiated thyroid cancer
    - Papillary thyroid carcinoma, Hurthle cell carcinoma, follicular thyroid carcinomas, and variants
    - Anaplastic thyroid carcinoma
    - Medullary thyroid carcinoma
    - Parathyroid adenoma and carcinoma
  - Salivary gland tumors
    - Pleomorphic adenoma
    - Warthin's tumor
    - Mucoepidermoid carcinoma
    - Adenoid cystic carcinoma
    - Acinic cell carcinoma
    - Salivary duct carcinoma
    - Carcinoma ex-pleomorphic adenoma
    - Adenocarcinoma

Infrequently encountered
- Neuroendocrine tumors, more frequently arising in sinonasal region
  - Small cell carcinoma
- Esthesioneuroblastoma, arises from cribriform plate
- Paraganglioma arising in the neck or skull base
- Schwannoma
- Merkel cell carcinoma
- Mucosal melanoma, most frequently arising in nasal cavity
- Hematolgoic malignancies
  - Non-Hodgkin lymphoma
  - Hodgkin's disease
  - Plasmacytoma
  - Extranodal NK/T-cell lymphoma, nasal type
- Sarcomas
  - Soft tissue sarcoma
    - Rhabdomyosarcoma, predominantly in children
    - Malignant peripheral nerve sheath tumor
  - Osteosarcoma, including periorbital region in retinoblastoma
- Primary tumors of the mandible
  - Odontogenic tumor
  - Ameloblastoma
  - Squamous cell carcinoma

one large analysis of more than 20,000 patients treated for head and neck cancer in Florida from 1998 to 2002 showed that African-American race and poverty are independent predictors of poor prognosis, even when controlling for demographics, comorbidities, clinical characteristics, and treatment approach (1).

A second remarkable trend that is currently transforming the field of head and neck cancer is a dramatic increase in the incidence of oropharyngeal squamous cell carcinomas. In fact, SEER registries have shown an annual increase in oropharyngeal cancers of 0.80% in the period from 1973 to 2004 in the United States. Further analysis of SEER data indicates that this trend is due to a major increase in the prevalence of human papillomavirus (HPV) in oropharyngeal cancers, even while smoking-related cancers are declining. This increase in oropharyngeal cancers is most notable in white men, and in people from the most recent birth cohorts studied, that is, people born in 1940s and 1950s. From 1988 to 2004, the incidence of HPV-associated oropharyngeal cancers climbed 225%, whereas HPV-negative oropharyngeal cancers declined in the same period by 50% (2). Should this trend continue, it is estimated that the number of HPV-associated oropharyngeal cancers will outstrip those of cervical cancers by the year 2020, and account for the majority of head and neck cancers by 2030. The reason behind the increase in incidence is most likely changing sexual behaviors in our population, with an increase in oral sex and oral HPV exposure over time. In fact, the prevalence of HPV infection in the U.S. population at present is approximately 7%. Prevalence is greater in men and independently associated with both the number of lifetime sexual partners and smoking (3). It is currently not known if routine HPV vaccination will be effective in the primary prevention of HPV-associated oropharyngeal cancers. Still, it is hoped that HPV vaccination, as recommended for females aged 9–26 years and males aged 9–21 to reduce anogenital malignancy and genital warts, will further mitigate the impact of HPV-related malignancy by reducing the incidence of HPV-associated oropharyngeal cancers in our population. Embedded in the bad news of the increasing incidence of HPV-associated oropharyngeal cancers is the good news that these cancers are, stage-for-stage, more curable than HPV-negative oropharyngeal cancers. To date, the largest study examining the outcomes of HPV-associated versus HPV-negative oropharyngeal cancers was performed by Ang and colleagues (4). They examined outcomes of patients enrolled in the Radiation Therapy Oncology Group 0129 study investigating accelerated-fractionated radiotherapy versus standard-fractionated radiotherapy with concurrent cisplatin chemotherapy in patients with locally advanced SCCHN, and found that patients with HPV-associated oropharyngeal cancers had better 3-year overall survival (82%) than those with HPV-negative disease (57%).

RISK FACTORS FOR HEAD AND NECK CANCER

Tobacco and alcohol remain important risk factors for this disease. The local effects of tobacco and alcohol carcinogens are both dose-dependent and synergistic. Ever-smokers are at an increased risk for SCCHN even at relatively low exposures, whereas among never-smokers, alcohol increases the risk of SCCHN only at high doses (i.e., three or more drinks/day).

Importantly, tobacco use also influences outcomes of HPV-associated SCCHN, increasing the risk of recurrence, distant metastasis, and death in this otherwise good-prognostic disease. Smokeless tobacco abuse results in a local exposure to carcinogens that promotes cancers of the oral cavity and to a lesser extent, the oropharynx, though the effect of smokeless tobacco alone is difficult to isolate as this form of tobacco is often used in combination with other products, such as betel nut, quid, slaked lime, and areca nut.

In addition to HPV, exposure to Epstein–Barr virus (EBV) is also associated with head and neck cancer. For both viruses, transient infection without long-term sequelae is common. Persistence of the viral genome and induction of malignant transformation is a rare event. While HPV is primarily associated with SCCHN of the oropharynx, (i.e., the tonsil and base of tongue tissues), EBV is associated with nasopharyngeal cancers. Nasopharyngeal cancer is rare in the United States and Europe, whereas nasopharyngeal cancer is endemic in Southern China, and seen with an intermediate incidence in Southeast Asia, the Mediterranean Basin, and the Arctic. EBV is a herpesvirus that is nearly ubiquitous worldwide. Most people infected with EBV will not, of course, develop cancer. Nonetheless, EBV viral proteins can have growth-transforming activity, and it is thought that disruption of the viral protein/host immune balance by modulation of the immune response can lead to the development of EBV-associated nasopharyngeal cancer.

Leukoplakia and erythroplakia are premalignant oral cavity lesions associated with a risk for transformation to in-situ and invasive cancers. Leukoplakia is a white, lacey-appearing lesion that may be posttraumatic and nondysplastic, with a low probability of malignant transformation. Persistent leukoplakia does, however, have malignant potential and should be sampled, preferably by excisional biopsy. Erythroplakia is a red lesion that harbors a greater malignant potential. This lesion should be surgically removed upon discovery. Not all patients with oral premalignant lesions will go on to develop an oral cancer. Clinical features that increase the risk of cancer include older age, lesions on the lateral or ventral tongue, and high-grade dysplasia. Molecular features associated with malignant transformation include increased epidermal growth factor receptor (EGFR) gene copy number and other genetic changes identified by gene expression profiling.

Lastly, one of the most important risk factors for developing SCCHN is having already had one. Compared to the general population, head and neck cancer survivors, particularly those with histories of tobacco and alcohol use, are at a significantly greater risk of developing a second aerodigestive tract primary malignancy, which occurs at a rate of approximately 2% per year. This has implications on both screening and risk modification for the long-term follow-up of SCCHN survivors.

MOLECULAR BIOLOGY AND NATURAL HISTORY

■ MOLECULAR BIOLOGY

Several recent advances in the molecular biology of SCCHN have led to new understandings of the pathogenesis of the disease, as well as new treatment strategies. EGFR is overexpressed in the majority of SCCHNs. Activation of this receptor tyrosine kinase (RTK) upregulates signaling pathways involved in proliferation, angiogenesis, invasion, and metastasis. As predicted by these mechanisms, EGFR overexpression correlates with poor prognosis and is thus an attractive therapeutic target. Indeed, two therapeutic strategies are available for targeting EGFR. Small molecule EGFR inhibitors, such as gefitinib and erlotinib, that target the intracellular RTK ATP-binding domain have been studied in SCCHN, yielding disappointing results, likely due to the absence of EGFR-activating mutations in SCCHN. Monoclonal antibodies, including cetuximab, which bind to EGFR's extracellular ligand-binding domain, have also been studied. While modest single-agent activity has been demonstrated in recurrent/metastatic SCCHN, an international phase III study comparing radiotherapy alone to cetuximab plus radiotherapy for definitive treatment of locally advanced SCCHN showed a 20-month improvement in median overall survival with the addition of cetuximab to radiotherapy (5). Cetuximab added to palliative chemotherapy for recurrent/metastatic SCCHN also improves outcomes compared to chemotherapy alone (6).

Further strides in our understanding of the biologic underpinnings of SCCHN were made by whole-exome sequencing of more than 100 SCCHN tumors carried out by two groups (7, 8). Several key findings were shared by these two studies. First, both confirmed the critical roles played by the previously identified tumor suppressor pathways governed by p53 and RB/INK4/ARF. Mutation in the tumor suppressor gene, *TP53,* was the most common alteration found, occurring in more approximately 50% of tumors. Rb pathway involvement was evidenced by frequent inactivation of *CDKN2A,* which encodes the cell cycle regulators p16/INK4 and p14/Arf/INK4B. *CDKN2A* mutations were found in approximately 10% of tumors, and additional tumors harbored copy number losses. Both groups further identified novel mutations in *NOTCH1* in approximately 15% of tumors. While activating mutations in *NOTCH* family members have been implicated in hematologic malignancies, these studies detected inactivating mutations, suggesting a tumor suppressor role for the gene in SCCHN. Notch signaling has been linked to multiple functions, including terminal differentiation in squamous epithelium. While molecular targeting of tumor suppressor pathways remains an unmet challenge in oncology, approaches that target activating mutations in other signaling pathways have met with greater success. To this end, alterations in the PI3K signaling pathway have also been identified in SCCHN. Six to eight percent of tumors were found to have *PIK3CA* mutations, while *PTEN,* which encodes a negative regulator of the pathway, is subject to frequent loss of heterozygosity in SCCHN. This PI3K pathway activation in SCCHN has exciting clinical implications given the multiple agents that inhibit this pathway currently being investigated in clinical trials.

■ NATURAL HISTORY

Squamous cell cancers of the head and neck are occasionally discovered during routine dental examination. More commonly, they are discovered after weeks to months of nonspecific, vague symptoms arising from the primary site, such as sore throat, dysphagia, otalgia, nasal congestion, or bleeding. Alternatively, many patients will present with isolated cervical adenopathy.

Such patients are often treated empirically for infection, and discovered to have head and neck cancer only later when the adenopathy does not resolve and the primary physician or a surgical consultant consequently performs a detailed examination of the head and neck region or biopsy of the neck mass.

The AJCC TNM staging system is used to define the extent of disease, and the majority of SCCHNs are locally advanced stage III or IVa/b at presentation. Distant metastatic disease at initial presentation is unusual, and symptomatic disease related to such is rarely seen. The AJCC TNM staging system has great clinical value, but it is understandably complex given the many anatomic subdivisions of the head and neck region, each with its own unique definition of T stage. N stage and the combined overall TNM stage are consistent for all mucosal sites, except in the case of nasopharyngeal cancer.

A site-specific review of the common presenting symptoms, natural history, and treatment of head and neck cancer is beyond the scope of this text. In general, squamous cell cancers of the head and neck region are locally aggressive and carry a moderate risk of spread to regional lymph nodes, but have a low probability of spread to more distant sites. This natural history has several site-specific exceptions. For example, certain primary sites are more likely associated with regional disease at presentation (e.g., the nasopharnyx, hypopharynx, base of tongue, and supraglottic larynx). In contrast, other sites have a relatively low risk for regional spread (e.g., paranasal sinuses and small true vocal cord primaries).

STANDARD EVALUATION AND TREATMENT

EVALUATION

It is important to obtain a surgical evaluation for patients with signs or symptoms relating to possible cancer in head and neck region. Depending on the setting, the initial interaction may be with a general surgeon or an otolaryngologist. Regardless of the specialty, the ultimate evaluation, diagnosis, staging, and follow-up must be undertaken by an otolaryngologist with sufficient training and expertise to achieve the following tasks.

A complete physical examination should include inspection of all visible mucosal surfaces of the head and neck including indirect mirror or fiberoptic laryngoscopy, as well as palpation of the floor of mouth, tongue and tonsil regions, and neck. Obvious tumor masses should be identified, along with potential second primary lesions and premalignant lesions. Suspicious lesions should be defined by primary site, extent of local involvement, and overall size. Associated cervical adenopathy should be assessed and if enlarged, the regional extent of disease should be quantified for staging purposes. Independent of whether surgical resection will be deemed appropriate, the potential for resection of suspected primary site and neck lesions should be determined. For example, lesions of the lateral tongue are often resectable while those of the nasopharynx or posterior pharyngeal wall are not. Neck lesions fixed to deep tissues or surrounding the carotid artery are not resectable.

In addition to physical examination, staging workup often includes computed tomography (CT) and/or magnetic resonance imaging (MRI) of the neck to characterize the extent of the disease. Patients with large T4 lesions or significant (>N1) lymph node involvement should also undergo chest CT to screen for distant metastases. PET/CT imaging is frequently performed, but is not always considered to be an essential component of the initial workup. One current important limitation to this modality is the lack of IV contrast available for the CT portion of the study, which is critical to evaluating the extent of both the primary lesion and nodal disease.

Examination under anesthesia is a key aspect of definitive staging for the majority of SCCHNs. Examination under anesthesia may include laryngoscopy, esophagoscopy, and bronchoscopy (a.k.a. triple endoscopy). During this procedure, biopsies are obtained to pathologically confirm a primary diagnosis, to define the extent of primary site disease, and to identify additional premalignant lesions or second primary cancers. An accurate description of anatomical involvement is critical to clinical staging as well to determining the expected morbidity of initial surgical resection.

Of special consideration is the evaluation of a neck mass of unknown origin. Supraclavicular neck disease should raise the question of a primary thoracic or thyroidal cancer, or perhaps an intra-abdominal cancer in the case of a left-sided supraclavicular lesion. Higher neck lesions are more likely to represent spread from a primary lesion in head and neck, including a possible cutaneous primary. Pathological confirmation of a squamous malignancy metastatic to a lymph node can usually be achieved by fine needle aspiration (FNA). A neck mass suspicious for regional metastatic disease can be approached by FNA if a potential primary mucosal abnormality of the upper aerodigestive tract or a salivary gland is not identified by a thorough physical examination. FNA specimens may also be sent for HPV and EBV analysis to potentially localize the primary site to the oropharynx or nasopharynx, respectively. Should an FNA prove inconclusive, an excisional nodal biopsy may be appropriate. In this case, consideration may be given to an immediate neck dissection at the time of this biopsy if frozen section indicates SCCHN or another nonlymphomatous malignancy. Such a neck dissection may assist in the control of extracapsular spread and additional malignant adenopathy, if present. However tempting, an incisional nodal biopsy should be avoided as it may compromise subsequent treatment and is associated with a lower probability of disease control.

■ PRINCIPLES OF TREATMENT

General Principles

Once a patient's primary diagnosis is established and initial staging studies are complete, secondary referrals are made to radiation and medical oncology, if not already done. The application of modern multidisciplinary treatments requires early input for all potential care providers. A team approach to care is clearly superior, and the team commonly includes head and neck cancer nurses, a speech and swallow therapist, a nutritionist, a social worker, and maxillofacial prosthodontist, among others.

As head and neck cancers differ greatly in locoregional stage and primary site, a detailed review of treatment options is beyond the scope of this chapter. However, a standard approach to treatment can be related. In general, all patients with untreated locoregional head and neck cancer are considered potentially curable if there is no evidence for distant metastatic disease.

Treatment decisions begin with an understanding of primary site extent and a decision as to whether the lesion is resectable (removable with a high probability of negative surgical margins). If a lesion is resectable, careful consideration must be given to the specific morbidity that would result from curative surgical resection. With few exceptions, primary lesions that are resectable with acceptable morbidity may benefit from primary resection; however, this varies by site and stage. Lesions that are classically unresectable (e.g., sinonasal lesions involving the skull base and lesions of the nasopharynx, posterior pharyngeal wall or encasing the carotid artery), or for which primary surgery would have significant morbidity (e.g., base of tongue necessitating total glossectomy) are typically approached with primary radiation plus concurrent chemotherapy. Exceptions to this general approach exist. For example, cancers of the hypopharynx and larynx are usually resectable, but chemoradiation is often offered as primary therapy in an effort to avoid laryngectomy and preserve the natural voice. In this case, laryngectomy is reserved for persistent or recurrent disease after radiation or in the primary setting of advanced disease with significant laryngeal destruction precluding acceptable posttreatment function. The oropharynx is another "resectable" site that is often suitable for an organ preservation approach, especially as HPV-related SCCHN is uniquely sensitive to radiation, although recent advances in transoral laser microsurgery and robotic surgery have renewed interest in upfront surgery for oropharyngeal cancer.

Regional nodal disease from head and neck cancer is strategically approached as a separate entity. With rare exception, all patients with defined nodal disease should receive radiation therapy, either before or after resection of the involved nodes. Traditionally, patients underwent neck dissection when nodal disease was advanced and not fixed to underlying structures. Exceptions include patients with nasopharyngeal cancers, which are uniquely sensitive to radiation, and patients with large unresectable primary site lesions who will be treated with definitive chemoradiation because of the extent of primary site involvement.

Advances in the multidisciplinary care of patients with chemotherapy have altered the historic paradigms for treating patients with head and neck cancer. For example, concurrent chemoradiotherapy has replaced traditional surgery and postoperative radiation for advanced lesions of the sites with high associated surgical morbidity, such as the hypopharynx, larynx, and oropharynx.

Management of metastatic cervical lesions has also changed with advances in chemoradiotherapy. Currently, the decision to resect regional nodes is often deferred pending reevaluation after definitive nonsurgical treatment with chemoradiotherapy. Patients whose regional disease has completely regressed on physical examination and imaging after combined chemoradiotherapy appear to have excellent outcomes with minimal to no added benefit from additional neck surgery. Should residual disease in the neck remain after chemoradiotherapy, salvage neck dissection should be undertaken.

Management of Limited Head and Neck Cancer

About one-third of patients present with limited T1 or T2 cancers without associated lymph node involvement or distant disease (stage I–II disease).

In general, these patients can be treated by a single modality, either surgery or radiation therapy alone, and have a projected 5-year survival of 70%–90%. Radiation doses range from 6600 to 7200 cGy, depending upon the site and stage. Comprehensive radiation treatment to the primary site and regional lymphatics carries a high risk of chronic morbidities such as mild to moderate xerostomia, dental decay, and mild dysphagia; and a low risk for more severe complications such as osteonecrosis of the mandible, chondronecrosis of the larynx, or accelerated atherosclerosis of the carotid artery.

Definitive surgical resection of limited cancers is preferred in several settings. For example, limited oral cavity lesions can often be resected with minimal impact on speech and swallowing. In this setting, patients often undergo primary site resection with a staging neck dissection for identification and treatment of possible occult spread to regional nodes. Indications for postoperative radiation include close or positive primary site margins, perineural spread, lymphovascular disease, or regional nodal involvement on the staging neck dissection. Positive primary site margins and/or extracapsular extension are clearly established high-risk features that warrant the addition of chemotherapy to adjuvant radiation.

Management of Locoregionally Advanced Cancer

More than half of all patients with head and neck cancer present with locoregionally advanced disease (stage III or IV disease with a T3 or T4 primary lesion and/or regional nodal metastases). In the absence of distant metastatic disease, such patients are also treated with curative intent. In the following sections, we outline options for combined modality regimens for locoregionally advanced disease.

Surgery followed by postoperative radiation ± chemotherapy When surgery is performed for stage III/IV disease, evidence from two randomized trials provides the basis for optimal postoperative treatment (9, 10). Both trials compared standard postoperative radiation to radiation plus 3 cycles of concurrent cisplatin in patients at high-risk for recurrence (i.e., positive margins at the primary site, perineural or lymphovascular spread of disease, multiple involved regional lymph nodes, or extracapsular extension of disease in the neck). While the toxicity of concurrent chemotherapy with radiation was greater than that seen with radiation alone, chemoradiotherapy was associated with improved locoregional control in both studies, improved overall survival in one trial, and a trend toward improved survival in the second. At this time, postoperative radiation is standard for all patients with resected stage III or IV head and neck cancer. Patients at high risk for locoregional relapse despite surgery should be considered for postoperative chemoradiotherapy. Ongoing clinical trials seek to identify additional radiation sensitizers (chemotherapy, anticancer antibodies, or small molecule inhibitors) that will enhance the effects of radiation to degrees similar or greater than cisplatin, but with less toxicity.

Definitive radiation with concurrent chemotherapy For the patient with locally advanced SCCHN, an alternative approach to primary site surgery is that of definitive radiation with concurrent chemotherapy. In this setting, primary site preservation is one of the therapeutic endpoints, and surgery is reserved for the salvage of recurrent or persistent disease after chemoradiotherapy. Multiple randomized trials have proven the validity of this approach (Table 67-3). Definitive standard fractionation radiation with concurrent high-dose cisplatin administered every 21 days is the regimen most frequently studied in SCCHN. However, additional chemotherapy regimens are commonly used during the typically 7-week course of radiation, such as cisplatin administered weekly, cisplatin with 5-flurouracil (5FU), carboplatin with 5FU, and weekly carboplatin and paclitaxel.

Another option for drug sensitization during radiotherapy has received FDA approval. Cetuximab is a chimeric IgG1a monoclonal antibody targeting EGFR, overexpressed in the majority of squamous cancers. In a phase III

TABLE 67-3 SELECTED RANDOMIZED TRIALS OF CHEMORADIOTHERAPY VERSUS RADIATION

Study	Treatment	Overall Survival (%)	Locoregional Control (%)
Jeremic, *Radiother Oncol*, 1997	RT	5Y: 15	5Y: 27
	RT + cisplatin	5Y: 32	5Y: 51
Brizel, *N Engl J Med*, 1998	Bid RT	3Y: 34	3Y: 41
	Bid RT + cis/5FU	3Y: 55	3Y: 61
Wendt, *J Clin Oncol*, 1998	Bid RT	3Y: 24	3Y: 17
	Bid RT + cis/5FU	3Y: 49	3Y: 36
Staar, *Int J Radiat Oncol Biol Phys*, 2001	RT	2Y: 39	2Y: 45
	RT + carbo/5FU	2Y: 48	2Y: 51
Adelstein, *J Clin Oncol*, 2002	RT	3Y: 23	NA
	RT + cisplatin	3Y: 35	NA
	RT + cis/5FU (alternating)	3Y: 27	NA
Denis, *J Clin Oncol*, 2004	RT	5Y: 16	5Y: 25
	RT + carbo/5FU	5Y: 22	5Y: 48
Bonner, *N Engl J Med*, 2006	RT	3Y: 45	3Y: 34
	RT + cetuximab	3Y: 55	3Y: 47
Ang, *ASCO*, 2011	RT (6 weeks) + cis	2Y: 80	NA
	RT (6 weeks) + cis + cetuximab	2Y: 83	NA

study, concurrent cetuximab with radiation improved locoregional control and overall survival by 20 months compared to radiation alone (5). Of note, the magnitude of improvement in survival with cetuximab compared to radiotherapy alone was similar to that seen in trials of concurrent chemotherapy and radiation versus radiation alone. That said, there has never been a trial comparing concurrent cetuximab plus radiotherapy to the standard of care for locoregionally advanced SCCHN. Therefore it is not known whether cetuximab plus radiotherapy is at least equivalent in efficacy to chemoradiotherapy in SCCHN. Further study of cetuximab in the curative setting for locally advanced SCCHN investigated the addition of cetuximab to cisplatin-based chemoradiotherapy in RTOG 0522 (11). This study randomized 895 patients with stage III-IV SCCHN to receive cetuximab plus cisplatin-based chemoradiotherapy versus cisplatin-based chemoradiotherapy alone. Patients in the cetuximab arm did experience more mucositis and dermatitis than those in the control arm, but neither progression-free nor overall survival improved.

The role of induction chemotherapy in SCCHN Historically, 40%–60% of patients with locoregionally advanced head and neck cancer were rendered disease-free by treatment and enjoyed good rates of long-term survival. Prior to the current era of combined modality approaches to SCCHN, locoregional relapse was the most common pattern of failure. Recent trials involving concurrent chemoradiotherapy have, however, shown a reversal in the traditional pattern of relapse such that distant metastases are now more common than locoregional failures.

This observation rekindled interest in the use of induction chemotherapy prior to chemoradiotherapy, in order to maximize treatment aimed at the potential presence of micrometastatic disease. Effective induction chemotherapy has the potential to downsize locoregional disease prior to definitive treatment, as well. Two randomized phase III studies further benefit from the incorporation of induction chemotherapy to definitive treatment in SCCHN (12, 13). Both studies investigated the addition of docetaxel to the prior standard induction regimen of cisplatin plus 5-FU in locally advanced SCCHN, and showed that the addition of the third drug was associated with an improvement in 3-year overall survival of 11% to 14%. Neither study, however, included a chemoradiotherapy alone arm. Thus, while it is clear that docetaxel, cisplatin, and 5-FU is the superior induction regimen, there was no definitive evidence that induction chemotherapy followed by chemoradiotherapy is superior to chemoradiotherapy alone. This question was investigated by two subsequent phase III studies of chemoradiotherapy with or without preceding induction of docetaxel, cisplatin, and 5-FU (14, 15). Both studies were terminated prior to enrollment of the originally planned full cohort and data are presently available only in abstract form, thus final conclusions cannot be drawn. Still, neither study showed a survival benefit to the addition of induction chemotherapy over chemoradiotherapy alone.

Management of recurrent or metastatic disease Up to 10% of patients will have distant metastasis at presentation, and another approximately 40% of patients will develop locoregionally recurrent and/or distant metastatic disease after definitive treatment. Those patients with distant metastasis at presentation who have a good performance status will frequently benefit from initial therapy, such as radiation or chemoradiotherapy, aimed at locoregional control of disease, so that impact on speech, swallowing, breathing, and overall comfort can be minimized. When patients experience locoregional recurrence and distant metastasis is ruled out, surgical salvage is always considered the best initial approach to treatment, unless the disease is unresectable. Regional recurrence is often easily addressed by neck dissection. Salvage surgery for primary site recurrence can be a greater technical challenging, but advances in reconstructive techniques utilizing vascularized free tissue transfers have vastly improved the morbidity of salvage surgery. Long-term disease control for patients with locoregional relapse that is deemed unresectable may still be possible with reirradiation, which is most frequently administered with concurrent chemotherapy. Patients with metastatic disease, poor performance status, and severe toxicity from previous radiation have typically been excluded from reirradiation trials. While there is no phase III comparison of reirradiation to palliative chemotherapy, outcomes with reirradiation appear favorable, at least in the subset of patients who achieve a complete response.

Unfortunately, most patients with recurrent or metastatic SCCHN are not candidates for surgical salvage or reirradiation, leaving palliative systemic therapy as the only remaining option. The standard approach for first-line treatment of recurrent or metastatic SCCHN in patients with a good performance status is platinum-based multiagent chemotherapy. The regimen supported by the best data available to date is cetuximab added to platinum (either cisplatin or carboplatin) plus 5-FU. In the phase III EXTREME trial, this regimen was compared to platinum plus 5-FU, and a 2.7-month improvement in overall survival was achieved (6). While the addition of a third cytotoxic agent to an established two-drug regimen is, in oncology, frequently precluded by unacceptable toxicity, the addition of the targeted agent, cetuximab, did not significantly detract from patient quality of life, as compared to quality of life with chemotherapy alone.

In the second-line recurrent or metastatic SCCHN setting, data from clinical trials are sparse. While there is no evidence that second-line chemotherapy in platinum-refractory SCCHN meaningfully prolongs survival, quality of life may be transiently improved or maintained. In general, single agents, such as paclitaxel, docetaxel, capecitabine or methotrexate, are used. Objective response rates are often less than 10%, and median survival is short. More effective treatments are clearly needed.

Molecularly targeted therapies are emerging in the treatment of SCCHNs, and are primarily under study in the recurrent/metastatic disease setting. Multiple drugs that target EGFR are under development in phase II and III studies, as are antiangiogenic agents. Other promising new therapies include agents that target signaling networks downstream from EGFR and VEGFR, agents that target the PI3K pathway in which driver mutations are known to be present in a subset of SCCHNs, HER3 monoclonal antibodies, and immunotherapeutic agents.

Cancer prevention therapy Considerable research has been devoted to the development of approaches to head and neck cancer prevention.

To date, several trials of *beta*-carotene and *cis*-retinoic have been performed which demonstrate regression of established premalignant lesions, such as leukoplakia. However, the effects of such treatments are only transient, and there is no evidence that such therapy reduces second primary cancers in high-risk patients. Small studies of other agents that might delay head and neck cancer formation, such as epigallocatechin-3-gallate from green tea and curcumin, have been recently completed or are underway.

It is generally accepted that cessation of tobacco and alcohol abuse will reduce the risk of primary head and neck cancer, but the impact of such cessation on second primary cancer formation is speculative.

Lastly, as described above, the incidence of HPV-associated oropharyngeal SCCHN is on the rise. Two HPV vaccines, Gardasil and Cervarix, are approved for the prevention of cervical cancer in women and of genital warts in both men and women. The impact of these vaccines reducing the incidence of HPV-associated oropharyngeal SCCHN has not yet been studied, but the potential is great.

Salivary gland tumors Malignant salivary gland cancers are primarily treated with surgery. Postoperative radiation is often advised to reduce the risk of locoregional relapse with indications being: positive or close surgical margins (a common occurrence necessitated by preservation of the facial nerve), an intermediate- to high-grade cancer, or nodal involvement. Many centers will consider the addition of radiosensitizing concurrent chemotherapy to radiation in high-risk patients, such as those with positive margins or high-grade histologies. Fortunately, a phase II trial testing adjuvant concomitant cisplatin plus radiation therapy versus adjuvant radiation therapy alone for high-risk salivary gland cancers is currently underway. Surgical resection without postoperative radiation is generally reserved for patients with benign salivary gland tumors or low-grade carcinomas that are resected with adequate margins.

Adenoid cystic carcinoma of salivary gland origin is an unusual cancer with a distinct natural history characterized by a high incidence of retrograde perineural spread along nerve tracts and frequent lung metastases that often are found years after the initial diagnosis. Postoperative treatment of adenoid cystic carcinoma usually requires radiation targeted not only to the primary site, but also along nerve pathways between up to the skull base.

For metastatic salivary gland cancers or refractory locoregional disease, clinical trials establishing the best standard of care are lacking. Therapy is given with palliative intent, usually often involves agents with relatively modest activity, such as doxorubicin, cisplatin or carboplatin, taxanes, vinorelbine, and gemcitabine. Recent findings regarding the molecular underpinnings of some salivary gland cancers may lead to new opportunities for treatment. For example a *MYB-NFIB* translocation has recently been identified in a number of adenoid cystic carcinomas (16). Identification of this translocation provides new targets for rationale drug development for the management of this rare tumor. Salivary duct carcinomas are another histologic subtype in which recent advances may translate into more effective therapies. Salivary duct carcinomas harbor frequent molecular abnormalities, including mutations in PIK3CA and BRAF as well as the overexpression of HER2 and androgen receptor, all potentially targetable with drugs that are currently available or in development.

ADVANCES IN SURGERY AND RADIATION THERAPY

Advances in head and neck surgery parallel those in other surgical oncology disciplines. In general, enhanced preoperative staging via CT and MRI scans has allowed identification of patients who should, or perhaps more importantly, should not undergo major ablative procedures. The trend to avoid unnecessarily morbid surgery has been supported by the increased effectiveness of concurrent chemoradiotherapy. Primary site preservation is now a well-established goal in multidisciplinary treatment programs designed to avoid relatively morbid procedures such as orbital exenteration or laryngectomy. Yet, surgery remains an integral and effective means of for many primary tumors, as well as in the salvage setting. When surgery is the appropriate primary treatment modality, procedures that preserve function are often possible, such as selective or modified neck dissection instead of radical neck dissection, and partial instead of total laryngectomy. There is growing experience with transoral laser microsurgery and transoral robotic surgery in select pharyngeal and laryngeal carcinomas. Single institution studies demonstrate excellent locoregional control rates, and acceptable functional morbidity. In the future, upfront resection of good-prognosis HPV-associated oropharynx primaries may allow for deintensification of the other treatment modalities, such as chemotherapy or radiation, and thus lead to improvements in the overall morbidity of treatment. When ablative surgery leads to unfavorable functional or cosmetic results, modern reconstructive techniques can be restorative. The use of microvascular free tissue transfer has led to significant strides in functional reconstruction with improved cosmetic appearance. These techniques have allowed for highly successful reconstruction of mandibular and pharyngoesophageal defects, as well as the management of wounds previously felt to be irreparable.

Advances in radiation therapy fall into two broad categories: improvements in targeting of the radiation fields and enhancements in radiation delivery. In the former category, improvements in anatomic staging of cancer by CT/MR scans and fused images allow precise definition of target tissues and delineation of adjacent normal structures. This has led to a more complete coverage of gross disease by radiation and a tighter correlation between dose and the extent of disease. In theory, the benefit from this is enhanced locoregional control of disease and reduced injury to normal tissues. Advances in radiation treatment delivery systems such as intensity-modulated radiation therapy (IMRT), image-guided radiation therapy, and tomotherapy take advantage of the advances in pretreatment target definition and deliver radiation therapy in a highly conformal way that further limits radiation exposure to adjacent normal tissue. The most compelling example of the benefit of IMRT in head and neck cancer is the ability to spare the major salivary glands. This has led to reduced xerostomia-related complications, such as dental injury, and profound improvements in the head and neck cancer patient's quality of life.

While most radiation treatments involve photons, neutron and proton beam therapy are alternative forms of treatment for selected patients.

Fast neutron beam therapy derives its benefit from a more effective biologic dose that overcomes radioresistant elements of a tumor, such as hypoxia. Clinical trials suggest that neutrons may be advantageous for treatment of unresectable salivary gland tumors. Normal tissues also experience the greater biologic effect of neutrons. The potential benefit in tumor control with neutrons must be weighed against an increase in normal tissue injury. Proton beam therapy takes advantage of the unique properties of protons that allow treatment to be exquisitely targeted. Because of the proton's positive charge, the depth of penetration can be manipulated so that radiation is not delivered beyond the intended target. This has obvious benefits and allows for even higher doses of radiation to be delivered than possible with techniques such as IMRT. Proton beam therapy is emerging as a preferred radiation treatment for an increasing number of head and neck sites, including periorbital and base of skull tumors, where adjacent normal tissue toxicity can result in blindness or brain or spinal cord injury.

ACUTE AND CHRONIC TOXICITIES OF TREATMENT

The side effects and potential complications of surgery are principally in the categories of pain, function (speech and swallowing), and cosmesis. In general, pain is transient and well managed. Dramatic improvements in posttreatment speech, swallowing, and cosmesis have been achieved by two means: the avoidance or limiting of surgical intervention in selected patients through the use of concurrent chemotherapy and radiation, and the use of novel reconstructive techniques. For example, up to 75% of patients who undergo total laryngectomy will regain intelligible speech, many via the surgical construction of a one-way tracheoesophageal fistula. This fistula allows diversion of exhaled air back into the pharynx with resultant oral speech. Palatal prosthetics and dental implantation into revascularized bone grafts after mandibular reconstruction can similarly augment functional oral rehabilitation.

Complications of radiation therapy are divided into acute and chronic toxicities. Acute toxicities principally relate to radiation dermatitis and mucositis with consequent issues of wound care, dysphagia, pain, thick oral secretions, and aspiration. These risks are not trivial, as recent trials of chemoradiotherapy report up to nearly 100% use of prophylactic gastric feeding tubes during treatment, and a 1%–2% rate of acute treatment-related mortality. Chronic radiation toxicities can vary from mildly disabling (abnormal taste, xerostomia, and accelerated dental disease) to severely disabling (soft tissue fibrosis with neck stiffness or tongue restriction, osteoradionecrosis, second primary cancers, accelerated carotid artery atherosclerosis, and permanent gastric tube dependence in up to 5% of patients).

Complications of chemotherapy vary depending on the specific agents used. Full-dose chemotherapy may bring expected risks of myelosuppression, mucositis, diarrhea, nausea and vomiting, alopecia, and nephrotoxicity. When weekly chemotherapy is used with radiation, chemotherapy-specific toxicities are often minimal. However, all forms of chemotherapy with radiation significantly increase the risk of radiation-induced dermatitis and mucositis. The latter increase has prompted clinical trials evaluating agents, such as keratinocyte growth factor, that may limit mucositis.

CONCLUSIONS

Cancers of the head and neck are a diverse collection of tumors, with multiple histologies and primary sites that govern not only the natural history of the disease, but also the approach to treatment. The field is rapidly evolving in several respects. HPV-associated oropharyngeal SCCHN is rising dramatically. This subset of SCCHNs has a unique biology and better prognosis compared to other SCCHNs. Current studies now stratify for HPV status, or are aimed specifically at deintensifying treatment for good-prognosis HPV-associated disease. Major advances in treatment are improving outcomes for survivors, particularly with improvements in surgical and radiation techniques that limit the impact of treatment on vital head and neck functions. Systemic approaches to head and neck cancers are also improving. The role of molecularly targeted treatment is firmly established in SCCHN, and more exciting developments are underway.

REFERENCES

1. Molina MA, Cheung MC, Perez EA, et al. African American and poor patients have a dramatically worse prognosis for head and neck cancer: an examination of 20,915 patients. *Cancer.* 2008;113: 2797–2806.

2. Chaturvedi AK, Engels EA, Pfeiffer RM, et al. Human papillomavirus and rising oropharyngeal cancer incidence in the United States. *J Clin Oncol.* 2012; 29: 4294–4301.

3. Gillison ML, Broutian T, Pickard RK, et al. Prevalence of oral HPV infection in the United States, 2009-2010. *JAMA.* 2012; 307: 693–703.

4. Ang KK, Harris J, Wheeler R, et al. Human papillomavirus and survival of patients with oropharyngeal cancer. *N Engl J Med.* 2010; 363 (1): 24–35.

5. Bonner JA, Harari PM, Giralt J, et al. Radiotherapy plus cetuximab for squamous-cell carcinoma of the head and neck. *N Engl J Med.* 2006; 354: 567–578.

6. Vermorken JB, Mesia R, Rivera F, et al. Platinum-based chemotherapy plus cetuximab in head and neck cancer. *N Engl J Med.* 2008; 359: 1116–1127.

7. Agrawal N, Frederick MJ, Pickering CR, et al. Exome sequencing of head and neck squamous cell carcinoma reveals inactivating mutations in NOTCH1. *Science.* 2011; 333: 1154–1157.

8. Stransky N, Egloff AM, Tward AD, et al. The mutational landscape of head and neck squamous cell carcinoma. *Science.* 2011; 333: 1157–1160.

9. Cooper JC, Pajak TF, Forastiere AA, et al. Postoperative concurrent radiotherapy and chemotherapy for high-risk squamous-cell carcinoma of the head and neck. *N Engl J Med.* 2004; 350: 1937–1944.

10. Bernier J, Domenge C, Ozsahin M, et al. Postoperative irradiation with or without concomitant chemotherapy for locally advanced head and neck cancer. *N Engl J Med.* 2004; 350: 1945–1952.

11. Ang KK, Zhang QE, Rosenthal DI, et al. A randomized phase III trail (RTOG 0522) of concurrent accelerated radiation plus cisplatin with

or without cetuximab for stage III-IV head and neck squamous cell carcinomas (HNC). *J Clin Oncol.* 2011; 29 (supplement): 5500.

12. Posner MR, Hershock DM, Blajman CR, et al. Cisplatin and fluorouracil alone or with docetaxel in head and neck cancer. *N Engl J Med.* 2007; 357: 1705–1715.

13. Vermorken JB, Remenar E, van Herpen C, et al. Cisplatin, fluorouracil, and docetaxel in unresectable head and neck cancer. *N Engl J Med.* 2007; 357: 1695–1704.

14. Haddad RI, Rabinowits G, Tishler RB, et al. The PARPDIGM trial: a phase III study comparing sequential therapy (ST) to concurrent chemoradiotherapy (CRT) in locally advanced head and neck cancer (LANHC). *J Clin Oncol.* 2012; 30 (supplement): 5501.

15. Cohen EW, Karrison T, Kocherginsky M, et al. DeCIDE: A phase III randomized trial of docetalec (D), cisplatin (P), 5-fluorouracil (F) (TPF) induction chemotherapy (IC) in patients with N2/N3 locally advanced squamous cell carcinoma of the head and neck (SCCHN). *J Clin Oncol.* 2011; 30 (supplement): 5500.

16. Persson M, Andren Y, Mark J, et al. Recurrent fusion of MYB and NFIB transcription factor genes in carcinomas of the breast and head and neck. *Proc Natl Acad Sci USA.* 2009; 106: 18740–18744.

INDEX

Note: Page numbers followed by *f* and *t* refer to figures and tables respectively.

849